Equine Clinical Nutrition

Equine Clinical Nutrition

Second Edition

Edited by

Rebecca L. Remillard, MS, PhD, DVM, DACVN
CEO
Veterinary Nutritional Consultations
Hollister, NC, USA, 27844

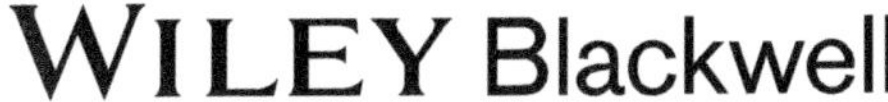

This second edition published 2023

Edition History
John Wiley, Blackwell Publishing Inc. (1e, 1995);

Registered Office
John Wiley & Sons, Inc., 111 River Street, Hoboken, NJ 07030, USA

For details of our global editorial offices, customer services, and more information about Wiley products visit us at www.wiley.com.

Wiley also publishes its books in a variety of electronic formats and by print-on-demand. Some content that appears in standard print versions of this book may not be available in other formats.

Library of Congress Cataloging-in-Publication Data is applied for
Hardback ISBN: 9781119303695

Cover Design: Wiley
Cover Image: Courtesy of Sandra L. Durkee

Set in 9.5/12.5pt STIXTwoText by Straive, Pondicherry, India

SKY10044257_031123

This work is dedicated to Dr. Donald E. Johnson and Dr. Lon D. Lewis, for, without their expert mentoring, thoughtful guidance, and collegial friendship, this textbook would not have been possible.

To Pat Parelli who introduced me to "love, language, and leadership" as a way of being with a horse that forever changed my relationship with horses.

And to all horses … who never forget but easily forgive, and only want freedom, forage, and friends.[1]

Editor's Philosophy on the Human-Horse Relationship:

Living with humans does not come naturally to horses but they benefit from the shelter, food, and health care we provide. Horses do not choose to live in our world but all the good we have to offer can only be realized when they have learned how to live with us and our unnatural 'things'. The training to live in our world must be appropriate as they have the cognitive ability and emotional fortitude comparable to a four-year-old human. We must teach them to move in and out of closed spaces (barns, stalls, trailers) which will not come naturally to a prey specie needing to watch the horizon for predators. We must teach them to eat our processed food of various forms, textures, and flavors that is different from the grass-like and broad-leaf plants they evolved to eat. We must teach them to allow close examination of their highly perceptive and most sensitive areas (ears, eyes, nose, mouth), and to accept blinding lights, injections, medications, and our machines (scopes, ultrasound, X-ray). We must teach them to yield a limb for examination and a hoof to the farrier, neither of which is inherently easy for a prey species whose primary defense is having control of all four feet for flight. The horse will acquiesce to all those necessities and more (ropes, saddles, bits) with thoughtful training from empathetic leaders. In turn, the horse provides us with incredible, sometimes deeply personal, experiences proving their strength, beauty, elegance and heart.

---

1 Fraser, L. 2012. The Horse's Manifesto. https://iaabc.org.

Contents

Contributors

Sarah K. Abood, DVM, PhD
CEO
Sit, Stay, Speak Nutrition, LLC
Dimondale, MI, USA

Simon R. Bailey, BVMS, PhD, FHEA, DECVPT, FRCVS
Veterinary and Agricultural Sciences
Melbourne Veterinary School
The University of Melbourne
Melbourne, Victoria, Australia

Géraldine Blanchard, DVM, PhD, DipECVCN
CEO
Vet Nutrition Coach SAS
Animal Nutrition Expertise SARL
Antony, France

Mieke Brummer-Holder, MS, PhD
Center for Animal Nutrigenomics & Applied Animal Nutrition
Senior Research Scientist
Alltech
Lexington, KY, USA

Kathleen Crandell, MS, PhD
Equine Nutritionist
Kentucky Equine Research
Versailles, KY, USA

Robert Coleman, PhD, PAS, Diplomate ACAS-Nutrition
Associate Professor
Department of Animal and Food Science
University of Kentucky
Lexington, KY, USA

Thomas Z. Davis, PhD
Research Molecular Biologist
Poisonous Plant Research Lab
U.S. Department of Agriculture
Logan, UT, USA

Sarah Dodd, BVSc, MS, PhD, DipECVCN, EBVS©
Dodd Veterinary Services
University of Guelph
Guelph, ON, Canada

Andy E. Durham, BSc, BVSc, CertEP, DEIM, DipECEIM, MRCVS
RCVS and European Specialist in Equine Internal Medicine
Liphook Equine Hospital
Liphook, UK

David A. Dzanis, DVM, PhD, DACVIM (Nutrition)
CEO
Regulatory Discretion, Inc.
Santa Clarita, CA, USA

Jesse M. Fenton, MS, PhD
Animal Science Food and Nutrition
School of Agricultural Science
Southern Illinois University
Carbondale, IL, USA

Nicholas Frank, DVM, PhD, DACVIM (LAIM)
Professor, Large Animal Internal Medicine
Associate Dean for Academic Affairs
Cummings School of Veterinary Medicine
Tufts University
North Grafton, MA, USA

Ashley Fowler, MS, PhD
Equine Nutritionist
Kentucky Equine Research
Versailles, KY, USA

Nicolás C. Galinelli, DVM
Department of Veterinary Biosciences
Faculty of Veterinary and Agricultural Sciences
Melbourne Veterinary School
The University of Melbourne
Melbourne, Victoria, Australia

Patricia Graham-Thiers, BS, MS, PhD
Professor and Department
Head of Equine Studies Program
Emory & Henry College
Emory, VA, USA

Richard Godbee, PhD, PAS, Dipl. ACAS-Nutrition
Founder, Equi-University
Reno, NV, USA

Patricia Harris, MA, PhD, DipECVCN, VetMB, MRCVS, RCVS specialist in Clinical Nutrition (equine)
Equine Studies Group
Waltham Petcare Science Institute
Melton Mowbray, UK

Katherine A. Houpt, VMD, PhD, DACVB
Professor Emeritus, Section of Behavior Medicine
Department of Clinical Sciences
College of Veterinary Medicine
Cornell University
Ithaca, NY, USA

Veronique Julliand, DVM, PhD
Professor of Animal Science
Univ. Bourgogne Franche–Comté, L'Institut Agro Dijon
Dijon Cedex, France

Jenna Kutzner-Mulligan, MS
Equine Nutritionist
Horse of a Different Color: Equine Management and Nutrition Counseling
Greenville, SC, USA

Laurie A. Lawrence, MS, PhD
Professor
Department of Animal and Food Sciences
University of Kentucky
Lexington, KY, USA

Nettie R. Liburt, MS, PhD, PAS
Senior Equine Nutrition Manager
Mars Horsecare US / BUCKEYE™ Nutrition
Dalton, OH, USA

Bridgett McIntosh, MS, PhD
Middleburg Agricultural Research and Extension Center
Virginia Polytechnic Institute and State University
Middleburg, VA USA

Stewart K. Morgan, PhD, DVM, DACVIM (Nutrition)
Food Animal Medicine
College of Veterinary Medicine
Western University
Pomona, CA USA

Jonathan M. Naylor, DVM, PhD, DACVIM
Saskatchewan Polytechnic, VetVisions
Large Animal Clinical Sciences
University of Saskatchewan
Saskatoon, Saskatchewan, Canada

Jacqueline M. Parr, DVM, MS, DACVIM (Nutrition)
Clinical Nutrition Service
Department of Small Animal Medicine & Surgery
College of Veterinary Medicine
University of Georgia
Athens, GA, USA

Erin Perry, MS, PhD
Associate Professor
Animal Science Food and Nutrition
College of Agricultural Sciences
Southern Illinois University
Carbondale, IL, USA

Meri Stratton-Phelps, DVM, MPVM, DACVIM (LAIM, Nutrition)
President
All Creatures Veterinary Nutrition Consulting, Inc.
Fairfield, CA, USA

Shannon Pratt Phillips, BS, MS, PhD
Professor, Equine Nutrition & Physiology
Department of Animal Science
North Carolina State University
Raleigh, NC, USA

Donna M. Raditic, DVM, DACVIM (Nutrition)
CEO
Nutrition and Integrative Medicine Consultants
Athens, GA, USA

Sarah L. Ralston, VMD, PhD, DACVN
Professor Emeritus
Department of Animal Sciences
Rutgers – State University of New Jersey
New Brunswick, NJ, USA

Rebecca L. Remillard, MS, PhD, DVM, DACVN
CEO
Veterinary Nutritional Consultations
Hollister, NC, USA

Megan Shepherd, DVM, PhD, DACVIM (Nutrition)
Veterinary Clinical Nutrition, PLLC
Christiansburg, VA, USA

Bryan Stegelmeier, DVM, PhD, DACVP
Poisonous Plant Research Lab
U.S. Department of Agriculture
Logan, UT, USA

Elizabeth M. Tadros, DVM, PhD, DACVIM (LAIM)
Department of Pathobiology and Diagnostic Investigation
College of Veterinary Medicine
Michigan State University
East Lansing, MI, USA

Jeanne van der Veen, MS
Equine & Specialty Nutritionist
Nutrition Department
Kent Nutrition Group
Muscatine, IA, USA

J. Scott Weese, DVM, DVSc, DACVIM (LAIM), FCAHS
Associate Professor
Department of Pathobiology
Centre for Public Health and Zoonoses
Ontario Veterinary College
University of Guelph
Guelph, ON, Canada

Preface

The first edition of Equine Clinical Nutrition: Feeding and Care was written by Dr. Lon Lewis and published in 1995. This referenced textbook for veterinarians and nutritionists provided details for understanding the prevention, diagnosis, and treatment of nutritional and feed-related equine diseases. The book was the first of its kind and became well established as a textbook for animal science and veterinary students. Since then there have been many advances in the nutritional management of both healthy horses and those with medical conditions. Numerous research and clinical studies have been published in the past 25 years, including the consensus-based Nutrient Requirements of Horses (2007) from the National Research Council and the Equine Nutrition: Nutrient Requirements, Recommended Allowances and Feed Tables (2015) from the Institut National de la Recherche Agronomique. Although much has been learned, we do not yet have all the information we need or would want in hand. We must be willing to practice comparative nutrition and adapt what we know from other species when applicable.

Dietetics is the study of diet and its effects on health, and the translation of scientific understanding of nutrition into practical applications. This second edition emphasizes the dietetic management of healthy horses in the prevention of nutrition-related diseases and the dietetic treatment of common diseases of horses including miniature, pony and draft sized animals.[1] The intended audience remains animal science students matriculating in equine science, animal nutrition, and pre-veterinary curricula, as well as veterinary students, enrolled in comparative and clinical nutrition courses <u>and</u> equine practitioners in need of feeding recommendations for specific medical conditions. This edition is organized utilizing an instructional approach to nutritional management with an iterative sequence of defined procedures as used in all of medicine.

Horses are presented to veterinary practitioners with one or more problems relating to health, productivity, or performance. Problems in medicine are much easier to resolve when they are well-defined. Evaluating each aspect of the case allows for the identification of problems, if any exist, and leads to a resolution. In clinical nutrition, problems are revealed using a repeating pattern of inquiry:

1) Assess the animal and develop a plan outlining the ideal ration and delivery of that diet.
2) Assess the diet. If different from the ideal, adjust the diet.
3) Assess the feeding method. If different from the ideal, modify the method.
4) After an appropriate period, re-assess the animal and repeat.

Therefore, the text is organized similarly in three sections: I. The Horse, II. The Diet, and III. Feeding Management.

Section I. Chapters 1–4 describe a healthy horse: elucidating from an evolutionary viewpoint the animal we have today, nutritional assessment of a horse with a physiological trip through the alimentary tract emphasizing the symbiotic relationship with the microbiome as knowledge of animal life stage and function determines nutrient requirements.

Section II. Chapters 5–9 define five essential nutrient groups: water, energy, protein, minerals, and vitamins in the diet of horses because knowledge of nutrient requirements determines the ration nutrient concentrations. Chapters 10–15 describe ration assessment, i.e. feedstuffs as ingredients, toxic plants, supplements, and regulation thereof, because knowledge of alimentary tract anatomy and physiology determines the feed ingredients in the ration.

Section III. Chapters 16–21, beginning with innate behaviors of alimentation, feeding management of all life stages of the horse are described because knowledge of animal behavior, not convenience, should dictate feeding practices and management. Chapters 22–28, the dietetics of managing 20 common disease conditions are described to bridge the current gap for students between production feeds & feeding courses and the management of common equine diseases in the United States.

1 The nutritional management of zebras and wild asses, including the donkey (Figure 1.1), are not specifically covered herein.

Additional features:

- Common examples of the basic calculations necessary in making sound feeding recommendations for each life stage of the horse are provided as sidebars in Chapters 17–21.
- Case in Point examples to illustrate an important concept or cite a common scenario with questions, and answers in Appendix A, have been provided in 24 chapters.
- Both USA customary and metric system units are used throughout the text because both systems are needed in clinical practice. Customary units (lb, cup) are common in commercial, personal, and social settings, and hence used when relaying feeding recommendations to clients. In science and medicine, metric units (Mcal, kg, L) are required in research, scientific publications, and ration formulations. At this time, nutritionists and practitioners must embrace and work within both systems. Common abbreviations used throughout the book are available in Appendix F.
- Topics are cross-referenced throughout the book either by chapter number and title or a specific chapter sub section to provide more specific or contextual information.

I am indebted to all contributors for their efforts, time, patience and willingness to see this project through to publication despite personal and world-wide difficulties. I have come to appreciate the depth and breadth of the knowledge, presented herein, acquired from the diversity of our training, work, and experiences. It is my intention and hope that the second edition of this book provides accurate and useful clinical nutrition information to those delivering health care services to horses and those who care for them.

Section I

The Horse

Animal Assessment

1

Feeding Horses

Back to Evolution

Rebecca L. Remillard

KEY TERMS

- Extinct refers to a species no longer in existence.
- Extant refers to a species still in existence; surviving today.
- Ungulates are even-toed or odd-toed hoofed mammals.
- The perissodactyls (odd-toed ungulates) extant examples are horses, rhinos, and tapirs.
- The artiodactyls (even-toed ungulates) extant examples are pigs, hippos, camels, deer, giraffes, antelope, cattle, and sheep.
- A "hand" is a non-international standard unit of measurement equal to 4 in. commonly used to measure the height of horses from ground level to the top of withers in many English-speaking countries.

KEY POINTS

- A review of equine evolution is essential to understanding their behavioral, nutritional, and dietary requirements.
- Horses evolved over the past 50 million years in response to environmental changes from dense humid forests to open arid grasslands.
- Extant horses adapted a form of cecal fermentation.
- The genus likely originated in North America and migrated to Old World and South America. The North American ancestors became extinct in the last American ice age but were re-introduced in the sixteenth century AD by European settlers.
- All breeds of *Equus ferus caballus* are derived from a 13–14 hand, gregarious, steppe-dwelling animal that thrived on high-fiber/low-protein/low-starch forages.

1.1 Introduction

Charles R. Darwin produced one of the first illustrations of an evolutionary "tree" in his seminal book *The Origin of Species* [1]. An evolutionary (phylogeny or phylogenetic) tree is a branching diagram outlining evolutionary relationships. Over 150 years later, evolutionary biologists still use tree diagrams to depict evolution because such figures effectively convey the concept that speciation occurs through adaptation and splitting of lineages. The tree is a visual representation of the relationship between different organisms, showing the path through evolutionary time from a common ancestor to different descendents. Important to note is that many lineages, or branches of the tree, are not successful when the environment changes and therefore become extinct. Ideally, each true species should have a name different from every other species. Specie classification has become more dynamic and may be automatically generated based on completely sequenced genomes [2]. The scientific classification of Equus, the horse, is outlined in Table 1.1 and Figure 1.1.

Within the family Equidae, Equus is the only recognized living genus with seven living species (Figure 1.1). All domestic horses (miniatures to draft size) are the same subspecies, *Equus ferus caballus*, including the feral horses of Australia, the Western United States, and Canada [4]. A true wild subspecies, *Equus ferus przewalskii*, is native to the steppes of Central Asia. Other extant members of the

Equine Clinical Nutrition, Second Edition. Edited by Rebecca L. Remillard.

Table 1.1 Taxonomic classification of equids.

Kingdom:	Animalia
Phylum:	Chordata
Class:	Mammalia
Order:	Perissodactyls
Family:	Equidae
Tribe:	Equini
Genus:	Equus
Living species and common names of Equus are:	
E. africanus (asses and donkey)	
E. ferus (wild, feral and domestic horse [draft, pony, miniature])	
E. grevyi (Grévy's zebra)	
E. hemionus (onager, kulan)	
E. kiang (kiang)	
E. quagga (plains zebra)	
E. zebra (mountain zebra)	

genus are wild asses and zebras. The domesticated donkey is *Equus africanus, subspecie asinus*. The other wild asses, kiang, onager and kulan, and zebras have not been domesticated. Equine species can crossbreed with each other. The most common hybrid is the mule, which is a cross between a male donkey and a female horse. A related hybrid, a hinny, is a cross between a male horse and a female donkey. Most hybrids are sterile and cannot reproduce. Other hybrids include the zorse, a cross between a zebra and a horse, and a zonkey or zedonk, a hybrid of a zebra and a donkey [5].

1.2 The Evolution of Equus

1.2.1 Environmental Changes

It is generally accepted that 66 million years ago (mya), an asteroid hit the earth and changed the atmosphere and vegetation. This ecologically devastating event was responsible for the loss of half of the species of plants and insects on the North American (NA) continent at that time. The subsequent colossal loss of vegetation was responsible for the eventual demise of the dinosaurs. However, small rodent-like mammals survived in part due to their small body size, living underground, and high reproductive rates. In the absence of dinosaurs, mammals thrived, evolved, and diversified to occupy land, sea, and sky in the millions of years following the asteroid. Around 56 mya, a massive volcanic rift opened in the north Atlantic sea increasing atmospheric greenhouse gases (CO_2, CH_4) which resulted in global warming. During this warming period, the NA continent became a lush, dense, rainforest reaching as far north as Alaska providing mammals with ample food and shelter for millions of years.

However as the volcanic rift cooled over 20–30 millions years, global temperatures decreased and the NA environment changed again from a tropical to the temperate climate we know today [6]. For the next several million years, still in the absence of human beings, mammals adapted to this temperate climate and again prospered. It was during this time when NA was changing from rainforest to grassland that Equus evolved from a small fox-size forest-dwelling creature to the large, odd-toed hoofed, prairie-dwelling herbivore we know today. The evolution of the horse during this time has

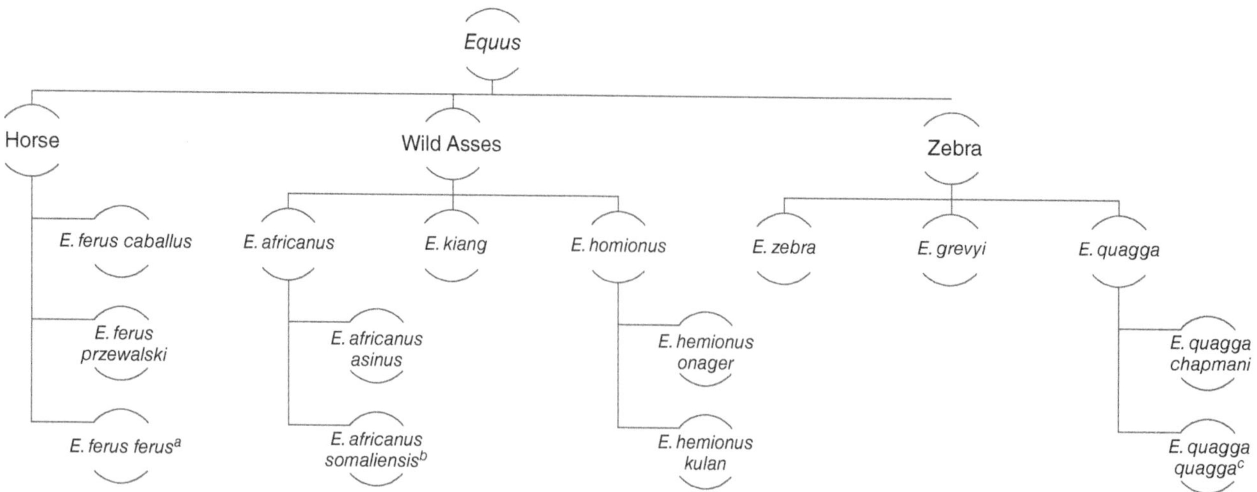

Figure 1.1 Cladogram of genus Equus speciation. *Source:* Based on Vilstrup et al. [3]. [a] Extinct in 1909, [b] Critically Endangered, [c] Extinct in 1883.

been described primarily based on changes occurring to their musculoskeletal and alimentary systems [7].

1.2.2 Musculoskeletal System Changes in Response to Predation on the Open Plains

The evolution of the horse began some 50 mya. See examples at specific points in time in Table 1.2. The common ancestor of the domesticated horse was Hyracotherium (Eohippus or the "Dawn horse"). Hyracotherium was a small mammal about 1 ft tall weighing about 15 kg, the size of a small dog, with large upper and lower canine teeth, four toes on the front limbs, and three on the hind limbs, appropriate for walking in the swamp-like rainforests of NA. See Sidebar 1.1. Eocene ancestors, Orohippus and Mesohippus, were larger and adapted to woodlands and meadow-like environments. Miohippus, Epihippus, and Parahippus

Table 1.2 A simplified version of Equus evolution in North America.

Name	Geological time periods	North American plant environment	Size/notable features
Unknown	Paleocene 56–66 mya[a]	Relatively warm temperatures worldwide gave rise to cacti, palm trees, and thick forests	Mammals only appear in the late Paleocene. Condylarths: ill-defined ancestor to the ungulates
Hyracotherium (Eohippus or Dawn horse)	Eocene 34–56 mya	In forests, while roaming the undergrowth and feeding on succulent leaves, fruits, flowers, and plant shoots, brachydont molars were changing to hypsodont molars	Height: 1 ft Weight: ~25 lb Had four toes on front three toes on rear limbs, had low-crowned teeth termed brachydont
Orohippus	Middle Eocene 45 mya	In forests, woodlands, and meadows, forest dwellers may have been browsing on plant leaves and shoots	Height: 2 ft Weight: ~50 lb Had enlarged middle toes on front and hind feet and low-crowned teeth
Mesohippus	Late Eocene 34–38 mya	In woodlands, meadows, and grasslands, forest dwellers may have been browsing leaves from bushes and small trees	Height: 2 ft Weight: ~75 lb Balanced on enlarged middle toe and had low-crowned teeth
Miohippus	Late Eocene – Early Oligocene	In meadows, grasslands, open plains, eating herbaceous plants bushes, young tree shoots, and grasses	Height: 2 ft Weight: ~100 lb Had a slightly longer skull, a large gap before the chewing teeth, and an increased tooth crown
Epihippus – a direct descendant of Orohippus	Oligocene 23–34 mya	In meadows, grasslands, open plains eating herbaceous plants, bushes, young tree shoots, and grasses	Height: 2 ft Weight: ~100 lb Had enlarged middle toes and a skull with 10 grinding molars
Parahippus – a direct descendant of Miohippus	Miocene 5–23 mya	In meadows, grasslands, open plains, adapting for quick locomotion; morphologically between brachydont and hypsodont grazing [8]	Height: 3–5 ft Weight: ~500 lb Had three visible toes but stood on one with more muscular legs adapted for forward motion, and higher tooth crown but cheek tooth wear indicates no shift to a complete grass diet
Merychippus	Miocene 15 mya	On grasslands grazing exclusively on grass – hypsodont molars	Height: 4–6 ft Weight: ~1 000 lb Had small toes surrounding enlarged middle hoof adapted for running. Incisors were better for cropping grass, and longer necks for grazing
Hipparion	Miocene 10 mya	Open grasslands of North America and Europe, and Steppe of Eurasia and Africa after migrating over the Siberian land bridge	Height: 5 ft Weight: ~500 lb Retained vestigial toes surrounding a hoof with a high-crowned compacted molar surface for grinding
Hippidion[b]	Pilocene 2.59–5.33 mya	Extinct in North America. Open grasslands in South America after the creation of the Isthmus of Panama	Height: 4–5 ft; weight: ~500 lb Direct link to modern horses

[a] Million years ago.
[b] Hippidion became extinct (~10 000 years ago) with the arrival of the first people in South America. European settlers re-introduced the horse into the Americas in the sixteenth century CE [9–12].

Sidebar 1.1: Hyracotherium Curated in Germany

The Welterbe Grube Messel (World Heritage Site Messel Mine) museum, near the village of Messel Germany, systematizes fossil findings from the abandoned Messel pit. The Messel mine contains a large and diverse number of fossils from life on earth 48 mya during the Eocene period. As a World Heritage Site, this museum has the same status as the Grand Canyon in the United States and the Galapagos Islands in South America [13]. And rightfully so as within this museum, there is a 40 million-year-old, near-complete skeletal of Hyracotherium (Eohippus or Dawn horse). The fossil remains are of a small dog-sized mammal with four distinct toes on the forelimb and rather large upper and lower canine teeth. Notably, the stomach contents of the animal's last meal, grapes, have also been well preserved. See Equus "Story of the Horse" [14].

(20–35 mya) were adapting to open grasslands as the forest and woodlands died off, and were, therefore, more vulnerable to predators. Anatomical adaptations for running became a matter of survival. The size of Miocene ancestors approached that of current day horses with an enlarged middle toe but two smaller toes on each foot. See Sidebar 1.2.

Sidebar 1.2: Limb Morphology Perissodactyls vs. Artiodactyls [7]

There are two main groups of hoofed ungulates: perissodactyls (odd-toed) and artiodactyls (even-toed). The two groups evolved independently from a common ungulate prototype (condylarths) and are differentiated today based on foot morphology. The foot evolved as the need for locomotion in search of food and escape from predators changed. The axis of symmetry in artiodactyls (example bovine) passes between the third and fourth metapodials. In perissodactyls (example equine), the axis of symmetry is through the third metacarpal and metatarsal.

Equini, one tribe of tridactyl horses, evolved to the monodactyl condition in the late Miocene. Differences in their foraging behavior and gait preference in Equini may have been a prime reason for the evolution of this monodactyl horse, at a time when tridactyl relatives predominated [9]. The second and fourth visible toes regressed to long thin vestiges (called splint bones today) as the third metacarpal and metatarsal elongated and then became muscular, hoofed, and developed a "spring mechanism" using musculotendons [15]. The spring mechanism adaptation reduces the work of galloping horses by 50% using the stored and returning elastic strain energy in spring-like musculotendons [16, 17]. The ability to cover longer distances at an energy-efficient trot gait in search of food and their rapid response to flee from predators were advantageous while living on the open grass plains of NA. Developing a critical sense of their surroundings (sight and smell) for the early detection of predators, primeval grassland horses banded together evolving a social behavior, i.e. herd mentality. Today, equines are odd-toed with slender legs, large eyes, and an acute sense of their surroundings. The biological need for a herd structure and the ability to flee became intrinsically linked to survival and are still very much present in our domesticated horses.

1.2.3 Alimentary System Changes in Response to a Changing Food Supply

Over time, natural selection leads to the expression of digestive features that approximately match the components and characteristics of the food supply. Jaw and skull musculature, stomach, and intestinal morphologies have all been shown to reflect dietary sources [18]. The morphological and functional features of the gastrointestinal tract (GIT) are unique to a species and can be explained by the interaction between the dietary chemical constituents, i.e. carbohydrates, proteins, fats, and principles of anatomy [19]. In other words, over millions of years of natural selection, GIT anatomy and physiology adapt to the food supply, or the specie dies out.

The expression of digestive enzymes and intestinal nutrient transporters also approximately match the dietary nutrient load consumed by the animal. Many of the nutrient transporters are the same across different animal phyla, though functional details may vary, e.g. glucose and amino acid transporters using K^+ vs. Na^+ exchange [20]. The digestive function also depends on the GIT microbiome. Feedstuffs resistant to endogenous enzyme digestion, e.g. cellulose, are fermented within a specialized chamber of the GIT, hosting a microbial population to digest cell wall polysaccharides. The mammalian bacterial population, as identified by 16S rRNA gene sequence data, is dominated the Bacteroidetes and Firmicutes phyla, each of which includes tens to hundreds of taxa [21]. The taxon richness of the microbiome is strongly influenced by diet.

As the NA environment changed from tropical forests to temperate grasslands, the types of forage changed; therefore, the form of energy changed, and hence, mammals adapted to the changing food supply for survival. Plant forms of carbohydrates contained within the cells are sugars and starch, and those contained in cell walls are cellulose, hemicellulose, and lignin. Plants contain little fat but will seasonally store starch in fruiting bodies (seeds/grain).

Structural parts of the plant contain large quantities of cellulose, hemicellulose, and lignin, primarily in stems, less so in leaves. The more upright fibrous the plant, the greater the proportion of cell wall to the cytoplasm, and the proportion of cellulose to the sugars and starch content. See Sidebar 1.3. Grasses have a higher cell wall to cell content ratio than the plants previously fed upon in tropical-like forests. Hence, as the plants changed due to climate change, the ratio of carbohydrate types changed, and accordingly, early mammals adapted their digestive processes to these new sources of energy.

Sidebar 1.3: Plant Cell Composition

Small herbivorous species eat primarily fruits, seeds, and berries. The **cell contents** of these fruiting bodies contain sugars and starches. Starch is a linear chain of several hundreds to thousands of D-glucose ($C_6H_{10}O_5$) units linked using α(1,4)-glycosidic bonds. The simplest form of starch is the linear polymer amylose; the branched form is amylopectin. Mammals endogenously synthesize intestinal α(1,4)-glycosidases to digest starch.

Large herbivores consume primarily the structural portions of plants, i.e. leaves and stems. The **cell walls** of these structural parts contain primarily the polysaccharide cellulose. Cellulose is a linear chain of several hundreds to thousands of D-glucose units but linked using β(1,4)-glycosidic bonds. Cellulose, hemicellulose, and lignin give rigidity to the cell wall allowing the plants (grasses, browse, and trees) to remain upright from the ground. No mammal synthesizes β(1,4)-glycosidases to digest these cell wall components. Any animal subsisting on a fibrous plant ration must therefore enter into a symbiotic relationship with cellulase-producing bacteria, and provide a fermentation chamber within the digestive tract to house the microbiota.

1.2.3.1 Evolution of the Digestive System in Perissodactyls

Mammals were successful at exploiting different ecological niches because they adapted to changing food supplies and diet composition. Anatomical changes in the Eocene and Miocene horses primarily occurred in the dental arcade and large intestinal tract as the NA food supply changed from fruits, seeds, flowers, leaves, and shoots to abrasive, upright grass forms containing more structural carbohydrates [7] (Table 1.2).

1.2.3.1.1 Dentition

Dental characteristics (tooth size and shape) respond evolutionarily to the physical properties of food because teeth are used in the mechanical processing of food [18, 22, 23]. The earliest mammals had relatively simple cheek teeth made up of three-pointed cusps lying nearly in a line. The highest cusp of the upper tooth occluded the space between adjacent lower teeth cusps, resulting in a vertical guillotine-like action that sliced or sheared food particles. These occlusal surfaces were suitable for holding, tearing, and shredding food pieces. Small mammals that consume primarily young plants and the reproductive parts of forest plants (fruits) eat a low cell wall to cell content ratio diet. These animals have brachydont molars because such plants require minimal mastication, only simple shearing or puncturing, to break open and release the cellular contents of a succulent food particle. See Sidebar 1.4.

Sidebar 1.4: Cheek Teeth Anatomy [10–12]

The primary function of teeth is to break down food without being broken or worn. In mammals, two distinctive types of teeth differ in the pattern of growth, morphology, and purpose:

Brachydont (Greek brachys meaning short) are low-crowned teeth as seen in man, pigs, dogs, and cats. The occlusal surfaces tend to be pointed, well-suited for holding prey and tearing and shredding. This type of tooth consists of a crown above the gingiva, a constricted neck at the gum line, and a root embedded in the jawbone. The crown is encased in enamel and the root in cementum. The earliest mammals had relatively simple cheek teeth made up of three cusps lying nearly in a line or low triangle. These cusps were surrounded by a cingulum on both labial and lingual sides. The highest cusp of the upper tooth occluded with the space between adjacent lower teeth, shearing food particles in a manner like that of pinking shears.

Hypsodont (Greek hypso meaning height) high-crowned teeth as noted in the permanent teeth of horses and cheek teeth of ruminants are well-suited for feeding on gritty, fibrous material. This type of tooth continues to erupt throughout life. Hypsodont teeth are usually described as having a body, much of which is below the gum line, and root, which is embedded in the alveolus of the jaw bone. Enamel covers the entire body of the tooth, but not the root. Hypsodont molars lack both a crown and a neck. The occlusal surface is rough and mostly flat, adapted for crushing and grinding plant material in a manner like that of millstones.

An estimation of when dietary fiber content impacted mammalian evolution can be made noting changes in molar teeth across geologic time periods. An adaptation by mammals to chewing abrasive and fibrous matter is evidenced by the development of a more millstone type of grinding surface [24]. Abrasive components such as silica and soil (grit) are consumed when grazing on grasses, and more so when grazing on plants lying close to the ground [25]. By the Miocene, these molars had become hypsodont, i.e. durable, robust, large, and flattened appropriate for grazing on high-cellulose plants [26]. Equid molars adapted to the consumption of grass or mature browse by increasing occlusal surfaces using two methods: increased complexity of the enamel pattern on occlusal surfaces, and premolars became molars. Increasing the root to crown length of the tooth is a hypsodontic change that does not directly increase molar surface area but does prolong the life of the tooth. Additionally, the direction of the wear facets on the molars of Eocene horses shows a greater transverse component to their jaw movement than previous specimens, which suggests consumption of a diet requiring a grinding motion [24].

1.2.3.1.2 Fiber Digestion

All members of perissodactyls had adapted to some form of primitive cecal fermentation in the late Paleocene (56–59 mya), that is, before Hyracotherium, before becoming a monodactyl, and before artiodactyls developed rumination [24]. However, the biochemistry of fermentation among ungulates is similar regardless of forage type or GIT site of fermentation, and the taxonomic composition of the GIT micro-organisms is broadly similar [24]. The volatile fatty acid products of cellulose fermentation (acetic, propionic, and butyric acid) are absorbed through the rumen wall of artiodactyls. Similarly, the same short-chain fatty acids are produced in the cecum and absorbed through the cecal and colonic epithelium of perissodactyls using a method of transcellular nonionic diffusion [20, 27].

Though the processes of fermentation appear to be similar within the cecum of horses and the rumen of ruminants, the site of fermentation with respect to the small intestine has important nutritional consequences with respect to protein and carbohydrate metabolism. In horses, available dietary protein and soluble carbohydrates (sugar, starch) are absorbed from the small intestine before reaching the cecum [28]. In ruminants, the rumen lies before the small intestine, and therefore dietary carbohydrates and protein are altered by microbes before the digesta reaches the small intestine. There are nutritional advantages and disadvantages to both systems.

The rate of digesta passing through the GIT of horses is not limited by particle size as in ruminants, hence when energy needs increase or forage quality decreases, food intake and the digesta rate of passage can be increased to meet the nutritional needs of horses [29]. However, for equines, the diet must contain all essential amino acids as the large quantity of microbial protein generated in the cecum is excreted in the feces and, therefore, not available to the host. Perissodactyls have not adopted a dependency on coprophagy most likely because they had very large home ranges (250–12 000 ac) and were cursorial, covering 12–50 miles daily while grazing or moving to water [15].

1.2.3.1.3 Feed Intake

The daily energy requirement for all mammals is based on metabolic body weight ($BW^{0.75}$), which is a function of body mass relative to the body surface area. Therefore, less energy is needed per kilogram of BW as animal size increases (Figure 1.2) [30]. For herbivores, as body size increased through the geologic time periods, less energy per kilogram of BW was required, and therefore surviving on a high-fiber/low-protein, fat, and starch diet became possible. Additionally, gut capacity increases linearly with body size and larger herbivores were able to accommodate a GIT fermentation chamber required to derive energy from fibrous feedstuffs, thereby not competing with carnivorous mammals. In summary, as herbivores evolved to larger body sizes, their energy requirement per kilogram of BW decreased and they were able to accommodate a GIT fermentation site, both of which allowed for the utilization of high-cellulose feedstuffs [24, 31].

As BW size increased in perissodactyls and food supplies increased in fiber content, hindgut cecal digestion was a significant adaptation that occurred about 28 million years ahead of rumen development in artiodactyls [24]. Ruminants adapted to a high-fiber diet in a later time period when they were of sufficient body size to physiologically accommodate a large foregut rumen for fermentation. The family Equidae continued to be successful even when ruminants dominated the landscape during the Miocene, Pliocene, and Pleistocene [24]. Today, Equus species are highly successful herbivores living on a diet with the highest fiber, and lowest protein content within a grazing community. Zebras have been reported to select the most fibrous part of the plant (tallest and oldest strands) [32]. Wild asses, onagers, zebras, Przewalski's horses, and feral horses (Mustangs, Assateague Ponies) in NA continue to live in areas with sparse, relatively low nutritional quality vegetation [33–35].

1.3 Equine Nutrient Requirements vs. Recommendations

The true nutrient requirements for any individual horse are determined by the animal's physiologic state; BW, life stage, physical activity and health. At best, based on equine feeding trials and extrapolations, daily nutrient intake recommendations have been published in the *Nutrient Requirements of Horses* [36]. Given the exact quantity of any nutrient required by an individual horse is not known, these are suggested initial nutrient intakes that would be adequate for most horses in the same category (BW, life stage, activity). This data should not be misinterpreted as setting nutrient minimums, maximums or even an estimate of optimal. Monitoring is

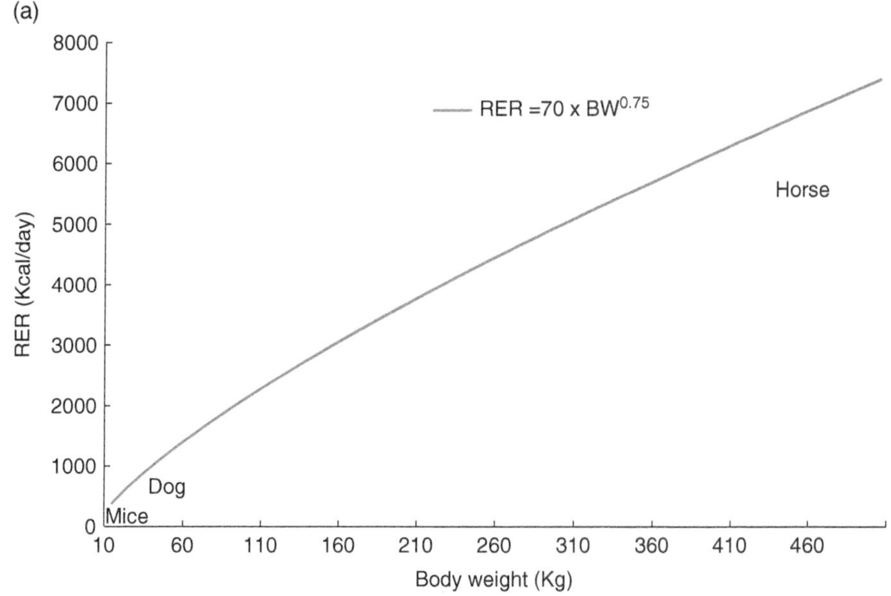

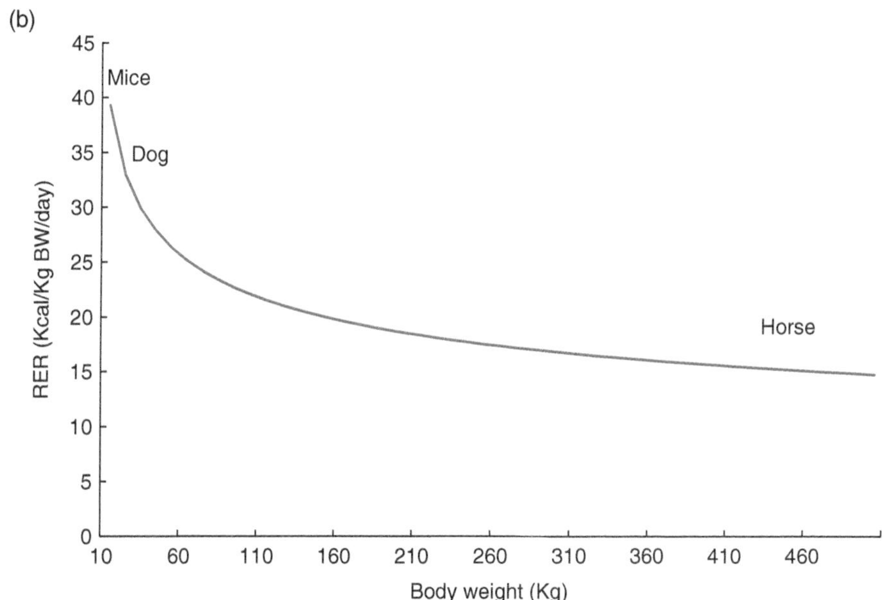

Figure 1.2 Relationship between body mass or weight and daily resting energy requirement (RER). Total RER increases as body mass increases (a) but RER per kilogram of BW decreases as body mass increases (b).

therefore essential as adjustments may be needed for an individual horse.

National Research Council (NRC) publications are the products of a temporary committee of members who have been invited to participate voluntarily. The invitations are extended to individuals considered to be experts in the broad field of equine nutrition and chosen based on their special competencies, and with due regard for an appropriate balance within the committee. The committee members hold advanced degrees (MS, PhD.) in animal nutrition and/or a Doctor of Veterinary Medicine, and additional American Veterinary Medical Association certifications in nutrition. These individuals have been actively involved in research within the field of equine nutrition with numerous scientific peer-reviewed publications to their credit. Collectively, they lend their knowledge and expertise to the NRC publication such that it represents the "best of our knowledge" at that time in the scientific literature. The first edition of NRC *Nutrient Requirements of Horses* was published in 1949. The 1989 fifth and 2007 sixth editions are available from the National Academies (www.nationalacademies.org). The publication is not revised at regular intervals. The next edition will likely be when it has been determined that there is sufficient new information available to warrant an update.

The 2007 NRC *Nutrient Requirements of Horses* is clearly the most frequently referred to source when estimating the nutrient needs for a healthy equine in the United States. This publication suggests the daily intake of 22 nutrients for horses with a healthy mature body weight of 200, 400, 500, 600, and 900 kg across 34 different physiologic states. Although that may appear to be sufficient data, there are gaps in the guidelines as there are no recommendations for horses with medical conditions. For example, how should the NRC nutrient profile recommendations for a healthy horse be adjusted for an obese pony when designing a weight-loss program, or for a 27-year-old horse with increased liver enzymes or chronic respiratory disease? Given the paucity of nutritional recommendations and data for the horse, both healthy and ill, clinical nutritionists then make their "best-educated guess" based on experience and resources when formulating the ration. See Appendix B. After a dietary recommendation has been implemented, the animal must be monitored and future adjustments are made as warranted. See Appendix C. Designing a ration for such cases that fall outside of the NRC recommendations requires expertise in both the science and the art of clinical nutrition.

Additional sources to be consulted include a review of the literature, e.g. scientific articles, abstracts, and proceedings, over the past 15 years as this information would not have been considered in the NRC 2007 publication. Another reasonable source of information on nutritional requirements may be found in the data of closely related species (Figure 1.1). Private research entities are another source as there are several involved in equine research, e.g. Kentucky Equine Research,[1] MARS Equestrian,[2] and Purina Animal Nutrition, LLC.[3] Unfortunately, industries rarely publish in-house nutritional studies in the scientific literature. However, it can be surmised that the nutrient concentrations of long-standing commercial products are safe and effective. By extension, reverse logic would suggest that if the nutrient concentration was found to be effective for one disease, it may be effective for a similar disease process. For example, if the ration concentration of omega-3 fatty acids were found to alter tissue concentrations in the blood of horses with arthritis, it would follow that the same concentration would be a reasonable starting point for a horse with chronic respiratory disease. Hence understanding the evolutionary and comparative aspects of clinical nutrition is an essential component of practice, still today, despite our endless push to specialize.

1 https://ker.com
2 https://www.marsequestrian.com/
3 https://www.purinamills.com/horse-feed

Case in Point

Patient Assessment

A 10-year-old Anglo-Arabian gelding in training for a 50-mile endurance race was reported by the owner to be exhibiting intermittent abdominal discomfort, not eating well, not always finishing all the feed offered, and had been somewhat resistant during training for the past 10 days or so. The horse is maintained on an unmanaged mixed grass/weed/wooded 10-ac pasture with a small herd of four other horses with an ad libitum water source and run-in shed for shelter. At the start of training about 30 days ago, a textured grain mix and a ration balancer pellet were added to the two meals/d of hay pellets routinely fed to the horse.

Body weight was estimated at 1300 lb using a weight tape, with a body condition score of 5/9, and weight loss had not been noted by the owner. Physical examination, complete blood count, and serum biochemical panel were within normal limits. Gastric ulceration was suggested and a standing gastroscopy procedure using a 2-m endoscope to visualize the stomach mucosa and margo plicatus was performed. There were two gastric lesions in the non-glandular mucosa, both with severity scores of 2/4 [37, 38]. The diagnosis was primary equine squamous gastric disease (ESGD) and treatment options were explained to the owner [38]. In addition to prescribing a proton-pump inhibitor, omeprazole for 28 d, a review of the ration and feeding method was recommended [39].

1) *What aspects of meal feeding pelleted feeds and grain concentrates likely relate to ESGD [42]?*

Assessment of the Ration and Method of Feeding:

The unmanaged pasture was assessed and determined to provide negligible nutrition other than a sparse low-quality fiber source. The owner considered the horse as doing "moderate" work and fed according to feed label instructions. The daily feeding offered consisted of:

Feed	lb fed/d	Mcal/lb	Mcal/d	Crude fiber%	Starch (Kg/d)
	as fed basis				
Hay stretcher pellets	15	1.1	16.5	18	1.43
Performance textured feed	9	1.65	14.85	9	0.92
Vitamin mineral balancer	2	1.7	3.4	5.5	0.05

2) *What are the total daily intakes of feed (lb/d), energy (Mcal/d), and starch (g/kg BW/meal)?*
3) *What would be a sound recommendation to the owner regarding the feeding management of this horse to prevent future ulcers?*
4) *What is the rationale for these feeding recommendations?*

See Appendix A Chapter 1.

References

1. Darwin, C.R. (1859). *On the Origin of Species*, 502. England: Easton Press.
2. Letunic, I. and Bork, P. (2021). Interactive tree of life (iTOL): an online tool for phylogenetic tree display and annotation. https://itol.embl.de (accessed 3 February 2021).
3. Vilstrup, J.T., Seguin-Orlando, A., Stiller, M. et al. (2013). Mitochondrial phylogenomics of modern and ancient equids. *PLoS One* 8 (2).
4. Cucchi, T., Mohaseb, A., Peigné, S. et al. (2017). Detecting taxonomic and phylogenetic signals in equid cheek teeth: towards new palaeontological and archaeological proxies. *R. Soc. Open Sci.* 4 (4): 160997.
5. Megersa, B., Biffa, D., and Kumsa, B. (2007). A mysterious zebra-donkey hybrid (zedonk or zonkey) produced under natural mating: a case report from Borana, southern Ethiopia. *Anim. Prod. Res. Adv.* 2 (3): 148–154.
6. Dix, R.L. (1964). A history of biotic and climatic changes within the North American grasslands. In: *Grazing in Terrestrial and Marine Environments* (ed. British Ecological Society), 71–89. London: Blackwell Publishing.
7. Janis, C. (2008). An evolutionary history of browsing and grazing ungulates. In: *The Ecology of Browsing and Grazing Ecological Studies*, vol. 195 (ed. I.J. Gordon and H.H.T. Prins), 21–45. Berlin/Heidelberg: Springer.
8. Hulbert, R.C. (1984). Paleoecology and population dynamics of the early Miocene (Hemingfordian) horse *Parahippus leonensis* from the Thomas Farm site, Florida. *J. Vertebr. Paleontol.* 4 (4): 547–558.
9. Janis, C.M. and Bernor, R.L. (2019). The evolution of equid monodactyly: a review including a new hypothesis. *Front. Ecol. Evol.* 7: 1–19.
10. Prehistoric Wildlife. http://www.prehistoric-wildlife.com (accessed 4 February 2021).
11. Strauss, R. 50 Million years of horse evolution. https://www.thoughtco.com/50-million-years-of-horse-evolution-1093313 (accessed 4 February 2021).
12. Strauss, R. 10 Prehistoric horses everyone should know. https://www.thoughtco.com/prehistoric-horses-everyone-should-know-1093346 (accessed 4 February 2021)
13. World Heritage Site Messel Mine. https://www.grube-messel. de. (accessed 5 February 2021).
14. Thompson, N. "Story of the horse" Episode 1: Origins. *Nature/PBS*. https://www.pbs.org/wnet/nature/equus-story-of-the-horse-about/16877.
15. Janis, C. (1976). The evolutionary strategy of the Equidae and the origins of rumen and cecal digestion. *Evolution* 30 (4): 757–774.
16. Waran, N.K. and Van Dierendonck, C.M. (2016). Ethology and welfare aspects. *Vet. Key* https://veteriankey.com/ethology-and-welfare-aspects (accessed 3 February 2021).
17. Wilson, A.M., McGuigan, M.P., Su, A., and Van den Bogert, A.J. (2001). Horses damp the spring in their step. *Nature* 414 (6866): 895–899.
18. Minetti, A.E., Ardigo, L.P., Reinach, E., and Saibene, F. (1999). The relationship between mechanical work and energy expenditure of locomotion in horses. *J. Exp. Biol.* 202 (17): 2329–2338.
19. Martin, S.A., Alhajeri, B.H., and Steppan, S.J. (2016). Dietary adaptations in the teeth of murine rodents (Muridae): a test of biomechanical predictions. *Biol. J. Linn. Soc.* 119 (4): 766–784.
20. Karasov, W.H., Martínez Del Rio, C., and Caviedes-Vidal, E. (2011). Ecological physiology of diet and digestive systems. *Annu. Rev. Physiol.* 73 (1): 69–93.
21. Karasov, W.H. and Douglas, A.E. (2013). Comparative digestive physiology. *Compr. Physiol.* 3 (2): 741–783.

22 Zaneveld, J.R., Lozupone, C., Gordon, J.I., and Knight, R. (2010). Ribosomal RNA diversity predicts genome diversity in gut bacteria and their relatives. *Nucleic Acids Res.* 38 (12): 3869–3879.

23 Michaux, J. (1971). Muridae (Rodentia) neogene from South-Western Europe. Evolution and relationship with current forms. *Cont. Paleobiol.* 2: 1–67.

24 Lucas, P. (2004). *Dental Functional Morphology: How Teeth Work*. New York: Cambridge University Press.

25 Dental anatomy. http://www.vivo.colostate.edu/hbooks/pathphys/digestion/pregastric/dentalanat.html (accessed 5 February 2021).

26 Kwan, P.W.L. (2007). Digestive system – the oral cavity. Open Courseware. https://web.archive.org/web/20120913162229/http://ocw.tufts.edu/data/4/531949.pdf (accessed 4 February 2021).

27 Myers, P., Espinosa, R., Parr, C.S. et al. (2013). Animal diversity web: the basic structure of cheek teeth. https://animaldiversity.org/collections/mammal_anatomy/cheek_teeth_structure.

28 Semprebon, G.M., Rivals, F., and Janis, C.M. (2019). The role of grass vs. exogenous abrasives in the paleodietary patterns of north American. *Front. Ecol. Evol.* 7: 1–23.

29 Janis, C.M. and Fortelius, M. (1988). On the means whereby mammals achieve increased functional durability of their dentitions, with special reference to limiting factors. *Biol. Rev. Camb. Philos. Soc.* 63: 197–230.

30 Giddings, J. and Stevens, C.E. (1968). In vitro studies of electrolytes and fatty acid transport across the epithelium of horse caecum. *First Equine Nutrition Symposium*. 15–16.

31 Hintz, H.F., Hogue, D.E., Walker, E.F. et al. (1971). Apparent digestion in various segments of the digestive tract of ponies fed diets with varying roughage-grain ratios. *J. Anim. Sci.* 32 (2): 245–248.

32 Edouard, N., Fleurance, G., Martin-Rosset, W. et al. (2008). Voluntary intake and digestibility in horses: effect of forage quality with emphasis on individual variability. *Animal* 2 (10): 1526–1533.

33 Kleiber, M. (1961). *The Fire of Life. An Introduction to Animal Energetics*, 179–222. New York: Wiley.

34 Parra, R. (1973). Comparative aspects of the digestive physiology of ruminant and non-ruminant herbivores. In: *Literature Reviews of Selected Topics in Comparative Gastro-Enterology* (ed. C.E. Stevens). Ithaca, NY: Department of Veterinary Science, Cornell University.

35 Bell, R.H. (1969). The use of the herb layer by grazing ungulates in the Serengeti. In: *Animal Populations in Relation to their Food Resources* (ed.British Ecological Society), 111–128. Oxford: Blackwell Publishing.

36 Groves, C.P. (1974). *Horses, Asses and Zebras in the Wild*, 1e, 91–133. Newton Abbot, London: David and Charles.

37 Ryden, H. (1972). *America's Last Wild Horses*, 73,89,90. New York: Ballantine Books.

38 Keiper, R.R. (1985). *Assateague Ponies*, 21–22. Centreville, MD: Tidewater Press.

39 National Research Council (2007). *Nutrient Requirements of Horses*, 6th Rev. Animal Nutrition Series, 1–341. Washington, DC: National Academies Press.

40 MacAllister, C.G., Andrews, F.M., Deegan, E. et al. (1997). A scoring system for gastric ulcers in the horse. *Equine Vet. J.* 29 (6): 430–433.

41 Sykes, B.W., Hewetson, M., Hepburn, R.J. et al. (2015). European college of equine internal medicine consensus statement-equine gastric ulcer syndrome in adult horses. *J. Vet. Intern. Med.* 29 (5): 1288–1299.

42 Reese, R.E. and Andrews, F.M. (2009). Nutrition and dietary management of equine gastric ulcer syndrome. *Vet. Clin. North Am. Equine Pract.* 25 (1): 79–92.

2

Nutritional Assessment of the Horse

Shannon Pratt Phillips and Meri Stratton-Phelps

KEY TERMS

- Allometric equations describe the relationship between body shape and weight.
- Body "fat" refers to triglycerides (TG) stored within adipocytes located in the subcutaneous tissue, peritoneum, and organs, whereas dietary fat is TG from oils in the diet.
- Diet is the feed and water provided to an animal, commonly within a 24-hr period, whereas a ration is the feed portion of the diet [1].
- Malnutrition is defined as any disorder (deficient, excessive, or an improper ratio) of nutrient concentrations.

KEY POINTS

- Nutritional assessment requires information about the patient, the ration, and the method of delivering the ration to the patient, and the cycle is repeated as often as needed to monitor the animal.
- A major consideration of nutritional assessment is the evaluation of body weight (BW) and composition.
- Laboratory tests are available to aid in the evaluation of the equine patient depending on the duration and etiology of the clinical signs.
- Clinical signs related to ration vitamin and mineral imbalances are a diagnostic challenge.

2.1 Introduction

Large animal veterinarians have long recognized that no aspect of production has more of an impact on health than nutrition [1]. A variety of animal factors, when taken together, provide a nutritional "snapshot" of the horse's nutritional status. To determine the role of nutrition under various veterinary circumstances, a systematic method is employed to ensure that all appropriate facets of nutrition are assessed. Nutritional assessment requires gathering information about the animal, the diet (ration and water), and the method of providing the diet to the animal. This cycle is repeated as often as needed to monitor the animal (Figure 2.1).

In contrast to animal nutritionists whose work begins with feedstuffs and formulating rations for a collection of livestock with specific production goals, veterinarians' work begins with the animal that requires treatment, management, or preventative care. The goal of nutritional assessment is to establish nutrient needs and feeding goals for the animal patient. The "patient" in the case of horses may be an individual animal, a pair, e.g. mare and foal, or the herd. See Appendix C Nutrition Competencies of Equine Veterinarians. Nutrient needs are then the benchmark by which to assess the ration and method of feeding. Assessment of animal factors is a process of gathering current and historical information from the owner and medical record, physical examination (PE) of the animal(s), and laboratory and/or diagnostic tests specific to the problem(s). Then, nutrient benchmarks or targets are established specifically for the patient's physiologic state and medical problem or diagnoses [2].

Equine Clinical Nutrition, Second Edition. Edited by Rebecca L. Remillard.

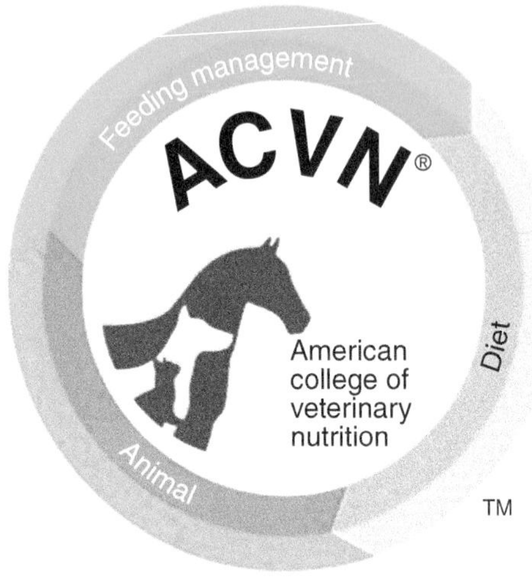

Figure 2.1 The ACVN logo illustrates the iterative process of veterinary clinical nutrition. This process involves a systematic evaluation of all three aspects affecting the nutritional status of a given animal or herd, and reiterating the process as often as needed to adequately monitor the animal. *Source:* Reprinted with permission from the American College of Veterinary Nutrition®

2.2 Obtaining a History

A medical record review provides objective historical information that documents the horse's previous health status and maintenance programs, or lack thereof, which will be useful in assessing the patient. Acquiring the animal's history includes the environment, such as the animal's housing and travel history, to better understand the problem.

Reviewing the medical record helps to determine the nutritional status of the patient. The signalment is part of the history, defines the horse's physiologic state, and includes age, breed, gender (mare, gelding, stallion), life stage (growth, maintenance, senior), and physiologic state (reproduction) and/or type of work performed. The nutrient requirements are determined directly from the horse's physiologic state. When a 500 kg adult horse is lactating, her nutritional requirements will be significantly greater compared with her requirements after weaning when the same 500 kg mare will be at "maintenance," i.e. neither gaining nor losing weight, or working. Similarly, a 500 kg gelding maintained as a pasture pet will have a lower energy requirement compared with the energy required when performing at rodeo events. Therefore, it is important to obtain a thorough description of the horse's past and present physiologic states, and possibly future expectations, when completing a nutritional assessment.

An accurate picture of the current feeding plan is necessary to assess the animal including a description of all feedstuff, commercial products, supplements, treats, and water, and how the feed and water are delivered or provided. Likewise, a description of the horse's appetite and eating behavior should be obtained. Knowledge of nutritional physiology in health and disease states, and nutritional pathophysiology, is essential to the diagnosis and treatment of nutritional diseases.

2.3 Physical Examination

Changes in a horse's weight and physical appearance (skin, hair, hoof), behavior, or productivity (performance, growth, milk production, reproductive efficiency), often provide the first indication of a ration imbalance. Unfortunately, these changes are usually nonspecific as most clinical signs are not pathognomonic for a particular nutrient. In some cases, when the nutrient imbalance is prolonged, clinical signs become more severe and, there may be more specific signs that may help identify the problem. When a nutrient is involved primarily with a single function or organ, e.g. iodine and the thyroid, abnormalities will be sufficiently specific to suggest the nutrient imbalance. However, most nutrients are involved in many metabolic reactions, functions, and organs. For example, while deficiencies in calcium, phosphorus, or vitamin D may produce bone abnormalities, inadequate intakes of copper, manganese, zinc, and vitamin A may also result in skeletal defects. Clinical signs associated with particular nutrient deficiencies and excesses are given in Table 2.1; however, most of these clinical signs have both nutritional and non-nutritional etiologies. Therefore, history, concurrent clinical signs, PE, diagnostic data, and procedures are necessary to narrow down and ultimately determine the etiology of a clinical sign.

Body weight is essential in assessing animals. It is imperative to know, or at least to have a good estimation of weight as daily nutrient requirements are primarily determined based on metabolic $BW_{kg}^{0.75}$. Ideally, a calibrated walk-on scale with a 1 ton (2000 lb) capacity should be used, but these are rarely available during farm visits. Monitoring a horse's BW over time is also an important nutritional assessment tool, particularly for growing horses, or identifying a disease or metabolic condition early.

Body condition is an overall assessment of body fat, less so muscling. While BW, age, and physiologic state are used to determine nutrient requirements, the horse's body condition is an important aspect of the nutritional evaluation when assessing the "big" picture currently and historically. For example, a mare in poor condition, i.e. low body fat reserves, at foaling will require a different ration for lactation compared with that required had her body fat stores been adequate before foaling.

Table 2.1 Clinical signs associated with nutrient imbalances in the horse.[a]

Clinical sign	Nutrient deficiency	Nutrient excess
Anemia	Vit A	Vit A, Se, Zn
Ataxia, Wobblers and/or posterior weakness	Mg, Vit E, thiamine	Na, Se, Vit A
Blindness	Vit A (night blindess)	Se
Colic	Fiber, Mg	CHO overload, Na, Vit K
Constipation	Na	
Convulsions/seizures	Vit A	Mg, Vit D
Decreased feed intake	Water, P, Na, K, Zn, Vit A, D, thiamine	F, Vit A, D
Decreased weight, growth, production and/or performance	Energy, protein, Ca, P, Na, K, Se, Zn, Vit A, D, E, thiamine	Fiber, Zn, F, Vit A, D
Dehydration	Water, Na	
Developmental Orthopedic Diseases	Protein, Ca, P, I, Cu, Zn	Energy, Ca, P, I, Zn
Diarrhea	Fiber, Se	CHO overload, Na, Se
Dyspnea, increased respiratory or heart rate	Se	Vit D
Excess lacrimation	Vit A	
Excess licking	Na, K, Cl	
Hematuria		Vit K
Hemorrhaging	Vit K	
Hoof defects, slow growth	Protein	Se, CHO overload laminitis
Impaired immunity	Se, Vit A	Fe
Lameness	Ca, P	Se, F
Muscle tremors	Mg, thiamine	
Nursing difficulty	Se	
Pica	Protein, Na, K, Cl, P	
Polyuria		Na, Vit D, K
Poor hair coat and/or hair loss	Protein, P, I, Zn, Vit A, E	Se, I, Vit A
Stiff movement	Se, Vit E, thiamine	Se, F, Vit D
Still born, weak and/or bone abnormalities	I, possibly Mn	I
Subcutaneous swelling and/or edema	Vit E	
Teeth mottled and/or pitted		F
Weakness, lethargy, fatigue, listlessness	K, Se, Vit A	Se, Vit A, K

[a] Calcium (Ca), Phosphorus (P), Magnesium (Mg), Sodium (Na), Potassium (K), Chloride (Cl), Selenium (Se), Zinc (Zn), Iron (Fe), Copper (Cu), Manganese (Mn), Iodine (I), Fluoride (F)

2.3.1 Determining Body Weight

The most accurate way to determine a horse's weight is by weighing on a calibrated scale. Scales give accurate readings, and depending on the scale quality, can give readings within 500 g. However, minor fluctuations in BW can be attributed to gut fill, defecations or urination, or water intake. It is recommended that when horses are weighed regularly, they should be weighed at the same time of day, ideally before a meal. An equine scale is a wise investment for those with growing horses to accurately track growth rates, or athletic horses to monitor BW changes closely, or to assess hydration, e.g. 1 L of sweat loss equates to 1 kg BW. Assessing BW, by scale or estimation, is not only important for addressing nutritional needs, but also for accurately dosing medications.

In the absence of a scale, equine practitioners used measurements of body length and heart girth circumference to estimate BW (Figure 2.2) [3, 4]. With the animal standing square, heart girth circumference should be measured from behind the elbow and perpendicular to the ground to hit the withers at the base of the mane hairs. Body length is

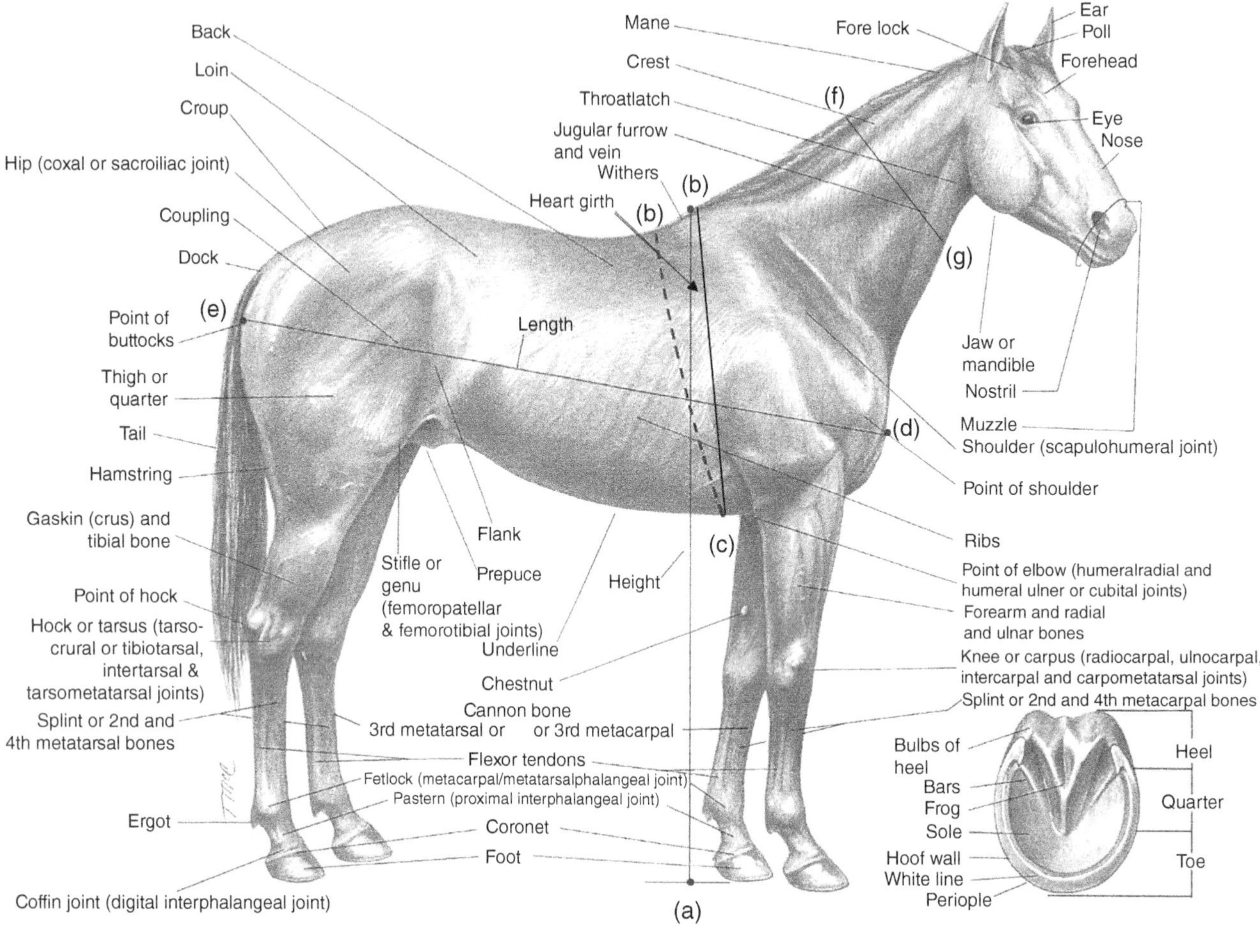

Figure 2.2 Estimate height by measuring from the ground (a) to the withers (b) where 4 in. = 1 hand. Estimate weight by measuring heart girth circumference (b)–(c) following weight tape instructions for specific placement over withers (b). A more accurate estimate of weight uses height, heart girth circumference, body length (d)–(e), and neck (f)–(g) in allometric equations. *Source:* Based on Milner and Hewitt [3]; Carroll and Huntington [4]; Carter et al. [5]; Catalano et al. [6].

measured with a horizontal line from the point of the shoulder, intermediate tubercle of the humerus, to the point of the buttock ischial tuberosity, i.e. not wrapped around the buttock. More recent published work has added measures of height and neck circumference [5, 6]. Height is measured at the peak of the withers, the third thoracic vertebra, from the ground. Neck circumference is located halfway between the poll and withers. Body weight can then be calculated from allometric equations for different types of horses (Table 2.2). Ideally, foals are weighed using a scale to very precisely track BW changes; however, these are not always available. Equations have been developed using Thoroughbred foals, ages 0–17 mos old, and this method includes carpus circumference and the left forelimb length (Table 2.2) [7].

Many horse owners do not have access to a scale, and, therefore, BW is then estimated most commonly using a weight tape. Weight tapes are an easy tool for owners but less accurate to estimate their horse's BW and there are several different types as there is no standardization of tapes (Figure 2.3). These are readily available from most feed stores and use only one measurement to estimate BW using one side of the tape. The horse should be standing square with the tape placed around the heart girth area (Figure 2.2). The tape must be lying flat around the horse with the weight side visible, and the BW estimate is read after pulling the tape snug. Placing the weight tape on the horse incorrectly according to tape instructions or inconsistently is a significant source of variation in obtaining the BW [10]. The difference between the BW tape estimates, under controlled conditions, averaged 66 kg below (13%) the actual weight of 110 horses ranging from 250 to 750 kg [11]. The same tape should be used each time, and following the directions on the specific weight tape, will yield useful information about BW changes and trends. The opposite side of the weight tape usually has linear demarcations in inches, cm or hands for measuring height at the withers.

Table 2.2 Body weight equations.[a]

Arabians/Arabian crosses	$BW = (girth^{1.486} \times length^{0.554} \times height^{0.599} \times neck^{0.173})/3596$
Stock[b]	$BW = (girth^{1.486} \times length^{0.554} \times height^{0.599} \times neck^{0.173})/3441$
Draft	$BW = (girth^{1.528} \times length^{0.574} \times height^{0.246} \times neck^{0.261})/1181$
Warmblood	$BW = (girth^{1.528} \times length^{0.574} \times height^{0.246} \times neck^{0.261})/1209$
Ponies	$BW = (girth^{1.486} \times length^{0.554} \times height^{0.599} \times neck^{0.173})/3606$
Thoroughbred foals	$M = [girth^2 \times length + 4(C^2 \times F)]/4\pi$ If $M < 0.27\,m^3$, $BW = M \times 1093$ If $M \geq 0.27\,m^3$, $BW = M \times 984 + 24$ C is carpus circumference; F is left forelimb length
Other horses	$BW = (girth^2 \times length)/11\,880$
Miniature (<147 cm)	$BW = (girth^2 \times length)/10\,787$

[a] Weight measures in kg; linear measures in cm.
[b] Paint, Quarter, Appaloosa, Appendix, Morgan, Mustang, and Colonial Spanish breeds of horses. For example, the BW of a mature Paint mare with 203 cm girth, 177 cm length, 150 cm height and 102 cm neck measurements would weigh 615 kg.
Source: Based on Catalano et al. [6]; Staniar et al. [7]; Martinson et al. [8]; Owen et al. [9].

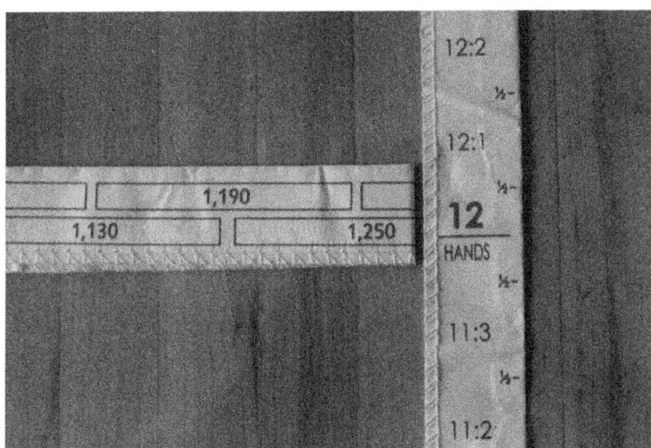

Figure 2.3 Two sides of a weight tape. Body weight in lb is indicated on one side (horizontal view), where the end of one side of the tape would be brought around the heart girth region to estimate weight. The other side has linear (hands) measurements (vertical view) to estimate height at the withers.

2.3.2 Estimating Body Composition

The "ideal" weight of a horse will depend largely on breed or body type (length and height), (Figure 2.2, Table 2.3). For example, a 16.2 hand Thoroughbred will likely weigh less than a 16.2 hand Clydesdale while both may be at their ideal BW. Therefore, the ideal BW estimated from the anatomical measurements of the length and height of various breeds has been developed (Table 2.3) [6, 8]. The difference between estimating BW (Table 2.2) and estimating ideal BW (Table 2.3) is the inclusion of girth and neck circumference for a specific animal. These additional measurements are affected by subcutaneous fat reserves. Comparing the actual BW with the ideal BW would indicate whether the animal was at ideal, under, or overweight relative to its skeletal size.

Table 2.3 Estimating ideal body weight equations.[a]

Arabians	Ideal $BW = (length \times 2.8) + (height \times 4.2) - 611$
Ponies	Ideal $BW = (length \times 2.8) + (height \times 4.2) - 606$
Stock horses[b]	Ideal $BW = (length \times 2.8) + (height \times 4.2) - 577$
Draft horse	Ideal $BW = (4.92 \times length) + (4.64 \times height) - 951$
Warmblood	Ideal $BW = (4.92 \times length) + (4.64 \times height) - 1016$

[a] Weight measures in kg; linear measures in cm.
[b] For example, the BW of a mature Paint mare with 177 cm length and 150 cm height measurements would have an estimated ideal BW of 549 kg.
Source: Based on Catalano et al. [6]; Martinson et al. [8].

2.3.2.1 Body Fat Content

Based on weight, the horse's body approximately consists of 60–65% water; 30–35% energy-supplying nutrients (protein, lipids, and glycogen), and 4% minerals [12]. However, body composition is characterized as a two-compartment model: fat-free mass vs. fat mass. The fat-free mass also called lean body mass includes muscle, bone, and organs. The fat mass is adipocytes within organs for immediate and short-term energy deficits, whereas, adipocytes storing fat surrounding the abdominal organs (peritoneal fat) and in the hypodermis (subcutaneous fat) is generally utilized during long-term energy deficits.

An important measure in determining the nutritional status of a horse is to quantify the fat stores relative to the known quantity of body fat associated with health. In dogs, body fat content of approximately 15–25% of BW has been considered healthy [13–15]. Excessively high and extremely low compositional fat reserves have been associated with increased morbidity and mortality in horses and ponies. Hence a horse with less than optimal body fat may be a clinical sign of malnutrition, disease, or poor management.

Conversely, a high total body fat content is a clinical sign of excessive caloric intake, which may predispose a horse to several metabolic and physiologic problems.

2.3.2.1.1 Carcass Fat

The "gold standard" of body fat quantification is carcass dissection and chemical fat extraction analysis [16]. White adipose tissue (WAT) is dissected from four regions: internal carcass – body wall-associated, internal carcass – organ associated, external carcass – palpable, and head and lower limb. White adipose tissue can also be categorized as external, which includes subcutaneous and intramuscular fat, or internal, which is body wall and organ fat. The weight of the dissected WAT is calculated as a percentage of empty body mass. Other quantifying methods of assessing carcass tissue fat are laboratory assays such as near-infrared spectroscopic or proximate analysis ether extract [16–18]. Carcass dissection and tissue analysis are performed only in deceased animals. A validated external evaluation system must be employed because the extent of internal (peritoneal and organ) fat depots cannot be assessed routinely in live animals. Carcass dissection and tissue fat assays, however, are used to validate external methods of assessing body composition.

2.3.2.1.2 Ultrasound

Accurately assessing body fat cover in live patients is desirable, and ultrasound can be used to measure subcutaneous fat based on a difference in density compared with the underlying muscle.

After clipping the hair and applying a conductive lubricant such as gel or corn oil, the probe is positioned at different locations to measure fat depth, and estimates are taken in triplicate. Common areas of measure include:

- Rump (middle gluteal): equidistant between the point of hip and the center of the tailhead [19]
- Rib-eye: Parallel with the 12th intercostal space, 15 cm lateral to the dorsal midline [19]
- Tailhead: parallel with the vertebral column, lateral to dorsal spinous processes of sacral/coccygeal vertebrae at the tailhead [20]
- Retroperitoneal: probe parallel and immediately lateral to the ventral midline, caudal to xiphisternum [20]

In an early study, live horses were evaluated for fat thickness by ultrasound, and then their carcasses were analyzed for chemically extractable fat. The rump fat ultrasound depth was well correlated ($r^2 = 0.86$) to carcass fat in eight horses [21]. Measures of subcutaneous fat may be used to estimate total body fat, but likely a better application for monitoring fat depth in horses over time, e.g. monitoring during weight-loss programs. The subcutaneous fat ultrasound depth, overlying the 12th intercostal space (rib-eye), was identified as an early marker of weight loss [19].

2.3.2.1.3 Body Water

Body composition can be determined by measuring the total body water (TBW) in an animal which estimates the fat-free mass. This method is based on Archimedes' principle, in which an object placed in water loses an amount of weight equivalent to the weight of the water that is displaced by the object's volume. Total body water, intracellular and extracellular water, is a significant component of the fat-free mass. Therefore, the quantification of TBW can be used to estimate fat-free mass, and thus by difference from BW, fat mass.

In humans, hydrostatic weighing is considered the gold standard of body composition analysis of a live subject. When a person is submerged in water and air from the lungs is exhaled, body density can be determined, and thus body fat can be calculated. This method is impractical in horses for obvious reasons. However, TBW can be quantified by deuterium oxide (D_2O) dilution. A blood sample is collected, and then deuterium oxide is administered to the horse at 0.12 g/kg BW intravenously one time. A second blood sample is taken 4 hrs after administration to allow for equilibration of the isotope within the body water spaces [17]. The TBW can be determined from the concentration of the isotope in the plasma. The fat-free mass is then calculated based on the assumption that lean tissue contains 73.2% water. This method has been validated for use in horses, with fat mass quantified by D_2O being linearly correlated with both WAT mass and lipid extraction from equine carcasses [17]. High correlations ($r^2 > 0.97$) have been found between TBW and body fat using both the proximate analysis and dissection methodologies, thereby validating the D_2O method as a means of determining total body fat in horses [22].

2.3.2.1.4 Bioelectric Impedance Analysis

Bioelectric impedance analysis (BIA) is another means to determine TBW and is based on the principle that electricity is conducted through the intracellular and extracellular fluids of the body, and that the majority of the body's water is within the fat-free mass. Bioelectric impedance analysis places one current drive electrode at the wing of the atlas, a voltage sense electrode 8 cm caudal toward the scapula, and a second current drive electrode at the ipsilateral tuberal ischia and the voltage sensor 8 cm proximal to the greater trochanter [23]. The electrodes measure resistance to the voltage sensors, to determine the opposition of the body to the current (impedance). While several studies have used BIA with some success to quantify hydration status, this procedure appears to be less useful for quantifying body composition, particularly fat mass [24, 25]. When body composition data derived from D_2O dilution was compared with BIA, the limits of agreement were low at 11.6% and fat mass was overestimated by 14.1%. The authors summated that the usefulness of BIA for determining body composition is limited [23].

2.3.2.1.5 *Morphometric Measurements*

In humans, the body mass index divides the BW by height. Both girth and abdominal ("belly") circumference against height has shown to be reasonably well related to fat coverage [6–8]. In horses and ponies, the girth to height ratio had the strongest associations with body condition score/scoring (BCS) and leptin [26]. Crest height and neck circumference to height ratio had strong associations with serum insulin [27]. These are some interesting relationships between external morphometric body measurements and hormones related to energy metabolism that warrant further investigation. Recently, a three-dimensional (3D) model was used to estimate body volume and muscle mass in horses. Using a hand-held 3D photonic scanner, the authors were able to successfully determine body volume within approximately 2 min. Muscle volume was not as well determined, though the technology may be able to track changes in muscle volume over time [28].

2.3.2.2 Body Muscle Content

Muscle mass is related to athletic performance and may be considered during a nutritional evaluation [29]. Many owners are interested in "building topline" or developing the hindquarters, and while nutrition can support these efforts, a larger impact will be due to exercise, training, and the horse's genetics. Free-fat mass includes muscle and can be quantified using dual-energy X-ray absorption, a derivation from TBW, bioelectric impedance, BCS, cadaver dissection, and ultrasound [30].

Muscle thickness has been measured using ultrasonography [30, 31]. There were low reproducibility and repeatability between examiners using ultrasound to determine equine muscle thickness, and there was difficulty locating the exact site for measurements [31]. Muscle mass has also been described using a subjective 1–5 scoring system, based on the definition and mass of major muscle groups that included gluteal, pectoral, and complexus muscles [32].

More recently, genetic testing has determined that some horses have more muscle mass as a result of a single nucleotide polymorphism g 66493737 at the myostatin gene (MSTN). Racing Thoroughbreds with two copies of the C base pair had more muscle mass as quantified by BW to withers height that presumed fat mass was low [33]. Knowledge of muscle mass and distribution may be considered when performing a nutritional assessment of a horse; however, more robust measures are required to evaluate muscle mass in the field.

2.3.3 Body Condition Scoring

Body condition scoring is a subjective estimate of body fat coverage in an animal because excessive or very low fat reserves in horses have major detrimental effects on health, morbidity, reproductive rates, work performance, and carcass quality [34, 35]. Typically, the Henneke Body Condition Scoring System is used [36] or as modified by Kohnke [37]. With the Henneke scale, the horse is assigned a score ranging from 1 to 9, where a BCS of "1" would represent a very low body fat content, while "9" would represent a very high body fat content. There are six external regions on the horse assessed for fat cover (Figure 2.4a and Table 2.4). These areas are the crest of the neck, the shoulder blade, and behind the shoulder, along the withers and ribs, and down the spine and tail head region. The Henneke system assigns an overall number to a horse based on the scale, while the Kohnke system scores each of six areas individually (neck, shoulder, withers, ribs, back, rump), and then these values are averaged to generate a score. The Henneke system was developed in American Quarter Horses and has been adapted to both Thoroughbreds and Warmbloods [38]; however, there is a greater variation between body condition scores when performed by horse owners compared with veterinarians [38–40].

A BCS of 5/9, corresponding to 10–15% body fat (BF), is typically considered a desirable score for most types of horses. Horses with a score of 4/9 are considered "moderately thin" (5–10% BF), while those with a score of 6/9 are considered "moderately fleshy" (15% BF), those with a score of 7/9 (20% BF) are considered "fleshy" or overweight, while those with a score of 8 or 9/9 are considered "obese" [36] (Figure 2.4b and Table 2.4). The Equine Guelph Center at the University of Guelph has developed a BCS chart, as a poster, using a color scale to indicate healthy scores (green), cautionary scores (yellow), and unhealthy scores (red) [41]. This provides clinicians with a visual aid to the body condition scale to help owners understand that there are negative significances to having excessive or low body fat scores.

There is not one perfect BCS to which all horses must be maintained. There is an acceptable range of scores between 4 and 6. A horse may have a BCS at different times due to changing physiologic states, e.g. gestation, lactation, and work. Evolutionarily, over months to years, the BCS in early horses most likely did change in response to the "feast vs. famine" availability of food. This would be exactly the reason for having a mobile energy reserve in the body. Today, most horses have a relatively constant supply of feed, and control over feed supply, in most cases, primarily lies with the horse owner.

Body condition score is determined by an external assessment of the subcutaneous fat[1] but must be correlated with internal fat depots to be meaningful as a whole animal assessment. Several studies have sought to compare and validate different measures of body fat with a

1 See https://www.purinamills.com/horse-feed/education/detail/body-condition-scoring-your-horse.

(a)

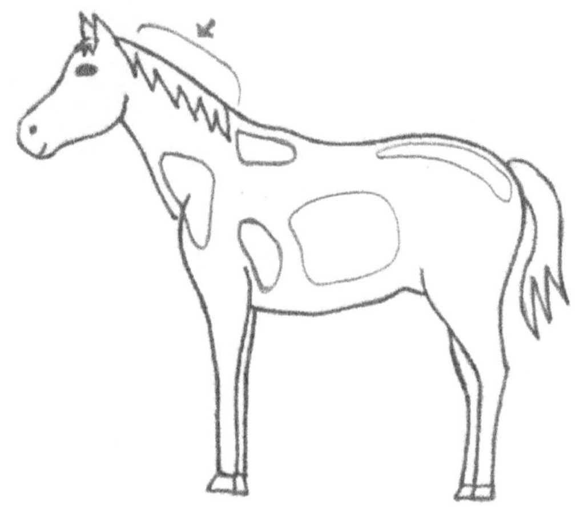

(b)

Body condition score of 1

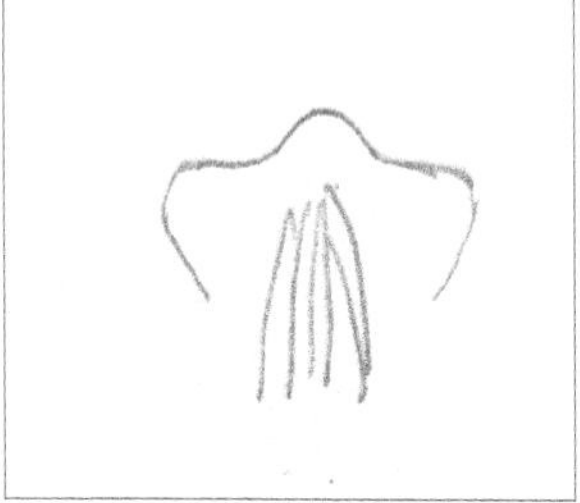

Body condition score of 3

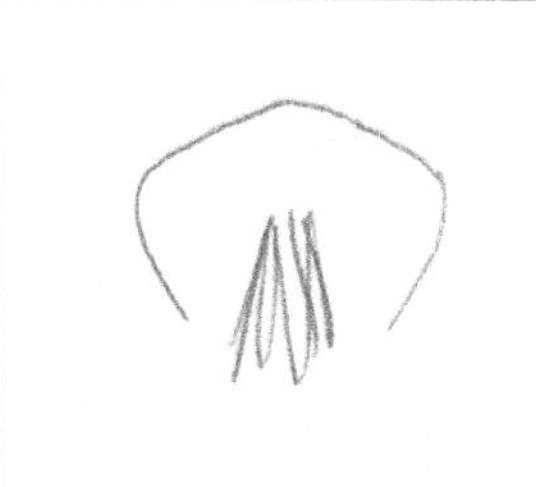

Body condition score of 5

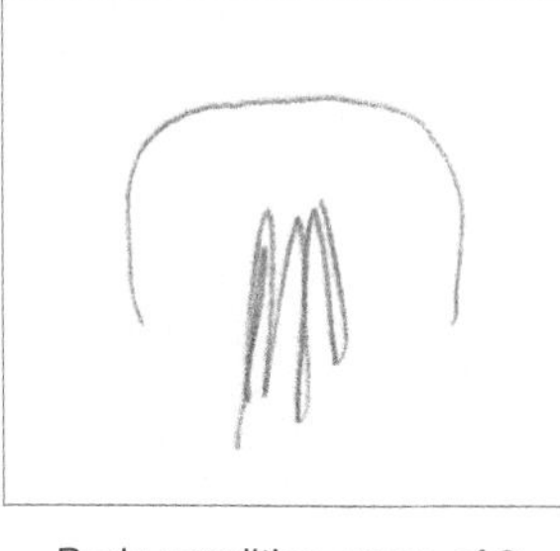

Body condition score of 7

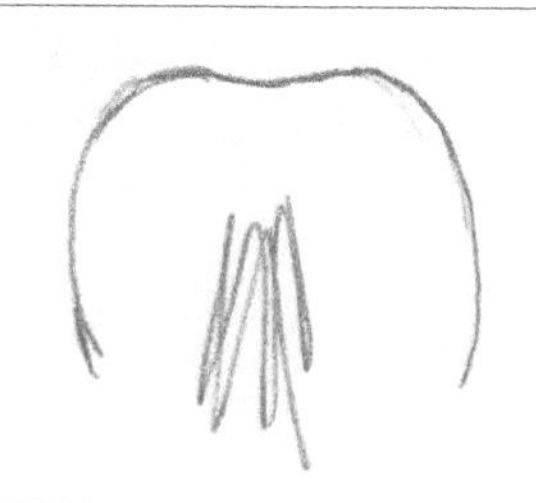

Body condition score of 9

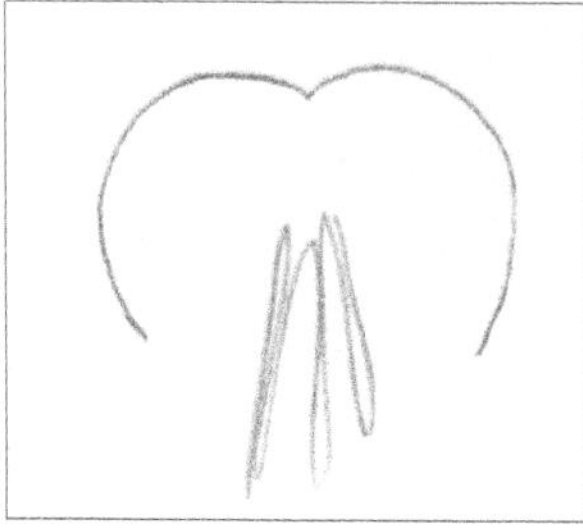

Figure 2.4 (a) Body condition scoring (BCS) sites (side view): crest of the neck (arrow); (b) BCS (rearview).
Source: Based on Henneke et al. [36].

BCS (Table 2.5). A few studies have independently verified that the association between BCS and body fat is nonlinear at higher scores [16, 47, 48]. In summary, BCS does estimate the body fat content of non-obese animals but may underestimate the fat content for those horses and ponies with a BCS >7. These animals have more body fat than a linear BCS system indicates, and, therefore, may be at a greater risk for the metabolic consequences of obesity than currently appreciated. See Chapter 28 Metabolic Syndrome.

2.3.3.1 Cresty Neck Scoring

Regional adiposity, such as fat accumulation along the neck, has been attributed to a higher risk for laminitis, and both crest height and neck circumference to animal height ratio had a statistically significant association with serum insulin concentrations [5, 49, 50]. Therefore, the cresty neck score was developed to describe neck crest adiposity (Figure 2.4a). Similar to the BCS method, a scale of 0–5 was established for neck scores, where 0 represents a neck with no palpable crest, while 5 describes a neck with an excessive amount of subcutaneous fat.

0 – No palpable crest

1 – No visual appearance of fat at the crest, some slight filling felt with palpation

2 – Noticeable appearance of a crest, but fat deposited evenly from poll to withers

3 – Crest enlarged and thickened, particularly in the middle of the neck (vs. the poll or withers)

4 – Crest grossly enlarged and thickened, may have crease or wrinkle

5 – Crest is so large it permanently droops to one side

The cresty neck score system was found to be well correlated ($r = 0.882$; $P<0.01$) with post-mortem nape fat measurements as a measure of carcass fat [35].

2.4 Changes in Body Weight

Monitoring a horse's BW over time, whether historically from the medical record, or ongoing to assess the efficacy of the feeding plan is undoubtedly an important nutritional assessment tool. Changes in BW of adult maintenance horses are a change in the fat mass, and to a lesser extent, the lean body mass. The fat mass is primarily a stored form of energy and changes proportionally with dietary energy intake, i.e. the fat mass will decrease when dietary energy intake is insufficient to meet daily energy requirements. At the extreme end of weight loss, there will be a loss in the

Table 2.4 Body condition scoring system based on Henneke et al. [36].

Score	General description	Neck area	Withers	Shoulder	Elbow	Ribs	Loin and tailhead
1	Poor	No fatty tissue felt, bone structure obvious	Very prominent	Scapula prominent	No fleshy tissue	Ribs obvious	Spine and hip bones prominent
2	Very thin	Prominent bone structure	Prominent	Prominent	Minimal fleshy tissue	Ribs clearly visible	Spine and hip bones visible
3	Thin	Lean	Lean	Obvious	Minimal fleshy tissue	Outline of ribs visible	Moderate visibility of hip bones
4	Moderately thin	Some fleshy cover	Some cover	Moderate blend into the body	Some fleshy tissue	Faint outline of ribs	Faint outline of hip bones
5	Moderate	Moderate fleshy cover	Moderate tissue cover	Blends into body	Moderate tissue	Not visible but easily felt	Back level, tailhead fleshy
6	Moderately fleshy	Fleshy cover	Fleshy cover	Well blended into the body	Extra fleshy tissue	Spongy cover over ribs	Soft tailhead
7	Fleshy	Fat deposited along the neck	Fat deposited along withers	Not obvious	Obvious fleshy tissue	Ribs felt with pressure	Soft tailhead, ridge beginning to appear
8	Fat	Obvious fat on neck	Not obvious due to fat coverage	Faint scapula	Fat	Barely felt with pressure	Crease down back
9	Extremely fat	Obvious fat and potentially cresty neck	Bulging fat, withers indiscernible	Bulging fat, scapula not visible	Bulging fat	Difficult to feel ribs due to excessive fat cover	Crease down back due to bulging fat on either side of the spine

Table 2.5 Body condition scores (BCS) correlation with body fat content determined by other means.

Horse breed (n)	Comparison methods	Correlation	Details	BCS range (References)
Garrano (27)	BCS and US	$r^2 > 0.74$	Subcutaneous fat + skin thickness, third lumbar vertebra	3–8 [42]
Light horse (24)	BCS and US	$r^2 = 0.75$	Subcutaneous fat at tailhead	3–9 [43]
Andalusian (127)	BCS and US	$r^2 = 0.63$	Subcutaneous at tailhead	3–9 [44]
Quarter horses, Thoroughbreds and Arabians (31)	BCS and US	$r^2 = 0.42$	Subcutaneous at tail region	4–7 [45]
Italian Saddler (25)	BCS and US	$r^2 = 0.549$	On croup, 11 cm cranial to tail head, 10 cm lateral to midline	1.5–4.5 on 5 scale [46]
Welsh × Dartmoore (75)	BCS and girth to height ratio	$r^2 = 0.83$		6–7.5 [5]
Welsh mountain (7)	BCS and white adipose tissue	$r^2 = 0.96$, exponential	Carcass dissection of fat	1–7 [16]

lean body mass (muscle and organs) as well. The animal will die when the fat mass has been depleted and approximately 25–30% of the body proteins have been catabolized for energy. Body protein catabolism is not random. Proteins providing structural support in the form of bones, ligaments, tendons, and cartilage are used after those in the plasma, viscera, and muscle. The extent of muscle loss is the primary determinant of survival because the loss of body protein compromises cardiac and pulmonary muscle function [51]. The cause of death is, usually due to cardiac and/or respiratory arrest as a result of heart, intercostal, and diaphragm muscle degradation and electrolyte imbalances. Conversely, the fat mass will increase when dietary energy intake is more than the daily energy need with seemingly no negative feedback loop to impose limits. There are no known limitations on the size of the body fat mass, although the fat mass begins to cause metabolic derangements and physically limits abdominal and thoracic organs, and the weight limits musculoskeletal mobility. At the extreme ends of obesity, there is little change in lean body mass.

Determining an accurate current BW is essential for nutritional assessment. Therefore, understanding the limitations of weight tapes, morphometric determinations, and BCS is necessary to appreciate the value of the weight data provided. Likewise, weight changes, i.e. a weight history, are important data that should be included in the assessment. Knowing the BW of a horse at some specific point in time previously and by what method(s) that measurement was obtained is important in the nutritional assessment. Body weight changes, decreases, or increases, may be observed in an individual animal or a group. Understanding whether weight changes have occurred in just one, some, or all of the horses in the herd helps rule out certain etiologies of the weight change.

2.4.1 Etiology of Weight Loss

Regardless of the reason for inadequate feed intake, the first and most noticeable effect is an energy deficiency. The majority (80–90%) of the feed ingested is catabolized for energy, 8–15% is needed for protein, 2–3% for minerals, and less than 1% for vitamins. Thus, with inadequate feed intake, the greatest deficit will be first in dietary energy, followed by protein, resulting in protein-calorie malnutrition (PCM). Unless there is a disease-related increase in the loss of specific minerals or vitamins, the signs and effects of deficiencies of these nutrients, during periods of inadequate feed intake, occur much later, to a lesser degree, and are masked by signs of energy and protein deficiency.

2.4.1.1 Foals

Low BW in a young growing foal is more often due to a poor rate of growth. A variety of nutritional and non-nutritional factors influence the growth rate in young horses. The most common causes include inadequate dietary intake of essential nutrients leading to PCM, parasitism, and systemic infection or inflammation. Other factors that will limit weight gain include genetic abnormalities and congenital malformations of the heart, kidney, or palate, toxicosis, and adverse environmental conditions, i.e. extreme cold, heat, and humidity.

Protein-calorie malnutrition is the most common clinical cause of decreased growth and poor weight gain in young foals. Foals are smaller in size, i.e. height and length, and their BW is lower than the normal minimum for the animal's age, breed, and gender. Inadequate intake of digestible energy, protein, and fat results in inadequate concentrations of amino acids, fats, and carbohydrates essential for normal metabolism and growth. Foals that grow slowly as a result of a protein-calorie deficiency may have a normal or increased appetite until they are terminally ill. Clinicopathologic data from foals with PCM often are within the normal range until the starvation process is well advanced.

The etiology of PCM in growing animals is more commonly due to insufficient quantities of feed to meet their nutrient requirements. The reason(s) for the insufficient intake of energy should become evident during a systematic review of the three facets of a nutritional assessment. If the foal has a congenital defect that limits suckling, this should be apparent after a PE. If the foal is offered an inadequate amount of feed, this should become clear after reviewing the feeding method. If the foal is receiving a poor quality diet (milk replacer, feed, or forage) that limits nutrient digestibility, this should become evident with an assessment of the ration.

Other indirectly related nutritional causes of poor foal growth are parasitism and infectious or inflammatory diseases that should become apparent on PE. Parasitism often affects foals and results in decreased growth and poor weight gains by increasing nutrient requirements, increasing nutrient losses, and/or decreasing nutrient absorption. In a heavily parasitized foal, inflammatory reactions associated with the intestinal parasites may also increase nutrient requirements and metabolic rate. Infections or inflammatory processes are important causes of decreased growth and poor weight gain in foals and may be associated with nutrient malabsorption, e.g. chronic salmonellosis, acute rotavirus diarrhea or equine proliferative enteropathy, anorexia as with pharyngeal abscess or systemic disease, increased nitrogen turnover, and direct protein losses from gastrointestinal disease. The decrease in a foal's growth may be of short duration followed by recovery and compensatory gain, e.g. *Rhodococcus equi* pneumonia or cryptosporidiosis, or may persist, e.g. chronic bronchopneumonia. Both energy and protein requirements may be increased as a result of chronic infection and inflammation.

2.4.1.2 Adult Horses

There are four reasons why an adult horse may not consume sufficient dietary energy:

- Feed quantity – the horse is not consuming enough dietary energy to meet the daily need
- Feed quality – poor feed digestibility limits quantity consumption or nutrient availability
- Physical limitation – the horse is physically unable to consume enough feed or water
- Anorexia – the loss of appetite or lack of desire for food

The reason(s) for the insufficient intake of energy, and hence weight loss, should become evident during a systematic review of the three facets of a nutritional assessment.

Weight loss due to insufficient quantities of feed available should become apparent while investigating the feeding method. Competition for feed and water between horses can have a profound effect when horses of different ages are mixed. The more dominant horses keep the more timid, older, or younger animals away from resources. Additionally, adverse environmental conditions, e.g. cold/snow/ice, heat/humidity/drought, flooding/mud, and biting insects can decrease access to feed. The quantity and quality of the water supply must always be considered as horses consume less dry feed when water is deprived.

Low-quality forages are often the cause of PCM, even when an unlimited quantity is available. As forage quality, i.e. digestibility, decreases, both dietary protein, and energy may be deficient despite what would normally appear to be an adequate intake of forage at 2–2.5% BW. Loss of weight in an adult horse may indicate a poor nutritional status caused by feeding poorly digestible forages, or a ration imbalance leading to PCM. Insufficient intake of digestible energy, protein, and fat results in inadequate concentrations of amino acids, fats, and carbohydrates for the metabolism and maintenance of tissues. The protein or calorie imbalance and poor diet digestibility should become evident while investigating the ration relative to the animal's age, size, and physiological needs. Healthy adult horses, including mares in late pregnancy or early lactation, and horses that are working under intense exercise conditions, may experience mild to moderate weight loss during these physiologic conditions. Conversely, pathologic weight loss can occur in pregnant and lactating mares if they are deprived of adequate calories and protein, and in severe cases, mare weight loss can affect milk quality, and hence, the health and growth of a nursing foal.

A physical limitation to obtaining sufficient dietary nutrients due to bodily injury, poor dentition, or parasitism should be considered during the PE. Poor dentition can affect a horse's ability to prehend and masticate feed, which limits feed intake or may lower nutrient digestibility. Parasitism should always be on the differential list in an animal that has lost weight. A chronic heavy parasite load may cause weight loss, but more often, it is a complicating secondary insult rather than the primary cause in adult horses. Parasitism can be further investigated by reviewing the deworming history and using appropriate laboratory tests.

Anorexia, the loss of appetite or lack of desire for food, usually occurs secondary to a primary disease and is regulated by cytokines, including interleukin and tumor necrosis factor-alpha that are released during an inflammatory response. The resolution of the primary disease process usually results in a return to voluntary food consumption. Increased nutrient demands occur with a variety of pathologic disease processes, e.g. sepsis, trauma, and burns, but have not been well defined in the horse to result in specific equine requirements during different disease states. Protein degradation and a negative nitrogen balance are hallmarks of the acute response to infection. Weight loss resulting from endogenous protein and lipid catabolism is often observed in horses with sepsis as a result of altered metabolic activity and nutrient requirements.

Other causes of poor feed intake and weight loss in an adult horse may be related to medical conditions that affect major organ systems involving, e.g. liver, renal, respiratory, and musculoskeletal systems. Weight loss is a frequent finding in horses with chronic respiratory disease that increases the rate and effort. Clinicopathologic data should be helpful in diagnosing liver, renal, or cardiac diseases in an adult horse. Chronic pain in other species is known to decrease appetite and might be in horses as well. However, as a prey species, the horse suppresses obvious signs of pain in the presence of possible predators, including humans. Many pain-assessment tools and scales currently in use in horses, e.g. the Obel grading system, rely on the evaluation while the horse is moving. There are efforts underway to understand how horses exhibit pain without having to move them. Such a tool may bring about a realization that some horses are experiencing chronic pain, which may explain poor appetite in some cases [52]. See Chapter 22 Pain and Discomfort Behaviors. Veterinarians play a key role in helping to identify diseases that can alter the weight and BCS of a horse, and should be consulted when a problem of weight loss is being investigated.

2.4.2 Weight Gain in Adult Horses

Excessive weight gain leading to an overweight or an obese body condition is a common problem in adult horses and develops when an animal consumes more calories than required at a particular life stage or level of activity. Obesity frequently develops in horses fed high-energy rations including grain and energy-dense commercial feed and can occur in horses grazing on highly digestible pastures. Even horses that are only fed hay may gain weight if they consume an excessive amount of energy. Obesity is recognized as an abnormal clinical condition that is related to a variety of difficult to manage metabolic, possibly life-ending diseases, e.g. insulin dysregulation (ID), equine metabolic syndrome (EMS), laminitis, and colic associated with strangulating lipomas and hyperlipemia. For example, a metabolic profile that included body condition differentiated laminitic vs. non-laminitic group ponies with a total predictive power of 78% [50].

Some horses are described as "easy keepers" and may require fewer calories than predicted by a maintenance energy equation to maintain ideal BW and BCS [53]. Certain breeds of equids, e.g. Arabs, Paso Finos, Morgans, and ponies, appear to be predisposed to obesity. Although direct genetic links have not definitively been made between obesity in different horse breeds, one study identified a genetically linked group of ponies that were predisposed to pasture laminitis and obesity, and show the potential role of genetics in excess weight gain and fat accumulation [50]. Leptin is an adipocyte hormone that provides information to the brain regarding body fat stores and reportedly promotes satiety and reduces food intake when the animal is in a positive energy balance [54]. One study in horses showed a positive correlation between serum leptin concentrations and BCS ($r = 0.64$; $p = 0.0001$) [26]. However, another study did not confirm the relationship between leptin concentration and BCS in horses [43].

2.5 Laboratory Tests

2.5.1 Weight Loss or Low Body Condition Score

The type of laboratory tests selected to aid in the evaluation of PCM in horses with weight loss differs based on the duration and etiology of the inadequate feed intake. Horses that have short-term anorexia (24–28 hrs) may show only a few abnormalities on a serum biochemical test. In cases of severe starvation, clinical signs and laboratory abnormalities may be more profound. A routine complete blood count (CBC) and serum biochemistry profile provide a variety of clues about the severity of PCM in an adult horse. Horses that experience weight loss due to a systemic disease or from a suspect parasitic infection should undergo additional diagnostic testing appropriate to rule out those particular diseases (Table 2.1).

2.5.1.1 Anemia

Horses with mild to moderate PCM often have a normal CBC. Anemia associated with a deficiency of iron, cobalt, or vitamin B_{12} is often only identified as a consequence of poor nutrition in a severely malnourished horse. If anemia is present, non-nutritional causes including blood loss due to internal bleeds, parasites, or insects, and that due to chronic disease should be ruled out before pursuing a diagnosis of nutritional anemia.

2.5.1.2 Hypoglycemia

Low blood glucose concentrations are a common complication in neonatal foals that are malnourished but is an uncommon finding in adult horses. Both neonatal foals and adult horses may develop glucose intolerance and hyperglycemia during periods of systemic illness, even if they are protein-calorie malnourished. An evaluation of the serum glucose must always be done with an evaluation of the patient's overall systemic health. Horses with glucose intolerance may require treatment with a therapeutic diet that will not exacerbate hyperglycemia.

2.5.1.3 Electrolytes

Derangements such as hypocalcemia, hypomagnesemia, hyponatremia, hypochloremia, hypophosphatemia, and hypokalemia may develop in anorectic systemically ill horses. Severe electrolyte derangements can also develop during the period of refeeding following PCM in chronically starved horses [55, 56]. Chronically malnourished horses must be closely monitored, and biochemical signs of the refeeding syndrome should be managed with appropriate electrolyte supplementation. See Chapter 24 Refeeding and Assisted Feeding.

2.5.1.4 Hypoproteinemia

Although hypoalbuminemia is occasionally observed in cases of malnutrition, it is not a specific finding, and often is associated with another primary disease process such as parasitism, protein-losing enteropathy, or hepatic disease. Severe protein malnutrition can result in an abnormally low serum urea nitrogen concentration and this finding is usually observed in horses with chronic malnutrition. Protein malnutrition can alter the serum amino acid profile. The excretion of 3-methylhistidine, a myofibril amino acid, in the urine is used as an indicator for muscle breakdown in dairy cows and may be an option in the future for horses [57].

2.5.1.5 Hyperbilirubinemia and Ketones

Partial to complete anorexia in adult horses often results in a mild unconjugated hyperbilirubinemia that resolves once feed intake resumes [58, 59]. Ketone bodies have a glucose-sparing effect in the body and are normally produced from the oxidation of fatty acids by the liver. The concentration of ketone bodies can easily be measured in the urine. Unlike ruminants, horses do not appear to develop severe ketosis following a period of food deprivation, so measurement of urine ketones is a less sensitive indicator of nutritional status than other biochemical measurements [59].

2.5.1.6 Hyperlipemia

Healthy adult horses that are in negative energy balance, even for a short period, rely on endogenous stores of lipid as an energy source. Non-esterified fatty acids (NEFAs) rise within 8 hrs of feed deprivation, and serum TG begins to increase after 36 hrs of withholding feed in healthy horses [60]. When a healthy horse is refed, serum concentrations of NEFA and TG gradually decline over 24–48 hrs and usually return to pre-fasting concentrations. More significant changes occur in the lipid profile of a horse that has been protein-calorie malnourished for greater than 48 hrs, where the concentration of serum triglyceride can be above 500 mg/dL, resulting in hyperlipemia. Pathologic elevations in serum triglyceride (>500 mg/dL) develop in some equine patients that are anorectic and that have a high daily energy requirement due to sepsis or their physiologic state, e.g. gestation and lactation. Miniature horses and ponies and some overweight and obese horses (BCS 7-9/9) may be at an increased risk of developing hypertriglyceridemia when they are malnourished. The prolonged elevation in serum triglyceride concentration may occur concurrently with hepatic lipidosis, a disease that requires aggressive dietary therapy to prevent permanent hepatocyte damage. Hypertriglyceridemia alone does not indicate an inadequate intake of calories but can also occur in horses with ID, renal failure, obesity, and in predisposed breeds (miniature horses, ponies).

2.5.2 Weight Gain or High Body Condition Score

The diagnosis of obesity in equids is currently made by a visual assessment of the patient and palpation of regional fat deposition rather than with laboratory testing. Horses that have gained an excessive amount of body fat, either externally or internally to the body wall, have an increased risk of developing derangements in glucose metabolism, i.e. ID and EMS. Diagnostic laboratory tests can be useful to help identify abnormalities in glucose regulation to help avoid more significant health problems. See Chapter 28 Metabolic Syndrome.

2.5.2.1 Hypertriglyceridemia

Triglycerides appear in the serum when tissue stores of triacylglycerol are broken down. While this often occurs in a fasted state during periods of early and late feed deprivation, hypertriglyceridemia may also appear in overweight/obese horses and those that have ID. In some breeds of horses, elevated serum TG is a useful predictor of pasture-associated laminitis [50].

2.5.2.2 Leptin

As a horse gains weight and has increased adipose tissue, the serum concentration of leptin also increases. Leptin is not diagnostic for ID or EMS and, at this time, the measurement of leptin in horses as a diagnostic tool related to obesity is not recommended.

2.5.3 Mineral and Vitamin Imbalances

While it may be easy to identify equids that are malnourished based on a low or high BCS and palpable fat deposition, identification of either deficiencies or toxicities of minerals and/or vitamins may not be obvious and can present a diagnostic challenge. In most instances, if the ration has not been specifically checked and balanced for minerals or vitamins, the ration will be deficient in more than one of these nutrients. The toxicity of these nutrients is more often iatrogenic related to excessive supplementation of the ration, and this information is often readily apparent in the diet history. Given these minerals and vitamins constitute less than 5% of the ration, during periods of inadequate feed intake, the clinical signs will occur much later, to a lesser degree, and are often overshadowed by the major clinical signs of energy and protein deficiency. In summary, it is plausible, but rare, for an animal to have a single mineral or vitamin deficiency or toxicity, and if so, is usually directly related to the dietary supplement or parenteral administration (Table 2.1).

In the nutritional assessment of the animal, a PE of the horse or several representatives of the herd is required. In particular, skin, hair, hooves, and lens provide an external historical picture of mineral and vitamin status given the longer turnover times of these tissues relative to blood or organs. For example, the hoof wall of a normal adult horse grows at a rate of approximately 6–10 mm/month with rates slower in cold months, higher in warm months, with asymmetrical growth around the hoof. To grow a new hoof from the coronet to the ground takes 9–12 mos at the toe, 6–8 mos at the quarters, and 4–5 mos at the heels; therefore, at ground level, the hoof horn material reflects the nutritional intake 6–12 mos previously (Figures 2.2 and 2.5) [61, 62].

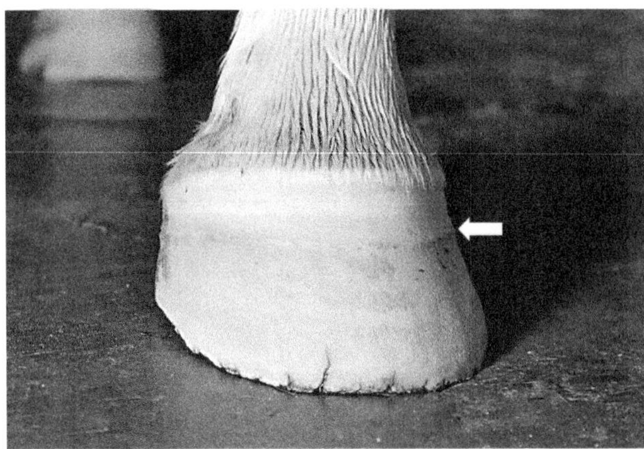

Figure 2.5 Physical examination revealed a distinct line of change in the hoof equidistance from the coronary band on all four hooves, and in all four horses fed the same ration that was changed 3 mos earlier during summer months. The line is not a pathognomonic sign for any particular nutrient change but rather a sign consistent with the ration change.

Table 2.6 In vivo nutrient concentrations and changes suggestive of imbalance.

Macro minerals	Units[a]	Normal range[b]	Suggestive of deficiency	Suggestive of excess	Test sample [62]
Calcium, ionized	mg/dL	5.4–6.4	na[c]	>13.5	Plasma, serum, FE[d]
Phosphorus[e]	mg/dL	2.5–5	<2–4	>6	Plasma, serum, FE
Magnesium	mg/dL	1.6–3	<1.6	>6–9	Plasma, serum, FE
Sodium	mEq/L	135–150	na	>160	Plasma serum, FE
Chloride	mEq/L	90–105	na	na	Plasma, serum, FE
Potassium	mEq/L	3–5	<2.8	>5	Plasma, serum
Micro minerals					
Copper	mg/dL	0.7–1.2	<0.6	>2	Liver, plasma, hair
Iodine	ug/L	16–27	na	>27	Serum T3, T4
Iron	ug/dL	120–210	na	na	Serum ferritin
Manganese	mg/L	0.1–11	<0.1	na	Plasma, serum
Selenium	mg/L	0.09–0.3	<0.065	>0.3	Plasma, serum, whole blood, hair
Zinc	mg/L	0.5–2	<0.5	na	Plasma, hair
Vitamins					
A	ug/dL	12–35	<10	>100	Plasma, serum, liver, relative dose response
D2 or D3	ng/mL	5–60	na	>100	Plasma, serum
E (Alpha-tocopherol)	ug/mL	1.5–10.5	<1	na	Plasma
Thiamin	ng/mL	20–40	<5	na	Erythrocytes
Riboflavin (blood)	ug/mL	0.11–0.17	na	na	na
Niacin (blood)	ug/mL	3–6	na	na	na
Pantothenate (blood)	ug/mL	0.41–0.82	na	na	na
Pyridoxine	ng/mL	26–33	na	na	na
Biotin (blood)	ng/mL	0.31–0.67	na	na	na
Folacin	ng/mL	5–17	<3	na	na
Cobalamin	ug/mL	2–7	na	na	na
Choline	ng/mL	0.11–0.22	na	na	na
Vitamin C	ug/mL	2–4	na	na	na

[a] Units in plasma except where noted in whole blood.
[b] See laboratory specific reference ranges.
[c] No known value available.
[d] Fractional excretion using plasma or serum and urine.
[e] Higher normal values during growth.

In cases where the etiology (deficiency or toxicity) of the clinical signs are not obvious, e.g. goiter or blindness, (Table 2.1), two options are available: [1] diagnostic testing of animal tissues, and/or [2] ration analysis, using laboratory assays, and/or computer assimilation. See Ration Analysis in Chapter 10. There is a common misunderstanding among owners that testing the blood for nutrients is quick, easy, efficient, and accurate. This, however, is often not true for minerals and vitamins because blood concentrations rarely reflect whole-body status, the testing can be expensive; there is often special sample handling precautions, and there is not a test for every nutrient (Table 2.6) [62]. The concentration of many nutrients in blood, plasma, and serum is regulated by hormones and do not accurately reflect whole-body status until there is an extreme deficit or excess. Additionally, the time of the sample relative to the last meal is important to note for some assays.

The urine concentrations of some major minerals, correlated with creatinine corrected for specific gravity, are a reasonable alternative (Table 2.6) [62]. The liver is the organ of choice when assessing micronutrients; however, obtaining a biopsy in the live horse is an invasive procedure that carries a high risk of harm while yielding a very small and limited sample relative to the organ's total size. Conversely, post-mortem liver assays are highly recommended when the liver has been fresh frozen and not preserved in formalin [62].

A word of caution about 'nutritional testing' is necessary. A laboratory offering an assay of a nutrient in body tissues or fluids should not be assumed to be valid as it is relatively easy to detect a nutrient. However, it is incumbent on the Veterinarian to first determine that a particular nutritional test has been independently certified to be appropriate and accurate for the patient's clinical condition [63]. For example, questions often arise about the validity of equine mane hair analysis to determine the mineral balance in the animal. In horses, to date, fewer published peer-reviewed studies have shown the accuracy of hair samples to correlate dietary intake with hair mineral results to determine the whole-body balance of macro, trace, or ultra-trace minerals. Mane and tail hair growth is 10–40 mm/month and may reflect the plane of nutrition 15–20 mos previously [64]. Hair may be a reliable assessment tool for dietary intake of copper, selenium, and zinc but only if the hair has not been treated with products containing these minerals [62]. Other mineral deficiencies or toxicities in horses have yet to be validated between serum, whole blood, other tissues, and hair, and should not be used for diagnostic purposes [64].

Case in Point

Patient Assessment

A 15-year-old Suffolk Punch mare, an English draft breed, presented for a routine PE. The mare was part of a 12-horse herd that did light work on a ranch. Concern about the over-condition of some of the horses and ID had been raised after one previously healthy horse developed bilateral forelimb laminitis and was diagnosed with EMS. The mare's PE was unremarkable except for a BW estimated at 1800 lb, using anatomical measurements (Table 2.2), and a BCS of 8/9. Her ideal BW using anatomical measurements was estimated at 1700 lb (Table 2.3). Routine CBC and serum biochemical panel were within normal limits except for a high serum TGs.

Assessment of the Ration

Total daily feed intake was 2% of the mare's BW [1800 × 2% = 36 lb] consisting of 30 lb of ranch-grown grass hay (0.93 Mcal DE/lb as fed) plus 6 lb of a commercial complete feed with an energy density of 1.2 Mcal DE/lb as fed. Water was provided from a trough, a salt block was present in the stall, and all essential nutrient requirements were met with the current ration. The horse consumed all feed offered.

Feed	lb fed/d	Mcal/lb	Mcal/d
		As fed	
Hay	30	0.93	27.9
Complete feed product	6	1.2	7.2
Total	36		

1) *What was the mare's daily energy intake based on the ration assessment?*
2) *What was the mare's recommended daily energy intake at her current BW doing light work? See NRC [53] pg 302.*
3) *What was the mare's recommended daily energy intake at her ideal BW doing light work?*
4) *How would you explain to the owner why the mare has a high BCS?*
5) *What recommendations would you suggest to the owner?*

See Appendix A Chapter 2.

References

1 Thatcher, C.D., Hand, M.S., and Remillard, R.L. (2000). Small animal clinical nutrition: an iterative process. In: *Small Animal Clinical Nutrition*, 4e (eds. M. Hand, C.D. Thatcher, R.L. Remillard, and P. Roudebush), 1–19. Topeka: Mark Morris Institute.

2 Grants, R. (1995). Veterinarians learn a lesson about nutrition. *Vet. Forum*: 82–84.

3 Milner, J. and Hewitt, D. (1969). Weight of horses: improved estimates based on girth and length. *Can. Vet. J.* 10 (12): 314–316.

4 Carroll, C.L. and Huntington, P.J. (1988). Body condition scoring and weight estimation of horses. *Equine Vet. J.* 20 (1): 41–45.

5 Carter, R.A., Geor, R.J., Burton Staniar, W. et al. (2009). Apparent adiposity assessed by standardised scoring systems and morphometric measurements in horses and ponies. *Vet. J.* 179 (2): 204–210.

6 Catalano, D.N., Coleman, R.J., Hathaway, M.R. et al. (2016). Estimation of actual and ideal bodyweight using morphometric measurements and owner guessed bodyweight of adult draft and warmblood horses. *J. Equine Vet. Sci.* 39 (4): 38–43.

7 Staniar, W.B., Kronfeld, D.S., Hoffman, R.M. et al. (2004). Weight prediction from linear measures of growing Thoroughbreds. *Equine Vet. J.* 36 (2): 149–154.

8 Martinson, K.L., Coleman, R.C., Rendahl, A.K. et al. (2014). Estimation of body weight and development of a body weight score for adult equids using morphometric measurements. *J. Anim. Sci.* 92 (5): 2230–2238.

9 Owen, K., Wagner, E., and Eller, W. (2008). Estimation of body weight in ponies. *J. Anim. Sci.* 86 (Supp 1): 431.

10 Ellis, J.M. and Hollands, T. (1998). Accuracy of different methods of estimating the weight of horses. *Vet. Rec.* 143 (12): 335–336.

11 Wagner, E.L. and Tyler, P.J. (2011). A comparison of weight estimation methods in adult horses. *J. Equine Vet. Sci.* 31 (12): 706–710.

12 Ensminger, M. and Olentine, C. (1978). Principles of nutrition. In: *Feeds and Nutrition*, 19–43. Clovis, CA: Ensminger Publishing.

13 Laflamme, D. (1997). Development and validation of a body condition score system for dogs. *Canine Pract.* 22 (4): 10–15.

14 LaFlamme, D., Kealy, R., and Schmidt, D. (1994). Estimation of body fat by body condition score. *12th Annual Veterinary Medical Forum*, 985. San Francisco, CA: American College of Veterinary Internal Medicine.

15 Burkholder, W. (1994). Body composition of dogs determined by carcass composition analysis, deuterium oxide dilution, subjective and objective morphometry and bioelectrical impedance, Virginia Poly Technic Institute and State University. http://hdl.handle.net/10919/40419 (accessed 2 January 2020).

16 Dugdale, A.H.A., Curtis, G.C., Harris, P.A., and Argo, C.M. (2011). Assessment of body fat in the pony: part I. Relationships between the anatomical distribution of adipose tissue, body composition and body condition. *Equine Vet. J.* 43 (5): 552–561.

17 Ferjak, E.N., Argo, C.M., Cavinder, C.A. et al. (2017). Comparison of horse body fat composition estimated by D_2O dilution, rump fat thickness, and tissue dissection. *J. Equine Vet. Sci.* 52 (5): 50.

18 Harris, L.E. (1970). Determination of ether extract. In: *Nutrition Research Techniques for Domestic and Wild Animals*, vol. 1, 2301. Logan, UT: Utah State University.

19 Dugdale, A.H.A., Curtis, G.C., Cripps, P. et al. (2010). Effect of dietary restriction on body condition, composition and welfare of overweight and obese pony mares. *Equine Vet. J.* 42 (7): 600–610.

20 Dugdale, A.H.A., Curtis, G.C., Cripps, P.J. et al. (2011). Effects of season and body condition on appetite, body mass and body composition in ad libitum fed pony mares. *Vet. J.* 190 (3): 329–337.

21 Westervelt, R.G., Stouffer, J.R., Hintz, H.F., and Schryver, H.F. (1976). Estimating fatness in horses and ponies. *J. Anim. Sci.* 43 (4): 781–785.

22 Dugdale, A.H.A., Curtis, G.C., Milne, E. et al. (2011). Assessment of body fat in the pony: part II. Validation of the deuterium oxide dilution technique for the measurement of body fat. *Equine Vet. J.* 43 (5): 562–570.

23 Ward, L.C., White, K.J., van der Aa Kuhle, K. et al. (2016). Body composition assessment in horses using bioimpedance spectroscopy. *J. Anim. Sci.* 94 (2): 533–541.

24 Fielding, C.L., Magdesian, K.G., Elliott, D.A. et al. (2004). Use of multifrequency bioelectrical impedance analysis for estimation of total body water and extracellular and intracellular fluid volumes in horses. *Am. J. Vet. Res.* 65 (3): 320–326.

25 Lindinger, M.I. (2014). Determining dehydration and its compartmentation in horses at rest and with exercise: a concise review and focus on multi-frequency bioelectrical impedance analysis. *Comp. Exerc. Physiol.* 10 (1): 3–11.

26 Buff, P.R., Dodds, A.C., Morrison, C.D. et al. (2002). Leptin in horses: tissue localization and relationship between peripheral concentrations of leptin and body condition. *J. Anim. Sci.* 80 (11): 2942–2948.

27 Carter, R.A., McCutcheon, L.J., George, L.A., Smith, T.L., Frank, N., and Geor, R.J. (2009). Effects of diet-induced weight gain on insulin sensitivity and plasma hormone and lipid concentrations in horses. *Am. J. Vet. Res.* 70 (10): 1250–8.

28 Valberg, S.J., Borer Matsui, A.K., Firshman, A.M. et al. (2020). 3 Dimensional photonic scans for measuring body volume and muscle mass in the standing horse. *PLoS One* 15: e0229656.

29 Kearns, C.F., McKeever, K.H., Kumagai, K. et al. (2002). Fat-free mass is related to one-mile race performance in elite standardbred horses. *Vet. J.* 163 (3): 260–266.

30 Kearns, C.F., McKeever, K.H., and Abe, T. (2002). Overview of horse body composition and muscle architecture: implications for performance. *Vet. J.* 164 (3): 224–234.

31 Lindner, A., Signorini, R., Vassallo, J. et al. (2010). Reproducibility and repeatability of equine muscle thickness measurements with ultrasound. *J. Equine Vet. Sci.* 30 (11): 635–640.

32 Graham-Thiers, P.M. and Kronfeld, D.S. (2005). Amino acid supplementation improves muscle mass in aged and young horses. *J. Anim. Sci.* 83 (12): 2783–2788.

33 Tozaki, T., Sato, F., Hill, E.W. et al. (2011). Sequence variants at the myostatin gene locus influence the body composition of Thoroughbred horses. *J. Vet. Med. Sci.* 73 (12): 1617–1624.

34 Burkholder, W. (2000). Use of body condition scores in clinical assessment of the provision of optimal nutrition. *J. Am. Vet. Med. Assoc.* 217 (5): 650–654.

35 Silva, S.R., Payan-Carreira, R., Guedes, C.M. et al. (2016). Correlations between cresty neck scores and post-mortem nape fat measurements in horses, obtained after photographic image analysis. *Acta Vet. Scand.* 58 S1 (60): 25–30.

36 Henneke, D.R., Potter, G.D., Kreider, J.L., and Yeates, B.F. (1983). Relationship between condition score, physical measurements and body fat percentage in mares. *Equine Vet. J.* 15 (4): 371–372.

37 Kohnke, J. (1992). *Feeding and Nutrition of Horses: The Making of a Champion.* Pymble, 197. Australia: Barubi Pacific.

38 Kienzle, E. and Schramme, S.C. (2004). Body condition scoring and prediction of body weight in adult warm blooded horses. *Pferdeheilkd Equine Med.* 20 (6): 517–524.

39 Suagee, J.K., Burk, A.O., Quinn, R.W. et al. (2008). Effects of diet and weight gain on body condition scoring in Thoroughbred geldings. *J. Equine Vet. Sci.* 28 (3): 156–166.

40 Mottet, R., Onan, G., and Hiney, K. (2009). Revisiting the Henneke body condition scoring system: 25 years later. *J. Equine Vet. Sci.* 29 (5): 417–418.

41 Guelph, E. (2020). Equine Guelph. Body Condition Scoring Chart Poster. https://equineguelph.ca/education/store.php (accessed 26 February 2020).

42 Silva, S.R., Payan-Carreira, R., Quaresma, M. et al. (2016). Relationships between body condition score and ultrasound skin-associated subcutaneous fat depth in equids. *Acta Vet. Scand.* 58 (1): 37–42.

43 Gentry, L.R., Thompson, D.L., Gentry, G.T. et al. (2002). The relationship between body condition, leptin, and reproductive and hormonal characteristics of mares during the seasonal anovulatory period. *J. Anim. Sci.* 80 (10): 2695–2703.

44 Martin-Gimenez, T., Aguirre-Pascasio, C.N., and De Blas, I. (2018). Development of an index based on ultrasonographic measurements for the objective appraisal of body condition in Andalusian horses. *Span. J. Agric. Res.* 15 (4): e0609.

45 Gobesso, A.A.O., Françoso, R., Toledo, R.A.D. et al. (2012). Evaluation of body condition score in horses by ultrasonography. *EAAP Sci. Ser.* 132 (1): 387–390.

46 Superchi, P., Vecchi, I., and Sabbioni, A. (2014). Relationship among BCS and fat thickness in horses of different breed, gender and age. *Annu. Res. Rev. Biol.* 4 (2): 354–365.

47 Martin-Rosset, W., Vernet, J., Dubroeucq, H. et al. (2008). Variation of fatness and energy content of the body with body condition score in sport horses and its prediction. In: *Nutrition of the Exercising Horse*, vol. 125 (ed. M.T. Saastamoinen and W. Martin-Rosset), 167–176. Wageningen: Academic Publishers.

48 Dugdale, A.H.A., Grove-White, D., Curtis, G.C. et al. (2012). Body condition scoring as a predictor of body fat in horses and ponies. *Vet. J.* 194 (2): 173–178.

49 Johnson, P.J., Messer, N.T., and Ganjam, V.K. (2010). Cushing's syndromes, insulin resistance and endocrinopathic laminitis. *Equine Vet. J.* 36 (3): 194–198.

50 Treiber, K.H., Kronfeld, D.S., Hess, T.M. et al. (2006). Evaluation of genetic and metabolic predispositions and nutritional risk factors for pasture-associated laminitis in ponies. *J. Am. Vet. Med. Assoc.* 228 (10): 1538–1545.

51 Matthews, D.E. and Fong, Y. (1993). Amino acid and protein metabolism. In: *Clinical Nutrition: Parenteral Nutrition*, 2e (ed. J.L. Rombeau and M.D. Caldwell), 75–112. Philadelphia, PA: WB Saunders.

52 Costa, E.D., Stucke, D., Dai, F. et al. (2016). Using the horse grimace scale (HGS) to assess pain associated with acute laminitis in horses (*Equus caballus*). *Animals* 6 (8): 47.

53 National Research Council (2007). *Nutrient Requirements of Horses*. 6th Rev. Animal Nutrition Series, 1–341. Washington, DC: National Academies Press.

54 Spiegelman, B.M. and Flier, J.S. (2001). Obesity and the regulation of energy balance. *Cell* 104: 531–543.

55 Witham, C. and Stull, C.L. (1998). Metabolic responses of chronically starved horses to refeeding with three isoenergetic diets. *J. Am. Vet. Med. Assoc.* 212: 691–696.

56 Crook, M.A., Hally, V., and Panteli, J.V. (2001). The importance of the refeeding syndrome. *Nutrition* 17 (7, 8): 632–637.

57 Houweling, M., van der Drift, S.G.A., Jorritsma, R., and Tielens, A.G.M. (2012). Technical note: quantification of plasma 1- and 3-methylhistidine in dairy cows by high-performance liquid chromatography-tandem mass spectrometry. *J. Dairy Sci.* 95 (6): 3125–3130.

58 Bauer, J.E. (1983). Plasma lipids and lipoproteins of fasted ponies. *Am. J. Vet. Res.* 44 (3): 379–384.

59 Naylor, J.M., Kronfeld, D.S., and Acland, H. (1980). Hyperlipemia in horses: effects of undernutrition and disease. *Am. J. Vet. Res.* 41 (6): 899–905.

60 Frank, N., Sojka, J.E., and Latour, M.A. (2002). Effect of withholding feed on concentration and composition of plasma very low density lipoprotein and serum nonesterified fatty acids in horses. *Am. J. Vet. Res.* 63 (7): 1018–1021.

61 Bowker, R.M. (2011). The concept of the good foot. In: *Rehabilitation and Care of the Equine Foot* (ed. P. Ramey), 2. Lakemont, GA: Hoof Rehabilitation Publishing.

62 Vervuert, I. and Kienzle, E. (2013). Assessment of nutritional status from analysis of blood and other tissue samples. In: *Equine Applied and Clinical Nutrition: Health, Welfare and Performance* (ed. R.J. Geor, P. Harris, and M. Coenen), 425–442. Edinburgh: Saunders Elsevier.

63 Murray, W., Peter, A.T., and Teclaw, R.F. (1993). The clinical relevance of assay validation. *Compend. Contin. Educ. Pract. Vet.* 15 (12): 1665–1675.

64 Davis, T.Z., Stegelmeier, B.L., and Hall, J.O. (2014). Analysis in horse hair as a means of evaluating selenium toxicoses and long-term exposures. *J. Agric. Food. Chem.* 62 (30): 7393–7397.

3

The Horse

Host

Veronique Julliand, Sarah L. Ralston, and Rebecca L. Remillard

KEY TERMS

- Aborad or distal is away from the mouth or opening.
- Orad or rostral is toward the mouth or opening.
- The alimentary tract includes the mouth (lips, tongue, teeth, and pharynx), esophagus, stomach, small intestine (duodenum, jejunum, and ileum), and large intestine (cecum, colon, and rectum).
- The gastrointestinal tract (GIT) refers to the stomach, small and large intestines.
- The foregut includes the stomach and small intestine.
- The hindgut includes the large intestines.

KEY POINTS

- The equine alimentary tract is uniquely adapted, anatomically and physiologically, to a high-fiber herbivorous diet.
- Understanding the functions of the digestive system will aid in the prevention and reduce the risk of diseases (choke, gastric ulcers, colic, colitis, and laminitis) due to improper feeding.
- Forages are critical for normal digestive function and provide nutrition, well-being, and health to the adult equine animal.
- The small intestine is the major site of soluble carbohydrates and protein digestion and absorption, whereas, the major sites of structural carbohydrate digestion are the colon and cecum.

3.1 Introduction

Equine veterinarians, in everyday practice, are regularly confronted with nutritional challenges and are expected to provide appropriate advice on nutrients, feeds, and feeding methods that benefit the horse. Nutrition is a major determinant of animal well-being, health, and performance. Improper feeds or feeding practices may lead to disturbances and, in extreme cases, death of the animal. For example, low-fiber and high-starch diets have been implicated in stereotypic behaviors such as cribbing, circling/pacing, and weaving, and metabolic diseases, such as insulin resistance, ulcers, laminitis, or developmental orthopedic disease. Specific knowledge of equine digestive physiology is essential to providing an informed feeding recommendation.

To understand how the equine digestive system works, each GIT segment will be described, starting at the mouth and ending at the rectum, with respect to structure, motility, endocrine and digestive secretions, and absorption of nutrients for the adult horse, which is useful in daily practice.

3.1.1 Function

The equine digestive system evolved to perform the primary function of breaking down feeds into nutrients that are then absorbed into the bloodstream and provide energy and essential nutrients in the form of simple carbohydrates, fatty acids, protein, minerals, and vitamins to the host. Given the herbivorous ration contains on average 35–60% cell wall carbohydrates (cellulose, hemicelluloses,

Equine Clinical Nutrition, Second Edition. Edited by Rebecca L. Remillard.

and pectins), i.e. "fibers," horses have developed huge distal fermentation chambers in the cecum and large colons that offer a propitious environment for commensal microorganisms. Whereas plant cell wall carbohydrates are resistant to the host's small intestinal hydrolytic enzymes, these fibers are hydrolyzed and fermented by the microbial enzymes, primarily in the large intestine. This leads to the production of short-chain fatty acids (SCFAs), amino acids, and some vitamins that are absorbed from the large intestine providing energy and nutrients to the host. The composition and activities specific to the microbial communities are detailed in Chapter 4 The Horse: Microbiome.

3.1.2 Morphology

The empty adult equine alimentary tract from the esophagus to the rectum constitutes 4.2–5.2% of body weight (BW) (Figure 3.1). The organs associated with the small intestine are the liver (1.1–1.4% BW), and the pancreas (0.9–1.0% BW) [3]. All organ weights decrease during exercise, probably because blood shunted is away from them, and all increase in weight, particularly the small intestine, when grain or feed concentrates are fed [4].

3.1.3 General Motility

A novel feature of our understanding of the digestive system is the enteric nervous system (ENS), referred to as the "second brain." Various gastrointestinal afferent and efferent pathways such as the vagus nerve and the hypothalamic–pituitary–adrenal pathway, ensure bidirectional communication between the ENS and the brain [5]. This regulates all aspects of motility, secretions, and homeostatic mechanisms such as satiety, hunger, and inflammation.

Gastrointestinal tract motility is predominantly stimulated by acetylcholine, via the parasympathetic (vagal) input, and to a lesser extent by substance P or the peptide motilin at the neuromuscular junction. On the other hand, GIT motility is inhibited by norepinephrine, which mediates the sympathetic (adrenergic) input, directly from the sympathetic ganglia. Other neurotransmitters such as nitric oxide, vasoactive intestinal peptide, or adenosine triphosphate also play an inhibitory role in motility. Calcitonin gene-regulated peptide and 5-HT serotonin subtype act to either up-regulate or down-regulate the activity. Secretory epithelia, endocrine cells, and vasculature within the GI tract are also under ENS control. Additionally, numerous peptide neurotransmitters (cholecystokinin, somatostatin, gastrin-releasing peptide, neuropeptide Y, orexin-A) and various opioids also are involved.

3.2 Oral Cavity

Prehension, mastication, and swallowing of foods by any animal are the first critical step in nutrient digestion and absorption. The critical factors affecting feed prehension, mastication, saliva production, deglutition (swallowing), and esophageal function are important aspects of the alimentary tract that are easily overlooked.

3.2.1 Prehension

The importance of the lips and tongue in the initial process of feed ingestion are often discounted. The horse's lips and tongue are essential for feed prehension, more so than the dental incisors [6–8]. The lips are prehensile and very mobile, used to select and draw the chosen particle into the mouth, usually with the assistance of both the rostral tongue and incisors. The overall importance of lip and tongue mobility is highlighted by the clinical signs in horses suffering from nigropallidal encephalomalacia caused by the ingestion of *Centaurea spp.* (yellow star thistle, Russian knapweed). This causes hypertonicity and paralysis of the lips and rostral tongue, which makes it difficult, if not impossible, to prehend loose hay [6, 7, 9]. The tongue and perhaps cheek muscles are necessary to propel ingested feedback to the cheek teeth (molars and premolars) for grinding and swallowing. Functional lips and distal tongue are essential to initiate the digestive process [10]. Anything that interferes with lip and/or tongue function will inhibit the ability of the horse to voluntarily take in feeds.

3.2.2 Feed Selection

The ability of horses to sort out components of textured feeds that have a variety of distinct feed components (processed grains, pellets supplements, powdered additives) is well recognized. They use their sense of smell, taste, and tactile cues from their lips, tongue, and perhaps whiskers to select what they want to ingest. Previous experience with the feeds offered and individual taste preferences will also markedly affect feed selection. Visual cues are of lesser importance, though horses learn to recognize sources of feed such as buckets, feeders, and hay bags. Horses with no experience with such devices are usually reluctant to approach unless they see other horses eating and/or drinking from the novel device.[1]

---

1 Ralston SL. Personal experience with feral horses 1999–2012.

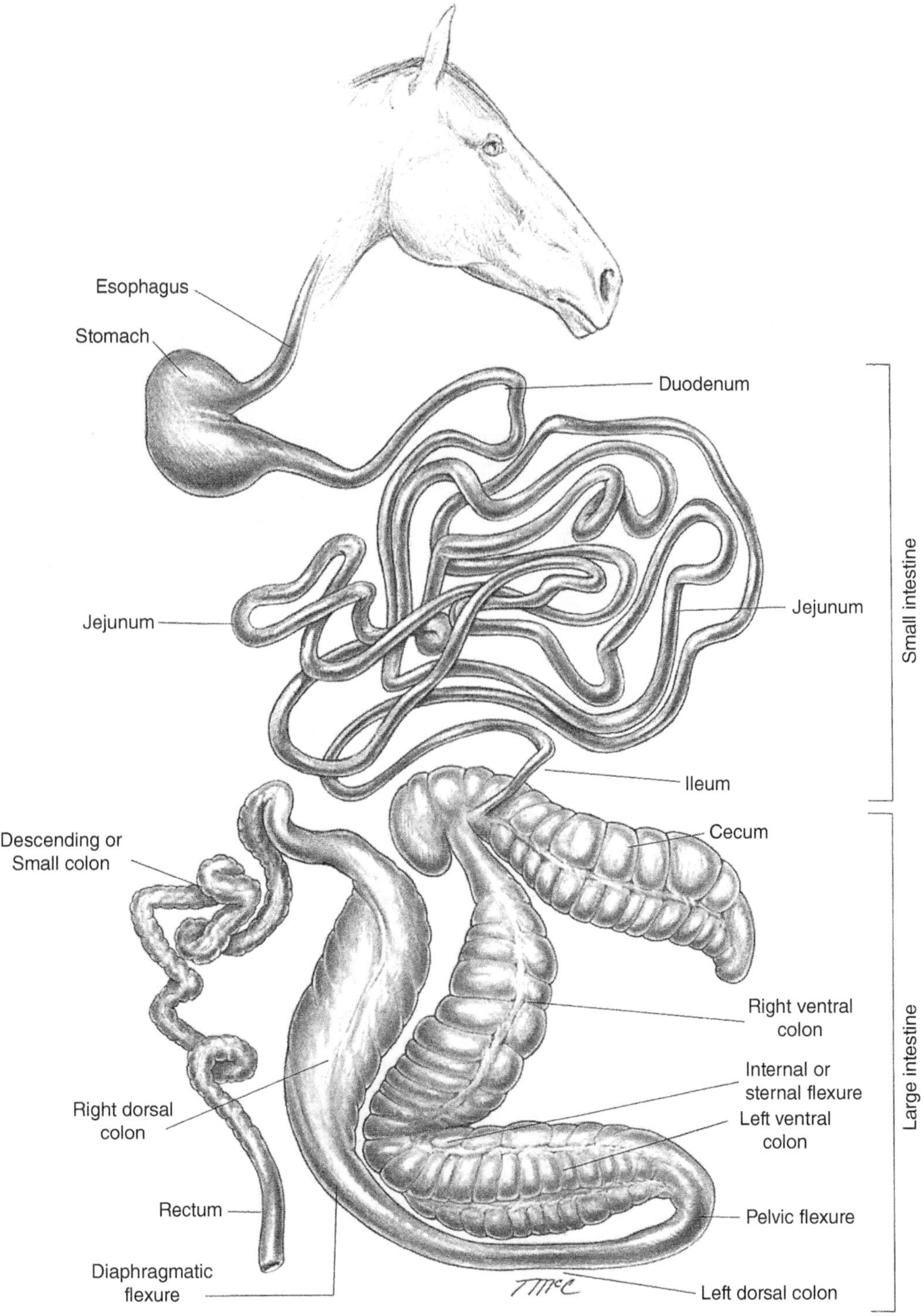

Figure 3.1 Gastrointestinal tract (GIT) of the horse. The stomach of the 1100 lb (500 kg) horse holds 7.5–15 L. Liquids pass from the stomach rapidly with 75% gone within 30 min after ingestion [1]. Of the feed DM ingested, only 25% has emptied from the stomach by 30 min, and more than 98% by 12 hrs following ingestion. Most of the feed dry matter ingested passes as a particulate matter to the small intestine.The small intestine is 20–22 m long, 7–10 cm in diameter, and holds 40–50 L. Liquids pass through the small intestine rapidly and reach the cecum 2–8 hrs after ingestion. In another 5 hrs, most of the liquid that reaches the cecum passes on into the colon. Passage of both liquids and particulate matter through the colon is slow and occurs over about 36–48 hrs.The cecum is 0.9–1.2 m long and holds about 33 L. The large, or ascending, colon is 3–3.7 m long with an average diameter of 20–25 cm and holds about 80 L. It consists of four portions: (i) the right ventral colon, (ii) the sternal flexure to the left ventral colon, (iii) the pelvic flexure to the left dorsal colon (common site of obstruction) and (iv) the diaphragmatic flexure to the right dorsal colon, which connects to the small or descending colon. The small colon is about 3 m long, 7.5–10 cm in diameter, and holds about 18–19 L. As the small colon enters the pelvic inlet, it is called the rectum, which is about 0.3 m long and opens to the exterior at the anus. *Source:* Based on Argenzio et al. [1]; Healy et al. [2].

3.2.3 Mastication

Dentition is also important in the initial digestion of feeds, particularly forages and annual inspections of dental health are recommended. Equine dentition is uniquely adapted to grinding forages and other fibrous feedstuffs into smaller particle sizes, which maximizes the surface area for subsequent enzymatic and fermentative activity in the digestive system [5]. In horses with normal dentition (Figure 3.2), long-stem (>50 mm) forages such as grass and hays, are usually reduced to particles between 0.1 and 1.8 mm in length [11, 12]. Processed feeds, such as pelleted feeds, forage-based cubes, and textured grains, are easily chewed to smaller particles and require less time masticating before being swallowed.

The unique aspects of equine dentition that are pertinent to the digestion of feeds include the continuous eruption of incisors and cheek teeth (premolars and molars) (Figure 3.3). Additionally, the side-to-side grinding of feeds wears down the occlusal surface of the teeth but not evenly [8]. The mandibular arcades are normally 30% closer together than the maxillary rami (Figure 3.4a) resulting in the mandibular teeth wearing more on the buccal (cheek) side, and the maxillary teeth wear more on the lingual (tongue) side. Sharp points, therefore, tend to develop on the outer edge of the maxillary and the inner edge of the mandibular cheek teeth (Figures 3.4b and 3.5). Counterintuitively, horses fed predominantly small particle feeds (pellets and grain mixes) have more uneven tooth wear and are more likely to have sharp tooth edges and points related to the less active lateral chewing activity.

The prevalence of dental abnormalities in adult equine animals has been reported to be 10–80%, depending on the population studied [8, 13, 14]. Common dental abnormalities include hooks on the rostral edge of the second premolars and the caudal edge of the last molar (Figure 3.5), stepped or cupped molars, and missing molars resulting in "wave mouth" (Figure 3.6) and incisor misalignments. Correction of these abnormalities, however, may not significantly improve digestion, body condition, or weight changes in horses that were in good body condition before the procedure was performed, regardless of the type of ration fed [12, 13, 15]. Though it is recommended that the correction of dental abnormalities should be done at least annually, it should be recognized that this may not be necessary for adequate digestion and absorption of nutrients. Horses with severe dental abnormalities (missing incisors, molars, premolars, wave mouth, severe malocclusions) can maintain good body condition if fed a balanced ration using processed feeds and delivered in a manner appropriate for their specific limitations.

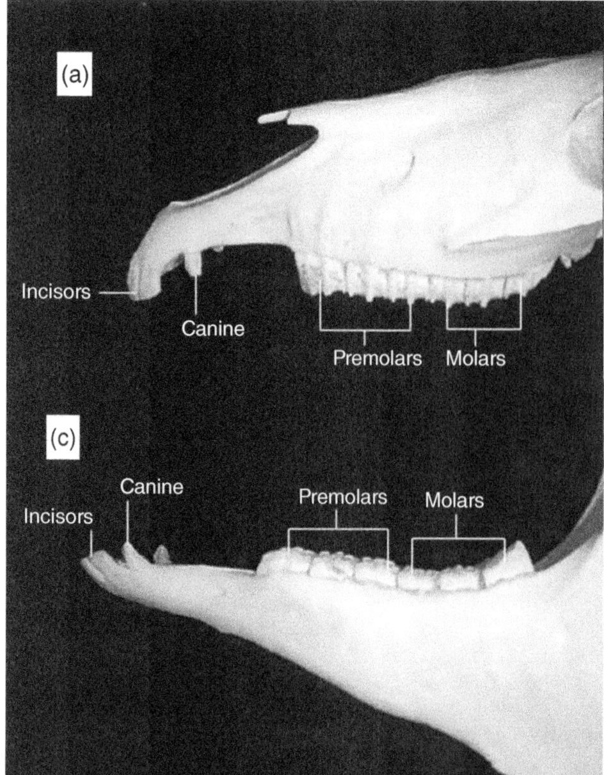

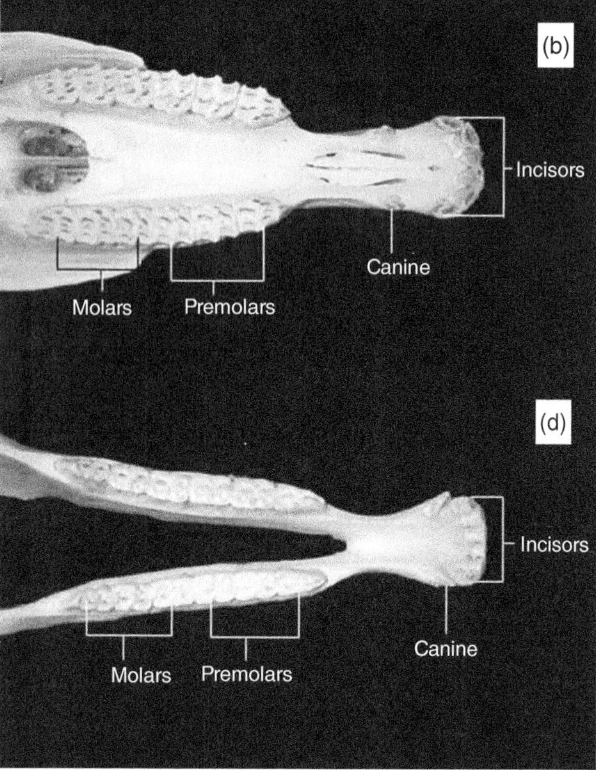

Figure 3.2 Equine dental arcade: maxillary arcade (a) lateral view; (b) dorsal view; mandibular arcade (c) lateral view; (d) ventral view. *Source:* From Melissa Rouge at Dental Anatomy of Horses with permission, VIVO Pathophysiology http://www.vivo.colostate.edu/hbooks/pathphys/digestion/pregastric/horsepage.html. Adult teeth are numbered 1 to 11 rostral to distal. Maxillary teeth are numbered 101 to 111 on the right or 201 to 211 on the left. Mandibular teeth are numbered 301 to 311 on the left or 401 to 411 on the right. The wolf tooth, absent in this specimen, is numbered appropriately xx5.

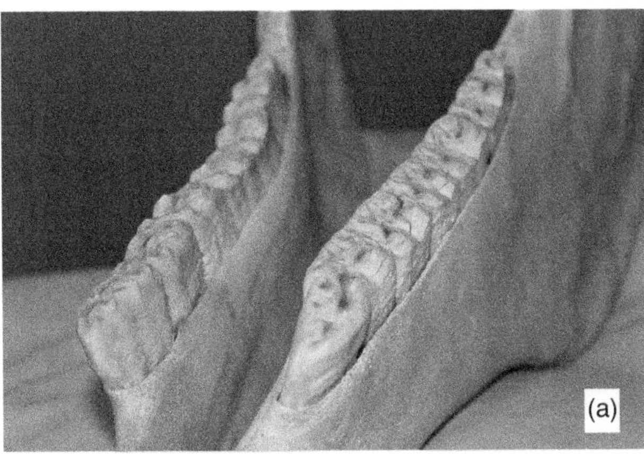

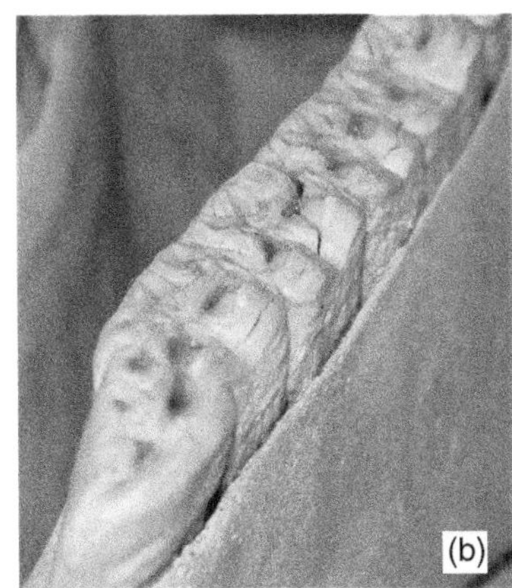

Figure 3.3 Mandibular arcade showing normal wearing premolars and molars (a). Equid molars adapted to the consumption of fibrous plants increasing the complexity of the enamel pattern on the occlusal surfaces (b).

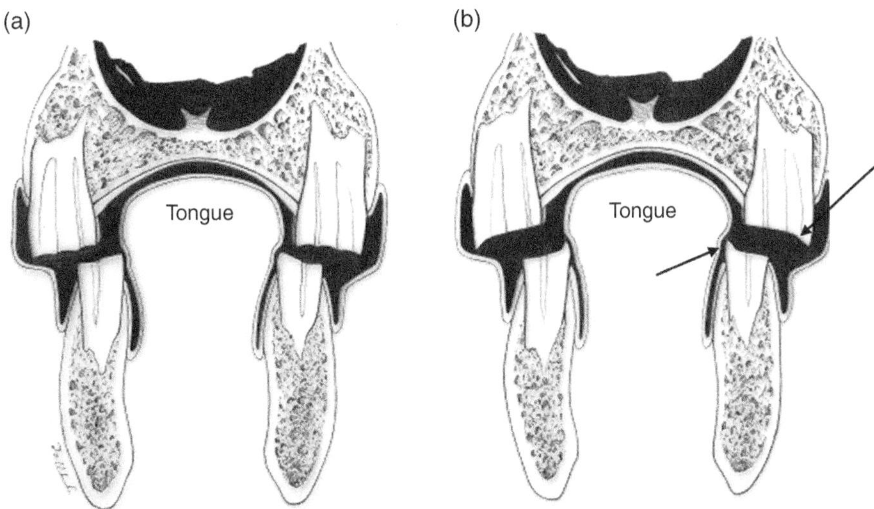

Figure 3.4 The mandibular arcade is normally 30% closer together than the maxillary rami to facilitate grinding across the occlusal surfaces of the cheek teeth. The horse's upper premolars and molars extend as much as one-half a tooth width outside the lower arcade. The teeth wear down the occlusal surfaces of each arcade, progressing from the shape shown in (a) to that shown in (b). The sharp points (arrow) on the upper arcade may lacerate the cheeks, and sharp edges (arrow) on the lower arcade may lacerate the tongue, making the mouth painful.

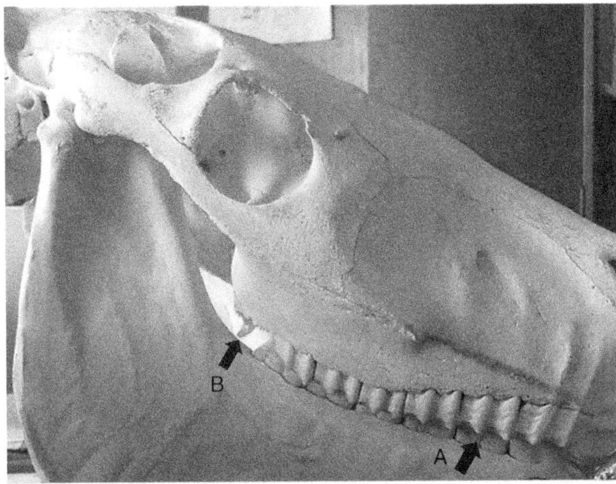

Figure 3.5 Skull of a horse with relatively normal dentition but visible "points" (a) on the maxillary molars and premolars, and a small hook (b) behind the last maxillary molar.

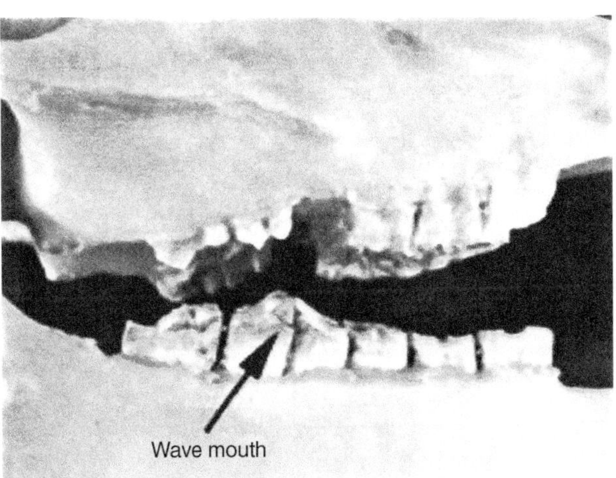

Figure 3.6 Skull of a horse with "wave mouth" due to tooth loss in the upper arcade.

3.2.4 Lubrication and Buffering

Saliva is secreted primarily from the parotid gland in horses and secretion is stimulated primarily by chewing activity. Equine saliva contains fairly high nitrogen (60 ± 18 mg/dL), sodium (162 ± 55 mg/dL), and potassium (76 ± 15 mg/dL) concentrations with lesser quantities of calcium (16 ± 6 mg/dL), magnesium (4 mg/dL), and phosphorus (2 ± 1 mg/dL) with traces of iron, zinc, and copper [5]. The primary functions of equine saliva are lubrication of feed boluses for ease of swallowing and buffering the ingesta to counter subsequent secretions of acid in the stomach. There is an insufficient concentration of amylase to significantly affect starch digestion. Average-sized adult horses may secrete 30–40 L of saliva/d with a pH of 8.6–9.1, depending on feed types consumed [5]. If excessive saliva loss occurs, as in clover-induced slaframine toxicity ("slobbers"), water and electrolyte losses can be clinically significant if water and salt are not freely available.

Long-stem hays and forages stimulate almost twice as much saliva secretion 400–700 L saliva/100 g diet dry matter [DM]) than pelleted feeds 206 L saliva/100 g DM). A horse can take between 9 and 38 min to consume long-stem forage but only requires 2–4 min to consume a comparable amount of pelleted feed. The chewing time difference and subsequent saliva production result in a drier bolus (21–34% DM) compared with boluses of long-stem forage (11–15% DM) [11]. The drier boluses and reduced saliva production with the pelleted feeds could contribute to an increased incidence of choke and reduced buffering of gastric contents, increasing the risk of gastric ulcers.

3.2.5 Absorption

While there is mucosal absorption of some drug preparations in the oral cavity, there is no known absorption of nutrients across the oral mucosa [16, 17].

3.2.6 Swallowing

Swallowing (deglutition) is a uniquely complex process in horses. When not actively swallowing, the rostral tip of the epiglottis lies dorsally over the soft palate, effectively blocking off the opening between the caudal oral cavity and oropharynx. This is why horses cannot breathe through their mouth and why regurgitated feed from a blocked esophagus comes out of the nasal cavity instead of the mouth.

During deglutition, a bolus of feed or fluid is propelled by the contracture of the base of the tongue in the oral cavity through the oral pharyngeal opening, pushing the epiglottis up to cover the laryngeal and tracheal openings, while the soft palate relaxes to facilitate passage of ingesta to the esophagus [10]. The vocal folds and arytenoid cartilages also adduct at this point, to further prevent aspiration. The pharyngeal musculature constricts in a caudal wave toward the esophagus, which is located dorsal to the larynx and trachea. During this phase of deglutition, respiration is not possible. The upper esophageal sphincter relaxes to allow passage of the swallowed substances and then constricts to initiate the esophageal phase of deglution, at which point the oropharyngeal structures return to resting positions and respiration resumes [5, 10]. All of this usually takes less than a second, so the restriction of respiration is normally not an issue.

3.2.7 Esophageal Propulsion

The esophagus is a flaccid tube that goes from the oropharynx to the stomach, usually located on the left side of the neck in the jugular groove above the trachea and adjacent to the jugular vein, carotid artery, and vagal nerves. Boluses of feed are propelled toward the stomach in a peristaltic wave, which culminates in the receptive relaxation of the sphincter at the gastric cardia, allowing passage to the stomach. The proximal two-thirds of the esophagus is composed of striated muscle and the distal third is smooth muscle. There is no reverse peristalsis, as in other species, and the horse cannot voluntarily vomit or expel stomach gas. Passive regurgitation is possible if there is an esophageal blockage, at which point the expelled substances will exit through the oropharynx and nostrils, increasing the risk of aspiration pneumonia if inhaled in the process. There is no known secretory or absorptive activity in the esophagus.

3.3 Stomach

The role of the equine stomach in the digestion of feedstuffs is often disregarded because it has a relatively small volume (8%) of the total GIT representing 8–15 L in the adult 500 kg horse [18]. However, the stomach plays a significant role in the initiation of digesting feedstuffs.

3.3.1 Acid Secretion

The major secretory product of the equine stomach is hydrochloric acid (HCl), produced by the parietal cells of the fundic mucosa. The fundic mucosa constitutes one portion of the glandular mucosa in the distal one-half of the stomach, which is demarcated from the squamous mucosa of the proximal one-half by the margo plicatus (Figure 3.7).

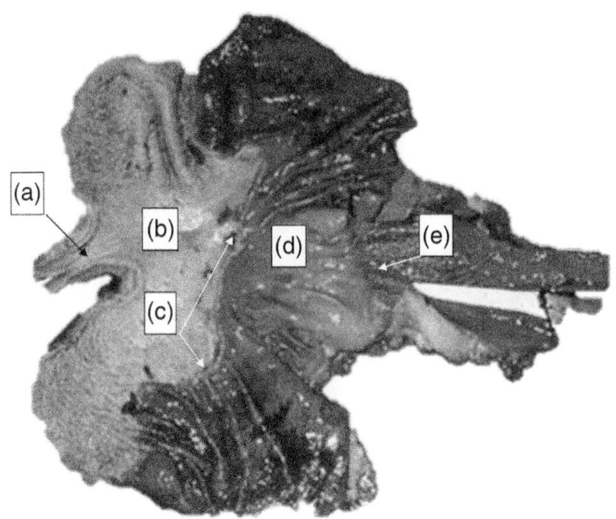

Figure 3.7 Equine stomach: (a) esophagus, (b) proximal, stratified squamous, non-glandular mucosa, (c) margo plicatus, (d) distal, glandular mucosa-secreting protective mucus and bicarbonate, and hydrochloric acid and pepsinogen for digestion, (e) pylorus.

An important characteristic of the equine stomach is that HCl acid secretion continues when the stomach is empty. If given free access to feeds, as is natural in free-ranging horses on pastures, horses eat multiple "meals" frequently throughout the day and night, most intensively in the early morning and evening. However, they rarely voluntarily go for more than 3 or 4 hrs without eating. It is assumed under free-range or ad libitum feeding circumstances that the stomach is never truly empty. On the other hand, when maintained in stalls, horses are not fed according to their natural feeding pattern but instead receive a limited number of meals, usually only 2 or three, often 6 to 8 hrs apart. The gastric glandular mucosa does secrete mucus and bicarbonate and, to a certain extent, can modulate acid secretion; however, acid secretion continues and can reduce the regional pH to dangerously low levels. However, the mucosa in the non-glandular gastric region is not protected, and thus is challenged by HCl acid and may ulcerate, causing equine squamous gastric disease (ESGD) [5, 19].

The secretion of gastric acid is regulated by the complex interplay of hormonal, paracrine, and neuronal components. The feedback loops are responsive to numerous factors, including feed intake and the size and nutrient composition of the ingested meal. In horses fed hay ad libitum, postprandial pH within the non-glandular region near the opening of the lower esophageal sphincter increased and reached a median value of 7.0 consistent with large volumes of saliva flowing to the stomach buffering the gastric acidity [20, 21]. In another study using six horses allowed free choice hay intake, a pH gradient of gastric contents had a median pH between 6 and 7 in the non-glandular portion due to the continuous exposure to saliva; however, the pH was between 1 and 2 within the glandular portion of the stomach where the acid is secreted [21]. In horses fed a pelleted 36% barley and 15% alfalfa concentrate meal in the morning and no hay, the bolus of feed within the stomach coalesced immediately into a bowl shape and remained within the glandular region for a couple of hours surrounded by acidic liquid [22]. The current recommendation is that long periods of fasting (>4 hrs) should be avoided if possible, and a horse should be fed frequent meals (4 to 6/d) or have free access to forage to prevent equine gastric ulcer syndrome (EGUS) [19].

3.3.2 Enzymatic Digestion

The fundic mucosa contains zymogen cells that secrete pepsinogen, which is converted to pepsin when the pH of the medium is <4.0. The role of pepsin in protein digestion is currently unknown in equine animals. Zymogen cells also secrete lipase that has an optimal range of pH between pH 4.0 and 6.0. The role of lipase in the digestion of fat within the gastric ingesta is not known in this species given the natural feedstuff consumed by horses have a low-fat content (4–6% DM).

3.3.3 Bacterial Fermentation

Fermentative activity does occur in the equine stomach. Research has confirmed that there is a large and varied gastric bacterial population in the stomach. There is a marked postprandial rise in bacteria, reaching up to hundreds of millions of colonies/mL of content 3 hrs after a meal. The overall gastric microflora impact on feed utilization is not well understood. Whereas hydrolysis and fermentation of fibrous carbohydrates are probably insignificant, the high proportion of starch-utilizing bacteria in the stomach does have implications in starch and sugar digestion, especially in horses fed grain-based concentrates.

Particle size and nutrient composition of rations appear to be important determinants of the degree of fermentation in the stomach. Starch digestion leads mainly to the production of lactic acid, and to a lesser extent, volatile fatty acids [23]. In horses fed a high-starch pellet, more lactate was fermented into SCFA in the stomach compared to animals fed a high-fiber pellet. This might impact the integrity of the non-glandular mucosa, as excessive production of SCFA is likely to contribute to squamous mucosal injury [24]. If the ingested feed is highly fermentable, the production of SCFA can cause gastric distension and discomfort, particularly if gastric emptying is delayed.

3.3.4 Gastric Accommodation

The elasticity of the gastric wall increases in response to meal ingestion. The gastric wall relaxation is a biphasic response; an initial "receptive relaxation" phase induced by mechanosensors within the pharynx and esophagus to receive the meal, and a secondary "adaptive relaxation" phase controlled by duodenal sensors to control the gastric ingesta exit [25]. Particle size and composition of the ration appear to be important determinants of the receptive relaxation phase. The duration of the receptive phase increased as the size of the hay meals increased from 0.5 to 1.0 g/kgBW [26]. The receptive phase was also shown to be more prolonged in horses fed a commercial sweet feed meal supplemented isocalorically with glucose than corn oil [27].

The secondary adaptive relaxation phase is controlled by the duodenum to regulate an appropriate amount of ingesta entering the small intestines. This interaction between the stomach and duodenum reconciles the difference between meal size held in the stomach and the need for a more consistent flow of ingesta to the smaller diameter intestines. Interestingly, the second adaptive relaxation was triggered only after the larger hay meal was consumed [26]. Therefore, the 1.0 g/kg BW meal size surpassed some threshold that then induced response to slow the delivery of gastric contents to the duodenum.

3.3.5 Gastric Emptying

Gastric emptying depends on slow waves initiated in the gastric corpus and propagated to the pyloric sphincter that generates gastric peristalsis. In the horse, the slow-wave frequency is ~3/min. The coarser contents are moved out primarily by peristaltic contractions that start at the mid-fundic level and move through the pyloric region with increasing rate and strength, i.e. "antral systole" to force the contents into the upper duodenum. The finer, more liquid contents collect within the pyloric region and are forced into the duodenum by a combination of increased proximal gastric tone and antral systole [25]. An interesting feature of equine gastroduodenal motility is that just before the commencement of phase I of the migrating motility complex in the proximal duodenum, the gastric antrum stops moving for a few minutes [28]. During this time, gastric emptying ceases, which may allow backflow of duodenal contents into the stomach.

The time needed for a meal to empty from the stomach depends on the latency period between the time of ingestion and the initiation of emptying, and the rate of emptying is dictated in part by feed composition. Overall, ingested solids leave the stomach more slowly than liquids. The time for emptying half (T½) of a small (200 mL) liquid meal in the horse is ±30 min, whereas small solid meals exit ±90 min [29]. However, isotonic solutions of saline cathartics (1.8% Na_2SO_4, 4.2% $MgSO_4$) did not influence the gastric emptying rate, whereas, hypertonic solutions of saline cathartics (25% Na_2SO_4, 25% $MgSO_4$) significantly delayed emptying [30].

Meal size and composition interact to affect gastric emptying and the effect of a combination may not be predictable. In horses fed a meal of glucose compared with an isocaloric 8% fat meal or 3% fat feed, there was no significant difference in emptying times [27]. However, the addition of soybean oil to an oat and bran mixture significantly decreased the gastric emptying time in ponies [31]. In another study, increasing the starch concentration in a meal significantly increased the gastric emptying time compared with a low-starch meal. Likewise, a small meal emptied faster than a large meal. However, when emptying rate in g/min and Kcal/min of large vs. small high-starch meals were compared, a large meal of high starch emptied at a significantly faster rate than a small meal of high starch [32].

Stress, either physical or psychological, will delay gastric emptying. It is not recommended to feed highly fermentable feeds in large volumes (>0.5% BW DM in a single meal) to a horse immediately before a potentially stressful event such as transport or competition [33, 34]. The current recommendation is that long periods of fasting (>4 to 6 hrs) should be avoided unless medically necessary and that no more than 0.5% BW in dry feed concentrates be offered per meal.

3.3.6 Absorption

It is not known how much, if any, of the end-products of fermentation, are absorbed across the gastric mucosa and thus what the contribution of gastric fermentation is to the nutrition of the host. *in vitro* preliminary studies showed that the stratified squamous mucosa neither absorbed nor transported SCFA in any significant amounts. The glandular gastric and pyloric mucosa absorbed SCFA from the lumen bath but transported very small amounts to the blood. Further results demonstrated that SCFA can penetrate the non-glandular submucosa if the mucosa is exposed to a pH of <4.0 [24]. However, this can be detrimental to the integrity of the mucosal barrier, and whether it allows significant movement of SCFA from lumen to blood *in vivo* remains to be determined.

3.4 Small Intestine, Pancreas, and Liver

The small intestine has three distinct segments (duodenum, jejunum, and ileum), all of which are vitally important to the adequate digestion and absorption of nutrients.

All segments are small in diameter relative to the stomach and large intestines, with a total length of about 25 meter in a 500 kg adult, representing 30% of the total GIT volume. Combined, all three segments have an enormous digestive and absorptive surface area [5]. There is an outer serosal layer with two distinct underlying muscular layers separated by a fascia. The outer longitudinal muscles aid in the mixing of the ingesta, whereas the inner circumferential layers are responsible for peristaltic (propulsive) action [5, 35].

The luminal mucosa of all three segments is lined with villi that are surrounded by crypts, from which the absorptive surface epithelial cells arise and migrate up the villi. These absorptive mucosal cells, along with other cells, such as mucous-secreting goblet cells and immune protective Paneth cells, form a continuous barrier that protects the underlying tissues, absorbs nutrients, and is self-renewing [36]. As these cells mature, they develop microvilli in the upper third of the villus, which produce several different types of digestive enzymes. Collectively, the microvilli are known as the small intestinal brush border with a vast array of digestive and absorptive capabilities. In the center of each villus, there is a circulatory network of blood vessels that receives the absorbed water-soluble nutrients, whereas lymphatic capillaries, primarily in the ileum, receive the absorbed fat-soluble nutrients. The total absorptive surface area due to these villi and microvilli is enormous, given the relatively lesser space occupied by the small intestine in the abdomen. In humans, the small intestinal surface area has been estimated to be 300 meter, which is approximately a 1-m wide path about the length of three football fields [37]. It is assumed the surface area in a 500 kg adult horse would be exponentially greater. Anything that disrupts the integrity of the villi and microvilli dramatically interferes with digestion and absorption of nutrients. Much of the fat and protein and about 50–70% of the soluble carbohydrate are digested and absorbed in the small intestine. All of the feed structural carbohydrates, i.e. fiber, and remaining soluble carbohydrates and other nutrients that escape digestion/absorption in the small intestine pass on into the cecum.

3.4.1 Duodenum

The duodenum is only 1–2 m long in the 500 kg adult horse. Actual nutrient absorption from the duodenum is low, due to the somewhat limited area, but it functions as the receptacle for the pancreatic and hepatic secretions, and orchestration of motility is critical [5, 35]. Enteroendocrine cells that are present in the duodenal mucosa interact with the ENS via neural and hormonal cues to help control motility and secretions throughout the digestive system. The proximal duodenum has been identified as an important "pacemaker" in the regulation of small intestinal peristalsis [35].

3.4.1.1 Mixing of Gastric Contents with Pancreatic and Hepatic Secretions

Digestion of protein, fats, and non-fibrous carbohydrates mainly begins in the duodenum. The pancreatic and hepatic bile ducts empty into the duodenal diverticulum, about 15–20 cm distal to the pylorus. There is a secondary pancreatic duct opening just beyond the diverticulum. Basal pancreatic digestive secretions in the horse have been reported to be copious and continuous, e.g. up to 20–25 L/d in a 500 kg adult horse [38]. Pancreatic "juice" has a high bicarbonate content (~30 mEq/L) and a pH of about 8.0, which serves to buffer gastric acid secretions and may enhance the activity of pancreatic enzymes amylase, trypsin, and lipase [38].

Horses do not have gallbladders to regulate the flow of bile into the intestine but have a continuous low flow on 3–5% fat forage rations [39]. Since horses can adapt to digesting two to three times as much fat as is present in forages, hepatic bile production and secretion can up-regulate. The bile production takes several weeks to fully adapt to a higher fat ration, but the mechanisms are unknown [40, 41].

3.4.1.2 Pancreas

Pancreatic secretions contain numerous hydrolytic enzymes responsible for the digestion of dietary macronutrients: protein, non-fibrous carbohydrates, and fat (Figure 3.8) [5]. Proteolytic enzymes, peptidases, hydrolyze the dietary proteins. There are two types of peptidases: endopeptidases that break bonds along the polypeptide chain, and exopeptidases that break bonds at either the carboxy- or amino-terminal peptide bond. Amylase hydrolyzes the alpha-1,4 and 1,6 glucoside bonds of starch and maltose. There are several different lipase enzymes produced by the pancreas. Lipase specific for dietary triglycerides is primarily responsible for dietary fat digestion but requires an oil–water interface, so only fatty acids emulsified with bile salts can be hydrolyzed and absorbed. Co-lipases facilitate the action of lipase and protect lipase from inactivation [42].

3.4.1.3 Liver

Hepatic contribution to the digestion and absorption of nutrients from food primarily involves the production of bile salts and the enterohepatic circulation of bile acids. Bile acids are conjugated with an amino acid to form water-soluble bile salts in the liver. The conjugated bile acids enter the proximal duodenum with pancreatic lipase and

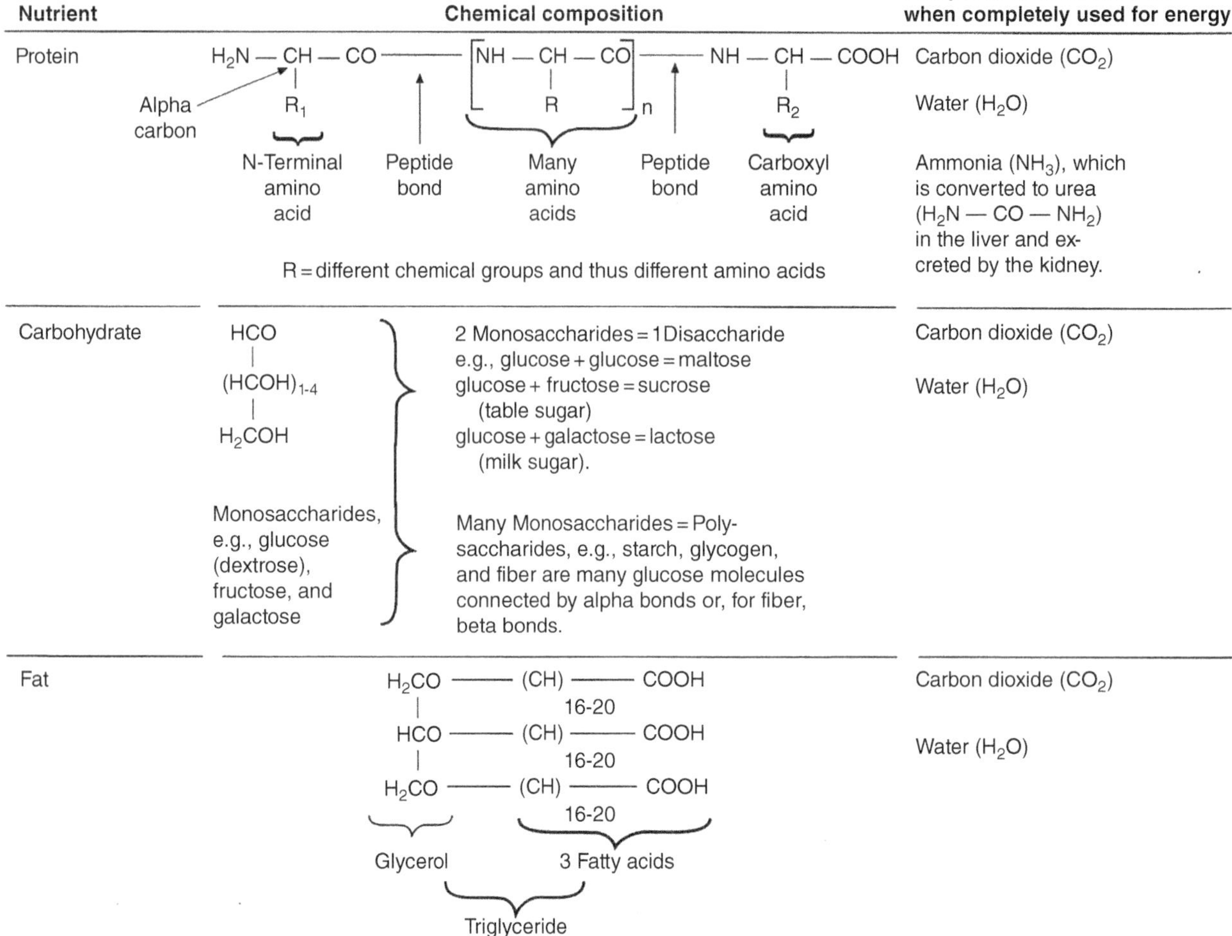

Figure 3.8 Chemical composition of energy-supplying nutrients. Reprinted with permission from Lewis LD, Morris M, Hand MS. Small Animal Clinical Nutrition, 3rd Edition Topeka, KS: Mark Morris Institute, 1987.

form mixed micelles surrounding dietary triglycerides, and the products of fat digestion; 2-monoglycerides and free fatty acids. Bile salts are not essential to fat digestion, however, the presence of bile acids favors smaller micelle formation (see Sidebar 3.1), and thereby, enhances lipase activity and fat absorption. Absorption of bile acids from the intestine occurs primarily in the ileum, by active transport, and are returned to the liver by the portal circulation. The enterohepatic circulation is efficient in the recycling of unconjugated bile acids [42].

Sidebar 3.1: Micelles

Given fat is hydrophobic and not soluble in the water medium of intestinal digesta, the digestion of dietary fat requires that the lipids be packaged into small micelles first, and then the micelles are dispersed, i.e. emulsified, throughout the digesta. Analogous to mixing 10 mL of corn oil into 100 mL of water and then shaking the container to see many small micelles of fat dispersed throughout the water. A micelle is a bilayer aggregate of hydrophobic and hydrophilic molecules in a water medium. The hydrophilic head is facing out and in contact with the water solvent, whereas the hydrophobic tail is facing the micelle center containing the lipid molecule. The micelle also contains lipase, which is directly in contact with the lipid molecules. Continuous mixing is essential to keep the micelles dispersed, just as leaving the corn oil in a water container still for an hour will allow a fat layer to coalesce on top of the water.

3.4.2 Jejunum

The middle and longest section of the small intestine is the jejunum measuring 18–20 meter long in a 500 kg horse. Despite the relatively narrow diameter, the villus/microvillus surface area is extensive [35].

3.4.2.1 Digestion of Dietary Nutrients

The jejunum is the primary site of dietary non-fiber bound starch and sugar, protein, and fat digestion. There is more than ample enzymatic digestive capability in this region in horses on most forage/concentrate rations, arising from both the pancreatic secretions and the enzymatic activity at the brush border surface. Enzymes required for the end-stage digestion of non-fibrous carbohydrates (sucrase, maltase, and lactase), are present in the brush border, as are co-lipases [5]. Ponies subjected to greater than 60% resection of the total jejunal length were unable to maintain adequate BW on standard hay and grain rations [43]. The majority of dietary structural carbohydrates (fiber) passes through the small intestine into the cecum.

3.4.2.2 Absorption of Nutrients

The absorption of the resultant nutrients from enzymatic digestion: mono- and disaccharides, di-and tri-peptides, and minerals (except calcium and phosphorus) occurs in the jejunum (Figure 3.8). It is not clear in the horse whether the absorption of free fatty acids, 2-monoglyceride, and fat-soluble vitamins occur only in the jejunum or in both the jejunum and ileum. Although water-soluble vitamins produced by microbial synthesis are absorbed across the large bowel mucosa, dietary sources of water-soluble vitamins are mainly absorbed in the jejunum. Almost 80% of the jejunal blood supply feeds the villi to transport absorbed nutrients directly to the liver. The blood supply to the jejunum is provided by an interconnecting series of 15–20 arteries that flow from the cranial mesenteric artery through the jejunal mesentery to the serosa and mucosa, where they anastomose with veins flowing back to the liver [18].

3.4.3 Ileum

The last segment of the small intestine is the relatively short, thick-walled ileum. Only a meter long in the average adult horse, this segment is where most, if not all, the fats, fat-soluble vitamins, and calcium are absorbed, based on studies of horses following jejunal–cecal anastomosis [44]. The intestinal lymph system receives absorbed fatty acids and fat-soluble vitamins that are transferred to the circulatory system at the thoracic duct. Significant amounts of phosphates are secreted into the lumen to provide further buffering to the cecal and colonic contents. If the ileum is bypassed surgically by jejunocecal anastomosis, the horse will require dietary (or parenterally) vitamins A and E supplemented in specialized water-soluble forms, and fat added to the ration should be avoided. Calcium absorption and phosphorus balance will also be of concern long term.

3.5 Cecum and Large Colon

The large intestine includes the cecum, large and small colons, and rectum, and represents about 60% of the total GIT volume in the adult 500 kg horse (Figure 3.1). The sacculated cecum accounts for an average volume of 33 L and the large colons can accommodate an average of 80 L [18]. The mucosa of the cecum and large colon forms deep cavities called crypts of Lieberkühn that open to the lumen, and lack villi. Cells within the crypts are involved in host defense and signaling and are the site of the stem cells that migrate up to replenish the mucosal epithelial cells. The epithelium is composed primarily of absorptive columnar cells, which have microvilli on their apical surface. The crypts are also lined with numerous goblet cells and single enteroendocrine cells within the basilar region but there are no Paneth cells [45].

The cecum and large colon absorb nutrients from the fermentation of ingested plant components that could not be digested or bypassed digestion/absorption in the small intestine, and phosphorus from ileal secretions. The sequential four compartments of the large colon are the ventral colons, right and left (RVC, LVC), and dorsal colons, left and right (LDC, RDC) (Figure 3.1). Each compartment creates an individual ecosystem as a dynamic entity composed of a distinct biological and environmental component. Here lies the key to the symbiotic relationship between the horse and the GIT microbiome. This relationship is very important to appreciate and understand. See Chapter 4 The Horse: Microbiome.

3.5.1 Microbial Utilization of Feeds

Endogenous enzymatic digestion in the large intestine has not been described and is probably negligible. On the contrary, the distal segments of the equine GIT are uniquely adapted to the microbial digestion of feeds. The environmental parameters of the hindgut are particularly favorable for the growth and activity of strictly anaerobic microorganisms. Hindgut pH oscillates around neutrality, with water content averaging 92% and 80% in the cecum and colon, respectively, is devoid of oxygen and temperature varies little from 39 °C [46]. The feeding conditions under which the horse evolved, i.e. a relatively continuous supply of fibrous feeds, are favorable to and drive the fermentation process in the large bowel. Conversely, abrupt changes in feed type and body temperature (hyperthermia and dehydration) can drastically and usually adversely affect the fermentation process, and subsequently, the nutrition derived from fibrous feeds.

Cecal and large colonic compartments have specialized in the digestion of plant structural carbohydrates, i.e. cellulose, hemicelluloses, and pectins, with conditions favorable to microbial populations capable of fiber digestion. Water-soluble carbohydrate that escapes foregut breakdown is digested within the cecum and colons. Some bacterial protein is also produced, digested, and absorbed from the cecum and colon.

3.5.1.1 Microbial Utilization of Dietary Complex Carbohydrates

Protozoans, fibrolytic, and amylolytic microorganisms hydrolyze carbohydrates into simple sugars of cellobiose, glucose, and xylose, which are then fermented leading to the formation of pyruvate, and subsequently to SCFAs, lactate, and gases, carbon dioxide (CO_2), hydrogen (H_2), and methane (CH_4). High concentrations of SCFAs within the hindgut contents, averaging 58 mmol/L in the cecum and 80 mmol/L in the colon, indicate intense hindgut fermentative activity [23]. The majority (75%) of SCFAs produced is acetate, with lesser concentrations of propionate (18%) and butyrate (6%), and total lactate concentration is relatively low, averaging 2.5–3 mmol/L although this is ration composition dependent [47]. Early work concluded that the majority of the total energy utilized by ponies fed forage-based feed was derived from SCFAs' metabolism [48]. It subsequently was estimated that approximately 30% of the digestible energy intake was supplied by cecal SCFAs metabolism in ponies fed a forage-based pelleted feed [49].

Additionally, the ratio of SCFAs [(acetate + butyrate)/propionate] is affected by ration composition. In horses fed 100% forage, the ratio ranged between 4.3 and 6.0, whereas lower values ranged from 3.1 to 4.3 in horses fed high-grain rations indicating that more carbohydrate from grain produces more propionate [23]. Likewise, as the proportion of barley increased in a hay ration, the concentration of lactate-utilizing bacteria increased in the colon but did not significantly alter the cecal population. These changes in the microflora were associated with a significant decrease in intestinal pH and [(acetate + butyrate)/propionate] ratio, and a numerical increase of lactate concentration [47]. This is noteworthy because propionate is a major hepatic gluconeogenic substrate. Acetate and butyrate do not contribute directly to the net synthesis of glucose [50].

3.5.1.2 Microbial Utilization of Dietary Fat and Protein

It is assumed that long-chain fatty acids (LCFAs) from dietary fats reaching the hindgut are fermented and converted to SCFA by the microbial populations. There has been some *in vitro* data suggesting that protozoa could contribute actively to triglyceride hydrolysis and that bacteria could utilize protein sources (gelatin, casein, peptones, amino acids, or ammonia) and to some extent urea [51, 52]. Little is known concerning the extent to which microflorae utilize dietary protein and non-protein nitrogen contributions to the amino acid pool in the horse.

3.5.2 Mixing and Emptying

Coordinated cecal-colonic motility is essential for optimal fermentative digestion and movement of ingesta through the compartments. Segmental motility contributes to the mixing of microorganisms with substrates and increases digesta retention time favoring the digestion and absorption of end-products and water. Propulsive motility contributes to large intestinal emptying, i.e. pushing the contents from one segment to the next. If intestinal contents move rapidly, optimal fermentative activity and water absorption are reduced, resulting in increased fecal water (diarrhea) or, if digesta moves slowly, fecal water is decreased and impaction may result.

In the cecum, which is essentially a blind sac with entry and exit orifices located dorsally in the abdominal cavity, electrical waves from the apex generate progressively defined rings of contraction toward the cecal base to push trapped digesta and some gas aborally into the RVC every 2–4 min. The orifice remains open for 20–40 sec during the cycle allowing some reflux of a small quantity of ingesta from the ileocecal area and RVC back into the cecal base. Other waves in the opposite direction happen along the whole cecal body and are orientated toward the apex. The turnover time of contents within the cecum is relatively short (less than 4 and 2 hrs for solid and liquid phases, respectively), which represents less than 10% of the transit time through the equine GIT. Fasting decreases cecal emptying and contents remain in the cecum for longer periods compared with regular feeding, which might increase the risk of impactions.

In the four large colon sections, there are three patterns of electrical waves: (i) distinct "slow migrating complexes" (SMCs) going aborally, that occur in 10–20 min intervals with cluster duration of 5–8 min and a propagation rate of 0.5–1.0 cm/min; (ii) random long spike bursts dispersed between the distinct SMC and happening up to 6 sec each in duration that rapidly propagates in either an orad or aborad orientation; (iii) very intense periodic "colonic migrating myoelectrical complex" (CMMC) of 5–8 min duration. This CMMC propagates rapidly (~3 cm/s) in an aboral direction and is followed by a period of relative electrical quiescence that lasts 5–15 min.

The motility of the equine large colon and its effects on digesta transit is not yet well identified. The average mean retention time in the cecum, RVC, LVC, LDC, RDC, and small colon was reported to be 2.9, 3.1, 5.9, 1.0, 4.0, and 4.0 hrs, respectively in Thoroughbred horse fed timothy hay and silage [53]. The DM content of the digesta plays an important part in the rate of passage, particularly through the various portions of the colon. Potential sites of decreased flow, particularly if the digesta contains larger particles or is dryer than normal, are at the pelvic flexure and the transverse colon where the lumen diameter becomes markedly smaller than that of the preceding LVC and RDC, respectively [54].

3.5.3 Absorption of Nutrients

3.5.3.1 Absorption of Short-Chain Fatty Acids and Lactate

The absorption of LCFAs from dietary fats in the equine hindgut has not been studied but they are likely fermented to SCFAs. Early work demonstrated that the rate of SCFAs absorption is inversely proportional to molecular weight, with the absorption of acetate > propionate > butyrate > lactate. The uptake of SCFAs across the apical membrane of colonocytes relies, in a small part, on passive diffusion of undissociated SCFAs but largely on the active transport of dissociated SCFAs anions using different competitive transporters [55].

Passive SCFA absorption is, unexpectedly, nearly independent of luminal pH. This is attributed to the presence of a nearly constant pH-microclimate at the epithelial surface [56]. It is unlikely that passive diffusion of the undissociated form plays a major role as SCFAs exist almost entirely in their dissociated, i.e. ionized, forms at the neutral pH in the cecum and large colon of horses.

The cellular entry of SCFAs is primarily dependent on specific carrier proteins on the cell surfaces, based on studies demonstrating that SCFAs transport follows saturation kinetics and is inhibitable. Acetate, propionate, and butyrate are transported across the equine colonic luminal membrane via a monocarboxylate/H^+ cotransporter. The transport of SCFAs from the lumen of the equine colon into the colonocytes occurs with sodium chloride (NaCl) and water absorption [57]. SCFAs absorption is accompanied by H_2CO_3 secretion into the lumen of the cecum and colons that buffers the content. The equine colonic monocarboxylate/H^+ cotransporter of SCFAs is inhibited by lactate [57, 58]. Additionally, alterations in the intracellular pH modulate the exchange of Na^+/H^+, which in turn influences salt, water, and nutrient absorption. In summary, when horses consume a ration that results in starch and sugars entering the large intestine, colonic lactate production increases, and pH decreases, which may alter bowel wall integrity. Horses fed a high-starch ration (11.4 g/kg BW) were found to have higher aerobic bacterial counts in mesenteric lymph nodes and liver compared with horses fed 2 g starch/kg BW [59]. The concentration and activity of fiber-degrading microorganisms become limited, and SCFAs production and water absorption decreases as starch intake increases [60, 61].

3.5.3.2 Absorption of Protein End-Products

From the 1970s, studies indicated that both protein and non-protein nitrogen (N) were used by the equine large intestine [62, 63]. It was suggested that identifying colonic N transporters may shed light on the nature of N absorption, including amino acids (AA), peptides, and N-end-products derived from microbial degradation. Since that time there has been very little research in horses on specific amino acid transporting systems in the equine large intestine.

However, more recent data revealed the presence of cationic and neutral amino acid transporter gene transcripts in the equine colonic mucosa. While some genes increased in abundance from cranial to caudal portions of the intestine, others decreased, and some remained relatively constant [64]. It was also reported that, *in vitro*, the large colon of ponies did transport L-lysine across the apical epithelial membrane with greater capacity but less affinity than the jejunum [65]. The large colon may, therefore, play a significant role in at least lysine absorption and homeostasis in horses.

The importance of the colon in nitrogen balance in horses was highlighted in studies of horses that had undergone surgical resection of the entire large colon, leaving only the cecum anastomosed to the small colon [66]. When the resected horses were fed an alfalfa-based ration with a high protein content (>16%), the animals maintained weight and condition, and one pregnant mare came to term and produced a healthy foal. When the same horses were placed on a low crude protein (7–9%) grass hay, the animals rapidly lost weight and condition. However, the quantitative and qualitative importance of microbial protein-derived AA from the large intestine in horses remains unknown.

3.5.3.3 Absorption of Minerals and Vitamins

Regarding calcium absorption in the equine large intestine, the mRNA expression of different proteins involved in transcellular calcium transport has been reported. Their expression is overall much lower in the hindgut than in the small intestine [67]. As for phosphorus, based on the resection studies conducted in the 1980s, the large colon appears important as a site of phosphorus absorption. Following major large colon resection, horses fed adequate rations were in negative phosphorus balance [66].

The mRNA expression of the vitamin D receptor is higher in the large colon (15–25-fold) than in the small intestine [67]. A recent study measuring the bioavailability of different forms of vitamin K administered orally concluded that the water-soluble form of vitamin K was the most efficiently absorbed. Since there is significant water-soluble vitamin production associated with fermentation, and horses that have not been shown to have dietary requirements for any of the water-soluble vitamins except, perhaps, thiamine, it is assumed these are absorbed efficiently in the large colon as well as the small intestine. However, the mechanisms of intestinal absorption of fat-soluble and water-soluble vitamins have not yet been described.

3.5.3.4 Absorption of Electrolytes and Water

There is also a net absorption of sodium, chloride, and water from the colonic lumen into the blood. Considerable liquid flows were measured from the cecum and the dorsal colon reaching respectively up to 54 and 49L/d [68]. In the four segments of the large colon, sodium absorption is primarily, though not exclusively, electroneutral, in exchange for H^+ that protonates the SCFAs. The large intestine is a major water reservoir that varies directly with the quantity of SCFAs produced by the microorganisms for the diffusion of substrates and microbial products [55, 69]. Thus food intake and meal composition have a strong impact on the hydration of horses through SCFAs.

3.6 Small Colon, Rectum, and Defecation

The equine small colon is a relatively short, narrow tube, the main function of which is to reabsorb the water from the ingesta arriving from the large colon and forming the fecal balls in the process to be excreted through the anus. It is rarely involved in pathology such as impactions except for one case where small colon impactions were associated with ingestion of hay containing hairy or common vetch seeds.[2]

3.6.1 Structure

The small colon is about 3 meter long, 7.5–10 cm in diameter, and holds about 18–19 L [18]. When it enters the pelvic inlet, it is called the rectum, which is about 0.3 meter long and opens to the exterior at the anus sphincter.

3.6.2 Motility

There are no data available on the control of motility in the equine small colon. However, defecation, i.e. the expulsion of feces from the rectum, is under voluntary control in equines. When psychologically stressed, horses will usually voluntarily defecate, and, if the stress is prolonged, do so repeatedly, the feces becoming more and more liquid, suggesting a much faster passage rate through the small colon.[3] This is probably an adaptation to the flight or fight response of prey animals. Additional weight has been well documented to slow a horse's speed and stamina, in flight or racing, and the average defecation of an adult 500 kg horse fed a primarily forage ration weighs 2–3 kg. Therefore, during stress and in preparation for flight, the horse will routinely defecate, presumably reducing bowel ballast.

3.6.3 Absorption

The primary absorptive function of the small colon is to remove water from the ingesta coming from the large colons, forming the fecal balls, which are normally 60–70% DM. There is the absorption of sodium from the small colon that is not coupled to SCFA absorption or acid/base adjustments but is moving down an electrochemical gradient to conserve sodium and water [69–72].

2 Ralston SL. Personal experience in one case.
3 Ralston SL. Personal experience with cases 1976–2020.

Case in Point

A 23-year-old Arabian gelding was evaluated for weight loss noticed in early spring by the longtime owner as the horse shed out from winter. The horse had been in good health but had a significant heart murmur (holosystolic). It had been fed local timothy hay offered ad libitum and 0.5 kg of a ration balancer fed once daily. Water and TM salt were available at all times. The owner had a younger horse in the same small dry lot with limited pasture that was not losing weight.

1) *Other information obtained before doing a physical examination:*
   a) *Can a deworming program be outlined?* Yes and determined to be adequate.
   b) *How are the horses fed?* Ad libitum hay as a group outdoors under a roof but individually stalled indoors for the concentrate once daily for about 30 min.

c) *Visual inspection of the hay and concentrate.* Feed appeared to be free of weeds, mold, and foreign materials and considered to be of good to excellent quality.
d) *Describe the horse's appetite?* It had been considered to be good and no change was noted.
e) *Is the ration known to be nutritionally balanced?* Yes, it had been checked the previous September after a hay analysis.
f) *What is the manure consistency and amount/d?* All considered normal by the owner.

2) *On physical examination, what areas are of particular concern in this case?*
The physical examination findings were unremarkable, except for the low BCS, cardiac murmur, and oral examination. The calculated ideal body weight based on body length and height (Chapter 2; Table 2.3) was 400 kg, but according to the estimated BW equations (Chapter 2; Table 2.2), this horse weighed 320 kg, 20% under an estimated ideal weight. The horse had a BCS 4/9, lower than ideal but not emaciated. An oral exam revealed that premolars #106 & #107 were missing; #108 and several #300 & 400 premolars were loose. The horse was able to consume the pelleted ration balancer with no problems when soaked in water but could not properly chew long-stem hay, dropping large, partially chewed boluses onto the ground (quidding). Laboratory data from a complete blood cell count and serum biochemistry were within normal limits.
3) *Summarize the problem(s) for the owner, suggest next steps and general dietary recommendations.*
4) *What specific changes to the ration could be made to provide more digestible calories to this horse?*

See Appendix A Chapter 3.

References

1 Argenzio, R., Lowe, J., Pickard, D., and Stevens, C. (1974). Digesta passage and water exchange in the equine large intestine. *Am. J. Physiol. Content.* 226 (5): 1035–1042.

2 Healy, H.P., Lawrence, L.M., Siciliano, P.D., and Blackford, J.T. (1993). Determination of gastric emptying rate of mature ponies. In: *Proceedings of 13th Equine Nutrition and Physiology Society Symposium*, 24–25. Gainesville, FL: Equine Nutrition and Physiology Society.

3 Meyer, H. (1987). Nutrition of the equine athlete. In: *International Conference on Equine Exercise Physiology* (ed. J.R. Gillespie and N.E. Robinson), 644–673. Davis, CA: ICEEP Publications.

4 Meyer, H., Coenen, M., and Stadermann, B. (1993). The influence of size on the weight of the gastrointestinal tract and the liver of horses and ponies. In: *Proceedings of 13th Equine Nutrition and Physiology Society Symposium*, 18–23. Gainesville, FL: Equine Nutrition and Physiology Society.

5 Merritt, A.M. and Julliand, V. (2013). Gastrointestinal physiology. In: *Equine Applied and Clinical Nutrition: Health, Welfare and Performance* (ed. R.J. Geor, P.A. Harris, and M. Coenen), 3–32. Edinburgh: Saunders Elsevier.

6 Knight, A. (1995). Plant poisoning of horses. In: *Equine Clinical Nutrition: Feeding and Care*, 1e (ed. L.D. Lewis), 447–502. Baltimore, MD: Williams and Wilkins.

7 Chang, H.T., Rumbeiha, W.K., Patterson, J.S. et al. (2012). Toxic equine parkinsonism: an immunohistochemical study of 10 horses with nigropallidal encephalomalacia. *Vet. Pathol.* 49 (2): 398–402.

8 Rucker, B.A. (2002). Diseases of the oral cavity and soft palate. In: *Manual of Equine Gastroenterology* (ed. T. Mair, T. Divers, and N.G. Ducharme), 69–77. London: W.B. Saunders.

9 Elliott, C. and McCowan, C. (2012). Nigropallidal encephalomalacia in horses grazing *Rhaponticum repens* (creeping knapweed). *Aust. Vet. J.* 90 (4): 151–154.

10 Lang, J.G. (2002). Differential diagnosis and evaluation of dysphagia. In: *Manual of Equine Gastroenterology* (ed. T.S. Mair, T.J. Divers, and N.G. Ducharme), 63–67. London: W.B. Saunders.

11 Meyer, H., Coenen, M., and Guer, C. (1985). Investigation on saliva production and chewing effect in horses fed various feeds. In: *Proceedings of the 9th Equine Nutrition and Physiology Society Symposium*, 38–41. East Lansing, MI: Equine Nutrition and Physiology Society.

12 Carmalt, J.L. and Allen, A. (2008). The relationship between cheek tooth occlusal morphology, apparent digestibility, and ingesta particle size reduction in horses. *J. Am. Vet. Med. Assoc.* 233 (3): 452–455.

13 Carmalt, J.L., Townsend, H.G.G., Janzen, E.D., and Cymbaluk, N.E. (2004). Effect of dental floating on weight gain, body condition score, feed digestibility, and fecal particle size in pregnant mares. *J. Am. Vet. Med. Assoc.* 225 (12): 1889–1893.

14 Nicholls, V.M. and Townsend, N. (2016). Dental disease in aged horses and its management. *Vet. Clin. North Am. Equine Pract.* 32 (2): 215–227.

15 Ralston, S.L., Foster, D.L., Divers, T., and Hintz, H.F. (2001). Effect of dental correction on feed digestibility in horses. *Equine Vet. J.* 33 (4): 390–393.
16 Bhati, R. and Nagrajan, R.K. (2012). A detailed review on oral mucosal drug delivery system. *Int. J. Pharm. Sci. Res.* 3: 659–681.
17 l'Ami, J.J., Vermunt, L.E., van Loon Johannes, P.A.M., and Sloet van Oldruitenborgh-Oosterbaan, M.M. (2013). Sublingual administration of detomidine in horses: sedative effect, analgesia and detection time. *Vet. J.* 196 (2): 253–259.
18 Nickel, R., Schummer, A., and Seiferle, E. (1979). Digestive system. In: *The Viscera of the Domestic Mammals*, 2e (ed. R. Nickel and A. Schummer), 21–69. Berlin: Verlag Paul Parey.
19 Sykes, B.W., Hewetson, M., Hepburn, R.J. et al. (2015). European College of Equine Internal Medicine consensus statement-equine gastric ulcer syndrome in adult horses. *J. Vet. Intern. Med.* 29 (5): 1288–1299.
20 Husted, L., Sanchez, L.C., Baptiste, K.E., and Olsen, S.N. (2009). Effect of a feed/fast protocol on pH in the proximal equine stomach. *Equine Vet. J.* 41 (7): 658–662.
21 Husted, L., Sanchez, L.C., Olsen, S.N. et al. (2008). Effect of paddock vs. stall housing on 24 hour gastric pH within the proximal and ventral equine stomach. *Equine Vet. J.* 40: 337–341.
22 Varloud, M., Fonty, G., Roussel, A. et al. (2007). Postprandial kinetics of some biotic and abiotic characteristics of the gastric ecosystem of horses fed a pelleted concentrate meal. *J. Anim. Sci.* 85 (10): 2508–2516.
23 de Fombelle, A., Varloud, M., Goachet, A.G. et al. (2003). Characterization of the microbial and biochemical profile of the different segments of the digestive tract in horses given two distinct diets. *Anim. Sci.* 77 (2): 293–304.
24 Nadeau, J.A., Andrews, F.M., Patton, C.S. et al. (2003). Effects of hydrochloric, valeric and other volatile fatty acids on pathogenesis of ulcers in the nonglandular portion of the stomach of horses. *Am. J. Vet. Res.* 64 (4): 413–417.
25 Kwiatek, M.A., Menne, D., Steingoetter, A. et al. (2009). Effect of meal volume and calorie load on postprandial gastric function and emptying: studies under physiological conditions by combined fiber-optic pressure measurement and MRI. *Am. J. Physiol. Gastrointest. Liver Physiol.* 297: 894–901.
26 Lorenzo-Figueras, M., Jones, G., and Merritt, A.M. (2002). Effects of various diets on gastric tone in the proximal portion of the stomach of horses. *Am. J. Vet. Res.* 63 (9): 1275–1278.
27 Lorenzo-Figueras, M., Preston, T., Ott, E.A., and Merritt, A.M. (2005). Meal-induced gastric relaxation and emptying in horses after ingestion of high-fat versus high-carbohydrate diets. *Am. J. Vet. Res.* 66 (5): 897–906.
28 Merritt, A.M., Campbell-Thompson, M.L., and Lowrey, S. (1989). Effect of xylazine treatment on equine proximal gastrointestinal tract myoelectrical activity. *Am. J. Vet. Res.* 50 (6): 945–949.
29 Lohmann, K.L., Roussel, A.J., Cohen, N.D. et al. (2000). Comparison of nuclear scintigraphy and acetaminophen absorption as a means of studying gastric emptying in horses. *Am. J. Vet. Res.* 61 (3): 310–315.
30 Snyder, A., Koeller, G., Seiwert, B. et al. (2014). Influence of laxatives on gastric emptying in healthy warmblood horses evaluated with the acetaminophen absorption test. *Berl. Munch. Tierarztl. Wochenschr.* 127 (3, 4): 170–175.
31 Wyse, C.A., Murphy, D.M., Preston, T. et al. (2001). The 13C-octanoic acid breath test for detection of effects of meal composition on the rate of solid-phase gastric emptying in ponies. *Res. Vet. Sci.* 71 (1): 81–83.
32 Metayer, N., Lhote, M., Bahr, A. et al. (2010). Meal size and starch content affect gastric emptying in horses. *Equine Vet. J.* 36 (5): 436–440.
33 Williams, C.A. (2016). Horse species symposium: the effect of oxidative stress during exercise in the horse. *J. Anim. Sci.* 94 (10): 4067–4075.
34 Julliand, V. and Grimm, P. (2017). The impact of diet on the hindgut microbiome. *J. Equine Vet. Sci.* 52 (5): 23–28.
35 Edwards, G. and Proudman, C.J. (2002). Diseases of the small intestine resulting in colic. In: *Manual of Equine Gastroenterology* (ed. T. Mair, T. Divers, and N. Ducharme), 249–265. Edinburgh: Elsevier.
36 Kararli, T.T. (1995). Comparison of the gastrointestinal anatomy, physiology, and biochemistry of humans and commonly used laboratory animals. *Biopharm. Drug Dispos.* 16: 351–380.
37 Gropper, S., Smith, J., and Groff, J. (2009). The small intestine. In: *Advanced Nutrition and Human Metabolism*, 5e, 43. Belmont, CA: Wadsworth.
38 Kitchen, D.L., Burrow, J.A., Heartless, C.S., and Merritt, A.M. (2000). Effect of pyloric blockade and infusion of histamine or pentagastrin on gastric secretion in horses. *Am. J. Vet. Res.* 61 (9): 1133–1139.
39 Gronwall, R., Engelking, L.R., Anwer, M.S. et al. (1975). Bile secretion in ponies with biliary fistuals. *Am. J. Vet. Res.* 36 (5): 653–654.
40 Rich, G.A. and Fontenot, J.P.M.T. (1981). Digestibility of animal, vegetable and blended fats by equines. In: *Proceedings of the 7th Equine Nutrition and Physiology Society Symposium*, 30–36. Warrenton, VA: Equine Nutrition and Physiology Society.
41 Kronfeld, D.S., Holland, J.L., Rich, G.A. et al. (2004). Fat digestibility in *Equus caballus* follows increasing first-order kinetics. *J. Anim. Sci.* 82 (6): 1773–1780.

42 Hornbuckle, W.E., Simpson, K.W., and Tennant, B.C. (2008). Gastrointestinal function. In: *Clinical Biochemistry of Domestic Animals*, 6e (ed. J.J. Kaneko, J. Harvey, and M. Bruss), 413–457. Elsevier Inc.

43 Tate, L.P., Ralston, S.L., Koch, C.M., and Everitt, J.I. (1983). Effects of extensive resection of the small intestine in the pony. *Am. J. Vet. Res.* 44 (7): 1187–1191.

44 Bertone, A.L., Stashak, T.S., Ralston, S.L. et al. (1992). A preliminary study on the effects of jejunocaecostomy in horses. *Equine Vet. J.* 24 (S13): 51–56.

45 Wille, K. and Nakov, C. (1999). Functional morphology of the large intestinal mucosa of horses (*Equus przewalskii f. caballus*) with special regard to the epithelium. *Anat. Histol. Embryol.* 28: 355–365.

46 Philippeau, C., Faubladier, C., Goachet, A.G., and Julliandi, V. (2009). Is there an impact of feeding concentrate before or after forage on colonic pH and redox potential in horses? In: *Proceedings of the Equine Nutrition and Training Conference*, 203–208. Madrid, Spain: Wageningen Academic Publications.

47 Julliand, V., De Fombelle, A., Drogoul, C., and Jacotot, E. (2001). Feeding and microbial disorders in horses: part 3 - effects of three hay: grain ratios on microbial profile and activities. *J. Equine Vet. Sci.* 21 (11): 543–546.

48 Argenzio, R.A. and Hintz, H.F. (1972). Effect of diet on glucose entry and oxidation rates in ponies. *J. Nutr.* 102 (7): 879–892.

49 Glinsky, M.J., Smith, R.M., Spires, H.R., and Davis, C.L. (1976). Measurement of volatile fatty acid production rates in the cecum of the pony. *J. Anim. Sci.* 42 (6): 1465–1470.

50 Engelking, L.R. (2015). Gluconeogenesis. In: *Textbook of Veterinary Physiological Chemistry*, 3e, 225–230. Elsevier.

51 Bonhomme-Florentin, A. (1976). Lipolytic activity of ciliates and bacteria of horse's caecum. *Anim. Physiol. Biochem.* 282: 1605–1608.

52 Baruc, C., Dawson, K., and Baker, J.P. (1983). The characterization and nitrogen metabolismof equine caecal bacteria. In: *Proceedings of the 8th Equine Nutrition and Physiology Society*. 151–156. Lexington, KY: Equine Nutrition and Physiology Society.

53 Miyaji, M., Ueda, K., Hata, H., and Kondo, S. (2014). Effect of grass hay intake on fiber digestion and digesta retention time in the hindgut of horses. *J. Anim. Sci.* 92 (4): 1574–1581.

54 Drogoul, C., Poncet, C., and Tisserand, J.L. (2000). Feeding ground and pelleted hay rather than chopped hay to ponies 1. Consequences for in vivo digestibility and rate of passage of digesta. *Anim. Feed Sci. Technol.* 87 (1, 2): 117–130.

55 Den Besten, G., Van Eunen, K., Groen, A.K. et al. (2013). The role of short-chain fatty acids in the interplay between diet, gut microbiota, and host energy metabolism. *J. Lipid Res.* 54 (9): 2325–2340.

56 Argenzio, R.A. and Southworth, M. (1975). Sites of organic acid production and absorption in gastrointestinal tract of the pig. *Am. J. Physiol.* 228 (2): 454–460.

57 Shirazi-Beechey, S.P. (2008). Molecular insights into dietary induced colic in the horse. *Equine Vet. J.* 40: 414–421.

58 Shirazi-Beechey, S.P. (1995). Molecular biology of intestinal glucose transport. *Nutr. Res. Rev.* 8 (1): 27–41.

59 Raspa, F., Colombino, E., Capucchio, M. et al. (2021). Effects of feeding managements on microbial contamination of mesenteric lymph nodes and liver and on intestinal histo-morphology in horses. In: *Proceedings 25th Congress of the European College of Veterinary and Comparative Nutrition*, 93. Vila Real, Portugal: European College of Veterinary and Comparative Nutrition.

60 Milinovich, G.J., Burrell, P.C., Pollitt, C.C. et al. (2008). Microbial ecology of the equine hindgut during oligofructose-induced laminitis. *ISME J.* 2 (11): 1089–1100.

61 Medina, B., Girard, I.D., Jacotot, E., and Julliand, V. (2002). Effect of a preparation of on microbial profiles and fermentation patterns in the large intestine of horses fed a high fiber or a high starch diet. *J. Anim. Sci.* 80 (10): 2600–2609.

62 Slade, L.M., Bishop, R., Morris, J.G., and Robinson, D.W. (1971). Digestion and absorption of 15N-labelled microbial protein in the large intestine of the horse. *Br. Vet. J.* 127 (5): xi–xiii.

63 Reitnour, C.M. and Salsbury, R.L. (1972). Digestion and utilization of cecally infused protein by the equine. *J. Anim. Sci.* 35 (6): 1190–1193.

64 Woodward, A.D., Holcombe, S.J., Steibel, J.P. et al. (2010). Cationic and neutral amino acid transporter transcript abundances are differentially expressed in the equine intestinal tract. *J. Anim. Sci.* 88 (3): 1028–1033.

65 Woodward, A.D., Fan, M.Z., Geor, R.J. et al. (2012). Characterization of l-lysine transport across equine and porcine jejunal and colonic brush border membrane. *J. Anim. Sci.* 90 (3): 853–862.

66 Sullins, K., Stashak, T., and Ralston, S. (1985). Experimental large intestinal resection in the horse: technique and nutritional performance. In: *Proceedings of the 31th Annual Convention of the American Association of Equine Practitioners*, 497–503. Toronto, Canada: American Association of Equine Practitioners (AAEP).

67 Rourke, K.M., Coe, S., Kohn, C.W. et al. (2010). Cloning, comparative sequence analysis and mRNA expression of calcium-transporting genes in horses. *Gen. Comp. Endocrinol.* 167 (1): 6–10.

68 Simmons, H.A. and Ford, E.J. (1990). Liquid flow and capacity of the caecum and colon of the horse. *Res. Vet. Sci.* 48 (2): 265–266.

69 Sneddon, J.C.C. and Argenzio, R.A.A. (1998). Feeding strategy and water homeostasis in equids: the role of the hind gut. *J. Arid Environ.* 38 (3): 493–509.

70 Giddings, R.F., Argenzio, R.A., and Stevens, C.E. (1974). Sodium and chloride transport across the equine cecal mucosa. *Am. J. Vet. Res.* 35 (12): 1511–1514.

71 Clarke, L.L., Roberts, M.C., Grubb, B.R., and Argenzio, R.A. (1992). Short-term effect of aldosterone on Na-Cl transport across equine colon. *Am. J. Physiol.* 262 (6): R939–R946.

72 von Engelhardt, W., Rösel, E., and Rechkemmer, G. (1995). Comparative views of electrophysiological parameters of large intestinal segments in pig, sheep, pony, guinea pig and rat. *Dtsch. Tierarztl. Wochenschr.* 102 (4): 157–159.

4

The Horse

Microbiome

Veronique Julliand and J. Scott Weese

KEY TERMS

- The term "microbiota" is synonymous with the former term "microflora."
- The microbiome is the collection of microorganisms and all their genetic material.
- There are seven main taxonomic units: kingdom, phylum or division, class, order, family, genus, species.
- Taxa (plural of taxon) are one or more populations of an organism or organisms seen by taxonomists forming a unit.
- Archaea are a group of single-celled prokaryotic organisms that have distinct molecular characteristics separating them from bacteria.
- "sp." is an abbreviation for species used when the actual species name cannot or need not or is not specified. "spp." is the plural form indicating "multiple species" within a genus.
- Bacteria can be further divided into subspecies indicated by subdivisions such as cultivar and serovar.
- Dysbiosis is an imbalance of intestinal microorganisms that may result in clinical disease.

KEY POINTS

- The equine gastrointestinal microbiota is rich, diverse, complex, and critically important for health and a range of digestive, immunologic, and metabolic functions, including fiber digestion, immune regulation, and vitamin production.
- The equine intestinal ecosystem is highly susceptible to dietary changes in high fermentable sugars. Dietary changes should thus be managed gradually to reduce the risk of dysbiosis and diseases such as colic, colitis, and laminitis, and potentially a wider range of conditions such as metabolic syndrome and inflammatory bowel disease.
- A wide range of other exogenous stressors are known to, or might, influence the microbiota, including antibiotic administration, transportation, and exercise.
- While the ability to define "normal" and "abnormal" is improving, individual-horse level assessment of the microbiota is challenging because of the degree of inter-horse variation and overlap in the microbiota composition between healthy and diseased horses.
- Methods to consistently and effectively manipulate the microbiota to prevent or treat disease are currently a challenge.

4.1 Introduction

The equine gastrointestinal tract (GIT) harbors a large and complex collection of microorganisms, something that has been recognized for over a century but is still poorly understood. Living "animalcules" and bacteria were described as early as 1843 and 1911, respectively, in the horse large intestine. In the early 1900s, functional properties of the cecal and colonic bacteria were demonstrated to be capable of utilizing starch, hemicelluloses, cellulose, and proteins; properties that are of importance for a monogastric herbivore. A century later, it is well

Equine Clinical Nutrition, Second Edition. Edited by Rebecca L. Remillard.

recognized that the large intestine microbial community (the microbiota) consists of a large diversity of prokaryotes, (bacteria, archaea, eukaryotes, protozoa, fungi) and viruses that support essential functions for their host.

The gastrointestinal microbiota has presumably evolved alongside the horse to enable the digestion of a specific diet. Horses have developed large intestinal fermenting compartments offering a favorable environment for the growth and activity of microorganisms. See Chapter 3 The Horse: Host. Within these compartments, microorganisms proficiently digest plant cell-wall carbohydrates, the host's hydrolytic enzymes did not digest in the small intestine [1, 2]. In the horse, an imbalance of intestinal microorganisms, i.e. dysbiosis, has been implicated in some diseases, such as colitis, colic, or laminitis. While certain microorganisms can potentially be harmful, others are considered beneficial and even vital for the host's health. Defining "harmful" and "beneficial" microbes can be a challenge based on our limited understanding of the functions of various microorganisms and how they interact with each other and the host.

The microbiota is critical for horses from a nutritional standpoint, but it also interacts closely with the host, locally and systemically. The microbiota can influence, and be influenced by most other body systems. In horses specifically, less is known if, and how, the equine intestinal microorganisms contribute to the host health and disease through metabolic and immune pathways. However, interactions between the gut microbiota and extra-intestinal host systems have been well studied in other mammalian species where impacts on metabolic, inflammatory, immune-mediated, neoplastic, and infectious diseases are well documented. As of yet, there is no reason to think the relationship would be different in horses versus other animal species.

Typically, the focus has been on specific microorganisms that have been implicated as pathogens. For example, much attention has been paid to clostridia as an important pathogen. Certainly, some *Clostridium* species such as *Clostridium (Clostridioides) difficile* and *Clostridium perfringens* are important pathogens. However, there are dozens of other *Clostridium* spp. present in horses, most of which probably play beneficial roles. Even known pathogens such as *C. difficile* and *C. perfringens* are commonly found in healthy horses and foals, indicating that there is much more to disease than the simple presence of a putative enteropathogen. Beneficial organisms, often members of the Class Clostridia, such as *Ruminococcus*, have received much less attention than potential pathogenic classmates. More likely, the balance between the beneficial and harmful microorganisms is the key to the overall health status of the host.

4.2 Microbiota in Adult Healthy Horses

Understanding the composition of the gastrointestinal microbiota in adult horses has changed dramatically in recent years because of advances in technology, but many gaps remain. Describing the "normal" microbiota is a challenge based on differences in study populations, GIT region, laboratory methods, and analysis. How those populations vary between horses and factors that impact the microbial composition of the GIT are only relatively superficially understood, but our understanding of this complex will likely improve greatly in the coming years.

For certain, the GIT comprises a complex population of microbes, including bacteria, archaea, fungi, viruses, and protozoa. Throughout the length of the GIT, the local environment, (enzymes, oxygen tension, and nutrients), varies greatly [3]. Unsurprisingly, the microbiota is variable throughout the GIT, i.e. different taxa are present in different portions of the GIT [3–5]. Microbial diversity is low in the stomach, increases somewhat in the small intestine, then markedly increases in the cecum; however, throughout the colon and rectum, the microbiome species are relatively unchanging [5].

The stomach has a surprisingly rich and diverse population, but one that is dwarfed by more distal GIT compartments. Taxa such as Bacilli are common, with acid-tolerant species being more adapted for this region. Genera such as *Lactobacillus*, *Streptococcus*, *Sarcina*, and *Actinobacillus* are common [4]. Transition to the small intestine results in a richer and more diverse population with composition changes occurring through the progression from proximal to distal regions. Proteobacteria increase over the length of the small intestine, with high but decreasing numbers of Bacilli and increases in Clostridia. The cecum functionally represents the start of the fermenting hindgut, and the microbiota undergoes a dramatic shift from the ileum to the cecum. Taxa of fiber-fermenting organisms including Spirochaetes, Verrucomicrobia, Clostridiales, and Bacteroidetes increase at this point with decreases in Proteobacteria [4, 5]. The change in the microbiota from the cecum to the large colon is more subtle, and the colonic microbiota is relatively similar from the proximal large colon to the rectum. Further increases in Clostridia occur, including important Clostridiales such as Ruminococcaceae and Lachnospiraceae.

Most studies of healthy horses report relatively similar results at higher taxonomic levels, (phylum or class) with greater deviation at lower levels. Commonly reported taxa among different studies are outlined in Table 4.1. Overall, the Firmicutes phylum predominates in feces, as well as colonic and cecal samples. This is a phylum of gram-positive bacteria that includes Clostridia, a dominant class, and

Table 4.1 Taxa most commonly reported in the equine fecal microbiota.

Phylum	Class	Order	Family	Genus
Firmicutes	Clostridia	Clostridiales	Clostridiaceae	*Akkermansia*
Verrucomicrobia	Gammaproteobacteria	Verrucomicrobiales	Lachnospiraceae	*Ruminococcus*
Spirochaetes	Verrocomicrobiae	Enterobacterales	Enterobacteriaceae	*Roseburia*
Proteobacteria	Bacilli	Pseudomonadales	Ruminococcaceae	*Oscillibacter*
Fibrobacteres	Alphaproteobacteria	Lactobacillales	Verrucomicrobiaceae	*Blautia*
Bacteriodetes	Negativicutes	Bacillales		*Alstipes*
	Erysipelotrichia	Bacteroidales		*Lachnospira*
				Treponema
				Fibrobacter
				Saccharofermentans
				Succinivibrio

Clostridiales, a leading order. In contrast to the common perceptions of Clostridia as pathogenic bacteria, there is increasing information that many Clostridia are key determinants of gastrointestinal health. While some *Clostridium* spp. are potential pathogens, many members of this group, particularly butyrate-producing genera such as *Lachnospira, Ruminococcus, Roseburia,* and *Faecalibacterium* are probably key determinants of gut health [6–8]. Proteobacteria is a varied phylum of gram-negative bacteria and overgrowth of this phylum has been associated with various gastrointestinal diseases in horses and other species [7–10].

Bacteria dominate the gastrointestinal microbiota and have been the most extensively studied population. The richness (i.e. the number of species present) of the equine GIT is high, with hundreds to thousands of different species being present [11–14]. Typically the distribution of species is very uneven, with a small number of individual species or genera accounting for a disproportionately large percentage of overall bacteria and a large number of species being present at very low numbers. Certain keystone species such as *Fibrobacter succinogenes* and *Ruminococcus flavefaciens* have the greatest impact on the herbivore due to their essential role in fibrolytic digestion (Figure 4.1) [15].

While most attention is paid to bacteria, other microorganisms are present and might play important roles. Anaerobic fungi, belonging to various species, play important roles in fiber degradation in the hindgut. Archaea is an unusual domain of single-celled organisms with similarities to both bacteria and eukaryotes. They tend to be

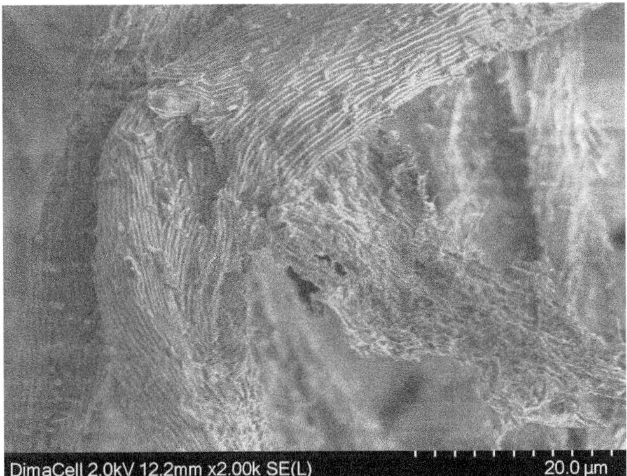

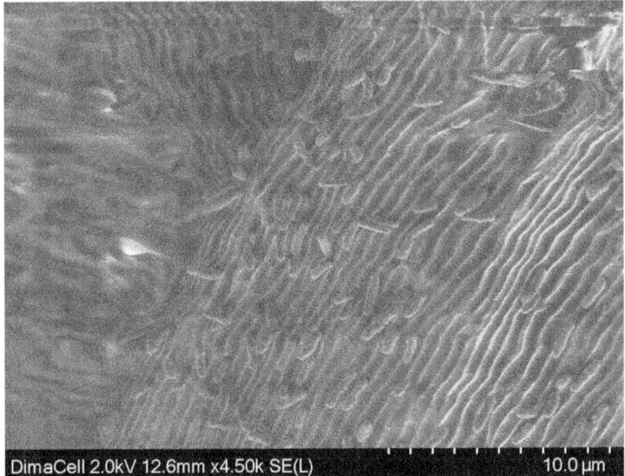

Figure 4.1 Scanning electron micrographs of *Fibrobacter succinogenes* during degradation of filter paper (scale = 20.0 μm on the left micrograph and 10.0 μm on the right micrograph). The *F. succinogenes* strain was isolated from a healthy horse at PAM Lab: Food and Wine Science & Technology. Adherent cells aligned along cellulose fibers. Removal of some adherent cells occurred during the preparation of cells for scanning electron micrographs. *Source:* Photo credits: Aline Bonnotte, Plate-forme DImaCell, AgroSup Dijon, INRA, Univ. Bourgogne Franche-Comté, F-21000 Dijon, France.

extremophiles (i.e. adapted living in extreme conditions such as in underwater thermal vents or high salinity environments) but some can be found as part of the gastrointestinal microbiota. They are minor components of the microbiota, their numbers being dwarfed by bacteria. Archaea have been reported incidentally in many sequence-based studies of the bacterial microbiota, and a variety of different genera can be present [16, 17]. This includes potentially clinically relevant methane-producing groups such as genera *Methanosphaera*, *Methanocorpusculum*, and *Methanobrevibacter* as methane directly impacts GIT motility and/or may play a role in colic through gas production [16–18].

While viruses have traditionally been approached as pathogens, there is a commensal "virome" that consists both of mammalian viruses, i.e. viruses that infect mammalian cells, and bacteriophages, i.e. viruses that infect bacteria [19, 20]. A preliminary study highlighted the potential complexity of the virome, with a large percentage of viral sequences potentially belonging to uncharacterized viruses [20]. Bacteriophages likely dominate the virome, with little understanding of their role in horse health. Lytic bacteriophages may impact bacterial numbers or distributions through lysis of specific bacteria, which may result in the transmission of genes (virulence factors, antimicrobial resistance genes) between bacteria in the equine intestinal tract.

Ciliated protozoa have long been studied and a relatively large population can be present. Fifteen genera, all belonging to the Litostomatea, were identified in one study, comprising a variety of species whose activities are largely unknown [16]. Various parasites may also be present, from single-celled protozoa to complex helminths. Clinically, parasites such as Ascarids are approached as pathogens, with structured programs to control or eliminate them. Less interest has been paid to the broader parasitic microbiota and the potential relationship with the host. The influence of parasitic populations on aspects such as inflammation and the development of immunotolerance is of increasing interest in various species. The interrelationship between the bacteria and parasitic microbiotas is another area of interest that needs further study, as differences in the fecal microbiota have been observed in horses with low vs. high fecal helminth egg counts [21].

These different components of the microbiota (bacteria, fungi, archaea, viruses, and protozoa) are typically studied individually. However, these groups live together in a complex microbial ecosystem, and interactions between them are poorly understood. The study of the overall microbiota is needed to assess potential interactions and their impact on equine health and disease.

4.3 Microbiota in Healthy Foals and Young Horses

The intestinal microbiota is not stable throughout the life of the horse. After birth, the intestinal tract undergoes a remarkable transition from the relatively sterile state of the fetus to the complex, rich and diverse microbiota that is required for proper development. The state of the intestinal tract at the time of birth is unclear. An average of 2.9 log10 colony-forming units (CFUs) of total anaerobes was measured per gram of freshly collected meconium, raising questions about the origin of commensal bacteria in the foal meconium of neonates [22]. Similar to other mammals, a bacterial mother-to-fetus efflux could exist during pregnancy, via the amniotic fluid and placenta, leading to the presence of bacteria in neonate meconium, although in equine species, the placenta is less permeable than in other species [23, 24].

Regardless of the status at the time of birth, the foal is exposed to bacteria from the mare and the foaling environment during and immediately after parturition. This results in exposure to a wide range of microorganisms that can potentially colonize the intestinal tract. Within 24 hrs of birth, hundreds to thousands of bacterial species can be present in feces, reflecting the massive initial maternal and environmental exposures [25]. Yet, many of these are probably transiently passing through the gut or residing there for a short time while the true commensal microbiota is being established. With culture-based approaches, the most abundant microorganisms identified during this initial period are aerobic and facultative anaerobic bacteria, such as enterococci, lactobacilli, staphylococci, and Enterobacteriaceae [26]. Sequence-based studies have identified more richness, and have also reported high relative abundances of those groups [25, 27, 28].

After the initial neonatal period, foals continue to be exposed to a wide range of bacteria from the mare's body, milk, the environment, and other horses. Milk contains up to 10^9 microorganisms/L of species, such as *Staphylococcus*, *Streptococcus*, *Corynebacterium*, *Lactobacillus*, *Bifidobacterium*, and *Propionibacterium*, taxa that are important components of the microbiota during the nursing period [25, 27, 28]. Coprophagia is a normal activity in young foals, providing further exposure to feces from the mare and other horses in the environment. As these exposures continue and as the GIT develops, the local microenvironments (nutritional sources, enzymes, oxygen tension) likely alter, along with the composition of the microbiota.

The early colonization by facultative anaerobic bacterial strains contributes to the development of an anaerobic environment that allows the establishment of a strictly anaerobic bacteria population. By the first wk of age, the ratio of facultative to strictly anaerobic bacteria is reversed and strictly anaerobic bacteria dominate [25]. During the first month of life, the increase in the detection of Bacteroidetes comprising strictly anaerobic bacteria was concomitant with the decrease of Enterococcaceae, which was likely attributable at least in part to a significant decrease in the genus *Enterococcus* and the decrease in both Enterobacteriaceae and Streptococcaceae. Despite a milk-based diet, cellulolytic bacteria are detected from the first wk of life along with the appearance of *F. succinogenes*, a major cellulolytic bacterial species [22]. The development of these populations happens concomitantly with the beginning of fiber consumption by foals. Further changes in the fecal bacterial structure take place until day 30 [22, 29]. The settlement of ciliates, which begins by day 11, reaches the level of an adult horse within the first month of age.

Interestingly a study on the age-related changes in fecal short-chain fatty acid (SCFA) or volatile fatty acid (VFA) concentrations in foals has shown that the bacterial fiber-degrading capacity begins at the end of the second wk of life and stabilizes at around two mos of age [22]. This suggests that by 60 d of age, the foal's fecal bacterial microbiota could have similar functions as that of adult horses, something that is consistent with a sequence-based study that determined that the microbiota in 2-mo-old foals more closely resembled the yearling microbiota than that of the neonate [25]. When the microbiota becomes an "adult" microbiota is unknown but the transition is likely almost complete by weaning [25]. No changes in the inter-individual variability of bacterial profiles and no shift in the bacterial community structure were detected after weaning when milk was progressively replaced by solid food before weaning [22]. This suggests that a progressive nutritional change leads to a gradual maturation of the fecal microbiota, rather than abrupt changes during major events such as weaning.

4.4 The Role of the Microbiota

4.4.1 Nourishment

The primary nutritional substrate from the cecum and colon are VFAs that may provide 50% or more of the host's digestible energy requirement, with possibly 30% provided by the cecum alone in 75% hay rations [30–32]. Hence, there would be no horse without hindgut microorganisms and feeding the horse a ration that in turn properly feeds the microorganisms is essential to the host's health (Figure 4.2).

4.4.1.1 Structural Carbohydrates

High-fiber rations provide more VFAs and subsequently contribute more digestible energy compared with low-fiber rations [33]. The major role of the microbiota is the

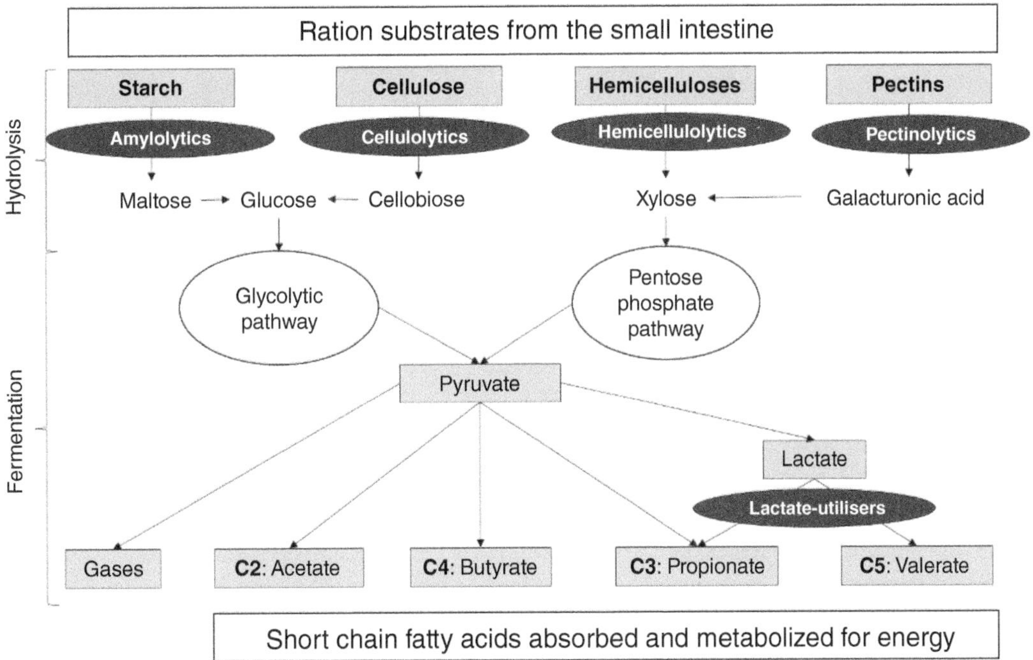

Figure 4.2 Catabolism of ration substrates by intestinal microbiota to short-chain fatty acids for host energy metabolism. Gases, predominately carbon dioxide (CO_2) and methane (CH_4), are expelled through the rectum and anus. *Source:* Julliand and Grimm [33] / With permission of Elsevier.

hydrolysis of complex plant cell walls, primarily composed of cellulose, hemicellulose, pectin, and lignin, also known as plant structural carbohydrates. These plant substrates typically comprise 35–60% of the equine ration dry matter (DM), and cannot be hydrolyzed by the host's endogenous digestive enzymes. Therefore, microorganisms that can efficiently digest structural carbohydrates, particularly the beta-glycoside bonds of cellulose, are critically important for the horse. Fungi and bacteria are involved in the fermentation process throughout the equine hindgut; however, cellulose and hemicellulose fermentation is greatest in the colon [34]. The major fibrolytic microorganisms identified are fungal species of Piromyces genus and bacterial species of the Ruminococcus and Fibrobacter genera. These microorganisms first attach to the plant cell wall and direct enzymes toward the structural substrates. Microbial polysaccharidases hydrolyze cellulose to glucose and hemicellulose and pectins to xylose that in turn are fermented by glycosidases into pyruvate and ultimately SCFAs and gases (CO_2 and CH_4) (Figure 4.2).

4.4.1.2 Non-fibrous Carbohydrates

The large intestinal microbiota is also responsible for the degradation of starch and water-soluble carbohydrates (WSCs) that escape small intestinal digestion. Water-soluble carbohydrates are polymers of glucose, fructose, galactose, and fructans that comprise 10–40% ration DM. In particular, fructans, a form of stored carbohydrate in many cool-season types of grass, are polymers of beta-linked sucrose (fructose and glucose), which may comprise 5–40% of the grass DM [35]. Fructans cannot be digested in the small intestine, are rapidly fermented in the equine hindgut, and have been associated with laminitis. The WSC portion that enters the cecal microbial ecosystem is first hydrolyzed into glucose by amylolytic bacteria belonging to the Streptococcus and Lactobacillus genera. Glucose is then fermented to ultimately SCFAs and gases (CO_2 and CH_4) (Figure 4.2).

The activity of fibrolytic microorganisms produces high levels of acetate (C2) and, to a lesser extent, butyrate (C4), whereas amylolytic microorganisms produce predominately propionate (C3). Therefore, hindgut fermentation can be evaluated in horses through the determination of the ratio [(acetate + butyrate)/propionate (C2 + C4)/C3] as a reflection of ration composition. The greater the fibrolytic activity, relative to amylolytic, will result in a higher C2 concentration and, thus, a higher ratio that is directly related to the ration fiber content. In horses fed 100% forage, the ratio ranged between 4.3 and 6.0, i.e. more fibrolytic activity; whereas lower values ranged from 3.1 to 4.3 in horses fed high-grain rations indicating more amylolytic activity [3].

4.4.1.3 Protein

Dietary crude protein comprises 6–20% of the diet DM but may reach 25% in some legume pastures during some times of the year [36]. Dietary protein may be within the cell contents or embedded with the cell walls of plants, but the total protein content of the ration does not indicate the availability of the protein. The overall estimate of digestible protein (DP) is about 30–75% of dietary crude protein in the horse [37–39]. Digestion and absorption of protein in the stomach and small intestine precede the microbial action in the cecum and colon. Therefore, protein from plant cell contents is digested in the small intestine by pancreatic pepsin and trypsin; however, that protein-bound within cell wall structures will not become available until cecal and colonic microbes dismantle the structural carbohydrates.

Nitrogen (N) disappearance from a GIT compartment is thought to be an estimate of protein digestion within that compartment. When an all hay ration was fed to ponies, only 16% of the N was absorbed anterior to the cecum [40]. In feeding studies where hay-grain combination rations were fed, 20–67% of the total net disappearance of N occurred primarily in the jejunum and ileum [41–43]. As As a result, 40–70% of the whole tract apparent nitrogen digestion appears to occur in the post-ileal compartments depending on the preceding pancreatic digestion and small intestinal absorption [44]. Therefore, the relative importance of protein digestion in the hindgut increases as more protein is bound in the plant structural carbohydrate fractions of the ration.

Evidence indicates the large bowel microorganisms play some role in protein balance in the horse but little is known of the exact fate of protein, amino acids, or nitrogen in the hindgut. If the sole site of digestion and absorption of intact amino acids was from the small intestine, then the horse would be susceptible to specific amino acid deficiencies, yet there is no evidence. Conversely, horses, after having undergone surgical removal of the large colon and fed a low-protein grass hay ration, lost weight and condition but were able to maintain weight and condition when fed a high-protein alfalfa hay diet [45]. Additionally, amino acid transporter gene transcripts have been reported in the colonic mucosa [46, 47]. Still, the quantitative importance of microbial protein-derived amino acids from the large intestine in horses remains unknown. The assumption is that microbial amino acid synthesis using substrates entering the cecum and colon is sufficient to complement dietary sources as needed when the ration contains an adequate concentration of a digestible protein [39].

4.4.1.4 Fat

Dietary fat represents, on average, about 4% ration DM. Lipolytic activity attributed to protozoa and bacteria has been demonstrated *in vitro* within cecal contents. In particular, the ciliate protozoa have been shown to contribute actively to triglyceride hydrolysis [48].

4.4.1.5 Vitamins

The water-soluble vitamins, i.e. B_3 (niacin), B_5 (pantothenic acid), B_6 (pyridoxine), B_{12} (cyanocobalamin), B_{15} (pantothenic acid), folic acid, biotin, choline, and vitamin C (ascorbic acid), are produced by the caecum and colonic microbiota, and therefore are not dietary essential nutrients for horses. Vitamins B_1 (thiamine) and B_2 (riboflavin) are also produced by the caecum and colonic microbiota; however, there are suggested dietary concentrations for these vitamins for different reasons [39, 49]. The thiamine derived from microbial synthesis is insufficient to prevent a deficiency if horses are fed a severely thiamine-deficient diet. Similarly, based on studies in Shetland ponies that evaluated growth and riboflavin, there is a minimum dietary riboflavin recommendation to ensure metabolic requirements are met.

4.4.2 Disease

The intestinal microbiota has been implicated in playing a role in a diverse range of diseases in other species, including inflammatory, allergic, infectious, metabolic, and neoplastic conditions. Studies in horses have been comparatively limited, but it is clear that the gastrointestinal microbiota is involved in at least a subset of these syndromes. Whether microbiota changes reflect causation or are rather a secondary effect is unclear, and differentiating cause vs. effect remains a challenge when studying the role of the microbiota in equine disorders.

4.4.2.1 Colitis

It has long been recognized that alteration of the gut microbiota is an important aspect of the pathophysiology of colitis. An increase in members of the Proteobacteria phylum and decreases in selected Firmicutes, particularly members of the Clostridiales, (Lachnospiraceae and Ruminococcaceae), that are increasingly associated with "gut health" in other species, has been identified in horses with colitis [8]. However, colitis is not a specific disease entity but is rather a clinical syndrome, and the study consisted of horses with idiopathic diseases. Different microbiota alterations may be present in different diseases, such as salmonella and *C. difficile* infections, but this has not been investigated.

4.4.2.2 Colic

Colic is an important cause of morbidity and mortality in horses, and while it is a non-specific syndrome with many potential causes, the intestinal microbiota could play an inciting role through mechanisms such as excessive gas production, acidosis, inflammation, and altered intestinal motility. Yet, investigations into the role of the microbiota in colic have been remarkably limited. As a sporadic disease, differentiating cause and effect is a challenge since samples for testing are usually only available at the time colic is underway.

One study was able to evaluate the microbiota in pregnant mares before the onset of post-parturient colic [7]. When fecal samples from mares that developed colic within a week after sample collection were compared with matched samples from mares that did not, differences that might indicate a risk of colic development were identified. This included a significant elevation in the relative abundance of Proteobacteria and a decrease in Firmicutes in mares that developed colic, along with differences in various measures of the microbial community membership and structure. Various Firmicutes members such as Lachnospiraceae, Ruminococcaceae, and other members of the Clostridiales order were reduced in mares that developed colic. While care must be taken to avoid over-interpreting the results of a single study of a specific population, the over-representation of Proteobacteria and depletion of various Firmicutes members, particularly Clostridiales, are consistent with alterations seen in various diseases in other species and suggest that a state of dysbiosis is present in at least some mares prior to the onset of colic.

While archaea have received limited study in horses, there is interest in methanogenic genera such as *Methanosphaera*, *Methanocorpusculum*, and *Methanobrevibacter* [16–18]. As methane producers, it is plausible (although not evaluated) that they could play a role in colic associated with intestinal gas production. Even less is known about the potential roles of viruses and parasites on the overall microbiota or potential influences on disease. Pathogenic parasites such as tapeworms have been associated with an increased risk of colic, but this is likely through direct impacts on intestinal motility and functional obstruction [50]. The role of other parasites, particularly the commensal protozoal microbiota, is unknown, yet worthy of study. The potential impact of the parasite burden on intestinal inflammation and/or the bacterial microbiota could be of clinical significance [21].

4.4.2.3 Laminitis

Influences of diet have long been recognized in the pathophysiology of pasture-associated and grain-overload laminitis, mainly through increases in colonic streptococci and other lactic acid-producing bacteria [51–57]. Changes in the cecal bacterial microbiota have been identified following carbohydrate infusion and experimentally produced early laminitis, including significant increases in Lactobacillus, Streptococcus, Veillonella, and Serratia [57].

Increased bacterial richness has been identified in horses with laminitis, along with significant differences in relative abundances of two unclassified Clostridiales, although the clinical relevance of those findings is unclear [58]. Cause and effect are hard to differentiate, and the changes in these taxa may represent both. Lactobacillus and Streptococcus are lactic acid bacteria that may be associated with the disease through the production of lactic acid in response to a carbohydrate overload, with corresponding local and systemic effects. In contrast, Veillonella can increase as lactate levels decrease, suggesting this could be a rebound growth in response to changes in the local environment after an inciting microbiota shift [59]. Defining the broad changes that occur during the development of laminitis and the range of bacteria that are involved is a challenge, but the microbiota does play a role in diet-associated laminitis.

4.4.2.4 Gastric Ulcer Disease

Gastric ulcer disease is a commonly diagnosed problem in competing horses. In humans, there is a strong link between *Helicobacter pylori* and gastric ulceration. A similar infectious etiology has not been identified in horses, and the pathophysiology of equine gastric ulcer disease remains complex, multifactorial, and not well understood. Yet, there is a distinct gastric microbiota, and management factors such as feeding that influenced this population [60–62]. Whether there is a direct or indirect role of the microbiota in gastric ulcer disease remains to be identified.

4.4.2.5 Metabolic Syndrome

Metabolic syndrome can cause various health effects in horses. The role of the microbiota in obesity and metabolic disease in humans is an area of intense study. Obesity is now recognized as, at least in part, an infectious disease, with the gut microbiota playing a major influencing role in energy conversion and weight gain. How the gut microbiota relates to equine metabolic syndrome (EMS) is unclear, but these horses had a different fecal microbiota compared with non-EMS horses. A decreased microbial diversity with enrichment of Verrucomicrobia and depletion of Fibrobacter has been identified [63]. The association of the phylum Verrucomicrobia with EMS was interesting as this relatively newly discovered phylum has been associated with obesity and metabolic disease in other species.

4.4.2.6 Grass Sickness

Equine grass sickness is a regionally important but devastating and enigmatic gastrointestinal disease. An opportunistic toxic infection by a particular strain of *Clostridium botulinum* type C. is thought to play a role but the etiology is not fully understood. A recent study identified decreases in Firmicutes and increases in Bacteroidetes in affected horses, along with changes in urine metabolites [64]. Whether these reflect potential causal changes or secondary effects of the disease remains to be determined.

4.5 Exogenous Impacts on and Manipulation of the Microbiome

4.5.1 Diet

In horses, the impact of the diet on the hindgut microbiome has long been recognized. Dietary components that are not digested by host enzymes in the foregut pass unchanged through to the hindgut and deliver a variety of growth-promoting and growth-inhibiting factors that influence the balance between species specialized for the fermentation of different substrates within the microbial community. A recent review summarized data from studies assessing the variations of the microbiome occurring in the hindgut under different dietary changes [33]. This showed that most studies have examined the impact of abrupt changes and changes between high-starch (HS) versus high-fiber (HF) diets, while the effect of feed form and processing or feeding frequency is rarely explored.

The abrupt change between forage and concentrate-based diets has a strong impact on the cecal and right ventral colonic microbiota (Figure 4.3). As early as five hours after incorporation of the concentrate in the hay diet, changes consistent with dysbiosis appear, with a marked increase of the starch-utilizing bacteria, leading to an increase in the lactate concentration followed by an increase of lactate-utilizing bacteria. Later, within the first days after the change, percentages of xylanolytic and pectinolytic bacteria decrease markedly. The increase of amylolytic activity and the decrease of fibrolytic activity were consistent with the decrease of the ratio [(C2 + C4)/C3] measured in the proximal hindgut.

A high-starch or high soluble carbohydrate diet induces a lower richness and diversity of cecal and right ventral colonic bacteria compared with a high-fiber diet. An increase of starch-utilizing bacteria and associated genera *Lactobacillus* and *Streptococcus* in the right ventral colon and the caecum is related to a marked increase in lactate concentration and, an overgrowth of lactate-utilizing bacteria (Veillonellaceae family). In turn, the concentrations of acid-intolerant fibrolytic bacteria e.g. cellulolytic, xylanolytic, and pectinolytic bacteria, decrease. Recent studies using culture-independent techniques have confirmed that the Lachnospiraceae and Ruminococcaceae families and the *Fibrobacter* spp. have lower abundance in the hindgut of horses fed a high-starch diet compared with

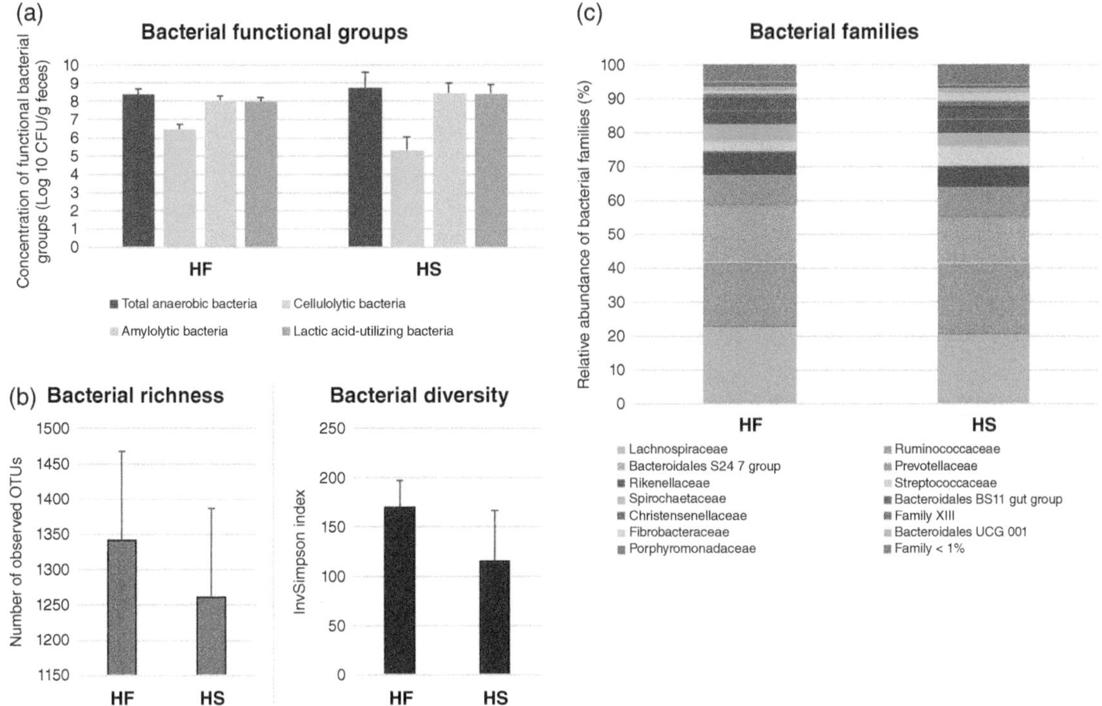

Figure 4.3 In six adult healthy horses fed a high-fiber diet (HF) and switched abruptly to a high-starch diet (HS), fecal modifications were observed for: (a) the functional groups regarding bacterial total anaerobes, cellulolytics, amylolytics, and lactic acid utilizers; (b) the bacterial richness and diversity assessed by the number of observed OTUs and InvSimpson indexes, variations between days for each supplementation; (c) the relative abundance of bacterial families. *Source:* Photo credits: Axelle Collinet and Véronique Julliand, Univ. Bourgogne Franche-Comté, AgroSup Dijon, PAM UMR A 02.102, Dijon, France; and Pauline Grimm and Samy Julliand, Lab To Field, Dijon, France.

those fed a high-fiber diet. These different alterations of the microbiota tend toward lower fibrolytic activity and higher amylolytic activity of the ecosystem with higher soluble carbohydrate intake reflected by the decrease of the ratio [(C2 + C4)/C3].

4.5.2 Probiotics

Probiotics, commonly named "direct-fed microbials", are live microorganisms that confer a health benefit on the host after oral administration at an appropriate dose. Thus to be recognized as probiotics, microorganisms must be viable within the gastro-intestinal tract and provide a beneficial effect on the host's health. The concept of probiotic therapy directly relates to the impacts of the gastrointestinal microbiota on host health. However, the complexity of the microbiota complicates effective probiotic therapy.

Two main approaches are used in horses, yeast-based and bacterium-based probiotics. Feeding yeast to horses fed high-starch, low-forage diets was associated with higher concentrations of lactate-utilizing bacteria in the large intestine compared with non-supplemented horses, resulting in a decrease in lactate produced by starch fermentation and limited the pH decrease [65]. Supplementing horses with yeast could thus reduce the hindgut microbiota disturbances caused by a high quantity of starch in the ration, and thus prevent acidosis and the appearance of digestive diseases. Feeding yeast to horses suffering from enterocolitis reduced both the severity and duration of their clinical signs compared with horses receiving placebo; however, the overall effect was relatively minor [66].

There has been limited study of prophylactic use of probiotics. One randomized clinical trial (RCT) reported no impact of a *Lactiplantibacillus plantarum, Lacticaseibacillus casei, Lactobacillus acidophilus*, and *Streptococcus faecium* [actually *Enterococcus faecium*] gel or *L. acidophilus, S. faecium, Bifidobacterium longum*, and *Bifidobacterium thermophilum* paste on post-operative diarrhea, salmonellosis, and *Salmonella* shedding in horses that underwent colic surgery [67]. Another RCT found no impact of a commercial probiotic containing *Lactococcus lactis, E. faecium*, and "yeast" on *Salmonella* shedding, fever, diarrhea, or leukopenia in horses admitted to a single facility for colic [68]. A study of an *Lactiplantibacillus plantarum, L. casei, L. acidophilus*, and *E. faecium* product found no impact on *Salmonella* shedding of "non-emergency" patients ≥6 m of age [69].

This study claimed a 65% reduction in *Salmonella* shedding but there was not a statistically significant difference, indicating little support for any suggestion of efficacy. Three other studies evaluated probiotics for the prevention of diarrhea in foals, with none showing a protective effect [28, 70, 71]. All identified potential adverse effects of probiotic treatment, with an increased risk of diarrhea or diarrhea that required veterinary intervention. A small RCT involving *Ligilactobacillus salivarius*, *Limosilactobacillus reuteri*, *Lactobacillus crispatus*, *Lactobacillus jonhsonii*, and *Ligilactobacillus equi* identified a significant decrease in diarrhea at one of the four-time points, yet no investigation of *Salmonella* was performed [72]. Quality control of commercial probiotics is another concern, as serious deficiencies in commercial products have been identified [73, 74].

4.5.3 Prebiotics

A prebiotic is "a substrate that is selectively utilized by host microorganisms conferring a health benefit." Dietary prebiotics must not be degraded by the target host enzymes. The most extensively documented prebiotics are the nondigestible inulin-type fructans (inulin, fructo-oligosaccharides, and short-chain oligosaccharides) and the galacto-oligosaccharides.

In horses, the impact of prebiotics on GIT tract microorganisms is not well documented. Short-chain fructooligosaccharides (scFOSs) supplementation was reported to increase starch-utilizing and lactate-utilizing bacteria in the gastric content as well as in the right ventral colon [75]. Since scFOS stimulates the immune system, there may be some impact of prebiotics on local and systemic immune responses, an area that warrants further study.

Inulin-type fructans have been related to laminitis. It is important to note that the dose used to induce laminitis in experimental studies was about 100 times higher than the doses currently recommended for prebiotic effects (10 kg vs. 0.1 kg/d). Therefore, the administration of prebiotics at commercial doses does not have a detrimental impact. Data on dosing interval and duration of administration are lacking.

4.5.4 Drugs

4.5.4.1 Antimicrobials

Impacts of antimicrobials on the equine GIT are well recognized, particularly given the relatively high susceptibility of horses to antimicrobial-associated colitis. However, a study of the impacts of antimicrobials on the fecal microbiota has been relatively limited. Former culture-based studies identified rapid and pronounced changes in some parts of the cultivable microbiota. For example, the administration of oxytetracycline was associated with rapid increases in coliforms, Bacteroides, *C. perfringens*, and *Streptococcus*, with the disappearance of Veillonella [76]. Corresponding changes were not identified following trimethoprim-sulfadiazine administration. Similarly, few changes were identified after intravenous or oral trimethoprim-sulfadiazine administration in another study, with only a transient decrease in coliforms [77]. Yet, a profound (>99%) decrease in cellulolytic bacteria, as well as decreases in lactobacilli and increases in *Salmonella* and *C. difficile*, was identified in horses treated with trimethoprim-sulfadiazine or ceftiofur, a third-generation cephalosporin [78]. A study combining culture and culture-independent methods reported no apparent impact of penicillin or anesthesia on the microbiota [79]. Whether these differences between studies relate to geography, diet, study methods, or other factors is unclear.

Next-generation sequencing-based studies have been limited. One study identified changes in the proportions of several taxonomic groups, along with changes in the overall bacterial community structure in response to treatment with trimethoprim-sulfadiazine, ceftiofur sodium, and procaine penicillin [11]. Changes were most evident with oral trimethoprim-sulfadiazine. The resilient nature of the microbiota in healthy adult horses was also demonstrated here by the return to a state similar to baseline within 25 d after cessation of treatment. However, some differences were still present at that time point. This suggests that the equine fecal microbiota rebounds fairly quickly but that there may be effects that linger for weeks, if not longer. This is consistent with humans, where subtle but prolonged changes have been noted after antimicrobial administration.

4.5.4.2 Other Drugs

Many other drugs could have an impact on the gastrointestinal microbiota, but the studies are lacking. These could include drugs that alter gastrointestinal motility, influence the immune system, or alter local environments (pH). One widely used drug class that could impact the gut microbiota is proton pump inhibitors (PPIs). Commonly used for prevention or treatment of gastric ulcers, this drug class raises the gastric pH, potentially resulting in changes in small intestinal pH, other aspects of the small intestinal microenvironment, and viability of ingested bacteria, i.e. survival of bacteria that would normally die during gastric transit in the naturally low pH. The clinical use of PPIs and nutritional impact on the GIT microbiota in horses is unknown, but the potential for negative impacts of PPIs on the GIT microbiota should be considered.

4.5.5 Other Factors

Any factor that affects the local gastrointestinal environment, directly or indirectly, can potentially influence the microbiota. The range of factors and situations that can do so in horses has received limited attention, and aspects such as the duration of effect and clinical relevance of changes are poorly understood. Yet, they provide insight into the response of the microbiota to exogenous influences and provide insight into the pathophysiology of conditions such as colitis and colic.

Acute exercise causes various physiologic stresses and can impact gastrointestinal mobility, so there are potential impacts on GIT microbiota. A relatively small study of horses undergoing incremental training on a treadmill identified rather modest impacts on the microbiota [80]. Interestingly, changes in beta-diversity (i.e. both the organisms that were present and their relative abundances) were noted during the exercise adaptation period, with a return to baseline by the end of the study. This suggests that changes in exercise, rather than the intensity of exercise, may be influencing factors.

Transportation has been implicated as a risk factor for colitis and colic and even short distances may result in changes in the intestinal bacterial community [81, 82]. Often, multiple potential influencing factors are encountered together, making it more difficult to study the impact of specific variables. One study evaluated the impact of transportation, fasting, and general anesthesia [82]. Changes in the relative abundances of various bacterial taxa were identified, with changes in potentially beneficial members of the Firmicutes phylum (*Roseburia, Ruminococcus*) being noteworthy. There were also broader changes in the overall microbial communities. While the duration of the study was limited, the changes may have been short-term as there appeared to be a return toward baseline by 72 hrs post-anesthesia, consistent with the resiliency in the microbiota noted in the exercise study [80].

Likely, many other factors can at least have short-term influences on the gastrointestinal microbiota. These could include vague and difficult to quantify variables such as stress. Additionally, there may be geographic influences. This has not been investigated in horses but there is evidence to suggest regional differences in the microbiota. For example, marked susceptibility of horses to *C. difficile* colitis in response to exposure to minute quantities of erythromycin from foals treated with that drug has been reported in Sweden but has not been identified elsewhere, despite widespread use of erythromycin in foals internationally [83]. There are also anecdotal differences in the apparent risk of colitis associated with the use of other antimicrobials. In humans, regional differences in the microbiota have been identified, but those studies have focused on groups with "western" vs. "traditional" diets. Understanding of the impact of broader geographic effects is limited.

4.5.6 Fecal Microbial Transplantation

Also referred to as transfaunation, fecal microbial transplantation (FMT) is the act of administering a slurry of feces or cecal contents from a healthy horse to a horse with enteric disease, via a nasogastric tube, and has been performed in horses for decades. While the microbiota was not understood at the time this practice was likely started based on an assumption that changes in the intestinal environment were associated with diseases. While objective data are lacking, FMT has been used with anecdotal success in horses with conditions such as chronic diarrhea.

There has been a resurgence in interest in FMT over the past decade, in part due to the attention it is getting as a highly effective treatment for recurrent *C. difficile* infection in humans, a disease that is associated with an altered gastrointestinal microbiota. Horses do not have clinical conditions similar to recurrent *C. difficile* infection or ulcerative colitis, so extrapolation must be done with care; however, acute colitis and chronic diarrhea are important problems with a presumed role of the gut microbiota. In the absence of objective data, preliminary guidelines for FMT in horses have been proposed [84]. As the beneficial components of the microbiota become better understood, key components could be part of a "synthetic feces" approach, using a cocktail of well-scrutinized beneficial microbes, resulting in a standardized FMT inoculum rather than administration of an undefined fecal or cecal slurry.

4.6 Assessment of the Microbiota and Microbiome

Because of the role of the microbiota in health and disease, there is an obvious desire to characterize the microbiota for reasons, such as identifying the risk of disease, diagnosing active disease, and monitoring response to treatment. Yet, the assessment of such a large and complex population is accompanied by many challenges. Cost, time, and complexity have been major barriers in the past. However, as taxa-sequencing costs and turnaround times decrease substantially, we are entering an era where a rapid sequence-based assessment of microbiotas will be possible. Currently, there are commercial sources that offer equine intestinal microbiota assessment. However, the nutritional or clinical use of any data generated through such testing is currently very limited based on the lack of individual horse-level data and scientific validation. There is currently inadequate information to interpret the results in the context of an individual patient, as opposed to comparing large populations. Individual animal microbiota data will likely be used as a clinical tool in the future, and if so, or for research studies, a variety of potential factors must be considered.

4.6.1 Sampling Sites and Types

Since fecal samples provide a good representation of the large colon, they are optimal for a disease that occurs in that region [4, 5]. Feces are a reasonable representation of the cecum (at least in healthy horses), so fecal samples are potentially useful for the assessment of cecal and large colonic disease [85]. However, as one moves more proximal, the agreement between feces and intestinal contents decreases. Changes that occur in proximal regions might still be reflected in feces, but there is no certainty that a lack of apparent changes in feces means there are no changes in the proximal GIT. A sampling of gastric fluid and contents from the proximal duodenum can be performed endoscopically if there is a need to assess those most proximal regions.

Another consideration is the collection of feces/intestinal contents versus intestinal mucous versus intestinal wall biopsies. While there is good general agreement between the bacterial composition of contents vs. mucosal samples in the colon of healthy horses, it is unknown if there are relevant differences during disease [4, 5]. Yet another consideration is whether testing should be performed on a homogenized sample or whether testing of a sample from the surface of a fecal ball is acceptable. This was assessed in one equine study, where there were no differences in the results from homogenized vs. surface samples [86].

4.6.2 Sample Handling

Sample handling can impact the results and must be considered when deciding to attempt to assess the microbiota. Culture techniques require fresh samples that are properly stored. If strict anaerobes are to be isolated, rapid transportation to the laboratory is required, with samples maintained in an anaerobic environment, if possible. For spore-forming anaerobes (*C. difficile*), the main target for isolation are usually the hardy spores, not the intolerant vegetative form. Therefore, handling conditions and time frame are less of a concern [87]. Handling conditions are less critical for facultative anaerobes such as *Salmonella* and *C. perfringens*.

Handling conditions can also impact culture-independent studies. One study identified significant changes in the microbiota of samples when aliquots were taken from the same fecal piles in the environment over time, perhaps related to high ambient temperatures (>30 °C) during the study period [86]. The results of this study highlight the potential impact of using feces collected from pastures or stalls when the time of defecation is unknown, as changes may have occurred, particularly at warm temperatures. The impacts of refrigeration or freezing, typical post-collection storage conditions, and the impact of storage time, have not been evaluated in equine samples. Additionally, freeze–thaw cycles can have an impact on some bacterial taxa [88].

4.6.3 Testing Methods

Culture is a commonly used clinical and research tool to evaluate targeted aspects of the microbiotas bacterial and anaerobic fungal components. Culture permits the enumeration and isolation of living microorganisms and the ability to explore the functional roles of isolates or microbial communities. For example, bacteria are classified as amylolytic or cellulolytic depending on their capacity to hydrolyze starch or cellulose. The main limitation of the culture-dependent technique is the fact that a large percentage of intestinal microorganisms are difficult or impossible to cultivate using conventional techniques. Many have never been isolated in the laboratory, but uncultivable organisms may still play key roles in gut health.

Cellulolytic bacteria are extremely oxygen-sensitive and thus highly difficult to cultivate, isolate, and study (Figure 4.4). However, they are considered "key-stones" for the host due to their capacity for degrading cell-wall polysaccharides. Some organisms may also be present at low levels that are clinically relevant and require selective culture techniques to isolate them. Thus, bacterial culture, especially using selective and enrichment methods, can be

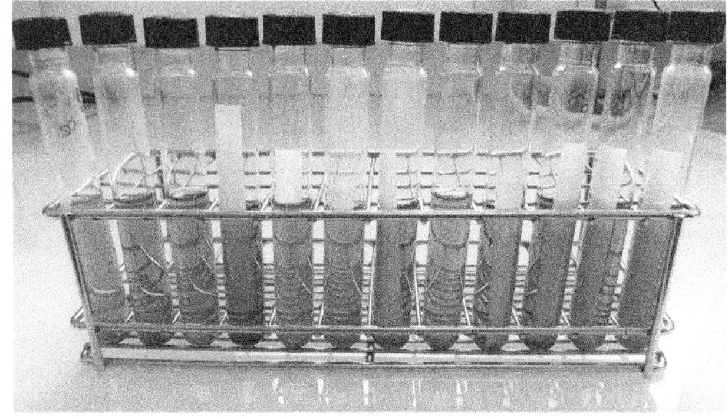

Figure 4.4 Horse feces have been inoculated in Hungate tubes containing a specific medium with filter paper strip as the only substrate. In some tubes, the filter paper disappeared indicating the presence of active cellulolytic bacteria in the feces. *Source:* Photo credits: Cécile Le Bras, 92 300 Levallois Perret, France.

a useful tool when there is a need to assess specific activities, to target species that are readily culturable *in vitro*, and to identify species that are difficult to detect with broader, (sequence-based), assays. Culture is commonly used for the diagnosis of enterocolitis, through the detection of a limited number of known pathogens (*Salmonella, C. difficile*).

While culture has important uses, it is not a highly effective tool for the broad characterization of such a large and complex microbiota environment. The past decade has witnessed revolutionary changes in our description, rather than understanding, of microbiotas because of advancements in next-generation gene sequencing and bioinformatics. It is now possible to identify thousands to millions of gene sequences from fecal, samples. However, sequence-based methods are still limited by gaps in reference datasets, given the huge proportion of unknown bacterial species in equine, unvalidated techniques, method biases, difficulties characterizing very rare components of the microbiota, and, importantly, difficulty interpreting what results mean. As laboratory and computing methods advance rapidly, our ability to generate data is outpacing our ability to interpret those results. Nonetheless, next-generation sequencing-based methods are providing exceptional new information and will be a core of gut microbiota assessment in the coming years. In summary, currently, no one method can provide all the answers so the approach to bacterial microbiota analysis depends on factors, such as the goals, access to different methods, ability to analyze results, and cost. The holistic approach combining both culturable and culture-independent techniques would currently be the most informative for assessing the microbiota composition and function.

Evaluation of microscopic fungi has mainly been assessed using the culturable technique. Similar to cellulolytic bacteria, due to their extreme sensitivity to oxygen, culturing is very laborious. Recent and rare studies have used next-generation sequencing and bioinformatics, which found that the majority of sequences obtained from horses represented novel taxa.

Evaluation of the virome is very limited in horses because of the time, technical difficulty, and cost, as well as limited ability to interpret results. Targeted testing, looking for specific viral pathogens (rotavirus) is used clinically and for research purposes. As with bacteria, this can involve viral culture, detection, and quantitation of virus particles by polymerase chain reaction or detection of the virus in tissue through immunofluorescence. Likewise, testing for archaea is rare. If performed, evaluation of these extremophiles would typically involve molecular methods. Similarly, the characterization of the protozoal microbiota is very rarely done as a research, not clinical, tool.

4.7 Summary

The equine intestinal microbiota is a complex, ever-changing microbial population that undeniably plays a crucial role in the health and disease of horses. As a monogastric herbivore driving energy from a diet that equids cannot, themselves, adequately digest, the horse requires a functional and adaptable gut microbiota. The microbiota also plays important roles in immune function, intestinal development, and pathogen exclusion, allowing the horse to live symbiotically with a GIT microbial population, and survive the onslaught of associated antigens. The high occurrence of diseases that could relate to the microbiota, such as colic, laminitis, and colitis, and the importance of many other diseases that could plausibly be affected by the microbiota, such as metabolic syndrome, obesity, and inflammatory disorders, highlight the need to better comprehend the equine gastrointestinal microbiota. While our understanding of the microbiota is still relatively superficial, as this field continues to rapidly advance, the role of the microbiota in health and disease, and methods to identify, prevent, and correct alterations to the microbiota may become a mainstay of horse management and veterinary medicine.

References

1 Julliand, V. and Grimm, P. (2016). Horse species symposium: the microbiome of the horse hindgut: history and current knowledge. *J. Anim. Sci.* 94 (6): 2262–2274.

2 Costa, M.C. and Weese, J.S. (2012). The equine intestinal microbiome. *Anim. Health Res. Rev.* 13 (1): 121–128.

3 de Fombelle, A., Varloud, M., Goachet, A.G. et al. (2003). Characterization of the microbial and biochemical profile of the different segments of the digestive tract in horses given two distinct diets. *Anim. Sci.* 77 (2): 293–304.

4 Ericsson, A.C., Johnson, P.J., Lopes, M.A. et al. (2016). A microbiological map of the healthy equine gastrointestinal tract. *PLoS One* 11 (11): 1–17.

5 Costa, M.C., Silva, G., Ramos, R.V. et al. (2015). Characterization and comparison of the bacterial microbiota in different gastrointestinal tract compartments in horses. *Vet. J.* 205 (1): 74–80.

6 O'Donnell, M.M., Harris, H.M.B., Jeffery, I.B. et al. (2013). The core faecal bacterial microbiome of Irish

thoroughbred racehorses. *Lett. Appl. Microbiol.* 57 (6): 492–501.
7 Weese, J.S., Holcombe, S.J., Embertson, R.M. et al. (2015). Changes in the faecal microbiota of mares precede the development of post partum colic. *Equine Vet. J.* 47 (6): 641–649.
8 Costa, M.C., Arroyo, L.G., Allen-Vercoe, E. et al. (2012). Comparison of the fecal microbiota of healthy horses and horses with colitis by high throughput sequencing of the V3-V5 region of the 16s rRNA gene. *PLoS One* 7 (7): 1–11.
9 Suchodolski, J.S., Dowd, S.E., Wilke, V. et al. (2012). 16S rRNA gene pyrosequencing reveals bacterial dysbiosis in the Duodenum of dogs with idiopathic inflammatory bowel disease. *PLoS One* 7 (6): 1–11.
10 Weese, J.S., Nichols, J., Jalali, M., and Litster, A. (2015). The rectal microbiota of cats infected with feline immunodeficiency virus infection and uninfected controls. *Vet. Microbiol.* 180 (1, 2): 96–102.
11 Costa, M.C., Stämpfli, H.R., Arroyo, L.G. et al. (2015). Changes in the equine fecal microbiota associated with the use of systemic antimicrobial drugs. *BMC Vet. Res.* 11 (1): 1–12.
12 Rodriguez, C., Taminiau, B., Brévers, B. et al. (2015). Faecal microbiota characterisation of horses using 16 rDNA barcoded pyrosequencing, and carriage rate of clostridium difficile at hospital admission. *BMC Microbiol.* 15 (1): 1–14.
13 Schoster, A., Arroyo, L.G., Staempfli, H.R., and Weese, J.S. (2013). Comparison of microbial populations in the small intestine, large intestine and feces of healthy horses using terminal restriction fragment length polymorphism. *BMC Res. Notes* 6 (1): 1–9.
14 Shepherd, M.L., Swecker, W.S., Jensen, R.V., and Ponder, M.A. (2012). Characterization of the fecal bacteria communities of forage-fed horses by pyrosequencing of 16S rRNA V4 gene amplicons. *FEMS Microbiol. Lett.* 326 (1): 62–68.
15 Julliand, V., De Vaux, A., Millet, L., and Fonty, G. (1999). Identification of *Ruminococcus flavefaciens* as the predominant cellulolytic bacterial species of the equine cecum. *Appl. Environ. Microbiol.* 65 (8): 3738–3741.
16 Fernandes, K.A., Kittelmann, S., Rogers, C.W. et al. (2014). Faecal microbiota of forage-fed horses in New Zealand and the population dynamics of microbial communities following dietary change. *PLoS One* 9 (11): 112846.
17 Dougal, K., Harris, P.A., Edwards, A. et al. (2012). A comparison of the microbiome and the metabolome of different regions of the equine hindgut. *FEMS Microbiol. Ecol.* 82 (3): 642–652.
18 Lwin, K.O. and Matsui, H. (2014). Comparative analysis of the methanogen diversity in horse and pony by using mcrA gene and archaeal 16S rRNA gene clone libraries. *Archaea* 2014 (1): 1–10.
19 Li, L., Giannitti, F., Low, J. et al. (2015). Exploring the virome of diseased horses. *J. Gen. Virol.* 96 (9): 2721–2733.
20 Cann, A.J., Fandrich, S.E., and Heaphy, S. (2005). Analysis of the virus population present in equine faeces indicates the presence of hundreds of uncharacterized virus genomes. *Virus Genes* 30 (2): 151–156.
21 Peachey, L.E., Molena, R.A., Jenkins, T.P. et al. (2018). The relationships between faecal egg counts and gut microbial composition in UK thoroughbreds infected by cyathostomins. *Int. J. Parasitol.* 48 (6): 403–412.
22 Faubladier, C., Julliand, V., Danel, J., and Philippeau, C. (2013). Bacterial carbohydrate-degrading capacity in foal faeces: changes from birth to pre-weaning and the impact of maternal supplementation with fermented feed products. *Br. J. Nutr.* 110 (6): 1040–1052.
23 Jacquay, E. and Kouba, J. (2017). Colonization and maturation of the foal fecal microbiota from birth through weaning and the effect of weaning method. Doctoral dissertation. Kansas State University. https://krex.k-state.edu/dspace/handle/2097/35563 (accessed 24 February 2020).
24 Quercia, S., Freccero, F., Castagnetti, C. et al. (2019). Early colonisation and temporal dynamics of the gut microbial ecosystem in Standardbred foals. *Equine Vet. J.* 51 (2): 231–237.
25 Costa, M.C., Stämpfli, H.R., Allen-Vercoe, E., and Weese, J.S. (2016). Development of the faecal microbiota in foals. *Equine Vet. J.* 48 (6): 681–688.
26 Julliand, V., DeVaux, A., Villaro, L., and Richard, Y. (1996). Preliminary studies on the bacterial flora of faeces taken from foals, from birth to twelve weeks. Effect of the oral administration of a commercial colostrum replacer. *Pferdeheilkunde* 12: 209–212.
27 Schoster, A., Staempfli, H.R., Guardabassi, L.G. et al. (2017). Comparison of the fecal bacterial microbiota of healthy and diarrheic foals at two and four weeks of life. *BMC Vet. Res.* 13 (1): 1–10.
28 Schoster, A., Guardabassi, L., Staempfli, H.R. et al. (2016). The longitudinal effect of a multi-strain probiotic on the intestinal bacterial microbiota of neonatal foals. *Equine Vet. J.* 48 (6): 689–696.
29 Earing, J.E., Durig, A.C., Gellin, G.L. et al. (2012). Bacterial colonization of the equine gut; comparison of mareand fal pairs by PCR-DGGE. *Adv. Microbiol.* 2 (2): 79–86.
30 Pethick, D.W., Rose, R.J., Bryden, W.L., and Gooden, J.M. (1993). Nutrient utilisation by the hindlimb of thoroughbred horses at rest. *Equine Vet. J.* 25 (1): 41–44.
31 Vermorel, M., Vernet, J., and Martin-Rosset, W. (1997). Digestive and energy utilisation of two diets by ponies and horses. *Livest. Prod. Sci.* 51 (1–3): 13–19.

32 Glinsky, M.J., Smith, R.M., Spires, H.R., and Davis, C.L. (1976). Measurement of volatile fatty acid production rates in the cecum of the pony. *J. Anim. Sci.* 42 (6): 1465–1470.

33 Julliand, V. and Grimm, P. (2017). The impact of diet on the hindgut microbiome. *J. Equine Vet. Sci.* 52 (5): 23–28.

34 Jouany, J.-P., Medina, B., Bertin, G., and Julliand, V. (2009). Effect of live yeast culture supplementation on hindgut microbial communities and their polysaccharidase and glycoside hydrolase activities in horses fed a high-fiber or high-starch diet. *J. Anim. Sci.* 87 (9): 2844–2852.

35 Hoffman, R.M. (2013). Carbohydrates. In: *Equine Applied and Clinical Nutrition: Health, Welfare and Performance* (ed. R. Geor, P. Harris, and M. Coenen), 156–167. Edinburgh: Saunders Elsevier.

36 National Research Council (1982). *United States-Canadian Tables of Feed Composition*. 3rd Rev. Nutritional Data for United States and Canadian Feeds, 1–148. Washington, DC: National Academies Press.

37 Slade, L.M. and Robinson, D.W. (1970). Nitrogen metabolism in nonruminant herbivores. II. Comparative aspects of protein digestion. *J. Anim. Sci.* 30 (5): 761–763.

38 National Research Council (1989). *Nutrient Requirements of Horses*. 5th Rev. Animal Nutrition Series, 1 -100. Washington, DC: National Academies Press.

39 National Research Council (2007). *Nutrient Requirements of Horses*. 6th Rev. Animal Nutrition Series, 1–341. Washington, DC: National Academies Press.

40 Gibbs, P.G., Potter, D.G., Kreider, J.L. et al. (1981). Partial and total tract protein digestion in ponies fed three forages. In: *Proceedings of the 7th Equine Nutrition and Physiology Society Symposium*, addendum. Warrenton, VA: Equine Nutrition and Physiology Society.

41 Gibbs, P.G., Potter, D.G., Kreider, J.L. et al. (1983). Partial and total tract nitrogen digestion in ponies fed soybean meal and cottonseed meal. In: *Proceedings of the 8th Equine Nutrition and Physiology Society*, 349. Equine Nutrition and Physiology Society.

42 Reitnour, C.M., Baker, J.P., Mitchell, G.E., and Little, C.O. (1969). Nitrogen digestion in different segments of the equine digestive tract. *J. Anim. Sci.* 29 (2): 332–334.

43 Glade, M.J. (1983). Nitrogen partitioning along the equine digestive tract. *J. Anim. Sci.* 57 (4): 943–953.

44 Gibbs, P.G., Potter, G.D., Schelling, G.T. et al. (1988). Digestion of hay protein in different segments of the equine digestive tract. *J. Anim. Sci.* 66 (2): 400–406.

45 Sullins, K., Stashak, T., and Ralston, S. (1985). Experimental large intestinal resection in the horse: technique and nutritional performance. In: *Proceedings of the 31th Annual Convention of the American Association of Equine Practitioners*, 497–503. Toronto, Canada: American Association of Equine Practitioners (AAEP).

46 Woodward, A.D., Holcombe, S.J., Steibel, J.P. et al. (2010). Cationic and neutral amino acid transporter transcript abundances are differentially expressed in the equine intestinal tract. *J. Anim. Sci.* 88 (3): 1028–1033.

47 Woodward, A.D., Fan, M.Z., Geor, R.J. et al. (2012). Characterization of l-lysine transport across equine and porcine jejunal and colonic brush border membrane. *J. Anim. Sci.* 90 (3): 853–862.

48 Bonhomme-Florentin, A. (1976). Lipolytic activity of ciliates and bacteria of horse's caecum. *Anim. Physiol. Biochem.* 282: 1605–1608.

49 Zeyner, A. and Harris, P.A. (2013). Vitamins. In: *Equine Applied and Clinical Nutrition: Health, Welfare and Performance* (ed. R.J. Geor, P.A. Harris, and M. Coenen), 168–189. Philadelphia, PA: Saunders Elsevier.

50 Back, H., Nyman, A., and Osterman, L.E. (2013). The association between *Anoplocephala perfoliata* and colic in Swedish horses-a case control study. *Vet. Parasitol.* 197 (3, 4): 580–585.

51 Milinovich, G.J., Burrell, P.C., Pollitt, C.C. et al. (2008). Microbial ecology of the equine hindgut during oligofructose-induced laminitis. *ISME J.* 2 (11): 1089–1100.

52 Milinovich, G.J., Trott, D.J., Burrell, P.C. et al. (2007). Fluorescence in situ hybridization analysis of hindgut bacteria associated with the development of equine laminitis. *Environ. Microbiol.* 9 (8): 2090–2100.

53 Milinovich, G.J., Trott, D.J., Burrell, P.C. et al. (2006). Changes in equine hindgut bacterial populations during oligofructose- induced laminitis. *Environ. Microbiol.* 8 (5): 885–898.

54 Milinovich, G.J., Burrell, P.C., Pollitt, C.C. et al. (2008). *Streptococcus henryi* sp. nov. and *Streptococcus caballi* sp. nov., isolated from the hindgut of horses with oligofructuose-induced laminitis. *Int. J. Syst. Evol. Microbiol.* 58 (1): 262–266.

55 Crawford, C., Sepulveda, M.F., Elliott, J. et al. (2007). Dietary fructan carbohydrate increases amine production in the equine large intestine: implications for pasture-associated laminitis. *J. Anim. Sci.* 85 (11): 2949–2958.

56 Garner, H.E., Moore, J.N., Johnson, J.H. et al. (1978). Changes in the caecal flora associated with the onset of laminitis. *Equine Vet. J.* 10 (4): 249–252.

57 Moreau, M.M., Eades, S.C., Reinemeyer, C.R. et al. (2014). Illumina sequencing of the V4 hypervariable region 16S rRNA gene reveals extensive changes in bacterial communities in the cecum following carbohydrate oral infusion and development of early-stage acute laminitis in the horse. *Vet. Microbiol.* 168 (2–4): 436–441.

58 Steelman, S.M., Chowdhary, B.P., Dowd, S. et al. (2012). Pyrosequencing of 16S rRNA genes in fecal samples reveals high diversity of hindgut microflora in horses and potential links to chronic laminitis. *BMC Vet. Res.* 8 (1): 1–11.

59 Biddle, A.S., Black, S.J., and Blanchard, J.L. (2013). An in vitro model of the horse gut microbiome enables identification of lactate-utilizing bacteria that differentially respond to starch induction. *PLoS One* 8 (10): 1–13.
60 Dong, H.J., Ho, H., Hwang, H. et al. (2016). Diversity of the gastric microbiota in thoroughbred racehorses having gastric ulcer. *J. Microbiol. Biotechnol.* 26: 763–774.
61 Perkins, G.A., den Bakker, H.C., Burton, A.J. et al. (2012). Equine stomachs harbor an abundant and diverse mucosal microbiota. *Appl. Environ. Microbiol.* 78 (8): 2522–2532.
62 Varloud, M., Fonty, G., Roussel, A. et al. (2007). Postprandial kinetics of some biotic and abiotic characteristics of the gastric ecosystem of horses fed a pelleted concentrate meal. *J. Anim. Sci.* 85 (10): 2508–2516.
63 Elzinga, S.E., Weese, J.S., and Adams, A.A. (2016). Comparison of the fecal microbiota in horses with equine metabolic syndrome and metabolically normal controls fed a similar all-forage diet. *J. Equine Vet. Sci.* 44: 9–16.
64 Leng, J., Proudman, C., Darby, A. et al. (2018). Exploration of the fecal microbiota and biomarker discovery in equine grass sickness. *J. Proteome Res.* 17 (3): 1120–1128.
65 Medina, B., Girard, I.D., Jacotot, E., and Julliand, V. (2002). Effect of a preparation of on microbial profiles and fermentation patterns in the large intestine of horses fed a high fiber or a high starch diet. *J. Anim. Sci.* 80 (10): 2600–2609.
66 Desrochers, A.M., Dolente, B.A., Ray, M. et al. (2005). Efficacy of *Saccharomyces boulardii* for treatment of horses with acute enterocolitis. *J. Am. Vet. Med. Assoc.* 227 (6): 954–959.
67 Parraga, M.E., Spier, S.J., Thurmond, M., and Hirsh, D. (1997). A clinical trial of probiotic administration for prevention of Salmonella shedding in the postoperative period in horses with colic. *J. Vet. Intern. Med.* 11 (1): 36–41.
68 Kim, L.M., Morley, P.S., Traub-Dargatz, J.L. et al. (2001). Factors associated with Salmonella shedding among equine colic patients at a veterinary teaching hospital. *J. Am. Vet. Med. Assoc.* 218 (5): 740–748.
69 Ward, M.P., Alinovi, C.A., Couëtil, L.L. et al. (2004). A randomized clinical trial using probiotics to prevent Salmonella fecal shedding in hospitalized horses. *J. Equine Vet. Sci.* 24 (6): 242–247.
70 Weese, J.S., Anderson, M.E.C., Lowe, A., and Monteith, G.J. (2003). Preliminary investigation of the probiotic potential of *Lactobacillus rhamnosus* strain GG in horses: fecal recovery following oral administration and safety. *Can. Vet. J.* 44 (4): 299–302.
71 Ströbel, C., Günther, E., Romanowski, K. et al. (2018). Effects of oral supplementation of probiotic strains of *Lactobacillus rhamnosus* and *Enterococcus faecium* on diarrhoea events of foals in their first weeks of life. *J. Anim. Physiol. Anim. Nutr.* 102 (5): 1357–1365.
72 Yuyama, T., Yusa, S., Takai, S. et al. (2004). Evaluation of a host-specific lactobacillus probiotic in neonatal foals. *Int. J. Appl. Res.* 18: 101–106.
73 Weese, J.S. (2002). Microbiologic evaluation of commercial probiotics. *J. Am. Vet. Med. Assoc.* 220 (6): 794–797.
74 Weese, S.J. and Martin, H. (2011). Assessment of commercial probiotic bacterial contents and label accuracy. *Can. Vet. J.* 52 (1): 43–46.
75 Respondek, F., Goachet, A.-G., Rudeaux, F., and Julliand, V. (2007). Effects of short-chain fructo-oligosaccharides on the microbial and biochemical profile of different segments of the gastro-intestinal tract in horses. *Pferdeheilkunde* 23 (March/April): 146–150.
76 White, G. and Prior, S. (1982). Comparative effects of oral administration of trimethoprim/sulphadiazine or oxytetracycline on the faecal flora of horses. *Vet. Rec.* 111 (14): 316–318.
77 Gustafsson, A., Båverud, V., Franklin, A., et al. (1999). Repeated administration of trimethoprim/sulfadiazine in the horse – pharmacokinetics, plasma protein binding and influence on the intestinal microflora. *J. Vet. Pharmacol. Ther.* 22 (1): 20–26.
78 Harlow, B.E., Lawrence, L.M., and Flythe, M.D. (2013). Diarrhea-associated pathogens, lactobacilli and cellulolytic bacteria in equine feces: responses to antibiotic challenge. *Vet. Microbiol.* 166 (1, 2): 225–232.
79 Grønvold, A.M.R., L'Abée-Lund, T.M., Strand, E. et al. (2010). Fecal microbiota of horses in the clinical setting: potential effects of penicillin and general anesthesia. *Vet. Microbiol.* 145 (3, 4): 366–372.
80 Almeida, M.L., Feringer, W.H., Carvalho, J.R.G. et al. (2016). Intense exercise and aerobic conditioning associated with chromium or l-carnitine supplementation modified the fecal microbiota of fillies. *PLoS One* 11 (12): 1–21.
81 Faubladier, C., Chaucheyras-Durand, F., da Veiga, L., and Julliand, V. (2013). Effect of transportation on fecal bacterial communities and fermentative activities in horses: impact of *Saccharomyces cerevisiae* CNCM I-1077 supplementation. *J. Anim. Sci.* 91 (4): 1736–1744.
82 Schoster, A., Mosing, M., Jalali, M. et al. (2016). Effects of transport, fasting and anaesthesia on the faecal microbiota of healthy adult horses. *Equine Vet. J.* 48 (5): 595–602.
83 Gustafsson, A., Båverud, V., Gunnarsson, A. et al. (1997). The association of erythromycin ethylsuccinate with acute colitis in horses in Sweden. *Equine Vet. J.* 29 (4): 314–318.
84 Mullen, K.R., Yasuda, K., Divers, T.J., and Weese, J.S. (2016). Equine faecal microbiota transplant: current knowledge, proposed guidelines and future directions. *Equine Vet. Educ.* 30 (3): 151–160.

85 Grimm, P., Combes, S., Pascal, G. et al. (2020). Dietary composition and yeast/microalgae combination supplementation modulate the microbial ecosystem in the caecum, colon and faeces of horses. *Br. J. Nutr.* 123 (4): 372–382.

86 Beckers, K.F., Schulz, C.J., and Childers, G.W. (2017). Rapid regrowth and detection of microbial contaminants in equine fecal microbiome samples. *PLoS One* 12 (11): 1–18.

87 Weese, J.S., Staempfli, H.R., and Prescott, J.F. (2000). Survival of *Clostridium difficile* and its toxins in equine feces: implications for diagnostic test selection and interpretation. *J. Vet. Diagn. Invest.* 12 (4): 332–336.

88 Cuthbertson, L., Rogers, G.B., Walker, A.W. et al. (2015). Implications of multiple freeze-thawing on respiratory samples for culture-independent analyses. *J. Cyst. Fibros.* 14 (4): 464–467.

Section II

The Diet

Nutrient Metabolism

5

Water

Jonathan M. Naylor

KEY TERMS

- Total dissolved solids (TDS) measure is the total amount of solids in water; these are mainly ions of common minerals that the water came in contact with.
- Hardness is the tendency to form precipitates on boiling; it is related mainly to the calcium content of the water.
- A closed water source is a body of water with no outlet, e.g. the Great Salt Lake in Utah.
- Open water sources flow, e.g. rivers.

KEY POINTS

- Total bacterial counts, coliform counts, TDS, and sulfates are the main indicators of water quality.
- Surface water is most likely to have bacterial contamination; pond or lake water is most likely to contain blue-green algae
- Well water and closed water sources (ponds and lakes with no outlets), particularly in arid areas, are most likely to have high mineral concentrations.
- Water requirement parallels energy requirements.
- As feed intake increases or digestibility decreases, water intake increases.
- Horses that have restricted access to water are more susceptible to impaction colic.

5.1 Water as a Nutrient

There are many different methods and conflicting opinions regarding the watering of horses. However, one of the five basic freedoms for livestock is freedom from thirst [1]. A review from the late 1970s concluded that "An obvious way to prevent trouble is to provide adequate water at all times when a horse is at rest and to allow sufficient opportunity to drink while working" [2]. This statement is the basis for most equine welfare codes of ethics and is consistent with decades of research. The actual daily water requirement of an individual horse is dependent on many factors, but an adequate supply of good-quality, palatable water is essential for horses. While information on the amount of water needed, how needs vary with age, life-stage, work, ration, environment, and the effects and causes of inadequate water intake is available, rarely is this needed as long as water is available ad libitum.

Water is hydrogen and oxygen (H_2O) in the ratio of two hydrogen atoms to one oxygen atom. Considered the second most important molecule, after oxygen, water is a solvent in which substances are dissolved and transported throughout the body and within cells. Water is essential to enzymatic digestion, is needed to regulate body temperature, and provides shape and resilience to tissues. As a major constituent of body fluids, water lubricates joints and eyes, provides protective cushioning for the nervous system, and aids in respiratory gas exchange [3]. There are three sources of water for animals. In order of decreasing volumes, these are imbibing liquid water, moisture in the ration, and water generated during metabolic reactions, aka metabolic water.

Equine Clinical Nutrition, Second Edition. Edited by Rebecca L. Remillard.

5.2 Body Water Content

The water content of the body ranges from 50% to 80% of the total weight depending on the age and body composition of the horse.

5.2.1 Age

The total body water in the average adult 500 kg horse is 60–70% while the total body water in a one-d-old foal is 65–80% (Table 5.1). In growing foals, water consumed per body weight (BW) unit is fourfold greater than a mature horse due to the higher demand for energy and feed consumed to sustain growth. Adult horses are larger but have less surface area resulting in lower evaporative losses from the skin per unit of BW than foals and yearlings. The mature horse requires less energy and consumes less feed per unit of BW, and hence, proportionately less water on BW basis than a young animal [8].

5.2.2 Body Composition

Lean body mass contains 70–80% water and 20–25% protein, whereas adipose tissue contains 10–15% water and 75–80% lipid. Two mature horses with the same BW but differing in body fat content will have different concentrations of total body water. Leaner and more muscular animals (body condition score (BCS) 5/9) have higher percent body water than those with a higher body fat content (BCS 8/9) [3].

Table 5.1 Body water compartments as percentage of body weight in mature horses and neonatal foals.

	Mature horse or pony	Neonatal (<1 d old) foal
Total body water	50–80%	74% +/− 2.4[a]
Blood volume	~7%	16%
Plasma volume	4% +/− 0.6	9.6% +/− 1.5
Extracellular fluid volume	25.3% +/− 1.7	36.3% +/− 1.4
Intracellular fluid volume	35.6% +/− 3.7	38.1% +/− 1.8

[a] 1 standard deviation.
Source: Based on Forro et al. [4]; Spensley et al. [5]; Brinkmann et al. [6]; Fielding et al. [7].

5.3 Water Requirement

Expected water intake helps when planning the capacities of water delivery systems and in determining if an individual has a medical problem related to water intake. Water intake varies with many factors including body size, physiologic life-stage, ration, and environmental factors. For many species, while at rest, the water requirement in liters/d is approximately equal to the energy requirement in Mcal/d because the water requirement is directly related to energy metabolism. For maintenance, the average adult horse energy requirement is 3.33 Mcal/100 kg BW/d and, therefore, a reasonable estimate of the amount of daily water required for maintenance is 3.3 L/100 kg BW/d plus an allowance for fecal water; however, there is considerable variation [9].

Voluntary water intake by the horse at rest in a moderate or cool environment while eating dry forage has been reported to be 2.5–7.0 L/100 kg BW/d [10, 11]. Voluntary freshwater consumption for horses fed dry feeds (hay and grain) is 5 L/100 kg BW/d for horses at rest, while higher amounts are required for those doing light exercise (6.4 L/100 kg BW/d). The total water intake from water in feed and drinking water by ponies at pasture under a variety of environmental conditions varied from 5 to 13.5 L/100 kg BW/d [12]. Horses of similar BW consuming the same ration, however, can differ in daily water intake, and for individual animals, it can vary from day to day [11].

5.3.1 Body Size

The total water volume consumed is primarily dependent on BW. All horses, including ponies and miniature horses, are considered one species (*Equus ferus caballus*). Although body weights range within the species 20-fold, the maintenance water requirement at rest in a thermoneutral environment is 3–5 L/100 kg BW/d. Circumstances (work, ambient temperature, and relative humidity) could increase the requirement threefold [8, 9].

5.3.2 Reproduction

In pregnant mares, the intake of water per unit of BW remains stable throughout gestation commensurate with energy needs. Most of the increased need for water during lactation is due primarily to the associated increased feed intake to meet the respective energy demands. Lactating mares had a 40% increase in water consumed mainly to meet the digestive and metabolic needs associated with the increased feed intake for energy, and only needed 20–30 mL/kg BW more water for losses in the milk [11].

5.3.3 Ration

The total quantity of water consumed must meet the physiological need and match losses. The total water intake equals the amount of water imbibed plus the quantity of water in the ration consumed, i.e. the amount taken in by drinking is less than the total daily water intake. Generally, as the ration water content increases, the quantity of water voluntarily consumed by the horse decreases.

Water balance is the relationship between total water consumed and total water losses (fecal, urine, skin, respiratory, and lactation). The quantity, type, and quality of the feed consumed directly affect the water balance. Horses, like other animals, consume feed for energy, and any difference between the water provided by the ration and water need is met by drinking. The water content of the ration varies considerably with the type of feed. In general, hay and grains contain about 10% moisture, silage or haylage contains 70% moisture while pasture grasses can vary between 30% and 85% moisture depending on the plant maturity [13, 14]. Feeds containing 40% or more moisture can supply enough water to meet the idle adult horse's needs in a moderate environment. A horse grazing a growing forage pasture may not need to drink any water, although most will drink if water is available and palatable [9]. In general, less digestible, fibrous feeds result in more fecal water loss and those higher in protein and minerals increase urine output; both increase water intake. Increased protein intake increases nitrogenous waste products that must be diluted and excreted in the urine, which increases urine water losses [15]. In horses, as in other species, water intake is directly correlated with sodium intake [16, 17]. Water intake was the same whether horses were fed grass or alfalfa hay, but how the water was lost differed; more water was excreted in the feces and less in the urine on grass hay because the alfalfa hay was more digestible but had a higher protein and mineral content [10].

Horses drink 3–4 L/kg of hay dry matter (DM) consumed [18, 19]. Water intake decreases as diet digestibility increases because higher digestibility decreases the volume of feces and, therefore, the amount of fecal water excreted. Therefore, as forage quality improves or as grain is added to the ration, the water consumed will decrease. For example, the amount of water consumed decreased to 2 L/kg feed DM when grain constituted more than 55% of the ration because fecal water content decreased from 72% to 66% [20]. In another estimate, horses fed hay had 84% more water in the intestinal digesta than horses fed a grain concentrate mix [10]. Conversely, as the proportion of grain in the ration is decreased and forage increases, more fiber is excreted in the feces, which increases the fecal mass and fecal water content, both of which increase fecal water excretion.

5.3.4 Climate and Activity

The ambient temperature and humidity, and physical activity of the horse affect the water balance of the body, which then directly affects the drive to drink. Water losses occur through the skin as sweat and the respiratory system as humid air to maintain normal core body temperature and prevent overheating in a hot environment and/or from physical activity. Water, sodium, and chloride requirements all increase as energy needs, sweat production, and heat stress increase. An increase in environmental temperature from only 55 to 70 °F (13 to 21 °C) can increase the horse's water requirements by 15–20% [21]. The amount of water needed may increase as much as 300–400% with work at high ambient temperatures [18].

Ideally, water at 45–65 °F (7–18 °C) should always be available to the horse. In winter, horses usually eat dry feeds, hay, or dried pasture grass and may require access to a water source with a water heater if freezing temperatures are possible. A decreased intake of water during cold weather increases the risk of intestinal impaction of dry partially digested feeds. Water consumption during cold temperatures can be encouraged by [1] removing ice to keep water open, [2] adding sodium chloride to the grain mix (1–2%), and/or [3] using a submersible water heater or tank de-icer (Figure 5.1). If an electric water device is used, the water should be touched daily to determine if a moderate water temperature has been maintained. An electrical "short" circuit will not likely create enough current to harm a horse but the resulting pain will prevent animals from drinking water at that source. Hot bran mashes are fed by some owners during the winter; however, the mash does little to keep the horse warm but does marginally increase water intake. Although snow is not recommended as a water source for horses, there are documented instances of Icelandic horses that continued to eat, remained healthy, and hydrated with no access to liquid water. A herd of 40 horses during a 9-d blizzard with free access to grass silage (70% moisture) and snow as the only source of free water during an average winter temperature of 14 °F (−9.8 °C) did not exhibit thirst or laboratory evidence of dehydration [22].

5.3.5 Competing Needs

The hypothalamus contains several regulatory centers including those for water, salt, food intake, and control of body temperature. The hypothalamus is also influenced

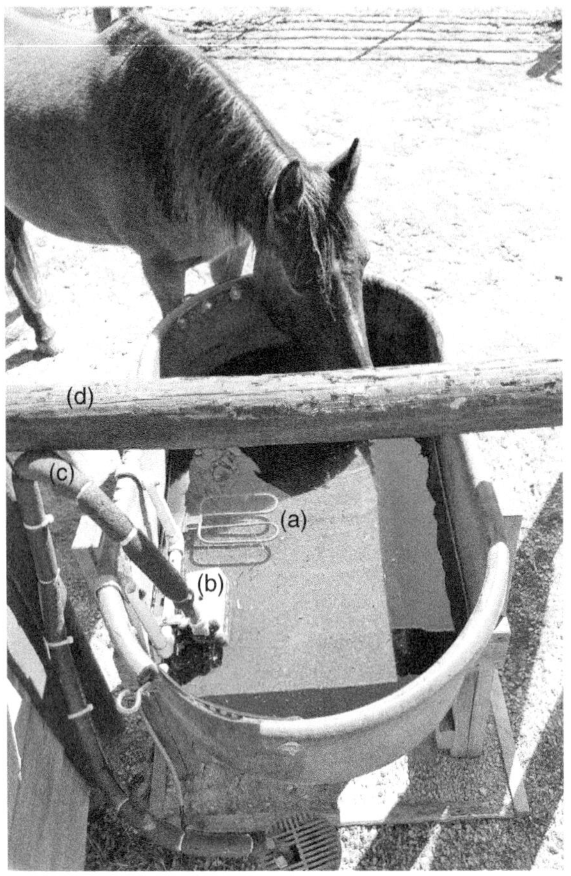

Figure 5.1 Winterized water tank with heater (a) submerged in the middle of the tank and a float valve (b) with an insulated heat-taped water line (c). The tank is straddled by a wooden fence (d) to minimize aggressive behaviors.

by inputs from other parts of the brain. Water intake appears to be regulated based on competing needs. For example, voluntary intake of cold water drops in horses housed outside in cold weather presumably to maintain body temperature more efficiently. Ponies maintained outdoors drank ~40% less water at near-freezing temperatures than heated water (66 °F [19 °C]), yet ponies maintained indoors at 60–80 °F (15–29 °C), drank similar amounts of warm 74 °F (23 °C) and cold 34 °F (1 °C) water [23, 24].

Another example is the relationship between water intake and feed intake. When water is deprived, horses consume less feed. In a 36-hr water deprivation study, feed intake by ponies decreased by 32% [25]. This is presumably to reduce fecal water losses and improve water balance. Free-roaming horses several miles from the nearest water source, reportedly return to drink once a day or as little as every other day presumably to reduce energy expenditure [26].

5.4 Water Deficiency

Water toxicity is rarely a clinical problem; inadequate water intake is the more common problem, which is detrimental. A deficiency of water produces death more rapidly than a deficiency of any other nutrient except oxygen. The drive to acquire water is strong. Thirst is initiated by a ~3% increase in plasma osmolarity and a ~5% increase in plasma sodium [27, 28]. In horses, the only obvious adverse effect of 3 d without water in either a thermoneutral or a hot environment is increased thirst. Horses can remain bright and alert for up to 8 d without water, although they are less active and some develop watery diarrhea after about 6 d [29]. This tolerance of water deprivation is in part due to the capacious large intestine in horses that acts as a reservoir during times of water deprivation [30]. This preferential reliance on the hindgut as a fluid reservoir may explain why individual horses on intermittent watering systems can appear systemically healthy as judged by behavioral and physiologic measures. Conversely, drying out of intestinal contents and alterations in gut flora as a result of water restriction are believed to increase the risk of intestinal impaction type colic [31].

Inadequate water intake occurs when water is inaccessible or unpalatable. Water may not be accessible for many reasons, such as a change in weather or physical conditions around the water site, herd dynamics, faulty wiring problems with electric heaters or fencing that cause animals to be shocked, empty and/or frozen water buckets, or mechanical problem with automatic waterers. Poor palatability may be due to poor water quality. Palatability is best determined by initially smelling and/or tasting the water, and laboratory water analysis, if needed. A change in the water source can change the taste. Ideally, horses should be trained to drink from a variety of sources and devices (streams, ponds, buckets, tanks, bowls). A horse may not drink as much following a move to new quarters, bringing water from the "home" source may help transition to the new environment. Other horses drinking from the new source is often enough to convince a horse that the water is safe. Flavoring the new water with molasses (0.5%; 1 tbsp. /5 gal) may be enough to render the new water source acceptable.

The first noticeable effect of inadequate water intake is increased episodes of colic, more severe restriction decreases dry feed intake, followed by decreased physical activity. Signs of dehydration, such as dry mucous membranes and mouth and sunken eyes (enophthalmos), are not evident until at least a 6% loss of body weight has occurred (Table 5.2). As water is lost from the body, the concentration of metabolites in body fluids increases with the greatest an increase in serum urea nitrogen concentration and smaller increases in serum electrolytes (Na, Cl, P, K, and Ca) [32].

Table 5.2 Estimating degree of dehydration and fluid needs.[a]

Percent dehydration	Physical findings
<5	No detectable abnormalities present
6	Slightly doughy inelasticity of the skin so that it remains in a pinched position longer than 1 s[b]
8	Definite skin inelasticity;[a] capillary refill time 2–3 s;[c] slight enophthalmos; mouth and mucous membranes dry; dry feces and decreased urine volume
10	Severe skin inelasticity;[a] capillary refill time over 3 s; marked enophthalmos; cold extremities; very weak; tachycardia
12	Previously listed signs worsen, unable to stand, shock, involuntary muscle twitching, tachycardia, and weak pulse generally present; death imminent if dehydration not corrected

[a] Liters of fluid needed to correct dehydration equals the percent dehydration present times kilograms body weight; e.g. 8% dehydration times 500 kg BW equals a fluid deficit of 40 L.
[b] Best evaluated in the skin over the shoulders, dorsal midline, or lumbar region and not loose skin, such as on the neck. A cachectic animal's skin, even without dehydration present, loses elasticity, whereas an obese animal tends to retain skin elasticity even when dehydration is severe.
[c] Normal capillary refill time is 1.5–2 s.

Urine concentration also increases as the kidney attempts to conserve water and decrease urine volume. Maximum urine concentration as measured by urine specific gravity and osmolality is 1.045 and 1310 mOsm/kg, respectively which occurs at 12–14% dehydration [32, 33]. Dehydration of more than 15% is lethal and can occur within seven days without water under moderate environmental conditions [8]. Water deprivation in hot environments results in more rapid weight loss and clinical signs of dehydration [32, 33].

5.5 Watering Devices

Feral horses' access to water is highly variable and rarely continuous, and therefore the ability to adapt is necessary for survival [34]. As evidenced in numerous studies, horses readily adapt to various water delivery systems and schedules [35]. Horses can obtain water from bowls, buckets, tanks, or natural features such as ponds and streams. For both horse health and environmental reasons, bowls, buckets, and tanks are preferred over natural water features. However, whichever method is chosen, water should be continuously available. A bucket, usually 5 gal (20 L) in capacity, with a wide brim is used by many owners. The most common problem with using buckets is keeping the buckets clean and filled in good and bad weather on a year-round basis. Two such buckets filled twice a day per horse are generally needed to have water readily available at all times. Reliably keeping water buckets filled is an important management issue because the lack of fresh unfrozen water is associated with a higher incidence of winter colic. Horses kept outdoors without a continuous supply of water were more than twice as likely to colic compared with horses that had an adequate supply of water [36, 37]. Horses allowed group drinking from a natural water source, other than tanks, buckets, and automatic waterers, had a significantly lower risk of colic as well [38].

Automatic waterers use a pressure valve (water is released when the horse presses on a plate to open the valve) or a float valve (water valve opens when the float drops) to provide a constant source of water. Pressure valve waters may be more reliable in the long term, although the flow of water should be relatively quiet and create little disturbance in the bowl. Float valve devices are more often used in watering tanks and can also be reliable if the water line pressure is adequate. A study comparing watering horses with buckets, pressure valves, and float valves noted that small or shallow bowls with a float valve delivered water too slowly and the water balance was negative in those horses. Additionally, buckets were preferred to pressure valves by horses [39]. In general, horses appear to prefer float valves to pressure valves, large over small bowls but prefer buckets over both types of valves [8]. Although many automatic watering bowls hold only 1–2 gal (4–8 L), the refill should be rapid and quiet. A flow rate of 8 L/min appears to be an ideal refill rate for adult 500 kg horses using small bowls [39]. If horses always have an automatic waterer readily available, one is physically sufficient for several horses, even during hot weather, because regardless of water needs, horses drink a relatively small amount at one time. With increased water needs, horses drink more frequently [26]. However, in pasture situations with a single watering bowl problems may arise when a horse low in dominance has not had a chance to drink before the herd moves off.

Feed and other debris should be removed from the water troughs and tanks daily, and they should be thoroughly cleaned as needed based on the appearance of algae and insect larva (mosquito wigglers). Water sources should be placed away from the feeding place to minimize contamination with feed, may require a thermostatically controlled heater to prevent the water from freezing, and if possible should be covered to minimize algae growth due to sunlight. The source should also be large enough to accommodate several horses drinking at the same time to avoid aggressive behaviors and injury around the water source (Figure 5.1). Whatever method is used, the critical factor is that there is clean palatable water in the container at all times and that a sufficient amount is available throughout.

5.6 Sources of Water

Although water makes up a very large portion of the earth's surface, most is locked up in the seas [40]. There are large areas across the United States and Canada where water quality and availability are a concern for horse owners. Water sources for horses can be treated or untreated and can originate from groundwater using wells or surface (flowing or closed) water sources.

5.6.1 Groundwater

Groundwater is obtained from deep or shallow underground aquifers brought to the surface by a well and pump. Groundwater composition is altered by dissolution, precipitation, ion exchange, and reduction/oxidation reactions of compounds from the soil and rock.

Well water can have high mineral content, particularly in the case of shallow wells in the middle parts of the United States and Canada [40]. These water sources should be tested periodically for minerals and toxic compounds to catch problems before serious illness occurs in animals (Tables 5.3–5.5).

5.6.2 Surface Water

Surface water sources are streams, rivers, lakes, ponds, dugouts, and sloughs (small pond, swamp or bog). Flowing water sources (streams, rivers, and most lakes) are known as open water sources, whereas lakes, ponds, and sloughs with no outlet are called closed water sources. Surface water takes on the characteristics of the environment and therefore, is a product of surrounding soil, runoff, farming practices, and nearby human and animal activity [9]. In general, flowing waters (rivers and streams) have relatively low mineral content. Arid areas have water with the highest concentrations of dissolved solids because minerals have not been leached from the area soils by heavy rainfall. In closed sources, because the water flows in but not out, evaporation concentrates the dissolved minerals and toxins. Small ponds and sloughs on the Great Plains of the United States and the Prairies of Canada are variable in TDS and can reach unacceptable concentrations, particularly in late summer [40].

Surface waters are more prone to bacteriological and parasitic contamination than groundwater. In addition, horses can erode the banks and contaminate the water

Table 5.3 U.S. total dissolved solid guidelines for the suitability of water for livestock.

TDS (ppm)[a]	Suitability and effect
<1000	Safe and should pose no health problems
1000–3000	Satisfactory for all livestock and poultry. May cause mild and temporary diarrhea in livestock not accustomed to it, but should not affect their health or performance
3000–5000	It should be satisfactory for livestock, although it might cause temporary diarrhea, or be refused at first by animals not accustomed to it
5000–7000	It can be used for livestock but there may be water refusal and decreased productivity, particularly in lactating dairy cows. It may be advisable to avoid water approaching the higher concentration for working, pregnant, or lactating animals
7000–10 000	Unfit for poultry and swine, a considerable risk may exist in using this water for pregnant, lactating, or young animals, or for any animals subjected to heavy heat stress or water loss. In general, the use of this water should be avoided, although animals other than young, working, and reproducing animals may subsist on it for long periods
Over 10 000	Not recommended for use by any animal under any condition

[a] Total dissolved solids, total soluble salts, or salinity in the water in ppm or mg/L.
Source: Based on NRC [9, 40].

Table 5.4 U.S. and Canadian water quality guidelines for horses.[a]

Parameter	Recommended upper limit (mg/L)
Total dissolved solids	6500
Calcium	500[b]
Sulfate	2500[c]
Nitrates	400[d]
Nitrites	10

[a] Conductance can be converted to TDS using the formula: TDS in mg/L ≈ 0.67 × Conductivity in μS/cm. However, depending on the type of water the conversion factor can vary from 0.54 to 0.96.
[b] Not toxic but at concentrations above the amount given may decrease water palatability.
[c] Or 833 ppm sulfur. Sulfate concentrations above 300–400 ppm can be tasted but a concentration below 2500 ppm has no effect on growing or reproducing cattle or swine. The highest no-effect concentration in horses is not known but is probably similar to that for cattle and swine.
[d] High nitrate concentrations in water occur most commonly as a result of fecal contamination.
Source: Based on NRC [40]; Olkowski [41].

Table 5.5 U.S., Canadian, Australian, and New Zealand mineral-safe upper limit guidelines for horses.[a]

Element	United States	CA	AU/NZ
	mg/L		
Aluminum		5	5
Arsenic	0.2	0.2	0.5
Boron		5	5
Cadmium	0.05	0.05	0.01
Chloride	3000[b]	3000	
Chromium	1	1	
Cobalt	1	1	
Copper	0.5[b]	0.5	0.5–5
Fluoride	2[c]	2	2
Iron	0.3[b]	0.3	
Lead	0.1	0.1	0.1
Magnesium	125[b]	125	
Mercury	0.01	0.01	0.002
Molybdenum		0.5	0.15
Nickel	1	1	1
Nitrate			
Potassium	1400[b]		
Selenium	0.01[d]	0.01	0.02
Sodium	2500[b]		
Vanadium	0.1	0.1	
Zinc	25[e]	25	20

[a] Blanks are no recommendations available.
[b] At concentrations above the amount given may decrease water palatability.
[c] Higher concentration may be safe for horses, as 2.5 ppm results in mottled enamel during teeth development in calves but no observable effects occur in mature cattle at concentrations of less than 8 ppm, and horses are reported to tolerate fluoride intakes two to three times greater than cattle. A concentration of 4 ppm is probably marginally safe for horses, but water with more than 8 ppm should be avoided.
[d] Although chronic selenium toxicosis has been reported as a result of consuming water containing 0.0005–0.002 ppm selenium, concentrations below 0.01 ppm are not generally considered harmful.
[e] High zinc concentrations may occur where galvanized pipes are connected to copper. This results in electrolysis, releasing zinc from the galvanized pipes into the water.
Source: Based on NRC [9, 40]; Olkowski [41]; ANZECC [42].

when defecating or urinating near the water edges. For these reasons, direct access to surface water is not desirable. Surface water should be fenced off and piped to a tank or trough for consumption (Figure 5.2). Placing the water inlet at least 1 yd (1 m) below the surface of clear water, not on the bottom, further reduces the intake of pathogens and toxic algae. Aeration, if possible, helps reduce both total and pathogenic bacterial load.

5.7 Water Quality

The quality of the water suitable for horses is assessed based on dissolved minerals, toxins, and the presence of pathogenic organisms. Ten substances account for 99% of the dissolved minerals in the water, these are sodium, potassium, calcium, magnesium, hydrogen, carbonate, bicarbonate, chloride, and sulfate and silicate ions. In North America, calcium and magnesium along with carbonates and bicarbonates are the major ions in most water sources. This type of mineral pattern produces "hard" water and develops when water percolates through limestone, a rock formed from the skeletal remnants of marine organisms. Less commonly, sodium, potassium, chloride, and sulfate ions dominate and accumulate when water percolates through salt and potash deposits from old sea beds [40]. Dissolved minerals are responsible for five types of water quality issues; TDS, hardness, pH, sulfates, and nitrates. However, only TDS and sulfate content appear to be important to horses. Recommendations for maximum mineral concentrations in water for horses can be found in Tables 5.3–5.5.

5.7.1 Total Dissolved Solids

Total dissolved solids are the most important indicator of water suitability. TDS is a measure of the combined total of organic and inorganic substances contained in a liquid. These solids are primarily minerals, salts, and organic matter, and are indicators of water quality. TDS is commonly reported as parts per million (ppm) or mg/L, the numeric values are identical. There are several related terms. TDS is sometimes referred to as salinity because waters high in TDS are high in saline ions. Salinity is the sum of all the salts dissolved in water (mostly Na and Cl) and is usually measured in parts per thousand (ppt). The average ocean salinity is 35 ppt and the average river water salinity is 0.5 ppt or less. If the units for the sum of ions for salinity are ppm or mg/L, the value is almost identical to TDS. Because electrical conductivity is easy to measure, water is often tested for conductivity. Formulae are often used to convert these values to an approximate TDS.

Signs of high TDS in order of increasing concentration are water refusal or increased water consumption and decreased production, performance, diarrhea, and death. Safe concentrations for horses have not been precisely established. Horses can tolerate concentrations up to 6500 mg/L although production problems in other species can be seen at lower concentrations [40, 41]. While horses can tolerate water high in TDS for maintenance purposes, based on other species, optimal performance including lactation and intense work or exercise may require lower TDS [40].

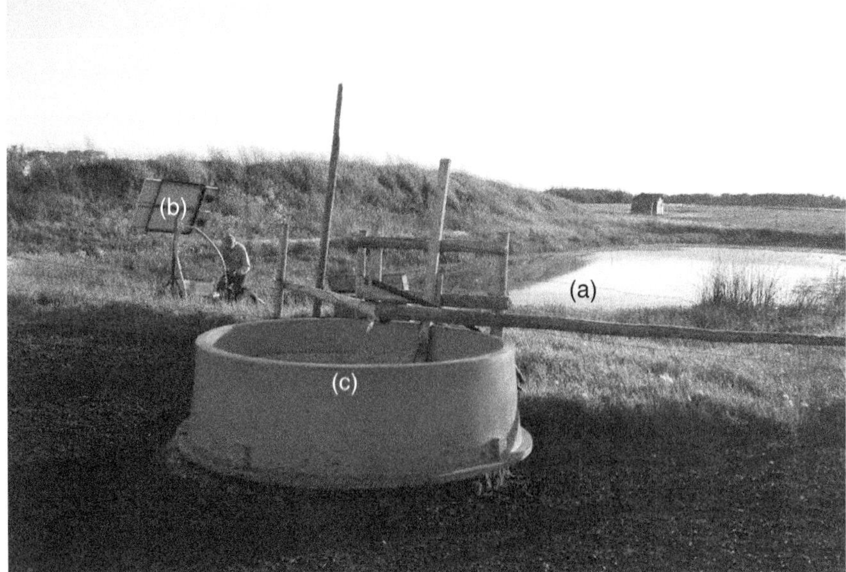

Figure 5.2 A wire fence (a) surrounds a pond to keep animals out of the pond. A solar-powered water pump (b) delivers water to a holding tank (c) within the animal area. *Source:* Reproduced with permission, Vet Visions Inc. 2006.

5.7.2 Hardness

Hard waters are high in calcium and magnesium carbonate and bicarbonates. These salts are relatively insoluble and form white precipitates when water is boiled, mixed with soap, or flows through metal pipes. Hard waters typically have only low or moderate TDS content because calcium and magnesium carbonates and bicarbonates are relatively insoluble. Compared with the diet, hard water contributes only a minor amount of calcium and magnesium. Hard water is generally not associated with problems in horses. Providing water that had been softened to remove most of the calcium and magnesium did not affect intestinal calcium and magnesium contents [43].

5.7.3 pH

Providing other guidelines are met, the pH of water is not a cause of concern. At one time, water high in TDS was sometimes said to be alkaline but there is a poor relationship between TDS and pH. TDS, not an alkaline pH, is detrimental to animals.

5.7.4 Sulfates

High sulfates in water are thought to be directly toxic although often found together with undesirably high TDS. The acceptable upper limit for sulfates in drinking water is 500 mg/L for people and up to 2500 mg/L for horses [41]. Water with 300–400 ppm sulfates has a different taste and odor that may reduce palatability. Water sulfate concentrations exceeding 1000 mg/L may cause diarrhea, although animals develop a tolerance to a constantly high concentration of sulfates and can tolerate two to three times this concentration after some time. Unlike cattle that metabolize sulfates to toxic hydrogen sulfide in their rumen, reports of problems in horses are rare. An outbreak of sudden death, neurologic signs, and diarrhea in a group of horses on the Canadian Prairies was associated with water sulfates >20 000 mg/L and TDS > 35 000 mg/L [44].

5.7.5 Nitrates

Nitrates (NO_3) are more harmful to ruminants than horses because ruminants convert nitrates to nitrites (NO_2) in the rumen, which is toxic. Horses probably absorb nitrates in the small intestine before conversion to harmful nitrites in the large intestine [45]. Nitrate concentrations are highest in shallow groundwater beneath agricultural land and are partly due to farm fertilizer runoff. An upper limit for nitrates of 400 mg/L has been proposed for horses [41]. However, nitrate toxicosis is rare in horses and is more often associated with high nitrate concentrations in forage, not water. The presence of nitrates in green feeds has been associated with hypothyroidism and dysmaturity in foals. The odds of a mare producing an affected foal when fed forage containing at least a trace of nitrate were 5.9 times greater than those of a mare fed nitrate-free forage [46].

Water high in bacteria is usually also high in nitrates as both are the result of surface contamination from manure and barnyard runoff. However, high nitrate water concentrations may come from other nitrate sources, such as crop fertilizers, and not high in bacterial count. Nitrates may build up in well water by leaching down through the soil but fluctuate widely, generally highest following wet periods and lowest during dry periods of the year. Since nitrates dissolve in water, they cannot be filtered out; however, commercially available anion exchange units remove both nitrates and sulfates.

5.7.6 Toxins and Pathogenic Organisms

In addition to mineral and compound contaminants, drinking water containing bacteria and algae can be harmful. In most areas and situations, bacteria in water pose a greater threat than mineral contaminants.

5.7.6.1 Bacterial Contaminants

Surface waters are more prone to bacterial contamination than water from deep aquifers. Well water, particularly those with shallow sources in permeable soils, can also have bacterial problems. The major source of bacterial contamination is from feces, and sometimes urine, of horses and other animals. This is particularly a problem when the animals (horses, cattle) stand in the water source to cool off in hot weather. Other sources of contamination include runoff from fields grazed by animals, fields fertilized with manure, seepage from slurry lagoons, septic tanks, and sewage outfalls.

Bacterial contamination is more of a problem following high rainfall when there is a heavy load of sediment in the water and warm temperatures that foster bacterial growth. If water nitrate or phosphate concentrations are low, the water probably does not contain excessive bacteria. However, if either nitrate or phosphate is high, bacterial concentrations may be elevated and should be checked. The criterion for sanitary water is the absence of coliform bacteria. Although only a few coliform bacteria are pathogens, the presence of coliforms indicates that other infectious bacteria and viruses may be present in the water. Bacterial and viral pathogens can survive for weeks to months in water depending in part on temperature and the concentration of organic matter present. The bacteriological quality of water is traditionally measured as the enteric coliform load and the recommended upper limit for agricultural use is 1000 CFU/100 mL [47]. Water with low fecal coliforms may have a low content of pathogens; however, the presence of pathogens does not always correlate with the enteric coliform load. A guideline of 100 thermotolerant coliforms/100 mL has been stated for livestock [42].

Escherichia coli is more commonly associated with enteric disease in people; however, horses do not appear to be affected [8]. Salmonella species are generally the bacterial contaminant in water most likely to cause disease in farm animals. Giardiasis is rare in adult animals but can be the cause of diarrhea in young animals [17]. The most common method of destroying bacteria in a water supply is chlorination, although iodine, ozone, exposure to ultraviolet rays or ultrasonic sound waves, and filters may be used. The objectionable chlorine taste and odor can be removed from water by an activated carbon filter.

5.7.6.2 Algae

Blue-green algae or phytoplankton, more accurately referred to as cyanobacteria, are a normal inhabitant of water because algae are an important first step in the conversion of inorganic to organic nutrients and support other aquatic life. The problems occur when they multiply rapidly and accumulate in the water source as a bloom. Cyanobacterial growth is driven by increases in the availability of nitrates and phosphates, sunlight, and warm water, most commonly during summer and fall. Nitrates and phosphates mainly enter the water source from animal feces and urine, slurry lagoons, and runoff from agricultural fertilizer application. In stagnant (closed) water sources, heat and drought concentrate these nutrients that favor cyanobacterial growth. Large numbers of algae make the water turbid and produce foul water odors and taste. Many blue-green algae make intracellular gas bubbles, float, and are visible as scum on the surface of the water. Steady prevailing winds may concentrate the algae at one end of the pond or lake, increasing the risk of toxicosis. Following the death of the algae bloom, a toxin is released into the water. Toxic species are *Oscillatoria agardhii, Nodularia spumingena, Aphanizomenom flos-aquae, Coelosphaerium kutzingianum, Gloeotrichia echinulata, Anabaena spiroides, Anabaena flos-aquae, Anabaena circinalis,* and *Microcystis aeruginosa* [17]. *Microcystis aeruginosa* is most often implicated and also associated with the greatest number of severe outbreaks.

The main concern for horse owners is the production of toxins. Only a few cyanobacteria species are toxic, and even then toxin production is intermittent. The major toxins are either neuro- or hepatotoxins and the clinical signs begin suddenly and are usually severe from the onset. Signs include nervous disorders, liver failure, and sudden death, which can occur within hours of drinking affected water. Bloody diarrhea, incoordination, muscle tremors, weakness, recumbency, excitability, convulsions, nasal discharge, and dyspnea have been reported [17]. Hepatic necrosis, serosal hemorrhages, and excess transudate in body cavities may be found at necropsy. Clumps of algae may be found in the gastrointestinal contents of animals that die suddenly. There are tests available; 11,500 cells/mL or toxin concentrations above 2.3 ug/L are used to delineate risk for horses; however, these guidelines were not determined using horses [8, 48]. Copper sulfate added to pond water, up to a concentration of 1 mg/L, has been used successfully to kill algae blooms but will probably harm other types of aquatic life [17].

5.8 Water as Habitat for Disease Vectors and Insects

5.8.1 Potomac Horse Fever

Potomac horse fever (PHF) is an acute enterocolitis syndrome with signs of mild colic, fever, and diarrhea in horses of all ages and does cause abortion in pregnant mares. The causative agent is *Neorickettsia risticii*. This disease is more common in horses at low altitudes in July and August. The original reports involved disease in horses that lived close (within 6 miles/10 km) to a large body of water such as a lake or river.

N. risticii has a complex life cycle, as it parasitizes trematodes (flukes) that in turn parasitize freshwater snails and aquatic insects. The main route of infection for horses is accidental ingestion of infected adult aquatic insects such as caddisflies, damselflies, mayflies, dragonflies, and stoneflies during times when these flies swarm. *N. risticii* is a gram-negative obligate intracellular bacterium that infects small and large intestine enterocytes, resulting in acute colitis. Clinical signs of PHF are initially mild depression and anorexia and then a fever of 102–107 °F (38.9–41.7 °C). Within 24–48 hrs, a moderate to severe diarrhea, with feces ranging in consistency from soft with no form to liquid develops in the majority of horses. The disease in some horses further develops to severe signs of sepsis and dehydration. Unfortunately, clinical signs are difficult to distinguish from those of Salmonella and other infectious causes of enterocolitis.

Horses with PHF can be treated successfully with oxytetracycline early with a positive response to treatment seen within 12 hrs [49]. Several vaccines based on the *N. risticii* are commercially available, although vaccination has been reported to protect 78% of experimentally infected ponies, there has been a marginal success in the field. Vaccine failure has been attributed to the fact that there are more than 14 different strains of *N. risticii* and there may be low antibody concentrations in the intestinal mucosa [49]. Reducing the chance of ingesting insects by turning barn lights off, which attract insects, has been suggested for stabled horses. Unfortunately, keeping horses in stables and/or applying fly sprays have not provided protection. The effectiveness of standard fly repellants against large aquatic insects is unknown.

5.8.2 Arbovirus Encephalomyelitis

Several types of equine encephalomyelitis are caused by arboviruses. There are three antigenically different alphaviruses causing specifically Eastern, Western, and Venezuelan equine encephalomyelitis. Since 1999, West Nile Virus, a member of the flavivirus genus, has been the most pathogenic arbovirus in horses in the United States. All have a life cycle that involves the multiplication of the virus in small mammals (rodents and rabbits) and birds with transmission to horses by mosquitoes. The transmission of the virus to horses occurs when birds are migrating out of the area and mosquitoes switch hosts. In more northern areas of North America this is late summer and early fall. The mosquito vector of these viral encephalitides requires water to breed. Horses in swampy areas with diverse habitats that can support high numbers of mosquitoes, birds, rodents, and rabbits are at an increased risk of contracting viral encephalitis. Protection involves vaccination, stabling horses indoors with a fan (dusk to dawn) that reduces contact with mosquitoes and controlling pools of water used by mosquitos. The initial clinical signs of encephalomyelitis are similar for the arboviruses; only the progression of clinical signs and severity of disease are the differentiating features. Many horses progress to recumbency within 12–18 hr of the onset of neurologic abnormalities. Most deaths occur within 2–3 d after the onset of signs. Treatment of viral encephalitis is supportive because there are no specific antiviral therapies [50].

5.8.3 Insects

All mosquitoes must have quiet waters for their life cycle and hence the best way to control the mosquito population and decrease the risk of equine encephalomyelitis is to remove potential egg-laying sites. This includes: (i) changing or circulating water in stock or holding tanks at least once a week, (ii) draining structures or containers that may trap water such as barrels, buckets, tires, and tarps covering hay or silage, (iii) stock ponds with mosquito-eating fish and thin out weeds, leaves, and debris from ponds allowing fish access to egg-laying areas, (iv) grade land areas to prevent standing water (potholes, ruts, and hoof prints). The use of pesticides or larvicides should be supplemental to controlling mosquito egg-laying sites in water [51].

Adult biting flies are not only a nuisance but certain types can transmit disease organisms carried on their legs and mouthparts. Adults lay their eggs in wet organic matter, such as wet manure, feed, bedding, and decaying material (leaves, vegetation) because moisture is needed to prevent the eggs, larvae, and pupae from drying out. Manure must be removed or disturbed once a week to dry out because the lifecycle for some species is less than two wks. Fly eggs only need about 1 in. of wet material to remain protected. Cleaning out feed bunks, troughs, and buckets of wet feed and removing wet bedding, and removing or harrowing manure piles reduces the fly burden. Controlling the sites suitable for laying eggs in moist material is an important step toward reducing the fly burden. Resistance to pesticides has occurred, so multiple strategies are needed. Appropriately used fly parasites, sprays, and well-placed bait and fly traps can be effective; however, no insecticide can overcome poor sanitation [52].

Case in Point

A rancher has recently drilled a new 400 ft. deep well on his Saskatchewan farm where he grazes cattle and several ranch horses. Some cattle are drinking water from the new well but most cows and the horses wait for the water to be trucked in from a different source several times a week. Several of the cattle have separated from the group, are behaving strangely, and appear to have facial and ear twitches. He submitted a water sample for analysis and the report indicates the water has a TDS of 5600 mg/L and sulfate content of 3600 mg/L.

1) *How does the water sample analysis compare with water quality guidelines for livestock?*
2) *How might the water analysis explain the clinical signs exhibited by the cattle?*
3) *What are the options for improving the quality of water from this well?*

See Appendix A Chapter 5.

References

1 Farm Animal Welfare Council (1979). *Report of the Technical Committee to Enquire into the Welfare of Animals Kept Under Intensive Livestock Husbandry Systems*. London: Her Majesty's Stationary.

2 Hinton, M. (1978). On the watering of horses: a review. *Equine Vet. J.* 10: 27–31.

3 Gross, K.L., Yamka, R.M., Khoo, C. et al. (2010). Macronutrients. In: *Small Animal Clinical Nutrition*, 5e (ed. M.S. Hand, C.D. Thatcher, R.L. Remillard, et al.), 49–105. Topeka: Mark Morris Institute.

4 Forro, M., Cieslar, S., Ecker, G.L. et al. (2000). Total body water and ECFV measured using bioelectrical impedance analysis and indicator dilution in horses. *J. Appl. Physiol.* 89 (2): 663–671.

5 Spensley, M.S., Carlson, G.P., and Harrold, D. (1987). Plasma, red blood cell, total blood, and extracellular fluid volumes in healthy horse foals during growth. *Am. J. Vet. Res.* 48 (12): 1703–1707.

6 Brinkmann, L., Gerken, M., and Riek, A. (2013). Seasonal changes of total body water and water intake in Shetland ponies measured by an isotope dilution technique. *J. Anim. Sci.* 91 (8): 3750–3758.

7 Fielding, C.L., Magdesian, K.G., and Edman, J.E. (2011). Determination of body water compartments in neonatal foals by use of indicator dilution techniques and multifrequency bioelectrical impedance analysis. *Am. J. Vet. Res.* 72 (10): 1390–1396.

8 Cymbaluk, N.F. (2013). Water. In: *Equine Applied and Clinical Nutrition: Health, Welfare and Performance* (ed. R.J. Geor, P.A. Harris, and M. Coenen), 80–95. Edinburgh: Saunders Elsevier.

9 National Research Council (2007). *Nutrient Requirements of Horses*, 6th Rev. Animal Nutrition Series, 1–341. Washington, DC: National Academies Press.

10 Cymbaluk, N.F. (1989). Water balance of horses fed various diets. *Equine Pract.* 11 (1): 19–24.

11 Groenendyk, S., English, P.B., and Abetz, I. (1988). External balance of water and electrolytes in the horse. *Equine Vet. J.* 20 (3): 189–193.

12 Brinkmann, L., Gerken, M., Hambly, C. et al. (2014). Saving energy during hard times: energetic adaptations of Shetland pony mares. *J. Exp. Biol.* 217 (24): 4320–4327.

13 Equi-Analytical Laboratories Services (2020). Common Feed Profiles. http://equi-analytical.com/common-feed-profiles (accessed 28 February 2019).

14 National Research Council (1982). *United States-Canadian Tables of Feed Composition*. 3rd Rev. Nutritional Data for United States and Canadian Feeds, 1–148. Washington, DC: National Academies Press.

15 Oliveira, C., Azevedo, J.F., Martins, J.A. et al. (2015). The impact of dietary protein levels on nutrient digestibility and water and nitrogen balances in eventing horses. *J. Anim. Sci.* 93 (1): 229–237.

16 Jansson, A. and Dahlborn, K. (1999). Effects of feeding frequency and voluntary salt intake on fluid and electrolyte regulation in athletic horses. *J. Appl. Physiol.* 86 (5): 1610–1616.

17 Naylor, J.M. (1991). Vitamins. In: *Large Animal Clinical Nutrition*, 1e (ed. J.M. Naylor and S.L. Ralston), 68–89. St. Louis, MO: Mosby.

18 National Research Council (1989). *Nutrient Requirements of Horses*. 5th Rev. Animal Nutrition Series, 1–100. Washington, DC: National Academies Press.

19 Pearson, R.A., Cuddeford, D., and Archibald, R.F. (1992). Digestibility of diets containing different proportions of alfalfa and oat straw in Thoroughbreds, Shetland Ponies, Highland Ponies and Donkeys. *European Conference on the Diet of the Horse*, 153–157, Hannover.

20 Cymbaluk, N.F. (1990). Comparison of forage digestion by cattle and horses. *Can. J. Anim. Sci.* 70: 601–610.

21 Caljuk, E.A. (1961). Water metabolism and water requirements of horses. *Tr. Vses Inst. Konevod.* 23: 295–305.

22 Mejdell, C.M., Simensen, E., and Boe, K.E. (2005). Is snow a sufficient source of water for horses kept outdoors in winter? A case report. *Acta Vet. Scand.* 46 (1, 2): 19–22.

23 Kristula, M.A. and McDonnell, S.M. (1994). Drinking water temperature affects consumption of water during cold weather in ponies. *Appl. Anim. Behav. Sci.* 41 (3, 4): 155–160.

24 McDonnell, S.M. and Kristula, M.A. (1996). No effect of drinking water temperature (ambient vs. chilled) on consumption of water during hot summer weather in ponies. *Appl. Anim. Behav. Sci.* 49 (2): 159–163.

25 Mueller, P.J. and Houpt, K.A. (1991). A comparison of the responses of donkeys and ponies to 36 hr water deprivation. In: *Donkeys Mules and Horses in Tropical Agricultural Development* (ed. D. Fielding and R.A. Pearson), 86–95. Edinburgh: Centre for Tropical Veterinary Medicine.

26 Crowell-Davis, S.L., Houpt, K.A., and Carnevale, J. (1985). Feeding and drinking behavior of mares and foals with free access to pasture and water. *J. Anim. Sci.* 60 (4): 883–889.

27 Ralston, S.L. (1986). Feeding behavior. *Vet. Clin. North Am. Equine Pract.* 2 (3): 609–621.

28 Sufit, E., Houpt, K.A., and Sweeting, M. (1985). Physiological stimuli of thirst and drinking. *Equine Vet. J.* 17 (1): 12–16.

29 Tasker, J.B. (1967). Fluid and electrolyte studies in the horse. 4. The effects of fasting and thirsting. *Cornell Vet.* 57: 658–667.

30 Sneddon, J.C.C. and Argenzio, R.A.A. (1998). Feeding strategy and water homeostasis in equids: the role of the hind gut. *J. Arid Environ.* 38 (3): 493–509.

31 Argenzio, R., Lowe, J., Pickard, D., and Stevens, C. (1974). Digesta passage and water exchange in the equine large intestine. *Am. J. Physiol. Content.* 226 (5): 1035–1042.

32 Brobst, D.F. and Bayly, W.M. (1982). Responses of horses to a water deprivation test. *J. Equine Vet. Sci.* 2 (2): 51–56.

33 Genetzky, R.M., Loparco, F.V., and Ledet, A.E. (1987). Clinical pathologic alterations in horses during a water deprivation test. *Am. J. Vet. Res.* 48 (6): 1007–1011.

34 Waring, G.H. (2003). *Horse Behavior*, 2e, vol. 138, 322. Norwich: Noyes Publications.

35 McDonnell, S.M., Freeman, D.A., Cymbaluk, N.F. et al. (1999). Behavior of stabled horses provided continuous or intermittent access to drinking water. *Am. J. Vet. Res.* 60 (11): 1445–1450.

36 Reeves, M.J., Salman, M.D., and Smith, G. (1996). Risk factors for equine acute abdominal disease (colic): results from a multi-center case-control study. *Prev. Vet. Med.* 26 (3, 4): 285–301.

37 Archer, D.C. and Proudman, C.J. (2006). Epidemiological clues to preventing colic. *Vet. J.* 172 (1): 29–39.

38 Kaneene, J.B., Miller, R., Ross, W.A. et al. (1997). Risk factors for colic in the Michigan (USA) equine population. *Prev. Vet. Med.* 30 (1): 23–36.

39 Nyman, S. and Dahlborn, K. (2001). Effect of water supply method and flow rate on drinking behavior and fluid balance in horses. *Physiol. Behav.* 73 (1, 2): 1–8.

40 National Research Council (1974). *Nutrients and Toxic Substances in Water for Livestock and Poultry: A Report of the Subcommittee on Nutrient and Toxic Elements in Water*, 1–94. Washington, DC: National Academy Sciences.

41 Olkowski, A.A. (2009). *Livestock Water Quality: A Field Guide for Cattle, Horses, Poultry and Swine*, 1e. Saskatchewan: Minister of Agriculture and Agri-Food Canada.

42 Australian and New Zealand Environment and Conservation Council (2000). Livestock drinking water guidelines. In: *Guidelines for Fresh and Marine Water Quality*, vol. 3, 9.3.1–32.

43 Hassel, D.M., Spier, S.J., Aldridge, B.M. et al. (2009). Influence of diet and water supply on mineral content and pH within the large intestine of horses with enterolithiasis. *Vet. J.* 182 (1): 44–49.

44 Burgess, B.A., Lohmann, K.L., and Blakley, B.R. (2010). Excessive sulfate and poor water quality as a cause of sudden deaths and an outbreak of diarrhea in horses. *Can. Vet. J.* 51 (3): 277–282.

45 Schultz, D.S., Deen, W.M., Karel, S.F. et al. (1985). Pharmacokinetics of nitrate in humans: role of gastrointestinal absorption and metabolism. *Carcinogenesis* 6 (6): 847–852.

46 Allen, A.L., Townsend, H.G.G., Doige, C.E., and Fretz, P.B. (1996). A case-control study of the congenital hypothyroidism and dysmaturity syndrome of foals. *Can. Vet. J.* 37 (6): 349–358.

47 North, R.L., Khan, N.H., Ahsan, M. et al. (2014). Relationship between water quality parameters and bacterial indicators in a large prairie reservoir: Lake Diefenbaker, Saskatchewan, Canada. *Can. J. Microbiol.* 60 (4): 243–249.

48 Wood, R. (2016). Acute animal and human poisonings from cyanotoxin exposure – a review of the literature. *Environ. Int.* 91: 276–282.

49 Madigan, J.E. (2018). Potomac horse fever – digestive system – Merck veterinary manual. In: *Merck Veterinary Manual*. Kenilworth, NJ: Merck Sharp & Dohme Corp.

50 Long, M.T. (2018). Overview of equine arboviral encephalomyelitis – nervous system. In: *Merck Veterinary Manual*. Kenilworth, NJ: Merck Sharp & Dohme Corp.

51 The Center for Food Security and Public Health (2008). *Mosquito Control Measures in Animal Shelter Settings*, 102. The Center for Food Security and Public Health.

52 The Center for Food Security and Public Health (2008). *Fly Control Measures in Animal Shelter Settings*, 101. The Center for Food Security and Public Health.

6

Energy

Richard Godbee and Robert Coleman

KEY TERMS

- Metabolism refers to the process of transforming food into the energy required for the body to function. Metabolism includes the entire range of biochemical processes that occur within a body that can be further divided into two types: anabolism and catabolism.
- Metabolic rate is the energy used by an animal, measured in Mcal in horses, per unit of time, most commonly 24-hr (day).
- Digestible energy (DE) is the gross energy (GE) in the feed minus the amount of energy lost through the feces. Most common energy measurement used in equine nutrition.
- Acid detergent fiber (ADF) comprises the least digestible plant fibers cellulose and lignin. As the percentage ADF increases, the digestibility of a plant decreases.
- Neutral detergent fiber (NDF) is a measure of hemicellulose, cellulose, and lignin, which make up the bulk of structural carbohydrates. As the percentage NDF increases, forage palatability decreases.

KEY POINTS

- The principle of storing excess energy in times of feasting and drawing on stored energy during times of fasting is similar in animals and plants. Animals derive energy from food; plants derived energy from sunlight.
- Energy intake meeting energy requirement is the first and foremost important principle of animal nutrition. Non-energy nutrients are consumed in balance with energy intake.
- Energy requirements are influenced by age, production, environment, feed type and digestibility.
- Dietary fats contribute 2.5 times more DE than carbohydrates or proteins.
- Hydrolyzable carbohydrates (α-1,4 and α-1,6 glycoside linkage) undergo endogenous enzymatic digestion in the small intestine to mono- and disaccharides; however, consumed excess will be fermented in the large bowel to lactate [1].
- Fermented carbohydrates (β-1,4 glycoside linkage) undergo microbial enzymatic digestion in the large bowel to volatile fatty acids (VFAs).

6.1 The Concept of Energy

Thermodynamics dictates that energy can be neither created nor destroyed but only converted into various forms. Nutritionally, energy is a property of nutrients that can be converted to perform metabolic work and body heat. Metabolism refers to the process of converting food energy into that which allows the body to function. Metabolism includes the whole range of biochemical processes that occur within a body that can be further divided into anabolism, which is the synthesis of new constituents (metabolites and structural tissues), and catabolism, which is the breakdown of body constituents of which some are recycled while others are expelled via the skin, lungs, urine, or feces. Metabolic rate is the energy used by an animal, measured in Mcal in horses per unit of time, most commonly per day (24 hrs).

Energy-supplying nutrients are primarily fats and carbohydrates (CHO), and to a lesser extent, protein. Protein

Equine Clinical Nutrition, Second Edition. Edited by Rebecca L. Remillard.

primarily provides amino acids for animal protein synthesis; however, protein can provide energy and nitrogen when completely oxidized. Protein, mineral, and vitamin concentrations are fed in proportion to the energy and total feed intake. In the truest sense of the word, energy is not a nutrient but a property of some nutrients (carbohydrates, fats, and proteins) possess. The primary source of all energy for all living things is sunlight. This energy is captured by plants using photosynthesis to change environmental carbon dioxide (CO_2) and water (H_2O) to carbon compounds. These compounds (carbohydrates, fats, and proteins) are used by the plant giving off oxygen (O_2) and water as by-products [6 CO_2 + 12 H_2O + sunlight goes to $C_6H_{12}O_6 + 6O_2 + 6H_2O$]. When nitrogen from the air or soil is added to carbon compounds, those become plant proteins. Therefore, fats, proteins, and carbohydrates in plants are storage forms of solar energy.

Animals consuming, digesting, and absorbing plant macronutrients (carbohydrates, fats, and proteins) transfer that stored energy to animal cells. Some carbon and nitrogen elements are used in the structural components of animal cells while some compounds are oxidized completely for energy. Within animals, these plant storage forms of energy are converted ultimately back to carbon dioxide and water by metabolic reactions. Anabolic reactions require energy whereas catabolic reactions release energy. Animals use a portion of the released energy in catabolic reactions as heat and another portion is transferred to compounds such as adenosine triphosphate (ATP), which then provide energy to drive anabolic processes. Estimated energy yields from fats, carbohydrates, and proteins to ATP are approximately 90%, 75%, and 55%, respectively [2]. Thus, plants and animals have a mutually sustaining relationship in which plants produce organic carbon compounds and oxygen that support animals, and animals produce end-products of carbon dioxide, nitrogen, and water, which in turn support plants. Thus, horses, plants, and all living things on earth are products of the air and the soil, and function solely as the result of solar energy.

Energy has no measurable dimension or mass, but can be converted to heat, which can be measured. Gross energy (GE) is the amount of heat produced when a feed undergoes complete combustion in the presence of oxygen. In a bomb calorimeter, the energy released upon complete combustion of a feed sample is measured by an increase in the surrounding water bath temperature [3]. Feed macronutrient composition largely impacts the gross energy a feedstuff may hold because fats (lipids) contain more energy per unit weight than protein or carbohydrates. The GE of fat, protein, and carbohydrate is 9.4, 5.65, and 4.15 Mcal/kg, respectively. A high-fat feed, therefore, will have a higher GE than a high carbohydrate feed. The carbohydrate type, structural or non-structural, has no bearing on gross energy because the GE of starch is the same as that for cellulose.

A 100% of the feed GE, however, cannot be captured by the animal. "A very considerable amount of energy must be expended in the separation of the indigestible matters from the digestible, and in the conversion of the latter into such forms as are suitable for the uses of the living cells in the body" [4]. Digestive processes are not 100% efficient and some of the energy consumed is lost in the feces. The digested fraction of the feed (consumed minus fecal content) is referred to as "apparent" digestible energy (DE) because feces contains endogenous material (unabsorbed intestinal secretions, bacteria, metabolites, sloughed mucosal cells, and mucus). Of that digested and absorbed, some energy is lost in the urine and gasses produced, primarily methane, and that remaining fraction of energy is called metabolizable energy (ME) (Figure 6.1).

There are additional losses of energy called the heat increment (HI) or specific dynamic action of food, which is the energy lost as heat due to the work of digestion, absorption, and metabolism [5]. The remaining energy at this point is referred to as net energy (NE), which can be further divided into that required for maintaining current body mass (NE_m) and that used for production (growth NE_g, pregnancy NE_p, lactation NE_l). Net energy is used first and foremost to maintain body tissues and metabolism (NE_m). During lactation or physical activity, over 50% of dietary energy is used for the maintenance of body mass. In growing horses, 60–95% of dietary energy is used for maintenance first before allowing the remainder to be used for growth. Maintaining body mass take priority over production (work, growth, lactation) when energy intake is limited.

Although metabolizable energy can be further compartmentalized into net energy for food-producing livestock, DE values are still in use for horses in the United States, Canada, United Kingdom, and Australia [6]. There are other energy systems for the horse; however, from a practical standpoint, regardless of the system used, the amount of feed to be offered to the average horse is similar [7]. Given that a large database of feed and animal DE estimates exists for horses, the use of DE, as opposed to the ME or NE systems, is more commonly used by equine nutritionists, veterinarians, feed producers, and owners.

In human and animal nutrition, the word "calorie," even if the "c" is not capitalized always refers to the kilocalorie (the capital C in Calories denotes kcal on food labels).

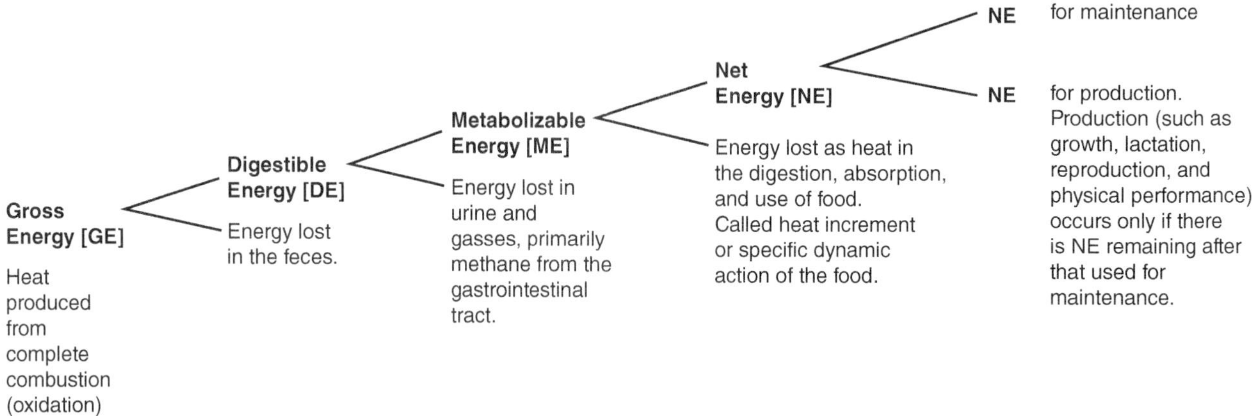

Figure 6.1 Dietary energy partition. *Source:* Reprinted with permission from Hand, M.S., Thatcher, C.D., Remillard, R.L. et al. (2010). *Small Animal Clinical Nutrition*, 5e. Topeka, KS: Mark Morris Institute.

One kcal or Calorie is defined as the amount of heat produced by oxidation (burning) that raises the temperature of 1 L of water by 1 °C, precisely between 14.5 and 15.5 °C, at a pressure of 1 atm. In large animal nutrition, such as in horses, the megacalorie (Mcal) predominates in the United States whereas megajoule (MJ) is used in Europe; 1 Mcal is equal to 4.18 MJ, approximately a fourfold difference. Total digestible nutrient (TDN) values are generally less used today yet values for many horse feeds are available and can be converted to DE; 1 kg of TDN is equal to 4.4 Mcal DE. When calculating the energy needed by an animal and/or the quantity of feed to be offered, any of the various energy terms or systems may be used as long as the same unit is used for both the feed content and the animal requirement.

For monogastric species, when the gross energy values of fat, protein, and carbohydrate (CHO) (9.4, 5.65, and 4.15 kcal/g, respectively) are multiplied by their respective coefficients of digestion (90%, 80%, and 84%), ignoring the very small gaseous losses but adjusting for urinary nitrogen losses, the resulting values of 8.5, 3.5, and 3.5 kcal/g are reasonable estimates of the ME derived from each dietary macronutrient fed to monogastrics [8]. However, the total metabolizability of fat, proteins, and carbohydrates by herbivores is much lower than in monogastric species primarily due to the lower energy efficiency of fermentation in the large bowel. Fermentation of CHO in the large bowel produces greater energy losses as heat and gas as compared with hydrolysis of CHO within the small bowel. The rounded-off modified Atwater factors (9, 4, 4 kcal/g) should not be used for horse feeds. A feeding trial using horses is the most accurate method of determining feed DE and ME in horses, and values are available for some common horse feeds; however, the number of digestibility trials completed in horses is limited compared with other production species. Therefore, attempts have been made to use equations knowing the chemical composition of the feed to estimate DE for the horse. See NRC 2007 Table 16-6 [6]. Ration digestibility is known to vary depending on the feed type, processing, and the specific combination of feed ingredients in the ration. Therefore, DE for horse feeds employs several different equations depending on the energy class of the feedstuff: [6]

$$\text{Concentrates}: \text{DE} = 4.07 - 0.055\text{ADF}$$

$$\text{Fats or oils: DE} = (-3.6 + 0.211\ \text{CP} + 0.421\ \text{EE} + 0.015\ \text{CF})/4.184$$

$$\text{Forages: DE} = 2.118 + 0.01218\ \text{CP} - 0.00937\ \text{ADF} - 0.00383\ (\text{NDF} - \text{ADF}) + 0.04718\ \text{EE} + 0.02035\ \text{NFC} - 0.0262\ \text{Ash}$$

where ADF is acid detergent fiber; CP is crude protein; EE is ether extract; CF is crude fat; NDF is neutral detergent fiber; NFC is non-fiber carbohydrate = 100−%NDF−%CP−%EE−%Ash.

The digestible energy of common horse feeds, on average, is about 60–70% of gross energy but the interactions between feed components can alter digestibility e.g. adding fat has been shown to reduce fiber digestibility in some but not all studies [9, 10]. Metabolizable energy in the horse is generally greater than 85% of digestible energy but varies with fiber content. Feed digested primarily in the large intestine will have higher heat and gas losses than that digested in the small intestine [11]. Therefore, feed DE calculations based on laboratory analyses and equations should be regarded as estimates.

6.2 Dietary Energy

Energy supplying nutrients are primarily fats and carbohydrates. Protein does provide energy; however, it is less efficient than fats and carbohydrates because handling the potentially toxic nitrogen is not optional and has an energy cost. Protein is preferentially used for providing essential amino acids and nitrogen, which is used for the synthesis of non-essential amino and nucleic acids. See Chapter 7 Protein.

6.2.1 Dietary Carbohydrates

The large class of nutrients called carbohydrates are characterized from several different perspectives. Carbohydrates may be divided by size into three categories: monosaccharides (glucose, fructose, and galactose); oligosaccharides (fructans composed of glucose and fructose), and polysaccharides (starch and cellulose composed of glucose chains). Monosaccharides are in relatively low concentrations in plants as the majority of these sugars are subunits of larger more complex CHO. Disaccharides commonly found in grass plants are sucrose (glucose + fructose), whereas maltose (glucose + glucose) is found in legume plants and lactose (glucose + galactose) is found in milk. Oligosaccharides are (<10) monosaccharides linked together e.g. small fructans, whereas a polysaccharide comprises (>10) monosaccharides linked together e.g. starch and cellulose.

Carbohydrates may also be characterized by the glycosidic bond between the monosaccharide units that ultimately determines the site of digestion in the horse. Saccharides linked by the 1,4-α glycosidic bond are hydrolyzed by mammalian enzymes in the small intestine while those linked with the 1,4-β glycosidic bond are hydrolyzed by bacterial enzymes in the large intestines. Starch that escapes small intestinal hydrolysis can be digested by bacteria in the large bowel and depending on the quantity, it may result in pH and water changes, diarrhea, or, at the very least, a change in the microflora population.

Carbohydrates may also be characterized by their cellular site and function within the plant. Structural carbohydrates are components of the cell wall and give rigidity to the plant whereas non-structural carbohydrates (NSC) contained within the cells are involved in plant metabolism (sugar, starch, and fructans). Historically, laboratory analysis of feeds was based on characterizing the plant cell wall components which worked well for ruminants with fermentation proximal to the small intestine. However, feed categorization based on plant cell constituents, rather than cell wall components, better characterizes feeds for horses with small intestinal digestion preceding large bowel fermentation. Metabolism of plant NSC beginning in the equine small bowel is energetically more efficient than large intestinal fermentation of cell constituents to VFAs [12]. Therefore, assaying for various cell components, i.e. sugar, starch, and fructan, in conjunction with structural CHO, is of significant importance in equine nutrition. See Figure 6.2.

6.2.1.1 Non-Structural Carbohydrates

Plant NSCs are simple sugars, starch, and fructan, and when plants produce NSC above immediate metabolic need, the excess is stored. In legumes and warm-season (C4) grasses, the excess sugar is stored as starch in the leaves. Starch, composed of linear or branched glucose molecules, is the primary storage form of energy in grains, legumes (alfalfa), and warm-season grasses (Bermudagrass). In cool-season (C3) grasses, the excess NSC is stored as fructan in the stem. Fructan, composed of sucrose (glucose + fructose) units that may be linear or branched, is the primary storage form of energy in cool-season grasses (fescue, orchardgrass, and timothy). The quantity of starch or fructan within the plant is dependent upon the plant species and resources (sun, water, and nutrients from soil and air). An important point for equine nutritionists is that plant sugar production via photosynthesis rises with sunlight (sunny days, summer) peaking in the afternoon. At suitable temperatures, with ample water and fertilizer, plants use these sugars for energy to grow and store the excess as starch and fructans. With no or low sunlight (overnight, cloudy days, winter), sugar production is slowed and plants then catabolize stored starch and fructans for energy with the storage nadir at dawn. Adding to this complexity, during sunlight but limited by low temperatures, low water and/or fertilizer, plants produce sugar but cannot grow resulting in increased starch and fructans stores. Therefore, NSC intake by horses can be somewhat controlled by when animals are allowed on pasture consistent with the time of day, local weather, season, and pasture management.

6.2.1.1.1 Sugars

Mono-, di-, and trisaccharides make up a small and variable portion (4–12% DM) of plant carbohydrates depending on the time of harvest. Monosaccharides require no digestion before absorption, whereas di- and trisaccharides with 1,4-α glycosidic bonds are hydrolyzed to monosaccharides by small intestinal brush border disaccharidases.

6.2.1.1.2 Starch

Starch is digested by amylase secreted by all animals primarily from the pancreas into the small intestine. Amylase digestion breaks starch down to the disaccharide maltose. Maltose, like the disaccharides sucrose and lactose, is split

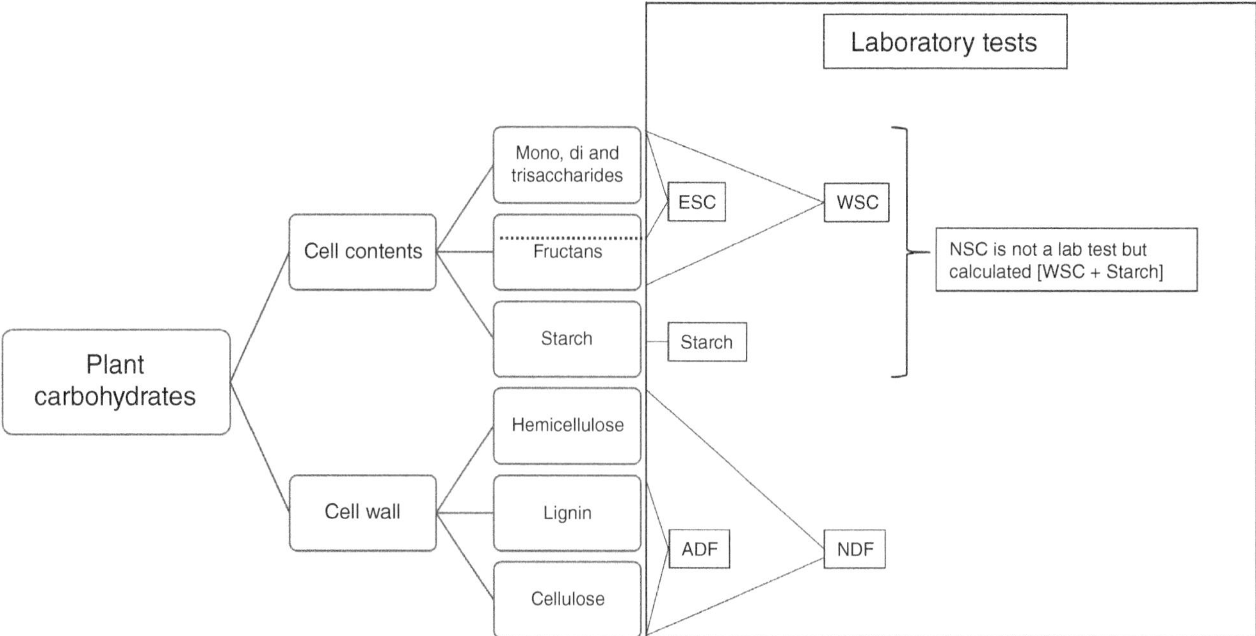

Figure 6.2 Relationship between plant carbohydrates, germane to feeding horses, and specific laboratory assays: ethanol soluble carbohydrate (ESC), water soluble carbohydrate (WSC), acid detergent fiber (ADF), neutral detergent fiber (NDF) and the calculated non-structural carbohydrates (NSC). Note: except for starch, laboratory procedures estimate more often a mix of plant carbohydrates.

into two monosaccharide units by the disaccharidase enzymes maltase, sucrase, and lactase at the intestinal brush border. If the brush border is damaged as with enteritis, end-stage carbohydrate utilization is impaired and the disaccharides enter the large intestine. Animals past nursing age lose lactase and, therefore, the ability to digest and absorb the milk sugar lactose [13]. As a consequence, the rapid introduction of lactose-containing ingredients to a mature horse may induce diarrhea.

Absorbed monosaccharides are used for energy; however, if not needed at the time of absorption, the sugar is held in the storage form of glycogen in the liver, kidney, and/or muscles, and when glycogen storage sites are full, these monosaccharides are converted to and stored as adipose tissue (body fat). These glycogen and fat stores can then be catabolized at any time to meet animal energy needs when feed energy is not available.

Resistant starch is a fraction of total starch that resists digestion within the small intestine. Physiologically resistant starch has several functions similar to soluble fiber in reducing the glycemic index of an ingredient because there is no associated blood glucose increase. Fermentation of resistant starch by bacteria produces butyrate that fuels colonocytes [14].

6.2.1.1.3 Fructan

Fructan is generally considered to pass through the small intestine undigested although some may be partially hydrolyzed or fermented in the foregut [15]. The majority of that consumed passes to the large intestine, digested by bacterial enzymes producing VFAs that are absorbed providing energy to the equine host.

Currently, the non-structural plant carbohydrates are analyzed using laboratory[1] enzyme hydrolysis and extraction methods. The assays involve three different procedures: (i) starch is estimated using an acid or enzyme hydrolysis, (ii) ethanol soluble carbohydrate (ESC) extraction estimates glucose, fructose, sucrose, and some fructans, and (iii) water-soluble carbohydrate (WSC) extraction estimates mono-, di-, oligo- and fructans [16, 17]. Fructans can be estimated using an expensive direct laboratory method or a colorimetric method that has been shown to underestimate fructans concentration. Therefore at present, the most practical estimate for fructans is WSC content minus ESC content, which may underestimate total content by the ESC fructan portion [18].

6.2.1.2 Structural Carbohydrates

Structural polysaccharides are pectins, hemicellulose, cellulose, and lignins. These are components that primarily compose the plant cell walls to give the plant a rigid upright form, i.e. a plant skeleton. Structural CHO is beta-linked and cannot be hydrolyzed within the small intestine but can only be

1 https://dairyone.com/download/forage-forage-lab-analytical-procedures.

fermented by the microflora in the large intestine of the horse. No animal produces the digestive enzymes necessary to break the beta bond linking the saccharides units in fiber. Microbes, however, possess the enzymes necessary to break beta bonds and, therefore, do digest and utilize fiber for the maintenance and growth of their populations. Animals are only able to utilize plant fiber with varying degrees of efficiency by hosting microbes within the gastrointestinal tract and then utilizing the byproducts of microbial fermentation.

Bacteria convert the fiber to short-chain, or volatile, fatty acids (acetic, propionic, lactic, isobutyric, butyric, isovaleric, and valeric). These VFA are absorbed and provide 30 to 70% of DE to the horse with low fiber/high grain and high fiber/low grain rations, respectively [19]. Bacterial fermentation of fiber occurs primarily in the rumen of ruminants (cattle and sheep), the cecum and colon of non-ruminant herbivores (horses, rabbits, and rats), and the large intestine of omnivores (people, pigs, and dogs), and to a limited extent in the large bowel of carnivores (cats).

Structural CHO can be further divided into soluble (pectins) versus insoluble (hemicellulose, cellulose, lignins) fibers based on solubility in water. Soluble fibers are the soft tissue portions and secretions of plants that include sap, resin, gums, pectin, and mucilages commonly found in fruits, cereal grains, and legume seeds (beans, lentils, and peas). Animals use nearly all of the soluble fiber ingested; however, common horse rations contain relatively small amounts of soluble fiber compared with the insoluble and NSC concentrations. Insoluble fiber (hemicellulose, cellulose) utilization is greatest for ruminants, comparatively less for horses, and least but still significant for omnivores. Horses and cattle are equally effective in digesting low fiber feeds; however, cattle are better able to utilize high fiber feeds [20]. Overall, fiber digestion by horses is only 65–75% of that by ruminants. In all species, as the fiber content of the diet increases, the digestibility of diet organic matter decreases, but the reduction in digestibility is greater for horses than for cattle [20]. Lignins are important in the formation of plant cell walls providing a high degree of rigidity to the plant (wood and bark), completely resistant to digestion and fermentation by animals and bacteria, and excreted in the feces. The undigested feed in the feces is primarily lignin that does have a purpose in maintaining normal gastrointestinal bulk and motility.

There are several laboratory methods used for determining the amount of insoluble fiber in the feed. The crude fiber method, as determined in the proximate analysis procedure, is the oldest and may be the only fiber value available for some horse feeds [21]. Unfortunately, crude fiber analysis is inaccurate because as much as 85% of the hemicellulose and 50% of the cellulose may be omitted, which underestimates the fiber content of the feed. The NDF and ADF methods were developed primarily for ruminant feedstuff [22, 23]. Neutral detergent fiber determination includes the structural fibers of cellulose, hemicellulose, and lignin, and hence is a mix of fibers that vary in digestibility based on several plant factors. In general, legume plants are lower in NDF than grasses, but invariably increase as the plant matures, which decreases feed palatability and digestibility, and so NDF is inversely a predictor of forage voluntary intake. ADF, a sub-fraction of NDF composed of cellulose and lignin, is currently the most accurate determination of the most poorly utilizable fiber component, lignin, which increases as the plant matures, and in turn, decreases ration digestible dry matter (DM). In general terms, NDF estimates how much forage will be consumed whereas ADF estimates forage digestibility in ruminants [24].

Although NDF content has been highly correlated with voluntary forage intake in cattle, DM intake of forages by horses does not appear to be specifically related to the NDF content [25–27]. As NDF concentration increased, forage DM digestibility decreased ($r^2 = 0.71$); however, individual horses showed different responses to declining forage quality in that some increased intake while others decreased intake but not enough to cause energy or protein deficiency [28]. From a practical standpoint, forage NDF concentrations below 40% are of excellent quality for horses but over 65% are unlikely to be consumed. ADF values below 45% are recommended for horses; excellent quality forage is below 31% (Table 10.3) [29]. Feeds containing 40–50% NDF and 30–35% ADF are considered preferable for working, young horses and broodmares with greater than adult maintenance energy needs [30]. Mature maintenance horses and easy keepers can be fed forage with slightly higher NDF (50–65%) and ADF (35–45%) values to lower ration energy density. Forages with an NDF >65% or an ADF >45% have little nutritional value for horses. For example, straw averaging 73% NDF and 50% ADF has been used to slow the rate of feed intake, extend meal feeding time, promote weight loss, and delay NSC intestinal absorption in obese, insulin-dysregulated, weight-loss resistant ponies. See Chapter 28 Metabolic Syndrome.

6.2.2 Dietary Fats

The caloric density of fats and the high efficiency (~90%) of utilization make this nutrient a valuable component (up to 20%) of the ration when additional calories are needed and/or as an alternative to NSCs [31]. Plant forms of fat occur as simple fats such as di- and triacylglycerols, free (non-esterified) fatty acids (FAs), and more complex fat compounds such as glycolipids and phospholipids. The fat content of forages is relatively low (2–3% DM) whereas grains are variable but intermediate (2–50% DM). Animal fat and plant oils, however, are 100% fat and only differ in their fatty acid composition [32].

Fats of interest in equine nutrition are triglycerides (TG) composed of one molecule of glycerol and three long-chain fatty acids that are carboxylic acids with long hydrocarbon chains. The hydrocarbon chain length may vary from 10 to 30 carbons; however, the three chains in the TG may be all the same or a mix of lengths between 16 and 20 carbon atoms. In contrast, short-chain or VFAs produced by bacterial fermentation have only two to five carbon atoms. Unsaturated indicates one or more double bonds between carbons whereas a saturated fatty acid has all carbons bound to hydrogen, i.e. no double bonds. The greater the number of double bonds in the FA, the lower the melting point of the triglyceride. When the melting point is less than room temperature, the triglyceride is referred to as oil and will be a liquid; however, when the melting point is greater than room temperature, it is referred to as fat and will be solid. Triglycerides are soluble in organic solvents such as ether. Most other constituents of plant and animal tissues are water-soluble and relatively insoluble in organic solvents. Therefore, ether extraction is the laboratory basis for determining the lipid concentration of a feed and may be referred to as ether extract. Fats or oils are used in horse rations as a source of calories but also for the absorption of the fat-soluble vitamins A, D, E, and K, and as a source of the unsaturated essential fatty acid (EFA) linoleic acid (LA).

Unsaturated fatty acids such as linoleic acid in feeds become oxidized (rancid) with increasing time, temperature, and humidity if sufficient protective antioxidants (preservatives) are not present. Rancid fats do not provide the linoleic acid needs of the animal and rancidity also impairs the utilization of vitamins A, D, and E, and decreases the feed palatability. Rancidity will occur if unsaturated fatty acids are not protected with antioxidants or preservatives. The time required for rancidity to occur decreases with increasing temperature and/or humidity.

Fat digestion in the horse is similar to that in other large mammals in that fats and oils must undergo digestion via enzymatic processes before they can be absorbed from the lumen of the small intestine [33]. Mechanical disruption of the dietary fat begins with chewing that results in large lipid droplets dispersed in the gastric chyme. Gastric chief cells secret lipase and begin the process of fat hydrolysis. Within the duodenum, the pH is neutralized and the digesta is mixed with pancreatic lipase and bile salts. The horse does not have a gall bladder and therefore, bile is continuously secreted by the liver directly into the duodenum. Pancreatic lipase cleaves fatty acids from the triacylglycerol, phospholipids, and cholesterol esters resulting in a mix of 2-monoacylglycerides and free FAs within an emulsified droplet. Bile salts on the outer surface of the lipid droplets interface between the water-soluble digesta and water phobic fat. In conjunction with pancreatic colipase, the actions of lipase continue to cleave triacylglycerol, phospholipids, and cholesterol esters. In the horse, the pancreas produces more lipase than amylase or trypsin, which is at odds with the relatively low-fat content of plants. The lipase activity in horses is similar to that in monogastric rats and pigs [32]. Within the small intestine, finely emulsified mixed micelles are formed with an outer layer of bile acid, monoacylglycerol, and lysophospholipids, surrounding a core of non-esterified FAs, cholesterol, and fat-soluble vitamins (Sidebar 3.1). The mixed micelles deliver and release the FAs, monoacylglycerols, and vitamins at the microvillus surface for enterocyte absorption.

6.2.2.1 Fatty Acids

Essential fatty acids are fatty acids considered necessary for "good" health that animals must ingest because EFAs cannot be synthesized endogenously. Linoleic acid (LA) is an essential omega-6 fatty acid (C18:2n-6) in the diet of all animals, although the concentration required by the horse has not been determined. Assuming linoleic acid is needed for the good health of horses, at least 0.5% LA in the diet DM is recommended for all equine life stages [34]. The horse can synthesize sufficient quantities all other fatty acids needed, including gamma-linolenic acid (GLA) and arachidonic acid (AA); therefore, fatty acids other than LA are not required in the ration. Arachidonic acid may upon stimulation produce the series 1 and 2 prostaglandins and thromboxanes and series 4 leukotrienes, via cyclooxygenase and 5-lipoxygenase, respectively, all of which are proinflammatory mediators in the body.

In most species, an EFA deficiency causes a dry, lusterless hair coat and scaly skin, and may predispose to a skin infection [35]. If the deficiency persists, hair loss, edema, and exudation from localized areas of the skin occur, resulting in moist dermatitis. Reproductive efficiency may be impaired, and there may be neonatal abnormalities and death. However, in the horse, an EFA deficiency has not been documented and reproductive failures associated with a fatty acid deficiency have not been known to occur. No clinical symptoms, visual indications of skin or hair coat alteration, or decreases in plasma concentrations of triglycerides or free fatty acids, including linoleic acid, occurred in ponies fed extremely low (0.05 and 0.22%) fat rations containing only 0.03 and 0.14% LA for seven mos [36]. The investigators suggested that a long biological half-life for LA in the fat stores of these ponies may be the reason that no clinical deficiency occurred. However, at the lowest fat intake (0.05%), tissue and plasma vitamin E concentrations fell significantly, perhaps indicating inadequate absorption of this fat-soluble vitamin due to the low content of the carrier fat in the ration. Horse feeds generally contain 2–6% fat, i.e. 10–30 times more than that present in the low fat (0.22%) ration study. Commonly used oils in horse feeds are also relatively high in linoleic acid (55% in corn oil and 73% in safflower oil). In contrast, coconut, palm, and olive oils are 1–2% whereas flaxseed (aka linseed) oil contains 14% LA. Thus, a dry, lusterless hair coat in the horse may occur but is unlikely to be due to a fatty acid deficiency. Instead, dietary concentrations of protein, energy, or Vitamin A should be further investigated.

One other fatty acid of possible benefit to the horse is alpha-linolenic acid (ALA), an omega-3 fatty acid (C18:3n-3) found at 55% in flaxseed oil. Alpha-linolenic acid can undergo a desaturation and chain elongation to eicosapentaenoic acid (EPA) (20:5n-3) and then on to docosahexaenoic fatty acids (DHAs) (22:6n-3), although the rate of conversion is most likely less than 20% as in other species [37, 38]. The 3 series prostaglandins and thromboxanes, and 5 series leukotrienes originating from an omega-3 EFA parent are considered to exert a weaker inflammatory response within tissues while those from an omega-6 EFA parent exert a relatively stronger pro-inflammatory response. The desaturation and elongation pathway of these two opposing fatty acid family types compete for several common desaturase and elongase enzymes. The first initial step using delta-6-desaturase is thought to be the rate-limiting step that may have a higher affinity for the n-3 family. The dermis of mice and guinea pigs, and presumably other species, lack delta-6-desaturase and is therefore dependent on dietary sources and/or hepatic synthesis of GLA, AA, and EPA [39, 40]. In addition to competing for the same enzymes, EPA and DHA are incorporated into cell membrane phospholipids in a time- and dose-dependent manner exchanging for AA and thereby changing the cell membrane fluidity and integrity [41].

Altering tissue concentrations of n-3 fatty acids has been possible in the horse, and so theoretically, altering the inflammatory response may be achievable in horses; however, the studies to date lack clinical significance. Feeding a marine n-3 source at 6 g n-3/100 kg of body weight (BW) for 70 d did increase the proportions of EPA and DHA in plasma and red blood cells compared with horses fed flaxseed [42]. Similarly, equine synovial explants pretreated with a range of ALA concentrations and then exposed to lipopolysaccharide (LPS) to simulate synovial inflammation demonstrated that ALA at the highest concentration (300 ug/mL) did inhibit prostaglandin E_2 production [43]. In another study, synovial fluid from six mature horses fed orally 36 g of marine oil for 90 d only tended to have a lower ($P = 0.10$) synovial PGE_2 concentration compared with controls [44]. In a more practical study, feeding 15 g/d EPA and 19.8 g/d DHA to horses for 90 d with preexisting arthritis in the knee, fetlock, hock, or stifle did have decreased ($P < 0.05$) synovial fluid white blood cell and plasma prostaglandin E_2 concentrations; however, based on force plate data there was no significant increase in weight-bearing on the arthritic limb [45]. By feeding horses with recurrent airway obstruction and inflammatory airway disease a polyunsaturated fatty acid omega-3-rich equine feed supplement, in a randomized controlled clinical trial for two mos, it was concluded that the supplement was an additional benefit to a low-dust ration [46].

In recent years conjugated linoleic acid (CLA) has been investigated as another source of LA because CLA has shown anti-inflammatory effects in some laboratory and food animal species. Conjugated linoleic acids are a family of isomers found mostly in meat and dairy products derived from ruminants. Conjugated linoleic acid contains both cis- and/or trans-fats and the double bonds of CLAs are conjugated but separated by a single bond between them. Horses fed CLA had greater plasma concentrations of CLA isomers compared with controls ($P < 0.01$), and plasma concentrations of AA were decreased in horses fed CLA ($P < 0.05$); however, the impact of the inflammatory pathway (Cyclooxygenase-II) was not investigated [47]. In a similar equine study, dietary CLA was incorporated into plasma and synovial fluid. Dietary CLA did not influence the inflammatory response to LPS stimulation but there was a reduction in cartilage degradation and an increase in cartilage regeneration reported [48]. In summary, several studies have demonstrated that feeding n-3 fatty acids and CLA can change plasma and cellular phospholipid membrane concentrations in horses; however, the physiologic and/or clinical importance of these cellular changes have not yet been clinically demonstrated.

6.3 Horse Energy Requirements

Animals must first maintain their condition or weight before any other type of activity is possible. The maintenance energy requirement, therefore, is calories of digestible energy that results in zero change in BW and composition while the horse is allowed routine daily activities. This does not include the energy needed for thermal regulation in adverse weather, work, gestation, or lactation. The energy required for maintenance was said in the 1800s to be related to BW raised to 0.667 power [$BW(kg)^{0.667}$]. One hundred years later, when the energy requirement of 25 different types of resting mature mammals ranging from a 25 g mouse to a 2000 kg elephant (an 80,000 fold difference in weight), was determined, by measuring oxygen consumed and carbon dioxide produced and plotted against BW, the relationship was determined to be $70.5 \times BW(kg)^{0.734}$ [49]. This equation was later amended and simplified to $70 \times BW(kg)^{0.75}$ and since has been widely accepted [50]. Hence the resting, or near basal, metabolic energy requirement for most species of domestic animals is estimated as kilocalories (kcal) or megacalories (Mcal) per kg of BW raised to ¾ power [51].

However, within the range of common mature horse weights, 275–1885 lb (125–856 kg – a sevenfold difference in weight), the maintenance energy requirement is practically linear to BW and so currently DE on a BW basis is used for horses [52]. There are three suggested DE equations for maintenance based on the horse's temperament, lifestyle, or extent of voluntary activity [6]. The suggested maintenance DE (DE_m) need for horses that are sedentary, docile, confined to a small area, have a non-reactive temperament, or have low voluntary activity even in a large area (often termed easy keepers or left-brained) minimal (DE_m) may be estimated at 30.4 kcal DE/BW(kg), which would be considered the minimum maintenance requirement, i.e. 15.2 Mcal DE/d for a 500 kg horse. The estimated average DE_m for horses with an attentive calm temperament and moderate voluntary activity regardless of the area available increases by 10% to that of sedentary horses to 33.4 kcal DE/BW(kg), i.e. 16.7 Mcal DE/d for a 500 kg horse. Horses that are more reactive, with an alert nervous temperament and high levels of voluntary activity regardless of the area available (often termed hard keepers or right-brained) have an elevated DE_m estimated at 36.4 kcal DE/BW(kg) or 18.2 Mcal DE/d for a 500 kg horse (Table 16-3 [6]). The basis for these personality factors affecting DE is that activity, exploration, boldness, and aggressiveness are energetically costly [53].

A confined DE (kcal/d) for horses has been estimated using $(21.28 \times \text{kg BW}) + 975$ based on measurements completed on four adult horses accustomed to standing in a straight metabolic stall, wearing respiratory calorimetry mask, and fed 50% of the daily ration [52]. This derived linear equation approximates 75% of DE_m and is used to initially estimate the resting energy requirement (RER) of a horse confined to a stall with limited activity and food intake, e.g. sick, hospitalized, or debilitated horses [54].

Within each temperament/activity category, body composition can affect the maintenance requirement. For example, a 500 kg horse with a greater lean body mass (low body condition score (BCS)) may require a 15% increase over average DE_m whereas another 500 kg horse carrying more body fat (high BCS) may need 10–15% less than average [55]. Additionally, if a 500 kg animal is not within the optimal BCS range of 4–6, each BCS unit is equal to about 16–20 kg and requires about a 10% change (plus or minus) in energy intake accordingly to gain or lose one BCS unit [6]. These equations should be used as starting guidelines with feeding adjustments made as needed based on the animal's response, i.e. BW, condition, and performance outcomes.

Another major variable factor not included in these DE_m estimates is environmental (seasonal) conditions. The ambient temperature, wind, solar radiation, precipitation, and relative humidity all affect horses and their energy requirement. The range of temperatures in which little or no additional energy expenditure is needed to maintain a normal body temperature is the thermoneutral zone (TNZ), below which metabolic rate increases and involuntary muscle activity (shivering) is required to maintain a normal body core temperature (99–101 °F; 37.2–38.3 °C). The highest temperature of the TNZ is called the upper critical temperature (UCT), above which there is an increase in metabolic rate and evaporative heat loss (vasodilation, sweating) to maintain a normal body core temperature. The TNZ is the range of temperatures to which a horse has been acclimated. Given adequate opportunity to adapt to their environment, horses can tolerate a wide array of environmental conditions. For example, Standardbreds adapted to an outdoor temperature of 50 °F (10 °C) had a TNZ range of 40–75 °F (5–25 °C) whereas Quarter horses with a natural hair coat adapted to winter had a TNZ range of 5–50 °F (−15 to 10 °C) [56, 57].

Age, body condition, breed, and time allowance for acclimation all influence the lower critical temperatures (LCT) and UCT for an individual horse. Acclimatization to either colder or hotter temperatures takes place over 21 d with nearly full acclimation in the first 10–14 d. The LCT of yearlings (−12 °F or −11 °C) and week-old foals (68 °F or 20 °C) is higher than that of adult horses whereas the UCT of young horses is more difficult to determine but probably is near to 95 °F (35 °C). Sweating (evaporative heat loss) in hot weather and increasing metabolic heat during cold weather both increase energy need; therefore, the TNZ becomes an important factor in determining the DE_m requirement. In feeding any class of horses, DE_m must first be met because the energy for growth, reproduction, lactation, or work is in addition to that needed for the horse to maintain current weight and condition.

Homeotherms, in general, have a narrow TNZ; however, wider temperature ranges and LCT have been associated with both greater body insulation and size [58]. Interestingly, the TNZ for humans is 77–86 °F (25–30 °C) for a naked man, standing upright, in still air. A "comfortable" temperature for humans is dependent on body composition, clothing, energy expenditure, age, and gender. With light clothing, indoors with radiation and convection losses controlled, the TNZ for humans is a narrow range of 65–72 °F (18–22 °C) [59, 60]. The wider 35 °F (20 °C) TNZ range in horses, compared with the relatively narrow range of 9 °F (5 °C) in humans, is likely due to the horse being a well-insulated large homeotherm. Thus a person's perception of comfort may be misconstrued when assessing horse comfort.

6.3.1 Cold Weather Care

Winter weather not only includes cold temperatures but also winds, rain/snow/sleet which are natural environmental stress factors. Horses should have access to shelter from storms and, in severely cold weather, will group closely together to provide mutual shelter and body heat or increase shelter-seeking behaviors. They may all take a run to increase body heat production, then come back together and stand in a close group to share the resulting increased warmth. Protected from wind and moisture, as within a three-sided shelter, horses may tolerate temperatures down to −40 °F (−40 °C) depending on their hair coat. In severe, stormy weather, horses stop grazing and will stand with their tail end to the wind. The tail is held close to the dock, shielding the hairless area of the perineum, the inguinal region, and the inner thighs, and hence a full, natural length tail is an important shield. The quantity and quality of hair in the mane and forelock are important in protecting the horse's ears and eyes from severe cold. A full mane, at a natural length and density, acts as a waterproof screen for the head, throat, and neck.

Weather combinations of cold temperatures, wind, and rain are particularly stressful. A long, thick hair coat is an excellent insulator and provides the first line of defense against the cold. The density of the hair coat and the direction in which the hair lies, especially over the hindquarters and back, act as an efficient weather shield such that a layer of ice may form on the back and rump of the horse without chilling or wetting the skin. The insulating value of the hair coat is lost when wet and/or matted down. In beef cattle, and therefore probably similar for horses, the LCT in cattle with summer, fall, or winter hair coats was 59, 45, 32 °F (15, 7, 0 °C), respectively [61]. Cattle with a dry, heavy winter hair coat were comfortable at 18 °F (−8 °C) and energy needs for maintenance increased only by 0.7% for each degree Fahrenheit (0.4 °C) of cold below the LCT. In contrast, an animal with a wet hair coat was comfortable only down to a temperature of 59 °F (15 °C), and energy needs increased by 2.0% for each degree ambient temperature decreased. Using these cattle estimates, a 1000 lb (454 kg) horse with a dry winter coat would need 18.6 lb (8.5 kg) of hay at 0 °F (−18 °C); however, the same horse with a wet hair coat would need 22.4 lb (10 kg) of hay at the same temperature to meet the DE_m requirement, i.e. 20% more hay was needed because the hair coat was wet vs. dry.

Blanketing is beneficial and very effective when a wet horse is shivering (muscles of the flank body wall will involuntarily contract and relax rapidly to generate heat) and if temperature or wind are expected to remain below the LCT and there is no opportunity for the horse to dry off. Blanketing and consuming average quality hay will often raise the core body temperature, dry the hair coat, and shivering will cease within 30–60 min. Above the LCT temperature, however, blanketing is not beneficial, does not provide increased comfort for the horse, and may cause sweating. Blanketing decreases hair coat adaptation to the cold and is uncomfortable for the horse during the warm time of day. Although blanketing the horse does induce shedding earlier in the spring, frequent grooming and an adequate diet may be preferable.

After the hair coat, the next line of defense against cold is subcutaneous adipose (fat) tissue. In cold climates, the horse ideally should have a BCS 5 to 6/9 when cold weather begins. In cold weather, more dietary energy is needed for the maintenance of a thin animal (BCS < 4/9) than an ideal (BCS 5/9) animal due to increased loss of body heat through the skin. Cold temperatures increase energy needs to maintain core body temperature and any increased activity required for winter grazing. Snow cover at depths >8 in (20 cm) decreases grazing activity because the energy cost of pawing through the snow to uncover poor quality grass was a net loss of energy for the horse. Hence horses on winter pasture need to be monitored and additional calories as hay and/or concentrate may be needed to maintain a BCS ≥ 5/9. If the additional feed is not available to provide the increased energy needed, BW and condition will decrease.

The effect of cold on nutritional requirements is an increased need for energy, and according to data in other domestic species, the requirements for the other non-energy nutrients is not changed during cold weather, e.g. protein, vitamin, and mineral requirements (unit/kcal) is not changed by cold weather. If the horse is allowed to consume an average or better quality forage ad libitum without wastage, additional dietary energy from cereal grains is not generally needed. In most cases, feeding more of a nutritionally balanced ration may be all that is needed during cold weather to maintain body condition. Forage feeding is preferable to feeding a concentrate because of the higher HI associated with hindgut fermentation; however, if the horse is unable to maintain BW on forage alone, then additional calories may be needed using a cereal grain or fat supplement to maintain adequate body condition. If the forage is a mature winter grass pasture or poor quality hay, less than 8% protein on a DM basis, a protein supplement should be fed to meet the maintenance protein need.

6.3.2 Hot Weather Care

The metabolizable energy required to maintain BW was 9% higher during the summer than during the winter, and high temperatures resulted in decreased grazing time [6, 62]. If feed intake does not increase sufficiently to provide the increased dietary energy needed during hot weather, BW, milk production, or growth rate will decrease. However, the heat-stressed animal decreases, rather than increases, feed intake to reduce the HI associated with digestion and fermentation. Therefore the decrease in feed intake coupled with the increased energy requirement during hot weather can result in weight loss, making it more difficult to maintain a performance or working horse at ideal BCS during hot weather. To prevent loss of weight and condition during hot weather, consider (i) providing a lower temperature, insect-free environment, (ii) maintaining a BCS of 4 to 5/9, and (iii) feeding a palatable high energy (fat), low fiber, minimally adequate protein ration.

Shade and air movement are quite beneficial in minimizing heat-induced discomfort and stress during hot humid weather. Trees, or even artificially constructed shades on a hill with an unobstructed surrounding view, are ideal. If sheds or stables provide the only shade, they should be well ventilated, ideally with an insulated high vented roof to let out (not trap) rising warm air. Ceiling or exhaust fans and those blowing across the top of the horse are beneficial in reducing heat stress. Hot weather also brings biting insects that can reduce or shift the routine feeding times of horses. The horse will change grazing times, places, and duration to avoid painful insect bites, which may result in decreased feed intake. For example, Tabanidae species are more active mid-day on hot, bright, low/no wind days. Providing a cooler, shaded area with air movement discourages some types of biting insects. Insect annoyance should be considered in cases of weight loss not explainable by a low quantity and/or poor quality pasture.

Although the insulation provided by subcutaneous adipose tissue is beneficial in cold weather, BCS >6/9 is a detriment during hot weather. Excess adipose tissue decreases the ability to cool the body. Secondly, the overweight horse requires more feed for maintenance than does the BCS 5/9 horse [63]. The greater amount of feed consumed to meet the higher requirement, in turn, increases heat production associated with digestion, and in hot weather, the net result increases heat stress. Overweight (BCS ≥7/9) horses have higher heart and respiratory rates, and higher plasma lactate concentrations before, during, and after exercise in hot vs. temperate weather. These same parameters at rest were higher in overweight horses than BCS <6/9 horses indicating a greater heat load and more heat stress directly related to the excess weight [63].

Rations that reduce heat load during hot humid weather are lower in fiber and contain minimally adequate protein because the heat of digestion and metabolism of fiber and protein is greater than the utilization of CHO and fat. A lower-fiber, higher-fat ration not only decreases HI but also increases the energy density of the diet. For the horse that tends to lose weight during hot humid weather, a palatable energy-dense diet containing 18–26% crude fiber, 8–10% protein, and 10–15% fat DM is preferred. Ideally, the diet during hot weather should meet the protein requirements but not exceed by more than a few percent because excess protein fed requires the additional metabolic work (heat) of eliminating the excess nitrogen as urea.

Given that appetite and feed intake decrease during hot humid weather, the ration should be highly palatable to encourage a sufficient amount consumed and should be high in energy density so that the horse will meet the energy needed in a smaller total quantity of feed. Total daily ration consumed in smaller frequent meals as opposed to one or two larger meals also reduces the HI after each meal. Both diet palatability and energy density can be increased and fiber decreased by feeding a higher grain, lower forage ration. However, to decrease the risk of colic and laminitis, the lowest amount of grain or a grain mix to maintain weight and condition should be fed, and should not be more than 50% by weight of the total ration. Corn (IFN 4-02-935) is a good cereal grain to feed and contrary to popular belief is not a "hot" feed in that corn is lower in fiber (2.6%) and protein (9.6%), and higher in fat (3.8%) and energy density (3.4 Mcal DE/kg DM) than other cereal grains [64, 65]. The energy content of corn may be greater than other cereal grains but the HI is lower. If needed, adding (1%) molasses or corn syrup to the grain mix will increase feed palatability for most horses.

If calories in addition to those supplied by a grain mix are needed to maintain body condition, dietary energy density can be increased, and HI decreased by adding fat (plant oil or animal fat) to the ration. Plant (vegetable) oils provide >2 times more energy than a similar weight of corn grain (9 vs. 3.4 kcal/g, respectively) [64]. Thus, adding fat to the grain mix increases the energy density of the ration without increasing the total volume of feed. Dietary fat has a very low HI as none undergoes fermentation. It is approximately 90% digestible and nearly 100% metabolizable. Although the horse can utilize a 20% fat ration DM, adding 10% fat decreased the total body heat production by 14% while dietary energy intake was unchanged [66, 67]. As a result, more DE was available for maintenance and over 60% more energy was available for physical activity, growth, or milk production. In a different study, when the ration fed was 10% fat, the amount of grain mix needed for weight maintenance was decreased by 25% [68]. Therefore, in hot weather, ration composition should be reconsidered and designed to minimize heat load. Feeding a ration higher in fat may be advantageous because fat: (i) will not increase the heat of digestion, (ii) will increase ration caloric density, (iii) allows for total feed DM consumed to decrease while (iv) providing the same or greater total energy intake thereby reducing heat stress in horses during hot weather.

In summary, during hot humid weather, particularly for horses that have a BCS less than desired: (i) feed a diet consisting of at least one-half grass forage (grass has a lower protein content than legume forages) and at the most one-half grain if needed to which up to 5% molasses and 20% of plant oil may be added; (ii) ensure that clean palatable water and salt are always readily available; (iii) provide shade ideally with some air movement, and (iv) maintain the horse in a 4 to 5/9 BCS. A minimum 16 d feed transitioning schedule (Sidebar 26.1) should be implemented before weather changes if a horse is known, or anticipated, to lose weight due to hot or cold weather.

Case in Point

Animal Assessment

A 6-year-old mustang mare was purchased 3 d ago from an auction and the owner, new to owning a horse, requests a checkup from the local veterinarian. After examining the horse, the vet finds the animal to be calm and confident despite being isolated from other horses, with an adequate hair coat and no medical issues. Given the unknown medical or diet history, the vet recommends a parasite control program beginning with a fecal egg count, and holding off on vaccinations because the animal has a low BCS of 3/9. The mare is housed in a two-acre pasture with a three-sided south-facing shed. The pasture is a thin stand of winter grass/weed mix and the nighttime temperatures average 30–35 °F (1–2 °C). The owner states the animal weighed 800 lb on the auction scales and but has an estimated optimal BW of 860 lb based on body length and height. He did purchase several 60 lb square bales of good-quality timothy grass hay best matching International Feed Number (IFN) 1-04-883 for the mare, but then, asks how much to feed.

How to make a ration recommendation?

1) *Assess the animal requirement:*
2) *Assess the available feeds:*
3) *Make a feeding recommendation by matching the feed available to animal requirement:*

See Appendix A Chapter 6.

References

1 Hoffman, R.M. (2013). Carbohydrates. In: *Equine Applied and Clinical Nutrition: Health, Welfare and Performance* (ed. R. Geor, P. Harris, and M. Coenen), 156–167. Edinburgh: Saunders Elsevier.

2 Flatt, J.P. (2001). Macronutrient composition and food selection. *Obes. Res.* 9 (S11): 256S–262S.

3 Harris, L.E. (1970). Determination of gross energy by using bomb calorimeter. In: *Nutrition Research Techniques for Domestic and Wild Animals*, vol. 1, 1901–1903. Logan, UT: Utah State University.

4 Armsby, H.P. (1903). Net available energy – maintenance. In: *The Principles of Animal Nutrition*, 1e, 394–443. New York: Wiley.

5 National Research Council (2007). *Nutrient Requirements of Horses*. 6th Rev. Animal Nutrition Series, 1–341. Washington, DC: National Academies Press.

6 National Research Council (2007). *Nutrient Requirements of Horses*. 6th Rev. Animal Nutrition Series, 1–341. Washington DC: National Academies Press.

7 Ellis, A.D. (2013). Energy systems and requirements. In: *Equine Applied and Clinical Nutrition: Health, Welfare and Performance* (ed. R.J. Geor, P.A. Harris, and M. Coenen), 96–112. Edinburgh: Saunders Elsevier.

8 Gross, K.L., Yamka, R.M., Khoo, C. et al. (2010). Macronutrients. In: *Small Animal Clinical Nutrition*, 5e (ed. M.S. Hand, C.D. Thatcher, R.L. Remillard, et al.), 49–105. Topeka: Mark Morris Institute.

9 Jansen, W.L., Geelen, S.N., van der Kuilen, J., and Beynen, A.C. (2007). Dietary soyabean oil depresses the apparent digestibility of fibre in trotters when substituted for an iso-energetic amount of corn starch or glucose. *Equine Vet. J.* 34: 302–305.

10 Bush, J.A., Freeman, D.E., Kline, K.H. et al. (2001). Dietary fat supplementation effects on in vitro nutrient disappearance and in vivo nutrient intake and total tract digestibility by horses. *J. Anim. Sci.* 79: 232–239.
11 Vermorel, M., Martin-Rosset, W., and Vernet, J. (1997). Energy utilization of twelve forages or mixed diets for maintenance by sport horses. *Livest Prod. Sci.* 47: 157–167.
12 Blaxter, K.L. (1989). *Energy Metabolism in Animals and Man*. Cambridge: Cambridge University Press.
13 Roberts, M.C. (1975). Carbohydrate digestion and absorption studies in the horse. *Res. Vet. Sci.* 18 (1): 64–69.
14 Topping, D.L. and Clifton, P.M. (2017). Short-chain fatty acids and human colonic function: roles of resistant starch and nonstarch polysaccharides. *Physiol. Rev.* 81 (3): 1031–1064.
15 Longland, A.C. and Byrd, B.M. (2006). Pasture nonstructural carbohydrates and equine laminitis. *J. Nutr.* 136 (Suppl 7): 2099s–2102s.
16 Hall, M.B. (2003). Challenges with nonfiber carbohydrate methods. *J. Anim. Sci.* 81 (12): 3226–3232.
17 Williams, C.A. (2013). Specialized dietary supplements. In: *Equine Applied and Clinical Nutrition: Health, Welfare and Performance Health, Welfare and Performance Health, Welfare and Performance* (ed. R.J. Geor, P.A. Harris, and M. Coenen), 351–366. Edinburgh: Saunders Elsevier.
18 Longland, A.C., Dhanoa, M.S., and Harris, P.A. (2012). Comparison of a colorimetric and a high-performance liquid chromatography method for the determination of fructan in pasture grasses for horses. *J. Sci. Food Agric.* 29 (3): 376–377.
19 Glinsky, M.J., Smith, R.M., Spires, H.R., and Davis, C.L. (1976). Measurement of volatile fatty acid production rates in the cecum of the pony. *J. Anim. Sci.* 42 (6): 1465–1470.
20 Olsson, N. and Ruudvere, A. (1955). Nutrition of the horse. *Nutr. Abs. Rev.* 25: 1–18.
21 Association of Official Agricultural Chemists (1965). *Official Methods of Analysis of the AOAC*, 10e . Washington, DC: Association of Official Agricultural Chemists.
22 Van Soest, P.J. (1963). Use of detergents in the analysis of fibrous feeds. 2. A rapid method for the determination of fiber and lignin. *J. Assoc. Off. Agric. Chem.* 46: 829–835.
23 Van Soest, P.J., Robertson, J.B., and Lewis, B.A. (1991). Methods for dietary fiber, neutral detergent fiber, and nonstarch polysaccharides in relation to animal nutrition. *J. Dairy Sci.* 74 (10): 3583–3597.
24 Rocateli, A. and Zhang, H. (2017). Forage quality interpretations. Oklahoma Cooperative Extension Service PSS-2117. Stillwater, OK. https://extension.okstate.edu/fact-sheets/forage-quality-interpretations.html.
25 Dulphy, J., Martin-Rosset, W., and Dubroeucq, H. (1997). Escalation of voluntary intake of forages trough-fed to light horses. Comparison with sheep. *Livest. Prod. Sci.* 52: 97–104.
26 Cymbaluk, N.F. (1990). Comparison of forage digestion by cattle and horses. *Can. J. Anim. Sci.* 70: 601–610.
27 Dulphy, J.P., Martin-Rosset, W., Dubroeucq, H. et al. (1997). Compared feeding patterns in ad libitum intake of dry forages by horses and sheep. *Livest. Prod. Sci.* 52 (1): 49–56.
28 Edouard, N., Fleurance, G., Martin-Rosset, W. et al. (2008). Voluntary intake and digestibility in horses: effect of forage quality with emphasis on individual variability. *Animal* 2 (10): 1526–1533.
29 Thunes, C. (2022). Hay analysis part III: carbohydrates. https://clarityequine.com/hay-analysis-part-iii-carbohydrates/ (accessed 28 February 2019).
30 Thunes, C. (2019). Horse hay analysis: what are 'ADF' and 'NDF'? https://thehorse.com/164773/horse-hay-analysis-what-are-adf-and-ndf/ (accessed 28 January 2019).
31 Bowman, V.A., Fontenot, J.P., and Webb, K.E. (1977). Digestion of fat by Equine. In: *Proceedings of the 5th Equine Nutrition and Physiology Society Symposium*, 40. St. Louis: Equine Nutrition and Physiology Society.
32 Warren, L.K. and Vineyard, K.R. (2013). Fat and fatty acids. In: *Equine Applied and Clinical Nutrition: Health, Welfare and Performance* (ed. R.J. Geor, P.A. Harris, and M. Coenen), 136–155. Edinburgh: Saunders Elsevier.
33 Brody, T. (1994). Digestion and absorption. In: *Nutritional Biochemistry*, 41–106. San Diego, CA: Academic Press Inc.
34 National Research Council (1989). *Nutrient Requirements of Horses*. 5th Rev. Animal Nutrition Series, 1–100. Washington DC: National Academies Press.
35 Roudebush, P., Allen, T., and Novotny, B. (2010). Evidence-based clinical nutrition. In: *Small Animal Clinical Nutrition*, 5e (ed. M.S. Hand, C.D. Thatcher, R.L. Remillard, et al.), 23–30. Topeka, KS: Mark Morris Institute.
36 Sallmann, H.P., Kienzle, E., and Fuhrmann, H. (1991). Metabolic consequences of feeding ponies with marginal amounts of fat. In: *Proceedings of the 12th Equine Nutrition and Physiology Society Symposium*. Calgary, Alberta. p. 81–82.
37 Burdge, G.C. and Wootton, S.A. (2002). Conversion of α-linolenic acid to eicosapentaenoic, docosapentaenoic and docosahexaenoic acids in young women. *Br. J. Nutr.* 88 (4): 411–420.
38 Burdge, G.C., Jones, A.E., and Wootton, S.A. (2002). Eicosapentaenoic and docosapentaenoic acids are the principal products of α-linolenic acid metabolism in young men. *Br. J. Nutr.* 88 (4): 355–363.

39 Campbell, K.L. (1990). Fatty acid supplementation and skin disease. *Vet. Clin. North Am. Small Anim. Pract.* 20 (6): 1475–1486.

40 Horrobin, D.F. (1989). Essential fatty acids in clinical dermatology. *J. Am. Acad. Dermatol.* 20: 1045.

41 Calder, P.C. (2009). Polyunsaturated fatty acids and inflammatory processes: new twists in an old tale. *Biochimie* 91 (6): 791–795.

42 Vineyard, K.R., Warren, L.K., and Kivipelto, J. (2010). Effect of dietary omega-3 fatty acid source on plasma and red blood cell membrane composition and immune function in yearling horses. *J. Anim. Sci.* 88 (1): 248–257.

43 Munsterman, A.S., Bertone, A.L., Zachos, T.A., and Weisbrode, S.E. (2005). Effects of the omega-3 fatty acid, α-linolenic acid, on lipopolysaccharide-challenged synovial explants from horses. *Am. J. Vet. Res.* 66 (9): 1503–1508.

44 Ross-Jones, T., Hess, M.V., Rexford, J. et al. (2014). Effects of omega-3 long chain polyunsaturated fatty acid supplementation on equine synovial fluid fatty acid composition and prostaglandin E2. *J. Equine Vet. Sci.* 34 (6): 779–783.

45 Manhart, D.R., Honnas, C.M., Gibbs, P.G. et al. (2016). Markers of inflammation in arthritic horses fed omega-3 fatty acids. *Prof. Anim. Sci.* 25 (2): 155–160.

46 Nogradi, N., Couetil, L.L., Messick, J. et al. (2015). Omega-3 fatty acid supplementation provides an additional benefit to a low-dust diet in the management of horses with chronic lower airway inflammatory disease. *J. Vet. Intern. Med.* 29 (1): 299–306.

47 Headley, S., Coverdale, J.A., Jenkins, T.C. et al. (2012). Dietary supplementation of conjugated linoleic acid in horses increases plasma conjugated linoleic acid and decreases plasma arachidonic acid but does not alter body fat. *J. Anim. Sci.* 90 (13): 4876–4882.

48 Bradbery, A.N., Coverdale, J.A., Vernon, K.L. et al. (2018). Evaluation of conjugated linoleic acid supplementation on markers of joint inflammation and cartilage metabolism in young horses challenged with lipopolysaccharide. *J. Anim. Sci.* 96 (2): 579–590.

49 Brody, S. and Lardy, H.A. (1946). Bioenergetics and growth. *J. Phys. Chem.* 50 (2): 168–169.

50 Kleiber, M. (1961). *The Fire of Life. An Introduction to Animal energetics*, 179–222. New York: Wiley.

51 Simons, J.C. and Naylor, J.M. (1991). Bioenergetics: basic concepts and ration formulation. In: *Large Animal Clinical Nutrition*, 1e (ed. J.M. Naylor and S. Ralston), 3–21. St. Louis, MO: Mosby.

52 Pagan, J.D., Hintz, H.F., and Equine energetics. I. (1986). Relationship between body weight and energy requirements in horses. *J. Anim. Sci.* 63 (3): 815–821.

53 Careau, V., Thomas, D., Humphries, M.M., and Réale, D. (2008). Energy metabolism and animal personality. *Oikos* 117 (5): 641–653.

54 Carr, E.A. (2018). Enteral/parenteral nutrition in foals and adult horses practical guidelines for the practitioner. *Vet. Clin. North Am. Equine Pract.* 34 (1): 169–180.

55 Coenen, M., Kienzle, E., Vervuert, I., and Zeyner, A. (2011). Recent German developments in the formulation of energy and nutrient requirements in horses and the resulting feeding recommendations. *J. Equine Vet. Sci.* 31: 219–229.

56 Morgan, K. (1998). Thermoneutral zone and critical temperatures of horses. *J. Therm. Biol.* 23 (1): 59–61.

57 Mcbride, G.E., Christopherson, R.J., and Sauer, W. (1985). Metabolic rate and thyroid hormone concentrations of mature horses in response to changes in ambient temperature. *Can. J. Anim. Sci.* 65: 375–382.

58 Cena, K. and Clark, J.A. (1979). Transfer of heat through animal coats and clothing. In: *International Review of Physiology Environmental Physiology III* (ed. D. Robertshaw), 1–42. Baltimore, MD: University Park Press.

59 Kingma, B.R.M., Frijns, A.J.H., Schellen, L., and van Marken Lichtenbelt, W.D. (2014). Beyond the classic thermoneutral zone. *Temperature* 1 (2): 142–149.

60 Kingma, B. (2012). The thermoneutral zone implications for metabolic studies. *Front. Biosci.* E4 (5): 1975–1985.

61 Ames, D.R. (1988). Adjusting rations for climate. *Vet. Clin. North Am. Food Anim. Pract.* 4 (3): 543–550.

62 Martin-Rosset, W. and Vermorel, M. (1991). Maintenance energy requirement variations determined by indirect calorimetry and feeding trials in light horses. *J. Equine Vet. Sci.* 11 (1): 42–45.

63 Webb, S.P., Potter, G.D., Evans, J.W., and Webb, G.W. (1990). Influence of body fat content on digestible energy requirements of exercising horses in temperate and hot environments. *J. Equine Vet. Sci.* 10 (2): 116–120.

64 National Research Council (1982). *United States-Canadian Tables of Feed Composition*. 3rd Rev. Nutritional Data for United States and Canadian Feeds, 1–148. Washington, DC: National Academies Press.

65 Equi-Analytical Laboratories Services (2020). Common Feed Profiles. http://equi-analytical.com/common-feed-profiles.

66 Hambleton, P.L., Slade, L.M., Hamar, D.W. et al. (1980). Dietary fat and exercise conditioning effect on metabolic parameters in the horse. *J. Anim. Sci.* 51 (6): 1330–1339.

67 Scott, B.D., Potter, G.D., Greene, L.W. et al. (1993). Efficacy of a fat-supplemented diet to reduce thermal stress in exercising Thoroughbred horses. In: *Proceedings of the 13th Equine Nutrition and Physiology Society Symposium*, 66–71. Gainesville, Fl: Equine Nutrition and Physiology Society.

68 Meyers, M.C., Potter, G.D., Evans, J.W. et al. (1989). Physiologic and metabolic response of exercising horses to added dietary fat. *J. Equine Vet. Sci.* 9 (4): 218–223.

7

Protein

Patricia Graham-Thiers

KEY TERMS

- Protein a large nutrient class essential to all plants (feed) and animals, composed of amino acids, which are complex compounds of carbon, hydrogen, nitrogen, phosphorus, and sulfur.
- Crude protein (CP) is a calculated estimate of the protein content of the feed, food, feces, or tissue sample using a laboratory determination of the nitrogen concentration in the sample times 6.25 as most proteins contain 16% nitrogen.
- Transamination is a chemical reaction that transfers an amino group (NH_3) to a ketoacid to form new amino acids converting essential to non-essential amino acids.
- Apparent protein digestibility is calculated by subtracting fecal protein from feed protein.

KEY POINTS

- Protein is a vital nutrient in the ration of a horse.
- Horses of all life stages and performance have responded to improved protein quality.
- The quality of a feed as a source of protein in the ration is a function of both the amino acid profile and the digestibility of that feedstuff.
- Foregut and hindgut digestion play different roles in maintaining the protein status of the horse.
- Further information is needed on the digestibility of various protein sources due to the interactions between protein and the various fiber components of the feedstuff.

7.1 Function and Composition

Protein, as a component of the body, is essential for the growth, development, and repair of all tissues in the body and performs a wide variety of functions. Proteins have structural functions, such as actin and myosin in muscle, regulate development as hormones, digestion of food as enzymes, and perform immune functions as antibodies. Proteins also have various macro and micro transport functions, such as albumin moving essential components via blood, and as carrier molecules within cell membranes.

Proteins are composed of various combinations of different amino acid units linked by a peptide bond. As an analogy, if amino acids were letters in the alphabet, proteins would be words. Just as different words consist of different numbers and combinations of letters, different proteins consist of different numbers and combinations of amino acids specific to the protein's function. Like carbohydrates and fats, amino acids contain many carbon molecules linked together, with hydrogen and oxygen attached to the carbon. However, all amino acids contain nitrogen (N), and some contain phosphorus and sulfur. There are approximately 20 amino acids categorized as either essential (indispensable) or non-essential (dispensable) to animals.

Essential amino acids are those that cannot be synthesized by hepatic transamination (conversion of one amino acid into another) in sufficient quantities or at an adequate rate compared with the body's need for that particular amino acid. Therefore, essential amino acids must be provided in the ration or produced by the microbiota within the intestinal tract. Although all of the amino acids are needed in the synthesis of new body proteins, non-essential amino acids are synthesized endogenously and do not need to be present in the feed or produced by the intestinal

Equine Clinical Nutrition, Second Edition. Edited by Rebecca L. Remillard.

microbiota. Non-essential amino acids are those that can be synthesized endogenously via transamination within the liver to meet the demand. In the typical feeds fed to horses, both essential and non-essential amino acids will be present; however, nutritionists are responsible for ensuring adequate essential amino acid intakes.

Additionally, different species have different essential amino acid requirements. Essential amino acids for a horse may have some in common with other species but are not entirely the same as those required by a ruminant (bovine) or monogastric species (canine). Within some species, the essential amino acid profile for growth is not the same as adult maintenance primarily because the demand for de novo tissue synthesis is greater during growth. Therefore, the animal requirement specifies the number and type of amino acids and is different across species and life stages. In summary, when formulating horse rations, meeting the essential amino acid requirement is of greater concern than a total ration CP concentration.

7.2 Dietary Protein

Most proteins contain 16 ± 2% nitrogen; therefore, the protein content of a feed is estimated by determining first the nitrogen concentration via one of several laboratory methods and then dividing the nitrogen by 0.16 (or multiplying by 6.25) [1]. The value obtained is the "crude" protein (CP) content of the feed because the protein concentration is only estimated from the average nitrogen content. Thus, a feed containing 1.6% nitrogen would have 10% CP (1.6/0.16). This calculation is not accurate for feeds containing non-protein nitrogen (NPN) substances, i.e. urea.

7.2.1 Protein Digestion

The total tract apparent protein digestibility (feed minus fecal protein) varies based on the sources of protein, other ration components, and the ratio of forage to concentrate in the ration. The apparent nitrogen digestibility as determined from a compilation of 85 studies was determined to be 79% for the total tract ($r^2 = 0.94$) [2]. Protein digestion is handled differently between the foregut (stomach and small intestine) and hindgut (cecum and large colon) of the horse. Digestion of grains in the foregut occurs enzymatically while digestion of forages in the hindgut occurs through fermentation. Additionally, the proportions of ration forage to grain affect the route of nitrogen excretion from the body. Higher forage diets demonstrated higher fecal excretion of nitrogen compared with higher urine nitrogen excretion with grain diets [3, 4]. This suggests that in all-forage rations, more protein may enter the hindgut affecting fecal N excretion. Concentrates in the ration increased the urine N excretion presumably due to greater absorption of N from the foregut.

7.2.1.1 Foregut

Pepsin and other proteinases break down protein into tri- and di-peptides (3 or 2 amino acid fragments) that are then actively absorbed across the small intestine into the blood. The plasma amino acid profile generally reflects the amino acid profile of the diet within the first few hours of digestion. Plasma amino acids are then utilized from the bloodstream for tissue building and repair, and synthesizing enzymes, hormones, transport carriers, and antibodies. The goal is to have the majority of the high-quality proteins digested in the foregut to enhance the plasma amino acid pool. Grains tend to have higher foregut digestibility due to a lower fiber content compared with forages and would, therefore, be the best source of amino acids to enhance the plasma amino acid pool. Apparent prececal digestion of protein from forages has been observed to be between 20% and 25% while grains have prececal protein digestibilities between 48% and 70% [5, 6]. Regression analysis of the available data (4 studies) suggests an average prececal protein digestibility of 51% ($r^2 = 0.83$) for mixed forage and concentrate rations [2].

7.2.1.2 Hindgut

When hay only was fed to horses, total tract protein digestion was 96% with only 37% occurring in the foregut. Therefore, the fiber content of the feedstuffs affects the site of digestion. The fiber "bound" protein results in less protein digestion in the foregut and more forage protein fermentation in the hindgut. When protein escapes digestion in the foregut and proceeds to the hindgut, the plasma amino acid pool appears to be less affected by the diet [7, 8]. This does not benefit the circulating amino acid pool for the horse and could be a problem for those with high essential amino acid requirements such as foals and lactating mares fed all forage rations.

Several studies have found correlations between crude fiber and CP digestibility, more specifically, an inverse relationship between the neutral detergent fiber (NDF) content and nitrogen digestion. In a comparison between timothy and alfalfa hay, the higher CP digestibility of alfalfa was due to a lower NDF [9, 10]. It may have also been related to higher CP concentrations or a combination of both. Hindgut microbial fermentation of dietary protein yields microbial protein (a structural component of microbes) and ammonia. There is some evidence that microbes also synthesize free amino acids.

There is continued debate regarding whether these amino acids can be absorbed and contribute to the circulating amino acid pool for the horse. Recently, several studies have reopened the debate on the absorption of amino acids from the hindgut. It has been shown in tissue brush border membrane from various segments of the horse's digestive tract that there are amino acid transporters in the cecum and large colon specifically for cationic and neutral amino acids. It is unknown, however, if this uptake would be limited to the brush border membrane and for use by the digestive tract epithelial cells or if this is evidence that microbes can contribute to the amino acid pool in the bloodstream [10, 11].

7.2.2 Protein Quality

The quality of a feed as a source of protein in the ration is a function of both the amino acid profile and the digestibility of that feedstuff. Feed proteins composed of a high proportion of essential amino acids, for a specific species, are referred to as high-quality proteins, while those lacking essential amino acids are considered low- or poor-quality proteins. Given essential amino acid requirements differ across species, a protein feed considered to be of high quality for one animal group may not hold for another. Therefore, high-quality protein feeds for the horse will be highly digestible and contain sufficient concentrations of equine essential amino acids.

Animal protein sources (eggs, milk, and meat) are generally of higher quality than plant protein sources; however, horses, as herbivores do not find animal proteins palatable. Within plant protein sources, grains have higher foregut digestibility coefficients and superior amino acid profiles compared with forage. Forages generally have lower essential amino acid concentrations and are fermented in the hindgut. Plant sources of protein considered to be of high quality are oilseed meals (soybean, cottonseed, sunflower meals) or concentrates of grain proteins (brewer's grain and gluten meals) with 20% CP or greater (Table 7.1). Forages, such as alfalfa meals with 20% CP, are relatively high in protein but are not necessarily of high quality due to the amino acid profile. All grains are not used as a source of protein, note other common types of cereal grains fed to horses, such as corn and oats are used in the ration as a source of calories and not as a source of protein. The amino acid content of common horse ration ingredients and forages are available [12].

7.2.2.1 Amino Acids

It is believed that there are 10 dietary essential amino acids for the horse: arginine, histidine, methionine, isoleucine, leucine, lysine, phenylalanine, threonine, tryptophan, and valine [2]. Many of these are assumed to be essential amino acids based on work completed in other monogastric species such as swine. Research in horses does conclude that lysine is the first limiting amino acid, i.e. most likely amino acid to be in short supply compared with demand.

Lysine has been demonstrated to be the first limiting amino acid for growing horses [13]. Growth and lactation have higher lysine requirements than maintenance and exercise as demonstrated by improvement in growth with lysine additions. Increasing the lysine content of the diet has resulted in an improvement in average daily gain (ADG) for growing horses of all ages (foals, weanlings, yearlings) [14, 15]. Ensuring an adequate lysine intake for the lactating mare, therefore, becomes important to not only meet the foal's lysine requirement but also help the mare maintain muscle mass throughout lactation [16].

Threonine is speculated to be the second limiting amino acid in growing horses again based on improved ADG observed in yearling horses. Three diets were fed with similar CP concentrations (12% CP) with varied lysine and threonine additions. Improved growth and reduced serum urea nitrogen concentrations were reported in yearlings fed lysine (127 mg/kg BW/d) plus threonine (110 mg/kg BW/d) compared with yearlings receiving no amino acid supplementation or only the supplemental lysine [17]. In a different study, there were improvements in muscle mass for exercising horses receiving both supplemental lysine and threonine [18]. Feeding growing horses higher-quality protein sources or improving quality through the use of synthetic lysine resulted in higher ADG. This was demonstrated using soybean meal (SBM) vs. urea, milk protein vs. SBM, milk protein vs. linseed meal, and utilizing both lysine and threonine supplemental amino acids [14, 17, 19, 20].

Branched-chain amino acids (BCAA) (leucine, isoleucine, and valine) are unique in that they are metabolized by muscle to yield energy. This may be particularly important for the exercising horse. Interest has centered on improving performance and stimulating glycogen resynthesis. However, research into the potential benefits of BCAA supplementation has been limited and inconclusive to date.

7.2.2.2 Digestible and Available Protein

Understanding protein digestibility in the horse enables protein requirements to be expressed in terms of digestible protein (DP) instead of CP. Interestingly, the National Research Council (NRC) 1949 expressed equine protein requirements in terms of % DP in ration dry matter. In the 1978 NRC, protein recommendations were stated in both CP and DP (kg/horse/d); however, in 1989, the DP estimate was replaced with an estimated percentage of lysine requirement [21]. When animal protein requirements and feedstuffs are expressed in terms of DP, the ration can be balanced according to DP. In France, protein requirements and the protein content of feeds are expressed in terms of

Table 7.1 Protein supplements: nutrient content and characteristics for horses[a].

Feed	Protein	Lysine	DE	Fiber	Fat	Ca	P	Comments
	%	%	Mcal/kg	%	%	%	%	
For comparison:								
Oats, whole grain	13	0.44	3.2	12	5	0.1	0.35	
Grass hay, good-quality	8–12	0.4–0.5	2.2	30	3	0.5	0.3	
Grass hay, fair-quality	5–7	0.3–0.4	1.65	36	3	0.3	0.15	Similar to straw
Alfalfa pellets (17%)[b]	19	0.9	2.36	24–28	2.5–3.5	1–2	0.2–0.3	Often used protein supplement
Oilseed meals:								
Canola or Rapeseed meal	35–44	2.3–2.5	3.1	10–13	3–4	0.5–0.8	1–1.4	Glucosinolates may cause goiter
Coconut or Copra meal	23	0.6	3.3[c]	15	5	0.2	0.65	
Cottonseed meal (41%)[b]	45	1.8	3.0	13	1.7	0.18	1.2	Must be low gossypol
Flax or Linseed meal (37%)[b]	40	1	3.0	9	1.6	0.4	0.9	May soften stools
Peanut meal (47%)[b]	53	1.7–2.3	3.25	8.5	1.5	0.2–0.3	0.65	
Safflower seed meal (42%)[b]	49	1.4	3.4[b]	9	1.9	0.3	1.8	
Soybean meal (44%)[b]	50	3.2	3.5	7	1.6	0.4	0.7	Most common protein supplement. Best plant-source protein in growth rations but must be cooked
Sunflower meal (44%)[b]	50	1.8	2.8	12	3	0.45	1	High concentration may decrease palatability
Oilseeds:								
Canola or Rapeseeds	20	1–2	4.3[b]	6	38	0.38	0.75	Glucosinolates may cause goiter
Cottonseeds	24	1.0	4.3[b]	18–20	24	0.15	0.7	Must be low gossypol
Flax or Linseeds	22.8	0.9	3.6	6.5	38	0.25	0.6	May cause cyanide toxicosis unless cooked
Safflower seeds	19.5	0.6	3.9[b]	31	19	0.25	0.75	
Soybeans	33–43	2.3–3.1	3.5	4–6	18–19	0.2–0.3	0.6–0.8	Raw suitable for adult but heated processed for young horses
Sunflower seeds with hull	18	2.3	3.6[b]	31	28	0.18	0.56	
Grain byproducts:								
Brewer's grains	25–28	0.95	2.7	15.6	7.4	0.33	0.55	
Distiller's grains	29–34	0.75–0.9	2.6	12–13	7–16	0.10–0.15	0.3–0.6	Palatable to horses >20%
Distiller's solubles	22–30	1.0	3.1	5–6	9–12	0.3–0.4	1.3–1.4	Palatable to horses
Gluten meal, corn	47	0.9	3.0	5	2.4	0.16	0.5	Not the same as gluten feed
Gluten meal, wheat	56	1.7	3.2	6.7	4.9	0.2	0.6	
Pulses:								
Beans and peas	21–26	1.3–1.8	3.6	5–7	1.5–1.8	0.1–0.2	0.4–0.6	Should be cooked before feeding
Animal sources:								
Fish meal, menhaden	60–70	4.4–5.7	3.1	0.9	10–14	5.6	3.2	Major fish meal fed in USA, low palatability unless flavored
Fish meal, white	60–70	4.0–5.0	3.3	0.8	2–8	8.0	3.9	Major fish meal fed in UK
Milk, bovine, skimmed	36	2.7	4.0	0.2	1.0	1.36	1.1	Excellent for young horse. High lactose content may cause diarrhea in adults
Milk, bovine, whole	27	2	5.6	0.2	27. 6	0.95	0.76	
Casein, dry	93	7.7	4.0	0.2	0.7	0.6	0.9	Excellent protein supplement
Single-cell sources:								
Yeast, brewer's	47–51	3.3	3.3	3–7	1.1	0.15	1.5	Used primarily as B-vitamin supplement
Yeast, torula	52.5	4.1	3.3	2–3	2.3	0.65	1.8	

[a] All values are average feed analysis on dry matter basis: Crude protein and Crude fiber, Calcium (Ca), Phosphorus (P).
[b] Guaranteed as fed minimum protein content.
[c] Ruminant value given. Equine value is likely 15% less from oilseeds and 20-30% less for seed meals.

Matières Azotées Digestibles Cheval (MADC) translated as "horse digestible crude protein." This system was developed to account for differences in the digestibility of various sources of protein and absorbable amino acids. The horse digestible CP (MADC) content of feeds is calculated from the estimated amounts of amino acids absorbed from the small and large intestines [22]. Several studies have determined DP values for a limited number of horse feeds, but as yet, insufficient data are available in the horse to be the standard for describing either the equine protein requirement or the wide range of feedstuff fed to them. At this time, the system is thought to be more complicated and not useful at the farm or barn level.

The quantity of CP is not 100% available to the animal, and adjusting CP content for that fraction of unavailable protein allows for an estimation of "available" protein (AP). The acid detergent insoluble nitrogen (ADIN) fraction of feeds is assumed to be indigestible except in ruminants through microbial fermentation. Available protein can be estimated by subtracting NPN and ADIN, which represent "bound" protein, from feed CP values. Thus, AP is a calculated estimate of protein that may be available to the horse while DP is based on whole tract digestibility studies that measured the amount of protein digested *in vivo*. A retro-respective view of studies that had evaluated protein digestibility in the horse was used to evaluate the concept of AP and the intake was compared with the DP intake. There was a high correlation between the two variables ($r^2 = 0.94$) [2, 5, 7–9, 23–27]. Comparisons of AP in feedstuffs can assist in selecting better sources of protein for the horse (Table 7.2). Additional research is required to evaluate this concept *in vivo* but it could be the next step in progressing from CP to DP in terms of expressing protein requirements for horses.

Table 7.2 Protein and nitrogen (N) composition of selected feedstuffs for calculation of available protein.

Feedstuff	Crude protein (%)	Acid detergent insoluble N (ADIN; %)	Non-protein N (NPN; %)	Calculated[a] available protein (AP) %
Bermuda grass	13.7	1.2	5.0	7.5
Oats	13.2	0.3	8.6	4.3
Soybean meal	49.9	0.4	11.2	38.3
Peanut meal	51.8	1.1	32.0	18.7

[a] AP = CP – ADIN – NPN.
Source: Based on NRC [28].

7.2.3 Ideal Protein

The ideal protein is a concept that states that amino acids need to be provided in adequate quantities and in the correct proportions to one another. This concept has been evaluated in swine through nitrogen balance studies. The resulting ideal protein for swine is also closely correlated to the major end-product, i.e. muscle (meat) amino acid profile.

The ideal protein for horses has not been well studied; however, estimating muscle amino acid profiles in animals at different life stages and performing various functions could be used to develop the ideal amino acid profile [29]. Skeletal muscle concentration of essential amino acids in horses at various life stages (maintenance, exercise, pregnancy, lactation, and growth) has demonstrated no difference except for lower phenylalanine in pregnant mares and lower methionine in exercising horses compared with maintenance horses [30, 31]. A follow-up study found no differences in total muscle amino acids except exercising horses that had lower histidine concentrations compared with all other life stages [32].

Young and aged exercising horses fed adequate amounts of dietary CP, based on 1989 NRC, were supplemented with lysine and threonine at concentrations recommended for growth to evaluate the horse's ability to build and maintain muscle mass [33]. The study reported lower plasma urea nitrogen and 3-methylhistidine (3MH) concentrations, as well as greater plasma creatinine and subjective muscle mass scores, for horses fed the amino acid fortified diets. The lysine intake of the control group was above the current recommendation for exercising horses [34]. The results suggest that supplementation of lysine and threonine favored exercising muscle metabolism. Additionally, the supplemented diet more closely resembled the ideal protein previously suggested [29].

It is therefore important to recognize differences in amino acid profiles, protein digestibility, and availability when selecting dietary protein sources for horses in various life stages. Equine protein requirements would be better met as an expression of dietary DP rather than CP. Ration protein sources compared based on DP would be closer to the metabolic ideal rather than CP. Individual amino acid requirements and ideal profile or balance of amino acids of the horse deserve closer attention.

7.2.4 Protein Supplements

Cereal grains and many forages do not contain enough protein to meet the requirements of the lactating mare or the growing horse, and some mature grass forages do not contain enough protein to meet maintenance horse requirements. A protein supplement is incorporated when the protein content of the ration is inadequate.

Protein supplements are feeds sufficiently higher in protein such that, when added to the ration, there is an increase in total ration protein concentration. Since most other horse feed contain <20% CP, a feed containing >20% when added to the ration would increase the protein concentration of the ration. As a result, a feed containing >20% CP is generally classified as a protein supplement. There are several different types of protein supplements classified according to origin: plant, animal, single-cell, or NPN. Any of the first three types of protein supplements are useful. In most rations, plant proteins are the most commonly used supplements for horses and other livestock. The major plant protein supplements used are oilseed meals, although grain protein supplements are also commonly used. Most plant protein supplements are not particularly palatable for most horses. For example, SBM (~50% CP) is a common feedstuff fed in the United States to increase ration protein concentration. SBM is slightly less palatable than wheat, barley, and rye, and considerably less palatable than oats and corn for most horses [35, 36]. Therefore, it is best to feed the protein supplement well mixed with cereal grains. When included as a loose dry mixture of feedstuff, wet molasses is beneficial and commonly used both to increase palatability and to prevent the protein supplement from sifting out, and hence referred to as textured feed products. See Chapter 13 Manufactured Feeds.

7.2.5 Non-Protein Nitrogen Sources

Rumen microbial organisms and those in the cecum and colon of the horse can use dietary nitrogen sources to synthesize protein, provided the animal also consumes sufficient nonfiber sources of dietary energy. Thus, a non-protein source of nitrogen, such as urea, fed to ruminants is incorporated into rumen microbial proteins. The protein produced by these microorganisms passes from the rumen to the small intestine, digested, and absorbed. However, feeding urea or NPN is of little value in providing protein to the horse. Most of the NPN fed to the horse is absorbed from the small intestine before reaching the cecum and colon [8]. That which reaches the hindgut may be used in microbial synthesis; however, most of the microbial proteins are excreted in the feces.

Excessive intake of NPN is toxic. Before microorganisms use NPN to synthesize protein, the NPN is converted to ammonia. If an excessive amount of NPN is ingested, toxic quantities of ammonia are absorbed. Initially, affected animals wander aimlessly and are uncoordinated. Following this, they may head press against fixed objects, become recumbent, become comatose, convulse, and die. Although ponies succumbed to single doses of 0.5 kg of urea, intakes of feed containing up to 5% urea in the total ration, providing as much as 0.25 kg of urea daily, did not have any detrimental effects on mature horses [31]. This is several times greater than the amounts that are toxic to cattle or sheep.

7.2.6 Protein Imbalance

7.2.6.1 Deficiency

Protein intakes below the horse's requirement will limit and challenge the amino acid demands of the body. A dietary CP concentration lower than recommended will result in a lack of specific essential amino acids, if not well formulated. Without adequate amino acids, a decrease in endogenous protein production will result. Examples of this would include slower or retarded growth in young horses, decreased milk production in lactating mares and potentially smaller foals, or fetal loss in pregnant mares, although this has not been specifically studied.

The most obvious manifestations of a protein deficiency are reduced growth in young animals, and in mature horses, weight loss, reduced performance, endurance, and decreased milk production. Hair growth and shedding are slowed, resulting in a rough, coarse, unkempt appearance (Figure 7.1). Hoof growth is slowed, which may result in increased hoof splitting and cracking. A protein deficiency in the horse may also cause appetite depravity and coprophagy, which are alleviated within 5 to 7 d after correcting the deficiency [37].

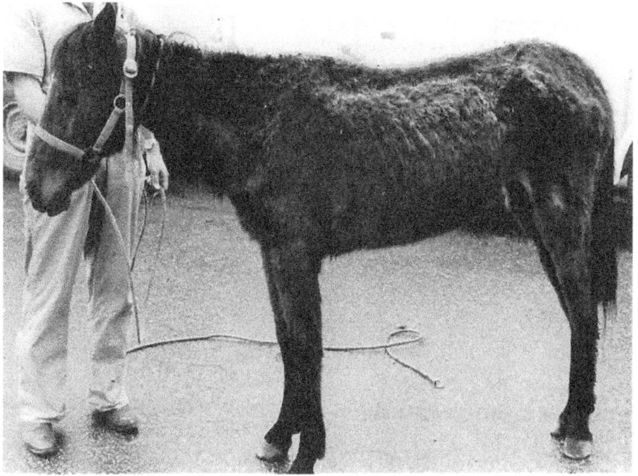

Figure 7.1 A three-year-old mare with a poor haircoat and muscling as a result of chronic protein and calorie deficiency. The horse was protein and energy-deficient as a result of an inadequate intake of a poor-quality (low protein) feed.

A protein deficiency may decrease feed intake, which not only worsens the protein deficit but in turn results in an energy deficit. An energy deficiency contributes to the clinical signs and further worsens the protein deficiency because most of the consumed protein will first be catabolized to meet energy and, therefore, cannot assist in tissue synthesis. It is futile to provide dietary protein if the animal's energy needs are not first met. As a result of either a protein or energy deficiency, or both, plasma albumin and total protein concentrations will decrease within weeks. If there is inadequate intake of energy sources (carbohydrates and fats), dietary protein will be catabolized for energy, and breakdown of body proteins will continue, i.e. muscle wasting.

A sufficient decrease in plasma protein concentration allows fluids to leave the plasma, resulting in edema and stocking up in the late stages of protein deficits. Loss of fluid from the plasma may increase globulin concentration, which, in conjunction with a decrease in albumin, decreases the albumin/globulin ratio below the normal. However, much before a significant decrease in the plasma protein concentration, or any clinical signs of a protein deficiency, the plasma or blood urea nitrogen (BUN) concentration will decrease. In horses, a BUN of less than 12–15 mg/dL (2–2.5 Mm/L) suggests inadequate protein intake, and less than 10 mg/dL (1.7 mM/L) suggests a deficiency. Blood urea nitrogen varies directly with protein intake but is also decreased by hepatic dysfunction and increased by renal dysfunction and dehydration. A decrease in pre-albumin, retinol-binding protein, and fibronectin are also used as indicators of a protein deficiency in people and may be useful in the horse, although this has not been investigated. A protein deficit may result in the following circumstances:

1) Inadequate concentrations of protein in the ration, e.g. horses eating mature grass forages.
2) Inadequate total feed intake regardless of the protein concentration, e.g. primary energy deficiency.
3) Adequate intake of poor-quality protein, e.g. essential amino acid deficiencies.

7.2.6.2 Excess

When more protein is ingested than needed, nitrogen is removed from the extra amino acids, forming ammonia. The carbon backbone of the amino acid is used for energy, or, if energy is not needed at that time, it is stored as fat or glycogen for later use. The ammonia that is removed from the amino acids is converted to urea (CH_4N_2O) by the liver. Blood urea nitrogen concentration is directly related to dietary protein intake and can be an indicator of excessive consumption of protein [8, 38].

The increased amount of urea produced is excreted in the urine. Urine nitrogen excretion increased in horses fed alfalfa diets as the protein intake exceeded the horse's protein need [39]. This increases urine volume and, subsequently, increases water consumption. It also increases the urine ammonia concentration and odor, which can be noticed in poorly ventilated barns. The increased urination due to the excess urea results in exceptionally wet bedding, which contributes to environmental nitrogen contamination and respiratory issues due to ammonia fumes. The increased BUN and water consumption to compensate for increased urination may resemble the early signs of kidney disease. Renal disease may be caused by several infectious organisms and toxins, but it is unlikely that chronic overfeeding of protein would cause renal or hepatic disease.

The protein intake must be in balance with total energy intake from carbohydrates and fats when evaluating a protein excess. The catabolism of protein for energy, in a low-energy ration, produces three to six times more metabolic heat than the utilization of carbohydrates or fats [40]. This may be beneficial in a cold environment but may contribute to excessive sweating and heat exhaustion during physical activity, particularly in a warm environment. In summary, feeding protein more than required provides no performance advantages; managing the excess urea is metabolically expensive and harmful to the environment [6].

7.3 Horse Protein Requirements by Life Stage

7.3.1 Maintenance

The amount of DP needed to achieve nitrogen balance has been estimated between 400 and 800 mg DP/kg BW/d in horses that are considered to be at maintenance (no imposed exercise) [8, 41–46]. Extrapolating data to a level of zero nitrogen balance using studies that measured nitrogen intake and nitrogen retention in horses was estimated to be 619 mg DP/kg BW/d (813 mg CP/kg BW/d) ($r^2 = 0.76$). Based on this result, the minimum DP intake for maintenance horses should be at least 620 mg DP/kg BW/d or 813 mg CP/kg BW/d. Evaluating the same data using a two-slope model to estimate the "break" point or ideal nitrogen intake to be 0.202 g N/kg BW/d, which would result in some nitrogen reserves in the body rather than a zero balance [2]. This concentration of nitrogen intake would be the equivalent of 1.26 g CP/kg BW/d or 630 g CP for the average 500 kg horse (Table 7.3).

Table 7.3 Daily crude protein and lysine requirements for horses at different life stages and performance.

Type	Crude protein	Lysine
	g/100 kg mature BW[a]	
Maintenance		
Minimum	108.0	4.64
Average	126.0	5.42
Elevated	144.0	6.20
Working		
Light	139.8	6.02
Moderate	153.6	6.60
Heavy	172.4	7.42
Very heavy	200.8	8.64
Stallions		
Nonbreeding	144.0	6.20
Breeding	157.8	6.78
Pregnant[b]		
Early	126.0	5.42
5 mos[c]	137.0	5.90
6 mos	140.8	6.06
7 mos	145.8	6.26
8 mos	151.8	6.54
9 mos	159.4	6.86
10 mos	168.2	7.24
11 mos	178.6	7.68
Lactation		
1 mos	307.0	16.96
2 mos	306.0	16.88
3 mos	293.6	16.06
4 mos	279.6	15.14
5 mos	266.0	14.24
6 mos	253.0	13.38
Growing[d]		
4 mos	133.8	5.76
6 mos	135.2	5.82
12 mos	169.2	7.28
18 mos	159.8	6.88
18 mos light exercise	170.6	7.34
18 mos moderate exercise	181.2	7.80
24 mos	154.0	6.62
24 mos light exercise	165.8	7.14
24 mos moderate exercise	177.6	7.64
24 mos heavy exercise	193.8	8.34
24 mos very heavy exercise	218.2	9.38

[a] Conversions to kilogram mature body weight basis was made using the protein and lysine required for a 500 kg mature horse from NRC [2], Table 16-3.
[b] Calculated based on pre-pregnancy weight.
[c] mos = months.
[d] Calculated intake based on expected mature weight. Example: a growing 4 m old with an expected mature weight of 500 kg requires [133.8 g CP × 5 (100 kg mature weight)] = 669 g CP/d.

Lysine requirements for maintenance horses have not been specifically studied. Utilizing data from studies that reported a lysine intake and nitrogen retention, an estimate of 36 mg lysine/kg BW/d would result in zero N retention. The ideal based on the two-slope model, identifying a plateau in N retention, would be an intake of 54 mg lysine/kg BW/d. This would make the minimum recommendation of lysine 18 g/d and an optimum of 27 g lysine/d for the 500-kg horse. If lysine is expressed as a percent of CP, this would be equivalent to 4.3% of the CP being lysine (27 g lysine/630 g CP). This may be useful when selecting sources of protein in the diet and recognizing when lysine may be deficient in the overall protein supply for horses in maintenance.

7.3.2 Growth

7.3.2.1 Weanlings

Protein in the growing horse would be used primarily for tissue formation and reflected in the horse's ADG. By combining data from several studies that evaluated growth in weanling horses, an estimated optimum intake of 3.98 g CP/kg BW/d for weanlings between 4 and 10 m of age with an expected mature body weight (BW) of 500 kg was observed. Therefore, a 4-mo-old (BW 168 kg) weanling would require 669 g CP per d. If the protein for maintenance is taken into account, the remaining CP would be available for gain and, based on previous studies, appears to have approximately a 50% efficiency of use for gain (presuming mainly muscle mass gain). Crude protein requirements for growth can be estimated from BW, rate of gain, digestibility, and efficiency of digested CP utilization (Table 7.3). Growth curves have been estimated from available growth data to estimate BW and ADG for growing horses of various ages [47–49].

7.3.2.2 Yearlings

Nitrogen retention was maximized at a protein intake of 3.2 g CP/kg BW/d (2.4 g DP/kg BW/d) for yearling horses [50]. The source of protein fed to yearlings (315–333 d of age) affected ADG with greater gains observed when yearlings were fed at least 3.3 g CP/kg BW/d using SBM and alfalfa compared with using SBM and bermudagrass hay [18, 20]. The efficiency at which the CP was used for weight gain in studies reporting CP intake, BW, and ADG was only 30% for horses over 11 m of age. So for example, a BW 321 kg yearling (12 m old) gaining 0.45 kg/d would require 846 g CP/d (Table 7.3) using 464 g CP/d for maintenance and 382 g CP/d for gain after adjusting for the efficiency of use and digestibility.

7.3.2.3 Lysine

Reviewing studies that evaluated needs of growing horses, lysine intake for weanlings (4–10 m of age) should be 33–42 g/d (151–179 mg lysine/kg BW/d) to improve ADG [13, 51, 52]. Applying the two-slope model to the data the lysine requirement is estimated to be 168 mg/kg BW/d. Therefore, the lysine requirement for a 4-mo-old BW 168 kg weanling would be 28 g lysine/d. Lysine requirement was equivalent to 4.3% of the CP requirement, which is similar to the relationship in maintenance horses. Based on these data, the suggested lysine requirement for both weanling and yearling horses is 4.3% of the CP requirement (Table 7.3).

7.3.3 Gestation

Protein and amino acid requirements for pregnant mares have received very little attention in the literature. The lower amount of acceptable protein intake for mares in early to mid-gestation has not been investigated thoroughly. It is generally accepted that mares in good condition are fed according to maintenance requirements until the later stages of pregnancy. Mares fed a CP to digestible energy (DE) ratio <35 lost weight and had a higher incidence of fetal loss compared with the groups fed CP : DE ratios ≥38 [53]. Likewise, a different study in mares fed a CP : DE ratio of 40 was observed to be in positive nitrogen balance [54]. The fetal growth rate has been estimated in the mare [55]. Foal body composition has been estimated at 20% protein. Considering the rate of fetal gain, estimates of protein needs above maintenance were made with an allowance for placental and uterine protein needs to be included [56]. This attempted to account for additional protein needs for gestation rather than simply assuming that increased caloric intake would provide adequate CP for the mare during pregnancy. It can be concluded that feeding mares in early- to mid-gestation at an average maintenance concentration of CP intake is adequate; however, additional research is needed to determine more precisely the needs of the mare in early- to mid-pregnancy. The current NRC (2007) recommends approximately 42 g CP/Mcal DE. Without any available data regarding the amino acid needs of the pregnant mare, the lysine requirement for pregnancy has been assumed to be 4.3% of the CP requirement (Table 7.3) [2].

7.3.4 Lactation

The quantity of milk produced by mares has been documented in several studies and reported to vary between 1.9% and 3.9% of the mare's BW up to 6 m of lactation. The same studies report the protein content of milk is 3.1% to 3.3% in early lactation (generally colostrum) but gradual declines to 1.6–1.9% in later lactation [56–59].

Therefore, based on milk production, milk protein concentrations, the efficiency of use of dietary protein for milk production and CP digestibility, an additional 50 g CP was determined to be needed per kg of milk produced above maintenance (Table 7.3).

There is reasonably good agreement between the amino acid profile in mare's milk and equine muscle, which potentially leads to formulating an ideal protein [16, 29]. Assuming an average lysine content of 1.7 g/kg milk and 65% utilization efficiency of the dietary lysine, the requirement was estimated to be 2.62 g digestible lysine/kg milk. Adjusting for protein digestibility, 3.3 g lysine is needed per kg milk produced in addition to that required for maintenance (Table 7.3). Both estimates for CP and lysine requirements for the lactating mare result in dietary intakes that may be difficult to provide in the short term. It is presumed that the lactating mare readily utilizes body reserves to overcome short-term deficiencies. Careful selection of protein sources during this demanding time is certainly warranted.

7.3.5 Work

Exercising horses are either developing muscle, repairing muscle, or both in comparison to maintenance horses. A description of workloads in horses ranging from "light" to "very heavy" has been proposed [2]. There is some evidence (and continued debate) regarding whether exercising horses require additional protein per kilogram of BW for developing or repairing muscle. Increased nitrogen retention has been reported for exercising horses as exercise load increased [60]. Horses retained an additional 0.37 g CP/kg BW/d during exercise compared with rest periods. However, this study did not account for all potential losses of nitrogen such as sweat. When an estimate is made on the potential protein lost in sweat in this study, not all of the retained nitrogen is accounted for. Therefore, the unexplained nitrogen retention (from measured losses) may represent an additional protein need over maintenance for exercising horses. The data from this study results in a recommendation of 1000 g CP for the 500 kg horse in very heavy work. Excess protein intake may be disadvantageous as studies have observed detrimental effects on acid–base balance [61]. It has been recommended that endurance horses should not be fed more than 2 g of DP/kg BW/d [18].

Exercising horses (heavy intensity) have been observed to have maximal nitrogen retention when fed a diet providing 1016 g CP/d [62]. Muscle protein turnover can be estimated using 3MH and this data predicted a CP requirement of 954 g/d [63]. Therefore, a recommendation of 1.9–2.1 g CP/kg BW/d for the heavily exercised horse has been suggested [60]. For the 500-kg horse, this would result in a requirement of 950–1050 g CP/d. The protein requirement for the exercising horse is therefore based on the fact that additional muscle appears to be gained during conditioning, additional muscle mass will result in increased CP needed for repair, and nitrogen is lost in sweat. Both muscle tissue gain, repair, and sweat loss are dependent on the intensity of exercise. The recommended requirements also have adjustments made for the efficiency of CP use and digestibility (Table 7.3).

There is little information about the influence of CP intake on glycogen and free pool amino acid concentrations in the muscle of horses in training. There has been some interest in how protein and amino acid concentrations may relate to performance in terms of lactic acid production as well as glycogen resynthesis after heavy exercise. A high-protein diet had no effect on exercise performance based on lactate concentrations during exercise; however, a diet by exercise interaction suggested a lower availability of glycogen in horses fed a high-protein ration (18.5% CP) [64]. Other studies have suggested lower dietary protein concentrations are sufficient for exercising horses and may improve conditions that may affect performance. Higher blood pH and strong ion difference (SID) were measured in exercising horses fed a 7% CP diet plus lysine and threonine compared with those fed a 14% protein diet [61]. A higher blood pH and SID may aid in performance through buffering oxidants produced during exercise that typically lower blood pH and alter the acid–base balance. Another benefit of exercise whether it be for growing or mature horses may be an improvement in overall protein digestibility [65]. Exercise has been shown to increase the digestibility of protein based on higher volatile fatty acids that suggest improved fiber digestion in the hindgut [66]. Exercise in growing horses has also been demonstrated to improve protein digestibility. Horses fed a low-protein (6–8%) diet and exercised performed, in terms of ADG, as well as those fed a high-protein (12–14%) diet [65].

Studies with appropriate data reported (diet composition and intake, lysine intake calculated) were utilized to evaluate the plateau for nitrogen retention based on a two-slope model in high-intensity exercising horses. The analysis resulted in a recommendation of 68 mg lysine/kg BW/d for the exercising horse. This would make the lysine requirement 37 g/d for a 500-kg horse in heavy exercise. If this same horse has a CP requirement of 862 g CP/d, a lysine requirement of 37 g/d is 4.3% of the CP requirement. Therefore, the requirement for lysine for the exercising horse is based on 4.3% of the CP requirement (Table 7.3).

Case in Point

Due to variations in amino acid profiles and digestibility related to fiber content and the site of digestion, it is important to ensure adequate protein and lysine intake for each horse. A 500 kg average adult horse at maintenance (BSC 5/9) requires 630 g protein/d [2] p 298.

1) How much of each feed (as fed basis) in the chart below will be required daily to meet the NRC suggested intake of 630 g protein?

	Crude protein	Feed[a]	Lysine	Lysine[b]
Feedstuff (Table 7.1)	(%)	kg/d	%	g/d
Grass hay (good quality)	8	?	0.4	?
Soybean meal (44%)[c]	45	?	2.9	?
Sunflower meal (44%)	45	?	1.6	?

[a] 0.630 kg protein/% CP = kg feed/d.
[b] Daily feed intake (kg/d) × % lysine × 1000 = g lysine/d.
[c] Guaranteed as fed minimum protein content.

2) Which feeds fed at the calculated daily rate to meet CP intake will also meet the NRC suggested intake of 27 g lysine/d [2] p 298 for the same horse?

See Appendix A Chapter 7

References

1 Harris, L.E. (1970). Determination of nitrogen and crude protein. In: *Nutrition Research Techniques for Domestic and Wild Animals*, vol. 1, 2501. Logan, UT: Utah State University.

2 National Research Council (2007). *Nutrient Requirements of Horses*. 6th Rev. Animal Nutrition Series, 1–341. Washington, DC: National Academies Press.

3 Jensen, R.B., Austbo, D., Bach Knudsen, K.E., and Tauson, A.H. (2014). The effect of dietary carbohydrate composition on apparent total tract digestibility, feed mean retention time, nitrogen and water balance in horses. *Animal* 8 (11): 1788–1796.

4 Graham-Thiers, P.M. and Bowen, L.K. (2011). Effect of protein source on nitrogen balance and plasma amino acids in exercising horses. *J. Anim. Sci.* 89 (3): 729–735.

5 Gibbs, P.G., Potter, G.D., Schelling, G.T. et al. (1996). The significance of small vs large intestinal digestion of cereal grain and oilseed protein in the equine. *J. Equine Vet. Sci.* 16 (2): 60–65.

6 Urschel, K.L. and Lawrence, L.M. (2013). Amino acid and protein. In: *Equine Applied and Clinical Nutrition: Health, Welfare and Performance* (ed. R.J. Geor, P.A. Harris, and M. Coenen), 113–135. Edinburgh: Saunders Elsevier.

7 Reitnour, C.M. and Salsbury, R.L. (1975). Effect of oral or caecal administration of protein supplements on equine plasma amino acids. *Br. Vet. J.* 131 (4): 466–473.

8 Hintz, H.F. and Schryver, H.F. (1972). Nitrogen utilization in ponies. *J. Anim. Sci.* 34 (4): 592–595.

9 LaCasha, P.A., Brady, H.A., Allen, V.G. et al. (1999). Voluntary intake, digestibility, and subsequent selection of matua bromegrass, coastal bermudagrass, and alfalfa hays by yearling horses. *J. Anim. Sci.* 77 (10): 2766–2773.

10 Woodward, A.D., Fan, M.Z., Geor, R.J. et al. (2012). Characterization of L-lysine transport across equine and porcine jejunal and colonic brush border membrane. *J. Anim. Sci.* 90 (3): 853–862.

11 Woodward, A.D., Holcombe, S.J., Steibel, J.P. et al. (2010). Cationic and neutral amino acid transporter transcript abundances are differentially expressed in the equine intestinal tract. *J. Anim. Sci.* 88 (3): 1028–1033.

12 National Research Council (1982). *United States-Canadian Tables of Feed Composition*. 3rd Rev. Nutritional Data for United States and Canadian Feeds, 1–148. Washington, DC: National Academies Press.

13 Ott, E.A. and Kivipelto, J. (2002). Growth and development of yearling horses fed either alfalfa or coastal bermudagrass: hay and a concentrate formulated for bermudagrass hay. *J. Equine Vet. Sci.* 22 (7): 311–319.

14 Borton, A., Anderson, D.L., and Lyford, S. (1973). Studies of protein quality and quantity in the early weaned foal. In: *Proceedings of the 3rd Equine Nutrition and Physiology*

Society Symposium. 19. Gainsville, FL: Equine Nutrition and Physiology Society.
15 Ott, E.A., Asquith, R.L., and Feaster, J.P. (1981). Lysine supplementation of diets for yearling horses. *J. Anim. Sci.* 53 (6): 1496–1503.
16 Wickens, C.L., Ku, P.K., and Trottier, N.L. (2002). An ideal protein for the lactating mare. *J. Anim. Sci.* 80 (Suppl 1 Abstr 620): 155.
17 Graham, P.M., Ott, E.A., Brendemuhl, J.H., and TenBroeck, S.H. (1994). The effect of supplemental lysine and threonine on growth and development of yearling horses. *J. Anim. Sci.* 72 (2): 380–386.
18 Harris, P. (2005). Feeding the endurance horse. In: *Applied Equine Nutrition: Equine NUtrition Conference (ENUCO)* (ed. A. Lindner), 61–84. Wageningen Academic Publishers.
19 Godbee, R.G. and Slade, L.M. (1981). The effect of urea or soybean meal on the growth and protein status of young horses. *J. Anim. Sci.* 53 (3): 670–676.
20 Hintz, H.F., Schryver, H.F., and Lowe, J.E. (1972). Comparison of a blend of milk products and linseed meal as protein supplements for young growing horses. *J. Anim. Sci.* 33 (6): 1274–1276.
21 National Research Council (1978). *Nutrient Requirements of Horses*. 4th Rev. Animal Nutrition Series, 1–33. Washington, DC: National Academies Press.
22 Martin-Rosset, W., Vermorel, M., Doreau, M. et al. (1994). The French horse feed evaluation systems and recommended allowances for energy and protein. *Livest. Prod. Sci.* 40 (1): 37–56.
23 Reitnour, C.M. and Salsbury, R.L. (1972). Digestion and utilization of cecally infused protein by the equine. *J. Anim. Sci.* 35 (6): 1190–1193.
24 Glade, M.J., Beller, D., Bergen, J. et al. (1985). Dietary protein in excess of requirements inhibits renal calcium and phosphorus reabsorption in young horses. *Nutr. Rep. Int.* 31: 649–659.
25 Gibbs, P.G., Potter, G.D., Schelling, G.T. et al. (1988). Digestion of hay protein in different segments of the equine digestive tract. *J. Anim. Sci.* 66 (2): 400–406.
26 Farley, E.B., Potter, G.D., Gibbs, P.G. et al. (1995). Digestion of soybean meal protein in the equine small and large intestine at various levels of intake. *J. Equine Vet. Sci.* 15 (8): 391–397.
27 Crozier, J.A., Allen, V.G., Jack, N.E. et al. (1997). Digestibility, apparent mineral absorption, and voluntary intake by horses fed alfalfa, tall fescue, and caucasian bluestem. *J. Anim. Sci.* 75 (6): 1651–1658.
28 National Research Council (2001). *Nutrient Requirements of Dairy Cattle*. 7th Rev. Animal Nutrition Series, 1–381. Washington, DC: National Academies Press.
29 Bryden, W. (1991). Amino acid requirements of horses estimated from tissue composition. In: *Proceedings of the Nutrition Society of Australia*, 53. Camden, Australia: Nutrition Society of Australia.
30 Graham-Thiers, P.M., Wilson, J.A., Haught, J., and Goldberg, M. (2010). Case study: relationships between dietary, plasma, and muscle amino acids in maintenance horses, exercising horses, and growing weanling horses. *Prof. Anim. Sci.* 26: 313–319.
31 Graham-Thiers, P.M., Wilson, J.A., Haught, J., and Goldberg, M. (2016). Case study: relationships between dietary, plasma, and muscle amino acids in maintenance, pregnant, and lactating mares. *Prof. Anim. Sci.* 26: 320–327.
32 Graham-Thiers, P.M.M., Wilson, J.A.A., Haught, J., and Goldberg, M. (2012). Relationships between dietary, plasma, and muscle amino acids in horses. *Prof. Anim. Sci.* 28 (3): 351–357.
33 National Research Council (1989). *Nutrient Requirements of Horses*. 5th Rev. Animal Nutrition Series, 1–100. Washington, DC: National Academies Press.
34 Graham-Thiers, P.M. and Kronfeld, D.S. (2005). Amino acid supplementation improves muscle mass in aged and young horses. *J. Anim. Sci.* 83 (12): 2783–2788.
35 Hintz, H.F. (1980). Feed preferences for horses. In: *Proceedings of the Cornell Nutrition Conference for Feed Manufacturers*, 113–116, Ithaca, NY.
36 Houpt, K.A. (1983). Taste preferences in horses. *Equine Pract.* 5 (4): 22–26.
37 Schurg, W.A., Frei, D.L., and Cheeke, P.R. (1977). Utilization of whole corn plant pellets by horses and rabbits. In: *Proceedings of 5th Equine Nutrition and Physiology Society Symposium*, 58–61. St. Louis, MO: Equine Nutrition and Physiology Society.
38 Connysson, M., Muhonen, S., Lindberg, J.E. et al. (2006). Effects on exercise response, fluid and acid-base balance of protein intake from forage-only diets in Standardbred horses. *Equine Vet. J.* 36: 648–653.
39 Woodward, A.D., Nielsen, B.D., Liesman, J. et al. (2011). Protein quality and utilization of timothy, oat-supplemented timothy, and alfalfa at differing harvest maturities in exercised Arabian horses. *J. Anim. Sci.* 89: 4081–4092.
40 Smith, R.R., Rumsey, G.L., and Scott, M.L. (1978). Heat increment associated with dietary protein, fat, carbohydrate and complete diets in salmonids comparative energetic efficiency. *J. Nutr.* 108 (6): 1025–1032.
41 Slade, L.M. and Robinson, D.W. (1970). Nitrogen metabolism in nonruminant herbivores. II. Comparative aspects of protein digestion. *J. Anim. Sci.* 30 (5): 761–763.
42 Harper, O.F. and Vander Noot, G.W. (1974). Protein requirements of mature maintenance horses. *J. Anim. Sci.* 62 (Abstr): 183.
43 Reitnour, C.M. and Salsbury, R.L. (1976). Utilization of proteins by the equine species. *Am. J. Vet. Res.* 37 (9): 1065–1067.

44 Meyer, H. (1985). Investigations to determine endogenous faecal and renal N losses in horses. In: *Proceedings of the 9th Equine Nutrition and Physiology Society Symposium*, 68. East Lansing, MI: Equine Nutrition and Physiology Society.

45 Patterson, P.H., Coon, C.N., and Hughes, I.M. (1985). Protein requirements of mature working horses. *J. Anim. Sci.* 61: 187–196.

46 Olsman, A.F.S., Jansen, W.L., Sloet van Oldruitenborgh-Oosterbaan, M.M., and Beynen, A.C. (2003). Assessment of the minimum protein requirement of adult ponies. *J. Anim. Physiol. Anim. Nutr.* 87 (5–6): 205–212.

47 Morel, P.C.H., Bokor, R.C.W., and Firth, E.C. (2007). Growth curves from birth to weaning for thoroughbred foals raised on pasture. *N. Z. Vet. J.* 55 (6): 319–325.

48 Brown-Douglas, C.G. and Pagan, J.D. (2020). Body weight, wither height and growth rates in thoroughbreds raised in America, England, Australia, New Zealand and India. *Adv. Equine Nutr.* IV: 213–220.

49 Jelan, Z.A., Jeffcott, L.B., Lundeheim, N., and Osborne, M. (1996). Growth rates in thoroughbred foals. *Pferdeheilkunde* 12 (3): 291–295.

50 de Almeida, F.Q., de Campos Valdares Filo, S., Donzele, J. et al. (1998). Apparent and true prececal and total digestibility of protein in diets with different protein levels in equines. *Rev. Bras. Zootec.* 27 (3): 521–529.

51 Ott, E.A., Asquith, R.L., Feaster, J.P., and Martin, F.G. (1979). Influence of protein level and quality on the growth and development of yearling foals. *J. Anim. Sci.* 49 (3): 620–628.

52 Breuer, L.H. and Golden, D.L. (1971). Lysine requirement of the immature equine. *J. Anim. Sci.* 33 (1): 227.

53 van Niekerk, F.E. and van Niekerk, C.H. (1997). The effect of dietary protein on reproduction in the mare. I. The composition and evaluation of the digestibility of dietary protein from different sources. *J. S. Afr. Vet. Assoc.* 68 (3): 78–80.

54 Boyer, J., Cymbaluk, N., Kyle, B. et al. (1999). Nitrogen metabolism in pregnant mares fed grass hays containing different concentrations of protein. *J. Anim. Sci.* 77 (Suppl 1): 202.

55 Platt, H. (1984). Growth of the equine foetus. *Equine Vet. J.* 16 (4): 247–252.

56 Doreau, M., Boulot, S., Martin-Rosset, W., and Robelin, J. (1986). Relationship between nutrient intake, growth and body composition of the nursing foal. *Reprod. Nutr. Dev.* 26 (2B): 683–690.

57 Smolders, E.A.A., van der Veen, N.G., and van Polanen, A. (1990). Composition of horse milk during the suckling period. *Livest. Prod. Sci.* 25: 163–171.

58 Martin, R.G., McMeniman, N.P., and Dowsett, K.F. (1992). Milk and water intakes of foals sucking grazing mares. *Equine Vet. J.* 24 (4): 295–299.

59 Mariani, P.A., Summer, A., Martuzzi, F. et al. (2001). Physicochemical properties, gross composition, energy value and nitrogen fractions of Haflinger nursing mare milk throughout 6 lactation months. *Anim. Res.* 50: 415–425.

60 Freeman, D.W., Potter, G.D., Schelling, G.T., and Kreider, J.L. (1988). Nitrogen metabolism in mature horses at varying levels of work. *J. Anim. Sci.* 66: 407–412.

61 Graham-Thiers, P.M., Kronfeld, D.S., Kline, K.A., and Sklan, D.J. (2001). Dietary protein restriction and fat supplementation diminish the acidogenic effect of exercise during repeated sprints in horses. *J. Nutr.* 131: 1959–1964.

62 Wickens, C.L., Moore, J., Shelle, J., Skelly, J. et al. (2003). Effect of exercise on dietary protein requirement of the Arabian horse. In: *Proceedings of the 18th Equine Nutrition and Physiology Society Symposium*, 128. East Lansing, MI: Equine Nutrition and Physiology Society.

63 Wickens, C., Moore, J., Wolf, C. et al. (2005). 3-Methylhistidine as a response criteria to estimate dietary protein requirement of the exercising horse. *In: Proceedings of the 19th Equine Nutrition and Physiology Society Symposium*, 205. Tucson, AZ: Equine Nutrition and Physiology Society.

64 Miller, P.A. and Lawrence, L.A.M. (1988). The effect of dietary protein level on exercising horses. *J. Anim. Sci.* 66 (9): 2185–2192.

65 Orton, R.K., Hume, I.D., and Leng, R.A. (1985). Effects of level of dietary protein and exercise on growth rates of horses. *Equine Vet. J.* 17 (5): 381–385.

66 Bergero, D., Assenza, A., Schiavone, A. et al. (2005). Amino acid concentrations in blood serum of horses performing long lasting low-intensity exercise. *J. Anim. Physiol. Anim. Nutr.* 89: 146–150.

8

Minerals

Ashley Fowler, Mieke Brummer-Holder, and Laurie A. Lawrence

KEY TERMS

- Apparent digestibility: determined by subtracting the amount of mineral that appears in the feces from the amount consumed, expressed as a percentage of the amount consumed.
- True digestibility: determined similarly to apparent digestibility except the mineral excreted in the feces is adjusted for the component that is of endogenous origin (epithelial cells, enzymes, etc.) as opposed to feed origin.
- Endogenous losses: mineral losses from intestinal cells, digestive enzymes, etc. that may appear in the feces (fecal endogenous losses) or urine (urinary endogenous losses).
- Mineral balance: determined using a balance trial to determine total intake and total excretion (losses). Zero balance occurs when intake equals losses. Negative balance occur when losses exceed intake; positive balance occurs when intake exceeds losses.
- Organic mineral source: minerals found in material harvested from living organisms (usually plants, but also yeast or bacteria) or that are attached to an organic compound such as a carbohydrate, amino acid, or protein.
- Inorganic mineral: minerals from inorganic sources (limestone, rock phosphate) or attached to another mineral (monocalcium phosphate, copper sulfate).

KEY POINTS

- Macrominerals are needed for body structure and maintaining acid–base balance, fluid balance, and transmembrane potentials for cellular function, nerve conduction, and muscle contraction.
- Most micro- or trace minerals are needed as components of metalloenzymes that are involved in controlling enormous numbers of diverse biological reactions.
- The goal in ration balancing is to meet the horse's nutrient needs, i.e. provide nutrients within the optimal range, based on sound scientific information of the highest possible grade while not harming the animal or the environment.
- The concentrations of many minerals in the blood are under homeostatic control so the best method to determine ration adequacy is a ration analysis based on properly collected and tested feed and water samples.

8.1 Introduction

Minerals are involved in a variety of body processes and are important components of body structure. The goal of all feeding programs is to provide nutrient-adequate rations, although some minerals may not be considered essential dietary components but can still affect body function or structure. The expected animal response to changing amounts of an essential nutrient in the ration is illustrated in Figure 8.1. Performance (growth, reproduction, etc.) is poor when the nutrient is deficient. A primary deficiency occurs when the diet contains an inadequate amount of a nutrient; a secondary deficiency occurs when the amount of the nutrient is adequate, but another dietary factor interferes with the absorption or use of the nutrient. For example, very high dietary zinc concentrations can interfere with copper absorption and thus cause a secondary copper deficiency. With increasing dietary mineral intake, performance improves until there is a peak or plateau in the response, indicating that the diet provides an adequate amount of the nutrient for that desired response. Once the peak or plateau is reached, there is no benefit to increasing the intake of the nutrient.

Mineral intakes exceeding the requirement may have negative effects on the animal (Figure 8.1). Feeding an

Equine Clinical Nutrition, Second Edition. Edited by Rebecca L. Remillard.

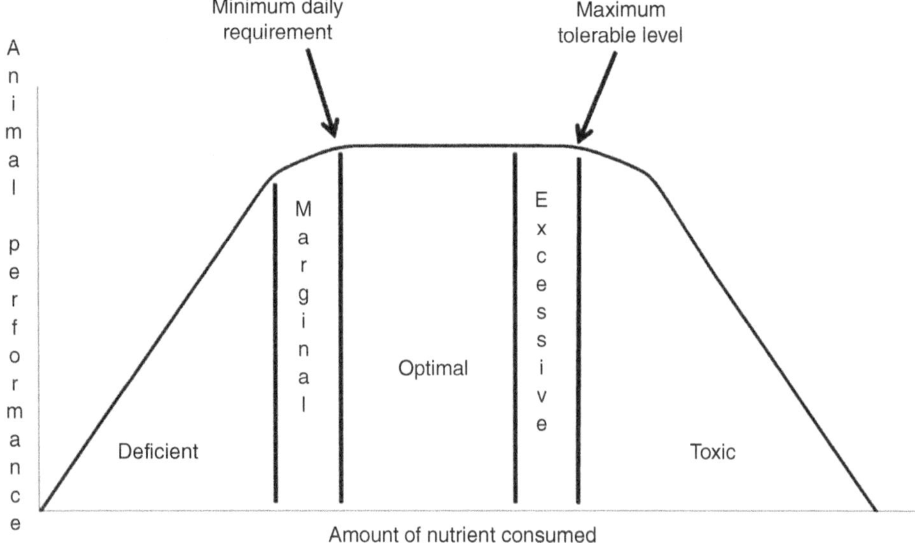

Figure 8.1 A general diagram of how nutrient intake affects animal response.

essential mineral at a concentration beyond that demonstrated to be effective is biologically inappropriate and not sustainable agriculturally. The detrimental effects of excessive mineral intake are not limited to the animal consuming the excess. Minerals that are fed more than an animal needs are almost always excreted by the animal into the environment. Phosphorus has received significant attention for its negative effects on water quality, particularly concerning run-off from animal-feeding operations. See Chapter 5 Water. Responsible stewardship of horse operations and ration formulation should avoid the over-supplementation of phosphorus and other minerals with potential environmental impacts. The goal in ration balancing is to meet the horse's nutrient needs, i.e. provide nutrients within the optimal range, based on sound scientific information of the highest possible grade while not harming the animal or the environment.

The major functions, sources, recommended ration concentrations of nutritionally relevant minerals, and then the clinical signs of inadequate vs. excessive intake of specific minerals, appropriate diagnostic test(s), and then a recommended course of treatment are presented. Whenever possible, estimates of the daily mineral requirements of horses will be reported (Table 8.1). Unfortunately, the number of studies examining the mineral requirements of horses are relatively few compared with other species, and for many minerals, optimum intakes have not been identified. Several factors are responsible for this lack of information. One issue relates to the practical aspects of conducting nutrient requirement studies that must utilize diets that span the range from deficient to excessive (Figure 8.1). The most common signs of mineral deficiencies and toxicities in horses are present in Table 8.2. Normal blood ranges of minerals are suggested in Table 8.3 as a guide only because most blood concentrations are under homeostatic controls, and may not accurately reflect whole-body or organ concentrations, and reference ranges may differ between laboratories. Nutritional assessment of the ration, either using laboratory assays or computer reconstruction, is often the best determinant of diet adequacy. See Ration Analysis in Chapter 10.

A bigger challenge is the identification of industry-relevant response variables for all horses. Maximizing average daily gain, milk production, and feed efficiency responses are important in many livestock but not in horses. Longevity, skeletal soundness, and athletic performance are important in horses but difficult to objectively quantify and would require large numbers of similar horses and several years, all of which are cost-prohibitive. Every effort is made to present recommendations based on research in horses, but in cases where horse studies were insufficient, estimates have been made from data in other species.

8.2 Macrominerals

Most of the body's minerals are the major, or macro-, minerals: calcium, phosphorus, sodium, chlorine, potassium, magnesium, and sulfur. So-called "macro" because they are required in larger amounts, i.e. grams, compared with "micro" or "trace" minerals. Typically, macrominerals are expressed as a percent (parts per hundred) in the diet. Macrominerals are needed for body structure and maintaining acid–base balance, fluid balance, and transmembrane potentials for cellular function, nerve conduction, and muscle contraction.

Table 8.1 Daily mineral requirements for horses at different life stages and performance.

	Ca	P	Mg	K	Na	Cl	S	Cu	Fe	Mn	Zn	Co	I	Se
Type	**g/100 kg mature BW[a]**							**mg/100 kg mature BW**						
Maintenance	4.0	2.8	1.5	5.0	2.0	8.0	3.0	20	80	80	80	0.10	0.70	0.20
Working														
light	6.0	3.6	1.9	5.7	2.8	9.3	3.0	20	80	80	80	0.10	0.70	0.20
moderate	7.0	4.2	2.3	6.4	3.6	10.7	3.4	23	90	90	90	0.12	0.80	0.23
heavy	8.0	5.8	3.0	7.8	5.1	13.3	3.8	25	100	100	100	0.12	0.88	0.25
very heavy	8.0	5.8	3.0	10.6	8.2	18.6	3.8	25	100	100	100	0.12	0.88	0.25
Breeding Stallion	6.0	3.6	1.9	5.7	2.8	9.3	3.0	20	80	80	80	0.10	0.70	0.20
Pregnant[b]														
<6 mos[c]	4.0	2.8	1.5	5.0	2.0	8.0	3.0	20	80	80	80	0.10	0.70	0.20
7–8 mos	5.6	4.0	1.5	5.0	2.0	8.0	3.0	20	80	80	80	0.10	0.70	0.20
9–11 mos	7.2	5.3	1.5	5.2	2.2	8.2	3.0	25	100	80	80	0.10	0.80	0.20
Lactation														
1 mos	11.8	7.7	2.2	9.6	2.6	9.1	3.8	25	125	100	100	0.12	0.88	0.25
2 mos	11.8	7.6	2.2	9.5	2.6	9.1	3.8	25	125	100	100	0.12	0.88	0.25
3 mos	11.2	7.2	2.2	9.2	2.5	9.1	3.8	25	125	100	100	0.12	0.88	0.25
4 mos	8.3	5.2	2.1	7.2	2.4	9.1	3.8	25	125	100	100	0.12	0.88	0.25
5 mos	7.9	4.9	2.0	7.0	2.3	9.1	3.8	25	125	100	100	0.12	0.88	0.25
6 mos	7.5	4.6	1.7	6.7	2.3	9.1	3.8	25	125	100	100	0.12	0.88	0.25
Growing[d]														
4 mos	7.8	4.3	0.7	2.2	0.8	3.1	1.3	8	42	34	34	0.04	0.30	0.08
6 mos	7.7	4.3	0.8	2.6	1.0	4.0	1.6	11	54	43	43	0.06	0.38	0.11
12 mos	7.5	4.2	1.1	3.5	1.4	5.3	2.4	16	80	64	64	0.08	0.56	0.16
18 mos	7.4	4.1	1.2	4.0	1.6	6.4	2.9	19	97	78	78	0.10	0.68	0.19
18 mos light exercise	7.4	4.1	2.3	4.6	2.2	7.4	2.9	19	97	78	78	0.10	0.68	0.19
18 mos moderate exercise	7.4	4.1	2.3	5.1	2.8	8.4	2.9	19	97	78	78	0.10	0.68	0.19
24 mos	7.3	4.1	1.3	4.4	1.8	7.1	3.2	21	107	86	86	0.10	0.76	0.21
24 mos light exercise	7.3	4.1	2.6	5.0	2.4	8.2	3.2	21	107	86	86	0.10	0.76	0.21
24 mos moderate exercise	7.3	4.1	2.6	5.6	3.1	9.4	3.2	21	107	86	86	0.10	0.76	0.21
24 mos heavy exercise	7.3	4.1	2.6	6.8	4.4	11.6	3.2	21	107	86	86	0.10	0.76	0.21
24 mos very heavy exercise	7.3	4.1	2.6	9.2	7.1	16.2	3.2	21	107	86	86	0.10	0.76	0.21

[a] Conversions to kg mature BW basis was made using the minerals required for a 500 kg mature horse from NRC [1]; Table 16-3.
[b] Calculated based on pre-pregnancy weight.
[c] mos = months.
[d] Calculated intake based on expected mature weight. Example: A growing 4 m old with an expected mature weight of 500 kg requires [7.8 g Ca × 5 (100 kg mature weight)] = 39 g Ca/d.

8.2.1 Calcium

Calcium (Ca) and phosphorus (P) make up about 70% of the mineral content of the body, and from 30% to 50% of the minerals in milk. About 99% of the Ca in the body is in the bones and teeth, with Ca comprising 35% of bone [1]. Calcium also is necessary for blood coagulation, cell membrane function, glandular secretion, temperature regulation, the regulation of the activity of many enzymes, and mitochondrial and neuromuscular functions. Blood Ca concentration is controlled within a narrow range and as such, blood Ca values say little about the Ca status of the animal [2]. Calcium homeostasis is mainly regulated by two hormones: calcitonin and parathyroid hormone (PTH). Calcitonin acts to reduce serum Ca concentrations

Table 8.2 Dietary cause and clinical effects of mineral deficiencies and excesses in horses.

Mineral imbalance	Dietary Cause(s)	Clinical Signs
Calcium deficiency	Diet Ca < req as in high grain-low legume, diet Ca:P < 0.6:1, or Ca:oxalate < 0.5:1 & oxalate > 0.5%	DOD[a], Dec density laminae dura dentes, then ribs & long bones last. Stiff, lame, Dec movement, bighead, lose wt & condition; fractures.
Calcium excess	Ca:P > 6-10:1 adult diet or 3:1 weanling diet due to excess added Ca	DOD, P def., poss Dec absrptn of Zn, Mn or Fe, Inc to normal bone density.
Phosphorus deficiency	Diet P < needs, no added P for growth, excess Ca or > 0.15% AI	Same as Ca deficiency. If long & severe, Dec bone density but laminae dura dentes not lost.
Phosphorus excess	Bran as the majority of diet or excess P added to the diet	Calcium deficiency
Sodium deficiency	No salt available or in feed	Dec sweating & performance, Dec food & water intake, wt. loss, weak, dehydration, excess licking & ± pica & constipation.
Sodium excess	Salt in only water, or feeding salt without adequate water available	Colic, diarrhea, polyuria, weak, staggering, posterior paralysis, recumbency.
Potassium deficiency	Excess sweating especially when on a high-grain (low-K) diet, diuretics, or diarrheic	Fatigue, weakness, lethargy, Dec feed and water intake & wt loss.
Potassium excess	Doesn't occur clinically except in horses with potassium-induced periodic paralysis	
Magnesium deficiency	Dec Mg & Ca in plasma rarely occur with transit	Muscle tremors, ataxia, collapse, sweating, convulsions
Magnesium excess	Does not occur clinically	
Sulfur imbalance	Does not occur clinically	
Selenium deficiency	In foals due to < 0.05 ppm Se in mare's diet	Dec immunity & growth. Stiff, listless, difficult nursing, dyspnea, lung edema, Inc HR, RR & salivation, "white muscle." The adult is stiff.
Selenium excess	Diet Se > 2-5 ppm from high-Se plants or mixing errors	"Blind staggers" or wt loss, listless, anemia, hair rough & loss from mane or tail, dark fluid feces, stiff, feet painful, abn. hoof growth & rings.
Iodine deficiency	Diet I < 0.1 ppm	Most often in the newborn. Stillborn or weak, DOD. Hypothyroidism & goiter with I excess & occasionally deficiency. Hair rough & loss, & myxedema rarely.
Iodine excess	Diet I > 5 ppm or 0.08 mg/kg BW/d due to I suppl, kelp, EDDI, or I salt in the feed	
Copper deficiency	Diet Cu adult < 5 ppm & weanling < 25 ppm. Diet Zn > 700 ppm or Cu:Mo of 1:8 but not at < 1:4	DOD. Uterine artery rupture in aged parturient mares. Anemia & Dec hair color in ruminants but not horses.
Copper excess	Adding 800 to 2800 ppm Cu to diet	Acute hemolytic anemia & icterus, lethargy & death. Hepatic & renal damage.
Molybdenum deficiency	Never reported	
Molybdenum excess	Contaminated or alkaline soils. Diet Cu: Mo of 1:8 but not at < 1:4	Cu deficiency
Zinc deficiency	< 15 ppm in adult & < 40 ppm in weanling diets	DOD, Dec feed intake, Dec growth, parakeratosis, and hair loss
Zinc excess	Diet Zn > 700 ppm. If > 3600 ppm	DOD, stiff & lame. Also get anemia & Dec growth.
Manganese deficiency	Diet Mn < 200 ppm, especially on limed soils	Possibly bone abnormalities in newborn
Manganese excess	Never reported	
Iron deficiency	Chronic or severe blood loss - Rarely due to a deficiency in the ration	Dec performance ability followed by anemia
Iron excess	Excess administered, esp. if vit E def in foals. Rarely diet	Death of neonate. Dec bacterial resistance
Cobalt deficiency or excess	Never induced or reported	Vit. B_{12} deficiency
Fluoride deficiency	Never induced or reported	
Fluoride excess	F in Phos suppl or industrial contamination. Diet F > 50-200 ppm or water > 8 ppm	Teeth slow coming in, mottled & pitted causing Dec fee & water intake & chronic debilitation. Stiff, Lame, Inc bone density.

[a]Developmental orthopedic diseases; Dec = decreased; Inc = increased

Table 8.3 Suggested normal ranges of minerals in blood components for adult horses.[a]

Mineral	Sample type	Range
Ca, mg/dL (total)	Serum	10.2–13.4 [2]
P, mg/dL	Serum	1.5–4.7 [2]
Mg, mg/dL	Serum	1.4–2.3 [2]
K, mmol/L	Serum	2.9–4.6 [2]
Na, mmol/L	Serum	128–142 [2]
Cl, mEq/L	Serum	93–109 [2]
Cu, mg/L	Plasma	0.7–1.5 [3] 1.02–1.78 [4]
Fe, μg/dL	Serum	50–200 [5, 6]
I, μg/L (protein-bound)	Plasma	16–27 [7]
Mo, ng/L	Serum	16–31 [8]
Se, ng/mL	Serum	130–160 [9]
Se, ng/mL	Whole blood	180–240 [10]
Zn, mg/L	Serum	0.5–2.0 [11]
Zn, mg/L	Plasma	0.327–1.308 [4]
Zn, mg/L	Whole blood	2.15–4.32 [12]

[a] Reference ranges may vary among laboratories. Reference ranges specific to the consulted laboratory should be used.

by inhibiting bone resorption [13]. Conversely, PTH increases bone resorption and renal reabsorption of Ca in response to low serum Ca [14].

Ionized Ca, or free Ca (Ca^{+2}), is the physiologically relevant form of Ca in the blood and normally constitutes about 50% of total plasma Ca. The remaining circulating Ca is bound primarily to albumin but also to citrate, nitrate, and sulfate. Because only ionized Ca is biologically active, only alterations in its concentration will affect the animal. For example, if the plasma ionized Ca concentration is significantly increased or decreased, the opposite effect occurs in muscle membrane excitability, i.e. hypercalcemia decreases muscle tone and hypocalcemia increases muscle tone. However, consideration of both ionized and total Ca is important for animals with alterations in plasma albumin or acid–base status. The binding of Ca to albumin in the blood is pH-dependent. During acidosis, the affinity between Ca and albumin is decreased, leading to an increase in ionized Ca with no change in total Ca [14]. Additionally, hypoalbuminemia will reduce the amount of bound Ca but not affect ionized Ca, causing total Ca values to decrease.

8.2.1.1 Sources and Factors Influencing Absorption

Grasses generally contain sufficient Ca for horses with lower requirements (i.e. non-breeding, non-working, mature horses). Legumes, such as alfalfa and clover, usually contain at least three times the concentration of Ca in grasses, and the inclusion of legumes into pasture or hay can substantially boost Ca intake for horses with greater requirements (growing, lactating, or working horses). Cereal grains and grain byproducts have low Ca concentrations and have inverted calcium to phosphorus ratios (Ca : P), meaning more P than Ca. Inorganic sources of Ca include calcium carbonate (limestone), calcium sulfate, dicalcium phosphate, calcium chloride, and calcium oxide. The availability of Ca from Ca-amino acid proteinates (organic source of Ca) does not appear to differ from inorganic Ca sources [15, 16]. Calcium supplements are incorporated into the grain or concentrate portion of the ration to ensure adequate Ca intake and a balanced Ca : P ratio.

If quantities of both Ca and P in the diet are adequate to meet the animal's requirements, the amount of Ca to P, or the Ca : P ratio, in the diet of the mature horse probably can vary from 0.8 : 1 to 8 : 1, and in the growing horse from 0.8 : 1 to 6 : 1, without resulting in problems [1]. However, a Ca : P ratio of less than 1 : 1 is not recommended for any horse, and a ratio of greater than 6 : 1 is not recommended for the growing horse, provided the total intake of both minerals are adequate. If the amount of dietary Ca or P is insufficient to meet the horse's requirement, or if the amount of one mineral to the other is outside of these ratios, skeletal alterations may occur. The majority of Ca is absorbed in the small intestine, whereas net P absorption occurs in the large intestine [17, 18]. Excess P in the diet can bind Ca and decrease its absorption in the small intestine. In contrast, excess dietary Ca has little effect on P absorption [19]. Most excess Ca ingested is absorbed from the small intestine and excreted in the urine, and therefore, is not present to decrease P absorption from the large intestine.

Dietary oxalates bind to Ca, decreasing its absorption, and can result in Ca deficiency. Typically, a diet with a total oxalate content over 0.5% dry matter (DM) basis and a Ca to oxalate ratio of less than 0.5 : 1 can cause Ca deficiency [1]. The Ca to oxalate ratio found in 33 samples of alfalfa taken from 14 states was 1.7 : 1 to 7.8 : 1. The true digestibility or availability of Ca from alfalfa with a Ca to oxalate ratio of 1.7 : 1 and 3 : 1 was 76% and 80%, respectively. Thus, even alfalfa with the lowest Ca to oxalate ratio had high Ca availability and was an excellent source of calcium for the horse [20].

The incidence and severity of oxalate-related Ca deficiency are highest in lactating mares and weanlings because, compared with other physiological states, these animals have a higher Ca requirement and with higher feed intakes, there is a greater intake of oxalates [21]. Additionally, the insoluble oxalate crystals may be deposited in the kidneys, causing renal damage [11]; however, decreased renal function from oxalates in feeds is rare. Consumption of large amounts of high oxalate plants (halogeton [*Halogeton glomeratus*], greasewood [*Sarcobatus vermiculatus*], *Rumex* species, or *Oxalis* species) may cause acute oxalate poisoning. The prevalence of Ca deficiency in herds grazing pastures containing these types of grasses varies widely. Up to 100% may be affected, with the onset of clinical signs varying from 2 to 8 m after being on the pasture while other cattle grazing the same pastures may remain healthy [21].

Phytate, the salt form of phytic acid, can bind positively charged minerals, such as Ca, preventing their absorption. In horses, phytase has been shown to improve Ca digestibility in diets with a Ca : P ratio of 1.6 : 1, but no effects of phytase on Ca digestibility were seen with diets containing Ca : P of 4.7 : 1 [22, 23]. These data suggest that phytase may be beneficial at improving Ca digestibility when the Ca : P ratio is low and Ca absorption is hindered by P.

A low dietary cation–anion difference (DCAD; defined as mEq (Na + K) – Cl/kg DM) has been shown to increase urinary Ca excretion and has been suggested as a potential cause of Ca deficiency in growing horses [24]. However, other studies have shown that horses can compensate for an increase in urinary Ca excretion by increasing intestinal absorption of Ca, resulting in little to no effect on overall Ca balance [25–27].

Proton-pump inhibitors (omeprazole) are used in horses to treat gastric ulcers. Because these compounds affect gastric pH, Ca solubility may decrease [28]. No changes in bone density, Ca balance, or serum Ca (neither total nor ionized Ca) were observed in mature, sedentary horses receiving omeprazole treatment for less than 2 m [29, 30]. However, the effects of omeprazole on Ca absorption in horses with greater Ca requirements (i.e. exercising, lactating, and growing) are unknown.

Furosemide is administered to racehorses to reduce the incidence of exercise-induced pulmonary hemorrhage. The administration of this drug stimulates urine and electrolyte excretion. Chronic administration of furosemide in sedentary ponies over 56 d caused an increase in the total amount of Ca excreted in the urine [31]. However, chronic (daily) administration of furosemide would be extremely unusual in horses. A single dose of furosemide in exercised Thoroughbreds did not influence the digestibility of Ca but did increase urinary Ca excretion, leading to a negative Ca balance that persisted for 72-h post-administration [32]. These results suggest that horses receiving furosemide may have an increased need for Ca, at least temporarily, to replace urinary losses; however, more research is needed before such a recommendation can be made.

8.2.1.2 Recommendations

For horses at maintenance, the Ca requirement serves to replace the endogenous losses of Ca while adjusting for the absorption efficiency. Endogenous losses are estimated to be 20 mg Ca/kg body weight (BW) for all classes of horses. While Ca digestibility can vary with age and other factors, true Ca digestibility may be as high as 70–80%. However, a true digestibility of 50% is used in calculating requirements to ensure adequate intakes [1].

Growth, gestation, and lactation all increase the Ca requirement over that of maintenance to support deposited Ca in new tissue or milk. Situations in which bone density is actively increasing, such as initiation of an exercise program, may also increase Ca requirements. Table 8.1 gives the recommended amounts of Ca for horses in various physiological states. In some instances, horses may enter training while still growing (2-yr-old), but the Ca requirement for these horses is suggested to be the same as the requirements for growth alone [1]. Additional research is needed to assess the Ca needs of growing horses initiating training.

8.2.1.3 Signs of Deficiency and Excess

8.2.1.3.1 Deficiency

Inadequate Ca absorption decreases plasma Ca concentration, causing the body to respond in a variety of ways to maintain Ca blood homeostasis. A lowered plasma Ca concentration inhibits calcitonin and stimulates PTH secretion, resulting in a net effect of increased bone resorption to release Ca into the blood. Long-term dietary Ca deficiencies and prolonged elevated PTH can result in a form of hyperparathyroidism and a calcium depletion of bone. Hyperparathyroidism may be primary or secondary. Primary hyperparathyroidism is caused by a functioning parathyroid gland tumor, which is rare in the horse [33].

Nutritional secondary hyperparathyroidism (NSH) is the most common form of hyperparathyroidism seen in horses. The overall effects of NSH are to maintain serum Ca concentrations by increasing bone resorption and stimulating renal Ca reabsorption. As bone minerals are mobilized, fibrous connective tissue (osteodystrophia fibrosa) increases. In younger mature horses, osteodystrophia fibrosa is frequently most noticeable as an enlargement of the facial bones above and behind the facial crests, giving rise to the name "bighead" for this condition (Figure 8.2); in older mature horses little or no facial bone enlargement may occur. Symptoms of enlarged facial bones include a cardboard sound when the facial sinuses are percussed, upper airway noise due to obstructed facial sinuses, and resorption of dental alveoli, which can result in loose teeth, painful, abnormal chewing, and decreased feed intake that could result in weight loss [35].

Other clinical signs of extensive bone demineralization may occur before an observable enlargement of the facial bones or the growing horse's metaphyseal growth plates. An insidious, shifting leg lameness and generalized bone and joint tenderness occur. Severely affected horses may have a gait similar to that of a hopping rabbit, and

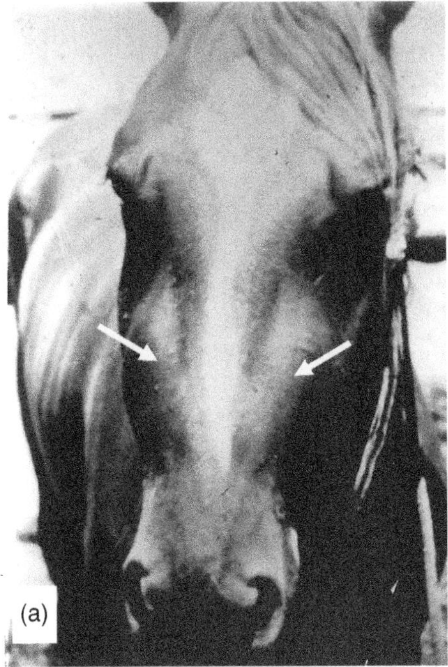

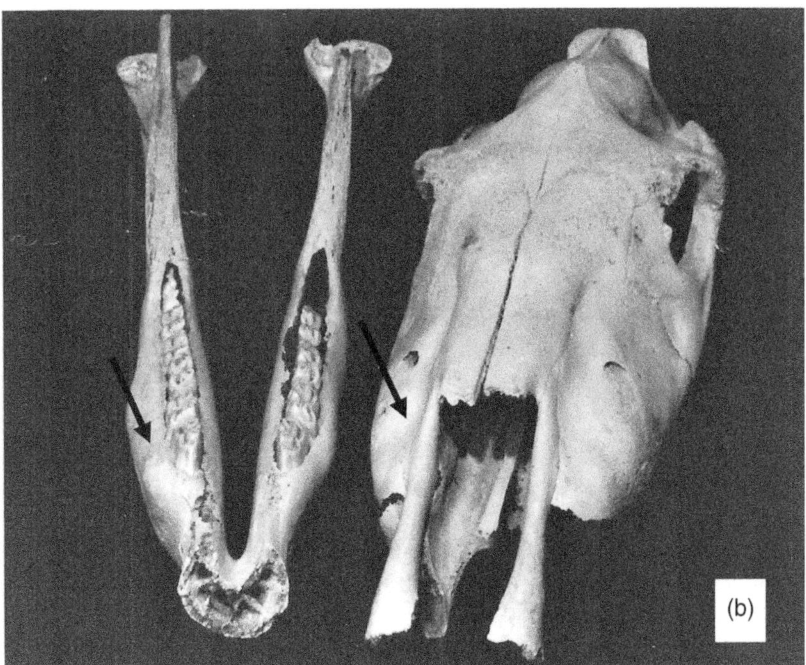

Figure 8.2 Skull bones of horses affected by calcium (Ca) deficiency or phosphorous (P) excess. Calcium deficiency, due to either inadequate dietary Ca, excess P or oxalate which decreases Ca absorption, causes nutritional secondary hyperparathyroidism. An increase in parathyroid hormone in response to low serum Ca causes Ca and P mobilization from the bone and increases urinary P excretion. Bone minerals are replaced by fibrous tissue, which increases the size of the bone. In mature young horses, as shown in (a), the increased bone size is often most noticeable on each side of the nose and the mandible, giving rise to the common name for the condition "big-head" disease. The skull of a 2-yr-old filly (b) shows these enlargements. *Source:* Reprinted with permission from the American Veterinary Medical Association [34].

reluctance to move. Exercise may induce or exacerbate the lameness. Although demineralization is generalized, different degrees of demineralization may occur in different areas of the skeletal system. However, lameness may be present for several months before radiographic changes are evident [36].

8.2.1.3.2 Excess

In the horse, the maximum tolerance concentration of Ca has been suggested to be 2% of the diet DM [37]. This recommendation is based on work in other species in which diets containing greater than 2% Ca resulted in reduced feed intake. However, no adverse effects of Ca intake up to 500% of Ca requirements have been reported in horses [38]. Excess dietary Ca has been proposed to cause hypercalcitonis-induced osteochondrosis in growing horses [39]. A review of more recent studies concludes that excess Ca is not a likely culprit in most cases of osteochondrosis [1]. Excess Ca has been shown to decrease some species' absorption of zinc, manganese, copper, and iron, and may contribute to deficiencies if the diet contains only marginal amounts of these minerals; however, it is unknown if this occurs in the horse.

There are a few reports of hypercalcemia in horses consuming calcinogenic plants [40]. These plants induce the release of $1,25(OH)_2D_3$ (calcitriol), which can substantially increase Ca absorption from the intestine, causing hypercalcemia. Calcinogenic plants known to induce calcinosis are *Cestrum diurnum* (day jasmine) and *Trisetum flavescens* (yellow oat grass); however, situations in which consumption of these plants result in calcinosis are rare.

8.2.1.4 Diagnosis and Treatment

8.2.1.4.1 Deficiency

If Ca deficiency is suspected, an inadequate Ca intake is best diagnosed and corrected by evaluating dietary Ca and P content. The total diet should include sufficient amounts of Ca and P relative to the horse's requirement (Table 8.1) and the Ca : P should be no less than 1 : 1. If dietary Ca and P appear adequate and the Ca : P is appropriate, the diet should be evaluated for excess oxalate concentration [41].

Plasma Ca, P, and alkaline phosphatase concentrations are of little benefit in diagnosing dietary Ca imbalances because changes in their values do not always represent either inadequate or excessive Ca consumption. Urine and fecal Ca and P concentrations on their own are also of little value due to a large amount of variation between samples within an individual horse. However, it has been suggested that Ca deficiency (or P excess) can be diagnosed by examining fractional excretion of Ca and P (using creatinine clearance ratios). A low dietary Ca : P usually results in elevated fractional excretion of P and inadequate Ca intake usually results in decreased fractional excretion of Ca [42]. During Ca deficiency caused by an imbalanced Ca : P, the fractional excretion of P will increase above 1% and the urinary creatinine to P ratio will be less than one [43]. Excretion of P increases as a result of Ca deficiency because the Ca deficiency induces hyperparathyroidism, which increases both Ca and P mobilization from the bone. The mobilized Ca remains in the body to maintain homeostasis and the mobilized P is excreted.

The fractional excretion of Ca in normal animals ranges from 5.3% to 40% [44]. A low fractional excretion indicates Ca deficiency and a high fractional excretion indicates Ca excess. However, in one study, the fractional excretion of Ca in 10 healthy mature geldings with free access to a nutritionally adequate, complete pelleted diet varied from −0.16 to 6.7 (95% confidence interval) with as much as a 30-fold variation in samples taken from the same horse [45]. This variation may have been due, at least in part, to variations in when the sample was taken relative to feed consumption. Thus, standardization of collecting samples must be observed to reduce variation in values. To minimize extraneous effects on sample analysis, urine samples for Ca or P analysis should be taken after at least one day of rest without transport, and after a 4- to 8-hr fast [42]. Urinary Ca excretion may be decreased by exercise and influenced by dietary Ca intake and the type of feed consumed within the previous 4 to 8 hrs [42, 46]. If a urine sample is obtained within 8 hrs of eating a high-Ca feed, such as alfalfa, but before eating a low-Ca feed, such as grain, urine Ca indicates adequate Ca intake and absorption, even if total dietary Ca intake was inadequate.

Measuring bone density to diagnose dietary Ca deficiency is likely of beneficial value only if interpreted with other data indicating Ca deficiency, such as ration evaluation. Bone density is typically evaluated using radiography, but quantitative computed tomography (QCT) has also recently been used successfully in horses [47]. The Ca content of bone can be determined by neutron activation or bone densitometry via dual-energy X-ray absorptiometry (DEXA) [48, 49]. However, QCT, neutron activation, and DEXA are not commonly used in a clinical setting and radiography remains the main method of evaluating bone density in horses. Most studies examining bone density were performed in growing horses and before digital radiography was available, so care should be taken when extrapolating results to mature horses evaluated using modern methods. No standards describe optimum bone density.

Parathyroid hormone is elevated in horses suffering from NSH [35]. If the plasma PTH and the plasma Ca concentrations are both increased, it is indicative of primary hyperparathyroidism and if only PTH is increased, it suggests NSH.

Dietary Ca deficiency (or P excess) can be treated by increasing Ca and/or decreasing P. Dietary Ca : P ratios should be at least 2 : 1 to ensure adequate Ca absorption. Prolonged excessive Ca intake (greater than five times maintenance requirements) during recovery has been suggested to result in excessive bone density and inadequate bone remodeling, which may prevent bone strength from returning to normal upon recovery [35]. Therefore, more moderate increases in Ca are recommended. Previous recommendations suggest feeding twice the required Ca [35]. If radiographic changes have been detected in the limbs, exercise should be limited until radiographic density returns to normal. Lameness may not completely disappear if the condition was very severe [35]. In many cases, there is little regression in enlarged facial bones [35, 36].

When the Ca deficiency is due to excess oxalate intake, the preferred treatment is to eliminate high-oxalate-containing feeds, and feed a diet with twice the Ca and P required at a ratio of 1 : 1 to 3 : 1. After two to three minutes, ensure that the diet meets the horse's Ca and P requirements. If lower-oxalate feeds are not available, both Ca and P intakes must be increased above normal requirements, to prevent negative Ca and P balances.

8.2.1.4.2 Excess

The only way to determine if the diet contains excess Ca is to evaluate the ration. Excessive Ca does not result in changes in the plasma Ca or P concentrations sufficient to be of diagnostic benefit. A urine creatinine/Ca ratio of less than 3.5 and a fractional excretion greater than 40% occur as a result of excessive Ca intake [44]. However, alterations in these parameters could be caused by other factors. Excess of Ca also generally has no significant effect on either plasma PTH concentration or urinary P excretion.

Excess Ca intake (along with other minerals) has been implicated in the formation of enteroliths. The presence of enteroliths is associated with high colonic pH, and greater concentrations of Ca, Mg, P, K, Na, and S compared with horses with no enteroliths [50]. Enterolith formation has also been associated with horses receiving a greater percentage of alfalfa in their diet and having less access to pasture compared with horses with no enteroliths [50, 51]. However, most horses consuming an alfalfa-based diet or a diet high in Ca do not form enteroliths, so the development of enteroliths is likely due to a combination of factors and cannot be attributed to one precipitating cause.

8.2.2 Phosphorus

Over 80% of the P in the body is in the bones and teeth, with P comprising 14–17% of the skeleton [1]. Phosphorus is also necessary as a buffer, as energy currency (i.e. ATP, phosphocreatine), in cell membranes as phospholipids, for nucleotide formation, and in numerous other cellular functions. Phosphorus concentrations in the blood are not controlled as strictly as Ca and can change with age and diet [52]. When the bone is mobilized to maintain normal blood Ca concentration, P is also released, which can affect blood P.

8.2.2.1 Sources and Factors Influencing Absorption

The P content of forages is influenced by growing conditions, such as soil P, season, and stage of maturity. Hay obtained from low P soils contains less P than hay from high P soils. Timothy hay from Alberta, Canada, where soil P is low may have a P concentration of 0.14% whereas grass hay from New England may contain 0.25% P [53, 54]. In Central Kentucky, where highly phosphatic limestone has produced phosphate-rich soils, P concentrations in cool-season forages may exceed 0.4% DM. Additionally, the phosphorus content of forages is higher in the earlier stages of plant growth compared with later stages. Independent of the effects of maturity, P content is also influenced by the time of the year, with the greatest concentrations of P occurring during periods of active plant growth. Legumes have a Ca : P ratio greater than 1 : 1 but inverted Ca : P ratios occurred occasionally in grasses grown on high P soils in Central Kentucky [55].

Unfortified grains are typically higher in P concentration than forages and usually have an inverted Ca : P ratio. Commercial grain-based concentrates are fortified with additional Ca to correct the Ca : P, and also often contain added inorganic P to ensure that P requirements are met if a low P forage is used. Inorganic P sources include phosphate rock (often defluorinated), dicalcium phosphate, ammonium phosphate, and sodium phosphate. While the addition of inorganic P to horse feeds may be warranted in some cases, phosphate is a limited resource and world reserves of phosphate are expected to be depleted within the next 50–100 yrs, so unnecessary supplementation should be avoided [56, 57].

Phytate, a hexaphosphate ester of inositol, which is found mainly in cereal grains and byproducts can bind P and negatively affect P digestibility in some monogastric species. For phytate-P, as well as minerals bound to phytate, to be absorbed, phytate must be broken down by the enzyme, phytase. While mammals cannot produce phytase, fungi (*Aspergillus* sp.), and bacteria, many of which are found in the equine gastrointestinal tract (*Klebsiella* sp., *Pseudomonas* sp., and *Enterobacter* sp) can produce phytase. Horses are capable of absorbing P from both the small and large intestines [18]. Thus even though phytate-P will not be available for absorption in the small intestine, it will become available in the large intestine where phytase activity from the microbiota appears to be high. Total tract degradation of phytate in the horse is around 95%, suggesting that the large bowel microbiota of the horse can liberate P from phytate [23, 58]. Exogenous phytase is available commercially for use in feeds for other monogastric animal species to increase P availability but has not been shown to improve P digestibility in horses [22, 23, 59].

Previously it was believed that inorganic P was more available than organic sources of P [1]. However, a ration fed to growing horses that contained only organic forms of P also had a true digestibility close to 45% [58]. These results suggest that organic P sources do not hinder P digestibility, at least in growing horses. The apparent digestibility of P is greatest in young horses and decreases with age [60]. Differences in observed P digestibility may be related to differences in P retained, as horses with increased P needs (growing, lactating) may retain more P and thus excrete less in the feces [55]. In horses retaining less P, absorbed but unneeded P is secreted into the gastrointestinal tract for excretion and results in a low observed P digestibility. Thus, P digestibility may be greater than previously believed, due to surplus absorbed P being secreted into the gastrointestinal tract.

Large amounts of dietary Ca to P may reduce P digestibility, but if dietary P is adequate, absorption of P appears to be sufficient to meet requirements. In one study, growing ponies were fed close to their P requirement and P digestibility tended to be lower in ponies fed diets containing a Ca : P of 4.3 : 1 compared with a ratio of 0.43 : 1 [61]. However, due to an increase in renal P excretion in the ponies fed an inverted Ca : P, P balance did not differ between treatments and was positive in both treatments. In mature ponies fed five times their P requirement, increasing dietary Ca from four times the requirement up to eight times the requirement (Ca : P increased from 1.2 : 1 to 2.5 : 1) decreased P digestibility from 25% to 11% [62]. Ponies in all treatments maintained a positive P balance despite depression in P digestibility, probably due to very high P intakes. Calcium is absorbed in the small intestine and P is mainly absorbed in the large intestine, with small amounts of P being absorbed in the distal small intestine [18]. Thus, the majority of Ca and P interactions will occur in the small intestine because less Ca is available in the large intestine to prevent P absorption. However, in situations where large amounts of Ca are fed, larger amounts of Ca are excreted in the feces, meaning that more Ca is available in the large intestine to interfere with P absorption as the dietary recommendations are exceeded.

Diets containing 2.6% and 4.3% oxalate were reported to cause negative P balances in ponies [63]. Feeding 4500 ppm aluminum (Al) to horses can reduce P absorption by 59% [64]. However, feeding a diet with 931 ppm Al (12 mg/kg BW/d) did not influence P absorption [65]. Concentrations of Al in the diet that exceed the maximum tolerable limit of 1000 ppm are likely to come from forages grown on high Al-containing soils or from environmental contamination of the feed [37]. On high-aluminum-containing acidic soils, forage may contain as much as 2500 ppm Al [66]. True P digestibility increased from 28% to 40% when dietary NaCl increased from 1% to 5%; however, all diets contained considerably more Na and Cl than required [67].

8.2.2.2 Recommendations

Table 8.1 suggests recommended daily P intakes for horses in various physiological states. Endogenous P losses used to calculate maintenance P requirements are 10 mg P/kg BW for mature horses. The P requirements of lactating and pregnant mares are estimated from maintenance endogenous losses and estimates of the P deposited in the fetus/placenta or milk. Likewise, the P requirements of growing horses account for P deposited in the body during growth as well as the maintenance component estimated from endogenous losses [1]. However, the endogenous P losses in growing horses have been estimated to be similar to those of mature horses or much higher at 18 mg/kg BW [68–70]. When growing horses were fed varying concentrations of Ca, ranging from 41% to 203% greater than required, endogenous losses were 18 mg/kg BW/d [68]. High concentrations of Ca (200% of requirement) have been shown to increase fecal endogenous P losses in growing horses, thus the high Ca concentrations fed may have caused greater endogenous fecal P losses [71]. If endogenous P losses are indeed lower for growing horses than currently suggested, then the current P requirement for growing horses may be overestimated.

True P digestibility is estimated to be 45% for growing horses and lactating mares and 35% for all other classes of horses, to account for the different forms of P consumed by these groups of horses [1]. Mature horses at maintenance have relatively low P needs that can be met primarily with forages containing organic P. However, lactating mares and growing horses have P needs that may not be met by feeding forages and unfortified concentrates, and thus will usually require additional P from inorganic sources. There may not be great differences in the availability of P from organic or inorganic sources in diets fed to horses. The estimate of true digestibility of diets based on organic P sources may be higher than 35%, which would result in an overestimation of P requirements for many horses. Horses fed over their P requirement will excrete the unneeded P into the environment where it can contaminate groundwater causing eutrophication and disruption of the aquatic ecosystems. Additionally, inorganic P is a limited resource with dwindling supplies worldwide [57]. Thus, when possible, oversupplementation with inorganic P sources should be avoided.

8.2.2.3 Signs of Deficiency and Excess

8.2.2.3.1 Deficiency

A dietary P deficiency results in bone demineralization and osteomalacia in mature horses and, as a result, an increase in both urinary and fractional excretion of Ca [72]. The increase in Ca excretion is indicated by a creatinine/Ca ratio of less than 3.5 but occurs as a result of either a P deficiency or a Ca excess [73]. However, with P deficiency, but not Ca excess, the plasma P concentration is usually decreased, although the decrease may not be diagnostically significant [72]. Urinary P excretion and dietary P intake are positively related, but urinary P excretion is relatively low in horses, with urinary P excretion of 1.5 mg P/kg BW in ponies fed slightly above their P requirement [61]. Thus, horses suffering from P deficiency should have little to no P in their urine, but urinary P concentration may not be informative of a P deficiency as horses fed up to three times their P requirement have little to no P in their urine as well [55].

8.2.2.3.2 Excess

The maximum tolerable concentration of dietary P is set at 1% of the diet provided the Ca : P is appropriate [37]. Feeding P at 1.2% of the diet has been shown to reduce Ca absorption and cause increased bone resorption [61]. Excess dietary P in any form binds Ca, preventing its absorption, which can cause Ca deficiency and NSH. Thus, the signs of P excess are signs of Ca deficiency. If sufficient Ca is supplied in the diet, excess P usually is not a problem. Rather, an inverted Ca : P ratio is the main cause of clinical symptoms. Excess P can also reduce the availability of Mg to the horse, which could potentially result in Mg deficiency.

8.2.2.4 Diagnosis and Treatment

8.2.2.4.1 Deficiency

The only way to confirm the presence of dietary Ca or P imbalances is to evaluate and correct the diet. Excess dietary P will increase plasma P concentration to some extent, although it will generally remain in the normal range and, therefore, the increase may not be sufficient to be of diagnostic benefit.

8.2.2.4.2 Excess

See 8.2.1.4 Calcium: Diagnosis and Treatment: Deficiency.

8.2.3 Magnesium

Approximately 60% of the body's magnesium (Mg) is located in bone. Another 30% of Mg is found in muscle, where it is important for muscle function [74]. Magnesium is an activator of many enzymes, is necessary for the activity of ATP, and is an important ion in the blood. Plasma Mg concentration is controlled primarily by intestinal absorption, renal excretion, and diffusion into body tissues. Only the ionized form of Mg is biologically active, thus ionized Mg (Mg^{2+}) rather than total Mg in the blood is informative about Mg status. Signs of hypomagnesemia may be present in animals with normal total Mg concentrations, but with lowered ionized Mg concentrations [75]. Red blood cells contain more Mg than plasma or serum and concentrations may be high as an artifact of a hemolyzed sample.

In humans, low-Mg status has been linked with diabetes mellitus and daily Mg supplementation has been shown to improve insulin-mediated glucose uptake [76]. Thus, Mg supplementation has been suggested for horses with insulin resistance [77]. One study fed laminitic, obese horses a supplement containing magnesium and chromium, but did not observe any changes in insulin sensitivity or resting insulin concentrations [78]. Insulin resistance in horses with a low-Mg status may be improved with Mg supplementation, but there are no studies to support this claim. Additionally, cases of low-Mg status in horses are rare as most feeds contain more Mg than required by the horse.

8.2.3.1 Sources and Factors Influencing Absorption

The Mg content of feeds commonly consumed by horses is 0.1–0.3%. The horse absorbs Mg primarily from the small intestine, but small amounts may be absorbed in the large intestine as well [64]. Absorption of Mg ranges from 40% to 60% in most feeds and maybe as high as 70% for inorganic sources [1]. Magnesium oxide (MgO), magnesium sulfate ($MgSO_4$), and magnesium carbonate ($MgCO_3$) are the most commonly supplemented forms of Mg, and differences in availability have been studied in other species [79, 80]. A limited number of studies have been comparing the utilization of various Mg sources by horses.

Magnesium absorption is not affected by dietary salt, Al, Ca, or oxalate [64, 67, 81]. Excess P can reduce the availability of Mg to the horse, which could potentially result in Mg deficiency [81]. However, the Ca : P was inverted in diets fed in that study, which may have played a role in the reduction in Mg absorption. While Mg digestibility was impaired by excess dietary P, apparent Mg digestibility remained between 41% and 45% when diets contained 125 mg P/kg BW [62, 64]. Exercise is not reported to influence Mg digestibility [82]. However, urinary Mg excretion was increased with exercise leading to lower Mg retention [83].

The main method of maintaining Mg homeostasis is through renal excretion. When Mg intake is low, the kidney conserves Mg so urinary excretion is minimal. However, when Mg intake is high, renal excretion of Mg increases proportionally to maintain normal concentrations in the blood. Hormones that increase renal reabsorption of Mg include PTH, PTH-related protein, vasopressin, aldosterone, insulin, and β-adrenergic agonists [75].

8.2.3.2 Recommendations

The endogenous Mg losses and true Mg digestibility used to calculate maintenance requirements for all classes of horses are 6 mg/kg BW/d and 40%, respectively [1]. However, a lower endogenous Mg loss of 2.2 mg/kg BW/d has been reported, which would result in a much lower daily requirement [84]. In either case, typical forages fed at 2% of BW would usually meet magnesium needs for horses at maintenance. Varying rates of Mg deposition in bone, tissue, and milk are reflected in the higher requirements for growing, exercising, gestating, and lactating horses (Table 8.1).

8.2.3.3 Signs of Deficiency and Excess

8.2.3.3.1 Deficiency

Neither Mg deficiency nor excess has been reported in horses fed common feeds. Hypomagnesemia (below 1.6 mg Mg/dL in serum) is uncommon in horses but has been experimentally induced in horses by feeding semi-purified diets containing 5–6 mg Mg/kg BW/d, which is about 35% of current maintenance requirements [85, 86]. Hypomagnesemia has also been reported with concurrent hypocalcemia in lactating mares during transport, presumably due to the fasting and stress of transport [84]. The signs of Mg deficiency include nervousness, muscle tremors, and ataxia, which may lead to collapse, hypernea, and death [1].

Supplemental Mg has been proposed to have a calming effect on horses, potentially due to a correction of Mg deficiency. However, some studies have combined Mg with other ingredients making it difficult to directly credit Mg with the calming effect [87, 88]. A pilot study reported a trend for horses supplemented with Ca and Mg to have reduced reactivity to stimuli, but no conclusions affirming the efficacy of the supplement were made [89]. A decrease in reaction speed to a startling stimulus was reported when mature Standardbreds received 10 g of Mg (as Mg aspartate in addition to the basal diet containing 11.2 g Mg/d) compared with control horses with no additional Mg [90].

In the horse, hypomagnesemia induces localized Ca and P deposition or mineralization in soft tissues, particularly the aorta, which can be detected histologically only 30 d after initiation of an experimental low-Mg diet and before clinical signs were detected [86]. These lesions are identical to those which occur as a result of vitamin D toxicosis.

Hypomagnesemia occurs most often in lactating cows (termed grass tetany) consuming lush, green pasture during periods of rapid plant growth. Green rapidly growing grasses are low in Mg and high in K, which decreases Mg absorption in ruminants [91]. Pastures conducive to causing hypomagnesemic tetany and death in ruminants do not affect horses similarly [1].

8.2.3.3.2 Excess

As part of the normal diet, excessive Mg intake by the horse is not known to be toxic. The maximum tolerable concentration of dietary Mg is set at 0.8% for horses based on a study that fed 0.86% of Mg in the diet as Mg oxide and observed no abnormalities in the ponies [37, 81]. Magnesium absorbed more than the horse's requirements is readily excreted in the urine, thus maintaining homeostasis in most feeding situations. In one case, an oral drench of 67–90 g of Mg (as Mg sulfate) was given to two horses suffering from colic and these animals experienced muscle tremors and severe hypermagnesemia, but renal function was compromised at the time of the drench, which may have inhibited the renal excretion of Mg from the blood [92]. Thus, concentrations of Mg in normal diets fed to horses with fully functional kidneys are extremely unlikely to cause Mg toxicity.

8.2.3.4 Diagnosis and Treatment

8.2.3.4.1 Deficiency

Serum ionized Mg concentration or urinary Mg concentrations have been used to diagnose Mg deficiency. Urinary Mg excretion correlates with Mg intake. A urine creatinine/Mg ratio of greater than 7.5 indicates marginal or inadequate Mg intake, while a ratio of less than 3.5 indicates sufficient to excess Mg intake [73]. The time of feeding does not influence Mg concentrations in spot urine samples [75]. However, it has been suggested that urine samples should be obtained on resting days, as urinary Mg excretion is decreased by exercise [46]. With a prolonged Mg deficiency, bone Mg content decreases below the normal range of 5.2–5.8 mg/g of rib bone ash content [86].

8.2.4 Sodium, Potassium, and Chlorine

Sodium (Na), potassium (K), and chloride (Cl) (the anion of chlorine) are intimately involved in whole-body homeostasis. Sodium is the major extracellular cation in the body while potassium is the major intracellular cation. Chloride is the most important extracellular anion. These ions regulate the distribution of fluid between the intracellular and extracellular spaces and contribute to strong ion difference, which influences systemic acid–base balance. Beyond these homeostatic roles, these electrolytes have many other essential functions. Sodium is essential for the transport of compounds across cell membranes and the conduction of electrical impulses in nerves and muscles. Potassium also has a role in neuromuscular activity, while chloride is an important component of gastric acid (as hydrochloric acid) and thus plays a role in the digestive process. The concentrations of Na, K, and Cl in the blood (Table 8.3) are tightly controlled, primarily through renal mechanisms.

8.2.4.1 Sources and Factors Influencing Absorption

On a DM basis, most forages contain less than 0.2% Na and may be less than 0.05% Na. Plain cereal grains (corn, oats) are also very low in Na, often less than 0.05%. Chloride concentrations in forages and grains are higher than Na concentrations, and K concentration in some feeds, such as forages, can range from 1% to 3% DM. Apparent Na digestibility was approximately 60% in horses fed forage and cereal grains with minimal salt (NaCl) supplementation and tended to decrease when 100 g of NaCl was added to the diet [93]. Previous studies have reported higher apparent Na digestibilities in horses even at intakes exceeding requirements. Overall, most of Na and Cl ingested by horses will be absorbed, with excess excreted primarily in the urine [67]. Urine Na and Cl excretion will vary directly with intake, whereas fecal excretion of Na and Cl may or may not be affected by intake. Apparent K digestibility may range from 50% to 99% [26, 94].

8.2.4.1.1 Salt

Plain salt contains 39% Na and 61% Cl by weight, and inclusion rates in most commercial concentrates usually range from 0.25% to 0.75% DM. Salt may also be supplied in a block or loose granular form. Iodized and trace-mineralized salts are also available. Additionally, commercially manufactured electrolyte supplements are available for horses. These supplements may provide K, Ca, and other components in addition to Na and Cl. Care should be taken to read the supplement label carefully to determine the amount of each electrolyte present in the supplement and appropriate dose rates.

8.2.4.2 Recommendations

For maintenance, a 500 kg (1100 lb) mature horse will require approximately 10 g Na, 40 g Cl, and 25 g of K/d, (Table 8.1) [1]. Most horses at maintenance will be receiving high-forage diets and thus the K requirement should be easily met by the forage. However, the amount of Na provided by a forage-only diet will often be below the estimated daily requirement, so it is customary to provide a source of free-choice salt (NaCl) available at all times or salt should be added to the grain mix. Horses' salt needs can be met by providing either block or loose salt. A wide variation in voluntary salt consumption has been reported. In one study, salt intake varied from 9 to 143 g/d among mature unexercised horses, and from 5 to over 200 g by the same horse on different days [67].

Lactation, pregnancy, and exercise all increase requirements. Commercially manufactured feeds for broodmares usually have added salt, and thus when fed in recommended amounts, these feeds will often meet Na and Cl requirements. Nonetheless, the provision of free-choice salt in addition to concentrate is typical. There is a greater effect of lactation on the K requirement than on the Na requirement. Mare milk contains two to three times more K than Na and the K requirement takes into account a lower availability of K than Na or Cl from most diets. Fortunately, lactating mares are typically fed significant amounts of forage, so the K requirement is usually met with a practical diet.

Sweating is the main thermoregulatory mechanism used by horses to dissipate heat. Fluid losses from sweating have been estimated to range from 0.25% of BW for horses in light work to 2% of BW for horses in very heavy work [1]. The main electrolyte in horse sweat is Cl, followed by Na, and K. Horse sweat is slightly hypertonic compared with plasma. The concentrations of Cl, Na, and K in horse sweat have been approximated at 5.3, 3.1, and 1.4 g/kg sweat, respectively [1]. Thus to replace sweat losses for a 500 kg horse in very heavy work, approximately 53 g of Cl and 31 g of Na would be necessary (above maintenance). The amount of dietary K needed to replace sweat loss in very heavy exercise is higher than the amount lost, as the availability of K has been estimated at 50%; thus, the daily K requirement above maintenance would be 28 g/d. Likely, the estimated requirements for daily intakes by horses in heavy work are higher than necessary [1]. While elite equine athletes may sustain high sweat losses during competition or on hard training days, it is not likely that these losses would occur every day. Supplementation strategies should be designed with the workload and environmental conditions in mind. Also, the effect of other thermoregulatory challenges on electrolyte losses should not be underestimated; for example, transportation in a hot trailer for several hours should also be considered. In addition to sweat losses, some equine athletes will have increased urinary electrolyte losses if treatment with a diuretic such as furosemide is administered prior to competition. Furosemide is used to reduce exercise-induced pulmonary hemorrhage and results in increased urination. The extent of electrolyte loss will be influenced by the amount and frequency of furosemide administration. Because of the large number of factors that can impact electrolyte losses in performance horses, no single dietary approach will meet the needs of all horses. Strategic use of electrolyte supplements might be a better approach to replacing sweat losses in equine athletes than daily dietary increases.

The relationship of major cations (Na, K, Ca, and Mg) to major anions (Cl, P, S) in the diet is often referred to as the dietary cation–anion balance or DCAD. The effect of DCAD has been studied extensively in dairy cattle. A large positive DCAD tends to be associated with an increase in systemic pH, while a low or negative DCAD is associated with a decrease in systemic pH. In dairy cows, manipulation of DCAD is used to alter calcium metabolism in the prepartum and immediate post-partum periods to reduce the incidence of hypocalcemia with the onset of lactation. In horses, diets with low DCAD have been reported to decrease systemic pH and increase urinary calcium excretion in some but not all studies [26, 27, 95–97]. There has also been some inconsistency in the method for calculating DCAD. Dietary DCAD can be calculated using only Na, K, and Cl, or can also include Ca, Mg, S, and P. It has been suggested that the concentrations of cations and anions in the diet should be adjusted for availability, as not all are absorbed to the same extent [98]. One study suggested that Cl had a stronger effect on systemic acid–base balance than S [27]. From a practical perspective, high-forage diets would be expected to have a high DCAD due to the large amount of K in most grasses and legumes; while low forage, high-grain diets would have a lower DCAD. Very few studies have been conducted on the effects of DCAD on horses during the past decade, but additional investigations are probably warranted as acid–base disturbances can occur in performance horses.

8.2.4.3 Signs of Deficiency and Excess

8.2.4.3.1 Deficiency

When salt intake is low, a lack of Na increases aldosterone secretion, which increases intestinal Na absorption and decreases renal Na excretion, so the short-term restriction of Na intake may not produce any observable effects. The greater the Na losses from the body, the shorter the time for a deficiency to occur. Thus, a deficiency is more likely to occur during lactation and increased sweating. Elimination of salt from the diet can also lead to a deficiency in Cl. The first effect of either a Na or a Cl deficiency is a tendency for affected animals to develop pica and to lick objects that might have salt on them [1]. A decrease in food and water intake, resulting in weight loss and dehydration may also occur.

Fatigue, muscle weakness, lethargy, exercise intolerance, and decreased water and feed intake are the major effects of a K deficit. Increased restlessness and timidity to noise have also been reported and a K deficiency may reduce growth in young horses [1, 99].

8.2.4.3.2 Excess

An excess intake of Na increases blood volume and the release of atrial naturetic factor, which increases urinary Na excretion. Diets providing NaCl above 6% of total intake are considered to be above the maximal tolerable limit [1]. Clinical signs of salt toxicosis include colic, diarrhea, frequent urination, weakness, staggering, paralysis of the hind limbs, recumbency, and death [100]. Most horses are relatively tolerant of high potassium intakes and can consume forages containing more than 3% K without apparent issue when adequate water is available. However, horses with hyperkalemic periodic paralysis (HYPP) are sensitive to high dietary K and should be fed diets containing 1% K or less [94].

8.2.4.4 Diagnosis and Treatment

Dietary history and ration analyses should be the first steps in evaluating whether deficiencies or excesses of Na, Cl, and K are present in a diet. Diets that contain forage and plain cereal grains are likely to be low in Na for horses with elevated requirements (lactating mares and heavily exercised horses). If horses have received this type of diet for an extended period without access to a salt source, and some of the deficiency signs described above are present, it is likely the conservation mechanisms for Na have been exceeded. Ideally, salt should be reintroduced to the diet gradually to prevent systemic or gastrointestinal disturbances.

If salt toxicity is suspected, a careful history should include an investigation into how, when, and how much salt (either as a block or loose) has been provided to the horse. Some horses develop an aberrant appetite for salt and can consume a small salt block (4 lb) in a day or less. If an aberrant appetite is present, free-choice access to salt should be prevented. If an aberrant appetite for free-choice salt is not present, feed analyses should be completed. If a mixing error has occurred resulting in excess salt being added to a concentrate feed, and horses are being given electrolyte supplements in their water, excess intake of Na and Cl could occur.

Horses affected by HYPP may exhibit muscle fasciculation, third eyelid prolapse, and involuntary recumbency when fed diets containing more than 1.1% K [94]. Feeds that are high in K should be avoided for horses affected by HYPP. When a low-K forage is not available, a high K hay can be soaked in water to reduce the K concentration before feeding. In one study, soaking hay in water for 1 hr reduced K concentration from 3% of DM to less than 1% [101].

8.2.5 Sulfur

Sulfur (S) makes up about 0.15% of BW (wet weight) and is needed as a constituent of S-containing amino acids (methionine, cystine, and cysteine), B vitamins (biotin and thiamin), as well as many other body constituents including coenzyme A, heparin, glutathione, lipoic acid, taurine, and chondroitin sulfate [44]. Sulfur-containing amino acids are used in synthesizing almost all body proteins and enzymes, including insulin and keratin, which are found in hair, skin, and hooves. In plasma, most S is associated with proteins.

8.2.5.1 Sources and Factors Influencing Absorption

The majority of ingested S is in the organic form of S-containing amino acids from plant protein such that the S feedstuff content can be crudely estimated based on the CP content of the feed. The percentage of S in plant CP ranges from 0.5% to 1.12% of total CP. Typically, grasses contain the fewest S-containing amino acids, and thus, the least amount of S in the CP fraction (0.54–0.59%). Legumes contain around 0.70% S in the CP fraction whereas grains and grain byproducts contain around 0.72–1.12% S in the CP fraction. Because the majority of dietary S is associated with amino acids, the digestibility of S is linked to protein digestibility in the small intestine. Absorption of S occurs in the small intestine. The apparent digestibility of S has been estimated to be around 81% based on a collection of 79 balance trials [44].

There is no research investigating the effects of water S concentration on equine performance, but in other species, S from drinking water can be significant enough to cause signs of S toxicity [37]. Additionally, some minerals (Mg, Zn, Cu, Mn) are often supplemented in the form of sulfate salts. This practice increases the inorganic S intake of animals along with the intake of the targeted mineral. Plasma inorganic sulfate concentrations may be responsive to fluctuations in dietary intake.

Many of the S-containing compounds in the body can be produced from methionine absorbed from the diet, except for thiamine and biotin [37]. However, horses cannot produce methionine from dietary inorganic S, so methionine is an essential amino acid and must be supplied in the diet. Dietary inorganic S can be used to synthesize sulfated carbohydrates, lipids and phenols, and other S-containing compounds, such as insulin, heparin, and chondroitin sulfate [1]. However, horses do not absorb inorganic S as efficiently as organic S (54% vs. 81%, respectively) [27, 44], and inorganic S is not used as efficiently in the body to produce all the necessary organic S compounds. In poultry, dietary inorganic S concentrations of 0.05% overwhelmed the body's ability to use inorganic S to produce organic S compounds [102]. Hindgut microbes can use inorganic S to produce the S-containing B vitamins, thiamine, and biotin, which the horse can absorb and utilize. However, the absorption of microbial S-containing amino acids in the hindgut is limited. See Chapter 7 Protein. Sulfur concentration may be reported as sulfate, sulfur (S), or sulfate-S. Concentrations reported as sulfur and as sulfate-S are the same. Sulfate is one-third S; therefore, divide the sulfate concentration by three to obtain the S concentration.

8.2.5.2 Recommendations

Sulfur requirements for the horse have not been experimentally determined. Most horse feeds contain at least 0.15% non-mineral or organic S, which appears to be adequate to meet the horse's S requirement. Requirements are based on an assumed dietary concentration of 0.15% S and varying intakes for different classes of horses. Therefore, for a 500-kg horse at maintenance, the S requirement is 15.0 g S/d or 30 mg S/kg BW [1].

Endogenous fecal losses of S are reported to be close to 6.9 mg/kg BW/d when examining data from more than 79 balance trials in four published papers [44]. Using a digestibility of 80% and endogenous losses of 7 mg/kg BW/d, the calculated S requirement would be 8.8 mg S/kg BW, which is lower than the current recommendation. However, due to lack of research, sufficient S supplied in normal equine diets, and no reports of deficiencies or excesses, the current recommendations seem appropriate [1].

8.2.5.3 Signs of Deficiency and Excess

8.2.5.3.1 Deficiency

An S deficiency has not been reported in the horse. It may be possible to achieve a marginal S intake if an extremely low-protein diet is fed (straw) or in cases of extreme restrictions of DM intake (<1% DM/kg BW) [44]. In other species, S deficiency decreases appetite, growth, hair or wool growth, and milk production, and in the mature animal results in weight loss. In the horse, it could be speculated that an S deficiency may result in impaired hoof strength due to a lack of S for disulfide bridging.

8.2.5.3.2 Excess

The maximum tolerable concentration of S intake for horses is set at 0.5% of DM, using data from other species [37]. However, no detrimental effect from excess S intake from high S-containing feeds has been reported in horses, except in one abnormal case. Mature horses accidentally fed 200 and 400 g of nearly pure inorganic S (as "flowers of sulfur") became lethargic within 12 hrs, exhibited colic, icterus, and labored breathing [103]. Two of the 12 died despite treatment. Chronic excess dietary S (greater than 0.3%) DM in swine and ruminants decreases copper absorption, but there is no evidence that this occurs in horses [37, 104]. Excess S is excreted in feces and urine, with fecal S excretion being closely correlated to S intake [105]. Sulfur is excreted in the urine, partly as Ca-sulfate, which has the potential to increase the risk of developing uroliths, especially when combined with the increased Ca intake [44].

8.3 Microminerals

Micro- or trace minerals are those for which dietary requirements are best expressed as parts per million (ppm or mg/kg), mg/d or ug/kg BW/d, or possibly per Mcal of digestible energy. Microminerals needed in the diet include selenium, iodine, copper, zinc, manganese, iron, and cobalt. Most trace minerals are needed as components of metalloenzymes that are involved in controlling enormous numbers of diverse biological reactions.

8.3.1 Selenium

Selenium (Se) can replace sulfur in the sulfur-containing amino acids, cysteine, and methionine. It can then be specifically incorporated into selenoproteins, where selenocysteine forms a part of the primary protein structure. Alternatively, Se-methionine can be non-specifically incorporated into a protein by replacing methionine, where it can also serve as a Se storage pool.

Nearly half of the selenoproteins that have been functionally characterized are thought to play a role in the antioxidant system of the body [106]. The antioxidant system combats free radicals generated by normal physiological processes. During energy metabolism, organic or carbon-containing nutrients are oxidized producing carbon dioxide and water. However, during this process, free radicals are also produced. These free radicals are powerful oxidizing agents that, if not neutralized, can damage living cells, notably their proteins and lipids. The antioxidant system includes fat-soluble antioxidants (vitamin E), water-soluble antioxidants (ascorbic acid), and antioxidant enzymes (glutathione peroxidase [GSH-Px]) that function as a team to control the effects of free radicals [107].

GSH-Px regulates hydrogen peroxide and hydroperoxide concentrations inside the cell [106, 108]. GSH-Px uses glutathione to reduce hydrogen peroxide to water, thereby limiting cell damage. GSH-Px activity is often used as an indicator of Se status where low concentrations of activity are typically associated with a low Se status [107]. GSH-Px also acts as a storage pool for Se, due to the four selenocysteine residues contained in each GSH-Px enzyme [109].

While GSH-Px functions in the intracellular fluid and removes lipid peroxides that form, the antioxidant protective mechanisms of lipid-soluble vitamin E, present in the cell membrane, decrease the formation of lipid peroxides. Consequently, Se and vitamin E are often described as having a sparing effect on each other. Optimal amounts of both, however, are necessary to minimize oxidation-induced tissue damage. Thus, Se and vitamin E should be considered together regarding the animal's requirements, and when addressing the effects and treatment of a deficiency of either. Some effects, however, are more prominent as a result of a deficiency of one than the other and are more responsive to the administration of the deficient nutrient.

There are approximately 25 selenoproteins and 35 proteins containing Se [107]. Some of the selenoproteins that are functionally better understood include thioredoxin reductase and iodothyronine deiodinase. Thioredoxin reductase is involved in the redox system of the cell [109]. Iodothyronine deiodinase is responsible for the conversion of the prohormone thyroxine (T4) to its active form, triiodothyronine (T3) [109–111]. Thyroid hormones are essential for health, as these hormones affect metabolism, growth, development, and differentiation [107].

8.3.1.1 Sources and Factors Influencing Absorption

Forages and grains commonly contain 0.01–0.3 mg Se/kg DM, while some plants are known to accumulate Se [1].

Soil and plant Se content varies geographically. Plants grown in most areas around the Great Lakes, in the eastern and western parts of the United States (Figure 8.3), and all of Canada (except the lower half of Manitoba, Saskatchewan, and Alberta) tend to be low in Se. See soil Se concentrations worldwide (1980–1999) and the effect of future climate changes [113]. Liming acidic soils, as well as adding Se and phosphorus to fertilizers, may increase forage Se content, as Se is taken up by plants more readily in alkaline soil compared with acidic soils [114–116]. Selenium naturally occurs in plants in the form of selenomethionine or selenocysteine. These two forms of Se are regarded as organic forms of Se [107]. To account for the generally marginal to low Se concentrations in forages, when compared with animal requirements, dietary Se supplements are typically added directly to the grain concentrate or ration balancer/supplement portion of animal feeds. Both organic and inorganic sources of Se supplements can be used in animal feeds to support adequate Se status. Inorganic Se is typically provided in the form of a mineral salt such as sodium selenite. Organic Se supplementation is usually provided in the form of selenomethionine, which, for example, is the main form in which Se can be found in Se-enriched yeast products. Sodium selenite is absorbed via passive diffusion in the small intestine, while selenomethionine is absorbed through sodium-dependent amino acid transporters. Studies conducted in other species have reported higher tissue Se concentrations when organic supplements were compared with inorganic supplements [117].

8.3.1.2 Dietary Recommendation

Table 8.1 provides Se recommendations on a kg BW basis for horses of all physiological classes [1]. The requirement estimates for mature horses that are idle, in light work, stallions, and pregnant mares are based on studies that evaluated blood response variables, such as GSH-Px activity, to different concentrations of Se supplementation, showing no benefit to these variables when exceeding 1 mg Se/d in mature horses. Selenium has a higher absorption rate than most trace minerals (59%), and when accounting

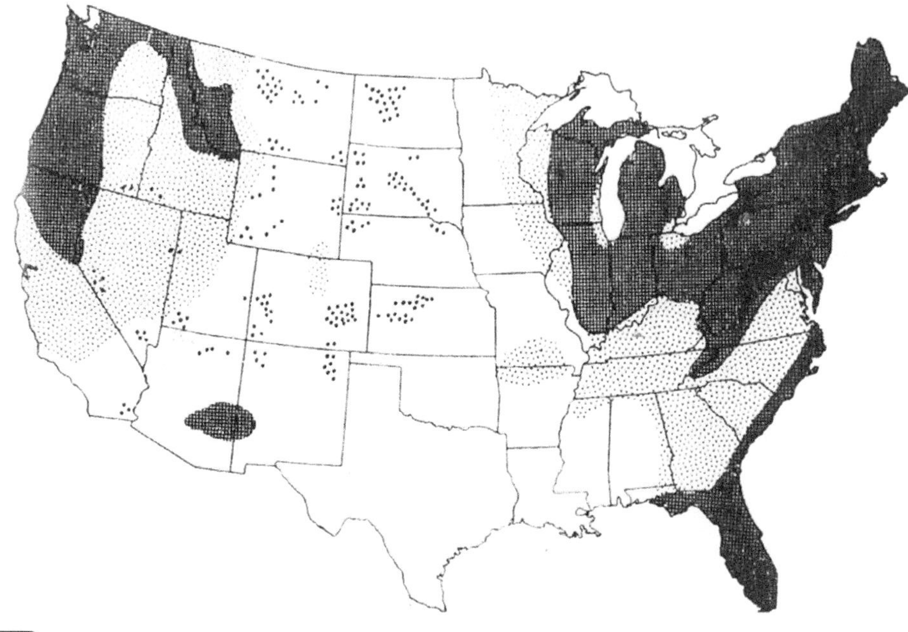

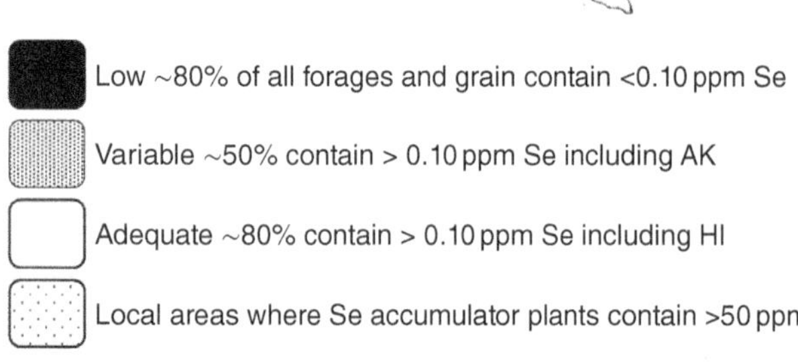

Figure 8.3 Regional distribution of forage and grain selenium content in the United States [112, 113].

for an estimated 37% of dietary Se being excreted in the urine, the calculated daily Se requirement for a 500 kg horse is 1.26 mg/d [44]. On a BW basis, the estimated requirements for Se are elevated for some performance horses, lactating mares, and growing horses.

Commercial horse feeds are often formulated to provide more than a total dietary Se concentration of 0.1 mg/kg DM. The inclusion of Se (or other minerals) at somewhat elevated concentrations in commercial feeds is often aimed at compensating for low concentrations of Se (or other minerals) in the forage component of the diet. However, because of its role in the antioxidant system, there has been increased interest in the potential benefits of elevated Se intakes. It should be noted that laws or regulations in many states and countries specify maximum inclusion concentrations for Se (and other minerals). The reader is therefore encouraged to look for the most current regulations available for their region.

Several research studies have evaluated the effect of higher concentrations of Se supplementation on indicators of Se status in the horse. Supplementation above the recommended intake may raise plasma, serum, or blood Se concentrations, but GSH-Px activity remains mostly unaffected. However, considering that there are at least 25 selenoproteins, other selenoproteins may be affected by an elevated Se intake. Some studies have used relatively short supplementation periods, which may limit the opportunity for the effects of additional Se to be recognized.

Red blood cell turnover takes approximately 140 d [118]. When horses were studied for 189 d, whole blood Se and whole blood GSH-Px activity were higher in horses receiving a total dietary Se intake of 0.3 mg/kg DM, compared with horses receiving a diet either below (0.06 mg/kg DM) or slightly above (0.12 mg Se/kg DM) the Se NRC recommendation of 0.1 mg/kg DM [119]. This study indicated that a total dietary Se concentration of 0.3 mg/kg DM did support higher concentrations of GSH-Px activity. Similarly, a study conducted with 18-m-old exercising horses also reported higher concentrations of whole blood GSH-Px in horses receiving 0.3 mg Se/kg DM, compared with 0.1 mg Se/kg DM. However, it was concluded from this study, considering all the exercise-specific variables measured, that Se supplemented above current recommendations were of limited benefit in horses subjected to a standard exercise test [120]. The role that Se plays in the antioxidant system makes it intuitive that exercise, which increases free radical production, could increase Se requirements. However, overall, results for exercise-based studies in horses evaluating Se have been inconsistent, potentially due to the body's ability to adapt to exercise.

Selenium is transferred both across the placenta and into the milk, the extent of which is dependent on the animal's Se status [121]. Broodmares fed diets with higher dietary concentrations of Se subsequently had higher Se concentrations in their colostrum and milk. Foals from mares receiving 3 mg Se/d had greater serum IgG concentrations at 2 wks of age than foals from mares receiving only 1 mg Se/d [122, 123]. Broodmares fed an organic Se-yeast supplement had higher milk and colostrum Se concentrations compared with broodmares fed sodium selenite [122]. However, Se injections given 14 d before foaling did not affect the foals' ability to obtain passive immunity from their dams [124].

Providing less than the NRC recommended amount of Se (0.06 vs. 0.1 mg/kg DM) over an extended period resulted in lower Se status as well as diminished immune responses, and an inability for GSH-Px activity to recover to pre-exercise concentrations following a mild exercise test [119, 125, 126]. Overall, the absolute dietary Se requirements of the mature, non-breeding horse must be close to the NRC recommended amount. Therefore, ensuring that the NRC (2007) minimum dietary Se recommendations are met is essential.

8.3.1.3 Signs of Deficiency and Excess

8.3.1.3.1 Deficiency

Most commercially manufactured horse feeds contain supplemental Se, but animals raised without supplemented feeds may be at risk of deficiency. In a survey of state veterinarians and diagnostic laboratories, Se deficiency was reported to be an important livestock problem in regions of 37 states, with mild or moderate deficiencies in nine additional states (Connecticut, Georgia, Louisiana, Mississippi, North Carolina, New Hampshire, South Carolina, Tennessee, and Texas) [127]. Only four states did not report Se deficiency problems (Delaware, Rhode Island, West Virginia, and Wyoming). In contrast, pasture forage grown in some areas of the Rocky Mountain and Great Plains states may contain toxic concentrations of Se. Toxicosis attributable to native plants was reported in eight states (California, Colorado, Idaho, Montana, Oregon, South Dakota, Utah, and Wyoming). However, in all of these states, except Wyoming, Se deficiency was also reported to be an important problem. This survey demonstrates that the evaluation of Se status in all livestock (including horses) is important. Although a low Se status has occasionally been observed in horses diagnosed with steatitis (or yellow fat disease), case studies indicate that it is primarily caused by low vitamin E status, more so than low Se status [128, 129]. When Se and vitamin E deficiencies occur in the mature horse, the muscles of mastication are affected, or those of the legs, resulting in a stiff, stilted gait [130, 131]. In adult horses, clinically apparent Se deficiency has been reported in the form of severe masseter myonecrosis, associated with low blood Se concentrations and/or low blood GSH-Px activity concentrations [132].

However, nutritional myopathy, often accompanied by vascular disorders, especially in newborn foals, is the predominant form of Se deficiency occurring in horses. See White Muscle Disease under Vitamin E deficiency in Chapter 9 and Nutritional Muscular Dystrophy in Chapter 25.

In foals, a Se deficiency is usually the result of inadequate Se intake by the dam during pregnancy or inadequate Se intake during lactation. Selenium is transferred across the placenta and is also secreted into the colostrum and milk [121]. Milk and colostrum Se content has been reported to be influenced by dietary sources of supplementation and dietary Se concentration [122]. Necropsy lesions evident in foals with myopathies include subcutaneous, intramuscular, and pulmonary edema and congestion, and a bilateral pallor and ischemic necrosis of affected cardiac and skeletal muscles, particularly those of the hind legs, neck, and tongue if involved, giving them a white appearance (Figure 8.4), leading to the name "white muscle disease." Histologically there is widespread tissue lipoperoxidation, leading to hyaline and granular degeneration, swelling, fragmentation, and calcification of affected muscle fibers, which give it a gritty feel when it is cut [133].

The only observable effect of a mild deficiency of Se may be a decrease in the animal's immune response to infectious diseases, and slower growth [134]. A long-term Se depletion and repletion study found that a low Se status and the length of time spent in a state of low Se status had more of an impact on the response of the immune system than supplementation exceeding requirements [126]. A decreased immune response increases the animal's susceptibility to, and the severity and duration of, infectious diseases, and decreases response to vaccinations [72, 135, 136].

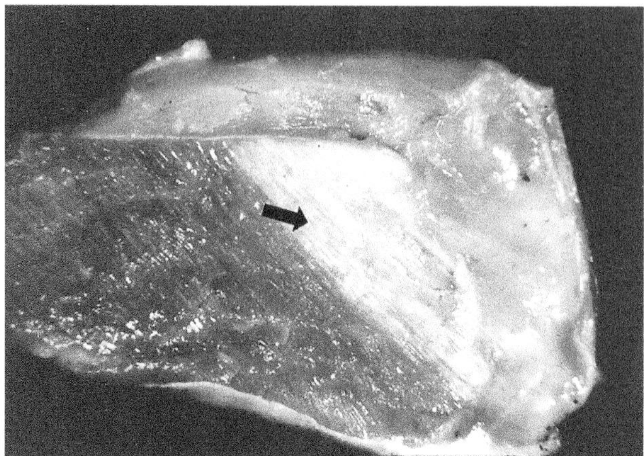

Figure 8.4 White muscle disease induced by selenium/vitamin E deficiency. A cross-section of muscle from an affected animal shows white areas of ischemic degeneration and calcification that give this disease this name.

8.3.1.3.2 Excess

Selenium toxicity can be classified as being either chronic or acute. Chronic toxicity is also referred to as alkali disease or blind staggers. Clinical symptoms of chronic toxicity include cracked hooves, ataxia, and hair loss from the mane and tail [137]. It is believed that the weakened hoof and hair structures are due to the replacement of sulfur with Se [138]. Chronic cases of Se toxicity have been reported for horses fed hay excessively high in Se, as well as mine-residue contaminated pasture/water sources [137, 139]. Acute toxicity, on the other hand, involves neurological signs, hyper-excitability, sweating, shortness of breath, fever, and, in some cases, death [138].

8.3.1.4 Diagnosis and Treatment

Serum Se concentration is generally considered sensitive to short-term dietary Se intake, while whole blood Se is a long-term indicator of Se intake. The GSH-Px activity can also be measured. Due to the sensitivity of GSH-Px to laboratory temperature and processing time, whole blood Se concentration is frequently the preferred indicator of Se status in the clinical setting [132]. A study evaluating hair Se content in 25 racehorses reported a range of 0.73–1.85 mg/kg although a normal reference range for hair samples has not been established [140]. Hair samples, however, may provide the opportunity to obtain a retrospective evaluation of a horse's dietary Se intake over multiple years [139].

A normal reference range for serum Se in adult horses of 130–160 ng/mL has been reported [141]. Serum Se concentrations in younger horses can be expected to fall between 70 and 90 ng/mL from birth to 9 days of age; 80–100 ng/mL from day 10 to 29; 90–110 ng/mL for 1–10 mos [141]. The reference range for whole blood Se in adult horses is 180–240 ng/mL [142]. A case study reported eight foals (<30 d old) diagnosed with white muscle disease, seven had whole blood Se concentrations below 99.5 ng/mL (1.26 um/L) [132]. GSH-Px activity is usually expressed in enzyme units (1 EU = 1 μmol NADPH oxidized/min) per mg of hemoglobin (Hb). For adult horses, normal whole blood GSH-Px activity usually ranges between 40 and 160 EU/g Hb [142].

Although reference ranges for Se in serum and blood have been reported, there are reports in the scientific literature where animals appear in good health despite being of marginal to low Se status according to blood Se concentrations [1]. In a study that involved the Se depletion of horses over a total of 18 mos, no clinical indications of Se deficiency were observed, regardless of whole blood Se concentrations and GSH-Px activity falling below reference ranges [119]. However, in these same horses, following a mild exercise challenge, GSH-Px concentrations did not recover to pre-exercise concentrations, as was the case for horses of adequate Se status [125]. Therefore, by considering the reference range guidelines determined for normal healthy animals, a sudden manifestation of clinical or subclinical symptoms in the event of adverse conditions can be avoided.

8.3.1.4.1 Deficiency

Severe Se deficiency can be treated by giving an intramuscular preparation containing Se. To maintain long-term adequate status, a total diet should be evaluated for Se, and supplemented accordingly to allow for adequate dietary Se intake discussed earlier. Whole blood Se concentration can be increased from low to adequate in horses of low Se status, within 28 d of receiving a diet with a total Se concentration of 0.3 mg Se/kg DM [119].

8.3.1.4.2 Excess

Whenever free access to a Se-containing salt is given, care should be taken to monitor salt intake. Salt intake tends to vary among horses, which can be problematic when dealing with a potentially toxic trace mineral. In the United States, salt containing up to 90 mg Se/kg (90 ppm) for sheep and 120 ppm for cattle is allowed by the FDA [143]. Most commercial horse feeds are formulated to provide a total dietary Se intake of up to 0.3 mg/kg DM when following the manufacturers' feeding instructions.

Cases of acute toxicity may occur in the event of incorrect doses of oral, intravenous, or intramuscular administration of supplements, and are less likely due to the consumption of natural, unfortified forages. For example, 20 polo ponies died when a calculation error led to the accidental intravenous administration of 2 g of Se to each horse [138]. The ingestion of plants containing high Se can also produce toxicosis. A lethal injectable amount of Se has been reported to be 1.49 mg/kg BW/d. The lethal oral dose for the horse is 3.3 mg/kg BW/d as compared with 10 mg/kg BW/d for cattle and 17 mg/kg BW/d for pigs [114, 144].

A case study evaluated mane and tail hair Se in three horses that grazed a pasture with access to a Se-contaminated stream from May to November for three consecutive years [139]. Pasture Se content ranged from <1.31 to 127.4 mg/kg DM. Their mane hair Se content ranged from 0.7 to 27.6 mg/kg, while tail hair Se ranged from 0.6 to 47.6 mg/kg and all three horses displayed hoof lesions. A fourth horse that only grazed this pasture for 45 d during the third year had no signs of hoof lesions, and mane and tail hair peak Se values were 3.1 and 3.2 mg Se/kg, respectively. In cases of chronic toxicosis, removal of the dietary source of Se (contaminated hay or removing horses from contaminated pasture) allowed horses to recover. In some cases, supportive care may be needed for hoof lesions [139, 142]. The prognosis will vary depending on the Se concentration, route, and time frame.

8.3.2 Iodine

The majority of iodine (I) can be found in the thyroid gland where it is oxidized and bound to tyrosine, forming mono- and diiodotyrosine, which are coupled to form the thyroid hormones triiodothyronine (T3) and thyroxine (T4) [9]. T4 is metabolically less active than T3, but T4 is released in larger quantities than T3. A large portion of T3 is derived from T4 in peripheral tissues using iodothyronine deiodinase type 1 and 2, which functions to convert T4 to T3. Conversely, iodothyronine deiodinase type 3 is involved in the conversion of T4 to reverse T3, which inactivates T3 and T4 [9, 107]. An increase in TSH causes a similar change in the production and secretion of T3 and T4, which then increases metabolic rate and consequent increases in oxygen utilization and heat production. An increase in T3 or T4 causes a decrease in TSH thus completing a classic negative feedback loop.

8.3.2.1 Sources and Factors Influencing Absorption

The I content of most horse feeds typically ranges from 0.05 to 0.2 mg/kg DM but can vary from 0 to 2 mg/kg [133]. Iodine-deficient areas are known to occur on every continent. In North America, iodine concentrations below those needed to meet the horse's requirement are most likely to occur in feeds grown in areas adjacent to the Great Lakes, and scattered areas of the western United States and Canada. Although soils low in iodine tend to produce I-deficient plants, there is sometimes little relationship between I concentrations in the soil and the plant. Soils in areas of recent glaciation, in areas distant from the sea, and areas of low annual rainfall, are most likely to be iodine deficient. Climate, soil type, fertilizer application, and many other factors are known to influence the I content of plants [10].

Iodine can also be supplied by the addition of iodized or trace-mineralized salt to the concentrate/grain portion of the horse's diet, or as a salt block for free-choice consumption. However, free-choice iodized salt alone may not suffice for some mares during pregnancy and lactation due to variable voluntary salt consumption. As a result, I deficiency may occur in some foals while not in others in the same herd, even though an I-containing salt is readily available for them and their dams [145, 146]. Inorganic sources of I include potassium- or sodium-iodates or iodides, while ethylene diaminedihydroiodide (EDDI) is an organic source of I. Additional sources of I may be found in supplements containing seaweed or kelp products.

Urinary I concentration closely follows that of dietary I intake, while fecal I content remains low regardless of increased I intake [147]. At times of excessive I intake, the ability of I to cross the placenta can result in hypothyroidism in foals at birth [9]. Similarly, high dietary I intake by the mare has been associated with high I content in mare's milk [44]. A high I diet fed to a broodmare can therefore result in I toxicity problems in the fetus and/or young nursing foals.

8.3.2.2 Dietary Recommendation

The current iodine dietary recommendation for an idle, adult horse, weighing 500 kg, is 3.5 mg/d (Table 8.1). This recommendation is based on work done in other species, combined with the reported endogenous I losses for horses of 7 μg/kg BW/d, and an assumption of a near 100% absorption [1, 147]. This iodine intake equates to a total dietary concentration of 0.35 mg/kg DM, assuming a DM intake of 2% of BW. A lower recommendation of 1.1 mg/d for the maintenance of a 500 kg BW horse has been made by others because the difficulty in quantification of forage iodine may lead to inaccurate assessment of I content [44]. This recommendation is similar to the I recommendation made in the previous edition of the NRC of 0.1 mg/kg DM [44, 133]. The maximum tolerable concentration of I in the horse's total diet is 5 mg/kg DM [37]. Dietary I recommendations increase with exercise, pregnancy, and lactation (Table 8.1).

8.3.2.3 Signs of Deficiency and Excess

The clinical signs of iodine or I deficiency and excess are similar. Iodine I deficiency or toxicosis may result in hypothyroidism and thyroid gland hypertrophy (goiter) (Figure 8.5). In iodine deficiency, there is insufficient iodide available to synthesize an adequate amount of I-containing thyroid (T3 and T4) hormones. In iodine toxicosis, the iodine excess inhibits the synthesis and release of thyroid hormones from the thyroid gland. In either case, the reduced concentration of thyroid hormones increases TSH secretion, which then stimulates thyroid gland hypertrophy and hyperplasia (goiter).

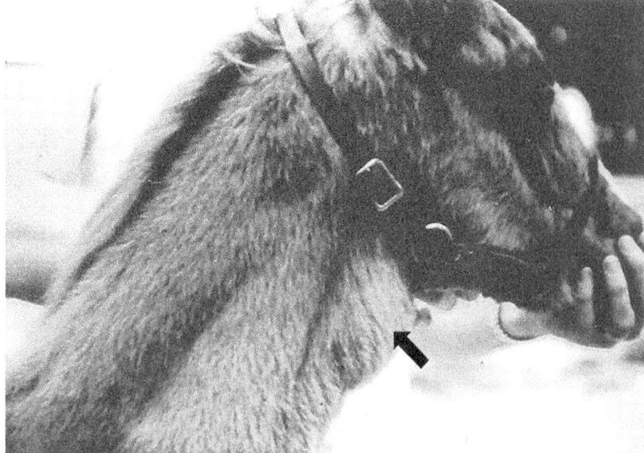

Figure 8.5 Goiter. Enlarged thyroid glands, which may occur as a result of either a deficiency or excess of iodine.

Although hair loss was reported in a mature horse fed excessive I, signs of I deficiency or toxicosis are more common in newborn foals than adults and are the consequence of either low or high dietary I intake by the dam [148]. Affected foals that are born alive are weak, have difficulty in standing, have a weak or poor suckle response, and generally have persistent hypothermia (rectal temperature less than 37.8 °C) [149, 150]. Thyroid hormones have a central role in the development and maturation of several organ systems, including the pulmonary system [151]. Therefore, affected foals may also have respiratory distress due to impaired or incomplete surfactant development [150]. The administration of a thyroid hormone treatment has been shown to enhance the synthesis of lung surfactant in other species [152]. Affected foals may also have angular limb deformities present at birth or occurring within the first few days of life, due to the collapse of inadequately ossified carpal or tarsal bones [146]. Thyroid enlargement may or may not be present while histological changes in the thyroid gland may be present.

Dams of affected foals may exhibit abnormal estrous cycles but usually do not have thyroid gland enlargement or show other signs of I deficiency [145, 146]. However, during toxicosis, I can cross the placenta, while milk I concentrations can increase, affecting the fetus and nursing foal [9, 44]. In mares given 350 mg of potassium iodide (76% I) approximately 266 mg of I/d daily (75 times their requirement) for one year, 17 of 39 mares aborted [7]. One stillborn foal and three foals that were very weak at birth had large goiters, whereas the remaining foals had weak fetlocks but no goiter. When I supplementation was stopped, foals born 6 to 8 wks later seemed to be normal. It has been suggested that I deficiency can result in a variety of non-specific signs (poor hair coat, poor growth, lethargy), while toxicosis can also affect disease resistance.

Iodine toxicosis in horses has been much more frequently reported than I deficiency. No cases of I toxicity from free-choice access to iodized salt were found in the literature, but adding more than 4–8% iodized salt to the total diet could exceed the upper tolerance for I intake. Over-supplementing horses with high iodine seaweed (kelp) could also lead to excess I consumption. Similarly, overfeeding organic or inorganic iodine sources can lead to toxicity [7, 148, 153].

8.3.2.4 Diagnosis and Treatment

Hypothyroidism reduces plasma T3 and T4 concentrations. Normal serum thyroid hormones are usually high in young foals compared with adult concentrations but decrease over time. It is also important to note that although these concentrations will become more similar to adult ranges by 1 m of age, they can remain high relative to adult ranges for the first year [154]. Therefore, it is important to make age-appropriate comparisons. In one study, plasma total T3 concentrations ranged from 26 to 733 ng/dL and total T4 concentrations from 4.4 to 25.1 ng/dL in 10 normal 1-d-old foals. Plasma T3 concentrations were found to increase for 24–48 hrs after birth, then declines during the following 2 wks [155].

The increase in plasma T3 concentration in response to TSH administration can be used to determine the presence of hypothyroidism. During the first few days of life, normal foals respond to the administration of either TSH (5 IU given IV) with a doubling or greater of plasma total and free T3 concentrations within 1 to 3 hrs, and a 16% or greater increase in total T4 concentration within 3 to 6 hrs [150, 155]. If a foal is diagnosed as hypothyroid, administration of T4 and T3 on a kilogram BW basis can be done to attain age-appropriate thyroid hormone concentrations in these foals. Supportive care should be provided, especially for weak foals, which may include exercise restriction to prevent damage to the skeleton and tendons [9]. With I toxicosis, the mare's plasma protein-bound I concentration may be increased above the normal range of 16–27 μg/L [149]. The foal, however, may be affected by I toxicosis even when the mare's plasma protein-bound I concentration is normal.

Treatment for primary I deficiency or toxicosis is to correct the dietary imbalance present. As both may cause hypothyroidism and similar symptoms, it is important to determine whether the horses have consumed too little or too much iodine. The best and surest way to do this is to evaluate the total diet. In a clinical setting, another way to estimate I intake is by determining urinary I concentration. Measuring urinary I content does require specialized laboratory analysis expertise and is therefore not commonly offered by all diagnostic laboratories. However, renal excretion of I was shown to closely reflect I intake in a study where horses were fed 0–80 μg I/kg BW [147].

If no supplemental sources of I (I-containing salt or supplements, organic I or seaweed) are being fed, the problem is likely a deficiency. It is important to realize, however, that an I deficiency may occur in some mares, and as a result affect their foals, while it may not occur in other mares in that same herd, when free-choice I-containing salt is the main source of supplemental I, due to differences in intake [145, 146]. Once symptoms due to an I deficiency occur, treatment is not generally very effective [133]. The nursing foal with I toxicosis must be fed an alternate source of milk low in I since the dam's milk will contain excess iodine.

If the dietary evaluation indicates that I intake is adequate, while signs of hypothyroidism are present, the diet should be evaluated for the presence of endocrine-disrupting substances, that can affect I uptake by thyroid tissues. These specific endocrine-disrupting substances include goitrin, nitrates, cyanate, perchlorates, or anti-thyroid substances. Therefore, the ingestion of large amounts of goitrogenic plants or the administration of anti-thyroid substances can cause hypothyroidism and goiter. Goitrogenic plants include kale, mustard, cabbage, and other plants of the Brassicaceae family, as well as uncooked soybeans [1, 44]. While linseed and rapeseed can be high in cyanide, some countries regulate these concentrations. Water (well water in particular) can be contaminated with perchlorates [44]. Although these plants and anti-thyroid substances probably have the same effects in horses as in other species, there are no reports in the literature on the occurrence of hypothyroidism or goiter due to plant/anti-thyroid substances in the horse. Awareness of the potential effects of these compounds on I metabolism, however, may be useful in situations of low to marginal dietary I intake.

8.3.3 Copper

Copper (Cu)-dependent enzymes are essential for many functions and are involved in bone collagen stabilization, elastin synthesis, the mobilization of body iron stores, superoxide detoxification, and melanin synthesis [1, 155]. The liver regulates Cu metabolism by storing Cu, incorporating Cu into the protein ceruloplasmin for vascular transport to the rest of the body, or excreting Cu in bile and urinary Cu excretion is minimal [133, 157–159].

8.3.3.1 Sources and Factors Influencing Absorption

The Cu content of common feeds can range from 1 to 80 mg/kg DM but is typically between 3 and 20 mg/kg DM. Plants low in Cu content usually grow in either sandy soils that are heavily weathered, or peat/muck soils that may have previously been swampy [1, 157].

Commercially available concentrates usually contain supplemental Cu from inorganic sources such as Cu sulfate, Cu chloride, or Cu carbonate, or an organic source such as Cu chelate. Studies evaluating different forms of Cu supplements have had contradicting outcomes. Some studies comparing inorganic and organic forms of Cu have indicated that the physiological class of the horse may play a role in the effectiveness or availability of a particular form of supplementation. Specifically organic supplements have been reported to have greater retention in growing horses, while the opposite appears true in mature horses [1, 159].

The percent Cu absorbed decreases with increasing intake, with reported values ranging from 5% to 50% [133, 158, 159]. In ruminants, Cu absorption is decreased if the diet contains more than 0.3% S, or 1–3 mg molybdenum (Mo)/kg DM, or a dietary copper to molybdenum (Cu:Mo) ratio of less than 2 : 1 [104, 161]. In the horse, Mo at 20 mg/kg DM, several times higher than generally present in horse feeds, did not appear to interfere with Cu utilization [104]. However, Cu absorption and retention were reduced when dietary Mo content was 107 mg/kg DM with 13 mg Cu/kg DM [161].

A diet containing 1000 mg zinc (Zn)/kg and 7.7 mg Cu/kg induced a secondary Cu deficiency in weanlings [162]. However, no effect of high Zn intake (1170 mg Zn/kg feed vs. 38 mg Zn/kg feed) was found on Cu metabolism or bone development in young horses fed diets containing approximately 9 mg Cu/kg feed [158]. The amount of Cu in the diet may, therefore, be an important consideration with regard to the influence that high dietary Zn may have on the overall Cu status of the horse.

8.3.3.2 Dietary Recommendation

The NRC 2007 recommends a dietary Cu intake of 0.2 mg Cu/kg BW or 100 mg Cu/d for a mature horse weighing 500 kg (Table 8.1). Other estimates have ranged from 86 to 106 mg Cu/d for a mature 500 kg horse [1, 44, 84]. The maximum tolerance concentration of dietary Cu is set at 250 mg/kg DM. Although higher concentrations have been tolerated according to scientific literature, lack of data, and possible genetic differences between horses, have resulted in the recommendation of this lower concentration [37].

Dietary Cu recommendations for the growing horse, the broodmare in late gestation, as well as the lactating broodmare, are in Table 8.1. The NRC concluded that the dietary Cu intake of the lactating mare does not appear to influence the Cu content of her milk. Therefore the current dietary Cu recommendation for the lactating mare serves to account for the Cu incorporated into the mare's milk (0.25 mg Cu/kg BW/d, assuming a DM intake of 2.5% of BW) [1].

8.3.3.3 Signs of Deficiency and Excess

8.3.3.3.1 Deficiency

Lysyl oxidase, an enzyme involved in collagen crosslinking, requires Cu as a co-factor [44]. Thus impaired collagen synthesis might be expected to occur during Cu deficiency. However, reports of naturally occurring primary Cu deficiencies in horses are scarce. Bone and joint problems in growing horses presumed to have altered Cu metabolism associated with excessive intakes of other minerals, particularly Zn, may occur [163, 164]. Studies investigating a possible connection between diet and developmental orthopedic disorders in horses are explored in Musculoskeletal System Disorders in Chapter 25. A sign of Cu deficiency is coat discoloration in cattle, and unpigmented bands in the wool of sheep, likely due to an impairment of melanin synthesis [10, 156]. Although cases of horse coat discoloration (specifically a yellowing of chestnut coats, and a rusty-brown undertone in dark coats) due to Cu deficiency have been mentioned in the popular press, it has not been documented in the scientific literature or controlled studies.

8.3.3.3.2 Excess

Horses are quite resistant to excess Cu intake. Ponies have been reported to tolerate dietary Cu as high as 791 mg/kg for 6 m although liver and kidney Cu content increased [165]. One of the ponies reportedly had a normal foal about 4 m after being fed this high amount of Cu. Additionally, 20 and 40 mg of Cu/kg BW as copper sulfate was given to mature ponies (equivalent to 1000–2500 mg/kg ration) without apparent adverse effect [165]. However, feeding a ration containing 2800 mg Cu/kg DM (125 mg copper sulfate/kg BW/d) for 6 m caused hypercupremia, hepatic and renal damage, and the death of horses 6 m after the start of the study [3]. Thus, the minimum dietary concentration at which Cu toxicosis occurs in horses is between 791 and 2800 mg Cu/kg diet DM. Nevertheless, the maximum tolerable total dietary Cu concentration for horse feed has been set at 250 mg/kg DM [37]. The horse's high tolerance to excess Cu ingestion may be in part due to the downregulation of Cu absorption with increasing Cu intake [161, 167].

8.3.3.4 Diagnosis and Treatment

Although the horse's plasma Cu concentration and dietary Cu intake have been reported to be positively correlated, the most appropriate way to confirm a dietary imbalance, and determine how to correct it, is to evaluate the diet involved [164].

Plasma, serum, or organ/tissue Cu concentrations may vary with age and physiological state. Copper concentrations in adult horses have been reported to range from 0.7 to 1.5 mg Cu/L in plasma, 6.5–10.5 mg Cu/kg wet weight in the renal cortex, and 2–3.6 mg Cu/kg wet weight in the pancreas in a group of five clinically healthy horses [163]. Another laboratory reported a normal equine plasma copper range of 1.02–1.78 mg Cu/L [168]. For foals, however, the normal plasma Cu concentration at birth is only 0.1–0.4 mg/L [169]. Plasma Cu concentration increases to adult concentrations by about 1 wk of age, and up to double that of the normal adult during the first year of life. Plasma Cu is also elevated in broodmares for approximately 1 m before and after foaling [169, 170].

Serum Cu concentration has also been reported to correlate with serum ceruloplasmin activity. However, ceruloplasmin synthesis in young animals is a maturation-dependent process that may be relatively insensitive to dietary influences [169]. A study evaluating Cu metabolism in ponies also found that ceruloplasmin reflected the degree of change in Cu metabolism, due to a change in dietary Cu intake, less accurately than serum Cu [167]. However, when Cu deficiency is present, liver Cu stores will decrease substantially before plasma Cu concentration decreases. Liver Cu concentrations have been reported to vary greatly in newborn foals ($n = 13$), ranging from 150 to 552 mg Cu/kg liver DM [170]. Liver Cu concentration of the foals declined over time and reached values (12–28 mg Cu/kg liver DM) comparable to that of their dams (0–39 mg Cu/kg liver DM) at 5 m of age. Other studies have reported fetal hepatic Cu concentrations ranging from 17 to 571 mg Cu/kg liver DM in yearlings [4, 171, 172]. The Cu concentrations for organs other than the liver have also been reported [158, 165, 173].

Mane hair Cu concentration ranged from 3.5 to 6.1 mg/kg hair in a group of healthy racehorses, and between 4.13 and 5.67 mg/kg hair for miniature horses fed four different diets ranging from below to above NRC requirements [1, 140, 172]. In another group of horses kept in industrial vs. non-industrial areas, the range of serum Cu concentrations was not reflected similarly in the range of hair Cu content. The industrial area horses had a wider range in serum Cu concentrations, but a narrower range for hair Cu content, while the opposite trend was observed for the non-industrial area horses [175]. Foal mane hair Cu concentrations have also been reported to be higher compared with their dams until about 90 d of age [176].

8.3.4 Zinc

The basic functions of zinc (Zn) can be divided into three categories: a catalyst for at least 300 enzymes, a structural component, and a regulator of gene expression [177]. Approximately 56% of the total Zn in the body is found in the muscles [44].

8.3.4.1 Sources and Factors Influencing Absorption

Common feedstuffs contain 15–40 mg Zn per kg DM. The common inorganic forms of supplemental Zn are Zn-oxide and Zn-sulfate, while organic forms of Zn include Zn-methionine, Zn-proteinates, and zinc polysaccharides.

The absorption of Zn is regulated by the animal's current Zn status and needs. For example, weanlings absorbed 89% and 6% from diets containing 38 and 1170 mg/kg DM, respectively [158]. In a study investigating the effect of high Zn intake on Cu absorption, the percent of Zn intake absorbed and retained by mature horses increased with increasing dietary concentrations from 73 to 400 mg Zn/kg DM but did not increase further with 540 mg Zn/kg DM [159]. Urinary Zn excretion was small and did not differ with increasing dietary Zn intakes, therefore the excess Zn was lost in the feces. True Zn digestibility has been reported to be lower in exercising horses, compared with idle horses [1]. It is not known whether phytate or excess Ca intake will decrease Zn absorption in horses, as is observed in several other species.

8.3.4.2 Dietary Recommendation

Zinc requirements vary with the physiological class (Table 8.1). Data collected from many studies over time report endogenous Zn losses to range from 0.10 to 0.16 mg Zn/kg BW/d. Similarly, true digestibility used to calculate daily intakes, range from 21% to 35% [84, 178]. This variation in data results in a daily Zn requirement for a 500 kg horse ranging from 236 to 420 mg/d. The NRC currently recommends 400 mg Zn/d for a 500 kg mature, idle, horse, while others opted for the higher recommendation of 420 mg/d for the same horse [1, 44]. The maximum tolerance concentration for dietary Zn in equine diets has been set at 500 mg/kg DM [37].

8.3.4.3 Signs of Deficiency and Excess

8.3.4.3.1 Deficiency

Hair loss, lethargy, diarrhea, decreased serum and tissue Zn concentrations, and decreased plasma alkaline phosphatase and lactic dehydrogenase activities (Zn-containing metalloenzymes) have been reported in foals fed an experimental diet containing 5 mg Zn/kg DM, while the foals receiving 40 mg Zn/kg appeared normal [179].

Mare's milk has been reported to contain 30 mg Zn/kg milk DM at foaling, decreasing to 18 mg Zn/kg milk DM at 2 to 5 m of lactation [133]. Feeding mares a ration containing 18 or 30 mg Zn/kg DM for 60 d before and after foaling, did not affect Zn concentration in milk or the serum of mares or foals and foal growth rate was similar between the two groups [180]. Young horses fed a diet containing 38 or 41 mg Zn/kg DM grew normally, maintained normal body-tissue Zn concentrations, and had no observed joint abnormalities [158, 181]. There was no difference in growth rate, plasma Zn, bone density, or bone total mineral content in weanlings fed 17, 40, or 50 mg Zn/kg DM for 4 m [182]. These results seem to indicate that growing horses could be fed diets with total dietary Zn concentration below 40 mg/kg DM without detriment. However, a better understanding of the complexity of the enzymatic systems supported by Zn makes it possible that these systems may be compromised long before obvious clinical signs are recognized. Therefore, supplying Zn per recommendations, especially for growing horses, is prudent as the long-term effects of low Zn diets have not been studied extensively.

8.3.4.3.2 Excess

Horses are thought to be tolerant of higher concentrations of Zn, as indicated by maximum tolerable concentrations [37]. Excess Zn decreases Cu absorption in ruminants, but diets containing 580 or 1 200 mg Zn/kg DM did not decrease Cu absorption by horses when dietary Cu concentrations were adequate [158, 183]. However, a dietary Zn intake greater than 700 mg/kg DM/d has been reported to interfere with Cu utilization by means other than decreasing its absorption [160].

Clinically, Zn toxicosis has been associated with industrial sources of Zn pollution [44]. For example, Gunson et al. investigated cases of chronic Zn/Cd toxicosis in horses and particularly foals born and raised near a smelting operation. Interviews with horse farms revealed that feeding hay imported from other areas allowed for normal development of foals, while feeding of locally grown forages resulted in severe lameness. Two foals and their dams fed local forage were evaluated. These foals shared similar signs of Zn toxicosis to that which has been previously described [163].

Signs of Zn toxicity in growing horses initially start with enlargements of the epiphyseal regions of long bones, followed by lameness with a stiff gait or reluctance to move. Severely affected foals will often stand with their head held low, have an arched back, and resist curving the spine laterally when turned to the side [163, 184]. Pathological evaluation of the two foals revealed osteochondrosis in all joints [163]. Decreased growth rate, poor condition, and progressive anemia may also occur. Foals fed 90 mg Zn/kg BW/d developed anemia and had decreased growth, enlarged growth plates of the long bones of the legs, stiffness, lameness, and increased blood and tissue Zn concentrations [185].

8.3.4.4 Diagnosis and Treatment

8.3.4.4.1 Deficiency

Circulating Zn concentrations are affected by many variables including age, stress, infection, hormonal alterations, and sample handling [186]. Blood collection vials that are manufactured to minimize trace mineral contamination should be used. Often Zn reference ranges use serum or plasma, however, most of the Zn in whole blood is found in the erythrocyte and one study found no relationship between whole blood Zn and plasma Zn [168, 187]. Any hemolysis during sample collection or handling could affect plasma or serum Zn concentration. Serum Zn has also been reported to be affected by the amount of time the clot remains in the serum [188]. Given the number of factors that can affect circulating Zn concentrations, reference ranges should be used with care. It has been suggested that under some situations (disease, stress) Zn can move between plasma and blood cellular components [187]. A decrease in the plasma Zn concentration from these causes can be differentiated from that due to a deficiency by measuring Zn in plasma along with erythrocyte metallothionein concentration. Metallothionein is present in most tissues and binds primarily Zn and/or Cu. Low concentrations of both metallothionein and Zn indicate a Zn deficiency; if metallothionein is not decreased, this indicates that the low Zn concentration may not be due to a deficiency [186]. In an induced Zn deficiency, a decrease in Zn concentration is greatest in bone and least in the liver and testes, whereas the heart, muscle, skin, and hair Zn content remain unchanged [186].

8.3.4.4.2 Excess

Weanling ponies fed a high 1 170 mg Zn/kg DM for 90 d had higher liver tissue Zn concentrations than weanlings fed the basal diet of 38 mg Zn/kg DM [158]. In post-mortem samples collected after feeding the two rations for 5 m, liver and kidney Zn concentrations were lower for ponies fed the basal diet than for those fed the high Zn diet. Spleen Zn concentrations, however, were similar for the two treatments.

Mane hair Zn concentration may reflect Zn intake. Feeding diets ranging from 15 to 201 mg Zn/100 kg BW did not affect serum Zn but resulted in higher mane hair Zn content in horses fed the highest amount of Zn [174]. Mane hair Zn concentration has been reported to range from 62 to 256 mg Zn/kg mane hair, but not all studies have reported Zn intakes, so the relationship between Zn intake and mane hair concentration is not well characterized [140, 174, 175].

Like all dietary nutrient imbalances, a dietary Zn deficiency or excess/toxicosis is best diagnosed by evaluating the complete diet as described in Ration Analysis in Chapter 10. Any deficiencies or excesses should be corrected with appropriate dietary changes. It may or may not be possible to reverse signs of Zn toxicosis, particularly those related to bone development in growing horses.

8.3.5 Iron

Iron (Fe) is distributed primarily in hemoglobin (60%) and in muscle myoglobin (20%) where it is involved in oxygen transport and use. It is a component of hemosiderin, transferrin, and ferritin, and is linked to the immune system as present in macrophages [44].

8.3.5.1 Sources and Factors Influencing Absorption

Forages can contain 50–400 mg Fe/kg DM, and cereal grains contain 30–90 mg Fe/kg DM. Supplemental Fe in both organic (chelated iron) and inorganic (Fe sulfate) forms are available; however, research comparing these forms as sources in horses is limited.

Iron absorption increases with increasing need, but Fe absorption can also decrease with excessive intake of cadmium, cobalt, copper, manganese, and zinc [189]. The hormone hepcidin is important in the regulation of Fe absorption. The basic mechanism of absorption involves uptake of Fe by enterocytes (divalent metal transporter 1 mediated) followed by phagocytosis of the sloughed enterocytes, containing the incorporated Fe [12, 44, 190].

However, although hepcidin functions to regulate absorption, excessive Fe intake is thought to have the ability to exceed the capacity of regulating mechanisms, particularly when mucosal damage is present [44]. Researchers investigating the mRNA expression of hepcidin in different tissues obtained from six healthy horses reported the highest expression of this hormone in the liver and stated that this was similar to findings in other species [191].

8.3.5.2 Dietary Recommendation

The NRC 2007 recommends 0.8 mg Fe/kg BW for mature idle horses (or 400 mg/d for a mature 500 kg horse). However, a more recent review using data from 69 trials provides a recommendation of 420 mg Fe/d for a 500 kg horse at maintenance [44]. Iron requirements increase for growing horses, horses in the last 3 m of pregnancy, and lactating mares; however, there is no agreement with regard to whether exercise increases the Fe requirement (Table 8.1).

8.3.5.3 Signs of Deficiency and Excess

8.3.5.3.1 Deficiency

A Fe deficiency can occur in horses if there is chronic or severe blood loss. The blood loss may be apparent, such as that due to severe lice infestation or intestinal parasitism. Bleeding gastrointestinal ulcers, exercise-induced pulmonary hemorrhage, and blood coagulation abnormalities can also be sources of chronic blood loss, resulting in depleted Fe stores and anemia [192].

Unless soil Fe concentrations are deficient, a clinically recognized Fe deficiency rarely occurs in healthy foals or mature horses at any performance level [1, 133, 193]. Foals are most susceptible to Fe deficiency as mares' milk contains 12–28 mg/kg milk DM at foaling decreasing to 5 mg/kg milk DM at 4 m postpartum. The foal's need for Fe increases as it grows with associated increases in blood volume and muscle mass. Only one case of severe Fe deficiency anemia is reported in the scientific literature in a newborn foal, and it occurred in conjunction with significant morphological red blood cell changes and septicemia [133, 194]. In this Fe deficient neonatal foal, microcytosis and hypochromasia were absent, even though the foal had serum Fe concentration of 1 μg/dL (reference range 49–288 μg/dL), ferritin 14 ng/mL (33–140 ng/mL), and total iron-binding capacity (TIBC) 449 μg/dL (437–777 μg/dL) [194].

In other species, the initial effect of an iron deficiency is a decrease in Fe storage in the liver, spleen, and bone marrow, paralleled by a decrease in the plasma ferritin concentration. The decrease in ionic Fe, a required co-factor in some enzymes, decreases exercise capacity. This decrease in exercise capacity occurs before anemia, and the iron-deficient anemic animal responds to Fe administration with an increase in endurance capacity before there is any significant increase in hemoglobin concentration [195]. If an iron deficiency persists, following a decrease in storage of Fe and endurance capacity, there is a decrease in transport of Fe characterized by decreased serum Fe and increased TIBC. The ratio of Fe to TIBC is the transferrin saturation, which is decreased at this stage of Fe deficiency. The final stage or effect of iron deficiency is anemia, which initially is normocytic normochromic, but becomes microcytic hypochromic if the Fe deficiency becomes moderate to severe. The anemia causes a further decrease in the Fe deficient animal's endurance capacity. As the supply of transport of Fe decreases, red blood cell protoporphyrin and distribution width increases, and hemoglobin production and mean corpuscular volume decrease [196]. Although preparations containing Fe are often given to improve performance; no studies have demonstrated the beneficial effects of Fe supplements to healthy horses receiving Fe-adequate diets [195, 196].

8.3.5.3.2 Excess

At birth, foals have a high plasma Fe concentration and transferrin saturation, and absorption of Fe is considerably higher in neonates than adults [197]. Iron-toxicosis-induced liver failure and death of foals have occurred due to the oral administration of a digestive inoculum containing iron [198]. To test the possibility of Fe toxicity, foals received 360 mg of Fe as ferrous fumarate on the first day of life or the same digestive inoculum. The condition was reproduced. Before death, the foals exhibited depression, diarrhea, icterus, dehydration, and coma. Morphological changes included erosion of jejunal villi, pulmonary hemorrhage, massive Fe deposits in the liver, and liver degeneration. It was suggested that a vitamin E and/or Se deficiency may increase the foal's susceptibility to acute Fe toxicosis, similar to baby pigs. These results along with previous studies by the same authors led them to conclude that neonatal foals should not receive oral Fe supplements in the first 3 d of life [198]. Ferrous fumarate toxicosis has also been reported in mature horses, but the toxic dose of Fe for the mature horse is as much as 25 times greater than that for the neonatal foal [199]. Feeding diets containing 436, 893, and 1400 mg Fe/kg DM/d for 3 m had no significant effect on weanling or yearling horses' feed intake, growth rate, red blood cell count, hematocrit; serum, liver, kidney, or spleen Fe, Ca, P, Cu, Zn, or Mn concentrations; serum unbound-iron-binding capacity; or TIBC [173]. These high Fe concentrations also did not affect Ca or P absorption, or third metacarpal bone mineral content, breaking strength, or size. The highest dietary concentration did increase the percent Fe saturation of transferrin from 36% to 42%. However, chronic Fe overload with hepatic toxicity and hemochromatosis has been reported in horses that consumed water containing high concentrations of Fe over several years [200].

Fe administration, in much smaller amounts than those necessary to induce Fe toxicosis, increases susceptibility to bacterial infections in most species. When bacteria invade mammals, one determinant of success or failure to establish an infection is the availability of the Fe needed to multiply. During a bacteria-induced inflammatory response, neutrophils release lactoferrin, which binds available Fe. The lactoferrin is then phagocytized, thus decreasing the availability of Fe for bacterial use. In mature horses, plasma Fe concentration has been shown to decrease with systemic inflammatory conditions. Clinical, as well as controlled studies, have indicated that plasma and serum Fe concentrations may be used as a sensitive indicator of systemic inflammation in horses [201, 202]. Corticosteroids dramatically increase the horse's plasma Fe concentration 48–72 hrs after their administration but do not affect serum Fe binding capacity or plasma ferritin concentration [203].

8.3.5.4 Diagnosis and Treatment

8.3.5.4.1 Deficiency

Diet-induced Fe imbalances are best diagnosed when the entire diet has been evaluated and total Fe intake determined. However, deficiency due to inadequate Fe intake is less likely than deficiency due to acute or chronic blood loss. Iron status may be evaluated with hemoglobin concentrations, red blood cell counts, mean corpuscular hemoglobin concentrations, serum/plasma Fe concentrations, serum ferritin, total Fe binding capacity, transferrin saturation, and unsaturated iron-binding capacity [193]. Low ferritin concentrations may be indicative of low body-Fe stores, while high ferritin concentrations suggest saturated body stores. Ferritin also plays a role as an acute-phase protein and may be impacted by inflammatory conditions or exercise.

As measures of Fe status, hematocrit and blood hemoglobin concentration are not very sensitive in horses. During excitement, anxiety, or exertion, the spleen contracts, releasing red blood cells, which can increase the hematocrit and hemoglobin concentration by more than 50%. Thus, splenic contraction can mask an iron deficiency-induced decrease in red blood cell number or hemoglobin concentration. Additionally, neither serum Fe concentration (normally 120–210 μg/dL in adults and 380 ± 20 μg/dL at birth decreasing to 70 μg/dL at 2 wks of age), serum TIBC (normally 370–470 μg/dL), percent Fe saturation (normally 30–50%) nor serum unbound-iron-binding capacity (normally 200–300 μg/dL) adequately indicate the horse's Fe status [204–206].

In contrast, the serum concentration of ferritin, the storage form of Fe, is an accurate measure of the horse's Fe status [206]. Its decrease is the earliest indication of inadequate body Fe. In people, the serum ferritin concentration increases in most chronic disease conditions but is not affected by stress, excitement, or exertion [207]. Anemia, which occurs with many chronic disease conditions, can be differentiated from anemia due to Fe deficiency by a normal to increased serum ferritin concentration. Erythrocyte sedimentation rate, zeta-sedimentation rate, and C-reactive protein are also useful in differentiation, as all increase with anemia due to chronic disease but not to Fe deficiency [196].

In normal, non-anemic horses, not known to have been given supplemental Fe, the serum ferritin concentration was 152 ± 55 ng/mL (mean ± SD, range 70–250 ng/mL) in one group of 28 horses, and 223 ± 13.4 ng/mL in a group of 103 horses that tended to be older [206]. In another group of 13 horses, serum ferritin concentration was 87 ± 53 ng/mL with a range of 33–139 ng/mL [205]. Thus, it appears that a serum ferritin concentration of less than 30 or greater than 250–300 ng/mL indicates that the horse's body-Fe status is abnormally low or high, respectively.

Mane hair Fe concentration was reported to range from 53 to 87 mg/kg hair DM but did not appear to closely reflect dietary intake in one study [174]. In healthy racehorses, mane hair Fe concentration ranged from 0 to 152 mg/kg hair DM, while a decrease in both mare and foal mane hair Fe concentration occurred within 90 d following parturition [140, 176].

Treatment of Fe deficiency due to blood loss is twofold: (i) correct the cause of the blood loss that resulted in the Fe deficiency, and (ii) give the nutrients necessary for increased red blood cell synthesis. An oral Fe supplement can be provided for these cases [192]. Intramuscular injection of Fe-dextran has been reported to result in the death of three horses, probably due to an allergic or anaphylactic reaction [208].

8.3.5.4.2 Excess

The only means of protection against excess Fe is decreased absorption, as the body has no means of excreting significant amounts of excess iron once absorbed. In cases of suspected toxicosis, the Fe content of the water should be evaluated and a ration analysis is recommended. Injected iron bypasses the body's only means of protection against Fe toxicosis, i.e. decreased intestinal absorption. Thus, a much smaller amount of Fe given by injection is more likely to cause toxicosis than an amount given orally.

8.4 Other Minerals of Interest

There are many other minerals (molybdenum, manganese, cobalt, fluorine, chromium, silicon, aluminum, vanadium, tin, nickel, and boron) present in the diet, but they are of relatively low nutritional importance in horses [37].

In general, heavy metal (arsenic (As), cadmium (Cd), lead (Pb), and mercury (Hg)) toxicity is associated with signs such as suppressed immune response, poor growth rates, and poor fertility [37, 209]. Heavy metals can enter the environment through industrial or mining wastes, fertilizers, soil correctives, livestock manures, wastewater irrigation, pesticides, and long-term applications of sewage sludge and are sometimes present in forages and feedstuff consumed by a horse [175, 209]. Researchers evaluating the trends for heavy metal contamination of animal feed components in Europe noted that feed material intended as sources of mineral in animal feeds frequently tested positive for heavy metal but below the maximum limit allowed in Europe [210]. However, researchers noted that marine-derived products in particular, for example, seaweed-derived products or fishmeal, were associated with heavy metal contamination. Studies such as these are helpful to the feed industry to continue expanding and improving the current quality control measures implemented in the animal feed manufacturing process.

Due to the different inclusion rates used by feed manufacturers, assessing the total dietary intake of heavy metals, across different feeds and manufacturers, is difficult [8]. However, if necessary, the accumulation of these metals can be tested by evaluating blood, milk, or hair. Blood may reflect more recent exposure, and hair or bone may reflect long-term exposure [209]. The maximum tolerance guidelines for total dietary concentrations of As, Cd, and Pb have been set at 30, 10, and 10 mg/kg DM, respectively. In the case of Hg, form plays a role in toxicity, and a maximum tolerance concentration has been set of 1 mg/kg DM for organic Hg, and 0.2 mg/kg DM for inorganic Hg [37].

Case in Point

Animal Assessment

A new client to your Michigan practice with six broodmares (BW ~1100 lb, BCS 6/9) explains, last year, she had one stillborn foal and two of the five foals born alive were weak, had difficulty standing and nursing even though each mare had adequate milk production. One foal with breathing problems was sent to the local Veterinary Hospital Intensive Care Unit and she would send those medical records. The broodmares all appeared healthy and had no abnormal physical findings.

Ration Assessment

Late gestation: she feeds the mares locally grown organic timothy grass hay at 3% BW with ~2 lb/horse/d of a local grain mix reported to be for lactating mares with 15% crude protein, 0.7% calcium, and 0.4% phosphorus. She would get the full nutrient profile of the grain mix but also has trace-mineralized salt blocks available to all mares ad libitum.

1) Does feeding 15 kg/H/d (500 kg BW × 3%) of mature grass hay and 2 lb of the grain mix meet the crude protein, calcium, and phosphorus requirements of late gestation mares?

Feed source[a]	Protein	Ca	P	Amount fed	Protein	Ca	P
	%	%	%	kg/d	g/d	g/d	g/d
Timothy hay IFN 1-04-881 [211]	17.0	0.66	0.34	15	?	?	?
Grain mix	15	0.7	0.4	1	?	?	?
Total daily intake					?	?	?
Mare requirements[b]							
Mare, 11-m gestation					893	36	26
Mare, 1-m lactation					1535	59	38

[a]All values are on as fed basis.
[b]NRC [1], p. 298.

2) The foal sent to the ICU was euthanized, and on necropsy was found to have histological changes consistent with thyroid hyperplasia. What is now the primary nutrient of concern?
3) What are the next steps to determine the imbalance in the mare's ration?

Feed source[a]	Iodine	Amount fed	Iodine
	mg/kg	kg/d	mg/d
Timothy hay IFN 1-04-893 [210]	0.04	15	?
Grain mix	0.1	1	?
Total daily intake			?
Mare requirements[b]			
Mare, late gestation			4.0
Mare, early lactation			4.4

[a] All values are on as fed basis.
[b] NRC [1], p 298.

4) What would be the recommendation for next year?

See Appendix A Chapter 8.

References

1 National Research Council (2007). *Nutrient Requirements of Horses*. 6th Rev. Animal Nutrition Series, 1–341. Washington, DC: National Academies Press.

2 Aiello, S.E., Moses, M.A., and Allen, D.G. (ed.) (2016). The Merck veterinary manual. In: *The Merck Veterinary Manual*, 11e, 2312–2329. Kenilworth, NJ: Merck & Co Inc.

3 Bauer, M. (1975). Copper sulphate poisoning in horses. *Vet. Arh.* 45: 257–268.

4 Eversole, D.E., Thatcher, C.D., Blodgett, D.J. et al. (1988). Repletion of blood selenium concentrations in weaned beef calves. *Cornell Vet.* 78: 75–87.

5 Smith, J.E., Cipriano, J.E., DeBowes, R., and Moore, K. (1986). Iron deficiency and pseudo-iron deficiency in hospitalized horses. *J. Am. Vet. Med. Assoc.* 188 (3): 285–287.

6 Harvey, J. (2008). Iron metabolism and its disorders. In: *Clinical Biochemistry of Domestic Animals*, 6e (ed. J. Kaneko, J. Harvey, and M. Bruss), 259–285. Amsterdam: Elsevier Academic Press.

7 Hintz, H.F. (1989). Iodine toxicosis. *Equine Pract.* 11: 5–6.

8 López-Alonso, M. and Miranda, M. (2012). Implications of excessive livestock mineral supplementation on environmental pollution and human health. In: *Trace Elements: Environmental Sources, Geochemistry and Human Health* (ed. D.A. de Leon and P.R. Aragon), 75–92. New York: Nova publishers.

9 Breuhaus, B.A. (2011). Disorders of the equine thyroid gland. *Vet. Clin. North Am. Equine Pract.* 27 (1): 115–128.

10 Underwood, E.J. (1981). *The Mineral Nutrition of Livestock*, 2e, 1–119. Slough: Commonwealth Agricultural Bureaux.

11 Walthall, J.C. and McKenzie, R.A. (1976). Osteodystrophia fibrosa in horses at pasture in Queensland: field and laboratory observations. *Aust. Vet. J.* 52: 11–16.

12 Muñoz, M., García-Erce, J.A., and Remacha, Á.F. (2010). Disorders of iron metabolism. Part 1: molecular basis of iron homoeostasis. *J. Clin. Pathol.* 64 (4): 281–286.

13 Rourke, K.M., Kohn, C.W., Levine, A.L. et al. (2009). Rapid calcitonin response to experimental hypercalcemia in healthy horses. *Domest. Anim. Endocrinol.* 36: 197–201.

14 Toribio, R.E. (2011). Disorders of calcium and phosphate metabolism in horses. *Vet. Clin. North Am. Equine Pract.* 27: 129–147.

15 Dundon, B., Baker, L., Pipkin, J., and Lawrence, T. (2011). Digestibility and balance of organic and inorganic sources of calcium and magnesium in exercised two and three year old geldings. *J. Equine Vet. Sci.* 31: 271–272.

16 Highfill, J.L., Potter, G., Eller, E. et al. (2005). Comparative absorption of calcium fed in varying chemical forms and effects on absorption of phosphorus and magnesium. In: *Proceedings of the 19th Equine Nutrition and Physiology Society Symposium*, 37. Tucson, AZ: Equine Nutrition and Physiology Society.

17 Schryver, H.F., Craig, P.H., Hintz, H.F. et al. (1970). The site of calcium absorption in the horse. *J. Nutr.* 100: 1127–1131.

18 Schryver, H.F., Hintz, H.F., Craig, P.H. et al. (1972). Site of phosphorus absorption from the intestine of the horse. *J. Nutr.* 102: 143–147.

19 Schryver, H.F., Hintz, H.F., and Lowe, J.E. (1974). Calcium and phosphorus in the nutrition of the horse. *Cornell Vet.* 64: 493–515.

20 Hintz, H.F., Schryver, H.F., Doty, J. et al. (1984). Oxalic acid content of alfalfa hays and its influence on the availability of calcium, phosphorus and magnesium to ponies. *J. Anim. Sci.* 58: 939–942.

21 McKenzie, R.A. (1985). Poisoning of horses by oxalate in grasses. In: *Plant Toxicology* (ed. A.A. Seawright, M.P. Hegarty, L.F. James, and R.F. Keeler), 150. Yeerongpilly, Brisbane: Queensland Poisonous Plants Committee, Queensland Department of Primary Industries, Animal Research Institute.

22 van Doorn, D.A., Everts, H., Wouterse, H., and Beynen, A.C. (2004). The apparent digestibility of phytate phosphorus and the influence of supplemental phytase in horses. *J. Anim. Sci.* 82: 1756–1763.

23 Lavin, T.E., Nielsen, B.D., Zingsheim, J.N. et al. (2013). Effects of phytase supplementation in mature horses fed alfalfa hay and pelleted concentrate diets. *J. Anim. Sci.* 91: 1719–1727.

24 Wall, D.L., Topliff, D.R., Freeman, D.W. et al. (1992). Effect of dietary cation-anion balance on urinary mineral excretion in exercised horses. *J. Equine Vet. Sci.* 12: 168–171.

25 McKenzie, E.C., Valberg, S.J., Godden, S.M. et al. (2002). Plasma and urine electrolyte and mineral concentrations in Thoroughbred horses with recurrent exertional rhabdomyolysis after consumption of diets varying in cation-anion balance. *Am. J. Vet. Res.* 63: 1053–1060.

26 Cooper, S.R., Topliff, D.R., Freeman, D.W. et al. (2000). Effect of dietary cation-anion difference on mineral balance, serum osteocalcin concentration and growth in weanling horses. *J. Equine Vet. Sci.* 20 (1): 39–44.

27 Baker, L.A., Topliff, D.R., Freeman, D.W. et al. (1998). The comparison of two forms of sodium and potassium and chloride versus sulfur in the dietary cation-anion difference equation: effects on acid-base status and mineral balance in sedentary horses. *J. Equine Vet. Sci.* 18 (6): 389–395.

28 Insogna, K.L. (2009). The effect of proton pump-inhibiting drugs on mineral metabolism. *Am. J. Gastroenterol.* 104 (Suppl. 2): S2–S4.

29 Caston, S.S., Fredericks, D.C., Kersh, K.D., and Wang, C. (2015). Short-term omeprazole use does not affect serum calcium concentrations and bone density in horses. *J. Equine Vet. Sci.* 35 (9): 714–723.

30 Nielsen, B.D., Eckert, S.M., Robison, C.I. et al. (2017). Omeprazole and its impact on mineral absorption in horses. *Anim. Prod. Sci.* 57: 2263–2269.

31 Houpt, K. and Perry, P. (2016). Effect of chronic furosemide on salt and water intake of ponies. *J. Equine Vet. Sci.* 47: 31–35.

32 Pagan, J., Waldridge, B., Whitehouse, C. et al. (2014). Furosemide administration affects mineral excretion in exercised Thoroughbreds. *Equine Vet. J.* 46 (Suppl. 46): 4.

33 Roussel, A.J. Jr. and Thatcher, C.D. (1987). Primary hyperparathyroidism in a pony mare. *Compend. Contin. Educ. Pract. Vet.* 9: 781–783.

34 Joyce, J.R., Pierce, K.R., Romane, W.M., and Baker, J.M. (1971). Clinical study of nutritional secondary hyperparathyroidism in horses. *J. Am. Vet. Med. Assoc.* 158 (12): 2033–2042.

35 Bertone, J.J. (1992). Nutritional secondary hyperparathyroidism. In: *Current Therapy in Equine Medicine* (ed. A. Śmieszek), 119–122. Philadelphia, PA: W.B. Saunders.

36 Krook, L. and Lowe, J.E. (1964). Nutritional secondary hyperparathyroidism in the horse: with a description of the normal equine parathyroid gland. *Pathol. Vet.* 1: 1–98.

37 National Research Council (1987). *Vitamin Tolerance of Animals*, 1–108. Washington, DC: National Academies Press.

38 Thompson, K.N., Jackson, S.G., and Baker, J.P. (1988). Equine applied and clinical nutrition: health, welfare and performance. *J. Anim. Sci.* 66: 2459–2467.

39 Krook, L. and Maylin, G.A. (1988). Fractures in Thoroughbred race horses. *Cornell Vet.* 78: 1.

40 Mello, J.R.B. (2003). Calcinosis – calcinogenic plants. *Toxicon* 41: 1–12.

41 McKenzie, R.A., Gartner, R.J.W.W., Blaney, B.J., and Glanville, R.J. (1981). Control of nutritional secondary hyperparathyroidism in grazing horses with calcium plus phosphorous supplementation. *Aust. Vet. J.* 57 (12): 554–557.

42 Harris, P. and Gray, J. (1992). The use of the urinary fractional electrolyte excretion test to assess electrolyte status in the horse. *Equine Vet. Educ.* 4: 162–166.

43 Caple, I.W., Doake, P.A., and Ellis, P.G. (1982). Assessment of the calcium and phosphorus nutrition in horses by analysis of urine. *Aust. Vet. J.* 58 (4): 125–131.

44 Coenen, M. (2013). Macro and trace elements in equine nutrition. In: *Equine Applied and Clinical Nutrition: Health, Welfare and Performance* (ed. R.J. Geor, P.A. Harris, and M. Coenen), 190–228. Edinburgh: Saunders Elsevier.

45 Morris, D.D., Divers, T.J., and Whitlock, R.H. (1984). Renal clearance and fractional excretion of electrolytes over a 24-hour period in horses. *Am. J. Vet. Res.* 45: 2431–2435.

46 Meyer, H., Stadermann, B., Schnurpel, B., and Nehring, T. (1992). The influence of type of diet (roughage or concentrate) on the plasma level, renal excretion, and apparent digestibility of calcium and magnesium in resting and exercising horses. *J. Equine Vet. Sci.* 12: 233–239.

47 Yamada, K., Sato, F., Higuchi, T. et al. (2015). Experimental investigation of bone mineral density in Thoroughbreds using quantitative computed tomography. *J. Equine Sci.* 26: 81–87.

48 Weaver, C.M. (1990). Assessing calcium status and metabolism. *J. Nutr.* 120: 1470–1473.

49 Donabedian, M., Delguste, C., Perona, G. et al. (2005). Third metacarpal bone mineral density assessment in the standing horse by dual X-ray absorptiometry. *Vet. Comp. Orthop. Traumatol.* 18: 26–30.

50 Hassel, D.M., Rakestraw, P.C., Gardner, I.A. et al. (2004). Dietary risk factors and colonic pH and mineral concentrations in horses with enterolithiasis. *J. Vet. Intern. Med.* 18: 346–349.

51 Cohen, N.D., Vontur, C.A., and Rakestraw, P.C. (2000). Risk factors for enterolithiasis among horses in Texas. *J. Am. Vet. Med. Assoc.* 216 (11): 1787–1794.

52 Pearson, P.B. (1934). Inorganic phosphorus of horse serum: the effect of age and nutrition. *J. Biolumin. Chemilumin.* 106: 1–6.

53 Coleman, R.J. (1983). Feeds and feeding in the northwestern United States and Western Canada. In: *Current Therapy in Equine Medicine* (ed. N.E. Robinson), 691–697. Philadelphia, PA: W.B. Saunders Company.

54 Hintz, H.F., Jacquay, J., and Sirois, P. (1983). Feeds and feeding in the northeastern United States. In: *Current Therapy in Equine Medicine*, 680–683. Philadelphia, PA: W.B. Saunders.

55 Fowler, A.L. (2018). Factors influencing phosphorus excretion by horses. Doctoral dissertation. Lexington, KY.

56 Smil, V. (2000). Phosphorus in the environment: natural flows and human interferences. *Annu. Rev. Energy Environ.* 25: 53–88.

57 Steen, I. (1998). Phosphorus availability in the 21st century: management of a non-renewable resource. *Phosphorus Potassium* 217: 25–31.

58 Fowler, A.L., Hansen, T.L., Strasinger, L.A. et al. (2015). Phosphorus digestibility and phytate degradation by yearlings and mature horses. *J. Anim. Sci.* 93: 5735–5742.

59 Hainze, M.T.M., Muntifering, R.B., Wood, C.W. et al. (2004). Faecal phosphorus excretion from horses fed typical diets with and without added phytase. *Anim. Feed Sci. Technol.* 117: 265–279.

60 Cymbaluk, N.F. (1990). Cold housing effects on growth and nutrient demand of young horses. *J. Anim. Sci.* 68 (10): 3152–3162.

61 Schryver, H.F., Hintz, H.F., and Craig, P.H. (1971). Phosphorus metabolism in ponies fed varying levels of phosphorus. *J. Nutr.* 101: 1257–1263.

62 van Doorn, D.A., Spek, M.E., Everts, H. et al. (2004). The influence of calcium intake on phosphorus digestibility in mature ponies. *J. Anim. Physiol. Anim. Nutr. (Berl).* 88: 412–418.

63 McKenzie, R.A., Blaney, B.J., and Gartner, R.J.W. (1981). The effect of dietary oxalate on calcium, phosphorus and magnesium balances in horses. *J. Agric. Sci.* 97: 69–74.

64 Kapusniak, L.J., Greene, L.W., and Potter, G.D. (1988). Calcium, magnesium and phosphorus absorption from the small and large intestine of ponies fed elevated amounts of aluminum. *J. Equine Vet. Sci.* 8: 305–309.

65 Roose, K.A., Hoekstra, K.E., Pagan, J.D., and Geor, R.J. (2001). Effect of an aluminum supplement on nutrient digestibility and mineral metabolism in Thoroughbred horses. In: *Proceedings of the 17th Equine Nutrition and Physiology Society Symposium*, 364–369. Lexington, KY: Equine Nutrition and Physiology Society.

66 Allen, V., Robinson, D., and Hembry, F. (1980). Aluminum in the etiology of grass tetany in cattle. *J. Anim. Sci.* 51 (Suppl. 1): 44.

67 Schryver, H.F., Parker, M.T., Daniluk, P.D. et al. (1987). Salt consumption and the effect of salt on mineral metabolism in horses. *Cornell Vet.* 77: 122–131.

68 Cymbaluk, N.F., Christison, G.I., and Leach, D.H. (1989). Nutrient utilization by limit-and ad libitum-fed growing horses. *J. Anim. Sci.* 67: 414–425.

69 Ögren, G., Holtenius, K., and Jansson, A. (2013). Phosphorus balance and fecal losses in growing Standardbred horses in training fed forage-only diets. *J. Anim. Sci.* 91: 2749–2755.

70 Oliveira, A., Furtado, C.E., Vitti, D. et al. (2008). Phosphorus bioavailability in diets for growing horses. *Livest. Sci.* 116: 90–95.

71 Kichura, T.S., Hintz, H.F., and Schryver, H.F. (1983). Factors influencing endogenous phosphorus losses in ponies. In: *Proceeding of the 8th Equine Nutrition and Physiology Society Symposium*, 60–65. Lexington, KY: Equine Nutrition and Physiology Society.

72 Greiwe-Crandell, K.M., Morrow, G.A., and Kronfeld, D.S. (1992). Phosphorus and selenium depletion in Thoroughbred mares and weanlings. In: *Europaische Konferenz uber die Ernahrung des Pferdes*, 96–98.

73 Meyer, H., Heilmann, M., Perez, H., and Comda, Y. (1989). Investigations of the post-prandial renal calcium, phosphorus, magnesium excretion in resting and exercising horses. In: *Proceedings of the 11th Equine Nutrition and Physiology Society Symposium*, 133–138. Stillwater, OK: Equine Nutrition and Physiology Society.

74 Grace, N.D., Pearce, S.G., Firth, E.C., and Fennessy, P.F. (1999). Content and distribution of macro-and micro-elements in the body of pasture-fed young horses. *Aust. Vet. J.* 77 (3): 172–176.

75 Stewart, A.J. (2011). Magnesium disorders in horses. *Vet. Clin. North Am. Equine Pract.* 27: 149–163.

76 Nielsen, F.H. (2010). Magnesium, inflammation, and obesity in chronic disease. *Nutr. Rev.* 68: 333–340.

77 Geor, R.J. and Harris, P. (2009). Dietary management of obesity and insulin resistance: countering risk for laminitis. *Vet. Clin. North Am. Equine Pract.* 25: 51–65.

78 Chameroy, K.A., Frank, N., Elliott, S.B., and Boston, R.C. (2011). Effects of a supplement containing chromium and magnesium on morphometric measurements, resting glucose, insulin concentrations and insulin sensitivity in laminitic obese horses. *Equine Vet. J.* 43 (4): 494–499.

79 Coudray, C., Rambeau, M., Feillet-Coudray, C. et al. (2005). Study of magnesium bioavailability from ten organic and inorganic Mg salts in Mg-depleted rats using a stable isotope approach. *Magnes. Res.* 18: 215–223.

80 Van Ravenswaay, R.O., Henry, P.R., Ammerman, C.B., and Littell, R.C. (1989). Comparison of methods to determine relative bioavailability of magnesium in magnesium oxides for ruminants. *J. Dairy Sci.* 72: 2968–2980.

81 Hintz, H.F. and Schryver, H.F. (1973). Magnesium, calcium and phosphorus metabolism in ponies fed varying levels of magnesium. *J. Anim. Sci.* 37: 927–930.

82 Pagan, J.D., Harris, P., Brewster-Barnes, T. et al. (1998). Exercise affects digestibility and rate of passage of all-forage and mixed diets in thoroughbred horses. *J. Nutr.* 128: S2704.

83 Stephens, T.L., Potter, G.D., Gibbs, P.G., and Hood, D.M. (2004). Mineral balance in juvenile horses in race training. *J. Equine Vet. Sci.* 24: 438–450.

84 Pagan, J.D. (1994). Nutrient digestibility in horses. In: *KER Short Course: Feeding the Performance Horse* (ed. J.D. Pagan), 127–136. Lexington, KY: Kentucky Equine Research.

85 Baird, J.D. (1971). Lactation tetany (eclampsia) in a Shetland pony mare. *Aust. Vet. J.* 47 (8): 402–404.

86 Harrington, D.D. (1974). Pathologic features of magnesium deficiency in young horses fed purified rations. *Am. J. Vet. Res.* 35: 503.

87 Grimmett, A. and Sillence, M.N. (2005). Calmatives for the excitable horse: a review of l-tryptophan. *Vet. J.* 170 (1): 24–32.

88 Barbier, M., Benoit, S., and Lambey, J.L. (2012). Effect of a complementary horse feed on nervous horse behaviour. In: *Applied Equine Nutrition and Training: Equine Nutrition and Training Conference (ENUTRACO) 2011* (ed. A. Lindner), 195–203. Wageningen: Wageningen Academic Publishers.

89 Nielsen, B.D. and O'Connor-Robison, C.I. (2014). A pilot study to determine if a dietary mineral supplement can affect reactivity to stimuli by horses in training. *Comp. Exerc. Physiol.* 10: 159–165.

90 Dodd, J.A., Doran, G., Harris, P., and Noble, G.K. (2015). Magnesium aspartate supplementation and reaction speed response in horses. *J. Equine Vet. Sci.* 35: 401–402.

91 Fontenot, J.P., Allen, V.G., Bunce, G.E., and Goff, J.P. (1989). Factors influencing magnesium absorption and metabolism in ruminants. *J. Anim. Sci.* 67: 3445–3455.

92 Henninger, R.W. and Horst, J. (1997). Magnesium toxicosis in two horses. *J. Am. Vet. Med. Assoc.* 211: 82–85.

93 Zeyner, A., Romanowski, K., Vernunft, A. et al. (2017). Effects of different oral doses of sodium chloride on the basal acid-base and mineral status of exercising horses fed low amounts of hay. *PLoS One* 12 (1): e0168325.

94 Reynolds, J.A., Potter, G.D., Greene, L.W. et al. (1998). Genetic-diet interactions in the hyperkalemic periodic paralysis syndrome in quarter horses fed varying amounts of potassium: IV. Pre-cecal and post-ileal absorption of potassium and sodium. *J. Equine Vet. Sci.* 18: 827–831.

95 Baker, L.A., Topliff, D.R., Freeman, D.W. et al. (1992). Effects of dietary cation-anion balance on acid-base status in horses. *J. Equine Vet. Sci.* 12 (3): 160–163.

96 Cooper, S.R., Kline, K.H., Foreman, J.H. et al. (1998). Effects of dietary cation-anion balance on pH, electrolytes, and lactate in standardbred horses. *J. Equine Vet. Sci.* 18 (10): 662–666.

97 Mueller, R.K., Cooper, S.R., Topliff, D.R. et al. (2001). Effect of dietary cation-anion difference on acid-base status and energy digestibility in sedentary horses fed varying levels and types of starch. *J. Equine Vet. Sci.* 21: 498–502.

98 Riond, J.-L. (2001). Animal nutrition and acid-base balance. *Eur. J. Nutr.* 40: 245–254.

99 Meyer, H., Gurer, C., and Lindner, A. (1985). Effects of a low K-diet on K-metabolism, sweat production and sweat composition in horses. In: *Proceedings of the 9th Equine Nutrition and Physiology Society Symposium*, 130–135. East Lansing, MI: Equine Nutrition and Physiology Society.

100 Hintz, H.F. and Schryver, H.F. (1981). Mineral nutrition in horses. *Compend. Contin. Educ. Pract. Vet.* 3: S18–S21.

101 Hansen, T.L., Fowler, A.L., Strasinger, L.A. et al. (2016). Effect of soaking on nitrate concentrations in Teff Hay. *J. Equine Vet. Sci.* 45 (10): 53–57.

102 Anderson, J.O., Warnick, R.E., and Dalai, R.K. (1975). Replacing dietary methionine and cystine in chick diets with sulfate or other sulfur compounds. *Poult. Sci.* 54 (4): 1122–1128.

103 Corke, M.J. (1981). An outbreak of sulphur poisoning in horses. *Vet. Rec.* 109 (11): 212–213.

104 Strickland, K., Smith, F., Woods, M., and Mason, J. (1987). Dietary molybdenum as a putative copper antagonist in the horse. *Equine Vet. J.* 19: 50–54.

105 Georgievskiĭ, V.I., Annenkov, B.N., and Samokhin, V.T. (1981). *Mineral Nutrition of Animals*, 475. Oxford: Butterworth-Heinemann.
106 Ferguson, L.R. and Karunasinghe, N. (2011). Nutrigenetics, nutrigenomics, and selenium. *Front. Genet.* 2 (Apr): 1–10.
107 Surai, P.F. (2006). *Selenium in Nutrition and Health*. Nottingham: Nottingham University Press.
108 Arthur, J.R. (1997). Selenium proteins. *J. Equine Vet. Sci.* 17 (Nov): 422–423.
109 Brown, K.M. and Arthur, J.R. (2001). Selenium, selenoproteins and human health: a review. *Public Health Nutr.* 4 (2B): 593–599.
110 Calamari, L., Ferrari, A., and Bertin, G. (2009). Effect of selenium source and dose on selenium status of mature horses. *J. Anim. Sci.* 87 (1): 167–178.
111 Muirhead, T.L., Wichtel, J.J., Stryhn, H., and McClure, J.T. (2010). The selenium and vitamin E status of horses in Prince Edward Island. *Can. Vet. J.* 51: 979–985.
112 National Research Council (1983). *Selenium in Nutrition*, Rev. 1–174. Washington, DC: The National Academies Press.
113 Jones, G.D., Droz, B., Greve, P. et al. (2017). Selenium deficiency risk predicted to increase under future climate change. *Proc. Natl. Acad. Sci. U.S.A.* 114 (11): 2848–2853.
114 Garner, R.J. (1967). Part two: mineral or inorganic substances. In: *Garner's Veterinary Toxicology*, 3e (ed. E.G.C. Clarke and M.L. Clarke), 37–132. London: Baillière, Tindall & Cassell.
115 Varo, P., Alfthan, G., Ekholm, P. et al. (1988). Selenium intake and serum selenium in Finland: effects of soil fertilization with selenium. *Am. J. Clin. Nutr.* 48: 324–329.
116 Montgomery, J.B., Wichtel, J.J., Wichtel, M.G. et al. (2011). The efficacy of selenium treatment of forage for the correction of selenium deficiency in horses. *Anim. Feed Sci. Technol.* 170: 63–71.
117 Vendeland, S.C., Butler, J.A., and Whanger, P.D. (1992). Intestinal absorption of selenite, selenate, and selenomethionine in the rat. *J. Nutr. Biochem.* 3: 359–365.
118 Shellow, J.S., Jackson, S.G., Baker, J.P., and Cantor, A.H. (1985). The influence of dietary selenium levels on blood levels of selenium and glutathione peroxidase activity in the horse. *J. Anim. Sci.* 61: 590–594.
119 Brummer, M., Hayes, S., Dawson, K.A., and Lawrence, L.M. (2013). Measures of antioxidant status of the horse in response to selenium depletion and repletion. *J. Anim. Sci.* 91 (5): 2158–2168.
120 White, S.H. and Warren, L.K. (2017). Submaximal exercise training, more than dietary selenium supplementation, improves antioxidant status and ameliorates exercise-induced oxidative damage to skeletal muscle in young equine athletes. *J. Anim. Sci.* 95 (2): 657–670.
121 Mahan, D.C., Moxon, A.L., and Hubbard, M. (1977). Efficacy of inorganic selenium supplementation to sow diets on resulting carry-over to their progeny. *J. Anim. Sci.* 45 (4): 738–746.
122 Janicki, K.M. (2001). The effect of dietary selenium source and level on broodmares and their foals University of Kentucky M.S. Thesis, Lexington, KY.
123 Karren, B.J., Thorson, J.F., Cavinder, C.A. et al. (2010). Effect of selenium supplementation and plane of nutrition on mares and their foals: selenium concentrations and glutathione peroxidase. *J. Anim. Sci.* 88 (3): 991–997.
124 Ji, L.L., Dillon, D.A., Bump, K.D., and Lawrence, L.M. (1990). Antioxidant enzyme response to exercise in equine erythrocytes. *J. Equine Vet. Sci.* 10: 380–383.
125 Brummer, M., Hayes, S., Harlow, B.E. et al. (2012). Effect of selenium status on the response of unfit horses to exercise. *Comp. Exerc. Physiol.* 8 (3, 4): 203–212.
126 Brummer, M., Hayes, S., Adams, A.A. et al. (2013). The effect of selenium supplementation on vaccination response and immune function in adult horses. *J. Anim. Sci.* 91 (8): 3702–3715.
127 Edmonson, A.J., Norman, B.B., and Suther, D. (1993). Survey of state veterinarians and state veterinary diagnostic laboratories for selenium deficiency and toxicosis in animals. *J. Am. Vet. Med. Assoc.* 202: 865–872.
128 Paulussen, E., Lefère, L., Bauwens, C. et al. (2017). Yellow fat disease (steatitis) in 20 equids: description of clinical and ultrasonographic findings. *Equine Vet. Educ.* 31(6): 321–327.
129 de Bruijn, C.M., Velduis Kroeze, E.J.B., Sloet van Oldruitenborgh-Oosterbaan, M.M. et al. (2006). Yellow fat disease in equids. *Equine Vet. Educ.* 18 (1): 38–44.
130 Owen, R.R., Moore, J.N., Hopkins, J.B., and Arthur, D. (1977). Dystrophic myodegeneration in adult horses. *J. Am. Vet. Med. Assoc.* 171: 343–349.
131 Wilson, T.M., Morrison, H.A., Palmer, N.C., and Finley, G.G. (1976). Myodegeneration and suspected selenium/vitamin E deficiency in horses. *J. Am. Vet. Med. Assoc.* 169: 213–217.
132 Streeter, R.M., Divers, T.J., Mittel, L. et al. (2012). Selenium deficiency associations with gender, breed, serum vitamin E and creatine kinase, clinical signs and diagnoses in horses of different age groups: a retrospective examination 1996-2011. *Equine Vet. J.* 44 (Dec): 31–35.
133 National Research Council (1989). *Nutrient Requirements of Horses*. 5th Rev. Animal Nutrition Series, 1–100. Washington, DC: National Academies Press.
134 Stowe, H.D. (1967). Serum selenium and related parameters of naturally and experimentally fed horses. *J. Nutr.* 93: 60–64.

135 Erskine, R.J., Eberhart, R.J., Grasso, P.J., and Scholz, R.W. (1989). Induction of *Escherichia coli* mastitis in cows fed selenium-deficient or selenium-supplemented diets. *Am. J. Vet. Res.* 50: 2093–2100.

136 Blythe, L.L., Craig, A.M., and Lassen, E.D. (1989). Vitamin E in the horse and its relationship to equine degenerative myeloencephalopathy. In: *Proceedings American College of Veterinary Internal Medicine Forum*, 1007–1010. American College of Veterinary Internal Medicine.

137 Hintz, H.F. (2001). The many phases of selenium. In: *Kentucky Equine Research Nutrition Conference for Feed Manufacturers*, 87–94.

138 Desta, B., Maldonado, G., Reid, H. et al. (2011). Acute selenium toxicosis in polo ponies. *J. Vet. Diagn. Invest.* 23: 623–628.

139 Davis, T.Z., Stegelmeier, B.L., and Hall, J.O. (2014). Analysis in horse hair as a means of evaluating selenium toxicoses and long-term exposures. *J. Agric. Food. Chem.* 62 (30): 7393.

140 Asano, R., Suzuki, K., Otsuka, T. et al. (2002). Concentrations of toxic metals and essential minerals in the mane hair of healthy racing horses and their relation to age. *J. Vet. Med. Sci.* 64 (7): 607–610.

141 Stowe, H.D. and Herdt, T.H. (1992). Clinical assessment of selenium status of livestock. *J. Anim. Sci.* 70: 3928–3933.

142 Stowe, H.D. (1998). Selenium supplementation for horse feed. In: *Advances in Equine Nutrition I* (ed. J.D. Pagan), 97–103. Nottingham, UK: Nottingham University Press.

143 Federal Drug Administration. 21CFR573.920. In: Code of Federal Regulations Title 21, Washington DC. https://www.accessdata.fda.gov/scripts/cdrh/cfdocs/cfcfr/CFRSearch.cfm?fr=573.920 (accessed 11 September 2021).

144 Néspoli, P.B., Duarte, M.D., Bezerra, P.S. Jr. et al. (2001). Aspectos clínico-patológicos da intoxicação experimental por selenito de sódio em eqüinos. *Pesqui. Vet. Bras.* 21: 109–116.

145 McLaughlin, B.G. and Doige, C.E. (1981). Congenital musculoskeletal lesions and hyperplastic goitre in foals. *Can. Vet. J.* 22: 130–133.

146 McLaughlin, B.G., Doige, C.E., and McLaughlin, P.S. (1986). Thyroid hormone levels in foals with congenital musculoskeletal lesions. *Can. Vet. J.* 27: 264–267.

147 Wehr, U., Englschalk, B., Kienzle, E., and Rambeck, W.A. (2002). Iodine balance in relation to iodine intake in ponies. *J. Nutr.* 132: 1767S–1768S.

148 Fadok, V.A. and Wild, S. (1983). Suspected cutaneous iodism in a horse. *J. Am. Vet. Med. Assoc.* 183 (10): 1104–1106.

149 Drew, B., Barber, W.P., and Williams, D.G. (1975). The effect of excess dietary iodine on pregnant mares and foals. *Vet. Rec.* 97: 93–95.

150 Murray, M.J. (1990). Hypothyroidism and respiratory insufficiency in a neonatal foal. *J. Am. Vet. Med. Assoc.* 197: 1635–1638.

151 Hitchcock, K.R. (1979). Hormones and the lung. I. Thyroid hormones and glucocorticoids in lung development. *Anat. Rec.* 194: 15–39.

152 Neufeld, N. and Melmed, S. (1981). 3,5-dimethyl-3′-isopropyl-l-thyronine therapy in diabetic pregnancy: stimulation of rabbit fetal lung phospholipids. *J. Clin. Invest.* 68: 1605–1609.

153 Baker, H.J. and Lindsey, J.R. (1968). Equine goiter due to excess dietary iodide. *J. Am. Vet. Med. Assoc.* 153 (12): 1618–1630.

154 Barton, M.H. (2015). How to interpret common hematologic and serum biochemistry differences between neonatal foals and mature horses. In: *Proceedings of the 61st Annual Convention of the American Association of Equine Practitioners*, 125–129. Las Vegas, NV: American Association of Equine Practitioners (AAEP).

155 Shaftoe, S., Schick, M.P., and Chen, C.L. (1988). Thyroid-stimulating hormone response tests in one-day-old foals. *J. Equine Vet. Sci.* 8: 310–312.

156 Bridges, C.H. and Harris, E.D. (1988). Experimentally induced cartilaginous fractures (osteochondritis dissecans) in foals fed low-copper diets. *J. Am. Vet. Med. Assoc.* 193 (2): 215–221.

157 Lofstedt, J. (1989). Comparative aspects of Cu metabolism in ruminants and horses. In: *Proceedings of the 7th American College of Veterinary Internal Medicine*, 501–505. San Diego, CA: American College of Veterinary Internal Medicine.

158 Coger, L.S., Hintz, H.F., Schryver, H.F., and Lowe, J.E. (1987). The effect of high zinc intake on copper metabolism and bone development in growing horses. In: *Proceedings of the 10th Equine Nutrition and Physiology Society Symposium*, 173. Fort Collins, CO: Equine Nutrition and Physiology Society.

159 Young, J.K., Potter, G.D., Greene, L.W., and Evans, J.W. (1989). Mineral balance in resting and exercised miniature horses. In: *Proceedings of the 11th Equine Nutrition and Physiology Society Symposium*, 79–84. Stillwater, OK: Equine Nutrition and Physiology Society.

160 Wagner, E.L., Potter, G.D., Gibbs, P.G. et al. (2011). Copper and zinc balance in exercising horses fed 2 forms of mineral supplements. *J. Anim. Sci.* 89 (3): 722–728.

161 Cymbaluk, N.F., Schryver, H.F., Hintz, H.F. et al. (1981). Influence of dietary molybdenum on copper metabolism in ponies. *J. Nutr.* 111: 96–106.

162 Bridges, C.H. and Moffitt, P.G. (1990). Influence of variable content of dietary zinc on copper metabolism of weanling foals. *Am. J. Vet. Res.* 51 (2): 275–280.

163 Gunson, D.E., Kowalczyk, D.F., Shoop, C.R., and Ramberg, J.C.F. (1982). Environmental zinc and cadmium pollution associated with generalized osteochondrosis, osteoporosis, and nephrocalcinosis in horses. *J. Am. Vet. Med. Assoc.* 180: 295–299.

164 Bridges, C.H., Womack, J.E., Harris, E.D., and Scrutchfield, W.L. (1984). Considerations of copper metabolism in osteochondrosis of suckling foals. *J. Am. Vet. Med. Assoc.* 185 (2): 173–178.

165 Smith, J.D., Jordan, R.M., and Nelson, M.L. (1975). Tolerance of ponies to high levels of dietary copper. *J. Anim. Sci.* 41: 1645–1649.

166 Stowe, H.D. (1980). Effects of copper pretreatment upon toxicity of selenium in ponies. *Am. J. Vet. Res.* 41: 1925–1928.

167 Cymbaluk, N.F., Schryver, H.F., and Hintz, H.F. (1981). Copper metabolism and requirement in mature ponies. *J. Nutr.* 111: 87–95.

168 McGorum, B.C., Wilson, R., Pirie, R.S. et al. (2003). Systemic concentrations of antioxidants and biomarkers of macromolecular oxidative damage in horses with grass sickness. *Equine Vet. J.* 35: 121–126.

169 Bell, J.U., Lopez, J.M., and Bartos, K.D. (1987). The postnatal development of serum zinc, copper and ceruloplasmin in the horse. *Comp. Biochem. Physiol. A: Comp. Physiol.* 87 (3): 561–564.

170 Cymbaluk, N.F., Bristol, F.M., and Christensen, D.A. (1986). Influence of age and breed of equid on plasma copper and zinc concentrations. *Am. J. Vet. Res.* 47: 192–195.

171 Van Weeren, P.R., Knaap, J., and Firth, E.C. (2003). Influence of liver copper status of mare and newborn foal on the development of osteochondrotic lesions. *Equine Vet. J.* 35 (1): 67–71.

172 Cymbaluk, N.F. and Christensen, D.A. (1986). Copper, zinc and manganese concentrations in equine liver, kidney and plasma. *Can. Vet. J.* 27: 206–210.

173 Lawrence, L.M., Ott, E.A., Asquith, R.L., and Miller, G.J. (1987). Influence of dietary iron on growth, tissue mineral composition, apparent phosphorus absorption and chemical properties of bone. In: *Proceedings of the 10th Equine Nutrition and Physiology Society Symposium*, 563–572. Fort Collins, CO: Equine Nutrition and Physiology Society.

174 Ghorbani, A., Mohit, A., and Kuhi, H.D. (2015). Effects of dietary mineral intake on hair and serum mineral contents of horses. *J. Equine Vet. Sci.* 35: 295–300.

175 de Souza, M.V., Fontes, M.P.F., and Fernandes, R.B.A. (2014). Heavy metals in equine biological components. *Rev. Bras. Zootec.* 43 (2): 60–66.

176 Brummer-Holder, M., Hayes, S.H., and Cassill, B.D. (2017). Trace element concentrations in mare and foal mane hair. *J. Equine Vet. Sci.* 100 (52): 92.

177 Wilson, D. (2011). *Clinical Veterinary Advisor: The Horse*, 1e. Edinburgh: Saunders Elsevier.

178 Hudson, C, Pagan, J., Hoekstra, K. et al. (2001). Effects of exercise training on the digestibility and requirements of copper, zinc and manganese in Thoroughbred horses. In: *Proceedings of the 17th Equine Nutrition and Physiology Society Symposium*, 138–140. Lexington, KY: Equine Nutrition and Physiology Society.

179 Harrington, D.D., Walsh, J., and White, V. (1973). Clinical and pathological findings in horses fed zinc deficient diets. In: *Proceedings of the 3rd Equine Nutrition and Physiology Society Symposium*, 51–54. Gainsville, FL: Equine Nutrition and Physiology Society.

180 Breedveld, L., Jackson, S.G., and Baker, J.P. (1988). The determination of a relationship between the copper, zinc and selenium levels in mares and those in their foals. *J. Equine Vet. Sci.* 8 (5): 378–382.

181 Schryver, H.F., Hintz, H.F., Lowe, J.E. et al. (1974). Mineral composition of the whole body, liver and bone of young horses. *J. Nutr.* 104: 126–132.

182 Thomas, M.L., Ott, E.A., Pagan, J.D. et al. (1987) Influence of copper supplementation and pelleted vs. extruded concentrate on growth and development of weanling horses. In: *Proceedings of the 10th Equine Nutrition and Physiology Society Symposium*, 165–172. Fort Collins, CO: Equine Nutrition and Physiology Society.

183 Hoyt, J.K., Potter, G.D., Greene, L.W., and Anderson, J.G. (1995). Copper balance in miniature horses fed varying amounts of zinc. *J. Equine Vet. Sci.* 15: 357–359.

184 Thompson, U. (1992). Heavy metal toxicosis. In: *Current Therapy in Equine Medicine* (ed. A. Śmieszek), 363–367. Philadelphia: WB Saunders.

185 Willoughby, R.A., MacDonald, E., McSherry, B.J., and Brown, G. (1972). Lead and zinc poisoning and the interaction between Pb and Zn poisoning in the foal. *Can. J. Comp. Med.* 36: 348.

186 King, J.C. (1990). Assessment of zinc status. *J. Nutr.* 120: 1474–1479.

187 Kolm, G., Helsberg, A., and Gemeiner, M. (2005). Variations in the concentration of zinc in the blood of Icelandic horses. *Vet. Rec.* 157: 549–551.

188 Baucus, K.L., Ralston, S.L., Rich, G.A., and Squires, E.L. (1989). The effect of copper and zinc supplementation on mineral content of mares' milk. *J. Equine Vet. Sci.* 9 (4): 206–209.

189 Underwood, E.J. (1971). *Trace Elements in Human and Animal Nutrition*, 3e. New York: Academic Press, Inc.

190 Muñoz, M., Villar, I., and García-Erce, J.A. (2009). An update on iron physiology. *World J. Gastroenterol.* 15: 4617–4626.

191 Oliveira Filho, J.P., Badial, P.R., Cunha, P.H.J. et al. (2010). Cloning, sequencing and expression analysis of the equine hepcidin gene by real-time PCR. *Vet. Immunol. Immunopathol.* 135: 34–42.

192 Schwarzwald, C.C. and Schuback, K. (2004). Abnormalities of the erythron. In: *Equine Sports Medicine and Surgery: Basic and Clinical Sciences of the Equine Athlete* (ed. K.W. Hinchcliff, A.J. Kaneps, and R.J. Geor). London: Saunders.

193 Assenza, A., Casella, S., Giannetto, C. et al. (2016). Iron profile in Thoroughbreds during a standard training program. *Aust. Vet. J.* 94 (3): 60–63.

194 Fleming, K.A., Barton, M.H., and Latimer, K.S. (2006). Iron deficiency anemia in a neonatal foal. *J. Vet. Intern. Med.* 20: 1495–1498.

195 Willis, W.T., Gohil, K., Brooks, G.A., and Dallman, P.R. (1990). Iron deficiency: improved exercise performance within 15 hours of iron treatment in rats. *J. Nutr.* 120: 909–916.

196 Johnson, M.A. (1990). Iron: nutrition monitoring and nutrition status assessment. *J. Nutr.* 120: 1486–1491.

197 Harvey, J.W., Asquith, R.L., McNulty, P.K. et al. (1984). Haematology of foals up to one year old. *Equine Vet. J.* 16: 347–353.

198 Mullaney, T.P. and Brown, C.M. (1988). Iron toxicity in neonatal foals. *Equine Vet. J.* 20: 119–124.

199 Arnbjerg, J. (1981). Poisoning in animals due to oral application of iron. With description of a case in a horse. *Nord. Vet. Med.* 33 (2): 71–76.

200 Theelen, M.J.P., Beukers, M., Grinwis, G.C.M., and Sloet van Oldruitenborgh-Oosterbaan, M.M. (2019). Chronic iron overload causing haemochromatosis and hepatopathy in 21 horses and one donkey. *Equine Vet. J.* 51: 304–309.

201 Borges, A.S., Divers, T.J., Stokol, T., and Mohammed, O.H. (2007). Serum iron and plasma fibrinogen concentrations as indicators of systemic inflammatory diseases in horses. *J. Vet. Intern. Med.* 21 (3): 489–494.

202 Corradini, I., Armengou, L., Viu, J. et al. (2014). Parallel testing of plasma iron and fibrinogen concentrations to detect systemic inflammation in hospitalized horses. *J. Vet. Emerg. Crit. Care.* 24 (4): 414–420.

203 Smith, J.E., DeBowes, R.M., and Cipriano, J.E. (1986). Exogenous corticosteroids increase serum iron concentrations in mature horses and ponies. *J. Am. Vet. Med. Assoc.* 188: 1296–1298.

204 Kaneko, J.J. (1981). Serum ferritin and iron metabolic parameters in the horse. In: *Proceedings of the Oregon Veterinary Medical Association*. Oregon Veterinary Medical Association.

205 Ott, E.A., Asquith, R.L., and Harvey, J.W. (1993). Influence of trace mineral intake of mares on the trace mineral status of suckling foals. In: *Proceedings of the 13th Equine Nutrition and Physiology Society Symposium*, 84–85. Gainsville, FL: Equine Nutrition and Physiology Society.

206 Smith, J.E., Moore, K., Cipriano, J.E., and Morris, P.G. (1984). Serum ferritin as a measure of stored iron in horses. *J. Nutr.* 114: 677–681.

207 McLean, L.M., Hall, M.E., and Bell, J.E. (1987). Evaluation of serum iron, total Fe binding capacity, unbound Fe binding capacity, percent saturation and serum ferritin in the equine. In: *Proceedings of the 10th Equine Nutrition and Physiology Society Symposium*, 443–446. Fort Collins, CO: Equine Nutrition and Physiology Society.

208 Wagenaar, G. (1975). Iron dextran administered to horses (author's transl). *Tijdschr. Diergeneeskd.* 100: 562–563.

209 Gall, J.E., Boyd, R.S., Rajakaruna, N. et al. (2015). Transfer of heavy metals through terrestrial food webs: a review. *Monit. Assess.* 187 (4): 201.

210 Adamse, P., Van der Fels-Klerx, H.J., and de Jong, J. (2017). Cadmium, lead, mercury and arsenic in animal feed and feed materials–trend analysis of monitoring results. *Food Addit. Contam. Part A Chem. Anal. Control Expo. Risk Assess.* 34 (8): 1298–1311.

211 National Research Council (1982). *United States-Canadian Tables of Feed Composition*. 3rd Rev. Nutritional Data for United States and Canadian Feeds, 1–148. Washington, DC: National Academies Press.

9

Vitamins

Sarah Dodd, Sarah K. Abood, and Jacqueline M. Parr

KEY TERMS

- Coenzymes are small organic molecules (nonprotein) required by enzymes (proteins) that assist or enhance enzymatic reactions.
- Micronutrients are dietary compounds required by the body in minuscule, i.e. IU, mg, μg, or ng per kg body weight (BW), amounts.
- Bioavailability refers to the ability of a dietary substance to be digested, absorbed, and utilized within the body of an animal.

KEY POINTS

- Vitamins are a heterogeneous class of nutrients that function as coenzymes in metabolic reactions found ubiquitously throughout the body.
- Vitamins A and E are essential dietary nutrients in horse rations.
- Vitamins C and D are synthesized de novo endogenously in the horse.
- All B vitamins and vitamin K are produced by the intestinal microbiome.
- There are dietary recommendations for vitamins A, D, E, thiamine, and riboflavin.
- Though manipulations in dietary vitamin concentrations have been attempted to improve performance, there is little evidence to suggest that supplementation above and beyond requirements provides any benefit to horse health or performance.
- Fresh forages and formulated feeds typically contain sufficient vitamins to meet horse requirements, thus feeding multiple vitamin supplements is rarely indicated.

9.1 Introduction

Vitamins are carbon-containing micronutrients produced by living cells required in minuscule concentrations, i.e. IU (international units), mg, μg, or ng per kg ration dry matter (DM) or body weight per day (BW/d), relative to the requirement of other dietary nutrients. In contrast to most other nutrients, vitamins are not composed of a single repeating building block, but are diverse in their structures, are different chemical compounds with widely varying biological activities, and within a single parent vitamin (vitamins K_1, K_2, and K_3) they may have different biological activities. Vitamins are classified as fat or water-soluble, determined by their absorption, storage, and excretion. Fat-soluble vitamins (A, D, E, and K) are absorbed in association with dietary fats, within chylomicrons, and stored within lipid tissues in the body, while dietary excess is excreted in feces. Water-soluble vitamins (B's and C) are absorbed directly from food sources, have no long-term storage within the body, and are excreted from the body in urine via the kidneys.

Water-soluble vitamins serve as coenzymes (catalysts) to promote and regulate a multitude of metabolic reactions and are neither catabolized for energy nor used as structuralconstituents to physically support the body (Table 9.1). Intermediary and energy metabolism ubiquitously require a multitude of B vitamins (Figure 9.1) [2]. The metabolic rate is directly related, but not linear, to body weight (BW). Within a species with a widely varying BW such as the horse (45–1100 kg), the metabolic rate and

Equine Clinical Nutrition, Second Edition. Edited by Rebecca L. Remillard.

Table 9.1 Water-soluble vitamins promote and regulate a multitude of metabolic reactions.

Vitamin	Name	Molecular function
Vitamin B_1	Thiamine	Thiamine plays a central role in the release of energy from carbohydrates, is involved in RNA and DNA production, as well as nerve function. Its active form is a coenzyme called thiamine pyrophosphate (TPP), which takes part in the conversion of pyruvate to acetyl coenzyme A in metabolism.
Vitamin B_2	Riboflavin	Riboflavin is involved in the release of energy in the electron transport chain, the citric acid cycle, as well as the catabolism of fatty acids (beta-oxidation).
Vitamin B_3	Niacin	Niacin is composed of two structures: nicotinic acid and nicotinamide. There are two coenzyme forms of niacin: nicotinamide adenine dinucleotide (NAD) and nicotinamide adenine dinucleotide phosphate (NADP). Both play an important role in energy transfer reactions in the metabolism of glucose, fat, and alcohol. NAD carries hydrogens and their electrons during metabolic reactions, including the pathway from the citric acid cycle to the electron transport chain. NADP is a coenzyme in lipid and nucleic acid synthesis.
Vitamin B_5	Pantothenic acid	Pantothenic acid is involved in the oxidation of fatty acids and carbohydrates. Coenzyme A, which can be synthesized from pantothenic acid, is involved in the synthesis of amino acids, fatty acids, ketone bodies, cholesterol [1], phospholipids, steroid hormones, neurotransmitters (such as acetylcholine), and antibodies.
Vitamin B_6	Pyridoxine	The active form pyridoxal 5′-phosphate (PLP) serves as a cofactor in many enzyme reactions mainly in amino acid metabolism including biosynthesis of neurotransmitters.
Vitamin B_7	Biotin	Biotin plays a key role in the metabolism of lipids, proteins, and carbohydrates as a critical coenzyme to four carboxylases: acetyl CoA carboxylase, which is involved in the synthesis of fatty acids from acetate; pyruvate CoA carboxylase, which is involved in gluconeogenesis; β-methylcrotonyl CoA carboxylase, which is involved in the metabolism of leucine; and propionyl CoA carboxylase, which is involved in the metabolism of energy, amino acids, and cholesterol.
Vitamin B_9	Folate	Folate acts as a coenzyme in the form of tetrahydrofolate (THF), which is involved in the transfer of single-carbon units in the metabolism of nucleic acids and amino acids. THF is involved in pyrimidine nucleotide synthesis, so is needed for normal cell division, especially during pregnancy and infancy, which are times of rapid growth. Folate also aids in erythropoiesis, the production of red blood cells.
Vitamin B_{12}	Cobalamin	Vitamin B_{12} is involved in the cellular metabolism of carbohydrates, proteins, and lipids, and is essential in the production of blood cells in bone marrow and for nerve sheaths and proteins. Vitamin B_{12} functions as a coenzyme in intermediary metabolism for the methionine synthase reaction with methylcobalamin and the methylmalonyl CoA mutase reaction with adenosylcobalamin.

requirements are best described based on metabolic BW ($BW^{0.75}$) [3–5]. See Chapter 6 Energy.

9.1.1 Sources

Horses with outdoor access and grazing on pasture grasses or fed fresh forage will generally consume their minimum requirements for vitamins A and E, vitamin D will likely be met with sun exposure, and all other vitamin requirements will likely be met by tissue and microbial synthesis. However, vitamin activity in dry feeds (hay and grains) is affected by factors such as sunlight, processing, temperature, air exposure, and nutrient interactions. Losses during storage are greatest for vitamins A, D, K, and thiamine. When fresh forage is unavailable, commercially processed feeds and supplements for horses should be formulated to contain vitamin concentrations sufficient to meet or exceed minimum requirements when fed at the manufacturer's recommended daily amounts. The vitamins should be considered viably active until at least 30 d after the manufacture date or until the printed expiration date or "best used by" date (Table 9.2). Therefore, feeding one or more vitamin supplements is often redundant, possibly incompatible, and not economical.

9.1.2 Requirements

Vitamin requirements are met by the provision of feedstuffs and supplements or endogenous synthesis in certain tissues or the microbiome. In horses, all but vitamins A

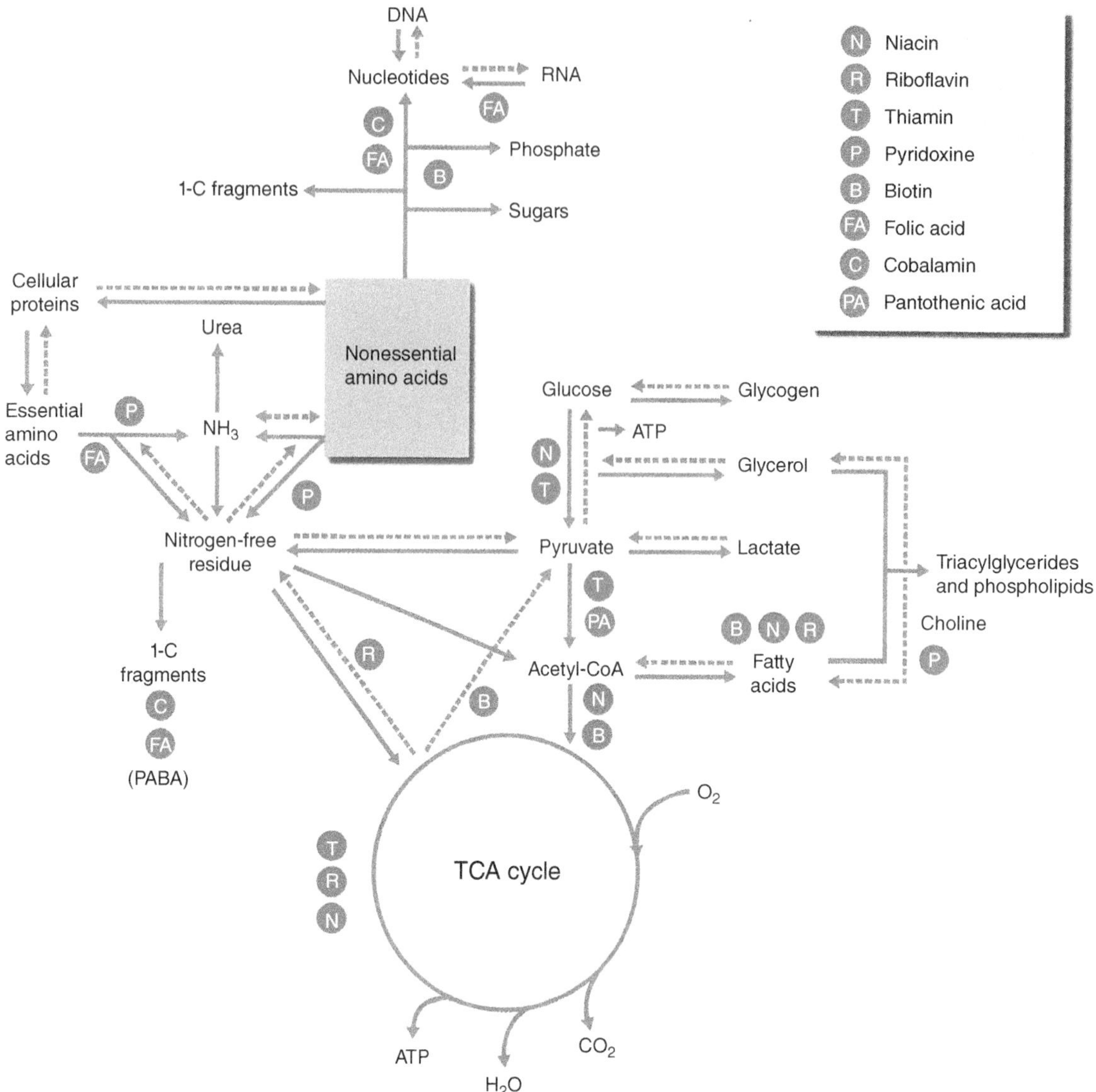

Figure 9.1 The role of B vitamins in intermediary metabolism. *Source:* Reprinted with permission from Hand MS, Thatcher CD, Remillard RL, Roudebush, P, Novotny, B. Small Animal Clinical Nutrition, 5th Edition Topeka, KS: Mark Morris Institute, 2010.

and E are produced endogenously [1]. Vitamins C and D are synthesized de novo in the horse's organs (liver and kidneys), while all B vitamins and vitamin K are produced by the intestinal microbiome. Although quantities of thiamine, riboflavin, pantothenic acid, nicotinic acid, pyridoxine, folic acid, and biotin are synthesized in the intestinal tract, studies in horses have demonstrated that the synthesis and absorption are inadequate to maintain skeletal muscle concentrations of most B vitamins when fed a deficient ration [7–11]. Absorption across the intestinal mucosa has not been directly documented for the B vitamins except for thiamine [12]. However, the absence of B-vitamin deficiencies in the majority of adult horses, fed under most management systems, indicates that metabolic requirements for B vitamins are adequately met through the sum of large bowel absorption, coprophagy, and fecal contamination of feed [11]. Therefore, only vitamins A and E are considered essential dietary nutrients in horse rations (Table 9.3). There are dietary recommendations for adding thiamine and riboflavin to horse rations to complement microbial synthesis (Table 9.3). The remaining B vitamins and vitamins C, D, and K are conditionally essential when requirements are greater during some life stages, disease processes, or therapeutic interventions [1].

The largest variances in determining the nutritional requirements of young and adult horses are those in

Table 9.2 Vitamin stability in forages.

Vitamin	% Loss/month	% of initial activity after stored properly for: 6 months	1 year	2 years
A (beadlet)	9.5	55	30	9
D3 (beadlet)	7.5	62	39	15
E acetate	2	88	78	62
K(MSDC)[a]	17	33	17	3
K(MDPB)[a]	15	38	23	5
B1 HCI	11	50	35	12
B1 mononitrate	5	74	54	29
B2 (riboflavin)	3	83	69	48
Niacin	4.6	75	57	32
Ca pantothenate	2.4	86	75	56
B6 (pyridoxine)	4	78	61	38
Biotin	4.4	76	58	34
Folic acid	5	74	54	29
B12	1.4	92	84	71
C (ascorbic acid)				
Uncoated	30	12	1	0
Coated[b]	7	65	42	17
Choline	1	94	89	78

[a] Menadione sodium bisulfite complex and menadione dimethyl pyrimidinol bisulfite.
[b] Coated with ethylcellulose.
Source: Based on Coelho [6].

"work," or what is more commonly referred to as "performance" in the horse world. Equine activities over and above maintenance would include recreational or competitive riding, driving, ranching, rodeo, and police work. Performance includes a range of work efforts from light work pleasure riding, to a quarter-mile sprint, to extreme exertion such as in a 100-mile/d endurance race. Given exercise, like work or performance, increases metabolic rate and requires additional calories, it would follow that vitamin needs should be increased proportionally to energy expenditure as coenzymes of metabolic reactions. Therefore, the dietary requirement for certain vitamins can vary greatly depending on the performance or work expected from the horse, but as of yet it has been difficult to quantify.

9.1.3 Deficiencies and Toxicities

When either inadequate or excessive amounts of vitamins are consumed or administered, the predominant effect will be specific to the metabolic processes dependent on that vitamin. Thus, knowing the function(s) is helpful such that vitamin imbalances can be recognized and corrected when noted. The causes, effects, and diagnosis of vitamin imbalances in horses are summarized in Tables 9.4 and 9.5. Under the majority of feeding situations, signs of deficiency are rare. Imbalances may occur when there is interference with normal vitamin synthesis or utilization, decreased feed intake, or a grossly inappropriate ration is fed. More often in a clinical setting, multiple deficiencies occur more frequently than a single vitamin deficiency [2]. There are vitamin–vitamin interactions that metabolically are mutually beneficial (one sparing the need for another), or symbiotic (one required for the optimal absorption of another), or cooperative (one protecting against oxidation of another), or detrimental (one interfering with the actions of another). See Sidebar 9.1. Vitamin interactions must be recognized to successfully resolve the clinical signs of vitamin deficiencies or toxicities.

Sidebar 9.1: Positive and Negative Interactions Between Vitamins [1, 2, 13]

Absorption or metabolic interference:
- Vitamin E interferes with vitamin K
- Vitamin B6 interferes with niacin
- Thiamine interferes with riboflavin

Optimizes absorption:
- Vitamin B6 for vitamin B_{12}
- Folate for thiamine

Incompatible within a supplement without protection:
- Thiamine is incompatible with riboflavin
- Thiamine and riboflavin are incompatible with B_{12}

Metabolic interdependence:
- Riboflavin needed for vitamin B6 and niacin
- Vitamin B6 needed for niacin

Obscure a deficiency:
- Folate deficiency obscures vitamin B_{12} deficiency

Protective of excess catabolism or urinary losses:
- Vitamin C spares vitamin B6

Protective against oxidative destruction:
- Vitamin E spares vitamin A
- Vitamin C spares vitamin E

Table 9.3 Daily vitamin requirements for horses at different life stages and performance

Type	Vitamin A	Vitamin D	Vitamin E	Thiamin	Riboflavin
Per 100 kg mature BW[a]	KIU	IU		mg	
Maintenance	3.0	660.0	100.0	6.0	4.0
Working					
light	4.5	660.0	160.0	6.0	4.0
moderate	4.5	660.0	180.0	9.3	4.5
heavy	4.5	660.0	200.0	12.5	5.0
very heavy	4.5	660.0	200.0	12.5	5.0
Stallions					
nonbreeding	3.0	660.0	100.0	6.0	4.0
breeding	4.5	660.0	160.0	6.0	4.0
Pregnant[b]	6.0	660.0	160.0	6.0	4.0
Lactation	6.0	660.0	200.0	7.5	5.0
Growing[c]					
4 mos[d]	1.5	748.0	67.4	2.5	1.7
6 mos	1.9	958.6	86.4	3.2	2.2
12 mos	2.9	1117.8	128.4	4.8	3.2
18 mos[e]	3.5	1232.2	155.0	5.8	3.9
24 mos[e]	3.9	1176.0	171.6	6.4	4.3

[a] Conversions to kg mature BW basis was made using the vitamins required for a 500 kg mature horse from NRC [1]; Table 16-3.
[b] Calculated based on prepregnancy weight.
[c] Calculated intake based on expected mature weight. Example: A growing 4 m old with an expected mature weight of 500 kg requires [1.5 KIU Vit A × 5 (100 kg mature weight)] = 7.5 KIU Vit A/d.
[d] mos: months.
[e] Vitamin recommendations are the same with exercise.

9.1.3.1 Deficiency

In situations where a single vitamin insufficiency is suspected, such as vitamins A or E, in horses stabled indoors and fed dry hay, supplementation with those specific vitamins is indicated. However, in instances where supplementation of multiple vitamins is needed, a balanced supplement providing complementary quantities of all vitamins is often the safest and least cost method, as opposed to feeding several different individual vitamin products. The provision of multiple individual vitamin-containing supplements increases the risk of unexpected vitamin interactions, an imbalance between vitamins, and possible toxicity. Many vitamins in unprotected forms are incompatible with other vitamins or nutrients, and are susceptible to destruction by air, light, and heat. Therefore, in all instances, vitamins must be protected to maintain their activity and efficacy. Commercial vitamin producers accomplish this by coating the vitamins with gelatin, wax, ethylcellulose, or sugar to protect them from degradation and vitamin–vitamin interactions [14].

9.1.3.2 Excess

Since fat-soluble vitamins are stored in body fat, toxicity is plausible and can be harmful to the horse's health. As with most domestic species, only vitamin A and D toxicities are of clinical relevance whereas toxicities of vitamins E and K have not been clinically relevant [15]. Conversely, there are no known maximum tolerable intake or safe upper limits of water-soluble vitamins stated for horses because the excess is easily eliminated from the body in urine.

Table 9.4 Fat-soluble vitamin imbalances.

Vitamin		Causes	Effects	Diagnosis
A	Deficiency	Insufficient forage	Decreased growth, poor haircoat, night blindness, keratin dysplasia	Relative dose–response >20%
	Excess	Excessive supplementation >20 000 IU/kg diet DM or >400 IU/kg BW	Decreased growth, poor haircoat, skeletal abnormalities	Plasma total vitamin A >40–60 μg/dL
D	Deficiency	Inappropriate diet	Decreased growth, poor bone mineralization, enlarged metaphyses	Decreased serum 25-hydroxyvitamin D, elevated PTH, decreased Ca, increased P
	Excess	Excessive supplementation	Decreased growth, stiffness, increased resting heartrate, polyuria, soft tissue calcification, seizures	Elevated serum 25-hydroxyvitamin D, low PTH, elevated Ca, decreased P
E	Deficiency	Genetic predisposition, insufficient fresh forage	Neuromuscular disorders: nutritional myodegeneration in foals, equine motor neuron disease, equine degenerative myeloencephalopathy, and vitamin E-deficient myopathy in adults	Serum plasma <1–2 μg/mL
K	Deficiency	Dicoumarol (from moldy hay) or warfarin ingestion	Hemorrhage	Elevated clotting times that normalize with parenteral administration of vitamin K
	Excess	Administration of excessive vitamin K IM or IV	Renal failure, colic, painful urination, hematuria	Proteinuria, isosthenuria, electrolyte abnormalities, history of vitamin K administration

Table 9.5 Water-soluble vitamin deficiencies.

Vitamin	Causes	Effects	Diagnosis
Thiamin	Decreased intestinal flora production, intake of thiamine antagonist	Decreased growth, neurological signs, hemorrhage	Serum thiamine <5 ng/mL
Biotin	Antimicrobial therapy, intake of biotin antagonist	Decreased growth, dermatosis, friable hooves	Whole blood biotin <0.3–0.7 ng/mL
Folate	Intake of folate antagonist	Anemia, bone marrow hypoplasia, oral ulceration	Serum folate <2–5 ng/mL, homocysteine >6.5 μmol/L
C	Advanced age, illness, chronic stress with insufficient fresh forage in diet	Collagen dysplasia, fatigue, pitting edema, hemorrhage	Plasma ascorbic acid <2 μg/mL, Serum ascorbic acid <4.5 μg/mL

9.1.4 Summary

The major functions, sources, recommended ration concentrations, and then the clinical signs of inadequate vs. excessive intake of specific vitamins, appropriate diagnostic test(s), and then a recommended course of treatment will be reviewed. Whenever possible, estimates of the daily vitamin requirements of horses will be reported. Unfortunately, as with the minerals, the number of studies examining the vitamin requirements of horses is relatively few compared to other species, and for many vitamins, optimal intakes have not been determined. Where data is lacking regarding requirements, or where deficiency or toxicity are not recognized, i.e. for most of the B vitamins, these sections of the narrative will be omitted.

The rationale for the recommendations made will be presented for each vitamin. However, there are significant limitations based on the available research regarding vitamin metabolism in the horse [1]. Large variability in metabolic BW, energy requirements, and physical demands placed on horses will affect their vitamin requirements [5]. Estimates of dietary requirements for vitamins A, D, E, B_1 (thiamine), and B_2 (riboflavin) have been suggested (Table 9.3). Inadequate data exists for definitive evidence-based requirements for the remaining B, C, and K vitamins because these are known to be synthesized endogenously [1].

9.2 Fat-Soluble Vitamins

9.2.1 Vitamin A

Vitamin A is an essential nutrient that is not synthesized de novo in the body. The preformed vitamin or its precursor, beta-carotene (β-carotene), must be consumed in the diet. The biologically active form of vitamin A is all-*trans*-retinol; however, the generic name vitamin A is given to several retinoids and provitamin carotenoid compounds. Retinol does not naturally occur in vegetation, though horses can meet their vitamin A requirement entirely from precursor dietary carotenoids, particularly β-carotene, present in plant material. β-Carotene is cleaved by intestinal enzymes in the wall of the small intestine to a retinyl ester (retinyl palmitate or retinyl stearate), before hydrolyzation to retinol. For each milligram of β-carotene ingested, the horse can attain approximately 400 IU of vitamin A activity. Upon absorption, retinol is transported in chylomicrons in lymph to the liver for storage and is released from the liver into circulating blood complexed with retinol-binding protein (RBP), or else is excreted as a glucuronide conjugate in the bile and then may enter enterohepatic circulation or be excreted in feces.

The primary role of vitamin A in the body appears to be related to the inclusion of its metabolites in the retina. As 11-cis-retinal, vitamin A combines with the protein opsin to form rhodopsin, a necessary component of the retina for vision, particularly night vision [1]. Vitamin A also plays a critical role in bone and muscle development, reproduction, immune function, and morphology of the skin, gastrointestinal (GI) mucosa, and cornea and is critical for epithelial cell differentiation and establishment of intracellular tight junctions [16].

In addition to providing a dietary source of vitamin A, β-carotene, the most common provitamin-A carotenoid, is also absorbed intact and has a biological function in horses. In the ovary, β-carotene serves as an antioxidant and is incorporated into the corpus luteum, and is involved in the control of progesterone secretion. Dietary β-carotene is thus not only required as a precursor of vitamin A but as a nutrient in its own right.

9.2.1.1 Sources

The concentration of carotenoids in horse feedstuffs varies greatly with most grains being almost devoid. Yellow corn has a small amount (2–6 mg/kg dry matter [DM]) while growing pasture grass and alfalfa have relatively large quantities (30–400 mg/kg DM). Carotenes are destroyed gradually by light, heat, and moisture, thus their concentration in conserved forages (hay and silage) can be unpredictable, ranging from only 4–5 mg/kg DM in poor-quality hay to 20–40 mg/kg DM in high-quality hay, making routine forage analyses necessary. During protected dry storage, vitamin A activity levels can decrease about 10%/month, while sun curing, high moisture, and/or high temperature accelerate the process, with less than half of carotene content in alfalfa hay detectable after 3 m of storage at warm ambient temperatures (Table 9.2). In one study, horse tissue stores of vitamin A were depleted within 2 m when fed hay with no access to pasture [17]. Thus, horses with limited access to growing pasture or fresh hay require additional dietary vitamin A either in a commercial feed or as a supplement. The major commercial forms of vitamin A are the salts of retinyl esters, retinyl acetate, and retinyl palmitate, which are more stable than retinol.

The bioavailability of β-carotene supplements may be variable. Daily feeding of a water-dispersible β-carotene failed to improve vitamin A status in deficient mares when retinyl palmitate was successful, and plasma β-carotene concentrations were unaffected by supplementation with dietary β-carotene [18, 19]. These findings have been disputed more recently, however, as a small cross-over study using four adult ponies demonstrated that daily feeding of β-carotene beadlets increased serum β-carotene concentrations significantly [20]. The difference in animal response may have been the form of the β-carotene fed; beadlets were developed to protect carotenoids against moisture and light destruction in processed feeds [14]. While the evidence for the essentiality of β-carotene in reproductively active mares is uncertain, the administration of highly bioavailable parenteral preparations of β-carotene may be of benefit to mares when access to fresh forage is limited, given no adverse reactions have been documented.

9.2.1.2 Recommendations

Vitamin A concentrations are expressed in IU/kg BW/d or kg ration DM where each IU is equivalent to 0.3 μg retinol or 0.6 μg β-carotene [21]. Horses with access to growing green pasture or fresh forage likely have adequate natural occurring carotene intake to maintain an adequate vitamin A status [22]. If old or low-quality forage or hay is being consumed for more than a few months, supplemental vitamin A is indicated to meet daily requirements (Table 9.3). Strong evidence for oral β-carotene supplementation has not been demonstrated, thus supplementation in the form of oral retinyl esters or intramuscular (IM) injection of vitamin A or β-carotene is recommended. Daily intake should not exceed the safe upper limit of 320 IU/kg BW/d [15]. Administration of a water-soluble emulsion of vitamin A given intramuscularly or subcutaneously (SC) one time at a dosage of 6000–7000 IU/kg BW/d will saturate the liver's storage capacity and does not need to be repeated for at least 3 m. Injection of four times that amount, or prolonged feeding of greater than 5–10 times that amount, may result in vitamin A toxicosis.

9.2.1.2.1 *Maintenance*

Determination of vitamin A requirement for maintenance has been based upon the minimum concentration of intake necessary to prevent night blindness in Percheron horses and adding two standard deviations [1]. Based on this outcome, the minimum amount of dietary vitamin A required for adult maintenance is 30 IU/kg BW/d and feeds containing 2000 IU vitamin A/kg DM are sufficient for maintenance. No requirements have been established at this time for dietary β-carotene.

9.2.1.2.2 *Reproduction and Lactation*

Vitamin A can affect reproductive performance in both male and female horses. In stallions, higher concentrations of dietary vitamin A have been found to maximize semen quality and quantity, and stallion reproductive behavior. In mares, vitamin A requirement is higher during pregnancy than for maintenance [23, 24]. A higher dietary requirement for vitamin A has been reported for pregnant mares based on research in Standardbred mares where measured outcomes included several serviced heats and the number of live foals [1]. Vitamin A requirement further increases at parturition, at least partially due to the presence of high concentrations of vitamin A and β-carotene in mare colostrum [25]. Vitamin A required for reproduction and lactation is suggested to be at least two times the amount required for maintenance, i.e. 60 IU/kg BW/d, so feeds containing 3000–4500 IU/kg DM are more appropriate for reproduction [1].

In addition to vitamin A, β-carotene has been suggested as a conditionally essential nutrient for mare reproduction. Indeed, β-carotene serves as an ovarian antioxidant and has a critical role in controlling progesterone secretion by the mare's corpus luteum, with supplementation reported to improve ovarian activity, produce earlier and stronger periods of estrus, improve conception rates, and reduce embryonic mortality in mares with no access to growing grass. However, in mares fed diets with sufficient β-carotene, additional β-carotene supplementation did increase β-carotene concentrations in plasma, colostrum, and milk, but did not improve measures of fertility [26]. No recommendations for β-carotene can be made at this time.

9.2.1.2.3 *Growth and Development*

Appropriate vitamin A intake is particularly essential for healthy skeletal development in the growing horse. As with the other fat-soluble vitamins, vitamin A is poorly transported across the placenta, and the foal relies on the vitamin-rich colostrum for its initial intake. Provided the mare's vitamin A status is adequate, milk is sufficient to meet the foal's requirements for the first months of life. Colostrum contains high concentrations of vitamin A (17–235 IU/mL) and β-carotene (0.2–7 μg/mL), which decrease rapidly in the first 48 hrs of lactation to provide a relatively stable intake (7–25 IU/mL vitamin A, 0.1–0.7 μg/mL β-carotene) until the foal is weaned [25–27]. From weaning to skeletal maturity, the growing horse should be provided with adequate vitamin A to prevent abnormalities in developing tissues and to decrease susceptibility to respiratory and GI infections. Hypovitaminosis A has been detected in weaned foals consuming poor-quality forage, demonstrating the necessity of appropriate dietary provision [28]. Vitamin A requirement for growth is between that for maintenance and reproduction and lactation, i.e. 45 IU/kg BW/d [1], thus feeds containing 3000–4500 IU/kg DM are appropriate for growth.

9.2.1.2.4 *Performance*

Requirements for vitamin A specific to performance and exercise have yet to be described in the scientific literature. Hypothetical recommendations for increased requirements of vitamin A have been proposed, based on the effect of exercise on connective tissue strain, GI permeability, and resistance to infection [5, 29]. It is recommended that horses receive the same minimum amount of vitamin A as for growth, 45 IU/kg BW/d during periods of high stress and exercise demands, met by feeds containing 3000–4500 IU/kg DM.

9.2.1.3 Signs of Deficiency and Excess

Signs of vitamin A imbalance are rare in healthy adult horses, as liver storage capacity can be saturated after four to six wks of grazing fresh green forage and will be sufficient to maintain serum retinol concentrations for three to six mos. Marginal deficiency resulting in liver store depletion, as indicated by decreased serum retinol concentrations and high relative dose–response (RDR) testing, has been demonstrated in unsupplemented horses fed poor-quality forage. However, longer periods of inappropriate nutrition are required to cause clinical vitamin A deficiency. Toxicity also manifests only after liver capacity has been exceeded and can only occur as a result of excessive vitamin A, not excess carotene, administration.

9.2.1.3.1 Deficiency

Clinical deficiency of vitamin A can present with signs ranging from night blindness to complete loss of vision, infertility, weight loss, loss of skin barrier integrity, poor growth, and immunocompromise. Night blindness is a condition pathognomonic for deficiency. Non-nutritionally associated night blindness occurs but is an uncommon condition present from birth that occasionally occurs primarily in Appaloosas. Differentiation is based on night blindness not being present at birth in vitamin-A-deficient foals, and the deficiency also causes hyperkeratinization of the cornea. Visual abnormality is the classical characteristic of vitamin A deficiency but only develops if the deficiency is sufficiently prolonged and severe. Due to large hepatic reserves and adaptive responses to low concentrations of carotene intake, horses are quite resilient to severe vitamin A deficiency [1]. More commonly observed signs, less specific to vitamin A deficiency but present in earlier stages, include reduced feed intake, poor growth, a dry or dull hair coat, reduced fertility, increased incidence and severity of muscle weakness, or respiratory and diarrheal diseases in foals. Vitamin A deficiency is of greater risk in growing horses than in adults. Far less common signs of vitamin A deficiency include sublingual salivary gland abscesses, squamous metaplasia of the parotid duct, seizures, and generalized weakness.

9.2.1.3.2 Excess

Just as a deficiency does not manifest clinically until hepatic reserves of vitamin A have been depleted, signs of toxicity do not occur until hepatic storage is exceeded. Vitamin A toxicity does not occur as a result of excess carotene intake, in part, due to the inverse conversion of carotene to vitamin A in proportion to intake, i.e. conversion decreases with high intakes. Since plants do not contain preformed vitamin A, true vitamin A toxicosis occurs only as a result of excessive iatrogenic supplementation with preformed vitamin A. Prolonged feeding of excessive vitamin A has been reported to cause bone fragility, hyperostosis, exfoliated epithelium, teratogenesis, and increased blood clotting times. Severe toxicosis (40 000 IU/kg BW/d) in ponies produced anorexia and unthriftiness by wk 15 and, shortly thereafter, rough hair coats, poor muscle tone, and depression [30]. By wk 20, young ponies had lost large areas of hair and epidermis, were periodically ataxic and severely depressed, spent much time in lateral recumbency with a failure to respond to external stimuli, and died shortly thereafter. Degenerative atrophy, fatty infiltration, and reduced hepatic and renal function also typically occur as a result of vitamin A toxicosis [15]. As with deficiency, toxicity is a greater risk in growing horses than in adults, resulting most often in developmental orthopedic disease [1, 30].

9.2.1.4 Diagnosis and Treatment

Serum vitamin A and β-carotene concentrations have wide normal ranges in healthy adult horses associated with seasonal intake, with vitamin A ranging from 12 to 35 μg/dL and β-carotene ranging from 8 to 250 μg/dL. Furthermore, serum vitamin A is not a sensitive indicator of vitamin A status, as substantial changes do not occur until liver storage capacity is either near depletion or exceeded. The hepatic reserve is sufficient to meet all the horse's vitamin A needs for three to six mos.

Variation in plasma vitamin A concentration within the normal range (12–35 μg/dL) is indicative of RBP concentration, the protein required for transport of vitamin A from the liver to peripheral tissues, and is not a good measure of vitamin A or β-carotene intake, or liver vitamin A stores. The concentration of RBP is most significantly affected by dietary protein intake and hepatic synthesis, not vitamin A or β-carotene intake. Retinol binding protein is always completely saturated unless liver storage is depleted and there is inadequate vitamin A to saturate RBP. Determination of vitamin A imbalance thus requires more than single serum measurements. The RDR test is an indirect measure of liver vitamin A and RBP stores, measuring the percentage increase in vitamin A concentration following administration of vitamin A, and is proportionate with the severity of the deficiency. The increase in RDR in horses with marginal vitamin A status occurs as a result of liver conservation of vitamin A. When vitamin A intake is sufficient, a relatively large proportion of dietary vitamin A is stored in the liver due to relatively low production and concentration of RBP. However, during deficiency, RBP synthesis and concentration are increased to distribute hepatic vitamin A to peripheral tissues. When vitamin A is orally administered to horses with vitamin A deficiency, a greater amount of RBP is released from the liver, which is correlated to the degree of vitamin A deficiency. The more RBP complex released from the liver, the greater the increase in the RDR value, corresponding to a larger deficiency of vitamin A. The RDR value is calculated from the following equation: $RDR = 100\ (SR_{15} - SR_0)/SR_{15}$, where SR_0 is baseline serum retinol and SR_{15} is serum retinol 15 hrs post oral administration of 123.5 mg retinyl palmitate in 5 mL of corn oil [17].

9.2.1.4.1 Deficiency

Suspicion of clinical vitamin A deficiency is confirmed by a total serum vitamin A concentration below 10 μg/dL, though a marginal deficiency may occur with serum concentrations within normal limits due to mobilization of hepatic reserves [5]. An RDR is still the most useful indicator of vitamin A status, even with its limitations. An RDR greater than 20% has been suggested to be indicative of vitamin A deficiency, based upon one study, in which thoroughbred broodmares ($n = 45$) and their offspring ($n = 23$) were fed varying concentrations of vitamin A [17]. After two years, RDRs of 20–30% were noted in horses with no clinical evidence of vitamin A deficiency [18]. Despite their prolonged insufficient dietary vitamin A intake, initial hepatic stores were sufficient to maintain adequate vitamin A activity for nearly two years.

The RDR test is affected by hepatic function and dietary protein, energy, and zinc deficiencies, and may also be affected by vitamin A absorption and hepatic mobilization of RBP and therefore may not be applicable if other nutritional deficiencies, hepatic dysfunction, or impaired fat or vitamin A absorption are present. A study using eight Shetland ponies found RDR to be an unreliable indicator of vitamin A status when ponies were fed adequate or increased vitamin A, suggesting that the RDR may only be of use in animals with a deficiency [31]. Instead, lipoprotein-bound retinyl esters were suggested to be a better index of vitamin A status, at least in ponies. Serum retinyl ester concentration is determined by dietary vitamin A but is also affected by age, breed, and individual variations in vitamin A metabolism. Although more sensitive than serum retinol concentrations, serum retinyl esters (retinyl palmitate and retinyl acetate) have not yet been validated as a determination of vitamin A status in equines, and no reliable reference ranges exist. Measurement of vitamin A concentrations from liver samples would be the most indicative of vitamin A intake and status, but liver tissue is rarely biopsied in the living horse due to the invasive nature of this procedure. Administration of a single water-soluble emulsion of vitamin A (IM or SQ) of 6000–7000 IU vitamin A/kg BW/d will saturate the liver's storage capacity and provide adequate vitamin A for several months, giving time for the ration correction to be implemented.

9.2.1.4.2 Excess

Serum total vitamin A concentrations greater than 40–60 μg/dL is indicative of toxicosis. Excessive supplementation >20 000 IU/kg ration DM or >400 IU/kg BW/d has been associated with vitamin A toxicosis. Toxicity is managed by the removal of the source of excess vitamin A in the diet and symptomatic therapy as required.

9.2.2 Vitamin D

In all species, the main role of vitamin D is in calcium (Ca) homeostasis in conjunction with parathyroid hormone (PTH) and calcitonin. When plasma Ca concentration is subnormal, calcitriol (1,25-dihydroxy vitamin D [1,25$(OH)_2$D]) and PTH production and secretion are upregulated, while calcitonin production and secretion are inhibited. Calcitriol, as well as PTH, increases the resorption of bone and release of the stored bone mineral, which is primarily composed of Ca and phosphorus (P). As stored minerals are released from bone, serum Ca and P become elevated. At the renal tubules, PTH acts to increase P excretion to mitigate increasing serum P. Calcitriol also acts to stimulate intestinal Ca, P, and magnesium absorption. Together, these actions cause an elevation in plasma Ca to bring concentrations back within the normal range.

Additionally, these mechanisms also regulate plasma P concentrations. In instances of P deficiency, the lower plasma P concentration results in less Ca being bound to P, resulting in a relative increase in ionized Ca, despite no change in total Ca concentration. This simultaneously stimulates calcitriol production and PTH suppression, which increases bone mineral resorption, decreases renal P excretion, and increases renal Ca excretion, resulting in increased plasma P with a minimal increase in plasma Ca. Vitamin D, as its activated form calcitriol, is thus the primary effector in Ca homeostasis, while PTH is the primary controller. Horses have active regulation of Ca and P serum concentrations, exhibit abnormalities in bone metabolism when deprived of sunlight and dietary vitamin D, and exhibit strong correlations between vitamin D receptors and vitamin D responsive gene transcripts [32]. However, in contrast to other grazing species studied, Ca and P homeostasis may not be as reliant on vitamin D status, and no signs of naturally occurring vitamin D deficiency have been described in horses. In addition to the well-known role in Ca, P, and bone metabolism, vitamin D has been demonstrated to have additional effects on cell proliferation and differentiation, inflammatory markers, and immune function, although these functions have not been described in the horse specifically [33].

9.2.2.1 Sources

Vitamin D occurs in two forms in nature: cholecalciferol (D_3), primarily present in animal tissues, and ergocalciferol (D_2), primarily found in plant (fungal) material. Ultraviolet (UV) sun rays with wavelengths of 295–315 nm convert 7-dehydrocholesterol to D_3 in the skin of animals, or ergosterol to D_2 in endophytes within the leaves of plants [34]. The content of vitamin D in forages, the natural dietary source for horses, is highly variable, depending on the method of preservation (sun-cured vs. artificially dried), species (clover vs. grass, alfalfa), and geographical location (latitude and sunshine hours). Ergocalciferol content in forages has been reported to range between 0.5 and 74 μg/kg DM [35–38]. The wide variation in reported D_2 content may be at least partially explained by differences in testing method, i.e. biological response in rat assays vs. measurement by high-performance liquid chromatography (HPLC) or liquid chromatography–mass spectrometry, geographical region (North Eastern United States, Denmark, Scotland, and Switzerland), time of year (spring, summer, and autumn), and changes in agricultural practices, forage species and forage quality over time (1958 vs. 2013). Vitamin D is sensitive to degradation during storage and is readily destabilized by heavy metals, low pH, and exposure to light and oxygen. Vitamin D activity reportedly decreases by 7.5%/m, leaving only around 39% present after one year of storage (Table 9.2).

Ingestion vitamin D is incorporated with lipids into chylomicrons and absorbed into the lymphatics. Both ingested and synthesized vitamin D are bound to vitamin D binding protein (DBP) in the blood and transported to the liver, and then converted to the most abundant metabolite, calcidiol (25-hydroxyvitamin D [25(OH)D]). This compound is also carried in the blood bound to DBP and is hydroxylated in the kidney to the active metabolite calcitriol ($1,25(OH)_2D$), which binds to vitamin D receptors in target organs [34]. Depending on vitamin D status and requirement, calcidiol may also be converted to the less active metabolite, 24,25-dihydroxy vitamin D, for excretion.

In addition to dietary vitamin D, many animals are capable of synthesizing vitamin D in their skin in response to exposure to UV radiation from the sun. As herbivores, the natural diet of horses includes vitamin D_2 exclusively, allowing for differentiation between dietary vitamin D_2 and endogenously synthesized vitamin D_3. Horses only need unshaded access to the outdoors for several hours a day, even when cloudy or overcast, to completely meet their vitamin D requirements. However, this concept has more recently been contested [39]. Relatively low concentrations of endogenously synthesized $25(OH)D_3$ have been reported in horses, compared with other animals, while dietary $25(OH)D_2$ appears to be the main, and more potent, vitamin D metabolite in equine serum [39–42]. Variable responses to UV exposure have been reported, with some studies finding seasonal alterations in serum calcidiol concentrations, yet others failed to demonstrate any seasonality [24, 39, 40, 42]. Another study demonstrated no difference in serum calcidiol or calcitriol between horses covered with horse blankets and a cohort without blankets, further supporting a greater role for dietary vitamin D_2 than endogenously synthesized vitamin D_3. The ability of the horse to maintain appropriate serum calcidiol, calcitriol, Ca, and P concentrations regardless of UV exposure may be explained by greater utilization of $25(OH)D_2$ compared to $25(OH)D_3$, given D_3 may vary but D_2 is relatively stable in the ration [24].

For horses with routine access to the outdoors, vitamin D requirements are likely met by a combination of endogenous synthesis of D_3 and dietary D_2 from natural sources. For horses without regular exposure to sunlight, vitamin D requirements may be met by feeding forage or a commercial diet containing added vitamin D. Dietary supplements containing vitamin D (typically as D_3) are available for addition to grain-based rations and may be offered, provided the horse's daily intake does not exceed the safe upper limit of 44 IU/kg BW/d [15].

9.2.2.2 Recommendations

Vitamin D concentrations are expressed in IU/kg BW/d or or kg ration DM, where each IU is equivalent to 0.025 mcg of vitamin D [21].

9.2.2.2.1 Maintenance

A true minimum dietary vitamin D requirement is still unknown. But for horses with sun exposure living below 55° latitude, cutaneous synthesis is likely sufficient. Horses living primarily indoors or above 55° latitude may require the dietary provision of vitamin D. A recommendation for horses living primarily indoors has been a minimum of 6.6 IU/kg BW/d recommended by the National Research Council [1]. At present, there is no data to suggest that vitamin D requirements are different for pregnant or lactating horses, particularly when mares have access to sunlight. Similarly, there are no reports of vitamin D deficiency in horses when maintained under practical common situations with some outside exposure to the sun.

9.2.2.2.2 Growth and Development

As vitamin D plays a role in skeletal development, the following recommendations have been made for growing horses based on age: 22.2 IU from birth to 6 m, 17.4 IU from 7 to 12 m, 15.9 IU from 13 to 18 m, and 13.7 IU from 19 to 24 m [1].

9.2.2.3 Signs of Deficiency and Excess

9.2.2.3.1 Deficiency

Naturally occurring vitamin D deficiency has not been described in the horse. In young ponies deprived of all sunlight and with no dietary vitamin D, a decrease in feed intake, growth, bone ash content, bone cortical area, and bone-breaking strength were reported [43]. However, no difference in feed efficiency or plasma Ca, P, or magnesium concentrations were observed when compared to a cohort also deprived of sunlight but fed 28 IU/kg BW/d, or those with sun exposure and no dietary vitamin D. Vitamin D deficiency has been postulated to contribute to proinflammatory states in sick foals and supported by findings of hypovitaminosis D in hospitalized foals, with hypocalcemia and hyperphosphatemia more prevalent in septic hospitalized foals [44]. Additionally, foals with low serum $25(OH)D_3$ and $1,25(OH)_2D_3$ were more likely to die than foals with vitamin D metabolites within the normal range.

9.2.2.3.2 Excess

Vitamin D toxicosis is likely the most commonly reported vitamin toxicosis in most species and occurs primarily as a result of improperly formulated feeds, excessive oral or parenteral administration of vitamin D, or ingestion of calcinogenic plants. Calcinogenic plants are a group of plants containing steroidal glycosides that are hydrolyzed by bacteria within the GI tract to release calcitriol [45]. These plants grow primarily in tropical and subtropical areas of the world, though *Cestrum diurnum* and *Solanum torvum* are found in the USA (*C. diurnum* in Florida; both species in Hawaii), whereas *Trisetum flavescens* is found in some European countries (Austria, Germany, and Switzerland).

Experimental induction of hypervitaminosis D was achieved by feeding a daily dose of 33 000 IU D_2 or D_3/kg BW/d for 30 d and resulted in variable clinical signs ranging from slight weight loss (8% BW), hyperphosphatemia, hypercalcemia, nonprogressive hyposthenuria, and soft tissue mineralization in the horse fed D_2, to severe weight loss (−29% BW), limb stiffness, tachycardia, anorexia, weakness, recumbency, polydipsia and polyuria, progressive hyposthenuria, bone fractures, and extensive soft tissue mineralization in the horse fed D_3 [46].

When dosed orally, clinical signs may take days to weeks of continuous oversupply of oral vitamin D to manifest, with D_3 being more toxic than D_2. However, when dosed parenterally, horses appear more susceptible to acute toxicity at lower doses. When 10 000 IU D_3/kg BW were injected IM for four consecutive days, ponies exhibited increased plasma Ca and P for six wks, with widespread moderate to severe soft tissue calcification [41]. Similar, but milder, findings were reported when the same protocol was repeated with horses, but their dietary Ca and P were restricted. A safe upper limit has been set at 44 IU/kg BW/d [15]. Hypervitaminosis is diagnosed by elevated plasma vitamin D or calcidiol; both are reliable indicators of toxicity in horses fed toxic quantities (33 000 IU/kg BW/d) of either D_2 or D_3 [46]. Typically, plasma Ca is high in the normal or mildly elevated range, whereas P is often moderately to markedly increased.

9.2.2.4 Diagnosis and Treatment

Vitamin D status may be determined by the measurement of calcidiol or calcitriol concentrations in blood plasma. Reported plasma concentrations in clinically normal adult horses have ranged from 1.9 to 18.0 ng/mL [34]. Independent measurements of 25(OH)D_2 and 25(OH)D_3 were also reported, with 25(OH)D_2 concentrations ranging from 0.1 to 5.1 ng/mL and 25(OH)D_3 concentrations ranging from 0.1 to 6.0 ng/mL. This wide range of values is complicated by geographical location (Finland, Denmark, Thailand, Mideastern USA, England, Germany, and Italy), time of year (January, March, May, June, July, September, October, and December), horse breed, supplementary dietary vitamin D (0–337.5 μg/horse), sun exposure, and detection method (multispecies enzyme immunoassay, HPLC, competitive protein-binding assay, and sheep antibody radioimmunoassay) [23, 24, 40–42, 47–50].

9.2.2.4.1 Excess

Treatment of vitamin D toxicosis includes immediate removal of all supplemental sources of vitamin D, Ca, and P and feeding a diet as low in these nutrients as possible. Typically, a diet rich in grains and low in forage has lower vitamin D and Ca, though the P content is generally higher, thus a diet consisting of an equal weight of grain and grass or artificially dried timothy hay (1 kg grain +1 kg grass/100 kg BW/d). Alfalfa hay, i.e. Lucerne, is contraindicated due to the high Ca content. Exposure to sunlight should be minimized. A cation chelator such as sodium phytate dosed orally may be beneficial to decrease intestinal Ca absorption. Increasing fluid intake can help to increase renal mineral excretion, so oral or intravenous fluid therapy could be administered, with or without diuretics provided no dehydration is present. Recovery can be slow, reportedly up to six mos for complete resolution of signs [46].

9.2.3 Vitamin E

The term vitamin E refers to a family of four tocopherols, α-tocopherol, β-tocopherol, γ-tocopherol, δ-tocopherol, and four tocotrienols, α-tocotrienol, β-tocotrienol, γ-tocotrienol, and δ-tocotrienol, with α-tocopherol (TOC) having the greatest endogenous biological activity [1]. Like the other fat-soluble vitamins, i.e. A and D, vitamin E is taken up by enterocytes and secreted along with lipids within chylomicrons into the lymphatic system. Circulating chylomicron triacylglycerols are hydrolyzed, and particles containing vitamin E are transported within lipoproteins to the liver and extra-hepatic tissues [51]. In the liver, TOC transfer protein binds TOC and acts to regulate plasma and tissue TOC concentrations, and excess is metabolized by side-chain degradation or excreted in bile. As the most important lipid-soluble antioxidant, vitamin E, incorporated into cell membranes, donates a hydrogen atom from the phenolic group to stabilize free radicals produced during cell membrane oxidation, resulting in stable lipid peroxide and stable tocopheryl radical [52]. Enzymatic degradation of lipid peroxides is then performed by superoxide dismutase or the selenium-dependent glutathione peroxidase (GHS) [52]. Vitamin E can donate two hydrogen atoms before requiring reduction back to its active form, a reaction that requires vitamin C. Thus, vitamin E, selenium (Se), and vitamin C have complementary activities. Additional roles of vitamin E in the modulation of gene expression, inhibition of platelet aggregation, and stabilization of plasma membranes have been described [53]. Supplementation with vitamin E has been demonstrated to improve both cellular and humoral immunity in aged horses [54].

9.2.3.1 Sources

Vitamin E is present in most equine feedstuffs, with fresh forages having the highest concentration (100–600 IU/kg DM), hay at a middle concentration (15–60 IU/kg DM), and dehydrated alfalfa pellets and grains at the lowest concentration (5–80 IU/kg DM) [55, 56]. The amount in forages decreases with plant maturity, i.e. 70–90% from early growth to maturity in grasses and 35–65% in alfalfa from bud to postflowering. From 30 to 80% of vitamin E activity is lost between cutting to baling hay and another 54–73% loss occurs in alfalfa hay stored at 97 °F (33 °C) for 12 wks [57]. A survey of 40 hays from various states showed that over 50% had a vitamin E content of less than 50 IU/kg DM, while 15% had over 80 IU/kg DM [58]. Whole oilseeds are good sources of vitamin E, but most vitamin E has been removed from oilseed meals. Commercial horse feeds often contain added vitamin E, typically as the more stable ester, α-tocopheryl acetate [1]. Differences in the activity of vitamin E supplements depend on the source, i.e. *RRR* stereoisomers, or a synthetic racemic mixture of stereoisomers, i.e. *all-rac*, [59]. Indeed, within RRR stereoisomers tested (acetate powder, alcohol powder, micellized alcohol powder, and micellized alcohol liquid), variability in vitamin activity has been reported, with micellized RRR-TOC having the greatest effect on plasma TOC concentration [59–61]. Natural-source *RRR* acetate provides 1.36 IU/mg, while synthetic *all-rac* provides only 1 IU/mg. Additional supplementation with TOC provides a greater vitamin E source equivalent to 1.49 IU/mg, though this must be added to the diet after feed processing, such as an addition to a meal [1].

Horses with access to pasture are likely to ingest adequate vitamin E to meet minimum maintenance requirements when pasture is actively growing [22, 62]. However, for horses confined indoors or with little access to pasture, and those in climates where pasture is dormant for certain seasons, i.e. temperate climates during winter or tropical climates with drought in summer, dietary provision of vitamin E is necessary to maintain an adequate status [24, 62]. There is some evidence that the fermentation of fresh forage to form silage or haylage preserves vitamin E better than drying to form hay, and thus these forages may be more appropriate for feeding to horses when growing pasture is unavailable [63, 64]. Regardless, dietary supplementation is recommended when access to pasture is minimal and in horses with increased requirements or risk of deficiency-associated diseases.

9.2.3.2 Recommendations

Vitamin E concentrations may be expressed in IU/kg BW/d or kg ration DM, where each IU is equivalent to 0.67 mg for naturally occurring D-alpha-tocopherol and 0.9 mg for synthetic DL-alpha-tocopherol [21].

9.2.3.2.1 Maintenance

The requirement for adult maintenance has been established based on the maximization of tissue stores (1.4–4.4 IU/kg BW/d) and support of immune function (1 IU/kg BW/d) [65, 66]. Rations containing a minimum of 50 IU vitamin E/kg DM will meet maintenance requirements. However, higher concentrations have since been reported for improved immune function (15 IU/kg BW/d), which would require rations to contain 750 IU vitamin E/kg DM [54].

9.2.3.2.2 Reproduction and Lactation

Though there have been many studies investigating the effects of vitamin E on fertility and reproductive health, there is little evidence in horses that requirements for pregnant or breeding mares are any higher than adult horse maintenance [1]. Requirements for mares in lactation, however, are greater. Plasma TOC increases from about two wks before parturition, likely reflecting mobilization of stored TOC in preparation for lactation; in particular, colostrum contains high concentrations of TOC [25, 27]. Due to the physiology of equine placentation, the transfer of fat-soluble vitamins preparturition is limited; therefore, a high concentration of vitamin E is required in the colostrum and milk to reach appropriate circulating concentrations in the foal [23, 27]. Furthermore, inadequate concentrations of vitamin E in broodmares may predispose their foals to nutritional myodegeneration. To support the needs of both mare and foal, the mare requires a higher dietary intake of vitamin E, at least double the maintenance minimum (2 IU/kg BW/d or a ration containing a minimum of 100 IU vitamin E/kg DM) [1].

9.2.3.2.3 Growth and Development

There is little evidence to support claims for vitamin E requirements specific to foal growth. Presently, the growth requirement is the same as the lactation requirement, 2 IU/kg BW/d [1]. Considering the safety of high concentrations of vitamin E, for foals at risk for equine degenerative myeloencephalopathy (EDM), a prudent recommendation is to provide the foal with 1000–2000 IU/d in their diet as a preventative measure until at least 12 m of age.

9.2.3.2.4 *Performance*

Exercise is known to contribute to lipid oxidation in horses, and exercise can decrease vitamin E in horses fed insufficient rations [67, 68]. Provision of dietary vitamin E greater than 1 IU/kg BW/d is likely to be beneficial in instances where oxidative stress may be greater than that in a maintenance sedentary horse and is known to be safe up to 20 IU/kg BW/d [1]. This may be beneficial when nutrient oxidation increases to satisfy energy needs that occur with exercise or exertion. This benefit was demonstrated by the absence of muscle soreness and lameness in horses and zebras following their capture and restraint when their diets contained 100 IU vitamin E/kg DM, whereas soreness and lameness occurred when their diet contained only 50 IU/kg DM [55].

Studies have reported on the effects of vitamin E supplementation above the minimum maintenance requirement on exercise and oxidative stress of horses undergoing various performance challenges by measuring parameters of the heart and skeletal muscle enzymes. Results have been variable as some studies have found that vitamin E supplementation at 1.6–2.7 IU/kg BW/d did not affect measures of oxidative injury in exercising horses [69, 70]. However, other studies have reported more favorable results when horses were supplemented with 2–7 IU/kg BW/d when compared to unsupplemented horses [59, 71–76]. Differences in the concentration of horse fitness, basal diet vitamin E content, control group vitamin E status, supplement form and dose, the intensity of work, and study design all account for some of the variability in the results. The current published recommendations for exercising horses are 1.6–2.0 IU/kg BW/d. This may be sufficient to maintain vitamin E status and avoid adverse effects of hypovitaminosis E, but the requirement is likely higher (6–7 IU/kg BW/d) for horses subjected to intense work.

9.2.3.3 Signs of Deficiency

Nutritional muscular dystrophy (NMD), aka white muscle disease and nutritional myodegeneration, is a vitamin E and selenium deficiency resulting in the degeneration of smooth, cardiac, or skeletal muscle in foals, calves, and lambs. A cross-section of muscle from an affected animal has white areas of ischemic degeneration and calcification. See White Muscle Disease under Selenium deficiency in Chapter 8 and Nutritional Muscular Dystrophy in Chapter 25.

Less commonly, generalized steatitis is primarily a vitamin E, rather than selenium, deficiency and may be present concurrent with muscle or neuronal diseases. This occurs particularly in older foals up to several months of age and may manifest as progressive emaciation and debilitation despite a good appetite. Affected horses have multiple indurated subcutaneous swellings composed of mineralized and necrotic adipose tissue, with sensitive, hardened nuchal ligaments. Fat deposits throughout the body are a yellowish-brown color due to ceroid accumulation, giving rise to the name "yellow fat disease." There may also be ventral subcutaneous edema due to capillary leakage and a rough, shaggy haircoat.

Considering the essential role of TOC as an intracellular antioxidant, signs of vitamin E deficiency manifest as neuromuscular disorders: equine motor neuron disease (EMND), neuroaxonal dystrophy (NAD), and EDM. The etiologies and diagnoses of these diseases can be complex, EDM and NAD are clinically indistinguishable, and there have been reports of concurrent NAD and EMND as well as theories that vitamin E deficiency myopathy may be an early stage of EMND or contribute to the vitamin-E-responsive recovery in horses who have been misdiagnosed as having EMND [77, 78]. See Chapter 25 Musculoskeletal System Disorders.

9.2.3.4 Diagnosis and Treatment

TOC concentration in blood has been used as an indicator of vitamin E status, with greater than 2 μg/mL considered adequate and less than 1.5 μg/mL considered deficient [53]. A prudent recommendation would be to repeat serum sampling in horses with marginal status (between 1 and 2 μg/mL) as variability in horses with deficient concentrations can be quite large [79]. Acute clinical deficiency has been described in horses with serum concentrations 0.04–0.56 μg/mL and chronic clinical deficiency with serum concentrations of 0.26–1.63 μg/mL [77]. Due to the storage of vitamin E in the liver, hepatic tissue samples can provide a robust indicator of vitamin E status, though these are typically only obtained postmortem. In adult horses, the reference range for hepatic vitamin E is 20–40 μg/g dry weight or 2.3–4.7 μg/g wet weight [65, 80]. Muscle biopsies may be of use in clinical settings for confirming vitamin E deficiency, as low muscle concentrations (0.43–1.14 μg/g, reference range 3.6–8.1 μg/g) have been documented in chronically affected horses [77].

A reasonable repletion dose for a vitamin-E-deficient horse would be at least double the maintenance minimum (2 IU/kg BW/d) for several months by allowing access to a green growing pasture if available or feeding a supplemented feed containing α-tocopherol. Horses with EDM respond better to therapy than do horses with NMD, EMND, or NAD, and though complete recovery is rare, the prognosis for return to function is fair to good [77].

9.2.4 Vitamin K

Vitamin K acts as a cofactor for vitamin-K-dependent carboxylase, an enzyme that catalyzes the synthesis of γ-carboxyglutamic acid (GLA) from glutamic acid, which is an essential component of proteins involved in blood clotting, bone metabolism, and vascular health [1]. The GLA residues in vitamin-K-dependent proteins bind calcium, which is critical in the activation of several blood clotting factors, synthesized as inactive precursors, including factors II (prothrombin), VII, IX, and X. Additional roles of vitamin K in other species have been identified in bone metabolism, vascular health, and sphingolipid metabolism in the brain [81].

9.2.4.1 Sources

Vitamin K exists in multiple forms: the natural forms phylloquinone (K_1), found in green leafy plants, menaquinone (K_2), produced by bacteria in the GI tract, and the synthetic form, menadione (K_3). Forages contain the highest concentration of vitamin K (3–20 mg/kg DM), while cereals contain little (0.2–0.4 mg/kg DM) [1, 82]. Provision of forage, either fresh or conserved, is likely to meet the dietary requirements of horses for vitamin K. As a fat-soluble vitamin, the natural forms, phylloquinone, and menaquinone are absorbed from the intestines into lymphatics by a process that requires the presence of both bile salts and pancreatic enzymes [83]. The synthetic form, menadione, is water-soluble. Regardless of the source, all forms of vitamin K are converted to the active form, hydroquinone, in the liver.

9.2.4.2 Recommendations

Phylloquinone content of forage, both fresh and conserved, and bacterially synthesized menaquinone are thought to equally meet the horse's requirements. Though vitamin K status, based on undercarboxylated osteocalcin, has been measured in growing foals and weanlings, there was no evidence for a dietary requirement for vitamin K in growing horses [84]. Mare's milk, and milk replacement, provides adequate dietary vitamin K without additional supplementation.

9.2.4.3 Signs of Deficiency

Unlike the other fat-soluble vitamins A, D, or E, little vitamin K is stored in the body, so deficiency may develop faster than other fat-soluble vitamin deficiencies. Vitamin K deficiency is characterized by decreased clotting ability, increased clotting times, and increased susceptibility to hemorrhage. Epistaxis may be the first sign in a horse, which must be differentiated from more common causes of epistaxis, such as exercise-induced pulmonary hemorrhage (EIPH), ethmoid hematoma, or guttural pouch mycosis. Other possible signs include hemorrhage into joints, the GI tract, or urinary tract, and hematomas in subcutaneous tissues of the neck, ventral chest, and abdominal walls or the muscles of the hind limbs. Cerebral hemorrhage may occur and result in neurologic signs such as blindness and paresis.

In theory, vitamin K deficiency could result from decreased feed intake, decreased bacterial synthesis, or impaired intestinal fat absorption (enteritis, colitis), extensive intestinal resection, disruption of normal GI flora by antibacterial drugs, lack of bile salts, pancreatic enzymes, and lymphatic obstruction. Due to minimal body stores and immature gut flora, neonates are at greater risk of deficiency if intake is inadequate. However, the only documented causes of vitamin K deficiency in horses have been secondary to vitamin K antagonism by dicoumarol ingestion or warfarin administration. Dicoumarol is a naturally occurring anticoagulant that acts by inhibiting hepatic synthesis of vitamin-K-dependent clotting factors. Some species of *Penicillium* molds produce coumarin from the precursors found in sweet clover hay or haylage. Clinical intoxication with dicoumarol may require weeks of ingestion of the affected moldy forage before vitamin K deficiency is evident. Warfarin is a synthetic dicoumarol derivative present in rodenticides and anticoagulants. It has been used in the past as a therapy for navicular disease because of its antithrombotic effects. In the blood, warfarin is highly protein-bound, and toxicity can be potentiated by concurrent administration of nonsteroidal anti-inflammatories or other highly protein-bound drugs that could displace the warfarin.

9.2.4.4 Diagnosis and Treatment

If clotting times are elevated as a result of both increased prothrombin time (PT) and activated partial thromboplastin time (APTT), a vitamin K deficiency should be suspected, as multiple clotting factors affecting both sides of the clotting cascade are reduced in cases with vitamin K deficiency. Definitive diagnosis requires the detection of the ingested or administered toxin in plasma, liver, kidney, or muscle, or the detection of dicoumarol in the feed; however, suspicion may also be confirmed if clotting times, PT and APTT, return to normal within 12–24 hrs of administration of vitamin K. Since vitamin K is required for vitamin-K-dependent carboxylase, vitamin K status may be inferred from the measurement of undercarboxylated osteocalcin [82]. In cases of suspected or confirmed toxicosis with a vitamin K antagonist, treatment consists of removal of the source of the toxin, immediate parenteral injection of vitamin phylloquinone 1–2 mg/kg BW/d IM, in divided doses, and addition of 3–5 mg phylloquinone/kg BW/d ration supplementation for three to four wks.

Supplementation of dietary vitamin K may be considered for horses with decreased hepatic function or dysregulation of intestinal flora. Impaired fat absorption greatly decreases the absorption of the natural forms of vitamin K but would not be expected to decrease the absorption of water-soluble forms of vitamin K_3. Parenteral vitamin K may be indicated in horses with chronic fat malabsorption. Vitamins K_1 and K_3 are available commercially, both in injectable and oral forms. Water-soluble forms of vitamin K_3 are the predominant form used for oral administration due to the lower cost.

9.3 Water-Soluble Vitamins

There are eight B vitamins: thiamine (B_1), riboflavin (B_2), niacin (B_3), pantothenic acid (B_5), pyridoxine (B_6), biotin (B_7), folate (B_9), and cobalamin (B_{12}). Except for thiamine, none of the B vitamins are essential nutrients for horses as they are all produced by microbes in the horse's caecum and large intestine. See The Role of Microbiota in Chapter 4. However, feeding the intestinal microbiome is essential to this symbiotic relationship. While thiamine is also produced by the microbiome, this may be insufficient to maintain adequate thiamine concentrations, thus there is a dietary recommendation for thiamine. Riboflavin has a suggested dietary concentration but lacks evidence for a strict dietary requirement, thus it is unlikely that horses require the dietary provision of riboflavin [1, 5].

9.3.1 Thiamine (B_1)

Thiamine plays an important role in carbohydrate metabolism, where thiamin pyrophosphate (TPP) functions in pyruvate dehydrogenase, α-ketoglutarate dehydrogenase, and transketolase reactions involved in the use of substrates such as glucose, lactate, and pyruvate [1]. Pyruvate dehydrogenase and α-ketoglutarate dehydrogenase are required for adenosine triphosphate (ATP) synthesis, with transketolase required for pentose phosphate metabolism (Figure 9.1). Thiamine is a critical nutrient for normal nervous system function, with classical signs of deficiency being predominantly neurological. Upon absorption from the intestine, which requires folate, thiamine is converted to an active coenzyme form TPP in the liver and kidney. Thiamine is one of the vitamins least stored in the body and rapidly excreted in the urine.

9.3.1.1 Sources

Thiamine is produced by bacteria in the GI tract of the horse and is also present in relatively high concentrations in green leaves, cereal grain germ, and yeast, though milling and feed processing decreases the amount present. Average forage (hay and pasture) contains 1–4 mg/kg DM and cereal grains contain 4–7 mg/kg DM, which would just meet the horse's requirement. However, thiamine activity decreases rapidly during feed storage, around 50% over 6 m, and low plasma thiamine concentrations have been reported in stabled horses not receiving fresh forage or supplemental thiamine. Yeast contains high concentrations of thiamine (150–160 mg/kg DM) and is often provided as a source of dietary B vitamins. Synthetic thiamine in the forms of thiamine hydrochloride and thiamine mononitrate can be added to feeds or supplements.

Healthy adult horses with access to good quality pasture or fresh forage may meet their maintenance requirements, assuming a minimum of 3 mg thiamine/kg DM with 50% absorption. This would achieve a minimum intake of 0.06 mg/kg BW/d for horses ingesting 2% BW on a DM basis. However, the addition of cereal grains, yeast, and/or a pelleted diet containing at least 5–10 mg/kg DM is recommended for any suggested intake above minimum adult maintenance.

9.3.1.2 Recommendations

Thiamine requirements are expressed as mg/kg BW/d or mg/kg ration DM. While horses are capable of using thiamine produced by GI microbes, however quantities are insufficient to prevent deficiency if horses are fed a thiamine-deficient diet. Microbial synthesis of thiamine appears to be adjunctive to dietary thiamine, as horses absorb about 50% of the thiamine present in unsupplemented feeds, and the efficiency of absorption decreases with increasing amounts ingested. There are no significant body stores of thiamine, the excess is rapidly excreted, and there is no evidence of toxicity at high doses, so thiamine supplementation is considered safe and effective.

9.3.1.2.1 Maintenance

The thiamine requirement recommended for adult maintenance is 0.06 mg/kg BW/d assuming 2% DM intake [1, 8, 55]. This requirement was determined by the diet concentrations necessary to maintain appetite [1].

9.3.1.2.2 Growth and Development

In pony weanlings, a faster growth rate was noted in those fed rations supplemented with thiamine as opposed to the basal diet without thiamine supplementation, recommending 0.165 mg/kg BW/d for growing horses.

9.3.1.2.3 Performance

Thiamine supplementation has been suggested to stimulate appetite, assist in the prevention of exertional rhabdomyolysis, and decrease anxiety in nervous horses, though there is little evidence supporting these effects. However, mean blood thiamine concentration and pyruvate dehydrogenase activity were demonstrated to be higher in exercising horses fed higher concentrations of thiamine than those fed diets with marginal thiamine concentration, leading to the establishment of a higher dietary thiamine requirement of 0.125 mg/kg BW/d. Parenteral administration of phosphorylated thiamine has been suggested to reduce serum lactate in exercising horses, though how this translates to dietary recommendations is not known [85].

9.3.1.3 Signs of Deficiency

Dietary thiamine deficiency is rare in adult horses, as a portion of the horse's needs is supplied by cecal and intestinal bacterial synthesis. In experimentally induced thiamine deficiency, clinical signs were reported, such as anorexia, bradycardia, muscle fasciculation, hyperesthesia, ataxia, and convulsions. Under normal circumstances, only foals with immature gut flora, performance horses with exceptional requirements, or horses with disruption of intestinal flora following prolonged oral antimicrobial therapy, decreased intake, and/or absorption with anorexia or colitis increased losses due to polyuria, intestinal parasitism, or ingestion of thiamine antagonists such as amprolium and bracken fern (*Pteridium aquilinum*), may be at risk of thiamine deficiency.

Amprolium is a coccidiostat commonly included in poultry and cattle diets; when ingested at high doses in horses, thiamine absorption and phosphorylation are decreased causing clinical thiamine deficiency. Bracken fern contains several antithiamine factors, including thiaminase and caffeic acid. Thiaminase cleaves thiamine into two inactive molecules, while caffeic acid inhibits intestinal thiamine absorption. Since thiamine is required for pyruvate and lactate metabolism, deficiency causes an increase in plasma pyruvate and lactate concentrations, with a concurrent decrease in plasma thiamine concentration.

9.3.1.4 Diagnosis and Treatment

Thiamine status can be determined by the measurement of transketolase activity in red blood cells (RBC-TK) and by percent stimulation of transketolase activity by exogenous TPP. An increase in RBC-TK activity *in vitro* in response to added TPP suggests thiamine deficiency, with an increase of 30–50% indicating subclinical deficiency, and 80–100% indicating severe deficiency. Alternatively, the ribose-5-phosphate activity can be measured, with a decrease of 15–25% indicating subclinical deficiency and a decrease greater than 25% indicating clinical deficiency.

In cases of thiamine deficiency, causative factors should be removed and supportive therapy initiated. Early repeated administration of thiamine parenterally is indicated, as the horse typically absorbs only about 50% of thiamine present in the diet, and efficiency of absorption decreases with the amount ingested, requiring much higher doses orally than parenterally. Extrapolation from data in other species suggests that 0.3–0.4 mg/kg BW thiamine may be given parenterally, or 0.6–1.2 mg/kg BW given orally, four times in the first 24 hrs, then once daily until one to two days after improvement of clinical signs.

9.3.2 Riboflavin (B_2)

Riboflavin is circulated bound to plasma proteins and functions in metabolic oxidation–reduction reactions essential to energy production (Figure 9.1). Riboflavin is the precursor to two coenzymes: flavin mononucleotide (FMN) and flavin adenine dinucleotide (FAD). Both coenzymes transfer electrons to the mitochondrial electron transport chain for ATP synthesis and also function in drug metabolism, lipid metabolism, and antioxidant defense mechanisms [1].

9.3.2.1 Sources

Like thiamine, riboflavin is produced in variable amounts by GI microbes and is present in relatively high concentrations in forage (7–17 mg/kg DM) but low concentrations in cereal grains (1–3 mg/kg DM). Riboflavin is also absorbed with decreasing efficiency with increasing amounts ingested; excess is excreted rapidly in urine and there is little body storage. Unlike thiamine, riboflavin is fairly resistant to moisture, oxidation, and heat during storage, but is sensitive to light. Riboflavin concentrations decrease only around 3%/month, meaning nearly 70% is still present 1 year after storage, and around 50% after 2 years of storage, making hay a suitable dietary source.

Considering the relatively high concentration of riboflavin in normal dietary constituents of horse rations, and robust resistance to degradation with storage, there is no recommendation for riboflavin supplementation for horses with access to pasture and/or conserved forage with or without commercially prepared feeds. These feed types are sufficient to provide horses with at least 2 mg riboflavin/kg DM. Were a horse to be fed cereal grains alone, riboflavin deficiency could potentially occur, although this would be of lesser concern than other conditions arising from such an inappropriate diet. The only horses considered to be at any risk of riboflavin deficiency would be foals unable to nurse and fed unsupplemented milk replacement. Milk replacement products may be deficient in riboflavin if not formulated for horses. Fresh or frozen mare's milk, or a commercial milk replacement designed for foals, should contain riboflavin and is the optimal feed for foals unable to nurse.

9.3.2.2 Recommendations

Considering the robust microbial synthesis of riboflavin, and a lack of evidence for a strict dietary requirement, it is unlikely that horses require the dietary provision of riboflavin. Studies in Shetland ponies conducted over 70 years ago evaluated growth and riboflavin status and are still cited by the NRC. Based on these studies, the horse's minimum dietary riboflavin requirement for maintenance is still considered at 0.04 mg/kg BW/d [1, 7, 55]. The minimum dietary requirement for growth is considered to be 0.05 mg/kg BW/d.

9.3.2.3 Diagnosis and Treatment

Research studies involving the determination of riboflavin status have used either a microbiological method of estimating riboflavin in urine and blood or coenzyme stimulation assays in the blood [10, 86].

9.3.3 Niacin (B_3)

The term niacin refers to two related compounds: nicotinic acid (pyridine-3-carboxylic acid) and the amide, nicotinamide (nicotinic acid amide) [1]. Dietary nicotinic acid is converted to nicotinamide and absorbed by the intestinal mucosa. Nicotinamide is incorporated into nicotinamide adenine dinucleotide (NADH) and nicotinamide adenine dinucleotide phosphate (NADPH). Like the riboflavin coenzymes FAD and FMN, NADH transfers electrons to the mitochondrial electron transport chain and is thus necessary for energy metabolism (Figure 9.1). Both NADH and NADPH are also used as reducing agents in several biosynthetic processes in the body. Therefore, niacin is critical for mitochondrial respiration and in the metabolism of carbohydrates, lipids, and amino acids. Similar to both thiamine and riboflavin, niacin has little retention in the body and is excreted rapidly in the urine. Niacin may also be synthesized from tryptophan in the horse's hepatic tissues as is known in other species.

9.3.3.1 Sources

As with thiamine and riboflavin, niacin is produced by microbes in the GI tract and is present in all living tissues. Leafy forages contain substantial amounts of niacin (24–42 mg/kg DM) as do cereal grains (16–94 mg/kg DM), though niacin in grains is a bound form and essentially unavailable [1]. Additionally, niacin can also be synthesized within the horse's liver from the amino acid tryptophan. This tryptophan–niacin conversion is affected by other factors in the diet, including intake of leucine, total protein, and pyridoxine. Cereal grains contain relative excesses of leucine and thus decrease tryptophan conversion to niacin. Niacin is fairly resistant to moisture, oxidation, reduction, heat, light, and pH alterations during storage, and activity in feedstuffs decreases only about 5%/month during normal storage conditions. Thus, hay stored for one year retains about 57% of its initial niacin concentrations. In addition to microbial and hepatic synthesis, normal equine feedstuffs (pasture, conserved forage, and commercial feeds) contain adequate amounts of niacin to prevent deficiency. Supplementation of dietary niacin is thus not required.

9.3.3.2 Diagnosis and Treatment

In research settings, the assessment of niacin status in horses has been performed using an enzymatic cycling method for measuring erythrocyte NADH and NADPH concentrations [1].

9.3.4 Pantothenic Acid (B_5) and Pyridoxine (B_6)

Pantothenic acid is incorporated into coenzyme A, acyl CoA synthetase, and the acyl carrier protein, which is all required for numerous metabolic pathways involving carbohydrates, lipids, proteins, neurotransmitters, steroid hormones, porphyrins, and hemoglobin (Figure 9.1) [1]. Pantothenic acid is absorbed and distributed through plasma as free pantothenic acid.

All forms of dietary pyridoxine are converted in the body to the active vitamin pyridoxal phosphate (PLP), which functions in most amino acid metabolic pathways (Figure 9.1), porphyrin, epinephrine and norepinephrine biosynthesis, glycogen utilization, and lipid and gamma-aminobutyric acid (GABA) metabolism. Pyridoxine naturally exists in three forms: pyridoxine, pyridoxal, and pyridoxamine, each with equal vitamin activity. The majority of microbial pyridoxine synthesis appears to occur in the caecum and colon, yet pyridoxine absorption primarily occurs in the small intestine [7, 15]. Therefore, horses likely rely more on the oral intake of pyridoxine than other B vitamins. As it is the characteristic of the water-soluble B vitamins, little pantothenic acid or pyridoxine is stored in the body, and excesses are rapidly excreted in the urine.

9.3.4.1 Sources

As with all B vitamins, pantothenic acid and pyridoxine are produced by microbes in the horse's GI tract and are present in typical feedstuffs. Pantothenic acid is naturally present in forage, grains, and yeast, as well as the salt calcium pantothenate. Forages and cereal grains typically contain 3–9 mg pyridoxine/kg DM, while yeast contains 30–50 mg/kg DM. Dietary supplementation of synthetic pyridoxine is generally in the form of pyridoxine hydrochloride. Like riboflavin and niacin, pantothenic acid and pyridoxine are relatively resistant to stress during storage, except for light and low pH. Activity in feedstuffs only decreases 2–4%/month, resulting in 70–75% retention in stored feeds after one year. In addition to microbial synthesis, normal equine feedstuffs (pasture, conserved forage, cereal grains), and commercial feeds, contain adequate amounts of these vitamins to prevent deficiency. No adverse reactions have been reported in any species following the ingestion of elevated concentrations of vitamins in the diet.

9.3.4.2 Diagnosis and Treatment

Responses to changes in dietary intake of pantothenic acid can be evaluated by changes in urinary excretion over time, though this is not routinely practiced in the clinical setting. In research settings, pyridoxine has been measured in equine blood samples using a coenzyme stimulation assay [86].

9.3.5 Biotin (B_7)

Biotin functions as a coenzyme for four carboxylase enzymes: acetyl-CoA carboxylase, pyruvate carboxylase, propionyl-CoA carboxylase, and β-methylcrotonyl-CoA carboxylase. These coenzymes are involved in fatty acid synthesis (acetyl-CoA carboxylase), gluconeogenesis (pyruvate carboxylase), amino acid metabolism (propionyl-CoA carboxylase and β-methylcrotonyl-CoA carboxylase), and metabolism of cholesterol and odd-chain fatty acids (propionyl-CoA carboxylase) (Figure 9.1) [1]. Based on its role in carboxylase enzymes, as well as roles in gene expression and biotinylation of histones, biotin is essential for cell proliferation.

9.3.5.1 Sources

Biotin is a sulfur-containing vitamin found widely in plant and animal tissues. Eight isomers of biotin are possible, but only D-biotin (cis) is physiologically active and the only form that occurs naturally or is synthesized for use in dietary supplements. Biotin is present in normal feedstuffs, such as forage (0.2–0.5 mg/kg DM), cereal grains (0.1–0.4 mg/kg DM), and legumes (0.2–0.5 mg/kg DM) [1]. Dietary biotin is highly protein-bound in the form of biocytin (ε-N-biotinyl-L-lysine) with variable bioavailability depending on the digestibility of the protein carrier. The biotin present in most cereal grains is poorly available to horses. Biotin is relatively resistant to degradation during storage, though somewhat sensitive to heat, low pH, and fat rancidity, and degrades at a rate of approximately 4.5%/month of storage, leaving about 58% present after one year (Table 9.2). Biotin is also produced by microbes in the horse's colon, where some are absorbed; however, most biotin absorption occurs more proximally in the small intestine. As it is the characteristic of the water-soluble B vitamins, little is stored in the body, and excesses are rapidly excreted in the urine.

9.3.5.2 Recommendations

Horses have no recognized requirement for dietary biotin; supplementation is only indicated in instances of poor hoof horn quality, in which case daily administration of biotin for 5 m or more may help. Once a hoof horn defect has been responsive to biotin supplementation, daily supplementation should be continued.

9.3.5.3 Signs of Deficiency

Biotin deficiency has not been described in horses. Biotin supplements are widely marketed and commonly used to "improve" horses' hooves; however, not all causes of poor hoof horn quality are responsive to biotin. Horses with thin brittle hoof walls, cracks in the weight-bearing border of the coronary horn with crumbling of the lower edges of the walls with thin brittle, tender soles, or open white lines that are prone to infection, may benefit from prolonged biotin supplementation. Multiple studies have demonstrated improved hoof horn in horses with abnormal hoof conditions when supplemented with biotin at 15 mg/d (thoroughbreds), 20 mg/d (Lipizzaner stallions), or 30 mg/d (draft horses) [87–89]. Responses were reported starting around 5–6 m, though improvement in white line condition and horn histology required 19 m of continuous supplementation [89]. Mean plasma biotin in the untreated horses was within the range generally considered normal, while plasma concentrations of biotin supplemented horses were elevated. Hence, the defects in these horses were not considered to have resulted from a biotin deficiency, but rather these horses were responsive to added dietary biotin. Similar findings have been reported in a study where horses without reported hoof horn abnormalities were fed either adequate biotin ration or the ration plus 15 mg biotin/d. Horses receiving the supplemental biotin reportedly had improved hoof growth rate and hardness [89].

Biotin supplementation may only be effective for horses with hoof defects involving the stratum externum. In one report, biotin supplementation alone was of benefit for three of three horses with stratum externum defects of the hooves but was of no benefit for any of 21 horses with stratum medium and stratum internum defects [90].

9.3.5.4 Diagnosis and Treatment

A normal biotin concentration in whole blood of horses is reported to be 0.3–0.7 ng/mL with decreased urine or blood biotin concentrations diagnostic for biotin deficiency. Horses with a stratum medium defect of the hoof wall responded to calcium and protein supplementation of a diet low in these nutrients, but not to biotin supplementation, whereas those with the stratum externum defect responded to biotin supplementation alone [90]. Since the two different structural defects cannot be differentiated clinically or by laboratory procedures generally available, prudence would dictate first ensuring the horse with clinical signs of poor hoof quality is consuming a ration adequate in protein and calcium, selenium below maximums, and is receiving regular appropriate foot care before initiating biotin supplementation.

On average, 9–12 m is required to grow a new hoof, i.e. for new tissue from the coronary band to reach the weight-bearing surface. Therefore, clinical treatments involving biotin supplementation for hoof improvement will take at least one, but more likely two years or more, to complete. Increased hoof strength may take 1.5 years to occur and continue to increase for up to three years with biotin supplementation. Biotin supplemented initially at 3 mg/100 kg BW/d for at least 12 m has been recommended, and with improvement, the supplementation could then be discontinued or fed at a lower dose (0.2–0.3 mg/100 kg BW/d) [87]. Others more recently, however, have recommended 5 mg/100 kg BW/d, and if there is hoof quality improvement, then continuation at that dose is warranted [91].

9.3.6 Folate (B_9)

Folate refers to several compounds with the biological activity of folic acid. Most dietary folates are polyglutamates that get hydrolyzed to monoglutamates before absorption and are then transported in the plasma to target cells. Within the cells, folate monoglutamates are reduced to the active coenzyme form 5-methyl tetrahydrofolate. Subsequent metabolism results in various one-carbon or methyl derivatives, which are carried on folate coenzymes 5-adenosyl methionine, vitamin B_{12}, and used to synthesize methionine, purine rings, and deoxynucleic acid (DNA) (Figure 9.1). Adequate dietary methionine can thus partially overcome folate insufficiency, while folate deficiency is worsened by a pyridoxine deficiency.

9.3.6.1 Sources

The predominant natural form of folate in animal and plant tissues is pteroyl-polyglutamates, while synthetic monoglutamates are used as dietary supplements. Folate can be found in relatively high concentrations in normal equine feedstuffs, including growing pasture and fresh forage (1.5–5 mg/kg DM), hay (0.5–4 mg/kg DM), and cereal grains (0.2–0.6 mg/kg DM). Folate is relatively sensitive to stresses during storage, particularly low pH, and its activity in feeds reportedly decreases with an average of 5%/month, with just over 50% present after one year of storage under normal conditions (Table 9.3). Additionally, folate is produced by microbes in the horse's caecum and colon. There is nominal folate storage in the equine liver as 5-methyltetrahydrofolate, and most excess folate is excreted in bile and enterohepatic circulation before being lost in feces.

9.3.6.2 Recommendations

Folate requirements are expressed as dietary folate equivalent (DFE) where 1 μg equals 1 μg naturally occurring folates or 0.6 μg of synthetic folic acid [15]. No dietary requirement for folate has been established in horses with access to pasture or fresh forage. In stabled horses, provision of 0.04 mg/kg BW/d dietary folic acid, a dose extrapolated from findings in other species, may be beneficial. For horses with particularly high folate metabolism, such as pregnant, lactating, and performance horses, supplementation with dietary folic acid around 0.04 mg/kg BW/d may be beneficial, though this has yet to be demonstrated.

9.3.6.3 Signs of Deficiency

Naturally occurring folate deficiency has not been well described in the horse. Although no folate is required in the diet of herbivores unless microbial synthesis is impaired, the inclusion of folate in the diet may be beneficial. Folate is essential for DNA and cellular replication, thus deficiency manifests first in actively replicating cell lines including bone marrow, GI epithelial lining, and epidermis. Initial signs of deficiency include a morphological change in peripheral white blood cells (neutrophil hypersegmentation), followed by leukopenia, macrocytosis, hypochromia, and finally anemia and pancytopenia. Steatorrhea and diarrhea due to intestinal mucosal atrophy may occur, and decreased growth is evident in young animals. Serum folate concentrations are lower in stabled horses than in pastured horses, and cases of horses in poor condition with low serum folate concentrations (5 ng/mL) have been reported.

Horses treated for long term with antimicrobials, such as sulfadiazine and pyrimethamine, are at risk of folate deficiency due to inhibition of microbial synthesis of folate (sulfadiazine) and folate absorption and metabolism (pyrimethamine). Three mares treated with sulfadiazine and pyrimethamine for equine protozoal myeloencephalitis (EPM) produced foals with congenital defects in the skin, kidney, bone marrow, and lymphoid tissues. All consequences are directly related to folate importance in DNA and purine synthesis during rapid cell growth [92]. A case report describing folate deficiency in a horse being treated for EPM with sulphadiazine and pyrimethamine concurrently for 9 m has been documented [93]. In this case, serum folate was below 5 ng/mL and the horse exhibited hematological defects, hypoplastic bone marrow, and dysphagia caused by oral ulceration and glossitis until antimicrobial therapy was changed and folic acid administered intravenously (IV).

9.3.6.4 Diagnosis and Treatment

Serum, plasma, and red cell folate concentrations may be measured directly, while homocysteine can be used as an indirect indicator of folate status. Serum, plasma, and red cell folate ranges reported in apparently healthy horses vary greatly, from 2 to 21.7 ng/mL (serum and plasma) and 35 to 986 ng/mL (red cell) [94, 95]. Horses fed diets low in folate have been documented to have plasma concentrations less than 5 ng/mL, which is considered a borderline deficiency in humans, indicating a potential requirement for the inclusion of dietary folate [96]. Plasma homocysteine concentration is negatively correlated with folate status, as homocysteine requires a B-vitamin-dependent enzyme for its metabolism. Normal plasma homocysteine in horses has been reported to be 5.1–6.4 μmol/L [95]. In horses with folic acid deficiency due to treatment with sulphadiazine and pyrimethamine, oral supplementation is contraindicated. In these cases, if signs of folate deficiency develop, antimicrobial therapy must be changed or discontinued, and parenteral administration of folic acid may be required with an initial injection of 0.11 mg folic acid/kg BW IV followed by injections of 0.055 mg folic acid/kg BW IV 24 and 48 hrs later [93].

9.3.7 Cobalamin (B_{12})

Cobalamin is required for the synthesis of methionine and thymidine, and for the uptake of folate into cells. Thymidine is necessary for DNA synthesis; thus, a deficiency of cobalamin can present similar to folate deficiency, with defective DNA synthesis resulting in macrocytic anemia. Cobalamin is also required for the metabolism of propionate, in the conversion of methylmalonyl CoA to succinate. Propionate is a major source of energy derived from bacterial fermentation of ingested carbohydrates, which is the primary source of energy for most horses (Figure 9.1).

9.3.7.1 Sources

Cobalamin is unique among vitamins in that it is synthesized in nature only by microorganisms, so sources of this vitamin for all animals come from microbial contamination of ingested feedstuffs, microbial production in the GI tract, or specific amounts added to feeds. Cobalt is an essential requirement for the microbial synthesis of cobalamin, so cobalt deficiency can manifest as cobalamin deficiency. Naturally occurring cobalamin is in the form of methylcobalamin or 5-doxyadenosylcobalamin, while cyanocobalamin is synthesized for feed supplementation. Unlike the other B vitamins, cobalamin is in relatively low concentration in yeast and is in low concentration in cereal grains as well. Due to microbial contamination, forages can be a rich source of cobalamin, compared to the horse's requirements, and the vitamin is stable during storage, decreasing only around 1.5%/month, with over 80% still present one year after storage (Table 9.2). In contrast to the other B vitamins, large amounts of cobalamin are stored in the liver, and this vitamin is well conserved by excretion in bile and efficient enterohepatic recirculation. Some storage of the vitamin may occur as well in the kidney, heart, spleen, and brain. Microbial synthesis of cobalamin primarily occurs in the horse's colon which is the main site of cobalamin absorption [97, 98].

9.3.7.2 Diagnosis and Treatment

As there are no recognized signs of cobalamin deficiency in horses, diagnosis and treatment must be based on clinical suspicion and confirmed by reduced cobalamin concentration in the blood. In horses, normal cobalamin concentrations range from 1.8–7.3 g/mL of plasma, 6.3–7.1 μg/mL of serum, or 0.7–1.8 g/mL of whole blood. Cobalamin can also be measured in urine [99]. Additionally, urinary methylmalonic acid can be used to diagnose cobalamin deficiency, as methylmalonyl CoA cannot be converted to succinate, resulting in increased excretion of methylmalonic acid in the urine.

9.3.8 Vitamin C

The term vitamin C refers to two compounds with equivalent biological activity: L-ascorbic acid and dehydro-L-ascorbic acid. Vitamin C is a chiral molecule, though only the L-isomer has biological activity and the D-isomer does not. Several other dietary compounds, ascorbate-2-sulfate, ascorbyl palmitate, sodium ascorbate, potassium ascorbate, and calcium ascorbyl-2-monophosphate, can also serve to provide vitamin C [1].

In horses, vitamin C is absorbed passively in the ileum, the efficiency of which appears to decrease with increasing ascorbic acid intake and increasing age. Otherwise, vitamin C is synthesized from glucose in the liver and is not an essential nutrient for horses, as is true for most, though not all, other mammals. Absorbed and synthesized vitamin C is distributed throughout the body water pool with a short half-life in plasma of only 3.6–8.7 hrs in the horse.

While not nutritionally essential for horses, vitamin C is physiologically essential for all species in scavenging free radicals in the water-soluble antioxidant system and is involved in several critical metabolic functions, such as regeneration of vitamin E; utilization of folic acid, vitamin B12, cholesterol, and glucose; enhanced intestinal absorption of iron and immune functions; synthesis of norepinephrine, tyrosine, carnitine, and steroids; and hydroxylation of tryptophan, lysine, and proline. Hydroxyproline is a major constituent of collagen, and abnormalities of vitamin C status are characterized by collagen dysplasia, as well as dysfunction of the redox system.

There are no recognized signs of vitamin C deficiency, as none have been described in the horse. Thus, diagnosis and treatment must be based on clinical suspicion and determination of vitamin C status. Normal plasma ascorbic acid concentration is reported to be 2–4.2 μg/mL, while serum ascorbic acid is 4.5–7.3 μg/mL [1]. Detection of vitamin C deficiency by plasma or leukocyte concentrations is poorly sensitive, with subnormal plasma and urine concentrations after oral vitamin C dosing, being a more sensitive, early indicator of depleted vitamin C stores.

Considering the demonstrably decreased vitamin C status of horses under marked stress, including illness, supplementation with vitamin C may be of benefit. A dose of 12–20 mg/kg BW/d has been demonstrated to be safe for long-term administration and reduced hemolysis and methemoglobin concentration in blood samples incubated with a known oxidizing agent [100]. Considering the lack of negative side effects, this is considered at least a safe, if not necessarily valuable, practice [101]. One study demonstrated acute administration of 200 mg/kg ascorbic acid improved erythrocyte fragility and hematological parameters in horses exposed to a road transportation stressor, and suggested that high-dose vitamin C be administered before known stressful events [102].

Case in Point

Animal Assessment

An eight-year-old Thoroughbred-cross gelding is presented during a barn call in February (2022) in upstate New York with the subjective complaint of "poor" performance and not being "right" under saddle for about 6 m. The owner rides the horse for pleasure (4–5 times/wk for an hour or two each session), trail riding during good weather, or in an indoor arena during winter months. The poor performance was described as the horse unwilling to move out freely, resistant with tail swishing when asked to trot, and the horse appeared to be stiff and often stood still in the stall after a session. The horse is stabled in a heated barn at night with access to a small (1/2 ac) dry lot for four to six hrs daily with two retired geldings. The horse is fed hay, grain, salt, and water in the stall and has no access to pasture or fresh-cut forage.

On physical examination, BW is 400 kg using a weight tape, BCS 4/9; however, the horse appears to be poorly muscled with a relatively dull, thin hair coat given the time of year. No abnormalities were noted on auscultation of the heart and lungs, and there was no evidence of joint pain after a brief lameness examination. The minimum database (complete blood count and serum biochemistry) indicated no abnormal findings. In particular, gamma-glutamyl transferase (GGT) indicative of liver dysfunction, and creatine kinase (CK) and aspartate transaminase (AST) associated with muscle disorders, were all notably within normal reference ranges. In general, the horse appeared healthy but was not thriving.

Ration Assessment

The gelding is fed local hay harvested during the summer of 2020. The square-baled mixed grass hay had been stored undercover year-round. Visual assessment of the hay, although not dusty or moldy, and lacked weeds, did contain more stalk (90%) than leaves (10%), was very dry and brittle, and pale brown. The horse was fed 14 kg of hay/d but rarely ate all that was offered. In addition, 1 kg of whole oats was fed twice daily which the horse did consume and had free access to a white salt block and an automatic waterer. The salt block showed evidence of consumption and the waterer was in good working order.

1) What would be your "next step" recommendation to the owner?
2) What vitamins are of greatest concern for potential deficiencies in this horse?
3) How could a suspected vitamin deficiency be diagnosed and treated?

See Appendix A Chapter 9.

References

1 National Research Council (2007). *Nutrient Requirements of Horses*. 6th Rev. Animal Nutrition Series, 1–341. Washington, DC: National Academies Press.

2 Wedekind, K.J., Kats, L., Yu, S. et al. (2010). Micronutrients: minerals and vitamins. In: *Small Animal Clinical Nutrition* (ed. M. Hand, C.D. Thatcher, R.L. Remillard, et al.), 122–141. Topeka: Mark Morris Institute.

3 Brody, S. (1974; 1945). *Bioenergetics and Growth. The Journal of Physical Chemistry*, 352–384. New York: Reinhold Publishing Co., Reprinted Hafner Press.

4 Kleiber, M. (1961). *The Fire of Life. An Introduction to Animal Energetics*, 179–222. New York: Wiley.

5 Zeyner, A. and Harris, P.A. (2013). Vitamins. In: *Equine Applied and Clinical Nutrition: Health, Welfare and*

Performance (ed. R.J. Geor, P.A. Harris, and M. Coenen), 168–189. Philadelphia, Pennsylvania: Saunders, Elsevier.

6 Coelho, M.B. (1991). Vitamin stability. *Feed Manage.* 42 (10): 24–35.

7 Carroll, F.D., Goss, H., and Howell, C.E. (1949). The synthesis of B vitamins in the horse. *J. Anim. Sci.* 8 (2): 290–299.

8 Carroll, F.D. (1950). B vitamin content in the skeletal muscle of the horse fed a B vitamin-low diet. *J. Anim. Sci.* 9 (2): 139–142.

9 Pearson, P.B. and Schmidt, H. (1948). Pantothenic acid studies with the horse. *J. Anim. Sci.* 7 (1): 78–83.

10 Pearson, P.B., Sheybani, M.K., and Schmidt, H. (1944). Riboflavin in the nutrition of the horse. *Arch. Biochem. Biophys.* 3: 467–474.

11 Naylor, J.M. (1991). Vitamins. In: *Large Animal Clinical Nutrition*, 1e (ed. J.M. Naylor and S.L. Ralston), 68–89. St. Louis, MO: Mosby.

12 Linerode, P.A. (1967). Studies on the synthesis and absorption of B-complex vitamins in the horse. *In: Proceedings of the 13th Annual Convention of the American Association of Equine Practitioners*, 283–314. New Orlean, LA: American Association of Equine Practitioners (AAEP).

13 Machlin, L. and Langseth, L. (1988). Vitamin–vitamin interactions. In: *Nutrient Interactions* (ed. L.E. Bodwell and J.W. Erdman), 287–306. New York: Marcel Dekker Inc.

14 Ward, N.E. (2019). Vitamin Stability during Pelleting. In: *Feed Pelleting Reference Guide* (ed. A. Fahrenholz, C. Stark, and C. Jones). Rockford, IL: WATT Global Media. https://www.wattagnet.com/ext/resources/uploadedFiles/WattAgNet/Feed_Pelleting_Guide/Section_4/4-16,_Vitamin_stability.pdf (accessed 19 February 2020).

15 National Research Council (1987). *Vitamin Tolerance of Animals*, 1–108. Washington, DC: National Academies Press.

16 Smith, A.D., Panickar, K.S., Urban, J.F.J., and Dawson, H.D. (2018). Impact of micronutrients on the immune response of animals. *Annu. Rev. Anim. Biosci.* 6: 227–254.

17 Greiwe Crandell, K.M., Kronfeld, D.S., Gay, L.A., and Sklan, D. (1995). Seasonal vitamin A depletion in grazing horses is assessed better by the relative dose response test than by serum retinol concentration. *J. Nutr.* 125 (10): 2711–2716.

18 Greiwe-Crandell, K.M., Kronfeld, D.S., Gay, L.A. et al. (1997). Vitamin A repletion in thoroughbred mares with retinyl palmitate or beta-carotene. *J. Anim. Sci.* 75: 2684–2690.

19 Watson, E.D., Cuddeford, D., and Burger, I.H. (1996). Failure of B-carotene absorption negates any potential effect on ovarian function in mares. *Equine Vet. J.* 28 (3): 233–236.

20 Kienzle, E., Kaden, C., Hoppe, P.P., and Opitz, B. (2003). Serum B-carotene and a-tocopherol in horses fed B-carotene via grass-meal or a synthetic beadlets preparation with and without added dietary fat. *J. Anim. Physiol. Anim. Nutr. (Berl.)* 87: 174–180.

21 National Institute of Health Office of Dietary Supplements. Unit Conversions. https://dietarysupplementdatabase.usda.nih.gov/Conversions.php (accessed 19 February 2020).

22 Gabe, A. and Männer, K. (2005). Is an extensive horse husbandry able to guarantee an adequate mineral and vitamin supply? *Pferdeheilkunde* 21 (2): 124–130.

23 Mäenpää, P.H., Koskinen, T., and Koskinen, E. (1988). Serum profiles of vitamins A, E and D in mares and foals during different seasons. *J. Anim. Sci.* 66: 1418–1423.

24 Mäenpää, P.H., Lappeteläinen, R., and Virkkunen, J. (1987). Serum retinol, 25-hydroxyvitamin D and tocopherol of racing trotters in Finland. *Equine Vet. J.* 19: 237–240.

25 Schweigert, F.J. and Gottwald, C. (1999). Effect of parturition on levels of vitamins A and E and of B-carotene in plasma and milk of mares. *Equine Vet. J.* 31 (4): 319–323.

26 Kuhl, J., Aurich, J.E., Wulf, M. et al. (2011). Effects of oral supplementation with B-carotene on concentrations of B-carotene, vitamin A and a-tocopherol in plasma, colostrum and milk of mares and plasma of their foals and on fertility in mares. *J. Anim. Physiol. Anim. Nutr. (Berl.)* 96: 376–384.

27 Gay, L.A., Kronfeld, D.S., Grimsley-Cook, A. et al. (2004). Retinol, B-carotene and B-tocopherol concentrations in mare and foal plasma and in colostrum. *J. Equine Vet. Sci.* 24: 115–120.

28 da Costa, M.L.L., de Rezende, A.S.C., Barbosa, I. et al. (2017). Retinol and mineral status in grazing foals during the dry season. *Braz. J. Anim. Sci.* 46 (2): 118–122.

29 Abrams, J.T. (1979). The effect of dietary vitamin A supplements on the clinical conditioning and track performance of racehorses. *Bibl. Nutr. Dieta* 27: 113–120.

30 Donoghue, S., Kronfeld, D.S., Berkowitz, S.J., and Copp, R.L. (1981). Vitamin A nutrition of the equine: growth, serum biochemistry and hematology. *J. Nutr.* 111 (2): 365–374.

31 Gück, T., Sallmann, H.P., and Fuhrmann, H. (2000). Influence of increased vitamin A supplements on a-tocopherol and retinoids in serum and lipoproteins of Shetland ponies. *J. Anim. Physiol. Anim. Nutr. (Berl.)* 84: 95–101.

32 Azarpeykan, S., Dittmer, K.E., Marshall, J.C. et al. (2016). Evaluation and comparison of vitamin D responsive gene expression in ovine, canine and equine kidney. *PLoS One* 11 (9): e0162598.

33 Khammissa, R.A.G., Fourie, J., Motswaledi, M.H. et al. (2018). The biological activities of vitamin D and its receptor in relation to calcium and bone homeostasis, cancer, immune and cardiovascular systems, skin biology, and oral health. *Biomed. Res. Int.* 2018 (May): 1–9.

34 Hymøller, L. and Jensen, S.K. (2015). We know next to nothing about vitamin D in horses. *J. Equine Vet. Sci.* 35: 785–792.
35 Kohler, M., Leiber, F., Willems, H. et al. (2013). Influence of altitude on vitamin D and bone metabolism of lactating sheep and goats. *J. Anim. Sci.* 91 (11): 5259–5268.
36 Jäpelt, R.B., Didion, T., Smedsgaard, J., and Jakobsen, J. (2011). Seasonal variation of Provitamin D2 and vitamin D2 in perennial ryegrass (*Lolium perenne* L.). *J. Agric. Food Chem.* 59 (20): 10907–10912.
37 Henry, K.M., Kon, S.K., Thompson, S.Y. et al. (1958). The vitamin D activity of pastures and hays. *Br. J. Nutr.* 12: 462–469.
38 Keener, H.A. (1954). The effect of various factors on the vitamin D content of several common forages. *J. Dairy Sci.* 37 (11): 1337–1345.
39 Azarpeykan, S., Dittmer, K.E., Gee, E.K. et al. (2016). Influence of blanketing and season on vitamin D and parathyroid hormone, calcium, phosphorus, and magnesium concentrations in horses in New Zealand. *Domest. Anim. Endocrinol.* 56: 75–84.
40 Pozza, M.E., Kaewsakhorn, T., Trinarong, C. et al. (2014). Serum vitamin D, calcium, and phosphorus concentrations in ponies, horses and foals from the United States and Thailand. *Vet. J.* 199: 451–456.
41 Harmeyer, J. and Schlumbohm, C. (2004). Effects of pharmacological doses of vitamin D3 on mineral balance and profiles of plasma vitamin D3 metabolites in horses. *J. Steroid Biochem. Mol. Biol.* 89–90: 595–600.
42 Saastamoinen, M. and Juusela, J. (1992). Influence of dietary supplementation on serum vitamin A and D concentration and their seasonal variation in horses. *Agric. Sci. Finl.* 1 (5): 477–482.
43 El Shorafa, W.M., Feaster, J.P., Ott, E.A., and Asquith, R.L. (1979). Effect of vitamin D and sunlight on growth and bone development of young ponies. *J. Anim. Sci.* 48 (4): 882–886.
44 Kamr, A.M., Dembek, K.A., Reed, S.M. et al. (2015). Vitamin D metabolites and their association with calcium, phosphorus, and PTH concentrations, severity of illness, and mortality in hospitalized equine neonates. *PLoS One* 10 (6): e0127684.
45 Mello, J.R.B. (2003). Calcinosis – calcinogenic plants. *Toxicon* 41: 1–12.
46 Harrington, D.D. and Page, E.H. (1983). Acute vitamin D3 toxicosis in horses: case reports and experimental studies of the comparative toxicity of vitamins D2 and D3. *J. Am. Vet. Med. Assoc.* 182 (12): 1358–1369.
47 Hymøller, L. and Jensen, S.K. (2011). Vitamin D analysis in plasma by high performance liquid chromatography (HPLC) with C30 reversed phase column and UV detection – easy and acetonitrile-free. *J. Chromatogr. A* 1218 (14): 1835–1841.
48 Breidenbach, A., Schlumbohm, C., and Harmeyer, J. (1998). Peculiarities of vitamin D and of the calcium and phosphate homeostatic system in horses. *Vet. Res.* 29 (2): 173–186.
49 Piccione, G., Assenza, A., Fazio, F. et al. (2008). Daily rhythms of serum vitamin D-metabolites, calcium ad phosphorus in horses. *Acta Vet. Brno* 77: 151–157.
50 Mäenpää, P.H., Pirhonen, A., and Koskinen, E. (1988). Vitamin A, E and D nutrition in mares and foals during the winter season: effect of feeding two different vitamin-mineral concentrates. *J. Anim. Sci.* 66 (6): 1424–1429.
51 Hacquebard, M. and Carpentier, Y.A. (2005). Vitamin E: absorption, plasma transport and cell uptake. *Curr. Opin. Clin. Nutr. Metab. Care* 8 (2): 133–138.
52 Buettner, G.R. (1993). The pecking order of free radicals and antioxidants: lipid peroxidation, a-tocopherol, and ascorbate. *Arch. Biochem. Biophys.* 300 (2): 535–543.
53 Finno, C.J. and Valberg, S.J. (2012). A comparative review of vitamin E and associated equine disorders. *J. Vet. Intern. Med.* 26 (6): 1251–1266.
54 Petersson, K.H., Burr, D.B., Gomez-Chiarri, M., and Petersson-Wolfe, C.S. (2010). The influence of vitamin E on immune function and response to vaccination in older horses. *J. Anim. Sci.* 88 (9): 2950–2958.
55 National Research Council (1978). *Nutrient Requirements of Horses.* 4th Rev. Animal Nutrition Series, 1–33. Washington, DC: National Academies Press.
56 National Research Council (1982). *United States-Canadian Tables of Feed Composition.* 3rd Rev. Nutritional Data for United States and Canadian Feeds, 1–148. Washington, DC: National Academies Press.
57 Lynch, G.L. (1991). Natural occurrence and content of vitamin E in feedstuffs. In: *Vitamin E in Animal Nutrition and Management* (ed. M.B. Coelho), 43–48. Parsippany, NJ: BASF Corporation.
58 Hall, R.R., Brennan, R.W., and Peck, L.M. (1991). Comparisons of serum vitamin E concentrations in yearlings and mature horses. In: *Proceedings of the 12th Equine Nutrition and Physiology Society Symposium*, 263–264. Calgary, Alberta: Equine Nutrition and Physiology Society.
59 Duberstein, K.J., Pazdro, R., Lee, K.C. et al. (2017). Effect of supplemental vitamin E form on serum a-tocopherol levels and blood oxidative stress parameters in response to a novel exercise challenge. *J. Equine Vet. Sci.* 57: 61–66.
60 Fiorellino, N.M., Lamprecht, E.D., and Williams, C.A. (2009). Absorption of different oral formulations of natural vitamin E in horses. *J. Equine Vet. Sci.* 29 (2): 100–104.
61 Brown, J.C., Valberg, S.J., Hogg, M., and Finno, C.J. (2017). Effects of feeding two RRR-a-tocopherol formulations on serum, cerebrospinal fluid and muscle

a-tocopherol concentrations in horses with subclinical vitamin E deficiency. *Equine Vet. J.* 49: 753–758.

62 Muirhead, T.L., Wichtel, J.J., Stryhn, H., and McClure, J.T. (2010). The selenium and vitamin E status of horses in Prince Edward Island. *Can. Vet. J.* 51: 979–985.

63 Ballet, N., Robert, J.C., and Williams, P.E.V. (2000). Vitamins in forages. In: *Forage Evaluation in Ruminant Nutrition* (ed. D.I. Givens, E. Owen, R.F.E. Axford, and H.M. Omed), 399–431. Wallingford: CABI Publishing.

64 Müller, C.E., Möller, J., Krogh Jensen, S., and Udén, P. (2007). Tocopherol and carotenoid levels in baled silage and haylage in relation to horse requirements. *Anim. Feed Sci. Technol.* 137: 183–197.

65 Ronéus, B.O., Hakkarainen, R.V., Lindholm, C.A., and Työppönen, J.T. (1986). Vitamin E requirements of adult Standardbred horses evaluated by tissue depletion and repletion. *Equine Vet. J.* 18 (1): 50–58.

66 Baalsrud, K.J. and Øvernes, G. (1986). Influence of vitamin E and selenium supplement on antibody production in horses. *Equine Vet. J.* 18 (6): 472–474.

67 Siciliano, P.D., Parker, A.L., and Lawrence, L.M. (1997). Effect of dietary vitamin E supplementation on the integrity of skeletal muscle in exercised horses. *J. Anim. Sci.* 75 (6): 1553–1560.

68 Saastamoinen, M. and Juusela, J. (1993). Serum vitamin-E concentration of horses on different vitamin-E supplementation levels. *Acta Agric. Scand.* 43 (1): 52–57.

69 Velázquez-Cantón, E., de la Cruz-Rodríguez, N., Zarco, L. et al. (2018). Effect of selenium and vitamin E supplementation on lactate, cortisol, and malondialdehyde in horses undergoing moderate exercise in a polluted environment. *J. Equine Vet. Sci.* 69 (10): 136–144.

70 Yonezawa, L.A., Machado, L.P., da Silveira, V.F. et al. (2010). Malondialdehyde and cardiac troponin I in Arabian horses subjected to exercise and vitamin E supplementation. *Ciência Rural.* 40 (6): 1321–1326.

71 Yonezawa, L.A., Barbosa, T.S., Watanabe, M.J. et al. (2015). Effect of vitamin E on oxidative and cardiac metabolism in horses submitted to high intensity exercise. *Braz. J. Vet. Anim. Sci.* 67 (1): 71–79.

72 Weigel, R.A., Silva Lima, A., Alberti Morgado, A. et al. (2013). Oxidative metabolism and muscle biochemical profile of polo horses supplemented with an ADE vitamin complex. *Pesqui Veterinária Bras.* 33 (Suppl. 1): 58–62.

73 Rey, A.I., Segura, J., Arandilla, E., and López-Bote, C.J. (2013). Short- and long-term effect of oral administration of micellized natural vitamin E (D-α-tocopherol) on oxidative status in race horses under intense training. *J. Anim. Sci.* 91: 1277–1284.

74 Duberstein, K.J., Johnson, S.E., McDowell, L.R., and Ott, E.A. (2009). Effects of vitamin E supplementation and training on oxidative stress parameters measured in exercising horses. *Comp. Exerc. Physiol.* 6 (1): 17–25.

75 Duberstein, K.J., Johnson, S.E., McDowell, L.R., and Ott, E.A. (2009). Protein carbonyl assay to measure oxidative stress in muscle of exercising horses supplemented with vitamin E. *Comp. Exerc. Physiol.* 6 (1): 1–5.

76 Williams, C.A., Kronfeld, D.S., Hess, T.M. et al. (2004). Antioxidant supplementation and subsequent oxidative stress of horses during an 80-km endurance race. *J. Anim. Sci.* 82 (2): 588–594.

77 Bedford, H.E., Valberg, S.J., Firshman, A.M. et al. (2013). Histopathologic findings in the sacrocaudalis dorsalis medialis muscle of horses with vitamin E-responsive muscle atrophy and weakness. *J. Am. Vet. Med. Assoc.* 242: 1127–1137.

78 Finno, C.J., Miller, A.D., Sisó, S. et al. (2016). Concurrent equine degenerative myeloencephalopathy and equine motor neuron disease in three young horses. *J. Vet. Intern. Med.* 30 (4): 1344–1350.

79 Vanschandevijl, K., Nollet, H., Deprez, P. et al. (2008). Variation in deficient serum vitamin E levels and impact on assessment of the vitamin E status in horses. *Vlaams Diergeneeskd Tijdschr* 78: 28–33.

80 Barigye, R., Dyer, N.W., and Newell, T.K. (2007). Fatal myocardial degeneration in an adult quarter horse with vitamin E deficiency. *J. Equine Vet. Sci.* 27 (9): 405–408.

81 Akbari, S. and Rasouli-Ghahroudi, A.A. (2018). Vitamin K and bone metabolism: a review of the latest evidence in preclinical studies. *Biomed. Res. Int.* 27 (2018): 1–8.

82 Siciliano, P.D. (2000). The effect of initiation of exercise training in young horses on vitamin K status. *J. Anim. Sci.* 78 (9): 2353–2358.

83 Shearer, M.J., McBurney, A., and Barkhan, P. (1974). Studies on the absorption and metabolism of phylloquinone (vitamin K1) on mares. *Vitam. Horm.* 32: 513–542.

84 Siciliano, P.D., Warren, L.K., and Lawrence, L.M. (2000). Changes in vitamin K status of growing horses. *J. Equine Vet. Sci.* 20 (11): 726–729.

85 Laus, F., Faillace, V., Tesei, B. et al. (2017). Effect of thiamine pyrophosphate (bicarbossilasi®) administration on the exercising horse metabolism. *Isr. J. Vet. Med.* 72 (2): 15–21.

86 McGorum, B.C., Jago, R.C., Cillin-Garcia, E. et al. (2017). Neurodegeneration in equine grass sickness is not attributable to niacin deficiency. *Equine Vet. J.* 49: 445–447.

87 Comben, N., Clark, R.J., and Sutherland, D.J. (1984). Clinical observations on the response of equine hoof defects to dietary supplementation with biotin. *Vet. Rec.* 115 (25–26): 642–645.

88 Josseck, H., Zenker, W., and Geyer, H. (1995). Hoof horn abnormalities in Lipizzaner horses and the effect of

dietary biotin on microscopic aspects of hoof horn quality. *Equine Vet. J.* 27 (3): 175–182.

89 Buffa, E.A., Van Den Berg, S.S., Verstraete, F.J.M., and Swart, N.G.N. (1992). Effect of dietary biotin supplement on equine hoof horn growth rate and hardness. *Equine Vet. J.* 24 (6): 472–474.

90 Kempson, S.A. (1987). Scanning electron microscope observations of hoof horn from horses with brittle feet. *Vet. Rec.* 120: 568–570.

91 Geyer, H. and Schulze, J. (1994). The long-term influence of biotin supplementation on hoof horn quality in horses. *Schweiz. Arch. Tierheilkd.* 136 (4): 137–149.

92 Toribio, R.E., Bain, F.T., Mrad, D.R. et al. (1998). Congenital defects in newborn foals of mares treated for equine protozoal myeloencephalitis during pregnancy. *J. Am. Vet. Med. Assoc.* 212 (5): 697–701.

93 Piercy, R.J., Hinchcliff, K.W., and Reed, S.M. (2010). Folate deficiency during treatment with orally administered folic acid, sulphadiazine and pyrimethamine in a horse with suspected equine protozoal myeloencephalitis (EPM). *Equine Vet. J.* 34 (3): 311–316.

94 Roberts, M.C. (1983). Serum and red cell folate and serum vitamin B12 levels in horses. *Aust. Vet. J.* 60 (4): 106–111.

95 Ordakowski-Burk, A.O., Kronfeld, D.S., Williams, C.A. et al. (2005). Temporal folate status during lactation in mares and growth in foals. *Am. J. Vet. Res.* 66: 1214–1221.

96 Seckington, I.M., Hunstman, R.G., and Jenkins, G.C. (1967). Serum folic acid levels of grass-fed and stabled horses. *Vet. Rec.* 81 (7): 158–161.

97 Davies, M.E. (1971). The production of vitamin B12 in the horse. *Br. Vet. J.* 127 (1): 34–36.

98 Stillions, M.C., Teeter, S.M., and Nelson, W.E. (1971). Utilization of dietary vitamin B12 and cobalt by mature horses. *J. Anim. Sci.* 32 (2): 252–255.

99 Wenzel, R., Major, D., Hesp, K., and Doble, P. (2018). Determination of vitamin B12 in equine urine by liquid chromatography-inductively coupled plasma – mass spectrometry. *J. Trace Elem. Med. Biol.* 50: 634–639.

100 O'Callaghan, D.K., Schall, S.A., Birmingham, S.S.W., and Lehman, J.S. (2015). Protective effects of ascorbic acid and α-tocopherol on the in vitro oxidation of equine erythrocytes caused by extracts of wilted red maple leaves. *J. Equine Vet. Sci.* 35 (11–12): 940–946.

101 Snow, D.H. and Frigg, M. (1989). Oral administration of different formulations of ascorbic acid to the horse. *J. Equine Vet. Sci.* 9 (1): 30–33.

102 Yaqub, L.S., Mshelia, W.P., and Ayo, J.O. (2014). Erythrocyte osmotic fragility and hematological responses of horses administered ascorbic acid and exposed to road transportation. *J. Equine Vet. Sci.* 34: 1324–1328.

Ration Assessment

10

Ration Assessment and Farm Investigations

Rebecca L. Remillard and Sarah L. Ralston

KEY TERMS

- See Appendix D Feed Glossary for common feed terminology [1].
- Nutrient concentration of equine feeds are commonly expressed on an 'as fed' (AF) basis which includes water and on a 'dry matter' (DM) basis excluding water.

KEY POINTS

- Malnutrition is any disorder of inadequate, excessive, or imbalanced nutrient intake.
- The basis for ration formulation is to supply energy and nutrients in a form and quantity an animal can utilize to meet essential nutrient requirements.
- The science and art of equine ration balancing provides energy and essential nutrients using available feeds in apposite quantities to support a specific life stage and promote health, productivity, or performance in horses.
- Forage quality and nutrient content are essential inputs in ration formulation; however, both are highly variable across different feed sources, types and forms that change over time due to weather, harvesting methods, transportation and storage conditions.
- Plant maturity at harvest is the single most important factor in determining the nutritive value of the forage because the nutrient profile cannot be improved by any subsequent harvesting or storage techniques.
- Manufactured feed and supplement nutrient profiles are relatively consistent over time; however, manufacturing errors are possible.

10.1 Introduction

Veterinary practitioners are presented with horses with one or more problems relating to health, productivity, or performance. The problem may be related to a disease process, malnutrition, inappropriate management, or a combination thereof. Nutrition may be part of the problem, part of the solution, or may not be related to the problem. To determine the role of nutrition in a given situation, nutritionists (i) assess the individual or group, (ii) assess the diet (ration and water), (iii) assess the feeding practices, and (iv) then devise a nutritional plan for the individual or group and re-assess [2]. The detection of nutrient deficiencies or excesses frequently involves the evaluation of several parameters. These include clinical signs, physical examinations, analysis of blood constituents and diet composition, radiographs, as well as tissue or urine examinations, dose–response tests, necropsy findings, and response to therapy. Some of these procedures apply to the diagnosis of some, but not all, nutritional imbalances. The greater the number of applicable inputs utilized to assess the case, the more likely the correct diagnosis will be made and appropriate treatment recommended.

10.2 Farm Investigation

The concluding nutritional assessment can be no better than the accuracy of the information obtained during the investigation, i.e. the outcome is only as good as the input. Investigating a nutrient- or ingredient-related problem requires the collection of a wide range of information and data, and care should be taken to be complete and thorough. Farm investigations involve assessing the animal, the feeds, and the method of feeding to provide essential

Equine Clinical Nutrition, Second Edition. Edited by Rebecca L. Remillard.

information. Ideally, an on-site visit by a nutritionist generally yields reliable, useful, and in-depth information most efficiently. First-hand observations and data collection by an experienced investigator (observing feeding methods and sampling of feeds) is recommended. Understandably, on-site investigations by experienced individuals may not be possible and information may be collected by a less-experienced individual (owner, farm manager, trainer). In such cases, an appreciation for possible lapses in the reliability of the data provided should be taken into consideration, e.g. feed sampling error, incorrect assessment of body weight and condition, a biased description of events, and/or the inability to assess forage quality.

10.2.1 Animal Assessment

A clear understanding of the horse to be fed is essential for assessing the adequacy of the ration. Animal input data includes life stage, body weight (BW), body condition score (BSC), health status, environmental factors (housing, individual vs. group management), temperament, and weather conditions. Additionally, owner expectations for the work or function to be performed by the horse must be well understood to establish the necessary nutrient profile of the ration (a pasture pet vs. a seasonal rodeo competitor vs. a group of broodmares or weanlings). See Chapter 2 Nutritional Assessment of the Horse.

In cases where a disease is under investigation, key nutritional factors are determined. The concept of key nutritional factors is the basis of clinical nutrition whereby specific dietary factors are known to be related to specific disease conditions. Examples would be low copper intake by broodmares and poor foal growth or high starch intake by a horse with metabolic syndrome. A key nutritional factor may be related to feed quality such as feeding molded hay that causes diarrhea or weight loss. Other key factors may be related to feeding methods such as providing a group of foals *ad libitum* feed or meal feeding grain to a horse with insulin dysregulation. The practitioner and clinical nutritionist must identify all key nutritional factors related to a disease process, low productivity, or poor performance in the horse or group of horses to address the owner's concern. See Appendix C Nutrition Competencies of Equine Veterinarians.

10.2.2 Ration Assessment

The ration includes all available forages, complementary feeds, supplements, water, and, increasingly so, treats. To complete a ration evaluation, the daily quantity consumed of each feed by a horse and the nutrient profile of that feedstuff must be known. See Sidebar 10.1.

Sidebar 10.1 Expression of Nutrient Concentrations in Equine Nutrition

A. Requirements vs. Recommendations

The animal requires nutrients. Ration nutrient concentrations are recommendations. For the same nutrient, there is an ingredient and ration concentration and then there is an animal requirement; for example, oats have 12% protein, the ration may contain 10% protein, and the animal may require 8% protein in the ration. The recommended ration nutrient concentrations to meet animal requirements are based on current knowledge and often greater than actual animal need to account for losses during digestion and metabolism. For example, the oral protein intake recommendation for an adult horse is 1.26 g/BW kg/d, whereas 1.0 g/BW kg/d is suggested for parenteral nutritional administration.

B. Common units used for horses and feeds:

- Animal body weight (BW) is expressed in lb or kg 1 kg = 2.2 lb.
- Feed dry matter (DM) and nutrient concentration may be expressed as % or ug, mg, g, or kg/unit of feed. Vitamins are often expressed as ug, mg, or international units (IU or KIU) per unit of feed.
- Digestible energy (DE) is expressed in Mcal or Mjoule for horses, where 1 Mcal = 1000 kcal = 4.187 MJ.
- In perspective, a 454 kg adult horse at maintenance requires ~15 Mcal/d or 7.5 times more energy than the average 70 kg man requiring ~2000 kcal/d.

C. Due to the wide range in BW and life stages for horses, nutrient intake recommendations are most efficiently expressed relative to BW, feed DM, or energy intake.

- Feed DM intake (DMI) is expressed as % BW where 2 kg DM/100 kg BW/d = 2% BW.
- If an adult horse requires 126 g protein/100 kg BW and eats 2 kg DM/100 kg BW, then the feed must contain 6.3% protein DM [0.126/2 × 100].
- If an adult horse requires 630 g protein and 16.7 Mcal DE/d, then the feed must contain 37 g protein/Mcal DE [630/16.7].

Animal example within a given life stage:

- The recommendation for an adult 10-mos gestating broodmare is 168 g protein and 4.04 Mcal DE/100 kg BW eating 2 kg/100 kg BW.
- These 10-mos gestating broodmares should receive 41.5 g protein/Mcal DE [168/4] and 8.4% protein DM [0.168 kg/2 kg DM × 100] whether she is an American Belgian Draft horse or a Shetland pony.

D. Due to the highly variable water content across different feeds, nutrients are expressed on a DM or energy basis to allow a direct comparison between feeds.

- Corn with 9.1% protein, 3.4 Mcal DE/kg as fed (AF) and 88% DM contains 10.3% protein DM [9.1/0.88] or 26 g protein/Mcal DE [91/3.4].
- Oats with 11.8% protein, 2.85 Mcal DE/kg AF and 90% DM contains 13.1% protein DM [11.8/0.9] or 41 g protein/Mcal DE [118/2.85].

These feeds can now be directly compared on a DM or energy basis.

Feedstuff example:

- Alfalfa hay contains 10% moisture, 90% DM, and 1.28% calcium (Ca) AF. On a DM basis, the hay contains 1.42% Ca DM [(1.28/0.90)]
- Alfalfa pasture contains 77% moisture, 23% DM, and 0.33% Ca AF. On a DM basis, the pasture contains 1.43% Ca DM [(0.33/0.23)].

This is the same feed (alfalfa) with different percentages of water at different stages of harvest, but both forms contain the same Ca concentration on a DM basis.

10.2.2.1 Forage

A basic understanding of forage quality coupled with nutrient analysis data helps guide the appropriate selection of hay and/or pasture for horses. However, one of the greatest unknowns to veterinarians and horse owners appears to be how to consistently subjectively assess hay or pasture quality. With organoleptic[1] evaluations coupled with some basic understanding of plant physiology and experience comes the ability to differentiate forage quality.

All forms of forage fed to the horse should be hand-inspected, sampled, and submitted for laboratory analysis. As the plant matures, the nutritional value declines. Plant maturity at harvest, either as hay or as pasture grass, is the single most important factor in determining the nutritive value of the forage, as the nutrient profile cannot be improved by any subsequent harvesting or storage techniques [3]. Forage quality and nutrient content differ with the stages of maturity at harvest, in cuttings from the same field within the same year, and in different years from the same field. Both subjective and objective evaluations should be made on all forages fed to horses.

10.2.2.1.1 Pasture

The evaluation of pasture requires a "walk about" through the area noting approximate percent of grass, legume, weed, and poisonous plant species. Pasture forage type, stage of maturity, and density should be recorded. The majority of pasture forages are either legumes or grasses and to a lesser extent cereal grain stubble. Within legume and grass types, plant species are further divided into perennials that regrow each year from roots that survive winter or annuals that complete a life cycle in just one growing season and must be reseeded. The plants are further divided into warm vs. cool seasons, which indicates the temperature, that is, the growing time of year, and the primary storage form of carbohydrates. Warm-season plants grow during the summer months, and cool-season plants grow in the spring and fall. Warm-season grasses store starch in leaves, and cool-season grasses store fructans in the stems, which are important differences in managing insulin dysregulation, laminitis, and obesity. See Chapter 11 Forages.

Information on recent pasture changes should be included in the ration history. A pasture stocking rate, as a general guide, is 2 ac/horse/yr [4]. When edible pasture forage is limited, horses may consume noxious weeds, although bitter and toxic, that otherwise would be avoided. See Chapter 12 Toxic Plants. Sampling pasture for nutritional content is advisable if pasture forage accounts for 20% or more of the horse's daily feed intake by volume. Estimating the percent of usable forage within a 1 × 1 ft^2 frame placed at given intervals while walking the field in a "W"" or "X"" pattern is recommended. There are several simple methods of collecting samples that minimize bias and represent the pasture area well [5–7].

10.2.2.1.2 Hay

Feeding dried preserved forage (long-stem, chopped, cubed, or pelleted hay) often comprises a major portion of the dry matter intake (DMI) of most horses. The quality of hay is highly variable, more so than in any other agricultural commodity [8]. Therefore, determining the acceptability of the hay based on features of quality and nutrient profile is an important aspect of ration assessment. Given the forage should be the foundation of the ration, at least 50% by weight, the formulation is easier with uniform lots (a single cutting, field or variety) of hay. The rate of hay turnover can be problematic for estimating feeding value. Assessing a large lot of hay from one source to be fed over several months is preferable to a high turnover of small lots from different sources. If consistent hay quality is necessary, feeding a bagged manufactured hay product from a large national company with labeled minimum guarantees may be considered.

Subjective Assessments Subjectively assessing forage quality involves using sight, smell, and feel, and requires some hands-on training and experience [8]. Ideally, hays fed to horses should: (i) be free of mold, dust, weeds, and foreign material; (ii) be leafy, with fine stems; (iii) be soft and pliable to the touch; (iv) have a pleasant, fragrant aroma; and (v) be green, brown, tan, or yellow as all hays lose color over time [9]. A plume of white talcum-like powder when the bale is moved is indicative of dust or fungal spores. The limitation to visual assessment is that these characteristics are subjective and difficult to standardize and may not accurately assess the acceptability to the horse [10].

1 Defined as involving the use of special sense organs, that is, sight, feel, sound, or taste.

Factors that most affect the nutritional quality of hay are plant species and variety, the stage of maturity at harvest, harvesting technique, and the duration and conditions of storage [11]. Higher quality hays are readily consumed, highly digestible, concentrated in available nutrients, and low in foreign material contaminants. Assessing hay quality at the time of harvest, at the time of purchase, or at the time of feeding may produce different results depending on how the hay is handled and stored. Hays are often subjectively evaluated based on the leaf-to-stem ratio, smell, softness, color, and purity [8]. Leaves are more nutritious than stems, and young plants are more nutritious than matured plants. The highly subjective assessments of smell and softness have relative importance based on the intended use of the hay. For example, odor and softness (or mouthfeel) are more heavily weighted for horses than for cattle [10]. Horses will refuse to eat hay with an unpleasant smell, regardless of the nutritional value, possibly to the point of losing weight, whereas a ruminant would consume the same hay; that is, "cow hay" may not be accepted by horses [8].

Harvesting and storage conditions must be considered before assessing hay color: green, yellow, brown, black, or tan. Green indicates sun-curing and keratin precursors to vitamins A and E, brown/tan may be indicative of exposure to rain, and black of mold or rot. Nutritious hay stored under cover may be sun-bleached yellow or tan on the outside but green on the inside. Purity refers to the lack of plant species variance in the hay, that is, presence of weeds, different stages of maturity, a mix of grass, or legume species [12].

Stage of Maturity Given that leaves contain two-thirds of the energy, three-fourths of the protein, and most of the other nutrients present in forages, plants should be harvested when leaf development has been completed, but not later. Leaf development is complete in legumes just before flowering, called bud or vegetative stage, and in grasses when seed heads show through the sheath, called early head or boot stage. As the plant matures, dry matter (DM) digestibility, energy density, and protein content decrease. Allowing the plant to stand after the vegetative or boot stage increases the fiber, reduces protein, and decreases digestible energy (DE) [13]. See Table 10.1. As legumes mature from full bud to full bloom and grasses mature from the boot stage to complete heading out, 50% of the protein and 30% of the energy content are lost. As the plant matures, yield measured in tons/ac will increase due to increasing plant fiber content, but nutritional quality, that is, digestibility, energy, and protein, decreases.

Contaminants The appearance of hay is the most commonly used and practical means of determining the presence of mold, dust, weeds, insects, foreign material (litter, paper, and plastic), leaves and sticks, metal, wood, animal carcasses (snakes, moles), stones, and broken machinery parts. It is difficult to completely avoid having some types of foreign material caught up in the baling of hay. Some species of weeds, tree leaves, and insects are toxic to horses; hence, when present in the hay, these should be identified and removed before feeding. Sharp objects made of metal, plastic, or glass may cause injury to the horse's lips and tongue. Horses, unlike cattle, rarely swallow foreign materials, although wire was the common foreign body found postmortem in three cases [15]. Foreign material swallowed may also serve as a nidus for enterolith formations. Removing the string, wire, netting, or wrap used to bale hay must be done before feeding as colic due to the

Table 10.1 Nutritional value (DE, protein, DMI, DDM and RFV) decrease as forage ADF and NDF increases with plant maturity.[a] [14].

Forage	Harvest	Stage	DE	Protein	NDF	DMI	ADF	DDM	RFV
			Mcal/kg	%	%	%	%	%	
Legume									
Alfalfa	Grazed	Late vegetative	2.94	22	31	3.9	24	70.2	211
		Full bloom	2.32	19	39	3.1	36	60.9	147
	Hay	Early bloom	2.48	20	39	3.1	32	64.0	152
		Full bloom	2.17	17	49	2.5	39	58.8	112
Grass									
Orchardgrass	Grazed	Early bloom	2.29	13	55	2.2	31	65.0	110
		Mid bloom	2.02	10	58	2.1	36	61.2	99
	Hay	Early bloom	2.17	13	60	2.0	34	62.6	98
		Late bloom	1.90	8	65	1.8	38	59.5	85

[a] All parameters are based on 100% dry matter (DM); DE: Digestible Energy; NDF: neutral detergent fiber; DMI: DM intake, ADF: acid detergent fiber; DDM: digestible DM; RFV: relative feed value.

consumption of bale netting and string foreign bodies have occurred in horses.

Feed hygiene is a broad term covering all measures necessary to minimize health risks due to physical, chemical, and biological contamination of feeds. Poisons ingested with feed intended for horses occur in both harvested and manufactured feeds. Sources of feed toxins include those produced by molds (mycotoxicosis), bacteria (botulism), plants (gossypol and nitrates), insects (blister beetle), environmental contamination (lead), or errors in feed preparation (ionophore and antibiotics) [16, 17]. See Contaminated Feed in Chapter 13.

Cubes and Pellets It is difficult to fully evaluate the quality of hay processed into cubes and pellets without a laboratory analysis. Good quality cubes and pellets are firm, not crumbly, and are free of mold, weeds, and foreign material. Visual inspection to evaluate the hay quality in cubes or pellets is limited to odor and color. Moist cubes or pellets will foster mold growth if left in a bag, bucket, or feeder. Water-soaked cubes and pellets fed to horses with dental disease should be limited to only that quantity consumed in one meal. Poorly made and old, dried-out pelleted feeds are crumbly and unpalatable and break down to a dusty material.

Hay Storage The storage site for both bagged forage and baled hay should be inspected to assess suitability in maintaining clean dry forage.[2] Hay should be kept out of the weather, stored off the ground and on a dry surface (gravel or pallets) but not over the heads of horses to minimize dust exposure. The moisture content of hay should be ≤14%. If hay with excessive moisture (>20%) is baled, spoilage, mold, and yeast growth will usually develop within a few days. See Sidebar 10.2. High moisture bales may overheat and combust, risking a barn fire.[3] Dried hay can reabsorb moisture from the soil and air in high humidity environments. Good airflow through the hay storage area minimizes mold and yeast growth in previously dried hay. The outer layers of bales exposed to sunlight will bleach to brown, yellow, or white as plant pigments are lost, but the nutritional value may be retained. Hay appropriately stored indoors under good conditions can be held for two to three years without losing significant nutrient content [18].

Sidebar 10.2 Hygienic Quality of Hay

Subjectively assessing forage quality involves using sight, smell, and feel [8]. It may be obvious when the hay is of poor hygienic quality due to a musty smell; patches of dark, wet rotting forage; or the rise of a white plume of fungal spores or dust when the bale is patted. Regardless of the laboratory nutrient analysis, poor hygienic quality forage should not be fed, although hay with such obvious contamination is rarely eaten by horses.

Forages contain some unavoidable concentrations of bacteria, molds, and yeast acquired during the harvesting, transportation, and storage of preserved forages. With particle sizes (5 μm) well below detection by the human eye (40 μm), laboratory assay methods are necessary to determine the "load" of microorganisms in a forage sample. Results are reported in colony-forming units (CFU) per g, and the highest acceptable counts have been suggested by feedstuff and microbial species [16]. For example, the highest acceptable concentration of Bacillus spp. in hay is 2×10^6 cfu/g, whereas 0.15×10^6 cfu/g is the highest for Streptomyces spp in hay, but lower concentrations are recommended for the same microbes in mixed and pelleted feeds.

Steaming hay at 212 °F can reduce bacteria and mold counts by 99%, reduce water soluble carbohydrate concentrations, but conserve the protein and mineral content [19].

Objective Assessments The objective laboratory or "hay" test results are most useful when sampled close to the point of sale or time of feeding. Using a correct sampling technique is key to obtaining a reliable estimate of the nutrient content of forages because sampling produces more variation in the results than does laboratory error [20]. The natural variation of analyzed nutrients within a forage sample might be 3–8% due to the differences between the proportions of leaf, stem, and weeds harvested, while lab-to-lab analysis variation on the same sample varies by 1–3% [20]. When proper sampling protocols are followed, the variation can be reduced to an acceptable level and an estimate of hay quality can be successfully predicted.

To perform a hay test, samples are collected using a commercial forage sampler or hay probe.[4] Submitting a "flake" or a grab sample is highly unlikely to represent the nutritional content of the hay accurately. "Hand-grab" samples from bales were significantly lower in estimated feeding value and quality than correctly sampled forage [20]. The recommended protocol for core hay sampling is to obtain cores from 15 to 20 bales randomly selected from the stack. These subsamples are then combined into a single composite for analysis that represents a particular lot of hay [7, 9].

2 Baled hay requires adequate (200 ft^3/ton) storage space. One 500 kg adult horse with a DMI of 2% will eat at least 3000 kg or 3.3 tons (as fed) of hay in 9 mos which will require 700 ft^3 of storage space, or a 12 × 12′ stall stacked 5 ft high [18].

3 Hay should be stored in a separate building in case of fire regardless of cause.

4 Listing of hay probes: https://www.foragetesting.org/hay-probes.

For hay lots of 100–200 tons or highly variable lots, taking 35 cores is recommended [20].

Long-stem hay does not come with a label or nutrient guarantee, although some hay brokers may provide a nutrient analysis. Bagged forages purchased as chopped, cubes, or pellets often do come with a product label. However, any information written about any hay product identifying the type of hay and/or any other information offered about the forage is considered “labeling” under the law and must not contain false or misleading information. See Basic Label Requirements in Chapter 15.

10.2.2.2 Complementary Feeds

Manufactured feeds, usually bagged or sacked, differ in the intended use and nutrient profile. These products may be referred to as concentrates, sweet or coarse-textured feeds, ration balancers, supplements, or treats. These products will contain variable quantities of cereal grains and/or fat for energy, protein and/or fiber sources, and vitamins or minerals. Occasionally, probiotics, enzymes, and nutraceuticals will be included. See Chapter 13 Manufactured Feeds. It is important to record each product fed and the amount offered to the horse daily by weight and, if possible, retain the label. The label information provides the targeted nutrient concentrations, ingredient list, use-by or manufactured date, and the manufacturer’s contact information. When labels are not available, information can often be obtained by contacting the feed company or reviewing website information. Samples of all complementary feeds should be obtained, although a laboratory analysis of each may not be necessary in every case. In general, sampling 5% is sufficient (2–3 lb sample of a 50 lb bagged feed and a ¼ to ½ lb sample of supplements and treats) using a grain or sack probe [7]. During sampling, the form, smell, texture, and hygienic quality should be noted. Although most sacked feeds are mixed thoroughly, fines or small particles do settle to the bottom and mixing the bag before sampling is recommended. The storage area for the complementary feeds should be inspected for suitability in maintaining clean, dry, uncontaminated feed. Feed storage areas ideally should be humidity- and temperature-controlled and rodent- and insect-free.

10.2.3 Water

Water should be continuously available to horses. For both horse health and environmental reasons, bowls, buckets, and tanks are preferred over natural water features. See Watering Devices and Water Quality in Chapter 5. The water supply should be inspected, sampled, and analyzed if suspected to be less than optimal. The number of watering devices and refill rate should be assessed, particularly if decreased feed intake has been reported. Water requirement parallels energy requirements, but feed consumption will decrease when water intake is limited. Conversely, water intake will decrease when feed is not available. Water intake can also be estimated when horses are provided individual buckets or metered devices; otherwise, intake from a communal tank is assumed to be adequate if there are no known medical problems.

10.2.4 Feeding Management Assessment

There are two methods of feeding: meal feeding and ad libitum, which is unlimited access with no feed quantity limitations. There are variations of both methods, such as providing an unlimited amount of feed for a limited time (pasture access limited to 4 hrs/d) or a limited amount of feed with unlimited access (hanging 25 lb of hay in a net for the day). There are individual vs. group feeding methods and variations thereof (group feeding of hay but individually meal feeding a complementary feed).

The delivery of feed to the horse(s) is ideally observed first-hand and quantification of each feed consumed (feed offered minus orts or feed remnants). Observing horses at feeding time, particularly if horses are group-fed, may reveal dominance behavior that limits feed intake by subordinate horses. Feeding stations for hay or concentrate must be far apart (10–50 ft) to discourage a horse from dominating the feeding area. Feeding stations should also be away from corners, gates, and blind spots that may trap a subordinate horse and pose a hazard when horses interact [21]. When ingestion of sand or dirt is of concern, mats can be placed under the feed bin.

Forage intake can be easily quantified when horses are fed individually and when waste is minimal (fed 5 kg of hay cubes twice daily in a bucket). When horses are group-fed, an estimate can be made using the quantity of hay offered and knowing the number of horses and days (900 lb bale lasting five horses (H) nine days is 20 lb/H/d). Voluntary intake of pasture intake is more difficult to estimate and variable. Intake is known to be dependent on the quality and quantity of forage, time spent on pasture, life stage of the horse, and whether horses turned out as a group or individually [22]. Often intake is estimated based on calculated DMI minus the known complementary feed intake for the life stage and BW of the horse. Horses on pasture full-time consume approximately 2% BW DMI [23]. Typically, the daily volume of complementary feeds, supplements, and treats fed (a scoop or cup) are known by the person feeding; however, the daily feed offered and orts must be quantified (lb or g/d) to estimate nutrient intake.

10.3 Ration Analysis

There are reference nutrient databases for various feedstuffs widely available [5, 14, 23], however, when investigating a problem specific to a farm or facility, laboratory analysis of 'on site' samples is advisable.

10.3.1 Laboratory Analysis

Feed samples should be sent to a laboratory that has demonstrated proficiency in forage and feed analysis. Laboratories certified by the National Forage Testing Association (NFTA) have shown the ability to produce accurate results using analytical methodologies approved by the Association of Official Analytical Chemists (AOAC) [24, 25]. Some feed-testing laboratories are connected to state universities and extension services, and some are independent commercial businesses. See Table 10.2.

Laboratory methods have been developed over several decades to analyze both organic and inorganic components of feeds for ration evaluation and formulation. An obvious logistical problem is that the laboratory analysis is performed on <2 g of dried forage, but the results are extrapolated to tons of hay or acres of pasture [3]. The laboratory analysis of a single feed (oats or timothy hay) should compare well with published averages, and analysis of complementary feeds should compare well with the company's targeted profiles. The laboratory analysis of the farm sample is a single point in time determination that represents the feedstuff on the farm at the time of sampling, whereas the manufacturer's nutrient profiles or published feedstuff nutrient averages often represent decades of similar samples from a variety of conditions. There are pros and cons to using one data set or the other, that is, lab vs. published data, usually dictated by the nature of the case, the problem being investigated, and the experience of the investigator.

If a feed sample analysis varies considerably from published average or the manufacturer's targeted concentrations, the sampling and analysis should be repeated. If the analysis is consistently different than expected, the discrepancy should be reviewed in light of the animal assessment. For example, if the trace mineral content of a supplement on analysis does not compare well with a company's stated concentration and if the young foals on the farm show signs of abnormal skeletal development after consuming the product, likely then the laboratory value is true and using product label concentrations in the ration evaluation would be misleading. Two laboratory techniques are used for analyzing feed nutrient content: (i) wet chemistries and (ii) near-infrared reflectance spectroscopy (NIRS).

10.3.1.1 Wet Chemistries

Traditional wet chemistry methods are the gold standard in determining nutrient content [26, 27]. Wet chemistry can be used for any forage or grains. Nutrient analysis of uncommon feedstuffs and for specific nutrients associated with a disease (non-structural carbohydrates and laminitis) should be determined using wet chemistry due to the importance of accuracy [7]. However, wet chemistries require more time and labor, and are hence more costly relative to NIRS.

10.3.1.2 Near-Infrared Reflectance Spectroscopy

The NIRS method uses a spectrophotometer to measure light scattered off of and through a sample, which is then compared to a feed database. Based on the molecular structure, the amount of light absorbed in the near-infrared wavelength is used to estimate the nutrient concentrations without altering the sample [28]. While a reliable method for some nutrients, the feed sample must be pure (100% oats or corn, aka "straights" or a single hay species with no weeds or other forage species) because NIRS is less reliable in mixed feed samples [7, 29, 30]. NIRS is safe, accurate, requires less time to perform than wet chemistry methods, and hence less costly. Many commercial laboratories offer NIRS for routine ration balancing involving healthy animals; however, when investigating a potential feed-related disease process or a mixed feed sample, wet chemistry analysis is recommended.

10.3.1.3 Laboratory Assayed Feed Values

An objective feed assessment requires data obtained from the laboratory analysis. The determination of water in the sample is necessary as all feed comparisons are done on a DM basis. A "proximate" analysis includes a specific set of laboratory procedures: crude protein (CP), ether extract (EE) of fat, crude fiber (CF), and ash. Ash estimates total inorganic minerals and is of limited value because individual mineral concentrations are not determined. Similarly,

Table 10.2 Forage testing laboratories for equine feeds.

Laboratory name	Web address
Equi-Analytical Laboratories, Inc	https://equi-analytical.com
Cumberland Valley Analytical Services	https://foragelab.com
Eurofins	https://www.eurofinsus.com
Midwest Labs	http://midwestlabs.com
National Forage Testing Association	https://www.foragetesting.org/proficiency-certification-program.

CF is not entirely an accurate assessment of the fiber for feeding hindgut fermenters. The Van Soest detergent system of assays, that is, neutral detergent fiber (NDF) and acid detergent fiber (ADF), have been used to further define the components of cell walls [23]. See Sidebar 10.3.

Sidebar 10.3 Feeding Value of Forage

Plant cells, as feed, are divided into intracellular contents vs. cell wall components. The cell contents (sugar, starch, proteins) are considered 98% digestible by all animals. Those animals with fermentative capabilities, in either the fore or hindgut, can digest significant portions, but not all, of the plant cell wall. There has long been an interest in finding an objective, rapid method of determining forage quality and feeding value to animals. The laboratory fiber assay system proposed by Van Soest has been considered the best indicator of *in vivo* forage voluntary DMI and digestibility. The acid detergent fiber (ADF) assay estimates cell wall cellulose and lignin, and the neutral detergent fiber (NDF) assay estimates cell wall cellulose, hemicellulose, and lignin. Animal studies have demonstrated a high negative correlation between ADF and DM digestibility, because ADF estimates indigestible lignin, i.e. higher the lignin content (ADF), the lower the DM digestibility. The voluntary feed intake by animals correlated negatively with the NDF assay, in that as NDF increased, voluntary DMI decreased due to the "gut filling" effect of fiber [23, 31].

Most laboratories can assay macro- and microminerals; however, vitamin assays are costly and the expense is rarely justified in equine ration formulations. Horses grazing on fresh forage or receiving a fortified complementary feed will likely consume sufficient vitamins A and E with all other vitamin requirements met by endogenous or microbial synthesis. When investigating a nutritional or dietary-related problem, determining at least DM, CP, NDF, ADF, EE, and macro- and microminerals using wet chemistry analysis is advisable. When investigating a problem related to dietary hydrolyzable carbohydrates: water-soluble carbohydrates (WSC) measuring simple sugars and fructans, ethanol-soluble carbohydrates (ESC) measuring simple sugars, and a separate starch analysis should be assayed.

10.3.1.4 Calculated Feed Values

From the fiber determinations, feed DE content is calculated using CP, ADF, NDF, EE, and ash [23]. Lysine and methionine are calculated from CP using conversion factors specific for feed or forage type. The non-fiber carbohydrate (NFC), including sugar, starch, pectins, and hemicellulose, is calculated by difference [100-(CP-EE-NDF-ash)]. Non-structural carbohydrates (NSC), not synonymous with NFC, are estimated by WSC + starch. Fructans are estimated by WSC minus ESC.

10.3.1.5 Comparative Forage Quality Estimates

Grades of hay were developed by the USA Department of Agriculture in 1946, based on organoleptic characteristics of maturity, leafiness, color, and proportion of foreign material present but did not include quantitative measurements of nutrient content. Working with forage quality and animal nutrition scientists to obtain objective measures of evaluating forage quality, the American Forage and Grasslands Council developed a system using laboratory data to assess the feeding value of hays [31]. The consensus of the council was that nearly all of the plant cell contents were digested by most animals regardless of gut fermentation and that plant cell wall content effectively limits feed intake. Based on forage data collected from northern and southern regions of the USA on alfalfa and seven different types of grass, most of which are fed to horses, the forage ADF value was highly correlated with DM digestibility and DM intake correlated best with forage NDF. Both voluntary feed intake and digestibility decreased with increasing forage NDF and ADF content, respectively [32, 33]. See Sidebar 10.4.

Sidebar 10.4 The Relationship Between Dry Matter Intake (DMI), Digestible Dry Matter[5] (DDM), and Plant Fiber

DMI and NDF:

NDF undergoes microbial fermentation in the hindgut of horses. As feed is fermented and hindgut digesta volume decreases, feed intake increases. Hence NDF content affects the rate of digestion and amount of forage the animal can consume. Maximum dry matter intake (%DMI) for forage can be estimated from 120/%NDF. As forage matures, the fiber content increases, NDF increases, and the maximum consumption rate as a %BW decreases. Hay cut at an immature stage with 40% NDF would have a maximum DMI of 3.0% BW, whereas the same forage cut later in the season as a mature plant with a 60% NDF would limit DMI to 2.0% BW. Forages with less than 65% NDF are recommended for horses unless weight loss is desirable. See Table 10.3.

DDM and ADF

ADF estimates the indigestible lignin portion and is considered the best chemical predictor of *in vivo* digestibility

5 Dry matter digestibility = [weight of feed dry matter consumed minus fecal dry matter weight]/weight of feed dry matter consumed × 100.

of forages. As forage matures, growing taller and heavier, the cell wall lignin content must increase to support the plant; hence, forage digestibility decreases as lignin increases. Digestible dry matter (%DDM) in forage can be estimated from (88.9 – [0.779 × %ADF]). Hay cut at an immature stage may contain 35% ADF and be 62% digestible, whereas the same forage cut later in the season may contain 45% ADF and be 53% digestible. Hence, as a forage matures, the feeding value decreases because digestibility decreases. Forages with less than 45% ADF are recommended for horses unless weight loss is desirable. See Table 10.3.

10.3.1.5.1 Relative Feed Value (RFV)

The RFV, a forage quality index quality index widely used in the USA, is calculated using %DDM from ADF and %DMI from NDF determinations[6] based on an average score of 100 for alfalfa hay containing 41% ADF and 53% NDF. The RFV grades were developed based on data from foregut fermenting, initially in sheep and later confirmed in cattle, and *in vitro* fermentation experiments [31]. Although horses are hindgut fermenters, the RFV does provide a basis for comparison between different lots of hay, particularly of the same type [37]. In the absence of any other objective measure, a relative feeding value is useful for horses; in that, the higher the RFV, the better the nutritional value. For example, with a choice between full-bloom alfalfa hay (RFV 100) or mid-bloom alfalfa hay (RFV 125), the latter hay should have a higher feeding value given all subjective assessments are equal.

Although not a perfect fit for horses, forage quality designations have been suggested using readily available forage relative feeding values. See Table 10.3. The RFV recommendations by life stage are suggested ranges because precision is not necessary when recommending or selecting hay for horses or when comparing two lots of hay. A good rule of thumb is to accept a calculated RFV within at least +/−5 points of the target value [38]. For example, if RFV 120 is the target value for an 18-mo-old horse, a forage value between 115 and 125 should be of equivalent feeding value. Due to the inherent variability of measuring ADF and NDF, the RFV values cannot be used in ration balancing but is one additional useful estimate of forage feeding value [39].

10.3.1.5.2 Relative Forage Quality (RFQ)

The RFQ is the qualitative index of hay quality that includes nutritional value and an estimate of intake based on

6 RFV = %DDM × %DMI × 0.775.

Table 10.3 Forage quality and relative feeding values recommended for various equine life stages [9, 34, 35].

Quality designation for horses *Example*	ADF[a]	NDF[a]	RFV[b]	Number of RFV samples[b]	Horse life stage
Recommendations for horses	**<45**	**<65**	**80–150**		
Excellent	<31	<40	>151		Working 18 to 24-mo-olds
Legume Hays	30.7	38.8	159	204 755	
High	31–35	40–46	125–151		Weanling, Late Gestation, Lactation
Mixed mainly legume (MML) Hays	34.9	47.9	124	20 131	
Good	36–40	47–53	101–124		12 to 18-mo-olds, Working adult, Stallion
Mixed mainly grass (MMG) Pastures	33.5	56.5	110	23 279	
Moderate	41–42	53–60	86–100		2 to 5-yr-olds, Adult <9 mos Gestation, Stallion
Grass Hays	38.5	61.9	90	93 370	
MMG Hays	38.1	59.6	95	60 516	
Grass Pastures	35.6	60.9	99	12 108	
Fair	43–45	61–65	77–85		Weight loss
Berumdagrass Hays	35.2	66.2	88	18 095	
Unacceptable	>45	>65	<77		
Straw	50.1	72.9	66	5946	

[a] Acid detergent fiber (ADF) and Neutral Detergent fiber (NDF) as % of forage dry matter.
[b] Equi-Analytical Feed Composition Library yrs. 2004–2020 [36].

digestibility measured at 48 hrs in ruminants and likely does not provide additional information over RFV for horses.

10.4 Ration Formulation

The goal in ration balancing is to meet the horse's nutrient needs, that is, provide nutrients within the optimal range, based on sound scientific information of the highest possible grade of evidence while not harming the animal or the environment. The goal should encourage sound management strategies that are biologically appropriate for the horse and agriculturally sustainable. All the information collected on the farm, from the caretaker(s), including subjective and objective assessments is synthesized to conclude if nutrition is playing a role in a given problem relating to health, productivity, or performance.

It is not the intention here to teach ration formulation, balancing, or how to correct an imbalance. Few practitioners need to know how to formulate equine rations. Horse nutrient requirements and feed nutrient profile data sets are readily available [23, 36, 40, 41]. However, ration formulation, software expertise, understanding nutrient bioavailability of various feedstuffs, knowledge of feed processing, acceptability, and palatability are complex issues acquired with formal training and experience. Some equine feed manufacturers employ veterinarians and equine nutritionists, and offer guidance within their product lines. There are equine veterinary nutritionist, working as independent consultants, offering farm investigation and ration evaluation services.

10.4.1 Initial Ration Assessment

Computer software for ration formulation is readily available. See Table 10.4. Based on the nutrient content of the feed and the quantity of each feed fed, daily nutrient intake is calculated and compared with the recommended daily intakes or allowances [23, 41]. Intakes are then compared with published nutritional recommendations. For example, for a 500 kg BW adult horse, eating 10 kg/d hay with 8% crude protein (CP) from lab analysis of hay sample is consuming 800 g CP/d, and this is compared to the recommended 630 g CP/d; hence, the CP intake of 800 g/d is more than adequate [23]. Assessing CP intake is one of 22 nutrient recommendations and relative parameters (caloric density, DMI, and Ca : P and forage to grain ratios) to be assessed.

10.4.2 Ration Balancing

When imbalances between nutrient recommendations and actual nutrient intakes occur, in cases involving a feed-related disease process, consultation with a veterinary nutritionist is recommended. When nutritional imbalances exist between recommended dietary and actual intakes, the difference should be resolved using hand calculations or ration balancing software, particularly for nutrients of concern. Corrections for these imbalances may require an additional supplement, a change in the complementary feed, or adjustments to the amount of feed fed. The corrections inevitably involve taking into consideration: (i) animal factors of signalment, feed intake, life stage, and health status; (ii) dietary factors of nutrient balance, availability, palatability, and hygiene; and (iii) management factors of feeding method, housing, and cost; therefore, suggested changes are often specific to the farm or animal.

10.4.3 Minimizing Feed Costs

Feed cost and logistics of obtaining certain types of feed are taken into account when recommending changes to a

Table 10.4 Ration formulation software.

Company name	Web address
Kentucky Equine Research	https://ker.com/tools/microsteed
National Research Council	https://nrc88.nas.edu/nrh
<u>Fee based:</u>	
Agricultural Software Consultants, Inc.	http://www.agriculturalsoftwareconsultants.com
Agriculture XPRT	https://www.agriculturexprt.com/software/concept5-animal-feed-software-366009
Cargill, Incorporated	https://www.formatsolutions.com/en/formulation
Creative Formulation Concepts	https://cfctech.com/products/horse-rationformulation.aspx
Equi-Balance	https://performancehorsenutrition.com/store
Feed XL	https://feedxl.com

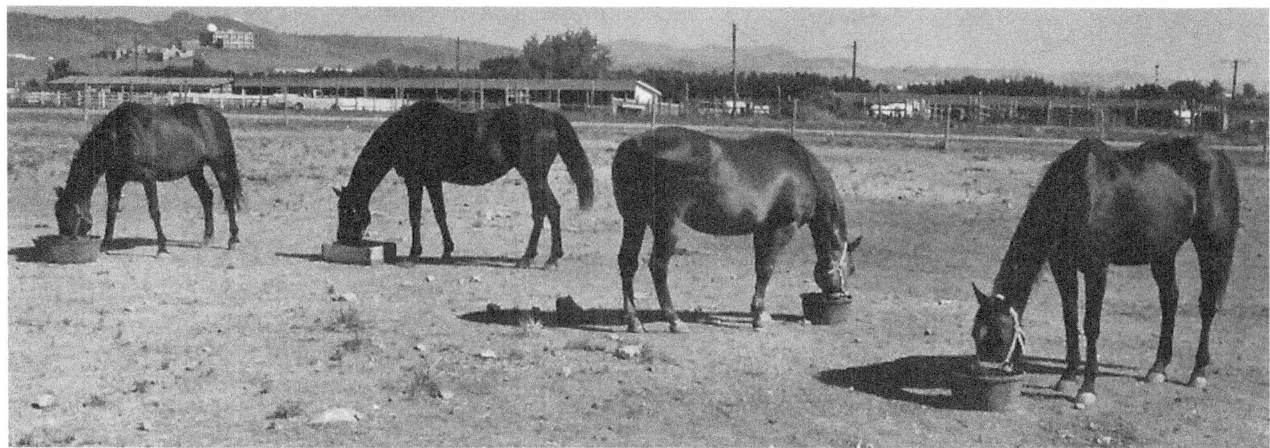

Figure 10.1 Providing feeding stations or training horses to consume complementary feeds individually is economical.

feeding program. As a general guide, the cost to feed a 1000 lb adult pleasure horse is approximately $2000/yr [42–44] See Case in Point in Chapter 13. Minimizing feed costs is done initially using least-cost ration balancing software, where product price is included in the data and the number of feeds to be used in the ration is minimized in addition to correcting any nutritional imbalances. Buying feeds in bulk is a cost-effective strategy keeping in mind a use-by date and storage space [9]. Weighing feeds, rather than estimating or feeding by volume, reduces feed waste and the cost of feeding. Forage waste can be minimized by (i) controlling pasture access (rotational grazing), because horses spot-graze, trample, and defecate large areas of edible forage; (ii) using hay nets to prolong intake in feeders with solid bottoms to catch leaves, as horses are unlikely to eat ground-soiled hay; and (iii) feeding complementary and supplement products individually, because more feed is required to allow subordinate horses access when group feeding [4]. See Figure 10.1.

10.5 Reassessment

Monitoring the implementation of dietary recommendations and clinical changes in the horses consuming the new ration brings the iterative process full circle. See Figure 2.1. Re-assessment of the ration and the horses should be performed at appropriate intervals to evaluate the effectiveness of the new feeding. The timing and frequency of re-evaluation are based on the life stage and nature of the problem, i.e. animal health, productivity, or performance. For young growing foals, re-evaluation every two wks may be appropriate, a recheck visit in 30 days may be appropriate for a horse with insulin dysregulation, or an annual assessment of the feeding plan may be sufficient for breeding programs. The reassessment involves the evaluation of diet and feeding factors in light of the horses' response to the implementation of recommendations, or lack thereof. Keep in mind that responses such as longevity, skeletal soundness, and athletic performance, although important in the horse industry, are difficult to objectively quantify.

Case in Point

The energy density (Mcal DE/kg DM) in any ration must be sufficient to meet the estimated daily energy requirement of the horse within a consumable volume. When the caloric density is too low (<1 Mcal DE/kg DM), the horse must consume more total food to meet the daily need for energy but likely will not be able to physically consume the necessary quantity of feed and may lose weight. Conversely, if the caloric density is too high, there is a minimum volume of food required to be satiated, and in eating to meet that volume, more calories will be consumed than are required for daily needs, resulting in weight gain. Most adult horses consume between 1.5 and 2% BW of feed DM/d. Ration or feed DM includes forage, complementary feeds, supplements, and treats.

Consider a 454 kg BW horse at maintenance requiring 15 Mcals DE/d:

Scenario 1: Offering a low energy (0.9 Mcal DE/kg DM) feed, the horse would have to eat 16.7 kg/d [15/0.9] to get 15 Mcal DE.

DMI would have to be [16.7/454 × 100] 3.7% BW. Feed intake would be limited by volume and the horse would likely lose weight in light of "eating a lot of hay" because the maximum daily DMI would be reached before the calorie need is met.

Scenario 2: Offering a high energy (3.0 Mcal DE/kg DM) feed, the horse would need to eat 5 kg/d [15/3.0] to get 15 Mcal DE.

DMI would be [5/454 × 100] 1.1% BW.

The horse would likely act hungry and, if fed more in response to acting hungry, would gain weight because caloric need would be met before volume satiation.

Scenario 3: What should the caloric density of the ration be to meet the daily energy need of 15 Mcal DE within a DMI of 2% BW for a 454 kg adult horse at maintenance?.

See Appendix A Chapter 10.

References

1 Association of American Feed Control Officials (2021). Official Publication AAFCO. Champaign, IL: Association of American Feed Control Officials, Inc. www.aafco.org

2 Thatcher, C.D., Hand, M.S., and Remillard, R.L. (2000). Small animal clinical nutrition: an iterative process. In: *Small Animal Clinical Nutrition*, 4e (ed. M. Hand, C.D. Thatcher, R.L. Remillard and P. Roudebush), 1–19. Topeka: Mark Morris Institute.

3 Redfearn, D.D., Freeman, D.W., and Hiney, K. (2017). Forage for horses. Oklahoma Cooperative Extension Service ANSI-3980. Stillwater,. https://shareok.org/bitstream/handle/11244/49954/oksd_ansi_3980_2013-08.pdf?sequence=1

4 Guthrie, T., Waite, K., and Cassida, K. (2014). Rotational grazing for Michigan horses E3200. Michigan State University Extension. https://www.canr.msu.edu/uploads/452/47497/E3200-Rotational_Grazing_for_Michigan_Horses.pdf (accessed 24 January 2022).

5 Equi-Analytical Laboratory. Taking a sample. https://equi-analytical.com/feed-and-forage-analysis/taking-a-sample (accessed 21 January 2022).

6 Kentucky Equine Research Staff (2014). sampling horse pasture for analysis. *EquiNews*. https://ker.com/equinews/sampling-horse-pasture-analysis.

7 Meehan, M. and Sedivex, K. (2018). Sampling feed for analysis AS1064. Fargo, ND: North Dakota State University Cooperative Extension. https://www.ag.ndsu.edu/publications/livestock/sampling-feed-for-analysis. (accessed 20 March 2020)

8 Rocateli, A. and Zhang, H. (2017). Evaluating hay quality based on sight, smell and feel – hay judging. Stillwater, OK: Oklahoma Cooperative Extension Service PSS-2588. https://shareok.org/bitstream/handle/11244/317990/oksa_pss_2588_2015-12.pdf?sequence=1

9 Undersander, D., Morrison, J., and Phillips, E. et al. (2002). Buying horse hay A3772. Michigan State University Extension. https://cdn.shopify.com/s/files/1/0145/8808/4272/files/A3772.pdf

10 van den Berg, M., Giagos, V., Lee, C. et al. (2016). The influence of odour, taste and nutrients on feeding behaviour and food preferences in horses. *Appl. Anim. Behav. Sci.* 184 (Nov): 41–50.

11 Ball, D., Hoveland, C., and Lacefield, G. (2007). Forage quality. In: *Southern Forages. Modern Concepts for Forage Crop Management*, 4e, 136–145. Norcross, GA: International Plant Nutrition Institute.

12 Becvarova, I., Pleasant, R.S., and Thatcher, C.D. (2009). Clinical assessment of nutritional status and feeding programs in horses. *Vet. Clin. North Am. Equine Pract.* 25 (1): 1–21.

13 Hintz, H.F. (1991). Feeds for livestock. In: *Large Animal Clinical Nutrition* (ed. J. Naylor and S.L. Ralston), 120–130. St. Louis, MO: Mosby.

14 National Research Council (1989). *Nutrient Requirements of Horses.* 5th Rev. Animal Nutrition Series, 1–100. Washington, DC: National Academies Press.

15 Lohmann, K.L., Lewis, S.R., Wobeser, B., and Allen, A.L. (2010). Penetrating metallic foreign bodies as a cause of peritonitis in 3 horses. *Can. Vet. J. La Rev Vet. Can.* 51 (12): 1400–1404.

16 Kamphues, J. (2013). Feed hygiene and related disorders in horses. In: *Equine Applied and Clinical Nutrition Health, Welfare and Performance* (ed. R.J. Geor, P.A. Harris, and M. Coenen), 367–380. Edinburgh: Saunders Elsevier.

17 Séguin, V., Garon, D., Lemauviel-Lavenant, S. et al. (2012). How to improve the hygienic quality of forages for horse feeding. *J. Sci. Food Agric.* 92 (4): 975–986.

18 Russell, M.A. and Johnson, K.D. (2007). Selecting quality hay for horses. West Lafayette, IN: Department of Agriculture Cooperative Extension Service.

https://www.agry.purdue.edu/ext/forages/publications/id-190.htm (accessed 5 July 2021).

19 Moore-Colyer, M.J.S., Taylor, J.L.E., and James, R. (2016). The effect of steaming and soaking on the respirable particle, bacteria, mould, and nutrient content in hay for horses. *J. Equine Vet. Sci.* 39 (4): 62–68.

20 Putman, D. and Orloff, S. (2003). Hay sampling protocols and a hay sampling certification program, 9. Davis, CA: University of California Cooperative Extension. https://www.foragetesting.org/exam-info (accessed 20 March 2020).

21 Lawrence, L. Equine feeding management ASC-143. University of Kentucky Cooperative Extension Service. http://www2.ca.uky.edu/agcomm/pubs/asc/asc143/asc143.pdf (accessed 20 January 2020).

22 Dunnett, C. (2013). Ration evaluation and formulation. In: *Equine Applied and Clinical Nutrition: Health, Welfare and Performance* (ed. R.J. Geor, P.A. Harris, and M. Coenen), 405–424. Edinburgh: Saunders Elsevier.

23 National Research Council (2007). *Nutrient Requirements of Horses*. 6th Rev. Animal Nutrition Series, 1–341. Washington, DC: National Academies Press.

24 National Forage Testing Association. Forage testing. National Forage Testing Association. www.foragetesting.org (accessed 22 January 2022).

25 A.O.A.C. International. Official methods of analysis. www.aoac.org (accessed 22 January 2022).

26 Harris, L. (1970). Chemical and biological methods. In: *Nutrition Research Techniques for Domestic and Wild Animals Part II*, vol. 1, 1401–3201. Logan, UT: Utah State University.

27 Undersander, D., Mertens, D.R., and Thiex, N. (1993). Forage analysis procedures. National Forage Testing Association. https://www.foragetesting.org/lab-procedures (accessed 22 January 2022).

28 Yan, X., Bai, S.-Q., Yan, J.-J. et al. (2012). Application of near infrared spectroscopy technology (NIRS) in forage field. *Spectrosc. Spectrom. Anal.* 32 (7): 1748–1753.

29 Plumier, B.M., Danao, M.C., Singh, V., and Rausch, K.D. (2013). Analysis and prediction of unreacted starch content in corn using FT-NIR spectroscopy. *Trans. ASABE*] 56 (5): 1877–1884.

30 Nieto-Ortega, B., Arroyo, J.-J., Walk, C. et al. (2022). Near infrared reflectance spectroscopy as a tool to predict non-starch polysaccharide composition and starch digestibility profiles in common monogastric cereal feed ingredients. *Anim. Feed Sci. Technol.* 285 (January): 115214.

31 Rohweder, D.A.A., Barnes, R.F.F., and Jorgensen, N.A.N. (1978). Proposed hay grading standards based on laboratory analysis for evaluating quality. *J. Anim. Sci.* 47 (3): 747–759.

32 Wells, L.A. (2015). The Applicability of NIRS to predict DMI and in vivo NDF digestibility in mature geldings consuming an all-forage diet. MS thesis. West Texas A&M University. https://wtamu-ir.tdl.org/handle/11310/66

33 Cuddeford, D. (2004). Voluntary food intake by horses. In: *Nutrition of the Performance Horse. EAAP #111* (ed. W. Martin-Rosset), 89–100. Wageningen, Netherlands: Wageningen Academic Publishers.

34 Swinker, A.M. (2014). Hay quality for different classes of horses. Pennsylvania State Extension Service; https://extension.psu.edu/hay-quality-for- different-classes-of-horses. (accessed 2 July 2021)

35 Thunes, C. (2015). Hay analysis part III: carbohydrates. http://summit-equine.com/hay-analysis-part-iii-carbohydrates (accessed 28 February 2019).

36 Equi-Analytical. Interactive common feed profile. https://equi-analytical.com/common-feed-profiles/interactive-common-feed-profile (accessed 7 April 2021).

37 Lawrence, L. (2011). Relative feed value of hay. University of Kentucky Cooperative Extension Service. http://equine.ca.uky.edu/news-story/relative-feed-value-hay (accessed 10 January 2022).

38 Rocateli, A. and Zhang, H. (2017). Forage quality interpretations. Stillwater, OK: Oklahoma Cooperative Extension Service PSS-2117. https://extension.okstate.edu/fact-sheets/forage-quality-interpretations.html

39 Martinson, K., Earing, J., and Sheaffer, C. (2011). Interpreting an equine forage analysis. 1–2 University of Minnesota. https://www.besthorsevet.com/Articles-FeedingandNutrition/Interpreting-an-Equine-Forage-Analysis.pdf.

40 National Research Council (1982). *United States-Canadian Tables of Feed Composition*. 3rd Rev. Nutritional Data for United States and Canadian Feeds, 1–148. Washington, DC: National Academies Press.

41 Martin-Rosset, W., Tavernier, L., Trillaud-Geyl, C. et al. (2015). Diet formulation. In: *Equine Nutrition: INRA Nutrient Requirements, Recommended Allowances and Feed Tables* (ed. W. Martin-Rosset), 97–120. Wageningen, the Netherlands: Wageningen Academic Publishers.

42 Ag Extension Service. Equine Facts: Guide to first-time horse ownership bulletin #1004 (2012). University of Maine Cooperative Extension Publication. https://extension.umaine.edu/publications/1004e (accessed 27 January 2022).

43 Renelt, T. (2011). Understanding the cost of horse ownership ExEx 2074. South Dakota State University Extension. http://openprairie.sdstate.edu/extension_extra/97 (accessed 27 January 2022).

44 Extension Foundation. (2020). Cost of horse ownership. USDA national institute of food and agriculture. https://horses.extension.org/cost-of-horse-ownership (accessed 27 January 2022).

11

Forages

Bridgett McIntosh

KEY TERMS

- Forages are seed heads, leaves, stems, and stalks of plants; harvested forage refers to hay, haylage, silages or green chop, whereas unharvested refers to pastures or crop residues that remain in the field, i.e. stalks, after harvesting a grain crop.
- The vegetative phase of plant development is the period of growth between germination and flowering. During the vegetative phase, plants are growing leaves and stems and accumulating resources needed later for flower and seed production.
- A lot of hay is defined as the bales from a single field that was harvested, cured, and stored in similar conditions.
- Hay is forage preserved by drying to a DM >85%; haylage is forage preserved by the exclusion of air stored with a DM ≥50%; silage is forage preserved by fermentation and acidification with DM below 50%.
- Green chop or soilage is fresh forage cut, chopped, and fed that day. For the best feeding value, the forage must be harvested at its optimum stage of growth or maturity which limits use, and therefore, is not commonly fed to horses.
- Drylot is a fenced grassless area of variable size.
- Forage and roughage are used interchangeably referring to the high fiber component of the ration. Forage typically refers to grass or legume feeds (fresh or dried); roughage often refers to hulls, straw, beet pulp by-products, or chaff.

KEY POINTS

- Forages are the foundation of the ration for all equine feeding programs. At least 1% BW in forages should be consumed daily.
- Assessing hay quality is essential in the assessment of equine rations.
- Relative feed value (RFV) is a widely indexed by which to assess forage quality across different forage varieties. Developed for ruminants, RFV estimates are not entirely accurate for horses but can provide a basis of comparison between hays.
- The type, quality, and amount of forage offered determines if type of other feeds are needed to balance the ration.
- When changing forage, at least two and possibly more than more than a three wks adaptation period may be required especially when energy, protein, and nonstructural carbohydrates are unknown or known to differ considerably.

11.1 Introduction

Forages fed to horses are primarily in the forms of hay and pasture, and the most important part of the diet for all classes of adult horses providing the fiber necessary for gastrointestinal tract (GIT) health and energy. Regardless of the class of horse, forages are the foundation of the equine diet. Well-managed pasture is economical, nutritious, and promotes healthy behavior, and therefore is the best way to provide forage to horses. Hay or other conserved forages can be fed to meet the horses' forage requirement when there is a lack of suitable acreage, when pasture is scarce, while traveling, or when horses cannot be turned out on pasture. The forage, the largest portion of the ration (>50%), should always be assessed for nutrient concentrations before adding grains, concentrates, or supplements into the diet.

11.2 Importance of Forages

Forages are extremely important feeds for herbivores, such as the horse, not only for the nutrients they provide but also for the stimulatory effects of forages on the muscle

Equine Clinical Nutrition, Second Edition. Edited by Rebecca L. Remillard.

tone and activity of the GIT, and feeding the GIT microbiome. Without adequate forage intake, colic, founder, and often an increase in stable vices may occur.

Pastures are the ideal environment for managing horses, providing optimal nutrition, access to exercise, and social interaction necessary for behavioral health. Under temperate climate growing conditions, 2 acres (ac) of pasture per horse is recommended to avoid overgrazing. Proper pasture management is necessary to ensure both horse and environmental health. Overgrazing pastures is detrimental to horse health and can lead to adverse impacts on the environment through erosion and waste runoff. If pasture acreage is limited, the primary purpose of pastures or paddocks is then to provide exercise. When the primary purpose of the pasture is exercise, hay and other alternative preserved forages are fed to provide the roughage necessary for digestive health and energy.

A minimum of 1–1.5% body weight per day (BW/d) as forage dry matter (DM) is required to avoid digestive dysfunction (10–15 lb for a 1000 lb horse). Grazing horses with ad libitum, i.e. unlimited quantity available at all times, access to productive pastures consume an average of 2–2.5% BW in forage DM/d (20–25 lb for a 1000 lb horse) [1]. As herbivores that naturally graze up to 18 hrs/d and rely on microbial fermentation of fiber to provide the majority of their energy requirements, forage is an essential component of the equine diet. The GIT digestion provides energy mainly through the production of short-chain fatty acids (SCFAs), i.e. acetate, propionate, and butyrate, also referred to as volatile fatty acids (VFAs) [2]. The whole digestive system is well adapted to the almost continuous intake of small amounts of fiber-containing feeds [3].

Most horses should be offered ad libitum access to forage, thus forage selection and feed management are fundamental components of equine nutrition. The nutritional content of forages is often adequate to meet many of the nutrient requirements of adult horses at maintenance (Table 11.1) [4]. However, forage nutrients can vary widely depending on the plant species, the environmental conditions during growth, the time of harvest, and the part of the plant ingested. Hay should be selected for horses based on both a visual assessment and chemical analysis, compared with the life stage or physiological state of the horses to be fed. Exceeding nutrient requirements for horses is not harmless and has potential for detrimental health effects, such as the acidogenic effect in performance horses caused by excessive protein, and the life-limiting metabolic consequences of obesity [6, 7].

Despite many advantages as a feed for horses, forage has several nutritional shortcomings compared with grains or concentrated feeds. Forages vary more in nutrient content and palatability, and more plant material and nutrients are lost in harvesting, storage, and feeding than other types of feeds. Forages have the following general nutritional characteristics compared with grains or concentrated feeds:

1) More bulk, i.e. low weight per unit of volume.
2) Higher in fiber and lower in digestible energy.
3) Higher in calcium and potassium but lower in phosphorus.

Table 11.1 Nutrient recommendations for adult horses and composition of pasture and hay forages (DM basis).[a]

	Digestible energy	Crude protein	NDF	ADF	Calcium	Phosphorus	Copper	Zinc
	Mcal/kg	%	%	%	%	%	mg/kg	mg/kg
Adult maintenance horse recommendations (average)	2.00	8.00	<65	<45	0.24	0.17	10	40
Forages								
Mixed mainly legume hay (MML)	2.35	19.1	47.2	35.4	1.17	0.3	9	24
Mixed mainly grass hay (MMG)	2.06	12.3	59.5	38.0	0.63	0.3	8	28
Cool-season								
Mixed grass pasture	2.39	26.5	45.8	25	0.56	0.44	10	36
Timothy hay	1.99	9.7	63.7	36.9	0.48	0.23	16	43
Warm-season								
Bermuda pasture	2.38	12.6	73.3	36.8	0.49	0.27	9	22
Bermuda hay	2.07	11.4	66.1	35.2	0.49	0.21	10	35

[a] NDF: neutral detergent fiber; ADF: acid detergent fiber. MML and MMG at mid-maturity.
Source: Based on NRC [4, 5] and Equi-Analytical Laboratory Services https://equi-analytical.com/common-feed-profiles.

4) Higher in vitamins A, E, and K, and vitamin D, if sun-cured.
5) Variable in protein content (legumes >20%, and grasses <4% crude protein (CP).

Unharvested forage (pasture) or harvested and conserved (hay) forage is the most natural, safest, and frequently least expensive feed for the horse. Feeding ensiled forages (haylage) to horses is common in the UK and Europe, and is just starting to become available in the United States; however, these products are often expensive and are not widely available in sufficient quantities for large numbers of horses.

11.3 Hay

The heads, leaves, and stems or stalks of plants immediately after cutting may be chopped and either fed that day as green chop or soilage or stored in an oxygen limiting facility (silo or bunker) and fed as haylage in 2 to 3 wks. However, most often, especially for horses, the forage following cutting is allowed to dry in the field, baled, stored, and fed as hay.

Hay dried to less than 20% moisture content before baling, stacking, or storage is by far the most common harvested forage fed to horses. Sun-curing hay is most common; however, drying time can be reduced by conditioning, i.e. crushing or crimping the plants, and/or adding drying agents (sodium or potassium carbonate) or potassium hydroxide solutions, at the moment of cutting. The faster the drying occurs, the lower the risk and extent of weather damage to the hay. Hay that is mowed and then rained on before harvest may lose 40% or more of the nutritional content [8]. If the moisture is too high, molding and heating that decreases protein utilization occur within the bale. Hay stored with excess moisture may heat to 175 °F due to fermentation within the bale and is then dangerously close to combustion and causing a fire within the haystack, loft, or barn [9]. However, hay containing less than 12% moisture before baling and storage is brittle and has a greater loss of leaves, particularly with legumes.

11.3.1 Types of Hay

There are three types of hay for horses: legumes, grasses, and less common, cereal grain hay.

11.3.1.1 Legume

The major legume harvested is alfalfa (lucerne or *Medicago sativa*). Other legumes less widely available include clovers (red, ladino, and sweet), bird's-foot trefoil, and lespedeza (Table 11.2). Legume hays are higher in nutritional value

Table 11.2 Classification of common forages in the United States.

Grasses			
Perennials		**Annuals**	
Cool-Season	**Warm-Season**	**Cool-Season**	**Warm-Season**
Tall Fescue	Bermudagrass	Barley	Crabgrass
Orchardgrass	Bahiagrass	Oats	Pearl millet
Kentucky bluegrass	Dallisgrass	Annual ryegrass	Teff
Timothy	Switchgrass	Wheat	
Reed canarygrass	Old World Bluestems	Rye	
Legumes			
Perennials		**Annuals**	
Cool-Season	**Warm-Season**	**Cool-Season**	**Warm-Season**
Alfalfa	Kudzu	Vetch	Cowpea
Bird's-foot trefoil	Sericea lespedeza	Ball clover	Korean lespedeza
Red clover		Hop clover	Soybean
White clover		Sweet clover	

than grass and cereal grain hays, generally containing two to three times more protein and calcium, and more soluble or nonfiber carbohydrates, beta-carotene, and vitamin E. Given the high concentrations of these nutrients, legumes are the preferred forage during growth, lactation, and the last three mos of pregnancy, if of good quality and available at a reasonable cost as compared to equal-quality grass or cereal grain hay.

The leaves are less firmly attached to the stem in legumes than in grasses. This can result in a greater loss of leaves from legumes if they are not cut at the proper stage of maturity, handled properly after cutting, or fed in a feeder that prevents their loss. Since leaves contain two-thirds of the energy, three-fourths of the protein, and most of the other nutrients present in forages, the loss of leaves greatly decreases the nutritional value, and therefore the quality of the hay. Most horses will generally consume more legume than grass hay, even if the legume hay is of poorer quality [10]. A particular risk of feeding alfalfa is the inadvertently feeding of Blister beetles. These beetles feed on weeds present in alfalfa fields and contain the toxin cantharidin, which causes GIT irritation and can be fatal to horses. Therefore, good pasture management practices involving weed and insect control are needed to ensure that alfalfa hay is free of blister beetles [11].

11.3.1.2 Grass

A variety of grasses are commonly fed, e.g. timothy, brome, fescue and orchard, Bermuda, blue, wheat, and ryegrasses (Table 11.2). The differences in their size and shape and a firmer attachment of the leaves in grass hay make leaf loss less of a problem than with legumes. This permits more latitude in the cutting and processing of grass hays with a lower risk of decreasing their nutritional value. Grass hays, compared with legumes, are usually less dusty, which results in less coughing for horses with chronic obstructive pulmonary disease or heaves and does not contain blister beetles. Within the same type of grass hay, the amount consumed is directly related to hay quality, i.e. the higher the hay quality the more hay the horse will consume. For equal-quality hays, the consumption of timothy by horses tends to be greater than brome, canary, and orchard grasses, which is greater than fescue and Bermudagrass [10]. Bahiagrass appears to be less palatable hay for horses [12].

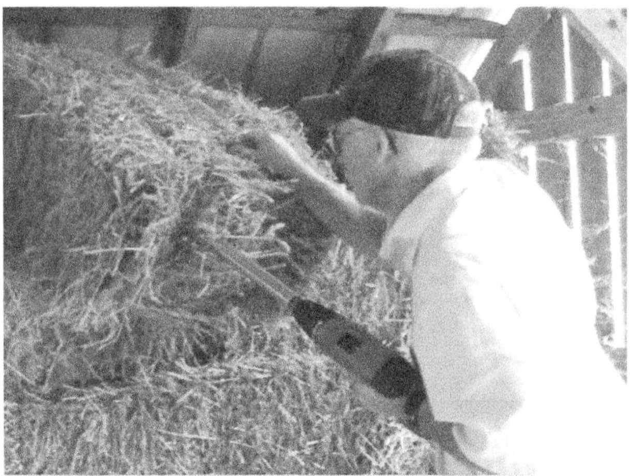

Figure 11.1 Collecting core hay samples for laboratory testing is performed using a 12 to 18 in probe attached to a drill which is inserted into the bale lengthwise. Sub-sampling 20% of the bales from each field or harvest should be composited into one representative sample for lab analysis.

11.3.1.3 Cereal Grains

Grain crops such as barley, wheat, oats, and triticale, a hybrid of wheat and rye, when still green and containing the grain, may be cut and used for hay (Table 11.2). The more grain they contain, the greater their nutritional value. Cereal grain hays are nutritionally similar to grass hays; however, if the seed heads, i.e. grain, are lost then only straw remains, which makes suitable bedding and a low-quality feed used as chaff.

11.3.2 Forms of Hay

Once sufficiently dried, the hay may be stacked loosely, baled, chopped, and/or compressed into cubes or pelleted for storage, transporting, and feeding. Dried long-stem hay may be processed into several different sizes of square or round bales. If long-stemmed hay is lacking in quality or availability, alternative sources of processed hay can be fed to horses to replace the forage in the ration. Alfalfa and grass hay further processing the into cubes or pellets are generally available year-round commercially. Several studies report no difference in DM, protein, fiber, energy, or any mineral digestibility, or in post feeding plasma glucose or insulin concentrations, in horses fed the same alfalfa hay either cubed, pelleted, chopped, or long-stemmed [13–15].

11.3.2.1 Square Bales

Small square bales weighing 45–70 lb are the traditional form of hay for horses (Figure 11.1), but more recently, medium square bales weighing 100–150 lb have become available [16]. Small square bales are easy to handle, suitable for traveling, and can be fed in stalls and the field. Small bales are better suited for feeding individual horses as the bale can be flaked apart and weighed for specific portion feedings (feed two flakes of hay q 4 hrs). Although small square bales can be handled by one person, overall these are more expensive to feed due to the low DM density, i.e. 11 lb hay/ft^3. Medium (900 lb) and large (1800 lb) rectangular bales with a higher DM density of 15 lb/ft^3 are more economical to transport and store. These larger bales are more suited for large horse operations but require larger storage facilities and greater horsepower (HP) tractors, i.e. 100–150 HP to maneuver [16, 17]. Some large rectangular balers combined small bales that may be appropriate for smaller horse operations. One advantage to large square bales over round bales is that large "flakes" can be fed to groups of horses managed in a field or paddock minimizing the risk of waste and molding with some degree of portion control.

11.3.2.2 Round Bales

Small (500–600 lb) and large (850–1900 lb) round hay bales have a DM density of 12 lb hay/ft^3 and may be wrapped with string, netting, or plastic for protection [17]. These bales are not suitable for feeding horses individually or while traveling but are appropriate for feeding groups of horses. The weight of these bales requires a medium or greater horsepower tractor, i.e. >30 HP) to maneuver. Although the shape does naturally shed water, these bales should be stored and fed

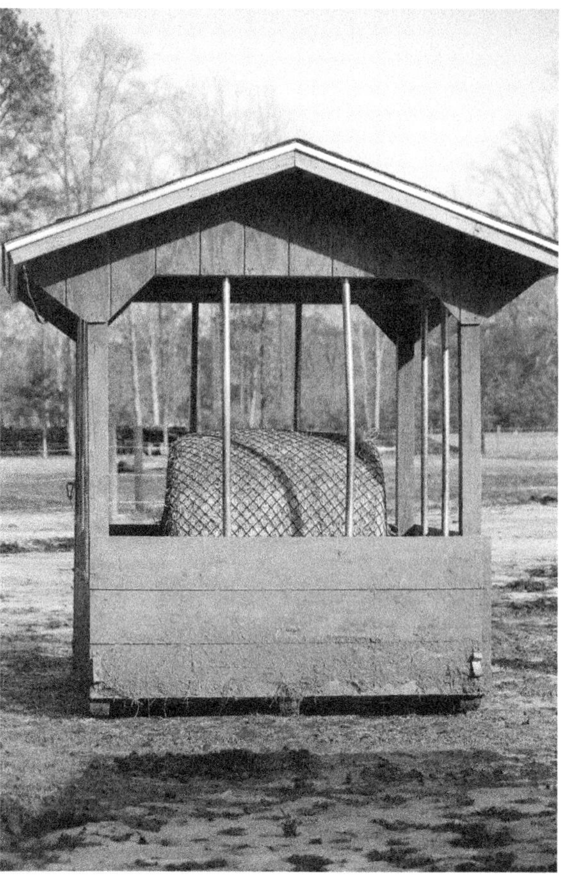

Figure 11.2 Round bale (600 lb) wrapped in a hay net fed undercover.

undercover (Figure 11.2) [16]. Round bales cannot be stacked as efficiently as square bales, and large round bales are susceptible to molding and bacterial contamination by *Clostridium botulinum*, which is a fatal disease.

11.3.2.3 Chopped

Most horses may prefer chopped to long-stemmed grass hay. The major advantage of chopping hay is to be mixed with grain and slow the rate of grain consumption; however, horses can easily separate the grain from chopped hay [18–20].

11.3.2.4 Cubes

In cubing, sun-cured hay is chopped and coarsely ground before being compressed into 1.25″ $(\text{in.})^2$ rectangular blocks that break apart every 2″–3″ in. to form a cube (Figure 11.3). Cubing is done by farm equipment that moves across hayfields picking up windrows of hay. It may take a few days for some horses to learn to eat hay cubes, and then the cubes will be consumed faster than loose hay. In one study, eating time was reduced from an average of 4.4–3.8 hrs by mares fed twice daily the same weight of the same alfalfa hay loose or cubed [21]. As a result of the more rapid rate of consumption, some horses may choke on cubed hay, but then these can be soaked in water before feeding. Wood chewing has been reported in horses fed cubes as the only form of forage [5]. However, there was no difference in the amount of wood consumed by mature mares when fed the same alfalfa hay loose or cubed either twice or three times daily [21].

11.3.2.5 Pellets

Hay is usually fed in a loose form, but could be compressed into pellets (Figure 11.3). Pelleting is agglomerated feed or feeds by compacting and forcing through die openings using a mechanical process (Figure 13.3). In pelleting, hay is finely ground and often artificially dehydrated before being compressed into small (0.25″×0.5″) or large (0.5″×1″) pellets using a pellet mill. Excessive heating of

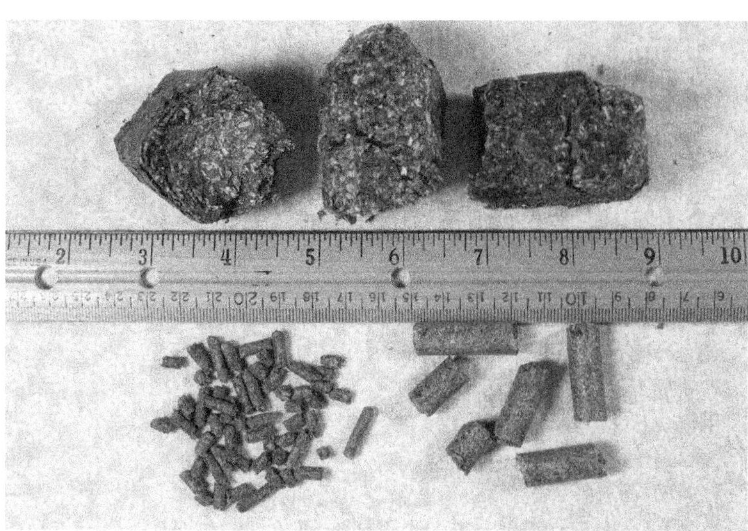

Figure 11.3 Alfalfa hay pressed into cubes (top). Grass hay compressed into large pellets (lower right). Vitamin mineral supplement compressed with soybean meal and wheat middlings into small pellets (lower left).

feeds generally lowers nutritional value by destroying vitamins and inducing the formation of indigestible protein–carbohydrate bonds. Although heat is used in dehydrating the hay, and some heat is produced within the pellet during production, pelleting does not affect the nutritional value of most hays. In one study, there was no difference in nutrient digestibility between loose, chopped, pelleted, or cubed alfalfa hay fed to horses [13]. However, the pellet form does result in a faster rate of food passage through the GIT and altered the rate of eating. Weanlings and yearlings consumed a pelleted ration more quickly than those fed the same ration not pelleted, 1.3 vs. 1.8 hrs, but with no difference in digestibility [22].

Wood chewing has been reported in horses fed pellets as the only source of forage [5]. In one study, nearly four times more wood chewed, i.e. 312 vs. 82 g of wood/H/d, occurred when pellets vs. long-stem hay were fed, respectively [23]. However, feeding pellets six times vs. once daily did decrease wood chewing by about 50%. Similarly, horses fed just hay pellets spent 3.5 hrs more foraging through wood-shaving bedding daily compared with long stem hay [24].

Fecal water content is lower when pellets vs. long-stem hay are fed, i.e. 75.2 vs. 81.5% [14]. The significance of lower fecal water on horse health is not known. Theoretically, there may be an increased risk of feed impaction in the intestines, although no data is supporting this association. Although impaction due to feeding pellets is not known to occur in horses, the recommendation to feed all horses at least 0.5 lb of long-stem hay or pasture forage/100 lb BW daily while feeding hay cubes or pellets has been made based on studies in cattle [25]. Feeding 25% of the forage as long-stem hay may decrease the risk of gastrointestinal problems and decrease wood chewing when pellets are fed.

The advantages of cubed and pelleted hay are the following:

1) Less wastage while feeding the horse. In cattle-fed baled hay, the wastage was 9% compared to a 4% loss when pelleted or cubed hay was fed. Similar losses might be expected for horses. Additionally, loss of leaves, particularly from legume hays, during harvesting and feeding, is lessened with cubes and pellets [14]. Since leaves contain most of the nutrients in the hay, decreasing their loss results in greater nutrient value being obtained from cubes and pellets than from long-stem hay. This was reflected in one study in which mares fed cubes gained 12 vs. 2 lb by matched mares fed the same weight of the same hay loose [21].
2) More feed can be consumed. When pellets are fed, intestinal fill may be reduced, so that as much as 20–30% more pelleted feed than loose forage can be consumed. This is of benefit if additional feed intake is needed. A decrease in intestinal fill also makes some horses look trimmer, with less of a "hay belly" appearance.
3) Less storage space. A ton of hay cubes occupies 60–70 ft^3, as compared with 200–330 ft^3 for each ton of baled hay and 450–600 ft^3 for each ton of loose hay [26].
4) Reduced transportation costs.
5) Ease of transport for feeding away from home.
6) Minimal dust when eaten, if made properly. This is an important advantage for horses, in which the dust or fungal spores in loose hay contribute to chronic obstructive pulmonary disease or heaves and coughing.
7) Facilitated automation in both harvesting and feeding.
8) Reduced manure production. If horses eating loose alfalfa were switched to pelleted alfalfa hay, the fecal output decreased from 37 to 28 lb manure/H/d [14]. However, digestibility was the same and, therefore, the lower amount of feces produced when pellets were fed was entirely due to lower fecal water content (75.2 vs. 81.5%). There was, therefore, no difference in fecal DM excreted.

11.3.3 Hay Cuttings

Depending on growing conditions, from one to as many as eight cuttings of hay may be obtained in a season in some areas. The first cutting of the season is generally high in nutritional value if harvested at the proper time and does not contain weeds that have grown up since the last cut in the previous season. Drying and baling the first cut of hay at the proper time and avoiding rain after cutting are more difficult earlier than later in the haying season.

Plant growth is generally fastest during the warmest part of the growing season if moisture is not a limiting factor. Rapid growth rates result in more stem and fewer leaves, which decreases the plant's nutritional value. However, later cuttings, when the temperature is cooler, generally have a higher leaf and nutrient content, the fewest weeds, and in many areas, the best opportunity of harvesting without raining on the cut hay, and, therefore, may have the highest feeding value. Thus, there is no reliable statement that can be made concerning which cut of hay has the highest nutritional value. In selecting hay, the major consideration is not the type of hay or the cutting, but the quality of the hay, availability, and nutritional content relative to cost and ease of handling.

11.3.4 Hay Grades and Relative Feed Value

The major factors that determine the quality of hay are the stage of maturity at harvest, weather and handling during harvesting, and the duration and conditions of storage.

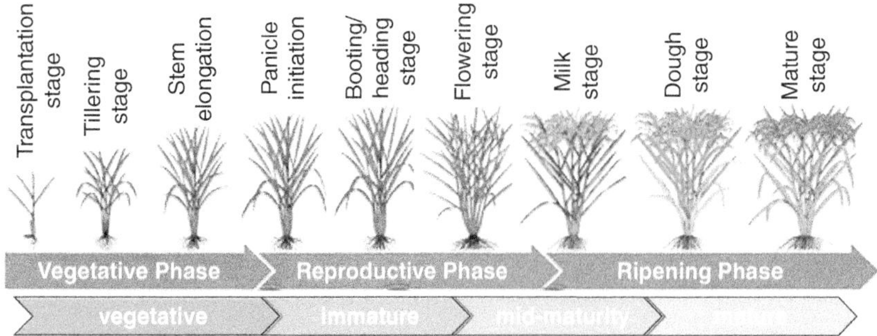

Figure 11.4 Growth stages of grass plants [28]. The forage should be harvested in the boot stage when the seed head begins to show through the sheath. *Source:* Kawamura et al. [28].

As the plant matures, energy and protein content and digestibility decrease. Just before the time legumes flower (the bud stage) or when seed heads become visible through the sheath of grasses (early head or boot stage), the leaf development has been completed and the forage should be harvested [27]. As legumes mature from full bud to full bloom, and grasses mature from the boot stage to complete heading out, one-half of the protein and one-third of the energy content are lost resulting in decreased total digestible nutrient intake and feeding value of that forage (Figure 11.4).

A measure of feeding, and market value of hay, was developed by the American Forage and Grasslands Council and shown in Table 11.3. Although this system is based on the feeding value of forages to ruminants and *in vitro* experiments, the overall grading scheme appears to apply to horses. As the plant matures, structural carbohydrates, i.e. ADF and NDF fractions, increase. These fiber fractions represent the indigestible parts of the plant that has been negatively correlated with voluntary feed intake and digestibility. The relationship between the feeding value of hay for ruminants, ADF, and NDF concentrations is as follows:

- Forage digestible dry matter (% DDM) = 88.9 − (0.779 × % ADF).
- Forage dry matter intake (% DMI) = 120/% NDF.
- Forage relative feeding value (RFV) = % DDM × % DMI × 0.775.

Although negatively correlated, forage NDF concentration is the best predictor of voluntary forage intake, whereas ADF concentration is the best indicator of forage digestibility in ruminants [29]. Relative feed value continues to be widely used as an index by which to assess forage quality and compare across different forage varieties and the pricing of hay [31].

It is usually best to select the highest quality hay available; however, for many horses, it is more important for the hay to be well preserved than to have a high nutrient content. Hay should be selected based on the needs of the individual horse. Growth, reproduction, and exercise require higher quality hay, but horses at maintenance may only require hay with a quality standard score of 3 or less (Table 11.3) [26]. Although feeding good-quality hay is certainly preferred and recommended, if the only feed available is poor, i.e. weathered (no mold, low dust), low leaf to high stem fractions, weeds, or nutritionally deficient hay, the recommendation is to offer larger quantities of the poor-quality hay. Horses will sort through the hay offered and eat only the better portions. If lesser amounts of poor-quality hay are offered, the horse is then "forced" to eat the poorer quality portions of the hay or consume less than an adequate quantity of feed to meet energy needs. Regardless of the hay grade, under no circumstances should moldy, dusty hay, or that containing poisonous weeds or insects should be offered to horses, i.e. low or poor hygienic hay. In other words, there is a distinct difference between feeding nutritionally poor-quality hay and that which may cause disease.

11.3.5 Feeding Management of Hay

Hay should be fed in a manner that minimizes nutritional leaf losses, fecal contamination of the forage, and dust inhalation, but allows for natural feeding behaviors of horses. As grazing animals, horses have an instinct to consume feed from the ground. Although consuming feed from the ground is the natural feeding position of the horse's head, feed losses are considerably higher compared with feeding forage from a feeder. Weanlings fed hay on the ground had an 18% lower average daily gain and feed efficiency than when fed an equal amount of the same hay in a feeder [32].

Feed losses when hay is fed on the ground are due to a greater loss of nutritious leaf material that is trampled and

Table 11.3 Marketing grades and relative feed value of forages[a].

Grade	Species and stage	Composition				
		Crude protein %	ADF %	NDF %	DDM %	RFV
Prime	Legume, prebloom	>19	<31	<40	>65	>151
1	Legume, early bloom, 20% grass-vegetative	17–19	31–35	40–46	62–65	125–151
2	Legume, mid-bloom, 30% grass-early-head	14–16	36–40	47–53	58–61	101–124
3	Legume, full bloom, 40% grass-headed	11–13	41–42	54–60	56–57	86–100
4	Legume, full bloom, 50% grass-headed	8–10	43–45	61–65	53–55	77–85
Fair	Grass, headed and/or rain-damaged	<8	>45	>65	<53	<77

[a] All quality parameters are based on 100% dry matter (DM); ADF: acid detergent fiber; NDF: neutral detergent fiber; DDM: digestible DM; DMI: DM intake, RFV: relative feed value is the relationship between the feeding and economic values of different forages. For example, grade prime hay would be worth at least 1.96 times (151/77) the price of grade fair hay. RFV = (DDM × DMI)/1.29, where DDM = 88.9 − (0.779 × % ADF) and DMI = 120/% NDF.

Source: Based on Ball et al. [26]; Rohweder et al. [29]; Rocateli and Zhang [30].

contaminated with urine and manure (Figure 11.5). Horses tend not to move off from the feeding area to urinate or defecate and mark the eliminations of herd mates with their feces, which creates piles of fecal material in and around the feeding area. When hay is placed in a feed bunk, most horses will pull mouthfuls of hay to the ground. Of the time spent eating in which all hay was initially placed in a feed bunk, horses spent 59% of the time eating from the ground vs. 42% from the bunk [34]. Although, horses prefer to feed on the ground, possibly > 50% is not eaten because horses have an aversion to feeding near fecal material regardless of the palatability of the forage [16, 34]. Hay nets with mesh openings from 1″ to 1.75″ do not allow horses to remove large wade of hay from the bale. Instead, horses must remove several strands of hay through the mesh openings using lips and teeth more similar to the grazing rate on pasture (Figure 11.5).

Harvested forages should be fed in a hay container or rack that catches leaves and loose forage, and that keeps as much forage as possible off the ground. Hay should not be fed in a deep-sided container where fine hay particles, dust, and mold collect at the bottom and then possibly inhaled while the horse's head is in the container. Yet the feed container should be high enough off the ground to prevent the horse from stepping into the bunk at the risk of injury, i.e. at or higher than the horse's elbow. Conversely, hay consumption from a feed bunk or feeder or net placed above the horse's withers increases material getting into the eyes, nose, and dust inhalation while eating, which in turn increases the risk and occurrence of respiratory problems such as coughing, emphysema, heaves, exercise-induced pulmonary hemorrhage, inflammatory airway disease, and increased susceptibility to infectious respiratory diseases [35]. Therefore, the recommendation is to feed harvested long-stem forages from hay racks designed to catch falling leaves and loose hay at a height between the horse's elbow and withers (Figure 11.6). Pellets and cubes can be fed from a bucket or trough in the same recommended height range.

11.3.5.1 Group Feeding

Feeding a large amount of hay to a group of horses is time, cost, and labor efficient. However, group feeding does allow an individual horse to overeat in that feed consumed per horses (H)/d may not be monitored or controlled. Monitoring for weight gain and condition in each horse will indicate a possible problem of excessive feed intake. Horses should be grouped by nutritional needs, such that low maintenance horses are not fed with horses requiring high-energy hay. A horse gaining weight within a group feeding situation may need to be removed from that group. Conversely, monitoring for losses in body weight and condition of the more submissive horses within the group will indicate a possible problem with access to the feeder. Within a group, a social hierarchy will exist and become apparent when resources, i.e. feed or water, become limited. See Chapter 16 Feeding and Drinking Behaviors. Therefore, hay feeders or racks, feed bunks, or troughs must have ample "head" room for all horses in the group to feed contentedly. Incidence of dominance, biting, and kicking should be minimal to lower the risk of injuries. The use of several feeding stations with sufficient space between feeders may be necessary to discourage a dominant horse from controlling more than one feeder at a time. Another option is to remove the low BW horse from the group once or twice daily to offer a high-energy feed separate from the group.

When feeding large round or square bales to groups of horses, the hay may only have to be fed out once or twice a week. Therefore, the hay should be placed in a covered feeder

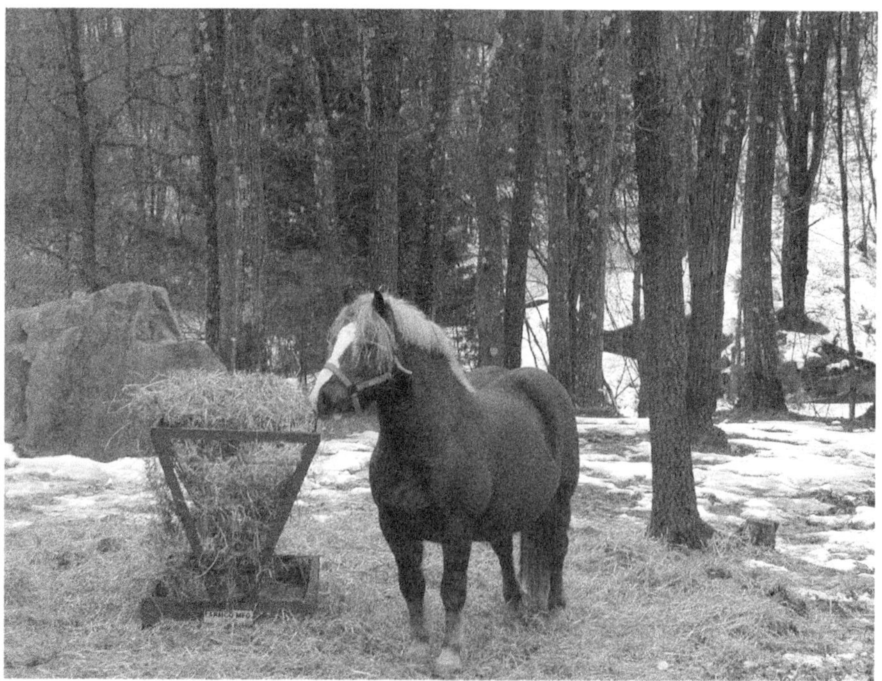

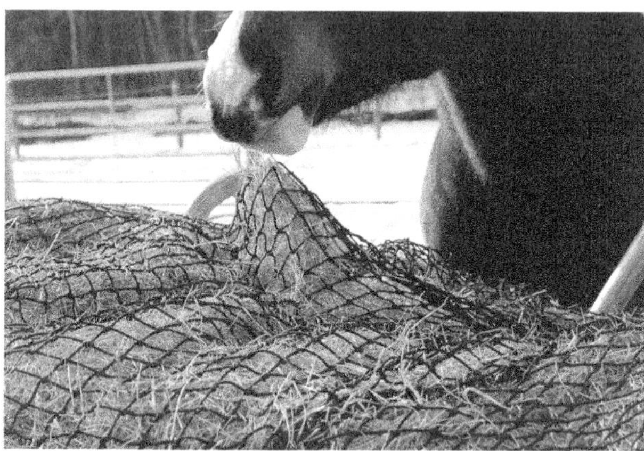

Figure 11.5 Top: Excess hay in an open feeder allows for waste due to weather, trampling, urine, and manure contamination. Bottom: Hay bale wrapped in hay net requires the horse to pull a few strands of hay at a time through the 1.25 in mesh openings minimizing waste.

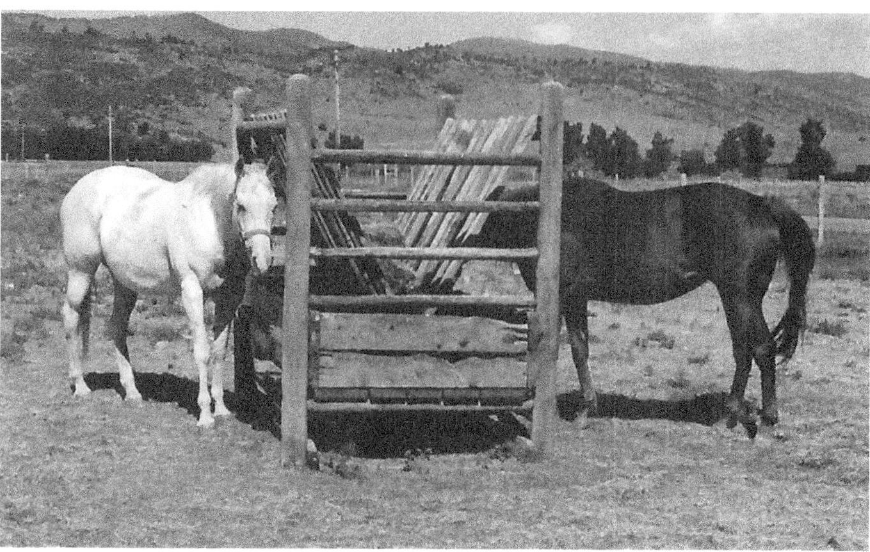

Figure 11.6 Hayrack feeders allow the horse to see while eating. The tray under the rack catches leaves and loose hay, minimizing loss and dust inhalation and could be used for feeding cubed or pelleted hay, or grain and supplement.

to keep the forage dry (Figure 11.2). The hay waste using eight different makes of round bale feeders, three covered and five uncovered, was compared to feeding horses on the ground. Horses wasted 57% of the hay fed on the ground, whereas 13–33% was lost from various uncovered types vs. 5–11% lost from covered feeders [36]. The specific feeder needed depends on the number of horses, shape, and size of the bale, and the equipment available to maneuver the bale [16].

11.3.5.2 Individual Feeding

There are advantages and disadvantages to all feeding systems. Feeding horses individually is labor-intensive, time-consuming, and more costly than group feeding; however, there are several advantages, such as portion control, customizing the ration, and the ability to monitor appetite and feed intake.

Portion control feeding, a specific quantity at specific time intervals to individual horses, is most commonly used to induce weight changes or in those horses with high-energy needs. Feeding a low-quality, or late maturity, hay at the minimum recommended quantities in frequent small meals is needed to promote weight loss [3]. Obese horses should be fed clean, weed-free hay that is low in digestible energy in small frequent meals throughout a 24-hr period. Feeding restricted quantities frequently will minimize waste as the horse will most likely eat all of the hay offered. See Feeding for Weight Loss in Chapter 23. Conversely, horses needing more calories to regain or maintain weight are likely to achieve maximum voluntary DM intake when hay is available at all times than those fed meals during daylight hours only. Feeding excessive amounts of hay once or twice daily does foster more waste as the horse will sift through the hay only consuming the more palatable parts and leaving the stems. Therefore, feeding appropriate amounts frequently rather than excessive amounts two or three times daily is recommended to minimize waste. See Feeding for Weight Gain in Chapter 23.

The feeding program and ration can be individualized for horses fed separately. Several different types and forms of hay may be fed in various quantities as needed. For example, a horse may feed on long-stem grass hay ad libitum while in the herd but then be separated each day to consume a specific quantity of cubed or pelleted alfalfa to achieve a specific protein intake. When horses are fed individually, appetite and feed intake can be monitored daily. Quantifying the feed intake is the first step to resolving a problem related to body weight. Feed offered minus that feed wasted must be quantified to accurately calculate the nutrient intake. Hence, when an obese horse is not losing weight as expected, knowing the current intake of calories is needed to adjust the weight loss feeding plan. Likewise, when a horse is losing weight or not gaining as expected, assessing appetite by quantifying the feed consumed and then calculating caloric intake is essential information when considering the next ration change. There is also valuable information in knowing that the caloric intake is appropriate, but the horse is still losing or not gaining weight, which then should lead to further investigation of the individual horse medically.

Many horses are permanently housed in individual stalls or small paddocks or dry lots (stallions, performance, and convalescing horses). Horses in highly populated areas where acreage or pasture space is limited or nonexistent may be housed in a stall with a few hours of outdoor socialization time daily in a drylot. Putting aside the ethical dilemma, housing horses in an isolated confined space presents several unique nutritional issues to consider. Horses will often consume all of the hay at once when fed a limited amount in confinement leading to long periods without access to feed. The lack of access to forage may lead to behavioral problems called stereotypies, including cribbing, wood chewing, and weaving [37].

The equine GIT is designed for a slow constant input of fibrous feeds. Horses naturally eat multiple "meals" frequently throughout the day and night, most intensively in the early morning and evening but never voluntarily go for more than 3 or 4 hrs without eating. When horses are fed only 2 or 3 meals/d, often 6 to 8 hrs apart, the secretion of gastric HCl acid continues and may ulcerate the stomach lining [2]. Stabled horses have been shown to have a low gastric pH during early morning hours (0100–0900) when the stomach tends to be empty [38]. Several nutritional risk factors, such as gastric ulcer syndrome, colic, and diarrhea, have been associated with a low long-stem forage intake. Therefore, it is recommended that horses have free choice access to hay when pasture is not available to avoid gastrointestinal disorders.

Horses maintained on pasture spend an average of 14–18 hrs/d grazing, thus attempts to mimic this natural feeding behavior of horses should be made for permanently or temporarily individually housed horses. Hay can be fed on the stall floor, from a rack or net, and the estimates of hay waste or loss will be the same as that for group feeding. Stalled horses defecate on average once every 90 min [33]. Therefore, fecal and urine contamination of long-stem hay on the stall floor is a substantial cause of hay waste for confined horses. Feeding cubes or pellets in the stall would decrease forage waste; however, given the propensity of horses to spend less time eating cubes or pellets and the risk of gastric ulceration, feeding long-stem hay would be advisable. Long-stem hay has been shown to result in greater chewing time and almost twice as much saliva secretion occurs compared with feeding pellets [39]. The rack or hanging net should be no higher than the horse's withers to avoid respiratory disorders and should have a bin or tray to catch hay material. Hay bins in the stall should be constructed such that the horse cannot step into the bin. In summary, stalled horses should have access to forage throughout the 24-hr period. Adjusting the hay quantity, quality, and digestibility as needed for the individual horse will be necessary to manage weight, body condition and stable vices.

There is no best feeding system for individually housed horses; however, the feeds and method of feeding must take foremost into account the nutrient needs, health, and safety of the horse, while the convenience and economics are secondary. Separating a horse daily from a herd for specialized feeding might be the best situation if plausible. Low body weight, young, old, or recuperating horses routinely running within a group of horses but needing a specialized ration could be separated from the herd for a short time each day to meal feed a specific quantity of a specific feed. If there is a size difference between horses in the herd, e.g. young horses and mares, a creep feeder may be useful. See Chapter 21 Feeding Growing Horses.

Sidebar 11.1: USA Geographic Distribution of Forage Species

The pasture grasses that generally produce the most forage and provide the best nourishment to the horse in different geographic regions of the United States are as follows:

Florida, Georgia, and the Gulf coast – pangola or other digitgrasses, Bahia varieties, and coastal Bermudagrass.
Middle Atlantic – coastal Bermudagrass, orchardgrass, bluegrass, tall fescue, and white, red, and ladino clovers.
Northeast – redtop, orchardgrass, reed canarygrass, Kentucky bluegrass, and timothy.
Midwest – smooth bromegrass, buffalo grass, bluestem, grama, and tall fescue.
Southwest – coastal Bermudagrass and ryegrass.
Northwest – fescue, bentgrass, bluestem, grama, and crested wheatgrass.
Far West – orchardgrass, coastal Bermudagrass, lovegrass, Rhodesgrass, and rescue bromegrass.

11.4 Pasture

Properly managed pastures provide the ideal environment for most horses both nutritionally and behaviorally. Pastures allow voluntary physical movement and social interactions which promotes healthy behavior. Feral horses evolved and still thrive, based on body condition and reproductive rates, on rangelands of low-quality forages [40]. However, this is not a fair comparison to domesticated horses in that feral horses travel (5–15 miles/d), to consume sufficient quantities of nutrients from thousands of acres of sparse vegetation and isolated watering locations [41]. Conversely, domesticated horses walk far less to obtain pasture grass or water. It is possible therefore for a domesticated horse to become obese on pasture given the considerably less exercise required to graze and the high-energy nutrient concentrations in cultivated pastures. The nutritional value of pasture for horses depends on the amount consumed and the quality of the forage. See Sidebar 11.1. When properly managed, even a small pasture can greatly decrease feeding costs, can provide all or a substantial amount of the feed and nutrients needed by a horse, reduced management chores such as cleaning stalls daily and feeding hay, and improve the horse's quality of life. However, poorly managed pastures that are overgrazed, have inadequate irrigation, fertilization, weed and insect control may decrease, possibly eliminate, all the benefits a pasture may provide.

Immature plants are nutritious and more palatable than older plants; however, quantity of feed per acre is lower. Digestible energy and protein content of tall fescue and orchardgrass decreased by 50% from spring to fall, and by winter, were negligible [42]. Many pastures begin to change from an emerald green color early on to a dark green to a slightly gray color at the best time for harvesting, and then with increasing maturity to yellowish brown. Proper pasture and grazing management are necessary if the horse is to obtain the maximum total amount of nutrients and, therefore, benefit from the pasture year after year. Most properly managed pastures contain several different types of forage and provide adequate concentrations of nutrients for the adult maintenance horse throughout most of the year depending on location and climate (Table 11.4). Differences between the forage concentration and that required by the horse based on life stage, training or imposed work should be provided in a supplement or complementary feed.

Horses are selective grazers and graze closer to the ground than cattle and tend to repeatedly graze the same areas of a pasture that challenges management in maintaining good vegetative cover. Intake of forage by horses with free access to pasture ranges from 1.5 to 3.1% BW/d with an average of 2% BW/d [4]. The class of horses may affect their forage intake. For example, lactating mares have been shown to have consumption rates higher than other life stages of horses given free access to pasture. The environmental conditions may also affect forage intake. For example, during hot days horses will seek shade and graze less whereas when temperatures are cooler at night, grazing time is increased. When relying on pastures to meet the nutrient requirements of horses, seasonal variation in available forage should be considered. Proper

Table 11.4 Nutrient content of mixed central Kentucky pasture forage[a] compared with adult horse requirement[b].

Nutrient	DM units	Adult maintenance requirement	Spring	Summer	Fall	Winter
Digestible energy	Mcal/kg	2.00	2.57	2.42	2.80	2.44
Crude protein	%	8.00	14.70	13.10	16.60	13.80
Calcium	%	0.24	0.37	0.40	0.43	0.47
Phosphorus	%	0.17	0.27	0.28	0.33	0.27
Magnesium	%	0.09	0.17	0.22	0.26	0.20
Zinc	mg/kg	40	28	20	31	28
Copper	mg/kg	10	15	10	17	20

[a] All values are the average in the forage dry matter from 11 pastures consisting of about 50% bluegrass, 30% tall fescue, and 20% orchardgrass. Seasonal variation was the same in all three kinds of grasses but different in degree: variation in energy, and protein content, being greatest in orchardgrass and least in fescue.
[b] 500 kg adult horse consuming 2% BW/d.
Source: Based on NRC [4, 5] and Jackson and Pagan [43].

pasture management increases the quality of the forage and is the best method for weed prevention. Well-managed pastures provide optimal nutrition for horses and prevent adverse environmental impacts from erosion and surface runoff. Maintaining healthy soil, appropriate forage species, plant management, weed control, and proper grazing strategies all play a role in pasture management [44].

11.4.1 Soil Testing and Fertility

Productive pastures start with healthy and fertile soil. A soil test is important for several reasons: optimize forage production, protect the environment from excessive applications of fertilizer which contaminate surrounding land and water, ensure the proper nutritional balance for the desirable species of pasture plants, and energy conservation of fuel in applying only the amount and type of fertilizer needed by farm equipment [45].

Soil testing is a simple and inexpensive first step to proper pasture management. Testing should be performed on soil from each pasture or field every 2–3 yrs to identify if pH should be adjusted and/or the correct type and amount of fertilizer, i.e. nitrogen (N), phosphorus (P), potassium (K), and trace minerals, are needed to provide nutrients for plant growth and health. Soil samples are collected by walking in a zigzag or "W" pattern across the field. Samples are collected using a probe to a depth of 4–6 in (Figure 11.7). The top one inch of plant material (leaves, stems, roots), if present should be discarded. For a pasture up to 10 ac, 20 samples should be collected and subsequently mixed

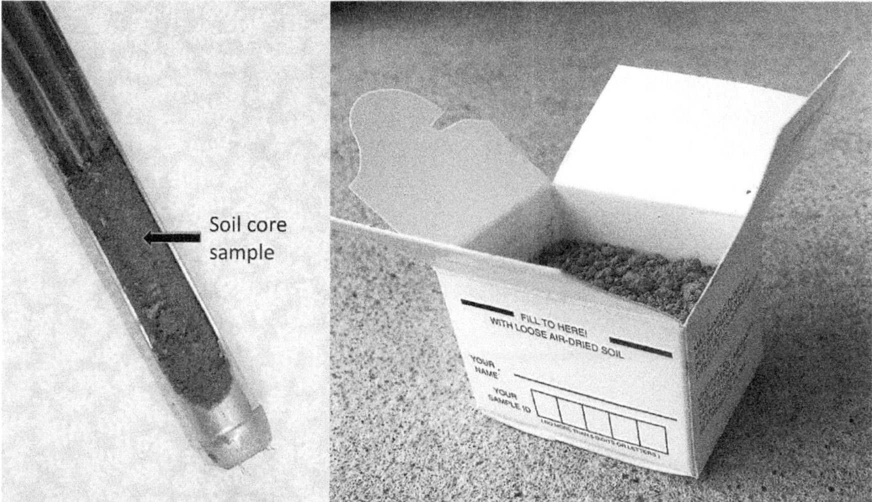

Figure 11.7 Soil probe with a core of soil (left). A single well-mixed and air-dried composite sample (right) from at least 20 randomized locations should be submitted for pastures of 10 or less. It is important not to overfill the box and to label distinctly such that the results refer to specific pastures or locations within a pasture.

thoroughly to form a composite sample removing stones, roots, insects, etc. A single well-mixed and air-dried sample, in approximately 1 cup volume, should be submitted for pastures that are 10 ac or less (Figure 11.7). Larger pastures or pastures with varying topography may require a greater number of composited samples. It is important to label the sample boxes so that the test results can easily be identified to a location. Soil sample boxes and supplies can be obtained from most land grant university agricultural extension offices or farm service retail providers.

Applying lime and fertilizer to pastures at rates indicated by the soil test is important to maintaining proper soil pH and fertility. Lime, i.e. ag-grade limestone, is applied to increase and maintain proper pH for the specific desirable plants in a pasture. Different forage has different optimal pH ranges; however, generally low soil pH reduces nutrient uptake by plants and binds some nutrients that render the nutrient unavailable to the plant. Lime is available in two forms, pulverized dust or pellets. Both work equally as well, although the pelleted form is easier to apply but more expensive. It is not necessary to remove horses from pastures after applying limestone as lime is not toxic, but horses can be removed until rain or after a heavy dew to avoid intake of the dusty pulverized form. Lime should be applied in the autumn because at least six mos is required to change the soil pH and foster nitrogen uptake in the following spring [46]. Fertilizers including N, P, and K should be applied to pastures when the forage is actively growing in the early spring and autumn. Warm-season grasses like bermudagrass should be fertilized in the late spring after regrowth begins, i.e. green-up. The recommendation is to remove horses from pastures until N, P, and K fertilizers have dissolved usually after 0.5″ rainfall or a few mornings of heavy dew.

11.4.2 Forage Selection

Pasture forage may be one or, often preferably, a combination of different types of plants. A combination of grasses may benefit each other, extend the grazing time in a pasture, provide a varied forage ration to horses, and create a more sustainable grassland ecosystem [47]. There are more than 60 species of forages that are grown in the southern USA alone [26]. There are three criteria for categorizing forages: [i] grasses vs. legumes; [ii] annuals vs. perennials; and [iii] cool season vs. warm season (Table 11.2).

11.4.2.1 Grasses

Grasses are herbaceous plants that produce one seed leaf, i.e. monocots, with parallel leaf veins, fibrous root systems, and a seed head on an elongated stem. Grasses can tolerate humid weather, cold weather, and poor soil conditions better than legumes, and can persist and maintain production with relatively less management.

11.4.2.2 Legumes

Legumes produce two seed leaves, i.e. dicots, produce seeds in pods, and many have a taproot system. Legumes, i.e. alfalfa, clovers, vetch, and birdsfoot trefoil, have a symbiotic relationship with bacteria that enables the utilization of atmospheric and soil nitrogen for the production of plant protein. The legumes grow during periods in which warm-season perennial pasture grasses grow little or not at all, thereby prolonging seasonal forage production from the pasture. Alfalfa and red clover are more palatable for most horses than equal-quality grasses.

11.4.2.3 Annual Plants

Annual plants that live for a single growing season reproduce only by seed, must be reseeded every year but are generally higher in nutrients than perennials, with the cool-season annuals generally being higher than warm-season annuals.

11.4.2.3.1 Cool-Season Plants

Cereal grains have high nutritional value for the horse for a short spring grazing period without decreasing yield when harvested for grain and straw later that summer. Winter wheat (*Triticum aestivum*) is commonly grazed by horses during early spring, and one to two additional months of grazing can be obtained if the wheat is not to be harvested. The forage obtained is higher in digestible energy and protein content than alfalfa, and is generally adequate in mineral content for all horses >18 mos old.

11.4.2.3.2 Warm-Season Plants

Sorghums, Sudangrass, and Johnson grasses are generally of limited value for horse pastures; however, pearl millet and Teff grass are especially useful as supplemental forage during some periods. Pearl millet appears to be a good pasture forage that is widely used in some areas for horses, with no problems reported. Teff grass may be grown to have a lower water-soluble sugar and starch content which may benefit some horses.

11.4.2.4 Perennial Plants

Perennial plants live for many years, reproduce by seed or rhizomes and stolons, and require the least investment to maintain.

11.4.2.4.1 Cool-Season Plants

Common grass hays for horses, i.e. timothy, orchardgrass, fescue, and bluegrass, produce two times of the year: spring and autumn when temperatures are cool, but go dormant in the summer and coldest winter months. Spring growth is about 60%, whereas fall growth is about 40% of the total annual yield.

11.4.2.4.2 *Warm-Season Plants*

Perennials, i.e. Bermudagrass and Bahiagrass, are most productive during the summer months and do not persist under cooling or cold temperatures. These grasses tolerate trampling, drought, and close grazing better than most other grasses. These high-yielding grasses often provide three or more cuttings per year, and the stand can be maintained indefinitely when properly fertilized and serve best as a hay crop or in a rotational grazing program.

11.4.3 Nutritional Considerations in Pasture Plant Selection

Grasses are the primary forage species used in horse pastures because; in general, grasses are persistent and more productive than legumes. Cool-season grasses are the dominant species in temperate climates and provide superior nutrition for most classes and types of horses. Overall, the nutritional value of warm-season grasses tends to be lower than cool-season grasses, largely due to the environmental conditions under which these grasses grow and develop. Warm-season grasses persist under hot temperatures and intense light, which increases the rate of growth and decreases the leaf to stem ratio, resulting in lower energy nutrient concentration and an increase in the structural carbohydrates and lignin. Still, warm-season grasses do provide excellent nutrition and some advantage to horses in hot climates where cool-season grasses will not grow (Table 11.1).

Cool-season forages adapted to cool, wet environments fix the carbon dioxide into a three-carbon compound and are called C3 plants. Warm-season forages adapted to hot, sunny environments fix the CO_2 into a four-carbon compound and are called C4 plants [48]. Cool-season C3 pasture grasses store energy as the sugar fructan in stems, while legumes and C4 plants store energy as starch in leaves. Fructan C3 grasses taste "sweeter," are more palatable and likely induce overconsumption relative to C4 grasses and legumes. See Nonstructural Carbohydrates and Figure 6.2 in Chapter 6. In addition to genetics, diurnal and seasonal variations in temperature, moisture, and sunlight affect the NSC content of the forage. Grazing patterns, pasture management, and haying techniques also affect the NSC content of the forage. However, overall, the NSC content in warm-season grasses is lower than cool-season species and is a better choice for horses at risk of metabolic and digestive disorders, such as insulin resistance, laminitis, obesity, and colic [7].

Legumes increase the nutritional value of grass forages. Under optimal growing conditions, legumes, particularly the leaves, are slightly higher in digestible energy, substantially higher CP, lysine, and calcium, and lower NDF, ADF, and phosphorus than grasses [34]. A pasture established with a mixture of grasses and legumes will be more sustainable because legumes effectively self-fertilize through nitrogen fixation [49]. For these reasons, seeding legumes with grasses or into established grass pastures is generally beneficial. A common practice is to overseed Ladino (white) clover into pastures. Alfalfa, fed alone or mixed with cool-season grasses, is suitable for horses with increased nutritional requirements. Blister beetles feed on weeds present in alfalfa fields, which causes deadly cantharidin poisoning in horses, hence monitoring for weed and the beetle is critical to horse health.

While both pasture and hay samples can be analyzed by commercial laboratories to determine nutrient content, pasture sampling, however, is challenging because nutrients fluctuate widely depending on environmental conditions, e.g. time of day, season, sunlight, and weather conditions. Sampling the pasture should be done in a manner resembling a horse's consumption. Observe the horse grazing to determine the grazing height, i.e. if the horses are leaving 4 in of grass stubble, the grazing height is 4 in. The grass sampled should then be any length of grass above 4 in. Similar to soil and hay sample collections, randomly collect subsamples from a minimum of 15–20 locations throughout a 10 ac or less pasture avoiding areas the horses would avoid, i.e. manure piles, trampled areas near gates, watering troughs, and weed patches. Larger pastures or pastures with varying topography may require several different composite samples. Cut the subsamples into 1–2 in pieces and then combine into one composite sample in a plastic bag, exclude the air, freeze immediately to stop plant respiration and minimize fermentation, and promptly mail, overnight, to the laboratory [50]. See Ration Analysis in Chapter 10.

11.4.3.1 Disease Considerations in Pasture Plant Selection

While Kentucky-31 (KY-31) tall fescue is an excellent grass for most horse pastures and is the predominant variety (35 million ac) grown in the USA, however, the majority of fescue is infected with a fungal endophyte [17]. The fungus and plant have a symbiotic relationship whereby the plant provides the endophyte with shelter and nutrients, and in turn, the endophyte produces alkaloid compounds that provide the plant with insect and drought resistance, grazing tolerance, and overall plant persistence. KY-31 is infected with a fungal endophyte called *Neotyphodium coenophialum* that produces toxic ergot alkaloids that also cause prolonged gestation, difficult birth, and lack of milk production in pregnant mares that graze infected pastures the last three mos of gestation. See Sidebar 11.2 and Fescue Toxicity in Chapter 20. Several endophyte-free varieties of tall fescue were developed, which eliminated the risk to pregnant mares, but the endophyte-free varieties only persisted for five years or less [51].

Sidebar 11.2: Tall Fescue and Mare Reproduction

Tall fescue (*Festuca elatior* or *Festuca arundinacea*) is often infected with the endophyte *Neotyphodium* (*formerly Acremonium*) *coenophialum*. The endophyte produces several ergot alkaloids; however, ergovaline represents more than 80% of ergopeptides in forage grass and more than 50% in seeds [52]. Fescue toxicosis is a commonly occurring problem in mares during the last months of pregnancy and in growing horses grazing fescue pastures infected by the endophytic fungus. Gestation in mares consuming infected fescue forage during late pregnancy may be prolonged to more than 13 m, during which signs of approaching parturition, such as udder development, may not occur while fetal size continues to increase [53]. The placenta is generally edematous with increased collagen and is difficult for the foal to break through at birth. The thickened tough placenta, poor relaxation of the pelvic ligaments and cervix, and large fetal size lead to dystocia, cervical tears, and soft tissue trauma to the mare's reproductive tract. Affected mares tend to gain less weight during pregnancy, and as a result, are in poorer body condition than those consuming noninfected fescue.

The concentration of these alkaloids in infected fescue grass is related to the degree of severity of fescue toxicosis effects. Although direct evidence that ergovaline toxin is responsible for fescue toxicosis is lacking, experimental administration of the synthetic ergot alkaloid, 2-bromo-α-ergocriptine, decreases mare plasma prolactin and progesterone concentrations [54]. The decrease in these endogenous hormones is thought to be responsible for the effects of fescue toxicosis. Removing mares from infected fescue pasture, or feeding noninfected fescue hay, is effective in rapidly alleviating fescue toxicosis effects. Pregnant mares showed signs of udder development within 48 hrs of being moved from an infected to noninfected pasture, delivered live foals within 7 d, and lactated normally. Conservatively, pregnant mares should be removed from endophyte-infected pastures before the last 90 d of gestation and fed endophyte-free forage.

Mares not removed from infected fescue should be monitored closely and provided assistance during parturition. Premature separation of the placenta may occur resulting in fetal suffocation. Regardless of placental separation, foals may be born dead, or weak and fail to breathe, although some are normal. The foal may be dead or weak at birth and may require respiratory assistance. As most affected mares are agalactic, the newborn foal must be given adequate quantities of colostrum and fed until the mare recovers sufficiently from the toxicosis to produce adequate milk. This will take about a week after the mare is consuming noninfected fescue. Pastures containing a significant amount of fescue should not provide the major part of the diet for growing horses unless known not to be infected.

More recently, researchers have inserted nontoxic endophyte strains into tall fescue varieties to give them the same benefits of persistence as KY-31. The nontoxic, also called novel, endophyte provides improved drought and pest resistance, and persistence similar to KY-31, if grazing management is similar, without the adverse effects on pregnant mares. It is important to kill off any KY-31 infected tall fescue and seeds in a pasture in the spring before planting a novel endophyte variety to ensure all of the toxic tall fescue is removed.

Grass species in the *Panicum* genus, including Fall Panicum, Kleingrass, and Switchgrass, contain steroidal saponins that cause liver damage to horses [55]. The plant has the potential to cause toxicity at all stages of maturity in both pasture and hay. The amount of grass intake required to cause toxicity is unknown, but there is some evidence from cases in Virginia on pastures and in hay that even small amounts can lead to elevated liver enzymes within days to two wks of consumption [56]. Plants of the genus *Sorghum* including Johnsongrass should also be avoided because they contain cyanogenic glycosides that are toxic to horses resulting in cystitis and ataxia [57]. See Table 12.1.

11.4.3.2 Weed Control

Weeds are classified as broadleaf or grass, winter or summer annuals, biennials, or perennials, and are most often the result of poor pasture management from either over- or under-grazing. Maintaining soil health, i.e. fertility and pH, grazing management, and mowing are the best and most environmentally friendly defenses against weeds. The strategic use of herbicides, however, may be a necessary component of pasture management. Several different types of herbicides can be used on pastures to control weeds. The type and amount of herbicide, as well as the timing of application, will depend on the type of weed(s) present. Therefore properly identifying the weed(s) is essential to selecting the most effective dose and timing of an herbicide. When several different weeds are problematic, control should be based on the emergence of the first or the most harmful to the horse. See Chapter 12 Toxic Plants. In cases where the weed type and density is greater than useable forage, complete pasture renovation may be advisable which involves killing all plants in the pasture, fertilizing and reseeding with the desired pasture forage.

Post emergent herbicides are most effective at a lower concentration when weeds are young, small and actively growing. The same herbicide may be less effective after the weed has matured and flowering. For example, buttercups, a commonly seen winter annual, can be controlled with herbicides in the autumn or early spring, before the flower appears. Post emergent herbicides should be applied following at least three days of ambient air temperatures above 60 °F when winds are calm and there is no chance of precipitation within 24 hrs, and allowing at least 2–3 days of weed growth before and after application. Adding a surfactant solution when applying herbicides increases uptake and results in a more effective weed kill. Removal of horses from pasture may not be required for some broadleaf herbicides, but following all herbicide label instructions and recommendations are important.

Pre emergent herbicides for weeds disrupt seed germination and must be present in the soil before the time of weed germination to be effective. For example, hare barley that appears in the pasture in late spring can be controlled with a winter herbicide application before weed seeds germinate in early spring. Due to the close similarities between pasture grass species (fescue) and weed grass species (Johnsongrass), controlling grass weeds is more difficult because the herbicide options are few.

Some chemicals may remain active in the soil after application and can reduce the productivity of clovers and other desirable legumes. Other herbicides may remain active in manure for up to 24 m when horses have consumed treated pastures or hay from a treated pasture. Picloram, clopyralid, and aminopyralid can remain active in the hay, fresh-cut grass, piles of manure, and in composted materials for several months to years before complete deactivation. It is important to know the properties of the active chemicals in all herbicides used, particularly, if manure will be used as fertilizer, either spread back onto the pastures or used in gardens [58]. Consulting with local county or state Agricultural Extension Services can be most helpful in pasture management, soil testing and weed control.

11.4.4 Grazing Management

The horse will eat, trample, or damage forage that is equivalent to at least 1000 lb of hay/month; hence, proper grazing management is essential for pasture providing optimal nutrition for horses efficiently. The carrying capacity of the pasture estimates the number of horses the pasture forage can nutritionally support over some specific period without damaging the pasture. This is not necessarily an easy estimation to make as several inputs revolving around the horses, land, management and environmental factors, are needed, hence consulting with the local Agricultural Extension Agent is advisable [59].

When more animals than the pasture can support are allowed to graze causing damage to the grasses beyond recovery, the pasture is overstocked. High stocking rates will lead to trampling, soil compaction, weed invasion, and overgrazing, which will result in the eventual loss of the forage stand. Too few animals are on pasture to keep up forage produced results in a patchwork of overgrown and overgrazed areas, the pasture is understocked. Understocking rates result in more mature forage growth of lesser nutritional value and weed invasion in overgrazed areas. Neither over nor under stocking is advisable for successful long-term pasture management. A minimum of 1–2 ac per horse has been recommended; however, a more practical guideline to ensure adequate feed is 2–4 ac per horse [59]. Therefore, a common recommendation across different pasture circumstances is approximately 2 ac of pasture is needed to provide adequate forage for each mature horse in temperate climates.

The nutritional value of pasture, and hence carrying capacity, varies widely with soil, climate, plant species, and management. Forage production of pasture in most areas occurs during a 5 to 7 month period. During this time, one ac of good, improved pasture receiving the optimum amount of water, either as irrigation or rain, may yield the equivalent of 5–7 tons of nutritious, high-quality forage. Thus, one ac of these types of pasture would support two mature light-breed horses during this period. In contrast, 30–60 ac of dry range pasture, typical of that in the USA Rocky Mountain Great Plains area, may be needed to support a single horse for one year.

Kentucky bluegrass, Bahia, fescue, and Bermudagrass are the most common pasture grasses in the southern United States. These grasses should be grazed at the time the feeding value meets or exceeds the requirements of the horses to be grazed (Tables 11.1 and 11.4). Although the horse on pasture will graze 14–16 hrs/d, if there are adequate quantities of good-quality pasture forage readily accessible, horses will consume a sufficient quantity to meet their maintenance energy need in 4 to 5 hrs of grazing. This illustrates why young horses grow rapidly, and mature horses may become overweight on lush, green growing pasture forage. Once the pasture forage is eaten down to the minimum recommended grazing height, all grazing animals should be removed to allow for a period of pasture rest, generally, 2–4 wks depending on environmental conditions.

11.4.4.1 Overgrazing

When plants are overgrazed without rest, die-off occurs because the plants do not have the opportunity or energy reserves in their roots for regrowth. An important management factor is the height at which grazing may start and should stop, which varies with species of forage, e.g. grazing of Bermudagrass may start at 4 to 6 in but should stop by 2 in, whereas orchardgrass may be grazed starting 8 to 10 in but should not be grazed below 3 in. The height of the pasture forage, either during a resting or grazing period, can be monitored using a grazing stick to measure, and then average the height of the forage in 10 or more locations throughout the pasture (Figure 11.8). Grazing any forage species below the recommended minimum height removes plant shoots, which causes a proportional shortening of roots and a decrease in the productive photosynthetic leaf area. During a pasture resting period, carbohydrates produced by photosynthesis will be restored in roots, stems, rhizomes, or stolons [60]. If a plant is overgrazed, additional time is then needed before growth rate and leaf area increase sufficiently to support photosynthesis and carbon fixation for rapid plant regrowth. Grazing then below the minimum height recommendations is harmful to the plants and slows regrowth so that over several years the average yearly yield is progressively less.

Overgrazing is therefore expensive and should be prevented. The short-term gain from the small amount of additional forage obtained by overgrazing is more than offset by the long-term loss of decreased forage growth. As a result, an increased amount of generally more expensive feed must be fed later. Overgrazing is a good example of being "penny wise and dollar foolish," i.e. to save a few cents you lose several dollars. Additionally, while overgrazed plants are slow to recover, weeds will invade the pasture and replace desirable plants, and then must be controlled with herbicides.

To prevent overgrazing, horses must be removed from the pasture. Offering additional feed while leaving the horses on the pasture will not prevent overgrazing. Horses offered grain and/or good-quality hay will continue to closely graze the preferred forage such that regrowth may not occur. The length of time horses may be maintained on pasture without overgrazing can be extended by closing the pasture off, having hay available for at least 4 hrs/d, and then allowing access to the pasture, i.e. a pattern of feeding hay while off the pasture such that the time/d on the pasture is shortened.

In summary, the keys to obtaining the greatest feeding value from pasture are to graze the forages while in the young growing stages of development, and then do not overgraze. As forages mature, palatability and utilizable nutrient content decrease (Table 11.4). As a result of the mature plants' reduced palatability, horses decline to consume older plants and instead overgraze the more palatable younger plants still growing. As younger plants die off early, weeds invade the overgrazed areas, while in the undergrazed areas the mature forage is wasted. Concurrently, most mature horses avoid grazing near fecal contaminated areas, yet the plants in these areas grow rapidly due to the fertilizing manure, producing lush but rapidly maturing forage in ungrazed areas. To correct a patched grazed pasture, the weeds must be killed by spraying an herbicide or mowing close to the ground, also mow the overgrown, mature forage areas short, and scattering the manure with a wire or chain drag or harrow. To avoid a patched grazed pasture, prevent any portion of the pasture to be overgrazed by either harvesting the excess growth, as hay, haylage, or green chop, or using rotational grazing.

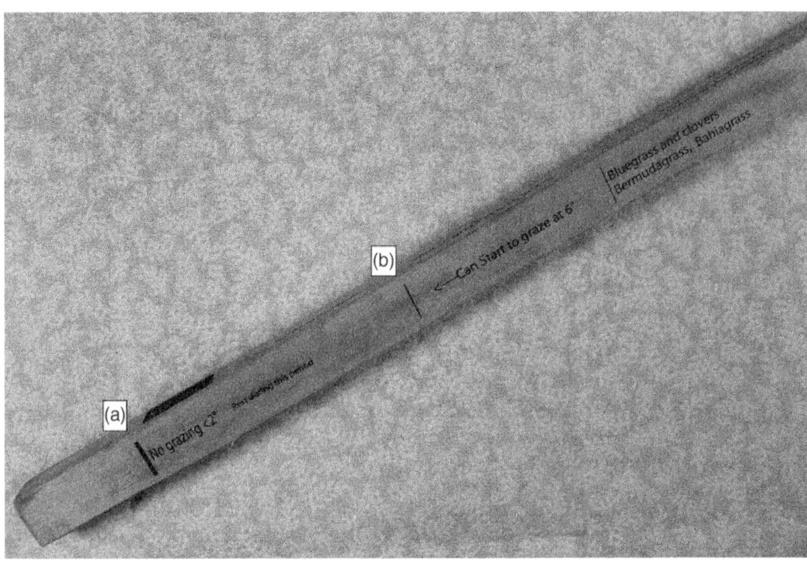

Figure 11.8 Grazing stick marking the minimum forage height to stop grazing (a) and the forge height to allow grazing (b) of Bluegrass, clovers, Bermudagrass, and Bahiagrass. Pasture is rested while forage heights are between points a and b.

11.4.4.2 Rotational Grazing

The best way to minimize overgrazing is through rotational grazing. Pastures can be divided into 4–30 paddocks or sections with permanent or temporary electric fencing, which are grazed one at a time (Figure 11.9). Grazing intervals on each paddock within a rotational system range from 5 to 50 d depending on forage height and maturity, and growing conditions, but 2–3 wks per paddock is typical during the growing season where there are at least four paddocks [59, 61]. Ideally, each paddock should be just large enough so that the horses will consume all the forage produced in that section within 14–21 days during the forage growing season. Following the short grazing period, the pasture should have about a month's rest for new forage growth to occur before the horses are rotated back.

The additional forage obtained by rotational grazing was well demonstrated in a study in which two groups of eight yearlings of similar BW and condition were each grazed on 5.2 ac of equal-quality alfalfa pasture with no other feeds fed [62]. One pasture was continuously grazed; the other pasture was divided into six similar-sized paddocks and rotationally grazed by eight yearlings, all of which were moved to a new paddock each time grazing available forage. The days of grazing were 25 on the continuous pasture, whereas 37 d of grazing were possible on the subdivided pasture of the same size. Yearlings grazing the paddocks sequentially had a 2.6-fold greater growth rate than those grazing the one pasture continuously. Based on the amount of digestible energy needed by yearlings for the growth obtained, about 2600 lb of early-bloom alfalfa was obtained from the continuously grazed pasture, as compared to over 5300 lb from the rotationally grazed paddocks. The greater forage production in the rotationally grazed pasture was due to (i) the forage growth that occurred when paddocks were rested and (ii) the fact that spot grazing was discouraged in the rotationally grazed paddocks but did occur in the continually grazed pasture. Additionally, spot grazing, i.e. portions of over-grazed and under-grazed sections, was prevalent in the continuously grazed pasture.

Grazing cattle or sheep with horses will also decrease patch grazing. Although horses and cattle show a large (77%) overlap in choice of forage, horses tend to graze only particular areas in the pasture while cattle and sheep graze more at random. Other types of livestock will also graze around manure piles left by horses, while most horses tend to avoid these areas. In contrast to cattle, there is little overlap between horses and deer in choice of forages and browse; thus, the presence of deer in the same pasture does not decrease the feed available for horses. Instead, a combination of livestock keeps pastures grazed more uniformly and helps maintain the pasture forage in the high-quality growth stage. The combination not only makes more efficient use

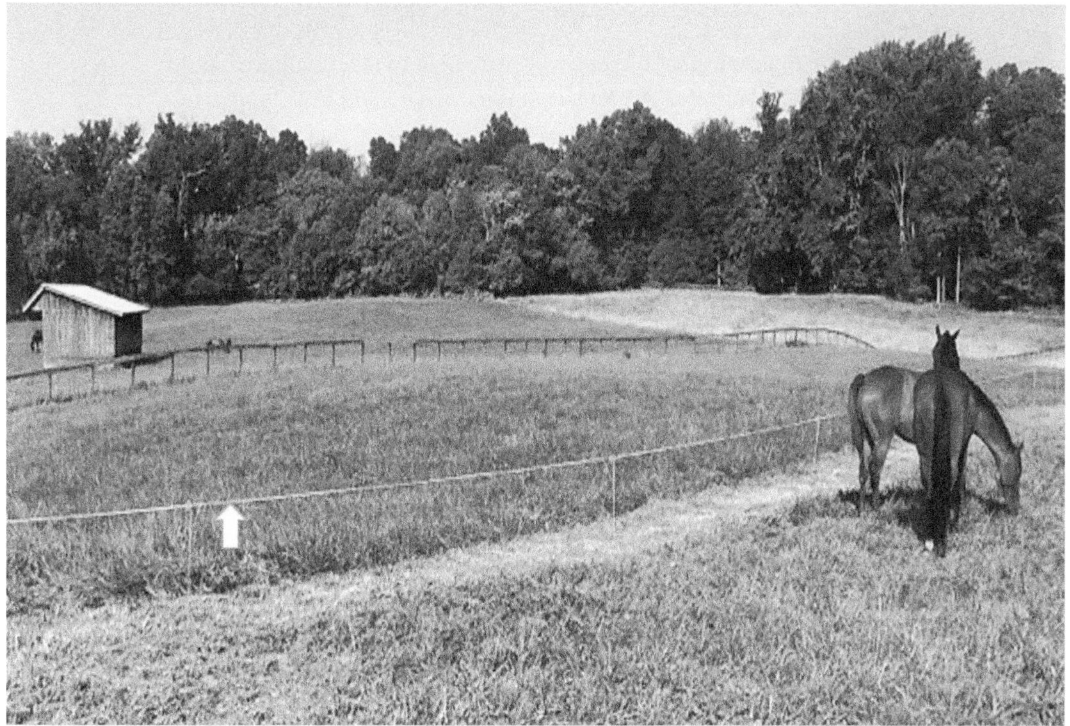

Figure 11.9 A rotational grazing system divides a pasture into multiple paddocks allowing forage plants to rest and recover. In this example, a single strand of an electric fence (arrow) is used to divide a pasture with permanent exterior fencing. When installed properly, electric fencing is an inexpensive and effective method for dividing pastures to create rotational grazing systems.

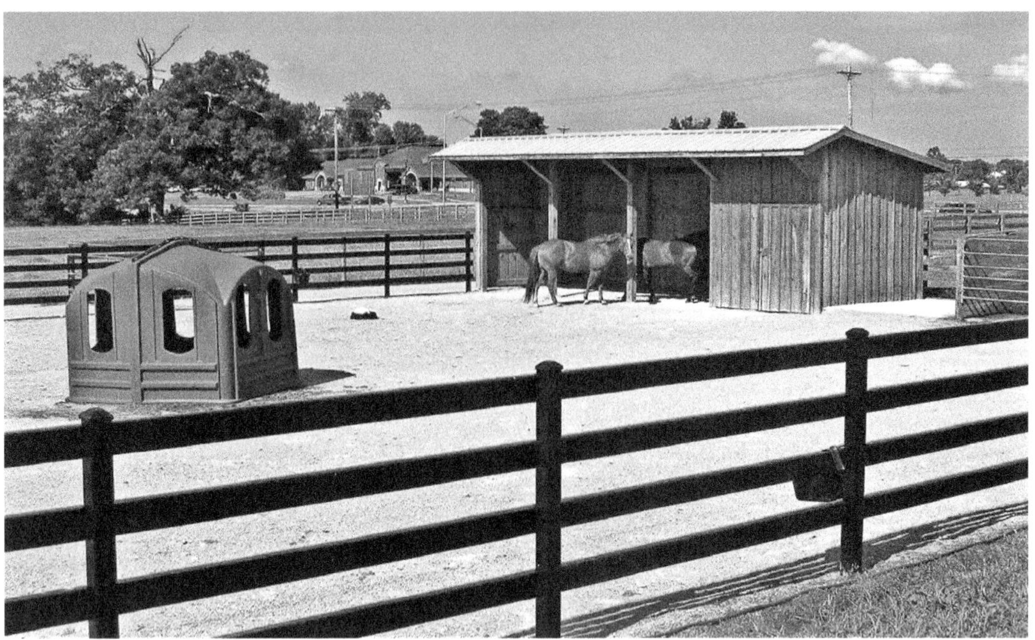

Figure 11.10 Heavy use areas constructed of nonerodible footing provide an area to house horses while resting pastures. Heavy use areas should include shelter, a source of water, and an efficient method of feeding hay (green hay hut).

of the pastures but also offers additional income from the pasture. Cattle, sheep, and horses may all graze the pasture at the same time, or the cattle or sheep may graze in the pasture after the horses have been removed.

It is ideal for both continuous and rotational grazing systems to include a heavy use area, i.e. drylot, constructed of footing that prevents erosion (Figure 11.10). The lot should be ample size to accommodate all horses, and space for minimal aggressive behavior, and should have a shelter, water source, and hay feeders or stations. Drylot areas provide a place to house horses when pastures need rest for regrowth, or under wet and muddy conditions to prevent pasture trampling. For maximum pasture forage production, horses should not be on the pasture during or shortly after precipitation or irrigation. Adequate time should be allowed for the drying of pastures to minimize trampling, plant injury, and soil compaction.

Case in Point

Animal Assessment

During March in Minnesota, a 29-yr-old Shetland gelding is reported to have lost weight over the winter. The owner did not appreciate the weight loss until early spring when he began shedding out and reports the previous autumn the pony was at good BW and BCS. The pony is kept as part of a small herd of 10 horses in 2 ac drylot at this time because fields are too wet and in the early growth stages. During the winter months, the herd was group-fed large round bales of grass hay under cover. The other horses' age ranged from 11 to 15 yrs, and all were shedding out normally and had body condition scores (BCS) ranging from 5 to 7/9. The last dental examination in this pony was 6 m previously, and there were no noteworthy problems at that time. The physical examination of the pony was unremarkable, except for a BW estimated at 340 lb, using anatomical measurements (Table 2.2) and a BCS of 3/9 (Table 2.4) in Chapter 2. The estimated ideal BW was at 400 lb (Table 2.3); therefore, the pony was 15% underweight. Routine complete blood count and serum biochemical panel were within normal limits.

1) What should be next investigated?
2) Given appetite appears to be good, and the pony had no physical problems eating a sample grain mix, and reportedly has no problems eating hay from the group feeder, what would be the next step in the investigation?
3) Hay DM analysis became available: DE 0.91 Mcal/lb, crude protein 9%, ADF 41.2% and NDF 69.1%, and RFV 76. Could this information explain the weight loss in this pony?
4) What would be your feeding recommendations for this pony?

See Appendix A Chapter 11.

References

1 Chavez, S.J., Siciliano, P.D., and Huntington, G.B. (2014). Intake estimation of horses grazing tall fescue (Lolium arundinaceum) or fed tall fescue hay. *J. Anim. Sci.* 92 (5): 2304–2308.

2 Merritt, A.M. and Julliand, V. (2013). Gastrointestinal physiology. In: *Equine Applied and Clinical Nutrition: Health, Welfare and Performance* (ed. R.J. Geor, P.A. Harris, and M. Coenen), 3–32. Edinburgh: Saunders Elsevier.

3 Harris, P.A., Ellis, A.D., Fradinho, M.J. et al. (2017). Review: feeding conserved forage to horses: recent advances and recommendations. *Animal* 11 (6): 958–967.

4 National Research Council (2007). *Nutrient Requirements of Horses.* 6th Rev. Animal Nutrition Series, 1–341. Washington, DC: National Academies Press.

5 National Research Council (1989). *Nutrient Requirements of Horses.* 5th Rev. Animal Nutrition Series, 1–100. Washington, DC: National Academies Press.

6 Graham-Thiers, P.M., Kronfeld, D.S., Kline, K.A., and Sklan, D.J. (2001). Dietary protein restriction and fat supplementation diminish the acidogenic effect of exercise during repeated sprints in horses. *J. Nutr.* 131: 1959–1964.

7 Longland, A.C. and Byrd, B.M. (2006). Pasture nonstructural carbohydrates and equine laminitis. *J. Nutr.* 136 (suppl): 2099s–2102s.

8 Hintz, H.F. (1991). Feeds for livestock. In: *Large Animal Clinical Nutrition* (ed. J. Naylor and S.L. Ralston), 120–130. St. Louis, MO: Elsevier.

9 Fetzer, L.M., Grafft, L., Hill, D.E. et al. (2019). Preventing Fires in Baled Hay and Straw. USDA AG Safety and Health. https://ag-safety.extension.org/preventing-fires-in-baled-hay-and-straw/#:~:text=The best way to reduce,moisture level%2C microbial activity decreases (accessed 18 March 2020).

10 Fonnesbeck, P., Lydman, R., Vander Noot, G., and Symons, L. (1967). Digestibility of the proximate nutrients of forage by horses. *J. Anim. Sci.* 26 (5): 1039–1045.

11 Campbell, J.B. and Ensley, S. (2002). Management of blister beetles in alfalfa. Lincoln, NE: University of Nebraska Division of the Institute of Agriculture and Natural Resources. NF551. https://digitalcommons.unl.edu/cgi/viewcontent.cgi?article=1091&context=extensionhist.

12 Lieb, S., Ott, E., and French, E. (1993). Digestible nutrients and voluntary intake of rhizomes peanut, alfalfa, bermudagrass and bahiagrass by equine. In: *Proceedings of the 13th Equine Nutrition and Physiology Society Symposium,* 98–99. Gainsville, FL: Equine Nutrition and Physiology Society.

13 Todd, L., Saucer, W., and Coleman, R. (1983). Voluntary intake and nutrient digestibility in cubes, pellets, chopped or loose alfalfa for mature horses. *J. Anim. Sci.* 57 (Supp 1): 273.

14 Pagan, J. and Jackson, S. (1991). Digestibility of long-stem alfalfa, pelleted alfalfa, or an alfalfa/Bermuda straw blend pellet in horses. In: *Proceedings of the 12th Equine Nutrition and Physiology Society Symposium*, 29–32. Calgary, Alberta: Equine Nutrition and Physiology Society.

15 Arana, M., Rodiek, A., and Stull, C. (1989). Blood glucose and insulin responses to four different grains and four different forms of alfalfa hay fed to horses. In: *Proceedings of the 11th Equine Nutrition and Physiology Society Symposium*, 160–161. Stillwater, OK: Equine Nutrition and Physiology Society.

16 Henning, J. and Lawrence, L. (2019). Production and management of hay and haylage. In: *Horse Pasture Management* (ed. P. Sharpe), 177–208. London: Elsevier Academic Press Elsevier Academic Press.

17 Ball, D., Hoveland, C., and Lacefield, G. (2007). Hay production. In: *Southern Forages: Modern Concepts for Forage Crop Management*, 4e, 151–156, 301. Norcross, GA: International Plant Nutrition Institute.

18 Hintz, H.F. (1983). *Horse Nutrition : A Practical Guide*, 228. New York: Arco.

19 Hintz, H.F. (1980). Feed preferences for horses. In: *Proceedings of the Cornell Nutrition Conference for Feed Manufacturers*, 113–116, Ithaca, NY.

20 Houpt, K.A. (1983). Taste preferences in horses. *Equine Pract.* 5 (4): 22–26.

21 Jackson, S., Rich, V., and Ralston, S. (1984). Feeding behavior and feed efficiency in groups of horses as a function of feeding frequency and the use of alfalfa cubes. *J. Anim. Sci.* 59 (Supp 1): 152.

22 Hintz, H.F. and Loy, R.G. (1966). Effects of pelleting on the nutritive value of horse rations. *J. Anim. Sci.* 25 (4): 1059–1062.

23 Hintz, H.F. (1977). Equine nutrition seminar. *Annual Conference for Veterinarians.* Fort Collins, CO.

24 Elia, J.B., Erb, H.N., and Houpt, K.A. (2010). Motivation for hay: effects of a pelleted diet on behavior and physiology of horses. *Physiol. Behav.* 101 (5): 623–627.

25 Ensminger, M. and Olentine, C. (1978). Feeding horses. In: *Feeds and Nutrition*, 919–971. Clovis, CA: Ensminger Publishing.

26 Ball, D., Hoveland, C., and Lacefield, G. (2007). Forage quality. In: *Southern Forages. Modern Concepts for Forage Crop Management*, 4e, 136–145. Norcross, GA: International Plant Nutrition Institute.

27 Department of Crop and Soil Science (2022). How does grass grow? Developmental phases. Corvallis, OR: Oregon State University. https://forages.oregonstate.edu/regrowth/how-does-grass-grow/developmental-phases (accessed 25 May 2022).
28 Kawamura, K., Ikeura, H., Phongchanmaixay, S., and Khanthavong, P. (2018). Canopy hyperspectral sensing of paddy fields at the booting stage and PLS regression can assess grain yield. *Remote Sens.* 10 (8): 1249.
29 Rohweder, D.A.A., Barnes, R.F.F., and Jorgensen, N.A.N. (1978). Proposed hay grading standards based on laboratory analysis for evaluating quality. *J. Anim. Sci.* 47 (3): 747–759.
30 Rocateli, A. and Zhang, H. (2017). Forage quality interpretations. Stillwater, OK: Oklahoma Cooperative Extension Service PSS-2117. https://extension.okstate.edu/fact-sheets/forage-quality-interpretations.html.
31 Jeranyama, P. and Garcia, A.D. (2004). Understanding relative feed value (RFV) and relative forage quality (RFQ). South Dakota State University Cooperative extension extra. Paper 352. http://openprairie.sdstate.edu/extension_extra/352 (accessed 21 March 2020).
32 Coleman, R., Milligan, J., and Burwash, L. (1989). The effect on daily gain in horses from feeding hay on the ground. In: *Proceedings of the 11th Equine Nutrition and Physiology Society Symposium,* 164–168. Stillwater, OK: Equine Nutrition and Physiology Society.
33 Sweeting, M.P., Houpt, C.E., and Houpt, K.A. (1985). Social facilitation of feeding and time budgets in stabled ponies. *J. Anim. Sci.* 60 (2): 369–374.
34 Ödberg, F.O. and Francis-Smith, K. (1977). Studies on the formation of ungrazed eliminative areas in fields used by horses. *Appl. Anim. Ethol.* 3 (1): 27–34.
35 Couëtil, L.L., Cardwell, J.M., Gerber, V. et al. (2016). Inflammatory airway disease of horses-revised consensus statement. *J. Vet. Intern. Med.* 30 (2): 503–515.
36 Martinson, K., Wilson, J., Cleary, K. et al. (2012). Round-bale feeder design affects hay waste and economics during horse feeding. *J. Anim. Sci.* 90 (3): 1047–1055.
37 McGreevy, P.D., Cripps, P.J., French, N.P. et al. (1995). Management factors associated with stereotypic and redirected behaviour in the thoroughbred horse. *Equine Vet. J.* 27 (2): 86–91.
38 Husted, L., Sanchez, L.C., Olsen, S.N. et al. (2008). Effect of paddock vs. stall housing on 24 hour gastric pH within the proximal and ventral equine stomach. *Equine Vet. J.* 337–341.
39 Meyer, H., Coenen, M., and Guer, C. (1985). Investigation on saliva production and chewing effect in horses fed various feeds. In: *Proceedings of the 9th Equine Nutrition and Physiology Society Symposium,* 38–41. East Lansing, MI: Equine Nutrition and Physiology Society.
40 Sharpe, P. (2019). Nutritional value of pasture plants for horses. In: *Horse Pasture Management* (ed. P. Sharpe), 37–64. London: Elsevier Academic Press.
41 Hampson, B.A., De Laat, M.A., Millis, P.C., and Pollitt, C.C. (2010). Distances travelled by feral horses in 'outback' Australia. *Equine Vet. J.* 42 (Suppl. 38): 582–586.
42 Moffitt, D.L., Meacham, T., and Fontenot, J. et al. (1987). Seasonal differences in apparent digestibilities of fescue and orchardgrass/clover pastures in horses. In: *Proceedings of the 10th Equine Nutrition and Physiology Society Symposium,* 79–85. Fort Collins, CO: Equine Nutrition and Physiology Society.
43 Jackson, S. and Pagan, J.D. (1993). Equine nutrition evaluation. *Large Anim. Vet.* 48 (2): 20–24.
44 Singer, J.W., Bobsin, N., Bamka, W.J., and Kluchinski, D. (1999). Horse pasture management. *J. Equine Vet. Sci.* 19 (9): 540–545.
45 Khan, H. (2018). Importance of Soil tests, 31 October. https://www.researchgate.net/publication/328631561_Importance_of_Soil_tests.
46 Wheeler, D.M. (1998). Investigation into the mechanisms causing lime responses in a grass/clover pasture on a clay loam soil. *New Zeal. J. Agric. Res.* 41 (4): 497–515.
47 Soder, K.J., Rook, A.J., Sanderson, M.A., and Goslee, S.C. (2006). Interaction of plant species diversity on grazing behavior and performance of livestock grazing temperate region pastures. *Crop. Sci.* 47 (1): 416–425.
48 Undersander, D.J. (2019). Forage plant structure, function, nutrition, and growth. In: *Horse Pasture Management* (ed. P. Sharpe), 1–10. London: Elsevier Academic Press.
49 Graham, P.H. and Vance, C.P. (2003). Legumes: importance and constraints to greater use. *Plant Physiol.* 131 (3): 872–877.
50 Equi-Analytical Laboratory Services (2019). Taking a pasture sample. https://equi-analytical.com/feed-and-forage-analysis/taking-a-sample/ (accessed 25 March 2020).
51 Rogers J. (2011) Clearing up some tall fescue misconceptions. *Agric. News Views* 29 (1): 7.
52 Guerre, P. (2015). Ergot alkaloids produced by endophytic fungi of the genus Epichloë. *Toxins (Basel)* 7 (3): 773–790.
53 Hintz, H.F. (1987). Tall fescue pasture for horses. *Equine Pract.* 9 (2): 5–6.
54 Zimmer, R., Loch, W., and Bennett-Wimbush, K. (1993). Effect of 2-bromo-α-ergocriptine on pregnant pony mares during late gestation. In: *Proceedings of the 13th Equine Nutrition and Physiology Society Symposium*, 326–327. Gainsville, FL: Equine Nutrition and Physiology Society.

55 Cornick, J.L., Carter, G.K., and Bridges, C.H. (1988). Kleingrass-associated hepatotoxicosis in horses. *J. Am. Vet. Med. Assoc.* 193 (8): 932–935.

56 Johnson, A.L., Divers, T., Freckleton, M.L. et al. (2006). Fall Panicum (*Panicum dichotomiflorum*) hepatotoxicosis in horses and sheep. *J. Vet. Intern. Med.* 20 (6): 1414–1421.

57 Adams, L.G., Dollahite, J.W., Romane, W.M. et al. (1969). Cystitis and ataxia associated with sorghum ingestion by horses. *J. Am. Vet. Med. Assoc.* 155 (3): 518–524.

58 Davis, J., Johnson, S., and Jennings, K. (2020). Herbicide carryover in hay, manure, compost, and grass clippings. North Carolina State Extension Publications AG-727. https://content.ces.ncsu.edu/herbicide-carryover.

59 Kenny, L., Burk, A., and Williams, C. (2019). Managing equine grazing for pasture productivity. In: *Horse Pasture Management* (ed. P. Sharpe), 141–156. London: Elsevier Academic Press.

60 Smith, R.S. and Lea, K.L. (2019). Pasture plant establishment and management. In: *Horse Pasture Management* (ed. P. Sharpe), 93–105. London: Elsevier Academic Press.

61 Undersander, D., Albert, B., Cosgrove, D. et al. (2014). Pastures for profit: a guide to rotational grazing. University of Wisconsin Cooperative Extension. A3529. https://learningstore.extension.wisc.edu/products/pastures-for-profit-a-guide-to-rotational-grazing-p96.

62 Freeman, D. (1987) Preliminary investigations of grazing horses on alfalfa. Oklahoma State University. Animal Science Research Report, pp. 127–130.

12

Toxic Plants

Bryan Stegelmeier and T. Zane Davis

KEY TERMS

- Weeds are undesirable or unwanted plants in particular human-controlled environments: rangelands [R], pasture/paddock [P], grain/hay [H], and manufactured feeds [M].
- A glossary of commonly used botanical terms is helpful in describing plants [1] pg 495.
- Photosensitization is radiation-induced dermatitis.
- Grayanotoxins are a group of closely related neurotoxins that bind to sodium ion channels on cell membranes and disrupt cell membrane transport.
- Neurotoxins adversely affect the nervous system by several mechanisms that inhibit neuron cellular processes.
- Toxalbumins disable ribosomes, inhibiting protein synthesis and producing severe cytotoxic effects in multiple organ systems.
- Reactive oxygen species (ROS) are highly reactive molecules as a result of the electron acceptability of O_2 (peroxides, superoxide, and hydroxyl radicals).

KEY POINTS

- Poisonous plants are found in nearly every plant community: rangelands, pastures, paddocks, and cultivated fields.
- Most poisonings occur in pastures during the spring and summer; however, feeding hay or manufactured feed containing a toxic weed may occur any time of year.
- Poisonous plants in pastures are common; however, consumption by horses resulting in poisoning is relatively infrequent. Recognition of common toxic plants reduces the potential of poisonings.
- Noxious plants add to the cost of having horses through the necessity for fencing, herbicides, mowing, and pastures reseeding where undesirable plants predominate.

12.1 Introduction

Plant poisoning of horses and other livestock in the United States has been recognized since these animals were introduced to North America (NA). As early as 1873, large numbers of horses were reported to have died from a neurologic disease appropriately named locoism, a name derived from the Spanish word meaning "crazy" [1]. The locoweeds (*Astragalus* and *Oxytropis* spp.) responsible for the losses of the horses were, and still are, abundant on many western rangelands. Similarly, in the early nineteenth century, settlers in the Midwestern states witnessed severe muscle tremors and deaths in their horses, sheep, and cattle after the animals ate white snakeroot (*Eupatorium urticaefolium*). People were also affected with similar signs if they drank milk from cows that had been eating white snakeroot [2].

Poisonous plants are found in nearly every plant community: rangeland [R], pasture and paddocks [P], and in cultivated grain and hayfields [H]. Certainly, early recognition of common toxic plants, reduces the potential for poisonings. Some are native plants with established stable populations, and others are noxious weeds that invade, dominate, and replace native species and nutritious forages. The invasive nature of some toxic plants can lead to contamination of fields cultivated for baled forages, pellets, mixed feeds, and grain. Factors such as drought, excessive moisture, fertilization, and soil mineral imbalances can

Equine Clinical Nutrition, Second Edition. Edited by Rebecca L. Remillard.

alter the amount of toxin in plants, making them more of a problem in some years than in others. The use of herbicides may also affect plant growth and alter the concentration of toxic substances such as nitrates in the plant. Although plant poisoning of horses continues to be a problem, the economic impact on the horse industry is not known. Relatively few poisonings are definitively confirmed, and losses due to subclinical intoxication have not been investigated. Additional losses due to the displacement of nutritious forages by noxious plants in pastures and rangelands are largely unknown. Indirectly, poisonous plants add to the cost of having horses through the necessity for fencing, herbicides, mowing, and reseeding of pastures where undesirable plants predominate.

Exposure to poisonous plants is common; however, poisoning is relatively infrequent. Horses are not at immediate risk if one or more poisonous plants are present in their pasture, paddock, or rangeland. For most toxic plants in many grazing situations, horses avoid eating toxic plants. However, when pastures are overgrazed, noxious toxic weeds can proliferate, and if alternative forages are not available or feeding competition is high, many unacceptable plants are eaten. The potential for plant poisoning increases if horses have the opportunity to eat large quantities (green plants at 5–10% body weight (BW)) of a toxic plant over several weeks or months. Rarely is a horse poisoned by a single mouthful of a plant, with the possible exception of the most toxic of plants, e.g. water hemlock (*Cicuta douglasii*) and yew (*Taxus* spp.). Some toxic plants are palatable and therefore dangerous whenever animals have access to them. At other times, poisoning has occurred when yard or garden prunings are tossed into horse corrals with mistaken good intentions, or when hungry horses are tied adjacent to plants. Although plant poisonings occur in horses on pasture during the spring and summer, many poisonings occur when hay or manufactured feeds [M] are contaminated with poisonous plants and fed to hungry animals. Additionally, some commonly used forages can become toxic if used inappropriately; if improperly fertilized; or if the plants are stressed by drought or frost.

It should be recognized that a plant toxin may exert effects on multiple organ systems, and therefore the clinical signs will reflect the variety and degree of organ involvement. For example, Tansy ragwort (*Senecio jacobea*) poisoning in horses may present as a neurologic disease. However, other poisoned horses may develop severe photodermatitis. For both processes the underlying problem is one of severe liver disease. In this review toxic plants that affect horses will be presented systematically, though other systems are certainly impacted and contribute to the disease process. Though these select poisonous plants are grouped by predominate organ system, secondary information relating to other affected systems, the source, conditions in which horses may be poisoned, and clinical signs will also be included. Certainly the tables will be useful as they sort the poisonous plants first by source, i.e. pastures (Table 12.1), rangeland (Table 12.2), and hay or manufactured feeds (Table 12.3), then by organ system affected and by a toxin and finally the most common clinical sign(s). The veterinary practitioner may find the tables more helpful in diagnosing a live case, whereas the text may be more useful to the diagnostician during a necropsy. Identifying the toxin and source often requires physically examining the horse's environment (pasture, paddock, range area) and hay. See Farm Investigations in Chapter 10.

12.2 Plants that Damage Dermal and Epithelial Tissues

12.2.1 Skin Photosensitization

Photosensitization is radiation-induced dermatitis that has heightened sensitivity when compared with sunburn or solar radiation-induced dermatitis. Increased sensitivity is due to photodynamic chromophores that when in or on the skin increase the efficiency of energy absorption and damage. Radiation energy reacts with the chromophores forming reactive intermediates that damage adjacent cellular proteins, membranes, and nucleic acids. These reactive intermediates may also react with oxygen, generating ROS intermediates such as superoxide anions, or singlet oxygen, and hydroxyl radicals that further damage cellular components. Oxidation of skin amino acids, such as histidine, tyrosine, and tryptophan provokes acute inflammation and necrosis. Depending on the chromophore source, photosensitization has been classified as primary chromophores of exogenous source or secondary where the chromophore is a metabolite of chlorophyll, phylloerythrin, that accumulates due to reduced hepatic excretion [3]. See Sidebar 12.1. Regardless of the source, the signs of poisoning are similar. Lightly pigmented areas with little hair protection that are exposed to the sun are severely damaged. The skin of the muzzle, ears, eyelids, face, tail head, vulva, and coronary bands are most often affected with red discoloration, photophobia, itching, erythema, edema, serous exudation, massive laminar necrosis, and scab formation. The inflammation is variable and related to radiation dose and duration. Severe lesions have extensive suppurative necrosis with massive crust and scab formation that often slough in layers. Horses with completely pigmented skin and heavily haired are relatively more protected as less radiation activates the photodynamic chromophores present in the skin capillaries. In such protected animals the only lesions may be periocular,

Table 12.1 Toxic plants found in cultivated pastures/paddocks [P] likely to poison horses.

Toxin/clinical sign	Toxic plant (*scientific name*)
Dermal tissues	
Unknown/laminitis	Black walnut (*Juglans nigra*)
hypericin, fagoyrun/photosensitization	St. John's wort (*Hypericum perforatum*), buckweed (*Fagopyrum esculentum*), wild parsnip (*Pastinaca sativa*)
Selenium toxicosis/hair, hoof	Two-grooved milkvetch (*Astragalus bisculatus*), golden weed (*Haplopappus engelmannii*), woody aster (*Xylorrhiza glabriuscula*), princes' plume (*Stanleya pinnata*), asters (*Aster* spp, gumweed (*Grindelia* spp.), saltbrush (*Atriplex* spp.), Indian paintbrush (*Castilleja* spp.), beard tongue (*Penstemon* spp.)
Gastrointestinal tract	
Awns/mechanical injury	Foxtail (*Hordeum jubatum*), bristle grass (*Setaria* spp.), wheat and rye (*Triticum secale* spp.)
Slaframine/slobbers	Red clover (*Trifolium* spp.)
Aesculin/diarrhea, colic	Horse chestnut and buckeye (*Aesculus* spp.)
Robin, phasin/diarrhea, colic	Black locust (*Robinia pseudoacacia*)
Tropane alkaloids Saponins/diarrhea, colic	Field bindweed (*Convolvulus arvensis*), Jimson weed (*Datura* spp.), pokeweed (*Phytolacca americana*), buttercups (*Ranunculus* spp.)
Solanine, hyoscine, hyoscyamine/diarrhea, colic	Nightshades (*Solanum* spp.), Jimson weed (*Datura* spp.)
Hepatopathy	
Phylloerythrin, indospicine pyrrolizidine alkaloid	*Senecio* spp., houndstongue (*Cynoglossum officiniale*), fiddleneck or tarweed (*Amsinckia intermedia*), rattlebox (*Crotalaria* spp.)
Indospicine/aflatoxin	Indigo (*Indigofera spicata*), alsike clover (*Trifolium hybridum*)
Carboxyactractyloside	Cocklebur (*Xanthium* spp.)
Saponin	Kleingrass, switchgrass (*Panicum* spp.)
Nervous system	
Stringhalt/abnormal hindlimb gait	Singletary pea (*Lathyrus hirsutus*), flatweed, or false dandelion (*Hypochoeris radicata*)
Benzofuran ketones/neuro and cardiac	White snakeroot, crofton, Jimmyweed, or burrow weeds (*Eupatorium* or *Ageratina* and *Haplopappus* spp.), coffee weed or coffee senna (*Cassia occidentalis*), avocado (*Persea americana*)
Repin, solistatin/facial, mouth dysfunction	Yellowstar thistle, knapweed (*Centaurea* spp.), sagebrush (*Artemisia* spp.)
Grayanotoxins/cardiac and GI	Laurel (*Kalmia* spp.), azalea (*Rhododendron* spp.)
Ricin/cardiac and GI	Castor bean (*Ricinus communis*)
Cyanosis/ataxia	Serviceberry (*Amelanchier alnifolia*), wild blue flax (*Linum* spp.), western chokecherry (*Prunus virginiana*), elderberry (*Sambucus* spp.), arrow grass (*Triglochin* spp.), Johnson, Sudan grasses (*Sorghum* spp.)
Sudden death	
Piperidine, cicutoxin, taxine, unknown	Poison hemlock (*Conium maculatum*), water hemlock (*Cicuta* spp.), yew (*Taxus* spp.), avocado (*Persea americana*)
Cardioglycoside	Foxglove (*Digitalis purpurea*), oleander (*Nerium oleander*), yellow oleander (*Thevetia* spp.), milkweeds (*Asclepias* spp.), pheasant's eye (*Adonis* spp.)
Systemic/nutritional	
Thiaminase/B_1 deficiency	Horsetail (*Equisetum* spp.), bracken fern (*Pteridium* spp.)
Hypercalcemia/vitamin D toxicity	Day-blooming Jessamine (*Cestrum diurnum*)
Oxalates/calcium deficiency	Buffel (*Cenchrus ciliaris*), pangola (*Digitaria recombens*), setaria (*Setaria sphacelata*), panic grasses (*Panicum* spp.), kikuyu (*Pennisetum clandistinum*)
Urogenital	
Hemolytic toxins/intra- and extravascular hemolysis	Red maple (*Acer rubrum*)
Tannins, gallic acid/renal tubular nephrosis	Oak (*Quercus* spp.)

Table 12.2 Toxic plants found on rangelands [R] likely to poison horses.

Toxin/clinical sign	Toxic plant (scientific name)
Dermal tissues	
Hypericin, Fagoyrun/ photosensitization	St. John's wort (*Hypericum perforatum*), buckweed (*Fagopyrum esculentum*), wild parsnip (*Pastinaca sativa*)
Selenium toxicosis/hair, hoof	Two-grooved milkvetch (*Astragalus bisculatus*), golden weed (*Haplopappus engelmannii*), woody aster (*Xylorrhiza glabriuscula*), princes' plume (*Stanleya pinnata*), asters (*Aster* spp.), broom, snake or match weed (*Guterrezia sarothrae*), gumweed (*Grindelia* spp.), saltbrush (*Atriplex* spp.), Indian paintbrush (*Castilleja* spp.), beard tongue (*Penstemon* spp.)
Gastrointestinal tract	
Awns/mechanical injury	Foxtail (*Hordeum jubatum*), bristle grass (*Setaria* spp.), wheat and rye (*Triticum* and *Secale* spp.)
Atropine-like tropane alkaloids/ diarrhea, colic	Field bindweed (*Convolvulus arvensis*)
Solanine, hyoscine, hyoscyamine/ diarrhea, colic	Nightshades (*Solanum* spp.), Jimson weed (*Datura* spp.)
Hepatopathy	
Carboxyactractyloside	Cocklebur (*Xanthium* spp.)
Saponin	Kleingrass, switchgrass (*Panicum* spp.)
Nervous system	
Benzofuran ketones/neuro and cardiac	Rayless goldenrod, white snakeroot (*Haplopappus* spp.)
Cyanosis/ataxia	Serviceberry (*Amelanchier alnifolia*), wild blue flax (*Linum* spp.), western chokecherry (*Prunus virginiana*), elderberry (*Sambucus* spp.), arrow grass (*Triglochin* spp.), Johnson, Sudan grasses (*Sorghum* spp.)
Stringhalt/abnormal hindlimb gait	Singletary pea (*Lathyrus hirsutus*), flatweed, or false dandelion (*Hypochoeris radicata*)
Swainsonine, nitrotoxins/ proprioceptive deficits, convulsions	Sagebrush (*Artemisia* spp.), locoweeds (*Astragalus* and *Oxytropis* spp.)
Thujone/hyper-reflexive, ataxia	Sand sage (*Artemisia filifolia*), bud sage (*Artemisia spinescens*), and fringed sage (*Artemisia frigida*)
Sudden death	
Cardioglycoside	Milkweeds (*Asclepias* spp.)
Systemic/nutritional	
Thiaminase/B_1 deficiency	Horsetail (*Equisetum* spp.), bracken fern (*Pteridium* spp.)
Urogenital	
Hemolytic toxins/intra- and extravascular hemolysis	Red maple (*Acer rubrum*)
Oxalate crystals/kidney disease	Halogeton (*Halogeton glomeratus*), black greasewood (*Sarcobatus vermiculatus*)
Tannins, gallic acids/renal tubular nephrosis	Oak (*Quercus* spp.)

ocular, oral perianal and mammary dermatitis. Common presenting clinical signs include increased lacrimation and photophobia. Some common plants that cause photosensitization are presented here.

12.2.1.1 St. John's Wort (*Hypericum perforatum*) [R,P,H]

St. John's wort (*H. perforatum*) [R,P,H] is a perennial European plant that grows in disturbed areas along roadsides, pastures, and waste places, and often is considered a noxious weed in NA, Europe, Australia, New Zealand, and South America [5]. All St. John's wort stages of growth, parts, and phenotypes are toxic Figure 12.1. Poisoning in horses at pasture is more likely when animals graze the more palatable, but toxic, early growth. Mature plants in pastures are generally not eaten if alternative forages are available. The toxin is not destroyed by drying and therefore, contaminated hay may also cause poisonings. Poisoning has been described in all seasons when the hay contains the mature

Table 12.3 Toxic plants found in hay [H] and manufactured concentrates [M] likely to poison horses.

Toxin/clinical sign	Toxic plant (scientific name)
Dermal tissues	
Unknown/laminitis	Black Walnut (*Juglans nigra*), Hoary Alyssum (*Berteroa incana*)
Hypericin/photosensitization	St. John's wort (*Hypericum perforatum*)
Selenium toxicosis/hair, hoof	Two-grooved milkvetch (*Astragalus bisculatus*), Golden weed (*Haplopappus engelmannii*), woody aster (*Xylorrhiza glabriuscula*), princes' plume (*Stanleya pinnata*), asters (*Aster* spp.), gumweed (*Grindelia* spp.), saltbrush (*Atriplex* spp.), Indian paintbrush (*Castilleja* spp.), beard tongue (*Penstemon* spp.)
Gastrointestinal tract	
Atropine-like tropane alkaloids/ diarrhea, colic	Field bindweed (*Convolvulus arvensis*), Jimson weed (*Datura* spp.), buttercups (*Ranunculus* spp.)
Awns/mechanical injury	foxtail (*Hordeum jubatum*), bristle grass (*Setaria* spp.), wheat and rye (*Triticum, Secale* spp.)
Slaframine/slobbers	red clover (*Trifolium* spp.)
Solanine, hyoscine, hyoscyamine/ diarrhea, colic	Nightshades (*Solanum* spp.), Jimson weed (*Datura* spp.)
Hepatopathy	
Carboxyactractyloside	Cocklebur (*Xanthium* spp.)
Phylloerythrin, indospicine Pyrrolizidine alkaloid	*Senecio* spp., houndstongue (*Cynoglossum officiniale*), fiddleneck or tarweed (*Amsinckia intermedia*), rattlebox (*Crotalaria* spp.)
Saponin	Kleingrass, switchgrass (*Panicum* spp.)
Nervous system	
Cyanosis/ataxia	Serviceberry (*Amelanchier alnifolia*), wild blue flax (*Linum* spp.), western chokecherry (*prunus virginiana*), Elderberry (*Sambucus* spp.), arrow grass (*Triglochin* spp.), Johnson and Sudan grasses (*Sorghum* spp.)
Fumonisins/ataxia, convulsions	Fungi (*Fusarium verticillioides, Fusarium moniliforme*)
Grayanotoxins/cardiac and GI	Laurel (*Kalmia* spp.), azalea (*Rhododendron* spp.)
Ricin/cardiac and GI	Castor bean (*Ricinus communis*)
Sudden death	
Piperidine, cicutoxin, taxine, Unknown	Poison hemlock (*Conium maculatum*), water hemlock (*Cicuta* spp.), yew (*Taxus* spp.), avocado (*Persea Americana*)
Cardioglycoside	Foxglove (*Digitalis purpurea*), oleander (*Nerium oleander*), yellow oleander (*Thevetia* spp.), milkweeds (*Asclepias* spp.), pheasant's eye (*Adonis* spp.)
Systemic/nutritional	
Dicoumarol/vitamin K Deficiency	Sweet clover (*Melilotus* spp.)
Hypercalcemia/vitamin D Toxicity	Day-blooming jessamine (*Cestrum diurnum*)
Thiaminase/B_1 deficiency	Horsetail (*Equisetum* spp.), bracken fern (*Pteridium* spp.)
Urogenital	
Hemolytic toxins/intra- and extravascular hemolysis	Red maple (*Acer rubrum*)

plant. St. John's wort toxin has been identified as hypericin, a potent chromophore that easily induces photosensitization [6]. Toxicity is characterized by photosensitivity with associated dermal necrosis affecting unpigmented and thinly haired skin. Poisoning appears between 2 and 21 days of ingestion. If exposure is discontinued, most lesions quickly resolve when animals are removed from sunlight and treated systematically.

12.2.1.2 Buckwheat (*Fagopyrum esculentum, Fagopyrum tataricum*, and Other *F.* Species) [P]

Buckwheat (*Fagopyrum esculentum, Fagopyrum tataricum*, and other *F.* species) [P] are Asian plants that were originally imported to many continents as a cover crop. Often it has escaped cultivation and expanded to dominate some plant communities. Preferring to grow in disturbed soils along field margins and fences, buckwheat historically

Sidebar 12.1: Primary and Secondary Photodermatitis [1]

Primary photosensitization develops when horses eat plants containing photosensitive pigments (polyphenolic compounds) that are absorbed and accumulate in the skin. Two plants historically associated with primary photosensitization in horses are buckwheat (*F. esculentum*) and St. John's wort (*H. perforatum*). Horses are also potentially at risk from plants such as spring parsley (*Cymopterus watsonii*) and bishop's weed (*Ammi majus*), which contain photoreactive furocoumarins that induce primary photosensitization in other livestock and poultry and, therefore, may do so in horses.

Secondary, or hepatogenic, photosensitization occurs more commonly in animals than primary photosensitization. Unlike primary photosensitization, liver disease is the underlying cause of secondary photosensitivity. The plant toxins themselves are not photoreactive but cause liver damage. Once 80% or more of the liver is affected, the elimination of phylloerythrin, a normal breakdown by-product of plant chlorophyll, is decreased and accumulates in the blood and skin. Phylloerythrin absorbs photon energy allowing it to damage dermal cellular structures resulting in photosensitization and dermatitis [4]. The prognosis for animals with secondary photosensitization is always far poorer than that for the primary condition because the underlying liver disease is frequently irreversible and eventually fatal in most affected animals.

poisoned livestock, pets, and humans; however, it did not compete well with newer invasive plants. Recently in most locations it has been replaced making poisoning relatively uncommon. A plant with simple, alternate leaves and blue-white perfect flowers is considered a low shrub or vine. The toxins have been identified as fagopyrin, photofagopyrin, and pseudohypericin have structures and toxicity similar to hypericin of St. John's wort. Poisoning was most frequent in cattle and goats, but occasionally poisons horses, consuming both the green and dried plant [1].

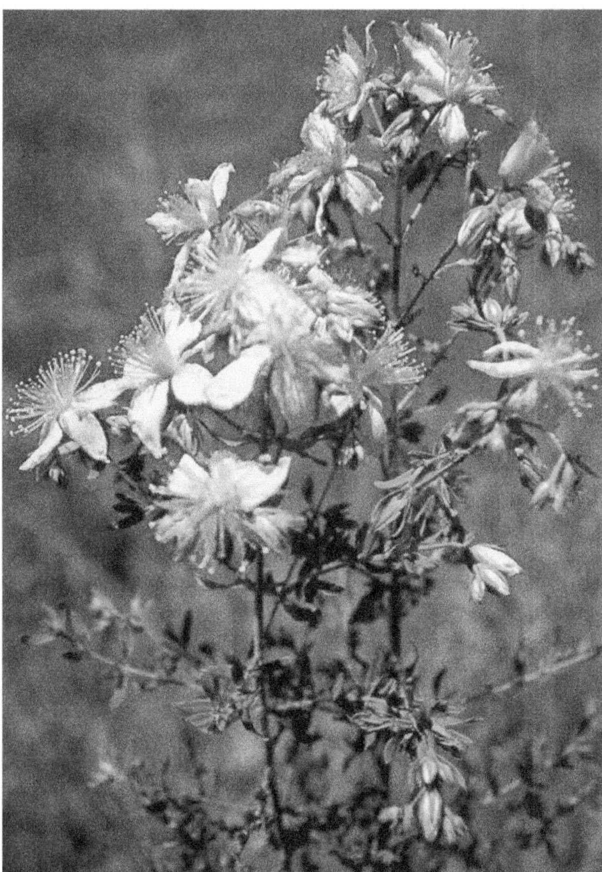

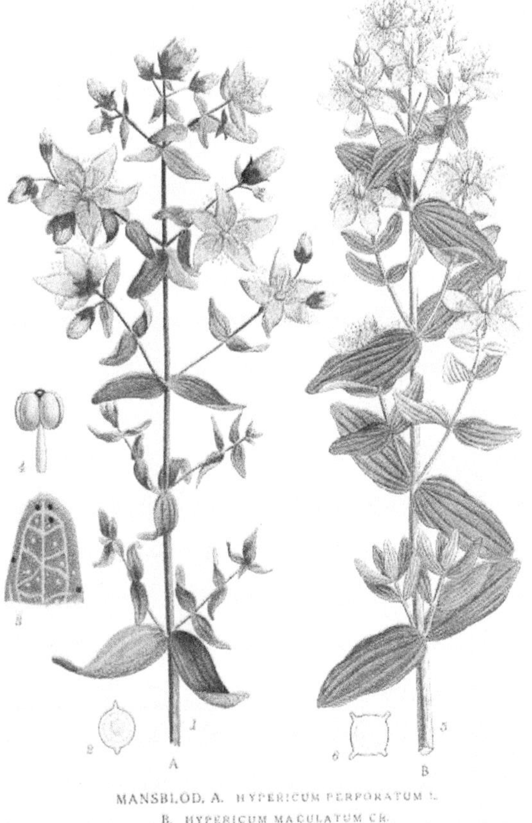

Figure 12.1 St. John's wort, goat weed, tipton weed, or klamath weed (*Hypericum* spp.) is a smooth-branched plant that can be up to two meters tall. The leaves are opposite, sessile, and elliptic to oblong not over 3 cm long. The flowers are bright yellow with flat-topped cymes and five petals. Spreading via seeds and runners, it often dominates pastures and rangelands. *Source:* Lindman [5].

12.2.1.3 Wild Parsnip (*Pastinaca sativa*) [P]

Wild parsnip (*Pastinaca sativa*) [P] is a biennial forb that grows to 1.5 m tall. It has pinnate leaves with several pairs of leaflets with toothed margins that can be up to 40 cm long. In the second year, the tall floral stem is hairy and mostly hollow with few branches and leaves. The yellow flowers are compound umbels about 20 cm in diameter with 5 to 25 pedicels supporting 3.5 secondary umbels. These form 4 to 8 mm flat oval fruits that are brown with several dark stripes. Wild parsnip is generally considered a nuisance as it displaces better forages, though sporadically it has been associated with photosensitization of livestock and humans [7, 8]. Several furanocoumarins, including xanthotoxin, bergapten, isopimpinellin, and imperatorin, were identified in wild parsnip, but oral dosing produced only minimal photosensitivity. However, dermal application of these compounds was highly photoactive, inducing extensive radiation-induced dermatitis similar to hypericin-positive controls [8]. These findings suggest dermal exposure is the most common cause of wild parsnip-induced photosensitivity.

12.2.1.4 Hepatogeneous and Idiopathic Photosensitivity

Phylloerythrin-associated photosensitivity is a common finding in many equine liver diseases including those of plant origin. The prognosis for animals with secondary photosensitization is always poor when compared with primary photosensitization because the underlying liver disease is frequently irreversible and eventually fatal. Normally hepatocytes conjugate and excrete phylloerythrin in the bile. Consequently, any disease that alters hepatic conjugation, decreases excretion, or reduces biliary flow increases phylloerythrin concentrations in the blood and skin that can result in photosensitivity. Plant-induced causes of liver disease in horses include dehydropyrrolizidine alkaloid-containing plants, alsike clover, and saponin-containing plants. All of these produce functional and morphologic hepatic lesions, producing clinical and biochemical changes, such as icterus, hyperbilirubinemia, hepatic encephalopathy, liver-related protein changes, and coagulopathies. These hepatotoxic plants also produce histological hepatic lesions confirming that the photosensitivity is due to altered liver metabolism and function. There are some horses with clinically normal liver function and morphology that have no known exposure to photosensitizing plants or chemicals, and yet develop photosensitivity (idiopathic photosensitivity). This generally occurs in young horses in the spring when solar exposure is high and forages are lush with abundant, quickly digestible plant carbohydrates and chlorophyll. Initial work suggests serum phylloerythrin concentrations in affected animals are marginally elevated. It has been suggested that this may be due to microbiome changes in response to the lush forage resulting in increased chlorophyll metabolism and phylloerythrin production. Alternatively, some young animals may be less capable of hepatic phylloerythrin excretion. More work is needed to determine the cause of these idiopathic photosensitivities.

12.2.2 Mechanical Injuries to Facial and Oral Tissues

Plants with awns and bristles can cause mechanical injuries to the lips, mouth, and eyes. Oral lesions may result in excessive salivation, difficulty in eating, and decreased feed intake. Less commonly, such plants may cause skin trauma and eye injury [1].

Awn-producing grasses [R,P,H]: foxtail (*Hordeum jubatum*), bristle grass (Setaria spp.), cheat grass (*Bromus tectorum*), wheat, rye, and many other grasses have awns that often cause ulcerative stomatitis resulting in salivation, slobbering, and anorexia. An awn is either a hair- or bristle-like appendage of a larger structure (such as a floret). They may be several centimeters long, straight or curved, single or multiple. Many such hairs result in a "hairy" appearance that is obvious in many of these grasses (Figure 12.2). The awn-induced oral lesions are common in the gingival recesses, under the tongue, and along the tooth margins. The plant material is often visible and can be manually removed. Other awns may be buried and hidden in the subsequent granulation tissue. Most horses quickly recover when exposure is discontinued, and embedded plant material is removed. Horses generally avoid eating such irritating plants while free-standing in pastures as most problems occur when these plants are included in hay and prepared forage.

12.2.3 Inflammation of the Hoof Laminae

Laminitis is a systemic condition that manifests in the foot resulting in varying degrees of pain, lameness, and debilitation. In the equine foot, there are two types of laminae: sensitive (dermal) highly vascularized laminae, and insensitive (epidermal) laminae that interdigitate with each other to form a bond that is responsible for holding the hoof wall onto the distal phalangeal bone (P3). Each hoof contains approximately 600 primary epidermal laminae (PEL). Each PEL, in turn, contains approximately 100 secondary epidermal laminae [9]. With lamellae inflammation, the bond between the dermal and epidermal laminae fails, and the inner hoof wall and P3 may separate with the weight of the horse and forces of locomotion [10].

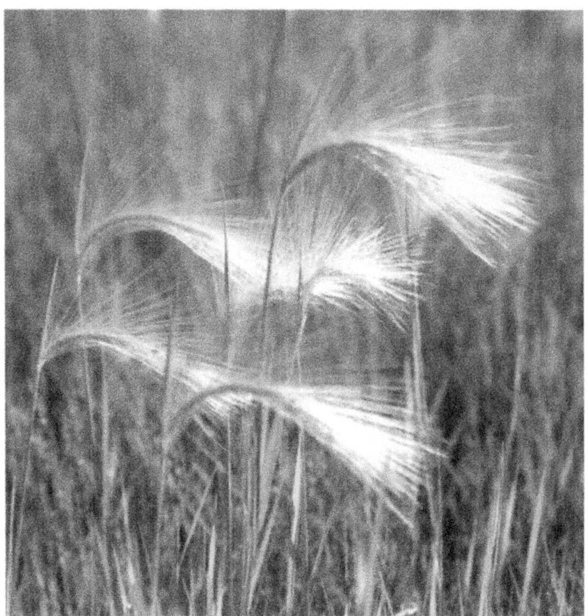
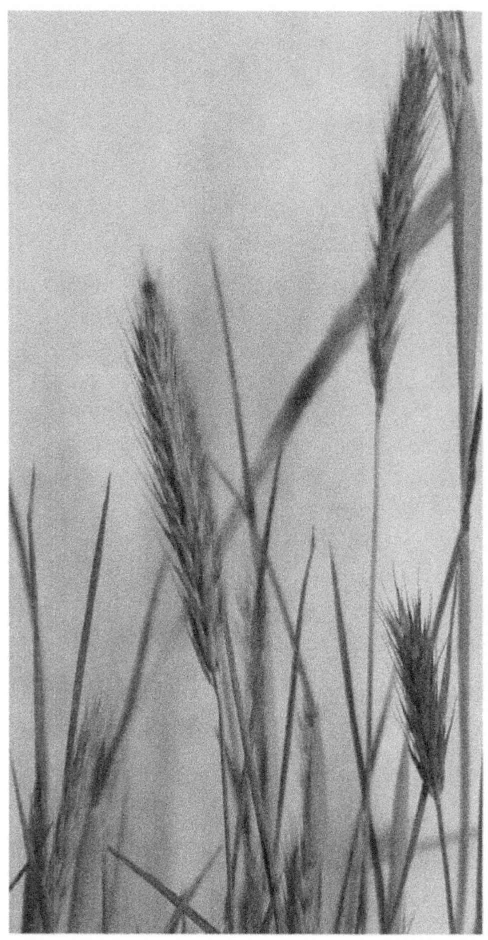

Figure 12.2 Foxtail, hare, and little barley (*Hordeum* spp.) seed heads with awns.

12.2.3.1 Walnut Trees: Black Walnut (*Juglans nigra*), English Walnut (*Juglans regia*) and Butternut (*Juglans Cinerea*) [P]

Several walnut trees (black walnut (*Juglans nigra*), English walnut (*Juglans Regia*) and Butternut walnut (*Jugulans cinerea*) [P] have been associated with equine laminitis [11]. Black walnut trees produce an edible spherical fruit with an encapsulated corrugated nut that is commonly grown in the Northeast and Midwest of NA. Toxicity is most often associated with percutaneous exposure when walnut shavings are used as bedding. Most horses develop the disease within several hours of exposure. The shavings range in color from purplish black to coffee-brown. When freshly cut or chipped they often have a distinctly sweet/ acrid odor. This is easily contrasted with the shavings of pine, fir, ash, oak, and most softwoods commonly used for bedding that are all light-colored. Bedding containing as little as 5 to 20% black walnut shavings can cause poisoning in horses [12]. Poisoning has on occasion been associated with the ingestion of walnut nuts or hulls. An allelopathic compound, juglone, has been suggested as the toxin; however, its toxicity has not been confirmed experimentally. Clinical signs include depression, limb edema, warm hooves, stiff gait, and painful hoof walls (laminitis). Most horses recover quickly when removed from the shavings and appropriate laminitis treatment is instituted.

12.2.3.2 Hoary Alyssum (*Berteroa incana*) [H]

Hoary alyssum (*Berteroa incana*) [H] is a European weed that is an erect, branching annual that grows up to 1 m tall. Its alternating leaves are narrow and smooth and the stems are haired. The flowers are white producing round, flattened seed pods that contain brown seeds. Hoary alyssum is originally an Eurasian plant that has been grown in many areas of NA. It can spread and is often considered a weed as it can grow in disturbed areas and it may invade pastures and hayfields. Most poisoning occurs when it contaminates prepared and dried hay. Within hours after exposure, horses develop fever, distal limb edema (stocking up), laminitis, colic, bloody diarrhea, abortion, dystocia, anorexia, dehydration, and death. Postmortem changes are those of laminitis [13]. Treatment includes removing exposure, treating laminitis, and monitoring pregnant mares for abortion.

12.3 Plants that Contain Gastrointestinal Toxins

12.3.1 Red Clover (*Trifolium* Spp.) [P]

During wet, cooler years, Red Clover (*Trifolium* spp.) [P] may become infected with a mold (*Rhizoctonia leguminicola*) and develop black patches on the leaves. These fungi can produce indolizidine alkaloids including slaframine. Slaframine is a secretagogue, resulting in an excessive salivary response called "slobbers" Orchard grass is highly susceptible to *R. leguminicola* infection, and it has been associated most often with poisoning. Slaframine, a potent parasympathomimetic, is fatal at high doses. Though the lethal toxicity is unknown in horses, the LD_{50} oral lethal dose in guinea pigs is 0.6–0.8 mg/kg BW [14]. Most clinical cases in horses involve much lower doses that produce excessive salivation (salivary syndrome) with few other lesions [15]. Most animals recover without complications when exposure is discontinued.

12.3.2 Black Locust (*Robinia pseudoacacia*) [P]

Black Locust (*Robinia pseudoacacia*) [P] is a 20–30 m tall tree native to NA. The bark, seeds, and leaves are toxic whether fresh or dried. Several toxalbumins, robin and phasin, have been identified and they have been proposed as the cause of poisoning as they are potent hemagglutinins. Signs of poisoning, that develop quickly after ingestion, include anorexia, colic, diarrhea, depression, laminitis, posterior paresis, dilated pupils, apnea, and death [16]. Horses are uniquely susceptible to black locust poisoning and all exposure should be avoided including using locust trees as fencing or hitching post materials.

12.3.3 Field Bindweed or Morning Glory (*Convolvulus arvensis*) [P,H,M]

Field bindweed or Morning Glory (*Convolvulus arvensis*) [P,H,M] is an extremely persistent, perennial, twining, or creeping weed with alternate leaves and white or pink funnel-shaped flowers. Field bindweed has invaded most continents including nearly all of NA (Figure 12.3). The plant reproduces readily from seed and it also expands from its extensive root system. Bindweed invades into pastures and fields tangling mechanical harvesters, contaminating hay and prepared feeds so it should be considered poisonous when grazed or when it is eaten in contaminated feed. All parts of bindweed contain atropine-like tropane alkaloids, e.g. tropine, pseudotropine, and

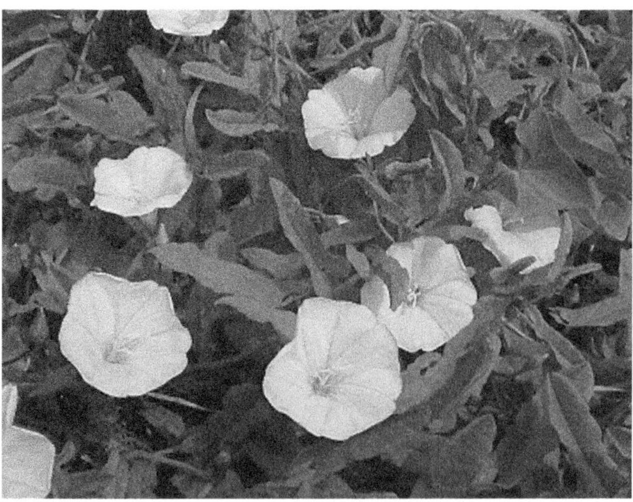

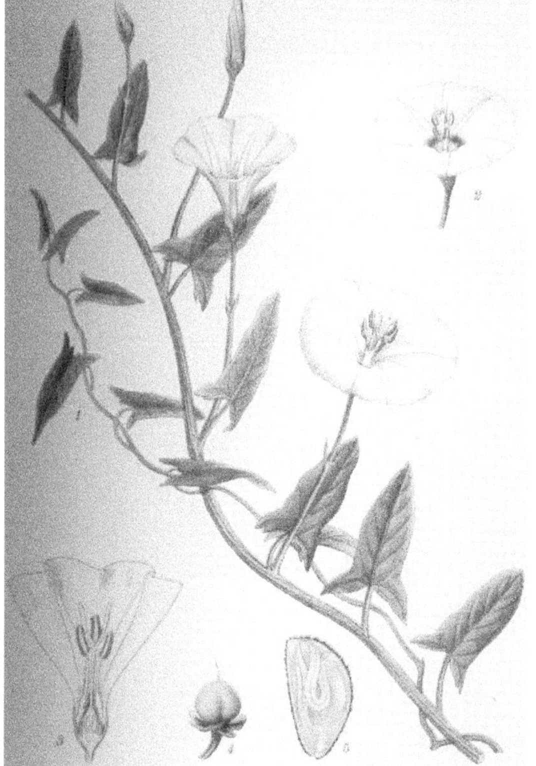

Figure 12.3 Field bindweed (*Convolvulus arvensis*) is a creeping perennial that has alternate leaves with white to pink funnel-shaped flowers, produces numerous seeds, and also spreads by an extensive root system. *Source:* Lindman [5].

tropinone that have parasympatholytic activities. In horses, this may result in colic resulting from intestinal fibrosis, stasis and flatulence. Poisoned horses may also have dilated pupils and bradycardia [17]. No specific treatment is known but symptomatic colic therapy is indicated until clinical signs resolve.

12.3.4 Castor Bean (*Ricinus communis*) [P,H,M]

Castor bean (*Ricinus communis*) [P,H,M] is an ornamental or weed found in many warm climates such as the southern United States and the Hawaiian Islands (Figure 12.4). Poisoning usually occurs when animals are fed concentrates that are contaminated with castor bean seeds. The toxin, ricin, inhibits ribosomal function in protein synthesis. It also may be antigenic, causing anaphylaxis in sensitive animals. The seeds or beans are highly toxic in that 0.1 mg/kg BW of well-chewed or ground seeds can be lethal to horses [19, 20]. This amount could be provided in a grain contaminated with only 1 to 2% castor bean. Castor oil extracted from the seeds is not toxic, as the ricin is insoluble in oil; however, it is a potent cathartic.

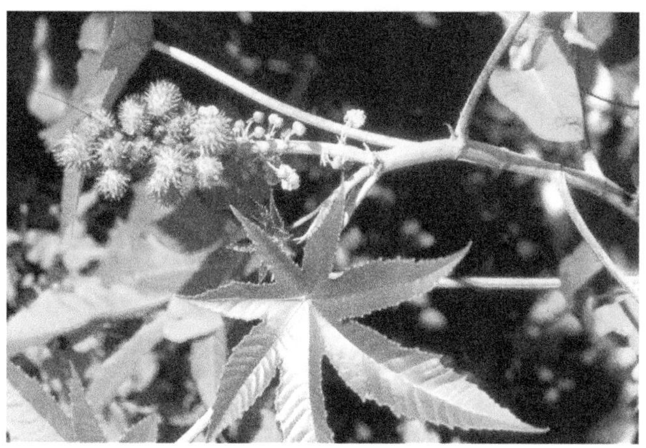

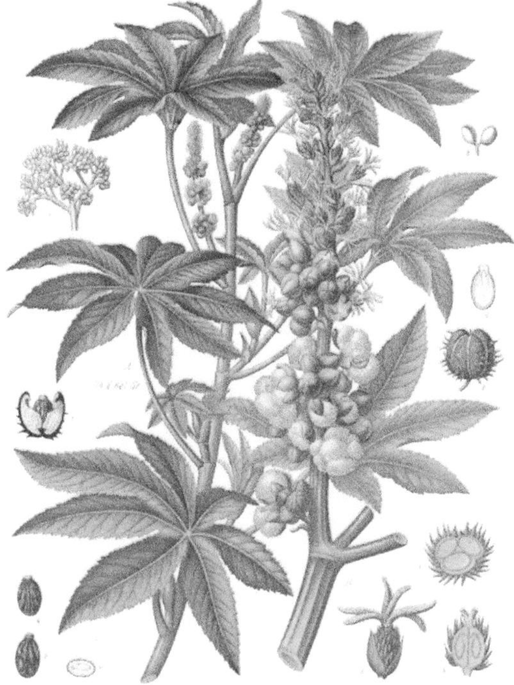

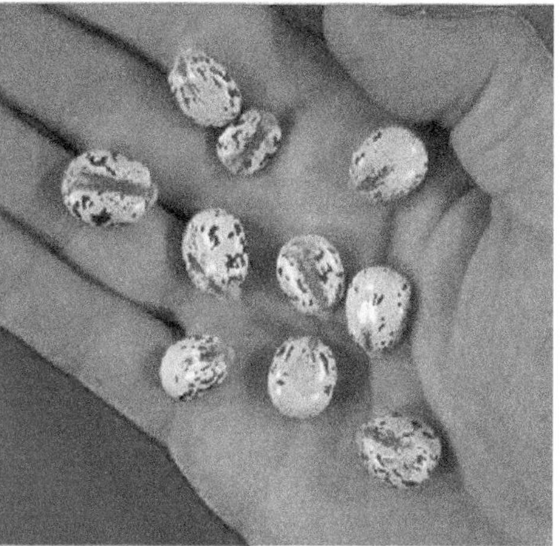

Figure 12.4 Castor bean (*Ricinus communis*) is a perennial tropical plant that grows from 1.5 to 3 m tall with a single, hollow, branching stem. The leaves are large, alternate with eight lobes. Each lobe has a central vein that radiates from the petiole attachment. *Source:* Brandt et al. [18].

Most animals develop clinical signs of poisoning 12 to 48 hours after ingestion of ground castor beans. Early signs of poisoning in horses include trembling, sweating, and incoordination. Signs advance to depression, anorexia, thirst, weakness, colic, trembling, sweating, incoordination, difficult breathing, progressive central nervous system (CNS) depression, fever, bloody diarrhea, convulsions, and death [20]. Treatment is palliative to reduce absorption, including activated charcoal, cathartics, and supportive care. Therapy should include aggressive administration of intravenous fluids to counteract signs of shock. Mineral oil (4 L/450 kg horse) followed 4 to 6 hrs later by activated charcoal (0.5 kg/450 kg horse) in a saline solution cathartic should be given by stomach tube to reduce further absorption of ricin. Poisoning often is fatal; many animals die without aggressive early intervention.

12.3.5 Grayanotoxins [P,H]

Grayanotoxins [P,H] are neurotoxins found in plants of the Ericaceae family including species of Azaleas (Rhododendron spp.), Kalmia (Mountain Laurel), Pieris, and Agarista genera. Of these only rhododendron is reported to have poisoned horses, although the others certainly have the potential [21]. These plants are used as ornamentals in many climates, but most are native to the Appalachian Mountains doing best in cooler climates. All parts of the plants contain andromedotoxin, a grayanotoxin, that binds to sodium ion channels depolarizing neurons, and some myocytes. The principal clinical effects are gastrointestinal (GI) irritation and disruption of myocardial electrical activity. Poisoning is characterized by tachycardia and dyspnea with decreased GI function, which in horses often results in hyper-salivation seen as green froth dripping from the mouth. Less-common changes include colic, frequent defecation, depression, weakness, and ataxia. If a sufficient quantity of laurel has been eaten, recumbency, coma, and death occur. There is no specific treatment. Mineral oil should be administered by stomach tube, and intravenous fluid therapy is administered as necessary. Poisoning in humans has increased as these toxins contaminate honey and have been associated with myocardial infarctions and sudden death.

12.3.6 Pokeweed (*Phytolacca americana*) [P]

Pokeweed (*Phytolacca americana*) [P] in NA Eastern and Southern states is a perennial branching herb that has become an invasive weed in Europe and other continents. In most areas, pokeweed is 1–3 m tall, has green to purple stems, and large alternate, ovate leaves. The flowers are small and white that mature into shiny purple berries. Saponins (phytolaccosides), oxalates, and nitrates have been suggested to be the pokeweed major toxins, but other toxins including histamine-like compounds and gamma-aminobutyric acid have been identified and may contribute to toxicity. Additionally several glycoproteins have been identified. These may cause immunomodulation and hemagglutination through the activation of B- and T-lymphocytes. Depending on the amount consumed, poisoned horses develop mild to severe colic followed by diarrhea. Mineral oil (4 L/450 kg horse) by stomach tube and intravenous fluids should be administered as needed. Although consumption is often fatal in other livestock, most horses generally recover with appropriate therapy [22].

12.3.7 Horse Chestnut and Buckeye (*Aesculus* Spp.) [P]

Horse chestnut and buckeye (*Aesculus* spp.) [P] are shrubs or small trees with large palmate leaves and white to red flower spikes on the ends of the branches, producing a spiny fruit that contains one to three brown nuts. The species that are reported to poison livestock and horses include *Aesculus glabra, Aesculus california, Aesculus pavia, Aesculus octandra,* and *Aesculus hippocastanum.* These toxic chestnuts are not related to edible chestnuts (Castanea spp.). The toxin has been identified as aesculin, a glycoside that is present in new growth, leaves, and nuts. Though colic is the main symptom, signs of poisoning also include muscle tremors, ataxia, incoordination, and paralysis [23]. There is no specific treatment, but administering mineral oil by stomach tube as a laxative, and supportive fluid therapy may be beneficial.

12.3.8 Alkaloids of the *Solanaceae* Family [R,P,H,M]

This large and diverse family of flowering annual and perennial plants range from herbs to vines, lianas, epiphytes, shrubs, and trees, and includes several crops (potato, tomato), medicinal plants, spices, and ornamentals. Horses have been poisoned by various genera within this family, notably nightshades (*Solanum* spp.), Jimsonweed or thorn apple (*Datura stramonium*), and less likely tomato (*Lycopersicon* spp.), potato (*Solanum tuberosum*), and jessamine (*Cestrum* spp.).

Within the genus *Solanum* (nightshades), there is *Solanum rostratum* (buffalo bur – a common hay contaminant), *Solanum ptycanthum* (black nightshade), *Solanum dulcamara* (bittersweet), *Solanum elaeagnifolium* (silver-leaf nightshade), *Solanum carolinense* (Carolina horse nettle), *Solanum dimidiatum* (western horse nettle), and

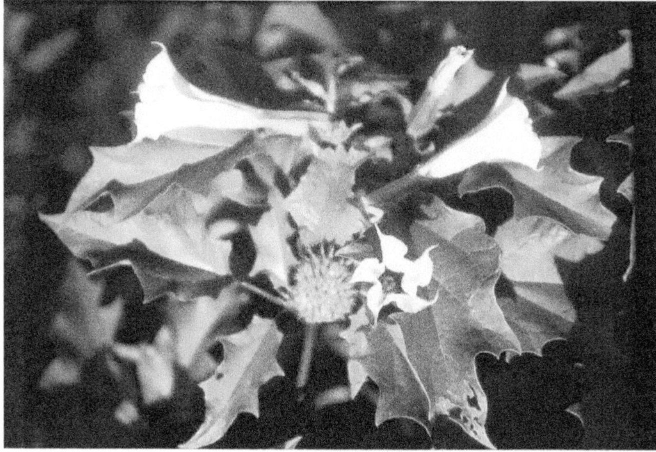

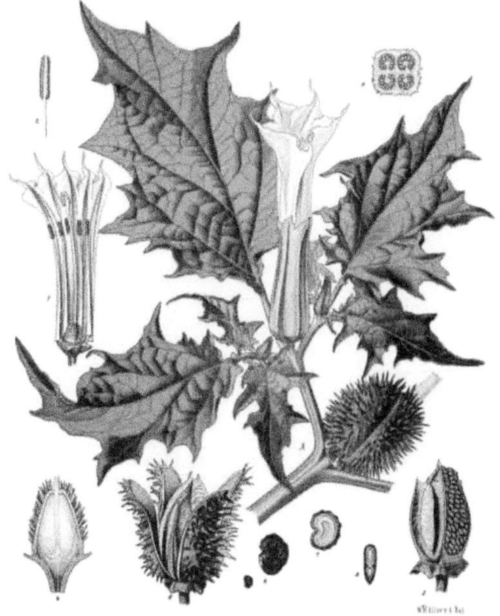

Figure 12.5 Jimson or Jamestown weed (*Datura* spp.) is an erect, branching annual that is 1–2 m tall. The large leaves are simple, alternate with large-toothed margins. The flowers are large, white, and funnel-shaped (6–10 cm). *Source:* Brandt et al. [18].

Solanum triflorum (cutleaf nightshade). Nightshade poisoning has been associated with several syndromes because these plants contain a variety of steroid alkaloids, especially in the green parts of the plant and the unripe fruits. The alkaloids, including solanine, hyoscine, and hyoscyamine, are similar to atropine in their effect on the autonomic nervous system and block the action of cholinesterase. This results in the accumulation of acetylcholine and, consequently, inhibition of the parasympathetic nervous system. The *Solanum* alkaloids are also potent mucosal irritants causing stomatitis and severe gastroenteritis. Solanine concentrations can be high, especially in the berries, and doses as small as 0.1–0.3% BW of silver leaf nightshade berries are toxic. Signs of poisoning include anorexia, salivation, abdominal pain, diarrhea, dilation of pupils, dullness, depression, weakness, progressive paralysis, prostration, but most intoxications are rarely fatal. Treatment generally is symptomatic and most animals quickly recover when exposure is discontinued.

Within the genus *Datura*, there are nine species of poisonous evening flowering plants and several of these are toxic. Jimsonweed (*Datura* spp.) contains toxic tropane alkaloids, atropine, and scopolamine and is fatally poisonous to horses (Figure 12.5). This plant is likely native to Eastern United States but is now found in many countries around the world. The highest toxin concentrations are found in the seeds. Horses are most often poisoned by the feeding of manufactured feeds and grains contaminated with Jimsonweed seeds. Nine horses died within one to three days of eating feed containing 60 to 300 g of *D. stramonium* seeds (0.1–0.7% BW) [24]. As little as 0.5% contamination in hay can be lethal. Such contamination in the feed or hay can cause an epidemic of colic in a barn affecting nearly all horses fed the same feed or hay. Clinical signs include anorexia, rapid heart and respiratory rates, pupil dilation, excessive thirst and urination, sweating, severe GI atony, and abdominal pain. Lesions are variable and mostly related to the cause of colic, due to obstruction, entrapment, and/or volvulus, all resulting in vascular compromise [25]. Most diagnoses are made by identifying the alkaloids in serum or ingesta, or finding the seeds or plant in the contaminated feed or ingesta taken at necropsy. Therapy is symptomatic as no specific treatment exists. Oral administration of activated charcoal (0.5 kg/450 kg horse) as an absorbent, along with a saline cathartic may be effective if given soon after the plants have been eaten.

12.4 Plants that Contain Hepatotoxins

12.4.1 Dehydropyrrolizidine Alkaloid-Containing Plants [P,H,M]

Over 3% of the flowering plants on nearly all continents contain dehydropyrrolizidine alkaloids (DHPAs). Consequently, DHPA-containing plants often poison

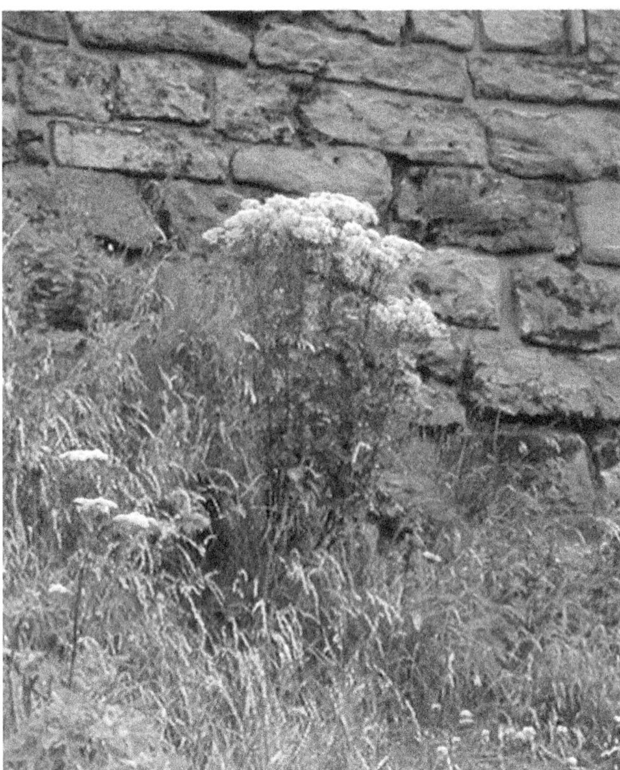

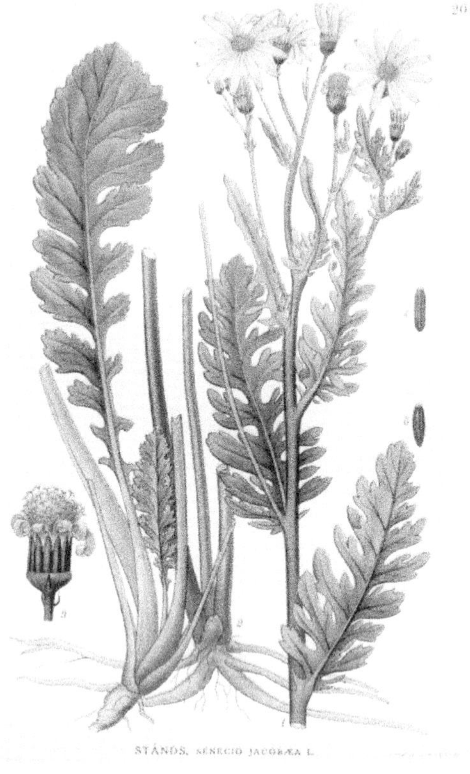

Figure 12.6 Tansy ragwort (*Senecio jacobaea*) is a noxious European weed that has infested many pastures, forests, and waste areas of Western Europe, South Africa, Australia, New Zealand, and North America. A tall (0.5–1.5 m), erect plant that is unbranched except at the inflorescence. In the spring, a tall, flowering stalk forms with composite heads that have terminal, flat-topped clusters about 1 cm tall and individual 1 cm long yellow rays. Each plant produces thousands of wind-dispersed seeds. Leaves are variably sized up to 22 cm long and 10 cm wide, with two or three deep pinnate divisions. *Source:* Lindman [5].

livestock, wildlife, and humans. When alternative forages are available, most horses avoid eating free-standing DHPA-containing plants due to their bitterness. However, in times of limited feed, increased herd-feeding pressure, or when contaminated hay and feeds are fed, many horses are poisoned. Common DHPA-containing plants that have been associated with equine poisoning include *Senecio jacobaea* (tansy ragwort, Figure 12.6), *Senecio integerrimus* (lamb's tongue groundsel), *Senecio longilobus* (wolly or treadleaf groundsel), *Senecio ridellii* (Riddell's groundsel), *Senecio spartioides* (broom groundsel), *Senecio vulgaris* (common groundsel), *Crotalaria sagittalis* (rattlebox), *Crotalaria spectabilis* (showy crotalaria), *Crotalaria retusa* (rattlebox), *Amsinckia intermedia* (tarweed or fiddleneck), *Echium vulgare* (viper's bugloss), *Echium plantagineum* (Patterson's curse or Salvation Jane), *Heliotropium europaeum* (Heliotrope), and *Cynoglossum officinale* (hounds tongue) (Figure 12.7) [1].

Dehydropyrrolizidine alkaloids poisoning in horses is dose and duration-dependent. High doses cause acute, severe, irreversible liver disease. Lower doses with intermittent or long duration may produce temporary clinical disease that may recur later when precipitated by additional damage from additional DHPA exposures or if the animal encounters some other hepatic stress. The toxicity of the various plants is related both to the concentration and type of DHPA. High doses that are generally produced by contaminated feed result in sudden, massive liver necrosis and failure. Low-dose exposure of extended duration generally occurs when animals are forced to eat standing plants or contamination is low. These chronic exposures often produce transient clinical disease characterized by weight loss or decreased gain with transient increases in serum enzymes. If damage is not extensive, these may resolve though liver failure and subsequent liver disease can recur months or years later when exposure is repeated or other stresses cause relapse, chronic liver disease and hepatic failure. Young animals are highly susceptible to poisoning and fetal and neonatal poisoning in foals can occur without maternal toxicity [26]. Signs of poisoning are related to liver failure and include weight loss, weakness, sleepiness, yawning, incoordination, neurologic derangement, icterus, photosensitivity, aimless walking, chewing motions, and head pressing. Histologically,

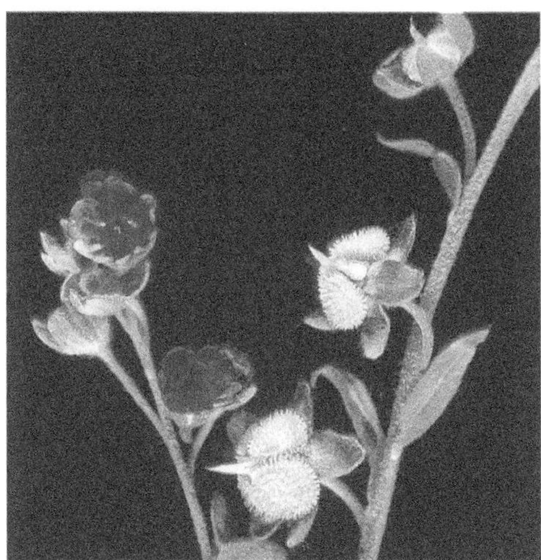
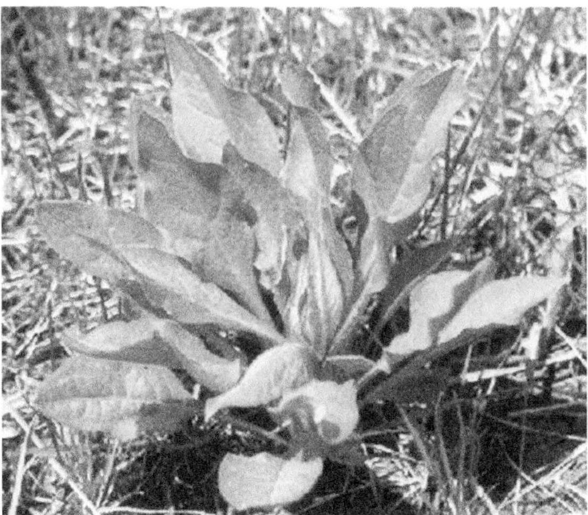

Figure 12.7 Houndstongue (*Cynoglossum officinale*), a Euroasia noxious weed, has spread in many continents including North America. A biennial that invades pastures, rangelands, and cultivated fields that may contaminate hay and prepared forages. Generally, in the first year, a leafy rosette forms, and in the second year, a flowering rosette develops. The plant is erect, usually 30–120 cm tall with large oblong-lanceolate leaves. The blue or purple flowers are terminal forming prickly nutlets (3–5 mm) which bind and entangle hair or clothing.

poisoned animals have hepatic degeneration and necrosis with fibrosis, biliary hyperplasia, and depending on the duration, may have megalocytosis. Diagnosis is made by associating exposure with the clinical disease and gross and histological lesions. To further confirm poisoning in some cases, DHPA metabolites or pyrroles can be extracted from the damaged liver and identified chemically. There are no recommended antidotes, treatments, or supportive care for liver damage or failure. As both contamination rates and varying DHPA concentrations make assessing risk difficult, avoiding exposure to any of these DHPA-containing plants is recommended.

12.4.2 Other Hepatotoxic Plants

12.4.2.1 Indigo (*Indigofera spicata*) [P]

Indigo (*Indigofera spicata*) [P] is a creeping legume that has become established in warm climates in many countries and has been associated with equine hepatic encephalopathy in Florida [27]. A similar disease called "Birdsville disease" has been identified in Australia and has been attributed to *Indigofera dominii* [28]. Creeping indigo is a prostrate plant composed of many branched runners that radiate from a white taproot. The pale green stems have alternate pinnate leaves and alternate ovate leaflets with a short petiole and pink flowers that project from the leaf axils that form clusters of pointed seed pods. It has been suggested that indospicine, a arginine antagonist amino acid caused indigo poisoning by inhibiting protein synthesis. The leaves may contain from 0.1% to 0.5% indospicine and the seeds as much as 2.0% (% dry weight) [27, 29]. Horses consuming high-protein meals, i.e., peanut meal or cottonseed meal both of which are rich in arginine (10–12% arginine of total protein), are relatively protected from the effects of indospicine [30]. Horses find the plant highly palatable and after several weeks of exposure, horses lose weight, develop depression, incoordination, ataxia, and difficulty in turning, backing up, or walking in a straight line. Some horses also develop apnea and corneal opacity. Most of the clinical signs have been attributed to liver disease and hepatic encephalopathy, as poisoned animals have extensive liver necrosis with nodular fibrosis. Affected pregnant mares may abort. Animals (dogs) eating meat from horses that have been poisoned by creeping indigo may suffer similar fatal poisoning [31].

12.4.2.2 Cocklebur (*Xanthium* Spp) [P,H,M]

Cocklebur (*Xanthium* spp.) [P,H,M] is a potent hepatotoxic plant that commonly affects livestock; however, there are only a few reports of poisoning in horses (Figure 12.8) [32]. The toxin, carboxyactractyloside, inhibits mitochondrial adenosine diphosphate translocase, inhibiting oxidative phosphorylation, which results in severe hepatic necrosis. Cockleburs are allelopathic (inhibiting growth of adjacent plants) allowing them to dominate some plant communities. The carboxyatractyloside, has been identified in all plant parts and has been used diagnostically when detected in GI contents of affected animals. Equine poisoning most often occurs when horses consume feed contaminated with seed or small seedlings. Doses of 0.3% BW have been suggested to be toxic. Common signs include neurologic

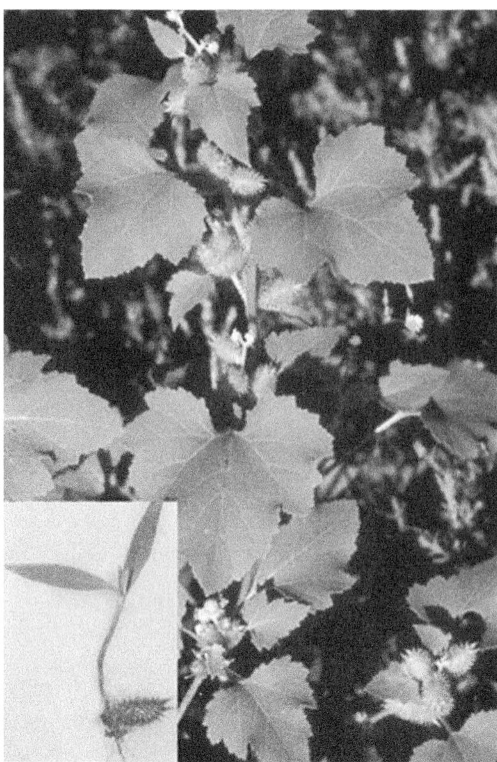

Figure 12.8 Cocklebur (*Xanthium strumarium*) is a summer annual that grows up to 1.5 m high. The ribbed stems may have purple spots with short white hairs, branched with large (~20 cm) alternate leaves one long purple petioles. A single spike-like flowering racemes composed of compound flowers that produce hundreds of bur covered seeds (inset) that often result in large colonies that can dominate pastures, fields, and disturbed areas along roads and fence lines.

disease related to liver failure, depression, weakness, prostration, abnormal eye position and movements, paddling, convulsions, and coma. Other changes include stocking up (swelling and edema of the feet and legs) and vasculitis. Serum biochemistry changes are dependent on disease duration and can include massive elevations in enzymatic activity and increases in serum bilirubin and bile acids. Gross lesions may include ascites, a pale swollen liver with a prominent red lobular mottling, e.g. nutmeg color. Severely poisoned animals generally die or develop chronic liver dysfunction and perform poorly. A small number of less severely affected horses may develop fibrotic hepatic lesions that are thought to progress to cirrhosis and chronic liver failure. Less severely poisoned animals appear to recover with little detectable permanent hepatic change [33]. Symptomatic treatment is usually unsuccessful as liver damage is generally extensive when animals become sick. Reducing exposure including herbicide application as well as mowing or removing cockleburs is recommended.

12.4.2.3 Alsike Clover (*Trifolium hybridum*) [P]

Alsike Clover (*Trifolium hybridum*) [P] has long been associated with liver disease and photosensitivity in horses. However, reproducing disease has been difficult making identifying its toxic components problematic. Poisoning often appears to be related to environmental conditions suggesting a fungus or aflatoxin may be involved. Occasionally, horses grazing clover, generally alsike clover (*T. hybridum*), during wet or humid weather, develop photosensitivity and hepatitis referred to as trifoliosis [20]. Exposures of weeks to months generally are required before horses develop the disease. Three syndromes have been identified. The first, called "dew poisoning," is characterized by photosensitivity (sunburn), colic and diarrhea, depression, or excitation. The second, called "big liver disease" is severe liver disease or recurrent bouts of liver disease that is seen clinically as icterus, weight loss, CNS depression, anorexia, incoordination, dark and discolored urine, and an enlarged fibrotic brown liver. The third is a slobbering syndrome and is probably related to fungal-produced slaframine as discussed with red clover poisoning. Alsike clover has also been associated with phytoestrogens as have many other clovers. Treatment includes removing horses from exposure to the plant, treating photosensitivity, and supportive care. Recovered animals often have chronic liver damage and are more susceptible to liver failure or other liver diseases. Horses may graze the same pasture again without a problem under different growing conditions in subsequent years or after the pasture dries out; however, alsike clover should not be included in pasture seed mixes for horses.

12.4.2.4 Crystalline Hepatopathy [R,P,H]

Liver disease associated with ingestion of *Panicum coloratum* (Kleingrass), *Panicum virgatum* (switchgrass), *Tribulus terrestris* (puncture vine), and *Nolinatexana (sacahuiste), Agave lechuguilla* (*lechugilla*) has been reported in most livestock species, including horses. Most of these plants are NA natives except for the *Panicum* spp. that were imported for use as cover crops or potential biofuels. Poisoning is often sporadic and at times does not appear to be related to dose or duration. Several saponins including diosgenin and yamogenin are thought to form crystals within ducts and cells damaging the liver biliary system. Because toxin concentrations vary and poisoning is sporadic, the risk is difficult to predict. Most animals never develop disease. Panicum grasses are not very palatable and are poor forages. In most cases, animals must be forced to eat them. Poisoning signs usually are related to sunburn or photosensitization with elevated serum biomarkers and enzymes suggestive of liver disease [34]. Lesions include severe sunburn with liver failure and characteristic histological changes of necrosis and bile-duct crystals and cholestasis.

As it is difficult to predict the dose or risk of poisoning, horses should not be fed monocultures of these forages. Treatment should include supportive care for both liver disease and sunburn.

12.5 Plants Containing Neurotoxins

12.5.1 Locoweed [R]

The locoweeds are composed of about 20 *Astragalus* and *Oxytropis* species that contain swainsonine and produce neurologic disease in livestock (Figures 12.9 and 12.10). Swainsonine inhibits several cellular mannosidases and sustained inhibition results in a plant-induced cellular storage disease similar to genetic mannosidosis. Horses readily eat locoweeds and are uniquely sensitive to poisoning. Though many locoweed lesions are reversible, chronic intoxication causes irreversible neuronal damage that limits their use as safe work animals. Signs of poisoning begin after several weeks of locoweed ingestion and include depression and reluctance to move. With continued exposure, animals develop intention tremors, proprioceptive deficits, loss of condition with irreversible neurologic changes. With stimulation, poisoned horses can become neurologically unstable, with fits ranging from anxiousness to maniacal aggressive bouts, which are dangerous for the poisoned animal and by-standing animals or caretakers. Many poisoned animals abort, have weak foals, or foals with birth defects. Many of the clinical signs and subsequent cellular lesions resolve when exposure is discontinued, but some neurologic lesions persist and previously poisoned animals may relapse with changes ranging from mild proprioceptive deficits to convulsive-like fits. Diagnosis is easily made by

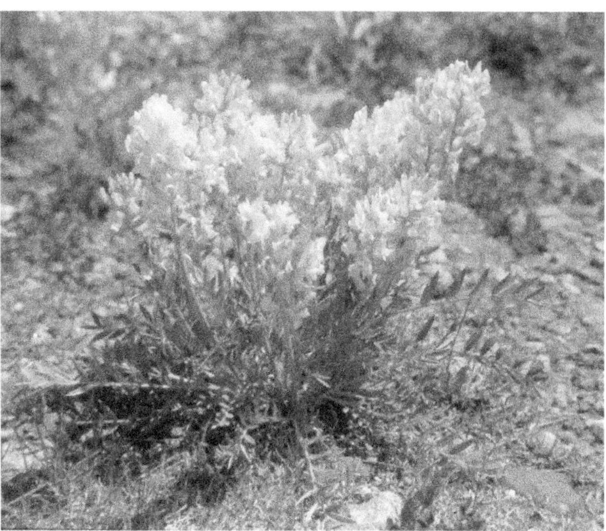

Figure 12.10 White locoweed (*Oxytropis sericea*) is a flowering perennial legume that grows from a deep taproot that provides considerable drought tolerance. This weed grows to about 30 cm and has white pea-like flowers that develop into 2–3 cm pods that are filled with numerous small 0.5 mm kidney-shaped seeds.

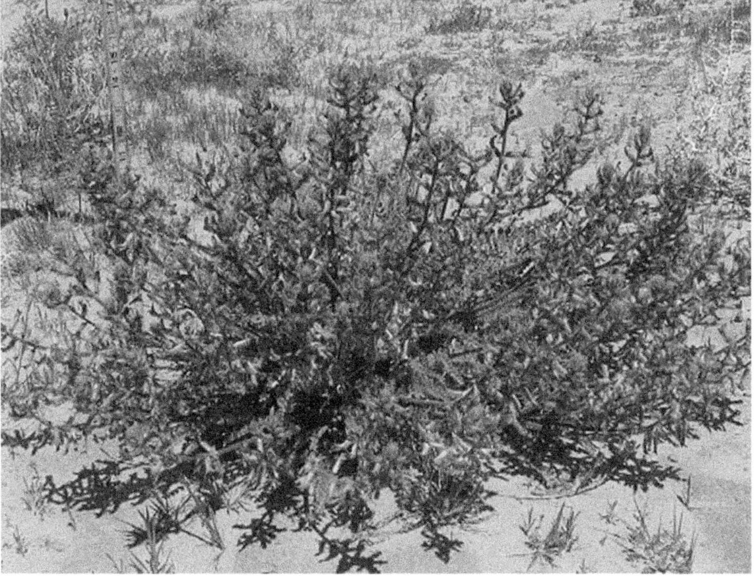

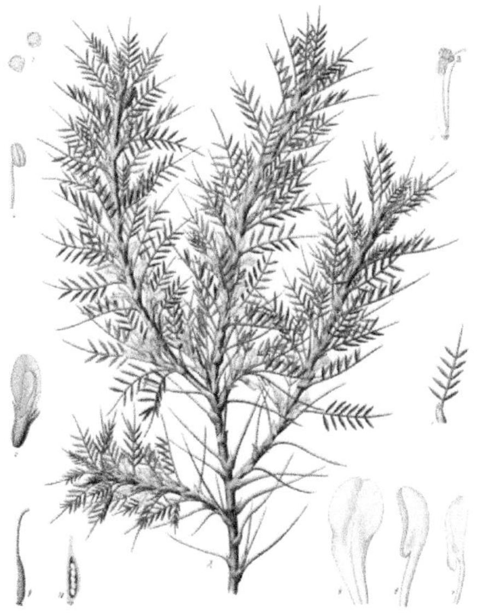

Figure 12.9 Locoweed (*Astragalus lentiginosus*) is a well-adapted native plant in the dry rocky areas of North America and is a prolific seed producer with long-lived seed banks. A perennial herb (~0.5 m) that has alternate and pinnately compound leaves, and pea-like flowers of variable numbers on axillary racemes. These develop into pods that contain small (2–4 mm) kidney-shaped seeds. Though growth patterns vary with location and precipitation, most germinate with the fall precipitation; remain green through the winter, and mature early in the spring when other green feeds may not be available. *Source:* Brandt et al. [18].

documenting exposure and identifying the characteristic histologic changes. Swainsonine can be identified in the blood and tissues of poisoned animals but is quickly cleared within days of discontinuing exposure. New biomarkers are being developed to better identify poisoning and predict recovery. There are no treatments for locoweed poisoning. As horses have to ingest locoweed for several weeks to be poisoned, avoiding prolonged exposures is essential. Many poisoned animals can recover and function as reproductive animals. However, any previously poisoned animal is likely to have permanent neurologic lesions that will likely impair function and should not be ridden or worked [35].

12.5.2 Nitrotoxins (*Astragalus* Spp.) [R]

Over 450 species of the *Astragalas* genera worldwide contain nitrotoxins or nitroglycosides. Nitrotoxins have also been identified in species of the *Cornoilla, Indigofera, Lotus,* and *Hippocrepis* genera and can be produced by certain fungi of the *Arthrinium*, *Aspergillus*, and *Penicillium* genera. In NA, a little less than 250 *Astragalus* species containing nitrotoxins have been identified. Many fewer species have historically poisoned cattle and sheep. Although clinical poisoning in horses has been documented, experimentally, reproduction using nitrotoxin containing *Astragalus* spp. has not been done. The nitrotoxins, 3-nitropropanol, 3-nitro propionic acid (NPA), and their glycosides inhibit succinate dehydrogenase, which is the only enzyme that participates in both the citric acid cycle and the electron transport chain. Succinate dehydrogenase catalyzes the rate-limiting step of oxidative phosphorylation and its inhibition results in a marked reduction of cellular energy production producing respiratory and neurologic damage. Clinical signs include depression, incoordination, and rear-limb weakness. With continued poisoning, animals become emaciated and severe incoordination causes gait changes and interference (limb-to-limb contact during movement).

Another equine disease that has been attributed to NPA is Australian "Birdsville disease" caused by the ingestion of *Indigofera linnaei*. Similar to NPA poisoned cattle, affected horses are weak, depressed, uncoordinated, and may shiver, twitch, and sway when standing. When severely poisoned, there is severe weakness and horses may drag their feet when forced to walk. The histologic changes have not been completely characterized but there also appears to be neuronal degeneration and necrosis in the basal ganglia [36]. *Indigofera linnaei* contains both NPA and indospicine. Indospicine is a toxic amino acid that causes severe hepatocellular degeneration and necrosis in dogs. Horses are not affected, but secondary poisonings have been documented in dogs fed indospicine-contaminated meat from horses and camels grazing *I. linnaei* [37]. More work is needed to better define NPA pathogenesis in horses, and how these similar equine neurodegenerative diseases are related.

12.5.3 Yellowstar Thistle (*Centaurea solstitialis*)

Yellowstar Thistle (*Centaurea solstitialis*) (Figure 12.11), Russian Knapweed (*C. repens*) (Figure 12.12), Maltastar thistle (*C. melitensis*) [P] poisoning produces a unique disease in horses, donkeys, and mules. Poisoning has not been recognized in other animals and no suitable model using experimental animals has developed with similar neurologic lesions. Various compounds including repin and solistatin have been identified as potential toxins, but none has been experimentally shown to produce this disease in horses. Intoxication with these plants is considered a disease of neglect. Most horses avoid eating these plants and poisoning generally occurs when horses are kept on a small

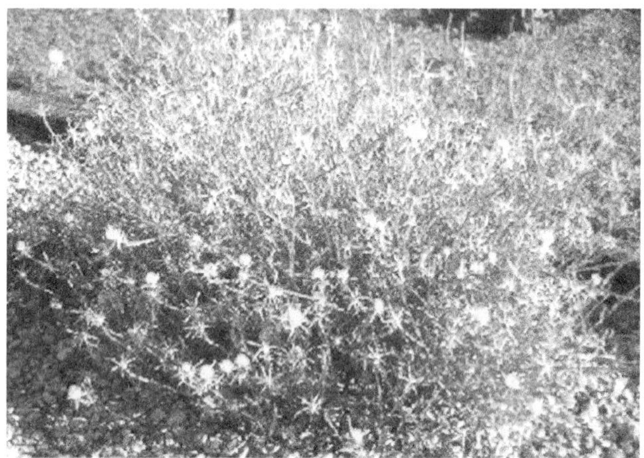

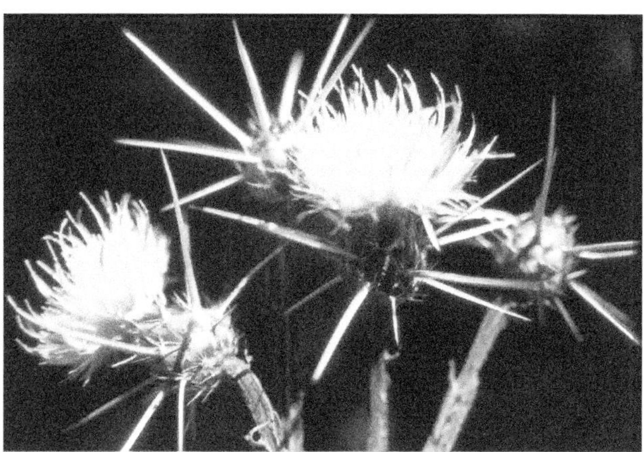

Figure 12.11 Yellowstar thistle (*Centauria solstitialis*) is a Mediterranean weed that has become established in many countries including western portions of North America dominating many roadsides and disturbed areas. Yellowstar thistle is a branching annual with finely haired leaves that are lobed basally and linear on the stem. The disc flowers are yellow and the bracts are tipped with stiff yellow spines.

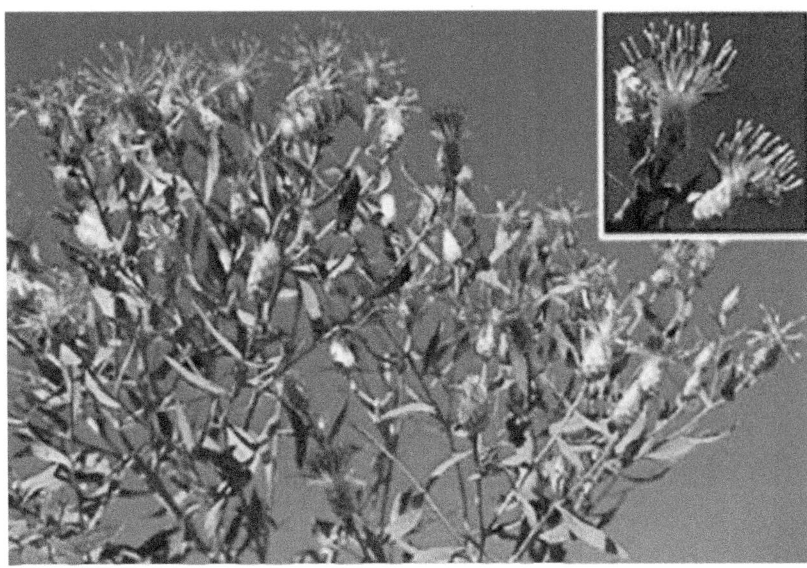

Figure 12.12 Russian knapweed (*Centaurea repens*) is a persistent, noxious allelopathic weed that grows in all soil types, invading fields, pastures, and roadsides spreading by both seeds and rhizomes. Perennial Russian knapweed is generally erect (~1 m tall) and the stems are covered with fine hairs. The leaves are alternate with serrated margins. The flowers form thistle-like heads (1 cm) and vary from white to purple. The paper-like bracts have no spines. Most seeds remain on the seed head, which is easily spread by animals.

pasture with limited feed. When other forages are exhausted, some horses develop a taste for the *Centaurea* spp. and these horses may continue eating these plants even when supplemented with other more nutritious forage. Doses between 50% and 200% BW over 30 to 90 days are required to develop the disease in horses. The clinical disease includes facial nerve dysfunction with impairment or loss of facial, mouth, and throat nerves and muscles. Affected horses try to eat and chew, but dysphagia results in quidding and nonproductive chewing. Continual chewing attempts have resulted in the disease being referred to as "chewing disease." As the disease progresses, there is facial-muscle hypertonicity, which causes "smiling," tongue lolling, protruding tongue, and head tossing. Horses unable to drink will "play" in the water, submerge their muzzle and face, and splash in an effort to drink. These early neurologic signs become worse and lead to lethargy, loss of interest in food, dehydration, malnutrition, difficulty breathing, incoordination, muscle tremors, and severe depression. Some die, but most affected horses have to be euthanized. Lesions include those of dehydration, starvation, and unique damage to brain stem *substantia nigra* and *globus pallidus* nuclei. This specific change resulted in the name of this disease, nigropallidal encephalomalacia [38, 39]. As there is no treatment and the disease is irreversible, avoiding exposure to the plants for prolonged periods is recommended.

12.5.4 Leukoencephalomalacia (Moldy Corn) [M]

This disease is caused when corn is infected with *Fusarium verticillioides* or *Fusarium moniliforme*. These fungi produce toxic fumonisins that alter sphingolipid synthesis and cell membrane integrity, resulting in severe, irreversible neurologic disease. This is seen histologically as liquefactive necrosis of the cerebral white matter characterized as leukoencephalomalacia. Clinical signs are neurologic and range from hypersensitivity, ataxia, and posterior weakness to convulsions. Lesions are not confined to the brain, as high fumonisin doses also produce liver necrosis. Most animals develop the clinical disease within 4 to 72 hours but occasionally 1 to 2 wks of eating contaminated grain. Concentrations at or above 8 ppm fumonisin B_1 in the feed are toxic, and horses rarely recover. As horses are uniquely susceptible to fumonisin poisoning, molded corn should not be fed to horses. Manufacturers of prepared feeds should be testing corn ingredients for contamination [40].

12.5.5 Sand Sage (*Artemisia filifolia*), bud Sage (*A. spinescens*), and Fringed Sage (*A. frigida*) [R]

Sand sage (*Artemisia filifolia*), bud sage (*A. spinescens*), and fringed sage (*A. frigida*) [R] are sagebrushes of the western United States that have been reported to poison horses. The sages are perennials that contain several different toxins. Most are volatile monoterpenoids that vary in species and season. Sand sage and fringed sage are common on the eastern slopes of the Rocky Mountains in the United States and Mexico. Bud sage is found on the western slopes in Nevada and California. All three have been associated with a neurologic disease that develops in hungry horses after several days of being forced to graze sage bushes. The sage toxins are thought to be similar to thujone, a monoterpene found in wormwood (*A. absinthium*). But none have been experimentally proven [41]. Many poisonings occur when other forages

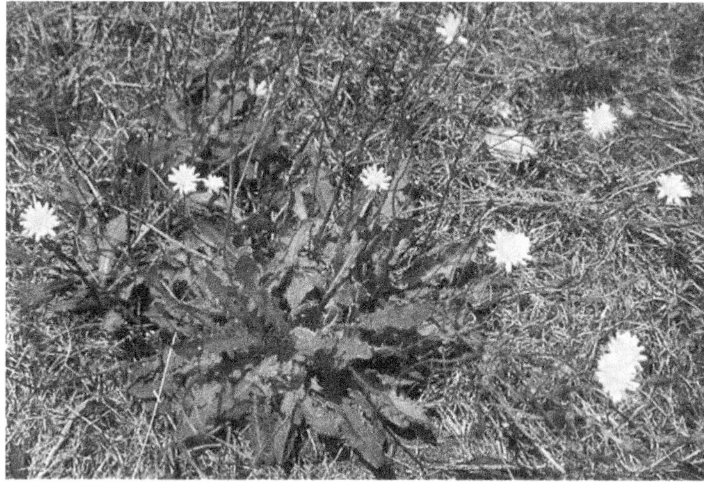

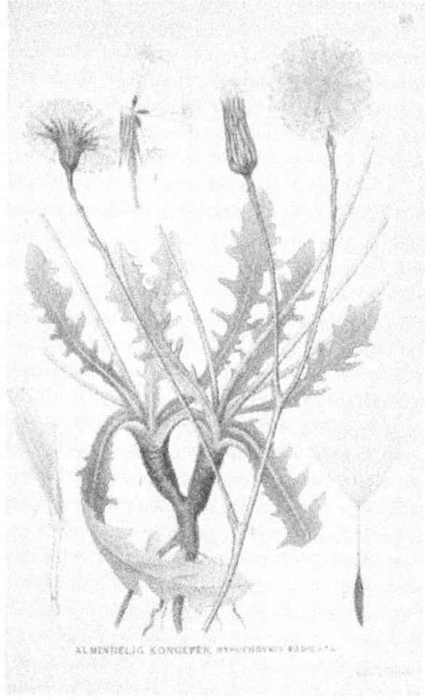

Figure 12.13 Flatweed or False dandelion (*Hypochoeris radicata*) is a perennial weed originally from Europe, commonly growing in disturbed soils or overgrazed pastures, resembling the common dandelion, with basal clusters of irregularly lobed 7–30 cm leaves. The branching, flowering stalks grow up to 0.5 m with a single yellow flower terminally. *Source:* Mentz and Ostenfeld [42].

are depleted or buried in snow. Clinically poisoned horses fall or may be hyper-reflexive to normal stimuli. Some animals may develop ataxia that may be more severe in the front legs. Others may circle or become excitable and unpredictable. The characteristic "sage" smell is noticeable on their breath and in the feces. Histological lesions are variable with non-specific degeneration in the medulla, brain stem, and cerebellum characterized by intraneuronal accumulation of pigment (lipofuscin). Poisoned animals generally recover when removed from exposure and fed better feed.

12.5.6 *Hypochoeris radicata* (Flatweed, False Dandelion) [R,P]

Stringhalt is an abnormal gait that generally is seen as goose-stepping or high-stepping of one or both rear legs. This abnormal gait probably has many different etiologies or causes. However, a few toxic plants have been associated with this disease. Chronic ingestion of *Lathyrus hirsutus* (singletary pea) seeds is thought to be one cause of stringhalt. *Hypochoeris radicata* (Flatweed, or false dandelion) (Figure 12.13) has also been implicated as the cause of stringhalt on several different continents. The lesions of stringhalt are non-specific and related to axonal degeneration in nerves that supply the pelvic limbs. Several surgeries have been used to minimize the hypermetric gait, but there is no proven treatment for the complete resolution of stringhalt.

12.5.7 Cyanogenic Neurologic Disease [R,P,H]

Many plants (>1000) contain cyanogenic glycosides. Examples include various berries, i.e. Serviceberry (*Amelanchier alnifolia*), Elderberry (*Sambucus* spp.), Western Chokecherry (*prunus virginiana*) and other cherries. Also, certain grasses and feed crops, i.e. wild blue flax (*Linum* spp.) and Sorghum, Johnson, or Sudan Grass, can accumulate cyanogenic glycosides. Poisoning in horses is often different from that of many other animals, although fatalities do occur where cyanide doses are high enough to result in sudden death. The more common presentation in horses is that of chronic poisoning. After exposures of a week to six mos (usually about eight wks), poisoned horses lose control of their hind legs and bladder (equine cystitis-ataxia syndrome). Affected animals stumble and fall with rear-limb paresis and proprioceptive deficits. The nerves that innervate the urinary bladder are damaged and the resulting paralysis is characterized by: loss of micturition reflexes, ballooning of the urinary bladder, and incontinence seen as urine dribbling and scalding of the hind legs. Abortions and fetal deformities (multiple arthrogryposes) also have been linked to these forages. Poisoned animals may not recover. The exact mechanism of poisoning has not been determined, though chronic exposure to hydrocyanic acid and lathyrogenic nitriles have been suggested as likely causes. Many of these forages are used safely for both pastures and hay; however, when stressed they have the potential to accumulate cyanogenic glycosides and nitrates. Although initially, the toxins remain in stored feeds and hay, there is some evidence that these cyanogenic glycosides degrade with time, and with proper sampling and analysis contaminated feeds might be considered safe, as the glycosides are hydrolyzed and the resulting cyanide dissipates. If there is a question of toxicity, most diagnostic laboratories have inexpensive assays to measure the cyanide-producing potential of feeds.

12.5.8 Neurotoxins Causing Sudden Death

The sudden death of horses due to plant poisoning with few or no previously occurring clinical signs is relatively uncommon. Determining the cause as quickly as possible to minimize further losses is important. Sudden death due to plants most often occurs when horses have been placed in situations where they have been compelled to eat unusual plants in hay or overgrazed pastures, or unintentionally when garden clippings or prunings are fed to horses. There are three major types of plant toxins that may cause sudden death: cyanogenic glycosides, cardiac glycosides, and alkaloids.

12.5.8.1 Cardioglycoside Containing Plants [P,H]

There are at least 34 plant genera that contain cardiac glycosides that are potentially toxic to man and animals, but relatively few have attained notoriety as causes of animal poisoning [21]. These include foxglove (*Digitalis purpurea*), oleander (*Nerium oleander*) (Figure 12.14), yellow oleander (*Thevetia* spp.), milkweeds (*Asclepias* spp.), dogbane (*Apocynum* spp.), and pheasant's eye (*Adonis aestivalis.*). (Figure 12.15) is an incomplete list of the plants that contain cardioglycosides, but includes most of those that have poisoned horses in NA. Many are ornamentals that are used in residential landscaping and as margin plants or hedges. Toxicity varies with the plant and growing conditions; however, all oleanders, foxglove, and milkweeds should be considered potentially poisonous. Most are rarely eaten fresh; however, horses are often poisoned after consuming clippings or discarded pruned plant material.

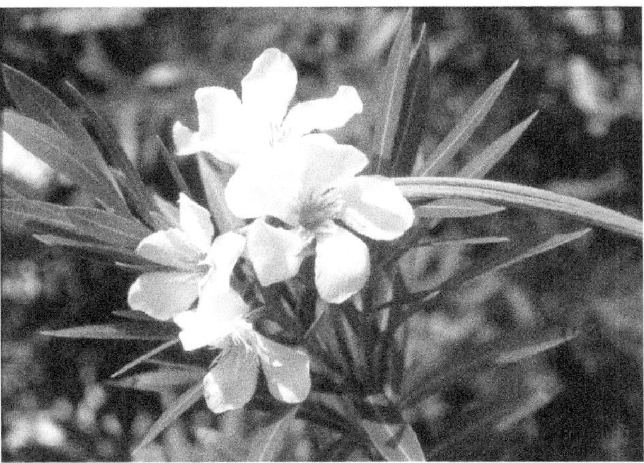

Figure 12.14 Oleander (*Nerium oleander*) is a Mediterranean evergreen perennial plant that has become naturalized in many warmer climates growing 2–6 m tall with white or pink flowers. Yellow flowers are *Thevetia peruviana*. The leaves are simple oblong to lanceolate, with prominent midrib and secondary veins. Most oleander poisonings occur when clippings are discarded into paddocks.

Still, others have escaped cultivation and have invaded fields and pastures. The cardiac glycosides are retained in dried plants, although in reduced quantities, oleander and milkweed pose the greatest threat if present in hay.

Most contain mixtures of toxins, including cardiac glycosides that are similar to digoxin and digitoxin. Toxicity varies according to the glycoside with lethal doses. In cattle and horses, as little as 0.005% BW of green oleander leaves or 0.05% BW of green labriform milkweed is reportedly lethal [6]. Cardioglycosides alter sodium/potassium channels and calcium homeostasis resulting in myocardial degeneration and necrosis, which is often seen as all types of cardiac arrhythmias and heart blocks that may be encountered at various stages of cardiac glycoside poisoning. Initial signs of poisoning that occur hours after ingestion include GI upset, salivation, anorexia, frequent defecation, diarrhea, colic, depression, weakness, incoordination, stupor, leg paralysis, weak heart rate, recumbence, coma, and death. The glycosides also act directly on the GI tract, causing hemorrhagic enteritis that results in vomiting, colic, and diarrhea. The milkweed cardiac glycosides also act on the respiratory and nervous systems, potentially causing dyspnea, muscle tremors, seizures, and head pressing. Low doses, when the initial myocardial necrosis is non-fatal, nearly always produce histological heart lesions (myocardial necrosis, fibrosis, and regeneration). Heart damage may lead to congestive heart failure (stocking up, ventral edema, jugular pulse, etc.). Little is known of possible sequelae of poisoning but sub-lethally poisoned animals are likely to have impaired endurance and performance. The duration of symptoms rarely exceeds 24 hours before convulsions and death occur. Animals consuming sufficient cardiac glycoside-containing plants to cause cardiac arrest are often found dead in 8–10 hours after ingestion and animals may die before developing the classic histological lesions. There is no specific treatment for counteracting the effects of cardiac glycosides. Horses should be given adsorbents such as activated charcoal (2–5 g/kg BW) by stomach tube with a saline cathartic to prevent further toxin absorption. The cardiac irregularities may be treated by administering antiarrhythmic drugs. Poisoned animals should be removed from the source of the plants; given fresh water, good-quality hay, and shade. They also should be kept as quiet as possible to avoid further stress on the heart. Animals that have not consumed a lethal dose of the plants recover over several days.

12.5.8.2 Plant Alkaloids

Plant alkaloids that may cause sudden death include Poison and Water Hemlock, Yew, Avocado, Larkspur (*Delphinium* spp.), Monkshood (*Aconitum* spp.), Death Camas (*Zigadenus* spp.) [1].

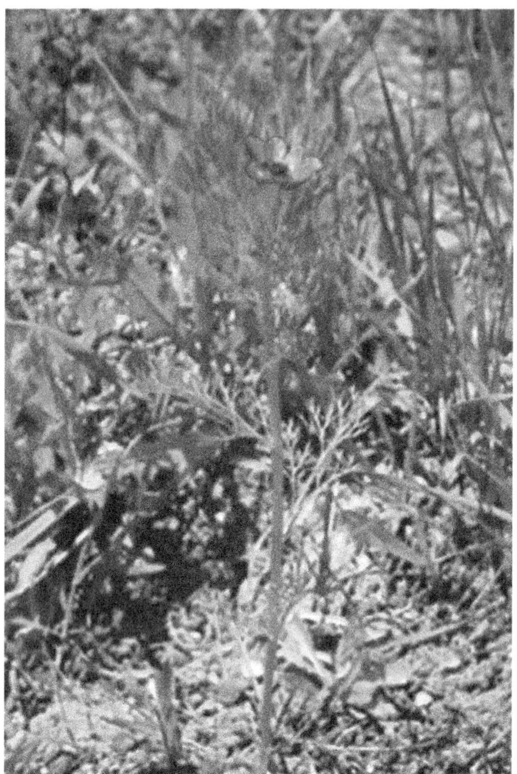

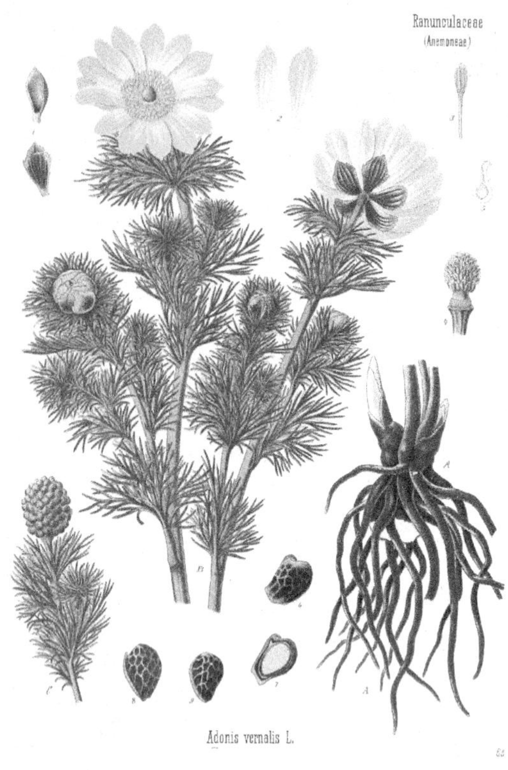

Figure 12.15 Summer pheasant's eye (*Adonis* spp.) is an introduced glabrous, 10–20 cm tall, with simple or branched stems species from Eurasia and has escaped cultivation in many parts of North America. The leaves are 2–6 cm long with narrow segments and the flowers are reddish-orange. An invading weed that grows in disturbed sites in pastures and fields, harvested with the forage and contaminating prepared feeds. Has become a serious problem in parts of northern Utah, and California. *Source:* Brandt et al. [18].

12.5.8.2.1 Poison Hemlock (Conium maculatum) [P, H]

Poison hemlock is a noxious weed that commonly invades pastures and fields (Figure 12.16). Poison hemlock is toxic to all animals, including people [20]. Horses often eat young vegetation in the early spring before other green forages are available. Later in the summer and fall, the more mature phenotypes are not palatable especially when free-standing. Hungry horses have been seen walking between tree-sized poison-hemlock plants when no other forages are available looking for something to eat. These mature plants do poison horses when hay or green chopped feed is contaminated. Poison-hemlock toxins have been identified as piperidine alkaloids: gamma coniceine, conine, and n-methyl conine. Although rarely eaten by horses or other livestock, sudden death will occur if consumed. Toxic doses in horses can be as little as 0.25% BW. Initially, poisoning produces CNS stimulation, followed by depression, muscle weakness, tremors, ataxia, excessive salivation, frequent defecation, excessive urination, abdominal pain, increased respiratory rates, weakness leading to muscular paralysis, recumbence, and death. Most horses that survive a couple of hours post-ingestion will recover. Although these piperidine alkaloids are teratogenic in other species, there are no reports of conine-associated birth defects in horses. No antidotes for conine poisoning are known. However, most horses become ill before ingesting a fatal dose. Consequently, most poisoned horses are weak and recumbent but recover if allowed to clear the toxin.

12.5.8.2.2 Water Hemlock (Cicuta Spp.) [P]

Water hemlock (*Cicuta* spp.) (Figure 12.17) [P] is an extremely toxic plant that produces violent convulsions and sudden death when eaten by livestock. Rare reports document poisoning in ponies and horses [43]. Water hemlock has been identified as cicutoxin and unsaturated alcohol that is extremely poisonous. Doses as small as 250 g of a plant (less than a handful) have been shown to poison an adult horse [44]. All plant parts are toxic, but the roots are especially poisonous as cicutoxin is concentrated in them. The plant remains toxic when dried suggesting that there is potential for toxicity if included in forages. However, inclusion is unlikely as these plants tend to grow along streams and ditches and are unlikely to be co-harvested with forages. Poisoned animals have severe convulsions with

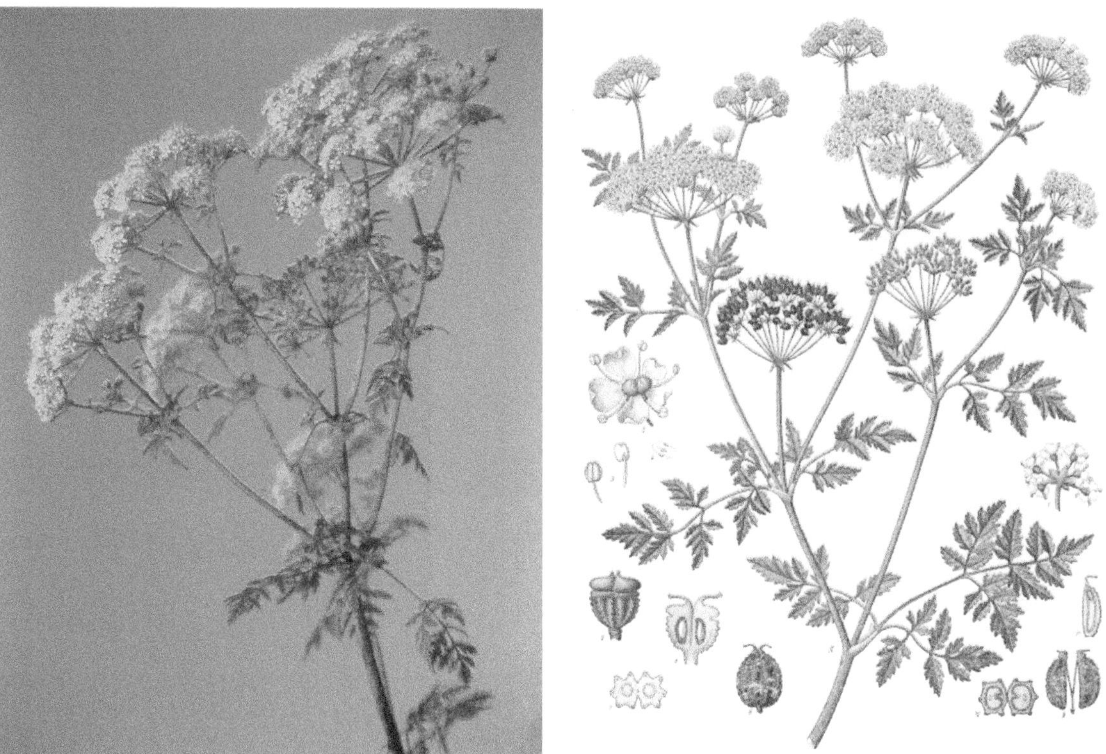

Figure 12.16 Poison hemlock (*Conium maculatum*) is a biennial, but in favorable locations, can be a perennial, growing along fence lines, in irrigation ditches, and other moist waste places. The plant has a 2–3 m tall hollow green stem with small purple spots and delicate leaves, like parsley, and a white taproot. Poison hemlock has white flowers that grow in small, erect clusters. Each flower develops into a green, deeply ridged fruit that contains several seeds. After maturity, the fruit turns grayish brown. *Source:* Brandt et al. [18].

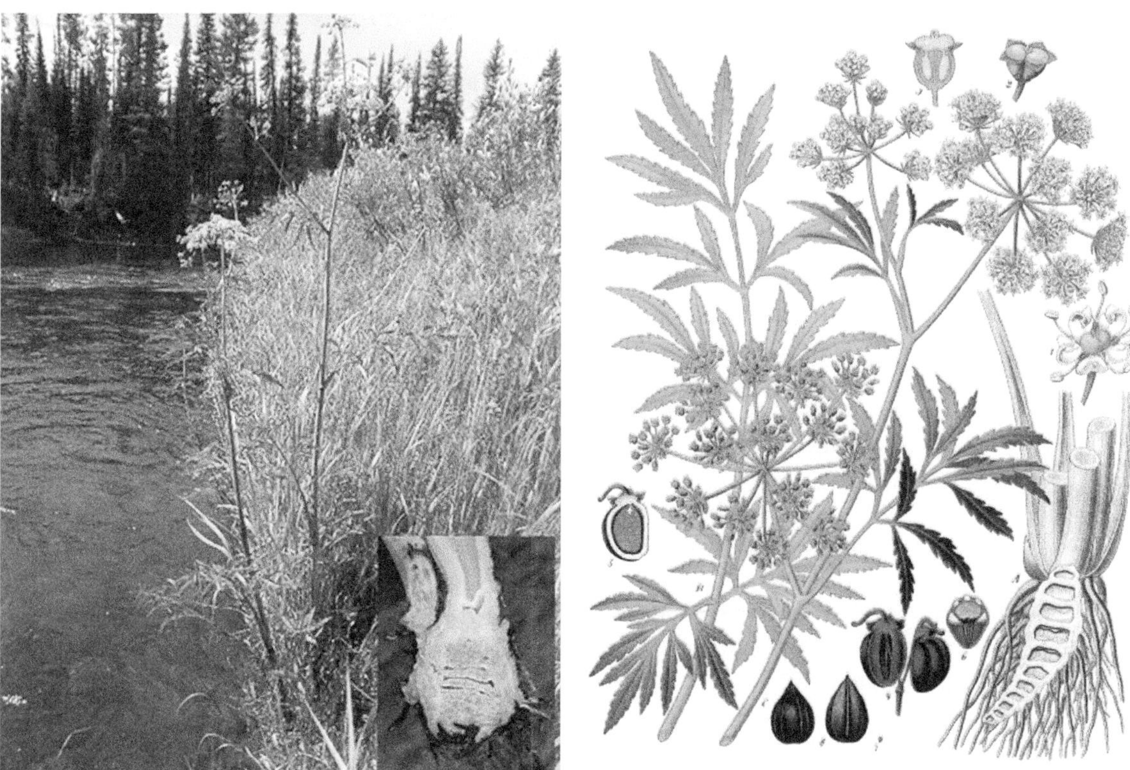

Figure 12.17 Water hemlocks (*Cicuta* spp.) is an erect, hairless plant perennial that grows in clusters from a thick tuberous root in moist areas along ditches and streams. The hollow stems grow to 1.8 m tall. The leaves are alternate and pinnate with lanceolate leaflets 3–10 cm long. The white flowers form compound umbels that form flat oval fruits with prominent ribs. *Source:* Brandt et al. [18].

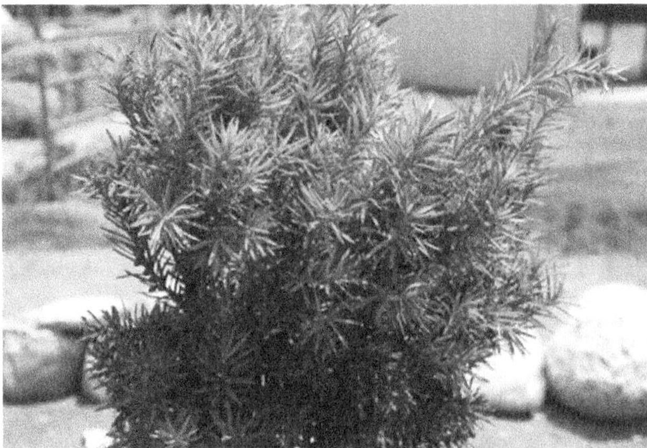
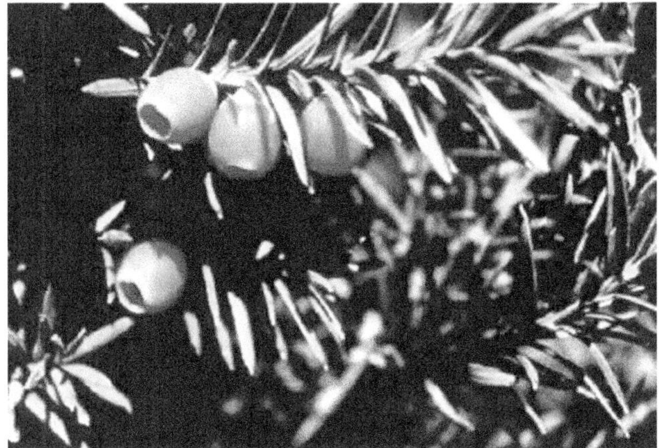

Figure 12.18 Yew (*Taxus* spp.) are evergreen ornamental shrubs that have glossy, rigid, green, linear leaves. The fruits are red to yellow, contain one seed, and grow best in moist, humid areas and most poisonings occur when livestock are allowed access to clippings.

tremors, salivation, chewing, and grinding of teeth. Poisoned horses have dilated pupils and the convulsions progress to coma as animals die of respiratory paralysis and asphyxia. Signs of poisoning develop within several hours of ingesting water hemlock. There are no specific antidotes, though heavy sedation can be used to reduce the convulsions and activated charcoal, mineral oil, and other laxatives to clear the toxin.

12.5.8.2.3 Yew (Taxus Spp.) [P]

Yew (*Taxus* spp.) [P] is an introduced ornamental that most commonly poisons animals when clippings are thrown into paddocks (Figure 12.18). Yew toxicity is attributed to taxine alkaloids but these plants also contain traces of cyanogenic glycosides, lignins, flavonoids, and volatile oils. The taxines and taxols alter myocardial calcium and electrolyte balance, resulting in systolic cardiac arrest (negative inotropes). All portions of the plant, green or dry, are toxic. Doses as low as 0.1% BW are lethal, e.g. just over 100 mg would be lethal for a 450 kg horse. Clinical signs are related to toxin disruption of cardiac function, including colic, sweating, incoordination, shallow and difficult breathing, muscle tremors, recumbence, diarrhea, bloody diarrhea, and death from cardiac arrest. Most poisonings result in sudden death, with none or minimal gross or histological lesions. Poisoned animals may have non-specific lesions of myocardial hemorrhage, pulmonary congestion, and edema. The diagnosis most often is made by associating sudden death with exposure and identifying plant parts in GI contents. As most cases are fatal, the prevention of ingestion of trimmed shrubs is paramount. If possible, treatments should include evacuation of the GI tract and minimization of absorption with activated charcoal, oil, and cathartics. As poisoned animals are likely to have compromised cardiovascular function, precautions should be taken to avoid stress and minimize animal exertion.

12.5.8.2.4 Avocado (Persea Americana) [P]

Avocado leaves, fruit, bark, and seeds contain persin and an unidentified cardiac toxin. Persin produces non-infectious mastitis and agalactia. Signs of poisoning in lactating mares are mastitis with occasional gastritis and colic. Other signs related to cardiotoxin-induced heart failure include dyspnea, coughing, and increased respiratory and heart rates. Other less-common changes include cardiac arrhythmias, edema of the neck and ventral abdomen, cyanosis, anorexia, general weakness, and recumbence. Postmortem findings include histological lesions in the heart, with generalized edema and congestion of many organs. As damage may be fatal and many of the cardiac changes are irreversible, preventing a horse's access to avocado groves is essential.

12.5.9 Thiaminase Inhibitors [R,P,H]

Bracken fern (*Pteridium* spp.) and horsetail (*Equisetum* spp.) (Figure 12.19): Bracken fern, more common in the Northwestern United States, usually is not eaten by horses, except when forage supply is inadequate or included in the hay. Bracken fern contains several toxins, including a radiomimetic carcinogen that causes bone marrow dysplasia and urinary epithelial cancer in livestock. In horses, the primary toxin is hypothesized to be thiaminase. This enzyme breaks down thiamine, vitamin B_1, causing neurologic disease [45]. Another toxic plant (*Equisetum* spp. or horsetail) contains similar thiaminases and produces similar diseases. Clinical signs require one to two mos of

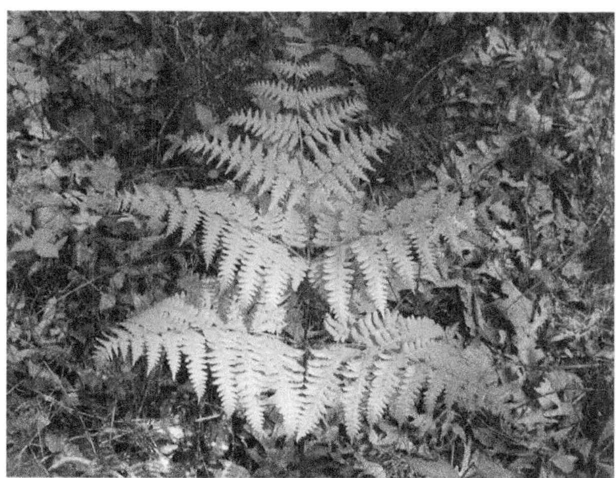

Figure 12.19 Bracken fern (*Pteridium aquilinum*) is found throughout the world in moist, open woodlands and will expand with fire and ground disturbances. A perennial fern with a branching root system that can extend for several meters to dominate areas with dense monocultures. The leaves arise from the rhizome up to 2 m high, forming large, triangular, bipinnately compound fronds. The underside of the leaf is haired with prominent brown spores around the leaf edges in late summer.

exposure to develop and, once initiated, will become markedly worse over two to three days. Changes include weight loss, incoordination, excessive staggers, wide base stance with arched back, muscle tremors, recumbence, inability to rise, and other injuries related to struggling. Some horses may live for up to 10 days without treatment, but treatment is essential if the disease is going to be reversed [20]. Sometimes the clinical signs and subsequent disease develop after the horse is removed from the bracken fern source. Affected horses should be given a bracken fern-free diet, and slowly injected intravenously with thiamin hydrochloride (5–10 mg/kg BW). Dilution of the dose in fluids will reduce the chances of adverse reactions. Daily doses of thiamin should be given intramuscularly for 5 to 7 days. Recovery is usually complete in 2 to 3 days.

12.6 Plants that Contain Muscle Toxins

12.6.1 White Snakeroot, Rayless Goldenrod, Crofton, Jimmyweed, or Burrow Weeds (*Eupatorium* or *Ageratina* and *Haplopappus* Spp.) [R,P]

White snakeroot (Figure 12.20) poisoning, or "milk sickness," is a historic disease that in the 1800s is suspected to have killed hundreds of early settlers in Illinois, Indiana, Kentucky, North Carolina, Ohio, and Tennessee. Nearly a century later, *Eupatorium rugosum* was identified as

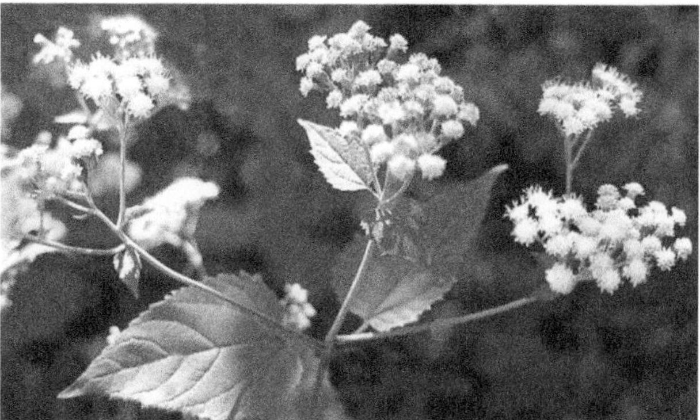

Figure 12.20 White snakeroot (*Eupatorium rugosum* or *Ageratina altissima*) is a perennial that grows from 100 to 140 cm tall. The leaves are ovate and opposite with long petioles. The leaf margins have marked serration with three distinct veins and pointed tips. The flowers are tubular and white. White snakeroot grows in low, moist areas along waterways and dense woodlands.

the cause. Though animal-husbandry improvements, feeding practices, and dairy quality-assurance programs have nearly eliminated human exposure, poisoning in livestock continues to be a problem throughout the Midwest and Eastern United States. Rayless goldenrod (Figure 12.21) contains similar toxins and consistently causes problems in Southwestern United States. Both white snakeroot and rayless goldenrod are toxic year-round and in stored feeds. However, most poisoning occurs in pasture and range animals in the summer and late fall when other forages are exhausted. The suggested toxins are benzofuran ketones (BFKs) such as tremetone [46]. Clinically, these toxins accumulate in tissues as these BFKs are lipid-soluble and transmammary poisoning has been reported in livestock and horses [47]. Poisoning in nursing neonates and people that drink the contaminated milk is commonly reported with no signs of toxicity in the lactating animal. Most studies suggest that doses of 1% or higher BW of the plant are toxic if ingested over several weeks. However, plant BFK concentrations vary within plant populations and phenotypes, and plant toxicity is not always related to BFK concentrations. Additionally, none of the BFKs have been identified in milk that poisoned nursing neonates. This suggests that there are yet some unidentified toxins or toxicity that may be due to unidentified BFK metabolite.

Clinical signs of poisoning include incoordination, muscle tremors, elevated heart rate, muscle weakness, congestive heart failure, jugular pulse, tachycardia, cardiac arrhythmias, profuse sweating, pitting edema, and quidding. As these plants directly damage muscle, especially heart muscle, poisoned animals often have chronic cardiac disease with decreased work capacity. Clinical blood changes are those indicative of muscle damage as

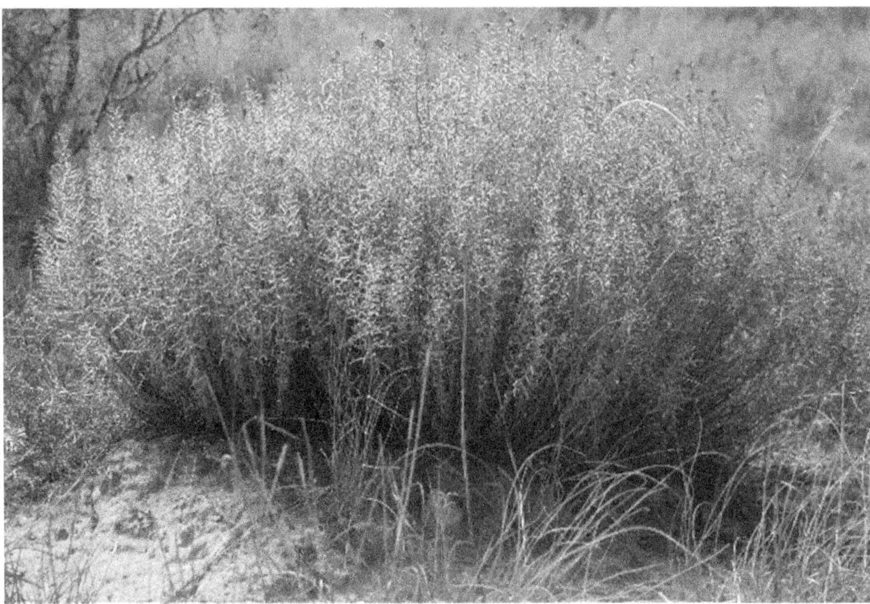

Figure 12.21 Jimmy or burrow weed, rayless goldenrod (*Isocoma pluriflora*, *Haplopappus heterophyllus*, Iscoma wrightii, Aplopappus) is an erect, branched perennial that grows up to 1 m tall. The leaves are linear and alternative with a sticky surface. The flowers are yellow with small clusters of 7–15 terminal flowers. Rayless goldenrod is commonly found in alkaline soils in arid rangelands of Texas, Arizona, and New Mexico.

evidenced by increases in serum enzyme concentrations of creatine kinase, troponin I, aspartate transaminase, and lactate dehydrogenase [48]. Most animals have increased myoglobin in the blood and urine. Treatment includes the use of activated charcoal and cathartics to prevent absorption and reduce exposure. Postmortem findings include patchy necrosis of the heart and skeletal muscle, liver necrosis, and myoglobin-induced kidney disease.

12.6.2 Two Day-Blooming Jessamine (*Cestrum diurnum*) [P,H]

Day-blooming Jessamine (*Cestrum diurnum*) (Figure 12.22) [P,H] is the NA version of the vitamin D-containing plants and produces a disease similar to *Solanum malacoxylon* in South America and *Trisetum flavescens* in Europe. The tropical plant is now commonly found in Florida, Texas, California, and Hawaii. These plants contain 1, 25 dihydroxycholecalciferol that increases calcium absorption, decreases excretion, and increases osteolysis resulting in marked hypercalcemia, hypoparathyroidism, metastatic calcification, and osteoporosis. Of these calcifying plants, only *C. diurnum* has been reported to poison horses.

Characteristic clinical signs of plant-induced calcinosis in horses are chronic weight loss despite normal appetite, and a generalized stiffness leading to severe lameness and prolonged periods of recumbency. Plasma calcium concentration in affected horses may be elevated while other blood parameters, including phosphorus concentrations, are generally normal. Radiographically, horses show marked osteopetrosis of the bones as increased bone density and decreased size of the medullary cavity. Increased

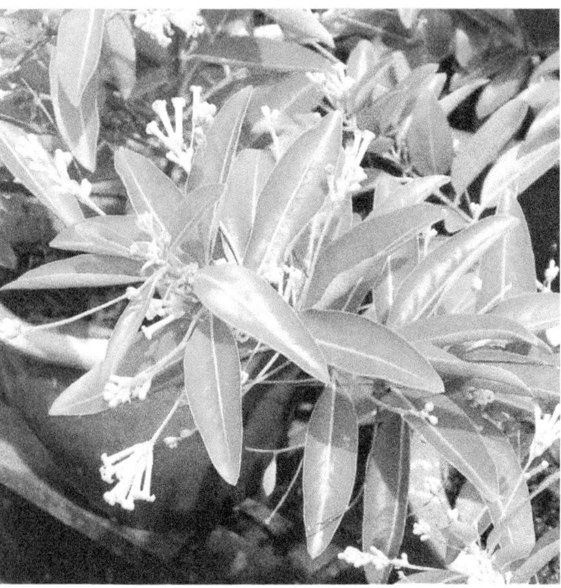

Figure 12.22 Day-blooming jasmine, night-blooming, or wild jasmine (*Cestrum diurnum*) grows 4–5 m high. The leaves are elliptic, with a dark-green, glossy upper surface. Flowers are white and clustered on the axillary peduncles, forming green berries that ripen black.

calcification of cartilage and increased metaphyseal and epiphyseal trabeculae are also evident radiographically [49]. Altered calcium metabolism causes mineral deposition or metastatic calcification to those tissues with elastic properties; tendons, ligaments, major arteries, heart, and kidney. Lameness is due to pain in the calcified ligaments and tendons of the legs and postmortem examination of affected horses confirms severe calcification of the tendons, ligaments, and elastic arteries. Recovery from plant-induced calcinosis is rarely reported, as animals are usually chronically affected. Recovery is likely in less severely affected horses if denied further access to the toxic plants and are given a balanced diet. Care should be taken to ensure that horses are not placed in pastures or pens that contain Cestrum species or other calcinosis-inducing plants.

12.6.3 Selenium Toxicosis [R,P,H]

There are a variety of high-selenium (Se) plants and poisoning is largely dependent on both dose and duration.

12.6.3.1 Indicator or Obligate Selenium Accumulator Plants

Indicator Se plants such as two groove milkvetch (*Astragalus bisculatus*), golden weed (*Haplopappus engelmannii*), woody aster (*Xylorhiza glabriuscula*), and princes' plume (*Stanleya pinnata*). The indicator plants can contain 1000's ppm Se but are mostly inedible, hence rarely are consumed and seldom poison livestock or horses.

12.6.3.2 Facultative Selenium Accumulator Plants

Facultative Se accumulator plants such as western aster (*Aster* spp.), gumweed (*Grindelia* spp.), and saltbrush (*Atriplex* spp.) generally contain 100's ppm Se and can poison livestock, but these also rarely poison equids because these too are unpalatable plants, and horses avoid eating them.

12.6.3.3 Plants that Passively Accumulate Selenium

Passive Se accumulator plants are forages (grass and alfalfa) that have elevated Se concentrations when grown in high Se environments. Consequently, most equine poisonings occur with relatively chronic consumption of grasses or alfalfa grown in high Se soils. Se concentrations as low as five ppm could potentially be toxic if grazed long enough, but most plants associated with equine poisoning have between 30 and 200 ppm Se [50]. Se poisoning follows several weeks to months of consuming a high-selenium diet.

Excess selenium consumption results in the substitution of sulfur in the keratin molecule by selenium. This results in the defective formation of the hoof and hair keratin protein. Initially, affected horses lose long hairs from the mane and tail. The hair shaft breaks at the site where selenium has replaced sulfur in the keratin. This gives the horse a roached mane and bobtailed appearance (Figure 12.23a). Lameness develops as a result of coronitis and abnormal hoof wall formation affecting all feet. Initially, affected horses walk stiff-legged followed by pronounced lameness. Horizontal rings or ridges that may progress to full-thickness cracks through the hoof wall causing severe lameness are characteristic of the condition (Figure 12.23b) [1]. Some horses may slough the hoof wall entirely. Initially, the diagnosis is suggested correlating Se lesions with access to high Se forages, but whole blood and postmortem hepatic Se concentrations are useful to confirm intoxication.

Successful treatment of selenium poisoning depends on early recognition and removal of horses from the source

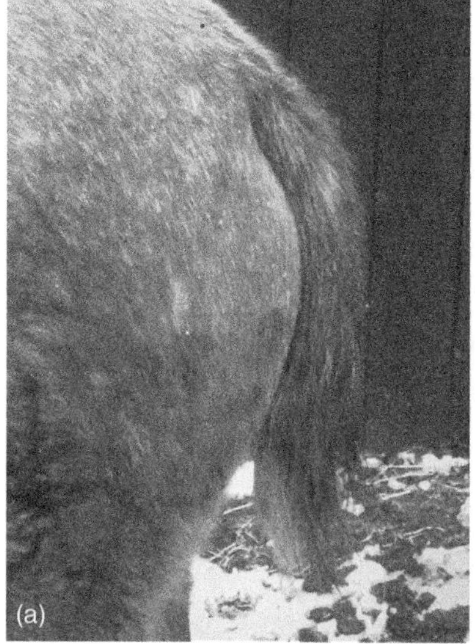

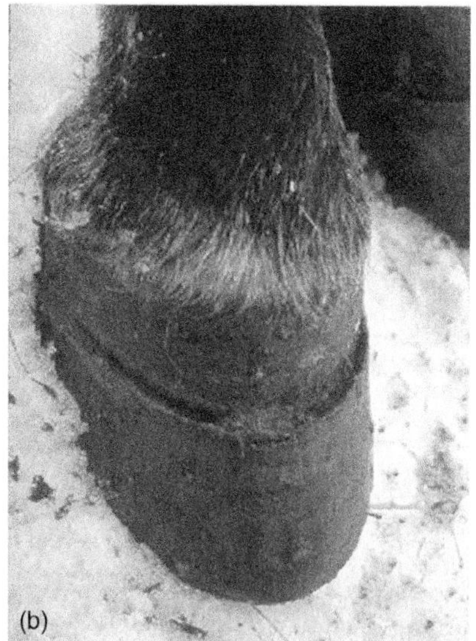

Figure 12.23 Clinical signs of chronic excess selenium consumption in a horse: bobbed tail (a) due to hair loss and circular horizontal cracks in the hoof wall (b).

of excess selenium. Feeding a low-selenium forages with a ratio more than adequate in the sulfur-containing amino acids cysteine and methionine will counteract most Se toxicity. For example, alfalfa hay, low in selenium concentration, is relatively high in protein, cysteine, and methionine when compared to grass hays. Feeding a cereal grain mix with 15–20% crude protein containing cottonseed, rapeseed, or fish meal will also provide an adequate intake of protein with adequate cysteine, and methionine. Additionally, ensuring the total ration contains 10–25 ppm copper will also reduce the toxicity [51]. Recovery from chronic selenium poisoning will occur gradually as the main, tail, and hoof walls grow out (~1 year). Providing feeds, such as grain or hay, known to be low in selenium when horses are grazing pastures containing high Se plants can assist in preventing selenium toxicosis.

12.7 Plants that are Toxic to the Urogenital System

12.7.1 Oak and Scrub Oak (*Quercus* Spp.) [R,P]

Oak and Scrub Oak (*Quercus* spp.) [R,P] contain toxic tannins, such as gallotannin. Not all tree parts contain enough tannins to be toxic, but animals have been poisoned from eating flowers, leaf buds, or acorns [52, 53]. Clinical signs of oak poisoning vary according to the number of oak leaves, bark, or acorns consumed or the tannin intake. Initially, poisoned animals stop eating, become depressed, and develop colic [54]. The feces are hard and dark, but this progresses and hemorrhagic diarrhea often occurs later in the progression. Some horses present as if choked with ingesta and saliva passing out through the nose, and oral ulcers may be present. Tannic and gallic acid causes severe renal tubular nephrosis and, therefore, clinical signs include dehydration, azotemia, hyperphosphatemia, hypocalcemia, and hypoproteinemia. Liver and kidney damage may also be evident seen as elevations in serum liver enzymes and blood urea nitrogen. Urine analysis may show low specific gravity, proteinuria, glucosuria, hemoglobinuria, and tubular casts. Horses may die within 24 hours after eating large quantities of acorns or may live for 5 to 7 days after the onset of clinical signs. On postmortem examination, mucoid hemorrhagic gastroenteritis, with edematous large-intestine mesentery are the predominant gross lesions occurring in horses that die from oak poisoning. Serosa hemorrhages on various organs and excessive amounts of fluid in the peritoneal and pleural cavities may also be present. The kidneys are usually found to be pale, swollen, and covered with small hemorrhages. Treatment should include extensive fluid therapy as is prescribed for acute renal or hepatic damage to maintain organ perfusion, correction of electrolyte and acid–base balances, and analgesics for colic pain relief.

12.7.2 Oxalate-Containing Plants [R]

Halogeton glomeratus (halogeton) and *Sarcobatus vermiculatus* (black greasewood) have relatively high oxalate concentrations (mostly sodium oxlates). If any horse consistently consumes a sufficient quantity of these plants, insoluble oxalate crystals may be deposited in the kidneys, causing renal damage. However, these plants are not very palatable to horses and renal damage from massive amounts of oxalates in feeds that fatally poisons other livestock is rare. Other plants that contain relatively high oxalate concentrations (mostly potassium oxalate) such as *Rumex crispus* (curly dock) or *Rheum* spp. (rhubarb) are generally mucosal irritates resulting in oral irritation, stomatitis, and gastroenteritis. Consequently horses generally avoid these plants also.

Given the opportunity horse commonly eat toxic doses of oxalate containing grasses, such as buffel (*Cenchrus ciliaris*), pangola (*Digitaria recombens*), setaria (*Setaria sphacelata*), panic grasses (*Panicum* spp.), kikuyu (*Pennisetum clandistinum*) (Figure 12.24). This result in chronic oxalate poisoning characterized by hypocalcemia as these oxalated chelate calcium. If the total dietary intake of oxalates is high relative to Ca intake, i.e. low Ca: oxalate ratio, clinical signs of calcium deficiency may develop. A prolonged relative calcium deficiency leads to nutritional secondary hyperparathyroidism seen clinically as lameness, bone pain, joint tenderness, loose teeth,

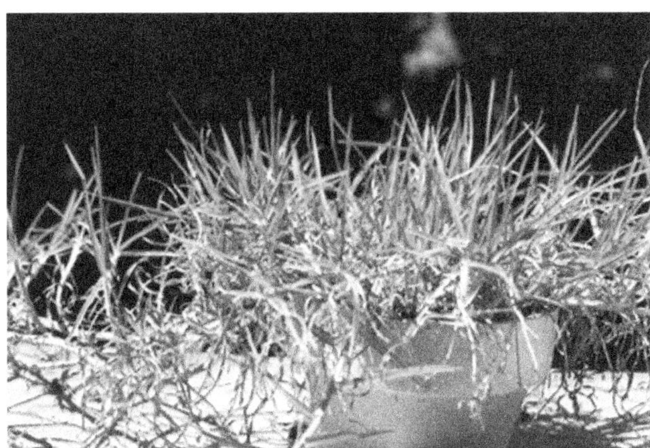

Figure 12.24 Kikuyu grass (*Pennisetum clandestinum*) is a tropical East African grass that has become a noxious weed and common lawn species in Australia, New Zealand, South Africa, North and South America, and the Pacific islands. It is a rhizomatous grass with green flattened leaves that can climb over and dominate other plants].

osteodystrophy, and emaciation [55]. This is likely to occur when horses consume a diet with a total oxalate content >0.5% dry matter, and with a Ca: oxalate ratio <0.45 [56]. Oxalate may increase and Ca decrease in pasture grass during the summer; however, 2 to 3 m of excess oxalate intake is unlikely to cause a problem in mature horses, although potentially harmful in growing horses [57]. A Ca deficiency from grazing plants high in oxalates and low Ca: oxalate ratio occurs in horses of all ages, but the incidence and disease severity are highest in lactating mares and weanlings because of their relatively higher calcium requirements. The prevalence of calcium deficiency in herds grazing pastures containing these types of grasses varies widely with up to 100% of animals affected. The onset of clinical signs varies from 2 to 8 mos after introduction to pastures containing high-oxalate grasses [56].

12.7.3 Red Maple (*Acer rubrum*) or Soft Maple (R,P,H]

Red maple (*Acer rubrum*) or soft maple (Figure 12.25) (R,P,H] is native to eastern NA. Maples have characteristic large (5–15 cm) palmate leaves with 3 to 5 lobes. The leaf margins are serrated or jagged and the leaf bottom is silver gray with red keys (winged seeds). Poisoning occurs most often in the summer and fall because fresh leaves do not appear to be toxic. Wilted red maple leaves commonly poison horses and ponies when leaves, branches, or prunings are accessible in pastures or paddocks. These prunings can remain toxic for up to 30 days [58, 59]. Ingestion of 1.5–3.0 g of leaves/kg BW has been suggested to cause hemolytic disease in horses.

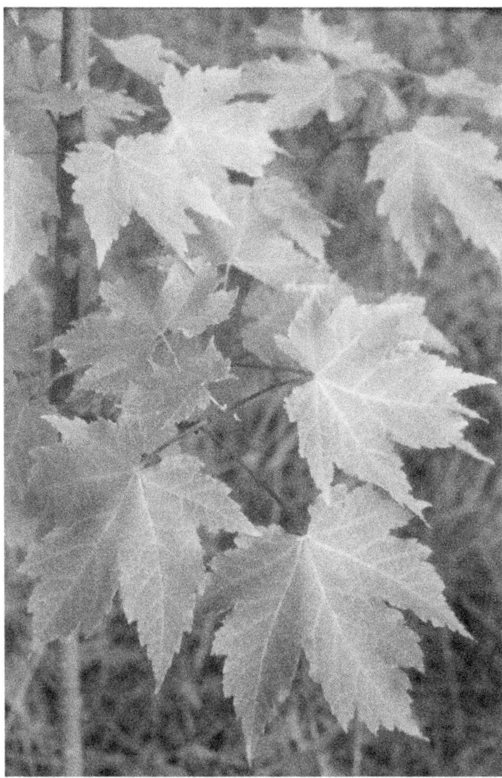

Figure 12.25 Red maple (*Acer rubrum*) or soft maple trees are common throughout most of eastern North America and south to Florida and Texas. The characteristic leaves are three- to five-lobed and shiny green above but turn a brilliant red in the fall. Poisoning occurs when horses eat wilted or dried red maple leaves.

Ingestion of dry leaves at a higher dose is usually fatal within 24 hrs. Removal of trees from paddocks is recommended and further avoiding exposure is recommended.

Signs of poisoning include depression with brown cyanotic mucous membranes. Intravascular and extravascular hemolysis results in hemoglobinuria (brown urine) and severe anemia. Hemolysis has been suggested to be caused by gallic acid-induced oxidative damage, which produces extensive methemoglobin. The prognosis is always guarded to poor for horses with red maple poisoning because of the rapid intravascular hemolysis, coagulopathy, hemoglobin nephropathy, and vascular thrombosis that commonly occur in clinical poisoning [58, 60]. Death is probably caused by cellular anoxia as a result of both anemia and methemoglobinemia. If poisoning is non-fatal, secondary lesions including laminitis and nephrosis are of clinical concern. Successful treatment of horses with red maple poisoning must be initiated as early as possible to counteract the hemolytic crisis and secondary effects. Appropriate intravenous fluid therapy to maintain cardiac output and renal function, and transfusions with packed erythrocytes, may be effective [61]. Although methylene blue is advocated as a treatment for oxidant toxicities of erythrocytes, use with considerable caution in the horse, as excessive treatment may result in a Heinz body hemolytic anemia.

12.7.4 Sweet Clover (*Melilotus* Spp.) [H] (Yellow and White)

Sweet clover (*Melilotus* spp.) [H] (yellow and white) was introduced in many countries as a forage for livestock and now grows as a weed in marginal land along roads, fences, and canals. It is a tall (1.5 m) biennial plant that has compound leaves with three leaflets and serrated edges. The flowers are yellow or white and they grow on axillary racemes that may be 10–12 cm long. The flowers mature into small pods that contain numerous hard-shelled 1 mm seeds. The clovers are not directly toxic, but if improperly cured in hay or haylage, they are frequently infected with various molds, e.g. *Penicillium* spp., which convert plant coumarin into dicoumarol. Dicoumarol is an anticoagulant that impairs the synthesis of vitamin K-dependent coagulation factors and prothrombin. The concentrations of coagulation factors are directly related to the dose and duration of dicoumarol exposure. As with many plant-associated toxins, animals can eat significant amounts of moldy sweet clover without developing the disease. Generally, horses have to ingest dicoumarol-containing forage for several weeks to develop hemorrhages from the nose, intestinal tract, urine, or into body cavities. Hematomas develop over trauma-prone areas and lacerations will bleed persistently and be difficult to control. Such extensive hemorrhage can be fatal and surviving animals have severe anemia. Horses will have signs and symptoms of hypovolemic shock with prolonged blood coagulation rates, i.e. prothrombin time, partial thromboplastin time, and activated clotting time.

Affected horses should be treated with whole blood transfusions as necessary. Ideally, vitamin K_1 should be administered; however, the cost may be prohibitive and often vitamin K_3 is considered. This is problematic as vitamin K_3 may cause a hypersensitivity reaction in horses. Vitamin K_1, has also been shown to be ineffective in treating moldy sweet clover poisoning in calves [62]. The response to vitamin K_3 therapy requires several days and results in pain and swelling at the injection site [63], whereas intravenous vitamin K_1 administration controls hemorrhaging in 3 to 6 hrs and returns prothrombin time to normal in 12 to 24 hrs.

Case in Point

Animal Assessment

A 26-year-old registered bay/tobiano Paint gelding (460 kg, BCS 3/9) (Figure 12.26) presented for skin lesions occurring initially in the white areas of his face and later on his neck. Initially, the owner thought the horse had rain rot, a superficial infection caused by *Dermatophilus congolensis* bacterium, and had been bathing the pruritic areas with anti-microbial soap. However, after treating the areas for more than 30 days, there was only minor improvement and more scabbing had recently appeared in the horse's white socks. On physical examination, the horse appeared healthy except for a serosanguinous exudate with edema and necrosis of the superficial non-pigmented areas of skin on his forehead, nose, coronary bands, and crest topline, which were painful to the touch.

1) The initial diagnosis is radiation-induced dermatitis. How would you determine if this is primary or secondary photodermatitis?
2) In taking a diet history, specifically what information would help confirm a primary vs. secondary photodermatitis diagnosis?
3) The presence of which weeds in the pasture or hay would refine the diagnosis?
4) What is your suggested initial treatment?
5) What is the prognosis for primary vs. secondary photodermatitis?

See Appendix A Chapter 12.

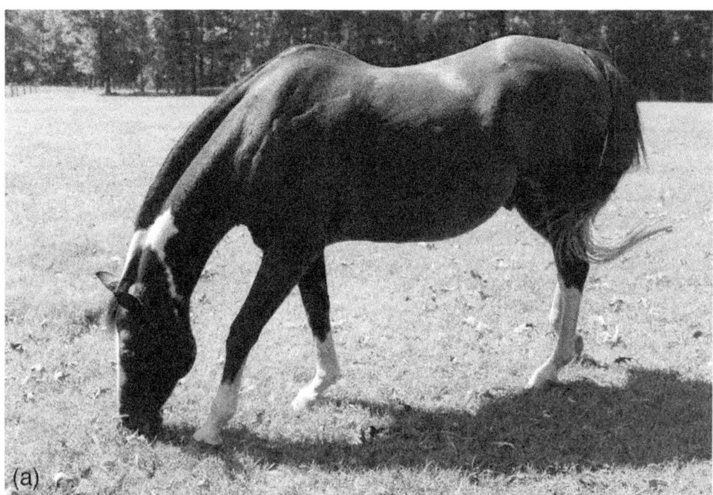

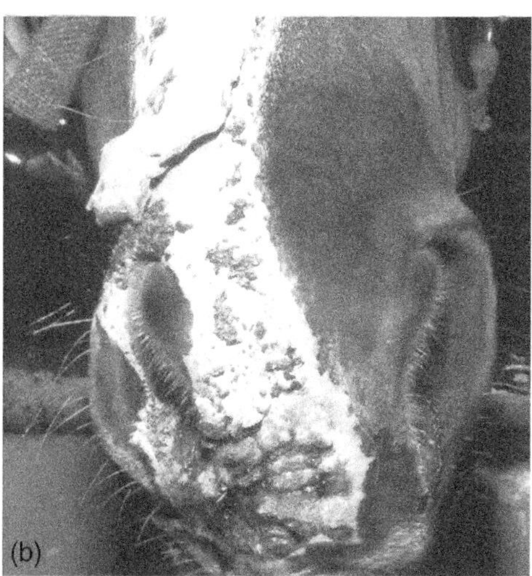

Figure 12.26 A registered Paint horse (a) one year before presenting with severe dermatitis affecting only non-pigmented skin areas (b).

Additional sources and photographs:

- Guide to Poisonous Plants. College of Veterinary Medicine and Biomedical Sciences, Colorado State University. https://csuvth.colostate.edu/poisonous_plants
- Poisonous Plants of the United States and Canada by JM Kingsbury, Prentice-Hall, Inc., Englewood Cliffs, NJ, 1964.
- Poisonous Plants of the Southern United States from the Agriculture Extension Service, University of Tennessee 1980.
- *Weeds of the West* by T.D. Whitson was published by the University of Wyoming in cooperation with the Western Society of Weed Science and the Western United States Land Grant Universities Cooperative Extension Services 1991.
- Plants Poisonous or Harmful to Horses in the North Central United States by KB Martinson, L Hovda, M Murphy from the University of Minnesota 2007.
- There are mobile 'apps' (computer software programs for mobile devices e.g. smartphone and tablet), specific for plant identification. Uploading a picture of the flower, leaf, fruit, bark or habit will help identify unknown suspect plants. Examples are 'PlantSnap' 'LeafSnap' and 'Pl@ntNet'.

References

1 Knight, A. (1995). Plant poisoning of horses. In: *Equine Clinical Nutrition: Feeding and Care*, 1e (ed. L.D. Lewis), 447–502. Baltimore, MD: Williams and Wilkins.

2 Mosley, E. (1906). The cause of trembles in cattle, sheep, and horses and of milk sickness in people. *Ohio Nat.* 6 (4): 463–470.

3 Rowe, L.D. (1989). Photosensitization problems in livestock. *Vet. Clin. North Am. Food Anim. Pract.* 5 (2): 301–323.

4 Ford, E.J.H. and Gopinath, C. (1974). The excretion of Phyllocrythrin and bilirubin by the horse. *Res. Vet. Sci.* 16 (2): 186–198.

5 Lindman, C.A.M. (1905). *Bilder ur Nordens flora: på grundvalen af Palmstruchs "Svensk botanik"*, vol. 3. Wahlström & Widstrand.

6 Cheeke, P.R. and Shull, L.R. (1985). *Natural Toxicants in Feeds and Poisonous Plants. Natural Toxicants in Feeds and Poisonous Plants.* Westport, CT: AVI Publishing Company Inc.

7 Kriazheva, S.S., Khamaganova, I.V., and Kolibrina, A.M. (1991). Dermatitis bullosa in children caused by cow-parsnip. *Pediatriia* 6: 88–90.

8 Stegelmeier, B.L., Colegate, S.M., Knoppel, E.L. et al. (2019). Wild parsnip (*Pastinaca sativa*)-induced photosensitization. *Toxicon* 167 (June): 60–66.

9 Bidwell, L.A. and Bowker, R.M. (2006). Evaluation of changes in architecture of the stratum internum of the hoof wall from fetal, newborn, and yearling horses. *Am. J. Vet. Res.* 67 (12): 1947–1955.

10 Geor, R.J. and Harris, P.A. (2013). Laminitis. In: *Equine Applied and Clinical Nutrition: Health, Welfare and Performance* (ed. R.J. Geor, P.A. Harris, and M. Coenen), 469–486. Edinburgh: Saunders Elsevier.

11 Minnick, P.D., Brown, C.M., Braselton, W.E. et al. (1987). The induction of equine laminitis with an aqueous extract of the heartwood of black walnut (*Juglans nigra*). *Vet. Hum. Toxicol.* 29 (3): 230–233.

12 Uhlinger, C. (1989). Black walnut toxicosis in ten horses. *J. Am. Vet. Med. Assoc.* 195 (3): 343–344.

13 Geor, R.J., Becker, R.L., Kanara, E.W. et al. (1992). Toxicosis in horses after ingestion of hoary alyssum. *J. Am. Vet. Med. Assoc.* 201 (1): 63–67.

14 Smith, G.W. (2018). Slaframine. In: *Veterinary Toxicology Basic and Clinical Principles*, 3e (ed. R. Gupta), 1029–1032. Academic Press.

15 Sockett, D.C., Baker, J.C., and Stowe, C.M. (1982). Slaframine (*Rhizoctonia leguminicola*) intoxication in horses. *J. Am. Vet. Med. Assoc.* 181 (6): 606.

16 Metzger, N., Eser, W., and Auer, J. (2006). Black locust (Robinia Pseudacacia) poisoning in 18 ponies and a mule. *J. Vet. Intern. Med.* 20 (3): 861.

17 Todd, F.G., Stermitz, F.R., Schultheis, P. et al. (1995). Tropane alkaloids and toxicity of *Convolvulus arvensis. Phytochemistry* 39 (2): 301–303.

18 Brandt, W., Gürke, M., Köhler, F.E. et al. (1887). *Köhler's Medizinal-Pflanzen in naturgetreuen Abbildungen mit kurz erläuterndem Texte*, vol. 1–4. Gera-Untermhaus: Fr. Eugen Köhler.

19 Challoner, K.R. and McCarron, M.M. (1990). Castor bean intoxication. *Ann. Emerg. Med.* 19 (10): 1177–1183.

20 Kingsbury, J. (1964). *Poisonous Plants of the United States and Canada*, 466. Englewood Cliff, NJ: Prentice-Hall.

21 Thiemann, A.K., Thiemann, A.K., Thiemann, A.K., and Thiemann, A.K. (1991). Rhododendron poisoning. *Vet. Rec.* 128 (17): 411.

22 Valle, E., Vergnano, D., and Nebbia, C. (2016). Suspected pokeweed (*Phytolacca americana* L.) poisoning as the cause of progressive cachexia in a Shetland pony. *J. Equine Vet. Sci.* 42: 82–87.

23 Tehon, L.R., Morrill, C.C., and Graham, R. (1946). Illinois plants poisonous to livestock. *Univ. Illinois College Ag Ext Service Circular* 599: 55–57.

24 Soler-Rodriguez, F., Martín, A., García-Cambero, J.P. et al. (2006). Short communications *Datura stramonium* poisoning in horses: a risk factor for colic. *Vet. Rec.* 158 (4): 132–133.

25 Binev, R., Valchev, I., and Nikolov, J. (2006). Clinical and pathological studies on intoxication in horses from freshly cut Jimson weed (*Datura stramonium*)-contaminated maize intended for ensiling. *J. S. Afr. Vet. Assoc.* 77 (4): 215–219.

26 Small, A.C., Keilly, W.R., Seawright, A.A. et al. (1993). Pyrrolizidine alkaloidosis in a two month old foal. *J. Vet. Med. Ser. A* 40 (1–10): 213–218.

27 Morton, J.F. (1989). Creeping indigo (*Indigofera spicata* forsk.) (Fabaceae) – a hazard to herbivores in Florida. *Econ. Bot.* 43 (3): 314–327.

28 Bell, A.T. and Hall, W.T.K. (1952). Birdsville disease of horses. *Aust. Vet. J.* 28 (6): 141–144.

29 Hegarty, M.P. and Pound, A.W. (1968). Indospicine, a new hepatotoxic amino-acid from *Indigofera spicata*. *Nature* 217 (5126): 354–355.

30 Hooper, P.T., Hart, B., and Smith, G.W. (1971). The prevention and treatment of Birdsville disease of horses. *Aust. Vet. J.* 47 (7): 326–329.

31 Kelly, W., Young, M., Hegarty, M. et al. (1992). The hepatotoxicity of Indospicine to dogs. In: *Poisonous Plants Proceedings Third International Symposium* (ed. L. James, R. Keeler, E. Bailey, et al.), 126–130. Ames, IA: Iowa State University Press.

32 Bela, F., Endre, B., Eniko, O. et al. (2008). Italian cocklebur (Xanthium italicum) poisoning of horses. *Magy Allatorvosok Lapja* 130 (5): 259–263.

33 Witte, S.T., Osweiler, G.D., Stahr, H.M. et al. (1990). Cocklebur toxicosis in cattle associated with the consumption of mature Xanthium strumarium. *J. Vet. Diagn. Invest.* 2 (4): 263–267.

34 Cornick, J.L., Carter, G.K., and Bridges, C.H. (1988). Kleingrass-associated hepatotoxicosis in horses. *J. Am. Vet. Med. Assoc.* 193 (8): 932–935.

35 Staley, E.E. (1978). An approach to treatment of locoism in horses. *Vet. Med. Small Anim. Clin.* 73 (9): 1205–1206.

36 Carroll, A.G. and Swain, B.J. (1983). Birdsville disease in the central highlands area of Queensland. *Aust. Vet. J.* 60 (10): 316–317.

37 Hegarty, M., Kelly, W., McEwan, D. et al. (1988). Hepatotoxicity to dogs of horse meat contaminated with indospicine. *Aust. Vet. J.* 65 (11): 337–340.

38 Cordy, D.R. (1954). Nigropallidal encephalomalacia in horses associated with ingestion of yellow star thistle. *J. Neuropathol. Exp. Neurol.* 13 (2): 338–342.

39 Young, S., Brown, W.W., and Klinger, B. (1970). Nigropallidal encephalomalacia in horses fed Russian knapweed (*Centaurea repens* L.). *Am. J. Vet. Res.* 31 (8): 1393–1404.

40 Wilson, T., Nelson, P., Ryan, T., and Rouse, C. (1985). Linking leukoencephalomalacia to commercial horse rations. *Vet. Med.* 80 (11): 63–69.

41 Burrows, G.E. (1986). Toxic plants. *Zimbabwe Vet. J.* 17: 1–2.

42 Mentz, A. and Ostenfeld, C. (1917). *Billeder af nordens flora*, vol. 1, 38. København: G.E.C. Gad's forlag.

43 Dijkstra, R.G.F.R. (1981). Een geval van cicutoxine-intoxicatie bij pony's (a case of cicutoxine poisoning in ponies). *Tijdschr. Diergeneeskd.* 106 (20): 1037–1039.

44 Panter, K.E., Keeler, R.F., and Baker, D.C. (1988). Toxicoses in livestock from the hemlocks (*Conium* and *Cicuta* spp.). *J. Anim. Sci.* 66 (9): 2407–2413.

45 Konishi, T. and Ichijo, S. (1984). Experimentally induced equine bracken poisoning by thermostable antithiamine factor (SF factor) extracted from dried bracken. *J. Japan Vet. Med.* 37 (11): 730–734.

46 Lee, S.T., Davis, T.Z., Gardner, D.R. et al. (2010). Tremetone and structurally related compounds in white snakeroot (*Ageratina altissima*): a plant associated with trembles and milk sickness. *J. Agric. Food Chem.* 58 (15): 8560–8565.

47 Smetzer, D.L., Coppock, T.W., Ely, R.W. et al. (1983). Cardiac effects of white snakeroot intoxication in horses. *Equine Pract.* 5 (2): 26–32.

48 White, J.L., Shivaprasad, H.L., Thompson, L.J., and Buck, W.B. (1985). White snakeroot (*Eupatorium rugosum*) poisoning clinical effects associated with cardiac and skeletal muscle lesions in experimental equine toxicosis. In: *Plant Toxicology* (ed. A.A. Seawright, M.P. Hegarty, L.F. James, and R.F. Keller), 411–422. Queensland: Queensland Poisonous Plant Committee.

49 True, R.G. and Lowe, J.E. (1980). Induced juglone toxicosis in ponies and horses. *Am. J. Vet. Res.* 41 (6): 944–945.

50 Buck, W.B. and Osweiler, G.D. (1976). Selenium. In: *Clinical and Diagnostic Veterinary Toxicology*, 2e (ed. G.A. Van Gelder), 345–354. Dubuque: Kendall/Hunt Publishing Company.

51 Stowe, H.D. (1980). Effects of copper pretreatment upon toxicity of selenium in ponies. *Am. J. Vet. Res.* 41: 1925–1928.

52 Anderson, G.A., Mount, M.E., Vrins, A.A., and Ziemer, E.L. (1983). Fatal acorn poisoning in a horse: pathologic findings and diagnostic considerations. *J. Am. Vet. Med. Assoc.* 182 (10): 1105–1110.

53 Warren, C. and Vaughan, S. (1985). Acorn poisoning. *Vet. Rec.* 116: 82.

54 Duncan, S.C. and Duncan, C.S. (1961). Oak leaf poisoning in two horses. *Cornell Vet.* 51: 159–162.

55 Stewart, J., Liyou, O., and Wilson, G. (2010). Bighead in horses – not an ancient disease. *Aust. Equine Vet.* 29 (1): 55–62.

56 McKenzie, R.A., Gartner, R.J.W.W., Blaney, B.J., and Glanville, R.J. (1981). Control of nutritional secondary hyperparathyroidism in grazing horses with calcium plus phosphorous supplementation. *Aust. Vet. J.* 57 (12): 554–557.

57 Blanco, J., Borras, F., Ouiroga, M., and Al, E. (1993). Crude protein: lysine, calcium: phosphorus and phytic: oxalic acids relationship in pastures used for weanlings in three different areas at Buenos Aires-Argentina. In: *Proceedings of the 13th Equine Nutrition and Physiology Society Symposium*, 88–89. Gainsville, FL: Equine Nutrition and Physiology Society.

58 Divers, T.J., George, L.W., and George, J.W. (1982). Hemolytic anemia in horses after the ingestion of red maple leaves. *J. Am. Vet. Med. Assoc.* 180 (3): 300–302.

59 Tennant, B., Dill, S.G., Glickman, L.T. et al. (1981). Acute hemolytic anemia, methemoglobinemia, and heinz body formation associated with ingestion of red maple leaves by horses. *J. Am. Vet. Med. Assoc.* 179 (2): 143–150.

60 Long, P.H. and Payne, J.W. (1984). Red maple-associated pulmonary thrombosis in a horse. *J. Am. Vet. Med. Assoc.* 184 (8): 977–978.

61 Semrad, S. (1993). Acute hemolytic anemia from ingestion of red maple leaves. *Compend. Contin. Educ. Vet.* 15: 261–264.

62 Alstad, A.D., Casper, H.H., and Johnson, L.J. (1985). Vitamin K treatment of sweet clover poisoning in calves. *J. Am. Vet. Med. Assoc.* 187 (7): 729–731.

63 Green, E. and Green, S. (1986). Vitamin K3: toxicosis and therapeutic considerations for use in horses. *Mod. Vet. Pract.* 67 (7): 625–628.

13

Manufactured Feeds

Erin Perry, Kathleen Crandell, Jeanne van der Veen, and Jesse M. Fenton

KEY TERMS

- Feed terminology – see the Feed Glossary in Appendix D [1].
- Feed is material consumed or intended to be consumed by animals, other than humans, that provides nutrition, taste, or aroma or has a technical effect on food, e.g. flavoring.
- Commercial feed is all materials, except unmixed whole seeds, distributed for use as feed or for mixing into a feed.
- Acceptability of a feed is assessed by measuring the daily consumption of a single feed to determine sufficient quantities will be eaten consistently and maintain BW, i.e. the one-bucket test.
- Palatability of a feed is the relative consumption (preference) for one feed when offered two simultaneously as measured by standardized methods, i.e. the two-bucket test.

KEY POINTS

- The process of manufacturing animal feeds is designed to increase nutrient density, ingredient variety, and consumer acceptance.
- The specific systems and equipment used to manufacture feed products vary between manufacturing plants; however, the basic principles of each method remain the same.
- Marketing concepts are strategies commonly utilized to affect the purchasing decision of the buyer.

13.1 Introduction

Significant scientific contributions in recent years have yielded an increased understanding of equine nutrition, and the diversity of ingredients utilized in equine feeds create a broad array of potential combinations to feed horses appropriately. Commercial horse feeds may be formulated for the maintenance of healthy adults, proper growth of young horses, or to aid in the prevention or management of specific conditions, e.g. weight gain, enteral nutritional support, or insulin dysregulation. Improvements in manufacturing technology have also resulted in advances in nutritional programs for equine athletes [2–4]. This increased product offering has resulted in greater choice for consumers, which can also mean greater confusion on the part of the horse owner. Additionally, veterinarians are tasked with educating horse owners on appropriate feed selection and feeding practices based on current knowledge and understanding of equine nutrition [5, 6]. Therefore, the intended purpose of any commercial feed and nutrient profile should be clearly defined on the label or tag. Ingredients and processes of manufacturing and subsequent effects on digestibility, palatability, quality control measures, packaging and labeling, and concepts in marketing manufactured feeds are reviewed.

13.2 Manufacturing Processes

The overall steps in producing animal feed products include purchasing and receiving ingredients from suppliers, creating a feed formula, processing and mixing ingredients to make a product, packaging, labeling, distributing, marketing, and selling of the product. In commercial

Equine Clinical Nutrition, Second Edition. Edited by Rebecca L. Remillard.

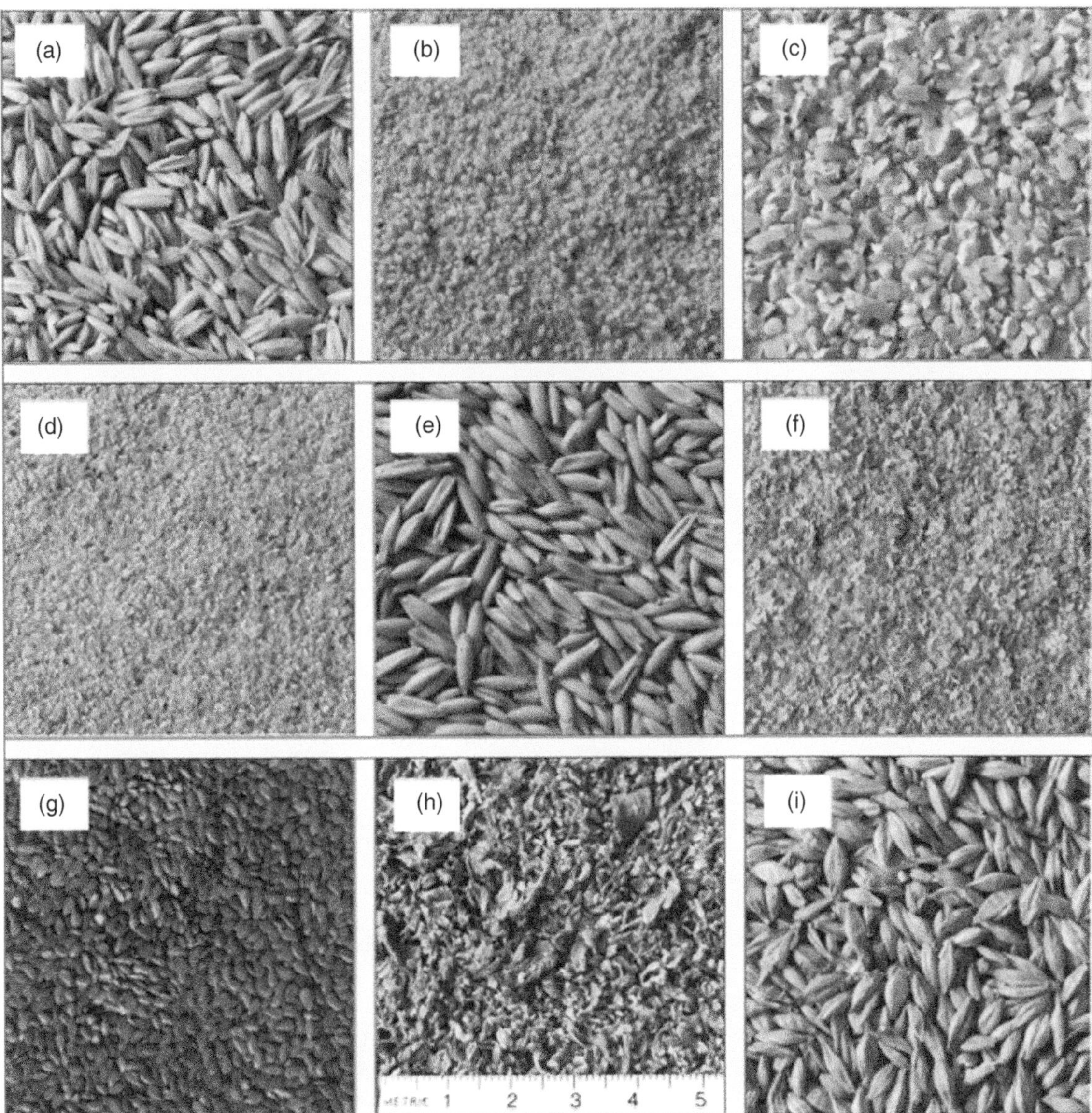

Figure 13.1 Commonly utilized ingredients in commercially manufactured horse feed. Ingredients listed from left to right and top to bottom: (a) crimped oats; (b) extruded soybean meal; (c) cracked corn; (d) soy hulls; (e) whole oats; (f) wheat middlings; (g) flax seeds; (h) dry beet pulp; (i) steam rolled barley. *Source:* Photo credit: Kathleen Crandell.

equine feed manufacturing, ingredients are commonly processed by pelleting, extruding, texturizing or a combination of these to produce a product. Pelleting and extrusion have both demonstrated impacts on digestibility in equine feeds [2, 7–9]. The finished product is packaged and labeled before distribution or sale.

13.2.1 Ingredients

Manufactured feeds use a variety of ingredients in their formulations that when combined are designed to make feeds that are balanced to complement forage for energy and nutrients, improve the well-being of the animal, and are safe (Figure 13.1). Among the ingredients typically used in manufactured feeds are grains, sources of protein, fiber and fat, minerals, vitamins, and additives. Ingredients are required to be listed in descending order of inclusion by weight. However, there are no routine methods by which to reverse engineer the exact ingredient formula or to distinguish specifically which ingredients have been included, so monitoring compliance with this law is not common.

13.2.1.1 Cereal Grains

Grains are seeds from cereal plants that are members of the grass family Gramineae. The seed is a nutrient store for the embryo or germ from which the plant develops. It consists

Table 13.1 Nutrient composition of cereal grains on dry matter basis.

Grains	Unground density	Digestible energy	Crude protein	Crude fiber	Neutral detergent fiber	Crude fat	Starch	Calcium	Phosphorus
Units	**kg/L**	**Mcal/kg**	**%**	**%**	**%**	**%**	**%**	**%**	**%**
Oats (regular)	0.4	3.23	11	14	36	5.4	41	0.11	0.36
Oats (heavy)	0.5	3.33	12.5	11	29	5.2	44	0.07	0.4
Oats (naked, hullless)	0.7	3.8	13	4.2	11.3	6.9	61	0.07	0.44
Corn	0.8	3.8	9	2.2	10	4.2	69	.04	0.3
Barley	0.7	3.6	12	5	21	2.2	54	0.06	0.39
Wheat	0.9	3.8	14	3	14	2.3	62	0.05	0.43
Rye	0.8	3.4	10.3	2.5	14	1.7	62	0.07	0.36
Rice	0.6	3.8	9	2	6.2	1.9	85	0.07	0.36
Grain sorghum (Milo)	0.8	3.75	10.8	2.8	11	3.4	74.5	0.03	0.33
Millet	0.7	3.3	11.5	9.5	21	3.5	45	0.8	0.3
Soybean (whole heated)	0.85	3.3	40	6	13.2	21	6.4	0.32	0.61
Lupins	0.6	3.4	32	14	27	6	2	0.2	0.3
Triticale	0.6	3.75	11.7	2.7	14.6	1.5	67.6	0.06	0.33

Source: Values compiled from: NRC [10], Equi-Analytical Lab [11], Feedipedia [12] and Dairy One Feed Composition Library (www.dairyoneservices.com/feedcomposition).

of a coat, starchy endosperm, and germ. Starch is the major component of a grain and its content varies greatly between the different types, depending on the amount of hull that is left remaining with the grain. Hulls are high in fiber; grains with hulls are therefore higher in fiber than those without hulls. The density and nutrient content of the most commonly available cereal grains are in Table 13.1. Historically, cereal grains have played a major role as a concentrated source of energy in the diet of the working horse. See Sidebar 13.1.

Total tract starch digestibility of cereal grains by the horse is 87–100% across different feeds; however, the site of digestion can differ and has consequences for the animal [13]. Ideally, when the starch content is within the capacity of amylase enzyme production for small intestinal hydrolytic digestion it will cause little to no problems in the horse. Research on acceptable starch levels indicate that less than 2 g starch/kg BW is a safe level [13]. Starch escaping small intestine digestion is digested by the hindgut microbiota, generating the short-chain fatty acid lactic acid which decreases the pH and can lead to hindgut acidosis. Hindgut acidosis if severe may result in diarrhea, colic, and laminitis. The risk of hindgut starch overload can be mitigated by feeding a higher forage and lower grain ration, pre-treating (heat and grinding) the grain to increase small intestinal digestion, and/or feeding grains with higher small intestinal digestibilities (oats > milo > corn > barley) [14].

Sidebar 13.1: General Characteristics of Cereal Grains

Highly palatable: most horses will preferentially consume cereal grains before forage

High DM[1] density: 4–8 times greater weight per volume unit compared with baled hay

High energy: 3.2–3.8 Mcal/kg DM which is about 50% more energy than hay

High starch: variable from 2% to 85% DM

Low fiber: 2%–15% DM which is 30% to 50% less fiber than hay

Variable protein concentration and quality: 9%–45% protein DM

Lack of sufficient concentrations of vitamins and minerals to meet horse requirements alone

1 Dry matter.

13.2.1.2 Protein Sources

Cereal grains and many forages may not contain sufficient protein to meet the requirements of the lactating mare or the growing horse, and some mature grass forages do not contain enough protein to meet adult maintenance requirements [10–12]. Protein supplements (>20% crude protein) are concentrated sources that when added to a grain mix, can adequately raise the total protein of the ration. Protein supplements are classified according to origin, i.e. plant, animal, single cell, or non-protein nitrogen (Table 13.2). Non-protein nitrogen is of little benefit because it is poorly utilized by the horse; however, plant, animal, and single-cell sources are beneficial. Plant proteins are more commonly used, and oilseed meals (35–50% crude protein) are the most common plant sources. Protein supplements are referred to according to their protein content, e.g. 44% soybean meal indicates that it contains 44% crude protein as fed. Soybean meal is by far the most widely used of all protein supplements for animal feeds. Plant protein supplements are not particularly palatable for most horses, i.e. soybean meal is less palatable than wheat, barley, rye, oats, and corn [15, 16]; therefore, protein sources need to be well mixed with cereal grains or palatable by-products[2]. When included in a loose mixture, wet molasses is beneficial and commonly used both to increase the feed's palatability and to prevent the protein supplement from sifting out. Current manufacturing practices for equine feeds commonly combine soybean meal or a comparable protein source with vitamins and minerals to produce a high protein mixing pellet for use in making textured feeds. This pellet may also be sold separately as a stand-alone low-intake feed called a "ration balancer."

13.2.1.3 Fiber Sources

Previously, performance horse feeds commonly contained large quantities of high-starch cereal grains, which have now been associated with alterations in the hindgut microbiota, elevated risk of laminitis, colic, gastric ulcers, and development of stereotypic behaviors [17]. In response to the negative effects of high grain concentrates, the use of energy-dense fibrous by-product ingredients has been considered a suitable alternative and has spawned the use of "high-fiber" or "low-starch" commercial feeds. These by-product ingredients are high in fermentable fiber yet easily incorporated into a textured, pelleted, or extruded feed (Table 13.3). Well-known by-products like beet pulp, alfalfa meal, soy hulls, and rice bran fed to horses were found to have a low glycemic index [18].

2 Although frequently perceived as less valuable or nutritious, by-products (secondary products) are the end-results of producing a primary or principal product, e.g. rice bran and beet pulp are by-products with specific nutritional attributes.

13.2.1.4 Fat Sources

Fats or oils are added to the manufactured feeds principally to increase the energy density of the ration but may serve other purposes as well: skin and coat conditioner, binding fine material in mixed feed, decreasing dust, and lubricate and lessen wear on feed preparation and mixing equipment. Fat, with the highest caloric density, is particularly well suited to increasing the energy density of a feed (Table 13.4). Plant or vegetable oils provide about three times more digestible energy than an equal weight of cereal grain and 3.5–6 times more than an equal volume of cereal grain [10–12]. The purpose of increasing ration energy density is to increase energy intake and/or decrease the amount of feed consumed to meet a high energy need, i.e. performance, milk production, reproductive efficiency, growth rate, or increase body weight (BW). Supplemental fats are well utilized by the horse (76–94% digestible) up to 20% of the concentrate portion of a ration [19, 20]. Fat digestibility was similar across oils but lower for animal and hydrogenated fats [21]. The effect of added dietary fat on the digestibility of the diet was determined by a meta-analysis over numerous studies and was shown to have no adverse effects on protein and neutral detergent fiber digestibilities, but had a significant negative effect on acid detergent fiber digestibility [22]. When feeding added dietary fat, the NRC recommends an upper limit of 0.7 g fat/kg BW to avoid potential negative effects on fiber digestion and potential loose stool [10].

13.2.1.5 Minerals

Inorganic or organic (chelated) forms of minerals are nutritional additives used to overcome specific deficiencies in the total ration. The macro minerals are usually added as individual ingredients, e.g. calcium carbonate. Micro minerals (copper, zinc, manganese, iron, iodine, selenium, cobalt) are commonly incorporated into the feed as a single premixed additive containing the minerals in appropriate proportion to one another. See Chapter 8 Minerals.

13.2.1.6 Vitamins

Vitamins are nutritional additives. Vitamins A and E are added to overcome the specific deficiencies in the total ration. Horses with access to fresh pasture will typically consume sufficient quantities of Vitamin A from carotenoids (chiefly β-carotene) present in fresh forage. Vitamin E functions as an antioxidant and is present in both fresh pasture and cereal grains. Vitamins D, C, K, and multiple B vitamins are synthesized endogenously in horses and therefore are added for specific feeding situations.

Although the fat-soluble vitamins A, E, and K are naturally occurring in fresh green forages, they can deteriorate

Table 13.2 Nutrient composition of protein supplements on dry matter basis.

Ingredients	Digestible energy	Crude protein	Lysine Feed/Protein	Crude fiber	Neutral detergent fiber	Crude fat	Starch	Calcium	Phosphorus
Units	Mcal/kg	%	%	%	%	%	%	%	%
Oilseed meals									
Canola meal (EA)	3.1	40	2.4/5.9	10	30.5	7.5	1.3	0.73	1.1
Coconut meal (copra)	3.3	23	0.6/2.5	15	56.4	5	>1	0.2	0.65
Cottonseed meal	3.0	45	1.8/4.1	13	27	1.7	3.3	0.18	1.2
Linseed (flax) meal	3.0	40	1.3/3.3	9	33.4	1.6	2.0	0.4	0.9
Peanut meal	3.3	42	2.0/4.2	9.6	19.5	2.3	10	0.2	0.47
Safflower seed meal	3.4	49	1.4/3.1	9	53.8	1.9	1.5	0.3	1.8
Soybean meal (44%)	3.5	46	3.16.3	7	22.0	1.6	1.3	0.4	0.7
Soybean meal (48%)	3.6	50	3.2/6.5	4.8	13.6	2.15	1.6	0.4	0.7
Sunflower seed meal (44%)	2.4	32.5	1.8/3.7	17	40.7	11.4	0.98	0.4	1.1
Oilseeds									
Canola or rapeseeds	4.3	20	1.5/5.9	6	20.4	38	3.7	0.38	0.75
Cottonseeds	4.3	24	1.0/4.1	18–20	48.6	24	2.1	0.15	0.7
Flax seeds (linseed)	3.6	23	0.9/4.1	6.5	21.7	38	5.2	0.25	0.6
Safflower seeds	3.9	19.5	0.6/3.3	31	46	32	5.8	0.25	0.75
Soybeans	3.5	38	2.7/6.5	5	18.6	18.5	2.4	0.25	0.7
Sunflower seeds with hull	3.6	18	2.3/4.2	31	13.2	28	6.4	0.18	0.56
Grain protein supplement									
Brewers grains	2.7	26.5	1.0/3.5	16	50	7.4	7.5	0.33	0.55
Distillers grains	2.6	31.5	0.8/2.6	12.5	34	7–16	5	0.13	0.45
Corn gluten meal	3.8	66	0.9/2.0	2	9.7	2.9	15	0.06	0.55
Corn gluten feed	3.4	23.5	0.65/3.0	8.6	36.5	4.2	14.7	0.09	1.06
Extruded soybean	4.0	39.9	2.8/6.6	6.8	17.5	13.2	1.3	0.3	0.67
Pulse proteins									
Beans and peas	3.6	21–26	1.3–1.8/5–8	5–7	20	1.5–1.8	42.7	0.1–0.2	0.4–0.6
Animal source protein									
Fish meal, menhaden	4.1	68.5	5.2/7.6	0.9	0	12	0	5.6	3.2
Fish meal, white	3.3	65	4.5/7.5	0.8	0	5	0	8.0	3.9
Milk, cows skim	4.0	35.6	2.7/7.6	0.2	0	1	0	1.36	1.1
Milk, cows whole	5.6	27	2.0/7.4	0.2	0	27.6	0	0.95	0.76
Casein, dry	4.0	93	7.7/8.5	0.2	0	0.7	0	0.6	0.9
Single cell protein									
Yeast, brewers	3.3	49	3.3/6.9	5	8.8	1.1	10.9	0.15	1.5
Yeast, torula	3.3	52.5	4.1/7.8	2.5	7.7	2.3	8.2	0.65	1.8

Source: Values compiled from: NRC [10], Equi-Analytical Lab [11], Feedipedia [12] and Dairy One Feed Composition Library (www.dairyoneservices.com/feedcomposition).

Table 13.3 Nutrient composition of by-products commonly used in manufactured feeds on dry matter basis.

Ingredient	Digestible energy	Crude protein	Crude fiber	Neutral detergent fiber	Crude fat	Starch	Total sugars	Calcium	Phosphorus
Units	Mcal/kg	%	%	%	%	%	%	%	%
Alfalfa meal	2.4	18.3	28.6	45.9	2.7	3.3	4.5	2.2	0.27
Almond hulls	2.9	6.5	11.5	36.8	2.9	3	28	0.23	0.11
Apple pomace	2.8	8	36	65.1	2.8	8.1	20[a]	0.6	1.4
Babassu meal (expeller)	2.7	21.8	16.1	65.5	5.5–10	0	2	0.2	1.0
Babassu meal (solvent)	2.4	18.7	29.0	38.5	1.8	0	2	0.12	0.84
Beet pulp	2.8	10	20	45.8	1.1	0.9	7.8	0.91	0.09
Citrus pulp	2.9	6.9	13	24.2	4.9	7.5	24.5	1.92	0.12
Coconut meal (copra)[b]	3.5	22.4	14.2	54.7	9.8	>1	11.4	0.12	0.58
Corn cobs	1.4	3	35	87.8	0.7	10.7	>1	0.12	0.04
Corn ears	3.3	9	9.5	27.9	3.7	56.4	2.5	0.07	0.27
Corn fodder	2.0	7.9	29	63.2	1.9	20.1	18.3	0.36	0.21
Corn stover	1.7	5.5	36	82.4	1.3	9.9	8.7	0.6	0.1
Cottonseed hulls	1.3	4	47	85	2	4.2	2.0	0.15	0.09
Lupin hulls	1.4	9	40	65.6	2.2	0.9	0.7	0.5	0.12
Molasses, cane	3.5	5.5	0.1	0.8	1	1.1	64.1	.92	0.1
Oat hulls	1.3	5.2	30.6	75.8	2.2	9.9	1.2	0.19	0.18
Oat mill feed	1.8	8.2	22.4	55.4	3.8	25	3.9	0.17	0.29
Peanut hulls	1.0	7.0	65.9	66.4	2.0	2.7	7	0.17	0.07
Rice bran	3.4	12.7	16.3	34.4	17.2	22.4	2.8	0.1	1.38
Rice hulls	0.5	3	43	65	1	5.3	6.6	0.1	0.07
Soybean hulls	2.25	13.1	39	64.4	2.2	5.2	1.8	0.55	0.15
Straw, wheat	1.6	4.2	41.5	77.5	1.4	1.0	1.2	0.48	0.1
Sunflower hulls	2.0	7	50.8	74.7	5.2	3.4	1.5	0.44	0.13
Wheat bran	3.2	17.3	10.4	45.2	3.9	23.1	7.2	0.14	1.27
Wheat middlings/ millrun	3.4	17.7	7.5	33.7	4.3	32.3	8.5	0.13	0.89

[a] Sum of total sugars (5.5% DM) and fructose (14.5% DM).
[b] Expeller extracted.
Source: Values compiled from: NRC [10], Equi-Analytical Lab [11], Feedipedia [12] and Dairy One Feed Composition Library (www.dairyoneservices.com/feedcomposition).

with harvesting and storage of conserved forages. As a result, all three are commonly added to manufactured feeds for those horses with no access to fresh forage. Vitamin D is synthesized with sun exposure and occurs in sun-dried forages but is commonly added to concentrates for horses maintained indoors or frequently blanketed. Vitamin K and the B complex vitamins are produced by the hindgut microbes but are commonly added to commercial mixes to counter dysbiosis. See Chapter 9 Vitamins.

13.2.1.7 Digestion Enhancers

A wide variety of substances are used to enhance feed utilization and promote health and well-being in the horse. Those substances include enzymes, prebiotics, probiotics, and yeast. In general, these enhancers aim to promote stability and balance within the gastrointestinal microbiota for horses with intestinal dysbiosis and may improve feed utilization. Overall, the stability of the intestinal microbiota and a strong mucosal barrier are key targets of these

Table 13.4 Digestible energy and density of fat and grain sources commonly utilized in commercial feed manufacturing.

Ingredient	Density		Digestible energy (as fed basis)		
Units	Lb/quart	kg/L	Mcal/kg	Mcal/L	Mcal/cup[a]
Oil, vegetable	1.92	0.92	8.98	8.3	1.95
Fat, animal	1.80	0.86	7.94	6.8	1.62
Corn, cracked	1.50	0.72	3.40	2.4	0.57
Oats, regular	1.0	0.48	2.88	1.4	0.33

[a] 8 oz or 237 mL/cup.

types of feed additives [23]. See Chapter 14 Dietary Supplements.

13.2.1.8 Non-Nutritive Additives

Micro quantities of non-nutritive additives are used to fulfill a specific technical requirement and some serve more than one function. All additives used in feeds must be an AAFCO approved GRAS (Generally Recognized As Safe) ingredient [1]. Some prevent caking and improve the flowability of the feed mix through the mixing equipment. Flavoring agents are commonly added to commercial horse feed to increase product palatability whereas others improve pellet quality and enhance animal acceptability. Other additives function as antifungal agents, mold detoxifiers, or antioxidants (preservatives).

13.2.2 Ingredient Processing

Although the term "processing" may have negative connotations to some, variations in processing techniques serve to provide better products with a wider range of use and does not necessarily relate to the nutritional adequacy of a product. Reasons for processing comprise the following: (i) an improvement in feed acceptability, palatability, and digestibility, (ii) improve cleanliness and sanitation, and (iii) ease of handling and storage. Examples of commonly utilized feed forms are shown in Figure 13.2.

Grain, like harvested forages, may be dried, ensiled, or acid-treated to prevent spoilage due to heating and molding during storage. Drying is most commonly accomplished by sun-curing in the field. Artificial drying or dehydrating may be used but generally substantially increases the cost of the grain. Although drying to a moisture content of less than 20% is adequate for hay, less than 13% is necessary for grain due to the higher fermentable soluble carbohydrate content. Moisture content below 10% stops the development of most insects. However, as moisture level decreases, especially below 12%, physical damage (breakage) to grain kernels increases.

Whole dried cleaned grains can be fed to horses as is or used in the manufacture of commercial horse feeds. Whole grains, not broken or exposed to air, may be less susceptible to spoiling. Researchers found no difference between whole unprocessed oats and chopped vacuum-cleaned oats, with or without the hulls, in the digestibility of dry matter (DM), protein, fat, acid detergent fiber, neutral detergent fiber, or gross energy when fed to mature quarter horses [24]. Horses fed whole oats had higher post-prandial glucose concentration when compared with feeding whole corn or barley, which is indicative of a higher prececal starch digestibility [25–27]. However, there was no difference in glycemic response when whole oats, corn, or barley were fed at or below 1.5 g starch/kg BW in a meal [28, 29].

Further processing of whole grain in any manner has been reported to increase the feeding value of that grain by 10–15% [30]. Dry grains may be processed using cold or hot temperatures. Cold processing involves milling, hammer, or roller mill grinding. Common hot processing includes steam flaking, rolling, or crimping (Figure 13.1), and also may include popping, micronizing, extruding, or pelleting. Heat accelerates the gelatinization of the starch granule structure, which increases starch digestion in the small intestine particularly for grains with a crystalline starch structure, such as barley and corn, sometimes called maize [7, 8, 31].

The primary reasons for processing grains are to improve consumption and increase small intestinal (prececal) digestibility. Prececal starch digestibility has been studied in fistulated[3] equines in conjunction with measuring serum glucose and insulin after feeding a meal [28]. While total tract digestibility of grain is over 90% for oats, corn, and barley, increasing prececal starch digestion decreases the quantity of starch reaching the cecum. Minimizing starch to the cecum lowers the risk of detrimentally altering the large intestinal microbial population [27, 32].

13.2.2.1 Common Manufacturing Processes [1]

13.2.2.1.1 Cleaning

Removal of material by methods such as scalping, aspirating, magnetic separation, or any other method. Cereal grains straight out of the field may be contaminated with large amounts of impurities, such as chaff, sticks, stones, broken grains, fine particles, and dust, and therefore should be cleaned before being fed to a horse or used in the manufacture of a feed. Cleaning involves scalpuration, separation, and aspiration of the grains done by passing the grains through some type of drum and screen sieves to separate the impurities from the grain. Blowing or aspirating air

3 A fistulated horse has been surgically fitted with a cannula that acts as a porthole device providing access into various gastro-intestinal segments.

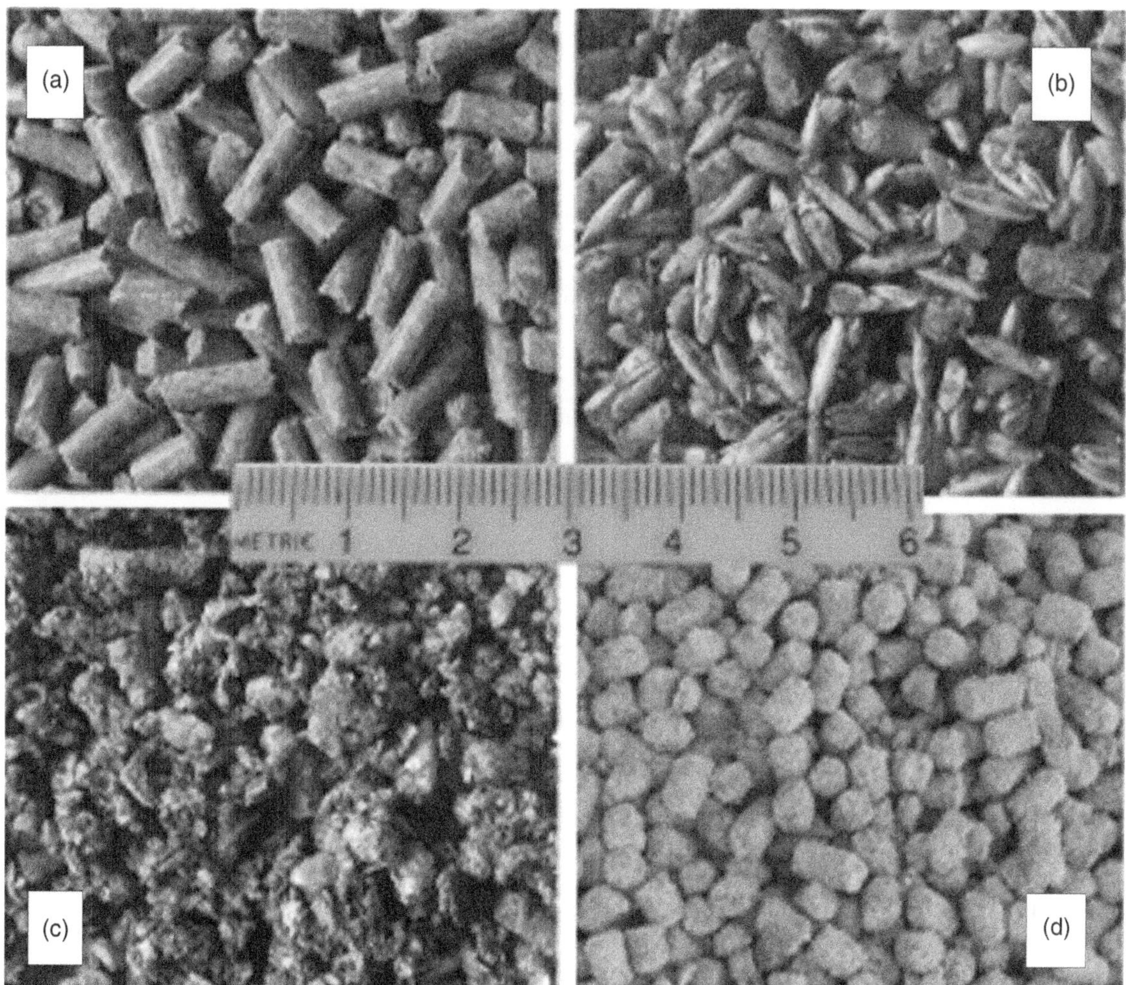

Figure 13.2 Commonly utilized feed forms in commercially manufactured horse feed. Feed types listed from left to right and top to bottom: (a) pelleted; (b) high grain textured feed; (c) high-fiber textured feed; (d) extruded. *Source:* Photo credit: Kathleen Crandell.

through the grains during the cleaning process eliminates nearly all the fine material and dust from the grains. Airborne particles were reduced by 70% after cleaning oats and barley [33]. Cleaning the grain will extend the product's shelf life. The more complete the cleaning, the higher the value of the grain. For example, triple-cleaned oats claim a premium price in the racetrack industry.

13.2.2.1.2 Rolling

A grain is run between rollers to change the shape and size; can be performed on cold grains or after conditioning.[4] The lowest serum glucose and insulin concentrations were observed after feeding horses rolled barley, as compared with feeding extruded and micronized barley at <1.5 and 2 g starch/kg BW [14]. However, the process of rolling is not necessarily protective against grain overload. Regardless of the source, feeding rolled barley, corn, naked oats, or oats, in conjunction with 1% of BW alfalfa cubes, decreased fecal pH relative to feeding alfalfa cubes alone. Additionally, two horses, in an experimental group of four, fed rolled barley with alfalfa cubes at 0.4% BW total non-structural carbohydrates developed acute laminitis [34].

13.2.2.1.3 Grinding

Reducing the particle size of grain by impact, shearing, or attrition. Grain should not be finely ground unless used in the preparation for pelleting or extrusion. Fine grinding decreases palatability, increases the dust, and may increase the risk of gastric ulcers and respiratory issues [35]. Although the starch structure of corn is relatively unaffected by grinding, the increased surface area exposed to digestive enzymes may improve digestibility [36]. Grinding has been demonstrated to improve prececal starch digestibility for oats, barley, corn, and wheat [7, 31, 37, 38].

4 Conditioning is having achieved pre-determined moisture characteristics and/or temperature of ingredients or a mixture of ingredients before further processing.

13.2.2.1.4 Cracking

Reducing the particle size of whole grain by a combined breaking and crushing action. Most horses prefer cracked over whole corn probably because it is easier to chew [15, 16]. Corn is the most common grain used in feeds in cracked form, albeit with similar small intestinal digestibility as steam flaking [39]. Preileal starch digestion of popped, ground, cracked, and whole corn has been reported as 90%, 46%, 30%, and 29%, respectively, and therefore, preileal starch digestion was increased threefold by popping and 50% by grinding but not at all by cracking [40]. The glycemic index from cracked corn was not different from rolled barley but 40% lower than glucose administration when fed at 2 g starch/kg BW [41].

13.2.2.1.5 Crimping

Using corrugated rollers, crimping is usually done with oats more often than any other grain fed to horses. Crimping did not affect DM, protein, or neutral detergent fiber digestibility of oats fed to ponies [30]. Crimping appears to be preferred over whole oats by horse owners, and prized for better palatability and fewer oats visible in the manure. Crimping may aid particle size reduction for the older horse with dental loss because the outer shell of the grain has been broken in the process.

13.2.2.1.6 Flaking

Grains can be flaked by rolling or cutting into flat pieces with or without prior steam conditioning. Steam flaked corn is a common ingredient in manufactured feeds as it improves starch gelatinization that facilitates prececal digestibility of starch [39, 42]. Feeding flaked barley resulted in significantly higher glycemic responses than rolled barley at 2 g starch/kg BW, suggesting that steam flaking increased starch digestibility [43].

13.2.2.1.7 Micronizing

Micronizing is a process where grains are moistened with steam, passed under infrared heat lamps until reaching the desired temperature, and then rolled, cooled, and dried. Micronizing barley, corn, and wheat yielded higher prececal digestibility compared with extruding [27]. In contrast, micronized barley did not result in as high of a glycemic and insulinemic response as extruded barley but higher than rolled barley that resulted in reduced cecal starch [14]. Feeding micronized barley minimized changes in hindgut fermentation patterns likely due to improved prececal digestion [44]. In addition to starch, protein digestion by the horse is 2–3% higher from both oats and milo when these grains are micronized as compared with crimping [45].

13.2.2.2 Commonly Utilized Manufacturing Processes to Make Concentrates

13.2.2.2.1 Texturizing

The process of texturizing or making a textured feed involves mixing ingredients to combine by agitation two or more materials to a specific degree of dispersion. A feed mixer is used for the production of a textured feed. The texturizing process involves weighing and mixing ingredients of different sizes, types, and forms. Primary ingredients for making equine textured feeds include any combination of whole, flaked, or cracked grains, beet pulp, molasses, and pellets containing protein, minerals, and/or vitamins. Other ingredients may be added depending on product purposes, such as to increase fat or fiber content. The feed mixer should be able to handle multiple sizes and forms of ingredients while maintaining structural integrity during mixing. Visibility of the different components in the feed is an important consideration in making a textured feed product. The manufacturer commonly incorporates molasses and/or oil during the mixing process to improve flavoring and dust control. Common names for textured feeds are sweet feed, coarse mix, grain muesli, loose mix, and compound feed. Textured feeds have the advantage of visible ingredients and excellent palatability. Glucose and insulin responses were least disturbed with textured feeds fed at <1.1 g starch/kg BW [46].

13.2.2.2.2 Pelleting

Pelleting is the mechanical process agglomerating feed by compaction and forcing it through die openings. See Sidebar 13.2. Pellet die openings range in size from 4 to 25 mm, the most commonly used for horse feed being 6–8 mm (Figure 13.3). Pellets are also called "cubes" outside the United States, although large (10–25 mm) diameter pellets are often called cubes or range cubes in the United States. Single ingredients can be pelleted, as in alfalfa pellets, or two ingredients, as in a fiber pellet of soy hulls and wheat middlings, or pellets can be made from a mixture of different ingredients to make a concentrate feed. Pellets are considered advantageous due to the homogeneity of the ingredients contained in the pellet and are thought to prevent horses from sorting the grains. Pellets also are easier to feed, particularly in freezing temperatures because they do not stick together or become hard as can happen in textured feeds with molasses, called "bricking." Pellet hardness does not appear to affect acceptability, although most horses dislike pellets that crumble too easily, and those that are excessively hard have been reported to increase the risk of choke when consumed rapidly (bolting food) without adequate mastication.

Factors that determine if a pellet is hard or soft, durable or crumbly are (i) time exposure to steam during conditioning (60–90 °C); (ii) retention time in the die, (iii) moisture

Sidebar 13.2: The Pelleting Process

Grinding: Machines such as hammer mills or roller mills are most often used in the grinding of ingredients. Large particle feed ingredients, such as whole grains, are ground to reduce their size for uniform mixing with other smaller particle-sized feed ingredients, such as soybean meal, minerals, and vitamins. The finer and more uniform the particle size of all the ingredients in the formula mix, the better the pelleting process and result. Grinding serves to break down hard seed coats and expose more surface area of the ingredients for enhanced nutritional characteristics such as digestibility.

Weighing and Mixing: A weighing system composed of one or more scales is used to measure out the desired quantity of each ingredient in a formula. A combination of computer-controlled scales and smaller hand-weighing scales may be used. The weighted ingredients are combined and mixed using a feed mixer producing a "mash." Mixing of the feed is essential for equal distribution of nutrients and producing a consistent product. To ensure proper mixing, mixing times are determined based on the characteristics of the ingredients that make up the feed mixture and the mixer type. The specific equipment used for weighing, combining, and mixing ingredients may vary depending on the manufacturing plant.

Conditioning: To prepare the ingredients for pelleting, heat and steam are added and mixed with the "mash" in a conditioning chamber. Liquid ingredients such as molasses or oil may also be added to the conditioning chamber. The increase in moisture and temperature of the mash is an important step in the pelleting process and serves to soften the feed particles for better compression into a pellet, activate natural binding agents in ingredients, and aid in lubricating the die that forms the pellet. The conditioning process may also result in partial starch gelatinization, increasing the availability of starch for prececal digestion. The amount of steam added varies depending primarily on the type and amount of the ingredients in the formulation. Temperatures may range from 60 °C to 90 °C.

Pelleting: Conditioned mash is fed into the pellet die chamber where it is compressed by rollers and forced through holes in a circular die (Figure 13.3). The friction and pressure involved in forcing the mash through the die holes further raise the mash temperature. The diameter and shape of the holes in the die determine the diameter and shape of the final dense pellet. Knives on the outside of the die are adjusted to cut the pellets to the desired length.

Drying and Cooling: The process of drying and cooling involves the circulation or movement of air through and/or around the pellets to remove moisture and heat generated during the conditioning and pelleting process. Proper drying and cooling are necessary to maintain feed quality and shelf life during handling and storage. The specific equipment used for drying and cooling will vary depending on the manufacturing plant.

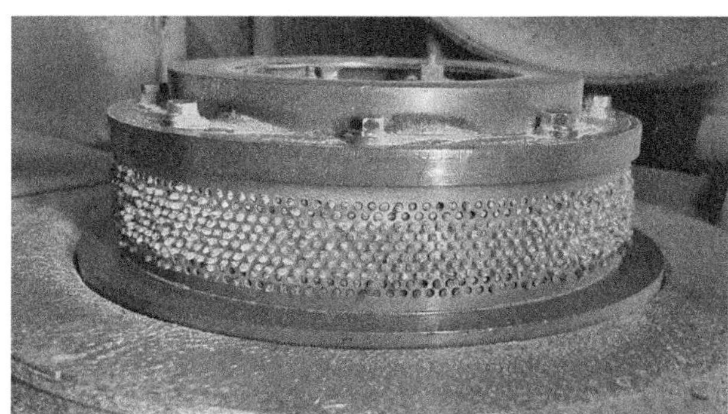

Figure 13.3 Manufacturing dies are commonly utilized for the production of equine feeds. The conditioned mash is fed into a die chamber where it is compressed by rollers and forced through holes in a circular die to produce the desired pellet size. *Source:* Photo credit: Kathleen Crandell.

concentration in the feed, (iv) ambient temperature and humidity, and (v) type and amount of pellet binder. The durability of the pellet is measured at the mill and if unacceptable, the feed will be reprocessed. The steam treatment in the conditioning period of pelleting helps to gelatinize a portion of the starch subsequently improving enzymatic hydrolysis. The degree of gelatinization may vary according to conditioning temperature. Pelleting barley resulted in a higher glycemic response than cracking indicating improved prececal starch digestion associated with pelleting [47]. Pelleting oats, corn, and barley improved prececal starch and protein digestion over ground grains [8]. Horses fed a single large meal compared to those fed three smaller meals had significant changes to cecal microbiota [48]. Weanlings fed a complete pelleted diet developed more gastric ulcers than when fed the same ingredients in hay cubes and sweet feed forms. However, the weanlings on the pelleted diet had a higher average daily gain [49].

13.2.2.2.3 Extruding

Extrusion is a process during which feed or a mixture of feed ingredients is pressed, pushed, or protruded through orifices under pressure. See Sidebar 13.3. Extruding a single ingredient is most commonly done with rice bran, corn or soy, but can be done using any ingredient with adequate starch content. A fully fortified concentrate feed can also be made using the extrusion process and a variety of extruded horse feeds are currently available. The extrusion

Sidebar 13.3: The Extrusion Process

Extrusion: The preconditioned mash enters the extruder where more steam is added as a large screw moves and mixes the mash along a cylindrical barrel creating a dough-like mixture. Extreme friction and pressure are created within the barrel as the dough is worked through the extruder. The cooking temperature can range between 90 °C and 150 °C for a very short time and results in more extensive starch gelatinization, and subsequent prececal starch availability, compared with pelleting. High temperatures also result in the destruction of potential microorganisms in the feed. The short-term exposure to heat minimizes the expected vitamin losses that are usually adjusted for in the formulation. Upon reaching the end of the barrel, the dough is forced out of the extruder through the openings of a specially shaped die. The size, thickness, shape, and number of openings in the die help determine the density, texture, and shape of the final product. A rapid drop in temperature and pressure as the extrudate leaves the extruder results in the expansion of the product, giving some extruded products their characteristic form and texture. Knives located on the outside of the die-cut the extrudate to the desired length.

Drying and Cooling: Drying of the high-moisture extruded product involves passing through a drying system in which varying temperatures of heated air slowly draw the moisture out of the product, much like an oven. Cooling is done through circulation or movement of non-heated air through or around the product. Proper drying and cooling are necessary to maintain feed quality and shelf life during handling and storage. The specific equipment used for drying and cooling will vary depending on the manufacturing plant.

process utilizes high temperature (90–150 °C), moisture, friction, and pressure to cook ground feed ingredients and work them into a dough-like mixture to be formed into a product of predetermined size, shape, and density. The advantages of extruded feeds are fewer fines (waste) and higher possible concentrations of fat as compared with pelleted feeds. The rate of consumption for an extruded product was 22–32% slower than the same grain mix when unprocessed or pelleted [30]. Slowing the rate of consumption lessens the risk of digestive disturbances and choking. The incidence of digestive disturbances, including gastric rupture, has been reported to decrease when young horses were changed from a pelleted to an extruded feed [50]. Extruding barley, corn, and wheat resulted in surprisingly lower prececal starch and protein digestibilities than pelleted or micronized grains [8]. Extrusion increased the availability of glucose in the small intestine of the horses and resulted in higher glycemic and insulinemic responses than from rolled or micronized barley [14]. Feeding extruded barley higher than 2 g starch/kg BW resulted in significantly higher glycemic responses than 1.5 and 2 g starch/kg BW flaked or rolled barley, and minimized changes in hindgut fermentation patterns [43, 44].

13.3 Palatability and Preference

The sensory perception of a feedstuff by the horse is generally referred to as palatability. Unfortunately, palatability is surprisingly underrepresented in the literature. Palatability has been characterized as the overall sensory perception of a feed with regard to smell, taste, texture, temperature, consistency, and appearance [2]. Horse preference of feedstuff is believed to be largely influenced by aroma, flavor, ease of prehension, and texture, while appearance is of less significance compared to their human counterparts [51, 52]. Palatability is often assessed using the paired preference test where the horse is offered two feeds at the same time for a specific duration, and the amount consumed is measured (Figure 13.4). The assumption is that the feed with greater consumption is the more palatable option.

There is an increased interest in the role of flavors on the acceptance and preferences of concentrate feeds offered to horses. Historically, there has been a relatively limited range of flavors marketed in concentrate feeds for horses, and many feed companies own patents controlling propriety mixtures for specific palatants (flavor enhancement) that are believed to increase acceptance of feed products. Data has demonstrated that anise, apple, fenugreek, banana, cherry, rosemary, cumin, carrot, peppermint, and oregano are preferred flavors, while orange and raspberry flavors are not preferred [2, 53–56]. However, there may be individual variations by horses.

Most horses prefer the type of feed to which they are accustomed and may develop conditioned feed preferences or aversions [15, 16, 57]. The initial lack of preference for newly introduced feedstuff does not, therefore, necessarily indicate that it is unpalatable. On encountering a novel feed, horses will accept the novel food sources more readily if accompanied by a familiar odor [58]. For example, a novel food, bamboo, was consumed when accompanied by the familiar lucerne (alfalfa) odor located underneath the feed bucket. After five days, both the plain bamboo and odor-treated bamboo were consumed equally [59]. Similarly, horses can learn feed aversion when associated

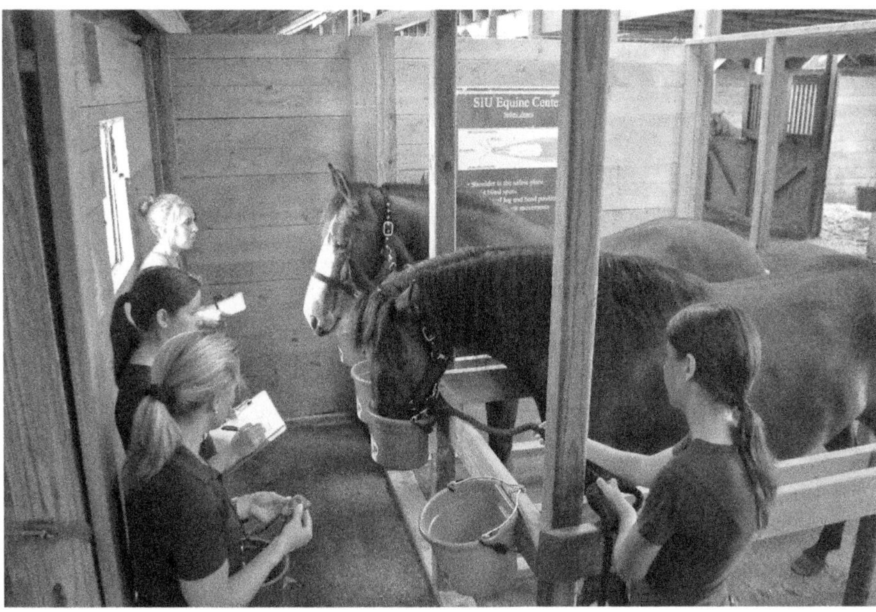

Figure 13.4 Palatability testing of equine feeds using side-by-side stocks using the two-bucket test in a standardized method. *Source:* Photo credit: Kelby Fenton.

with the onset of illness within 30 min of consumption, though the aversion behavior may be compromised if the feed is highly palatable [16].

Pellet size and density have also been investigated for their impact on horse intake. Pellet size (0.4–1.9 cm) did not impact consumption but less dense pellets were eaten faster [60]. Faster consumption of pelleted feed has been associated with esophageal obstruction (choke) in horses and is commonly mitigated by feeding smaller meals, adding water to the pellets, adding a softball or other round object in the feeding bucket to decrease bite-size, and by feeding with a grazing muzzle [61].

13.4 Quality Control Measures

Scientific validation of label claims through research and innovation is an expensive and time-consuming process. Many companies simply do not have the needed resources to complete this type of testing. As a result, vague language and puffy claims with no evidence are frequently used on feed packaging materials. To understand what has been scientifically validated through testing and research, it is important to understand the legal standards for the wording used.

13.4.1 Regulatory Compliance

Commercial horse feeds are regulated at two levels in the United States: at the federal level by the Food and Drug Administration (FDA) and then states exercise authority over horse feeds distributed within their respective borders. The Association of American Feed Control Officials was formed in 1909 to provide legal definitions for feeds, ingredients, label information, quality control procedures, and other manufacturing-related recommendations across the states. The organization comprises regulators from the state and federal levels and publishes guidelines annually outlining the regulations. AAFCO is responsible for maintaining the list of ingredients that are approved for use in animal feeds. AAFCO and FDA work jointly on the enforcement of the regulations. According to federal law, ingredients used in a feed must be approved by the FDA or listed as Generally Recognized As Safe (GRAS), and facilities manufacturing animal feed are required to be registered with the FDA. See Chapter 15 USA Feed Regulations and Safety.

13.4.2 Quality Assurance Programs

The National Grain and Feed Association recommends a model containing six areas of quality assurance as follows [62].

13.4.2.1 Purchasing and Receiving Ingredients

Many of the ingredients utilized in commercial equine feeds are by-products of other manufacturing processes. Variability in ingredients has been reported to contribute to as much as 40–70% of the nutrient variation in finished feeds [63]. Ingredient standards and expectations should be communicated to suppliers to maintain consistency within the supply. Deficiency claims should be filed if ingredient standards are not met.

13.4.2.2 Feed Manufacturing and Process Controls

These areas of quality assurance involve personnel, equipment, and procedures. Personnel must be properly trained with a commitment to quality as a priority. Equipment repair and maintenance must occur with regular inspections. Protocols for operating procedures are critical. Lack of process controls may result in unsuitable products and/or unsafe levels of specific ingredients, some of which have been attributed to the deaths of horses [64].

13.4.2.3 Finished Feed Sampling, Inspection, and Labeling

Industry officials recommend one to two feed samples per shift to monitor nutrient content. Most feed manufacturers maintain a sample of each batch run for analysis in case of customer complaints. Labeling requirements vary from state to state and thus each manufacturer should employ a quality assurance group that has responsibility for compliance with labeling guidelines.

13.4.2.4 Feed Shipment and Delivery

This area should contain procedures for sequencing and flushing feed at the farm or in the mill when one product is finished and another begins. This is especially critical for products designed for different species that may utilize medications or other ingredients that may be fatal for horses, e.g. ionophores used in cattle feed.

13.4.2.5 Sanitation and Pest/Rodent Control

Insects, birds, mice, rats, and other rodents may contribute to the contamination of ingredients. Proper steps must be taken to ensure that ingredients are protected from exposure to potential pathogens introduced by the presence of pests and rodents.

13.4.2.6 Feed Product Investigations and Recalls

In the event of a customer complaint, recall team members should be trained to handle all components of the claim.

13.4.3 Safety and Testing

Laboratory testing is a critical component of quality assurance for manufactured feeds. Tests may be chemical, physical, or electronic to obtain data on the ingredients received at the plant, which are then compared with an acceptable standard. Typical analyses include measurements of moisture, protein, fat, fiber, starch, mycotoxins, pathogens, and other factors that may impact product quality.

13.4.4 Contaminated Feed

13.4.4.1 Mycotoxins

Mycotoxins are secondary compounds commonly found in grains and forages. Feed spoilage can be a potentially fatal problem [65]. Horses are particularly susceptible to mycotoxicoses and may present with a variety of symptoms making proper diagnosis difficult. See Sidebar 13.4. Exposure may occur over time as evidenced by work done in Germany demonstrating low concentration commonly present in many cereal grains used for equine feed formulation [66]. Confirming a diagnosis of mycotoxin poisoning should include direct testing of suspect feedstuffs using an accredited laboratory, in addition to collating clinical signs, physical examination, animal laboratory data, and necropsy findings.

Sidebar 13.4: Commonly Occurring Mycotoxins and Associated Symptoms

Aflatoxins	Ataxia, tremors, fever, anorexia, inappetence, weight loss, icterus, hemorrhage, bloody feces, brown urine, death
Ochratoxins	Kidney damage
Deoxynivalenol	Inappetence, weight loss, liver damage, reduced immunity
Fumonisins	Depression, lethargy, head pressing, ataxia, staggers, stupor, seizure, lameness
Zearalenone	Vaginal prolapse, abortion, internal hemorrhage, flaccidity of male genitalia
Ergot alkaloids	Prolonged gestation, agalactia, red bag placentas, fetal loss

13.4.4.2 Blister Beetles

Blister beetles contain a toxin (cantharidin) that is very irritating to the digestive system and potentially fatal to horses [67]. Blister beetles are found in alfalfa fields and thus may be harvested with alfalfa. Dead beetles are still toxic when contained in feedstuff ingested by horses. Drought conditions cause the beetles to migrate and may result in greater concentrations for some areas given different agricultural conditions at harvest.

13.4.4.3 Animal Feces

Animal feces can carry organisms that may contaminate feed or hay if not properly stored [68]. Equine protozoal myelitis is a neurological disease transferred by wildlife droppings such as those of raccoons, rats, and opossum. Grain and hay should be protected from rodents during storage to prevent fecal contamination.

13.5 Package and Label

Packaging serves to protect feed products from environmental contamination, increase shelf life, facilitate handling and distribution, and convey product information. The packaging process is usually automated using equipment that handles various types and sizes. After drying and cooling, the finished feed product is weighed directly into a designated package to meet the guaranteed weight on the label.

The primary form of packaging for equine feed is the bag. Bags are typically constructed of paper, plastic (polyethylene commonly referred to as "poly"), or a combination of paper and plastic. Packaging material has a large impact on the shelf life of feed products. For example, baked horse treats stored in unlined paper packaging had a reduced shelf life and visible mold growth and subsequently reduced palatability, when stored for 12 m compared with treats stored in polyethylene packaging for the same duration [69]. The deciding factor about the type of bag material and construction that must be used would vary depending on the characteristics of the feed product, plant bagging equipment capabilities, economics, and marketing preferences and demands. For example, products containing a large amount of liquid such as molasses or oil require specialized plastic liners to minimize seepage. Other packaging forms include plastic buckets with resealable lids. These are often used for packaging small quantities of low-feeding rate products such as specialized equine supplements.

Manufactured feed products are labeled to convey the purpose of the feed, ingredients, and all necessary details for the safe and effective use of the feed [70]. Label information for horse feed is either incorporated into the package design or a feed tag is applied independently to the packaging at the point of closure. The process of applying labels or tags is usually automated. Date code information along with the associated production lot code, although not required, may also be automatically stamped on the package. This information is essential in the event of an adverse event and product recall.

Laws and regulations determine the specific information that is required to be on a feed label and will vary from around the world. In the United States, feed labels must meet federal labeling requirements set by the FDA as well as labeling requirements set by individual states. Most states (~two-thirds) have adopted the feed regulations outlined in the Association of American Feed Control Officials Model Bill [1]. AAFCO lists the recommended content on a feed label as product name, brand name (if applicable), a product purpose statement, levels of nutrients provided, the ingredients used to make the feed, feeding directions (adequate directions for use), cautions and/or warnings, manufacturer/distributor information (the person or firm responsible for the feed), and net weight of the package, or contents of the container, if applicable [1]. The regulations in states that have not adopted the AAFCO Models usually address similar aspects. Adopting AAFCO regulations provides uniformity in appearance and information on equine feed labels from state to state. This helps regulatory officials with uniform enforcement of regulations, and horse owners when attempting to compare different feed products. To provide proper feeding recommendations to equine clients, veterinarians should know how to read a feed label, understand the limitations, and be able to differentiate between objective information and romance copy. See Chapters 14 and 15.

13.6 Equine Marketing Concepts

Equine owners have been segmented into different groups (amateur, experienced, and expert) with different purchasing characteristics for each [71]. Purchasing characteristics change often and companies may employ multiple strategies to appeal to a wider target group. An understanding of equine feed marketing concepts helps veterinarians evaluate the advertised use of products to assist clients in making informed decisions. Veterinarians should bear in mind that horse owners frequently lack basic knowledge regarding equine nutrition and thus may require guidance so that product selection is based on content rather than product packaging [6].

Some common equine marketing concepts are stated here.

13.6.1 Specific Purpose

The "specific purpose" concept is based on a product being designed for a specific use. Feed products may be marketed to meet specialized nutritional requirements or they may contain special additives known or believed to be beneficial or serve a particular purpose. There may also be some other aspect of the product that is associated with a specific purpose. Products advertised for a specific purpose, however, may or may not be beneficial or necessary for that purpose. It is important to know and understand the actual nutritional needs of the horse and verify that a product will be suitable, regardless of the advertised purpose. Examples of "specific purpose" concepts are presented.

13.6.1.1 Horse Type

A package claim may suggest the product has been designed for specific breeds or types of horse, i.e. a miniature horse, pony, standard, or draft size horse. However, complete nutritional requirements have not been scientifically evaluated or defined for all horse types or breeds. Recommended nutrient intakes have been established by BWs (200, 400, 500, 600, 900 kg) [10] by the NRC [10].

13.6.1.2 Life Stage or Stage of Production

A package claim may suggest the product has been designed for a specific life stage, i.e. maintenance, growing, breeding, lactating, adult, or senior horse. As in other species, nutritional needs do vary based on life stage. NRC recommended nutrient intake has been established specifically for idle adults, working horses, stallions, pregnant and lactating mares, and for growing horses (4–24 m with exercise) [10]. No universal recommendations have been established for senior horses. More often the case, older horses have medical conditions for which a veterinarian is expected to make the dietary recommendations.

13.6.1.3 Activity or Performance Type

A package claim may suggest the product has been designed for a specific level of work activity or type of performance such as dressage, hunting, jumping, endurance, or racing. Nutritional requirements have been identified for increased levels of work but not different types of work.

13.6.1.4 Special Metabolic or Health Needs

A package claim may associate the product with a specific health condition, i.e. colic, rhabdomyolysis, laminitis, ulcers, or joint health. Claims that a product is intended for the diagnosis, cure, treatment, prevention, or mitigation of disease is a "drug" claim per the FDA. Such claims made on the label or other materials, websites, or advertisements risk enforcement action by the FDA. On the other hand, it is advantageous to have products with specific nutrient or ingredient profiles available in the market for veterinarians to recommend for specific patients.

It is important to note that products advertised with "specific purpose" strategies may be nutritionally adequate for more than one category or type of horse. For example, a geriatric horse feed designed to meet the forage requirements may be fed to several other types of horses as well, e.g. those with poor dental health, poor access to consistent quality forage, or those recovering from colic. Based on the nutrient profile or ingredient composition, a product may likely be fed to more than one equine type, class, or life stage. Conversely, an individual horse may properly fit into more than one type or have more than one medical condition, e.g. a geriatric, BCS 3/9 horse with laminitis, tooth loss, and oral pain. Manufactured feed products should be viewed as an array of dietary tools that can be utilized to design a ration explicit to a patient's needs.

13.6.2 Price and Ingredients

It is important to remember that commercial feeds are prepared from a wide array of ingredients designed to meet a targeted nutrient content. The concept of differentiating products based on price is associated with specific ingredients and the perceived value of those components. Specific ingredients, either included or excluded, are commonly targeted on higher-priced products, e.g. "no corn" or "with beet pulp." Ingredients associated with specific nutrients are also emphasized on higher-priced packages, e.g. "contains omega 3 fatty acids." Legally, the ingredient statement in the information panel must be accurate and the romance copy in the display panel cannot be false or misleading; however, it is difficult, to verify the inclusion or exclusion of specific ingredients at the advertised concentration. See Chapter 15 USA Feed Regulations and Safety.

13.6.3 Nutrients

Concentrations of specific nutrients are often stated on package claims. The use of this advertising strategy requires the addition of that nutrient to the guaranteed analysis on the package tag, in addition to the other required nutrients. Examples of products with claims regarding specific nutrients are "added biotin," "lower starch and sugar," or "added fat." Nutrients contained within most commercially manufactured feeds are designed to complement forage or hay and are not to be the sole source of nutrition. Products labeled as a "complete feed" are designed to be nutritionally adequate feed as the sole ration, except for water, capable of maintaining life.

13.6.4 Features and Benefits

Traditional marketing concepts focus on highlighting the functions of the product by calling attention to specific features and the perceived related benefits to the horse. This strategy is particularly effective; however, very little substantiation is required for such claims, and consumers may find themselves overwhelmed with perceived health benefits from bold packaging claims. For example, horses and humans do not necessarily share preferences for horse treats. In a study comparing horse and horse-owner preference for two different treat products, horses showed no preference for either product while humans showed a marked preference for one of the products based on appearance, texture, size, and purchase intent [52]. Features and benefits are subject to various laws and regulations governing animal feed and supplement claims. Horse feeds can only have claims on taste, aroma, or nutritive value. If claims express or imply the intended use is to "cure, treat or mitigate disease" then it would be considered an illegal drug. In certain circumstances, the use of the term "prevents" can be acceptable, but unfortunately sometimes illegal claims slip through regulatory scrutiny.

13.6.4.1 Complete and Balanced

This phrase is commonly used to refer to either the inclusion of all required fiber or the inclusion of all required energy, protein, vitamins and minerals to fulfill shortcomings of forage. Unfortunately, this term is not legally defined for horse food and so has an ambiguous interpretation.

13.6.4.2 Researched

Once again, this term is widely used with no standardized definition. It may refer to rigorous experimental examination with subsequent publication of results in peer-reviewed literature, or based on anecdotal evidence. See Figure 14.2.

13.6.4.3 Organic

AAFCO provides a legal definition for organic as "A formula feed or specific ingredient within a formula feed that has been produced and handled in compliance with the requirements of the USDA National Organic Program (7 CFR Part 205)" [1]. The USDA provides comprehensive guidance on the process for achieving organic status and the use of it as an advertising claim (https://www.usda.gov/topics/organic). Producers must follow guidelines for the management of land, soil, pest control, the origin of livestock, and animal healthcare. Prohibited substances are clearly defined, e.g. genetically modified organisms (GMO), some synthetic and non-synthetic ingredients.

13.6.4.4 All Natural and Holistic

Natural is defined as a feed or ingredient derived solely from plant, animal, or mined sources, either in its unprocessed state or having been subject to physical processing, heat processing, rendering, purification, extraction, hydrolysis, enzymolysis, or fermentation, but not having been produced by or subject to a chemically synthetic process and not containing any additives or processing aids that are chemically synthetic except in amounts as might occur unavoidably in good manufacturing practices. The European Union includes non-GMO in their definition of "natural." Holistic is another advertising claim that appeals to a consumer perception with no defining standards.

13.6.4.5 Low or Controlled Starch

Many products make claims of low or controlled starch. This claim must be weighed carefully. Analyses for starch and sugar content can include water-soluble carbohydrates (monosaccharides, disaccharides, and fructans), ethanol-soluble carbohydrates (monosaccharides and disaccharides), and non-fiber carbohydrates (starch, sugar, pectin, and fermentation acids). The claim of "lower" is a relative term that begs for a standard or value to which the comparison was made, but is often not stated. "Controlled" likewise is a vague term that does not define the concentration for the horse owner. However, products highlighting starch/sugar content, must state the starch or sugar concentration within the guaranteed analysis on the label. The horse owner must then decide if the concentration is appropriate for the horse.

13.7 Calculating Cost of Feeding

Simple calculation of the cost of feeding a horse takes into consideration only the forages, feeds and supplements. There are other elements that play into the actual cost of feeding a horse that are difficult to calculate but do factor into the true expenditure when they apply, such as: pasture maintenance, feeding equipment, delivery costs of the feed/forage, feed storage facilities, salaries for workers, hay harvesting equipment, etc. Maintaining a horse on pasture is normally more economical than having to purchase all the forage, however, it may be dependent on how much input goes into maintaining the pasture, the size of the field, productivity of the soil and the stocking rate (horses/ac).

If purchasing hay, the costs are not solely the price paid for the bale but also the weight/density of the bales and the suitability to the horse (palatability and amount of undesirable hay in the bale). These should be taken into consideration when selecting a forage. Paying a premium for good quality hay may end up being more economical in the end if the hay will be totally consumed with little waste and the horse maintains weight with less input from concentrate. A similar principle can be seen with concentrate feeds, buying a higher quality feed may end up being more economical if the horse can maintain weight/condition consuming less feed.

Calculating the cost of feeding involves knowing the price of the product and feeding rate. Rather than making a purchasing decision on the price of the product alone, calculating the price per dose or day will give the actual cost. For example, the cost of a bag of performance horse feed may be less than a bag of ration balancer, but since the daily recommended feeding rates are much lower for the ration balancer the cost/d will be less. Figuring out cost per dose is especially important when comparing supplements because that will give the true cost of using that product. There are no standards for recommended feeding rates or scoop size on any horse feed or supplement and the dosing recommendations are determined by the individual manufacturer. If trying to make a purchasing decision between manufacturers, figuring out the cost per dose or day may be enlightening. For example, joint supplement #1 is $150.00 for 1500 g with a recommended dose of 16 g/d will cost $1.60/d, while joint supplement #2 is the same price $150.00 but for 1200g but recommended at 4 g/d which will cost $0.50/d. Calculating cost/horse/d is helpful to determine the true cost of feeding and providing supplements. Calculations for cost/horse/d have been shown with product weight but can also be calculated using a density measurement, such as quarts or liters. For example, if a $15 bag contains 30 quarts of feed and the horse gets 2 quarts/d, then the cost would be $15/30 x 2 = $1.00/d to feed.

Case in Point

Given the following factors, calculate the cost per horse per day and per month:

Example #1

8-yr-old BW 450 kg BSC 5/9 average temperament Paint gelding used for team penning. Current feeding regimen is:

- Hay
  - Cost is $60 fescue hay/400 kg bale = $?/kg hay
  - Fed 8 kg/d = $?/d for fescue hay
- Ration balancer
  - Cost is $25/20 kg bag = $?/kg ration balancer
  - Fed 1 kg/d = $?/d for ration balancer
- Rice bran
  - Cost is $36/18 kg bag = $?/kg rice bran
  - Fed 0.25 kg/d = $?/d for rice bran
- Flax seed
  - Cost is $24/4 kg bag = $?/g flax seed
  - Fed 60 g/d = $?/d for flax seed

Total cost/d =

Total cost/30 d =

Example #2

3-yr-old BW 500 kg BCS 4/9 elevated temperament Thoroughbred stallion in race training. Current feeding regimen is:

- Hay
  - Cost is $15 timothy hay/25 kg bale = $?/kg hay
  - Fed 4 kg/d = $?/d for timothy hay
  - Cost is $540 alfalfa/metric ton (1000 kg) = $?/kg hay
  - Fed 2 kg/d = $?/d for alfalfa hay
- Sweet feed
  - Cost is $18/20 kg bag = $?/kg sweet feed
  - Fed 6 kg/d = $?/d for sweet feed
- Joint Supplement
  - Cost is $120/1.5 kg bucket = $?/g joint supplement
  - Fed 30 g/d = $?/d for joint supplement
- Electrolytes
  - Cost is $22/2 kg bucket = $?/g electrolytes
  - Fed 60 g/d = $?/d for electrolytes

Total cost/day =

Total cost/30 d =

See Appendix A Chapter 13.

References

1 Association of American Feed Control Officials (2021). *Official Publication AAFCO*. Champaign, IL: Association of American Feed Control Officials, Inc. www.aafco.org.

2 Hill, J. (2007). Impacts of nutritional technology on feeds offered to horses: a review of effects of processing on voluntary intake, digesta characteristics and feed utilisation. *Anim. Feed Sci. Technol.* 138 (2): 92–117.

3 Rich, G.A. and Breuer, L.H. (2002). Recent developments in equine nutrition with farm and clinic applications. In: *Proceedings of the 48th Annual Convention of the American Association of Equine Practitioners*, 24–40. Orlando, FL: American Association of Equine Practitioners (AAEP).

4 Harris, P.A. (1998). Developments in equine nutrition: comparing the beginning and end of this century. In: *Waltham International Symposium on Pet Nutrition and Health in the 21st Century*, 2698S–2703S. Orlando, FL: American Society for Nutritional Sciences.

5 Roberts, J.L. and Murray, J.-A. (2014). Equine nutrition in the United States: a review of perceptions and practices of horse owners and veterinarians. *J. Equine Vet. Sci.* 34 (7): 854–859.

6 Hoffman, C.J., Costa, L.R., and Freeman, L.M. (2009). Survey of feeding practices, supplement use, and knowledge of

equine nutrition among a subpopulation of horse owners in New England. *J. Equine Vet. Sci.* 29 (10): 719–726.

7 Julliand, V., De Fombelle, A., and Varloud, M. (2006). Starch digestion in horses: the impact of feed processing. *Livest. Sci.* 100 (1): 44–52.

8 Rosenfeld, I. and Austbø, D. (2009). Effect of type of grain and feed processing on gastrointestinal retention times in horses. *J. Anim. Sci.* 87 (12): 3991–3996.

9 Brøkner, C., Bach Knudsen, K.E., Karaman, I. et al. (2012). Chemical and physicochemical characterisation of various horse feed ingredients. *Anim. Feed Sci. Technol.* 177 (1): 86–97.

10 National Research Council (2007). National Research Council (2007). *Nutrient Requirements of Horses*. 6th Rev. Animal Nutrition Series, 1–341. Washington, DC: National Academies Press.

11 Equi-Analytical Laboratories Services (2020). Common Feed Profiles. www.equi-analytical.com/common-feed profiles (accessed 28 February 2019).

12 Feedipedia – Animal Feed Resources Information System. Feedipedia: an online encyclopedia of animal feeds. www.feedipedia.org (accessed 8 April 2021).

13 Kienzle, E., Radicke, S., and Wilke, S. (1992). Preileal starch digestion in relation to source and preparation of starch. In: *Proceedings of the European Conference on Nutrition for Horses*, 103–106.

14 Vervuert, I., Voigt, K., Hollands, T. et al. (2008). Effects of processing barley on its digestion by horses. *Vet. Rec.* 162 (21): 684–688.

15 Hintz, H.F. (1980). Feed preferences for horses. In: *Proceedings of the Cornell Nutrition Conference for Feed Manufacturers*, Ithaca, NY, 113–116.

16 Houpt, K.A. (1983). Taste preferences in horses. *Equine Pract.* 5 (4): 22–26.

17 Richardson, K. and Murray, J.-A.M.D. (2016). Fiber for performance horses: a review. *J. Equine Vet. Sci.* 46: 31–39.

18 Rodiek, A.V. and Stull, C.L. (2007). Glycemic index of ten common horse feeds. *J. Equine Vet. Sci.* 27 (5): 205–211.

19 Potter, G.D., Hughes, S., Julen, T., and Swinney, S. (1992). A review of research on digestion and utilization of fat by the equine. *Pferdeheilkunde Sonderh.* 1(September): 119–123.

20 Potter, G. (1999). Fat-supplemented diets for horses. *J. Equine Vet. Sci.* 19 (10): 616.

21 Markey, A.D. and Kline, K.H. (2006). Effects of dietary fat and yeast culture supplementation on total tract digestibility by horses. *Prof. Anim. Sci.* 22 (3): 261–266.

22 Sales, J. and Homolka, P. (2011). A meta-analysis of the effects of supplemental dietary fat on protein and fibre digestibility in the horse. *Livest. Sci.* 136 (2): 55–63.

23 den Hartog, L., Smits, C., and Hendriks, W. (2016). Feed additive strategies for replacement of antimicrobial growth promoters and a responsible use of antibiotics. *Feedipedia* 34: https://www.feedipedia.org/sites/default/files/public/BH_034_feed_additives_strat.pdf (accessed 7 April 2021).

24 Lopez, N.E., Baker, J.P., and Jackson, S.G. (1988). Effect of cutting and vacuum cleaning on the digestibility of oats by horses. *J. Equine Vet. Sci.* 8 (5): 375–378.

25 Arana, M., Rodiek, A., and Stull, C. (1989). Blood glucose and insulin responses to four different grains and four different forms of alfalfa hay fed to horses. In: *Proceedings of the 11th Equine Nutrition and Physiology Society Symposium*, 160–161. Stillwater, OK: Equine Nutrition and Physiology Society.

26 Radicke, S. and Meyer, H.K.E. (1994). Über den Einfluß von Futterart und Fütterungszeitpunkt auf den Blutglucosespiegel bei Pferden (Influence of feeding and time of feeding on blood values in horses). *Pferdeheilkunde* 10: 187–190.

27 Rosenfeld, I. and Austbø, D. (2009). Digestion of cereals in the equine gastrointestinal tract measured by the mobile bag technique on caecally cannulated horses. *Anim. Feed Sci. Technol.* 150 (3): 249–258.

28 Vervuert, I., Coenen, M., and Bothe, C. (2003). Effects of oat processing on the glycaemic and insulin responses in horses. *Anim. Physiol. Anim. Nutr. (Berl.)* 87 (3–4): 96–104.

29 Vervuert, I., Coenen, M., and Bothe, C. (2004). Effects of corn processing on the glycaemic and insulinaemic responses in horses. *J. Anim. Physiol. Anim. Nutr. (Berl.)* 88 (9–10): 348–355.

30 Hintz, H.F., Schryver, H.F., Mallette, J., and Houpt, K. (1989). Factors affecting rate of grain intake by horses. *Equine Pract.* 11 (4): 35–42.

31 Philippeau, C., Varloud, M., and Julliand, V. (2014). Mobile bag starch prececal disappearance and postprandial glycemic response of four forms of barley in horses. *J. Anim. Sci.* 92 (5): 2087–2093.

32 Hansen, T.L., Fowler, A.L., Strasinger, L.A. et al. (2016). Effect of soaking on nitrate concentrations in teff hay. *J. Equine Vet. Sci.* 45 (10): 53–57.

33 Hessel, E.F., Garlipp, F., and Van den Weghe, H.F.A. (2009). Generation of airborne particles from horse feeds depending on type and processing. *J. Equine Vet. Sci.* 29 (9): 665–674.

34 Hussein, H.S., Vogedes, L.A., Fernandez, G.C.J., and Frankeny, R.L. (2004). Effects of cereal grain supplementation on apparent digestibility of nutrients and concentrations of fermentation end-products in the feces and serum of horses consuming alfalfa cubes. *J. Anim. Sci.* 82 (7): 1986–1996.

35 Hedde, R.D., Lindsey, T.O., Parish, R.C. et al. (1985). Effect of diet particle size and feeding of H2-receptor antagonists on gastric ulcers in swine. *J. Anim. Sci.* 61 (1): 179–186.

36 Kienzle, E., Pohlenz, J., and Radicke, S. (1997). Morphology of starch digestion in the horse. *J. Vet. Med. Ser. A* 44 (February): 207–221.

37 de Fombelle, A., Varloud, M., Goachet, A.G. et al. (2003). Characterization of the microbial and biochemical profile of the different segments of the digestive tract in horses given two distinct diets. *Anim. Sci.* 77 (2): 293–304.

38 de Fombelle, A., Veiga, L., Drogoul, C., and Julliand, V. (2004). Effect of diet composition and feeding pattern on the prececal digestibility of starches from diverse botanical origins measured with the mobile nylon bag technique in horses1. *J. Anim. Sci.* 82 (12): 3625–3634.

39 Hoekstra, K.E., Newman, K., Kennedy, M.A.P., and Pagan, J.D. (2001). Effect of corn processing on glycemic response in horses. In: *Advances in Equine Nutrition II* (ed. J. Pagan and R. Geor), 105–110. Nottingham: Nottingham University Press.

40 Meyer, H. and Radicke, S.K.E. (1993). Investigations on preileal digestion of oats, corn and barley starch in relation to grain processing. In: *Proceedings of the 13th Equine Nutrition and Physiology Society Symposium*, 92–97. Gainesville, FL: Equine Nutrition and Physiology Society..

41 Jose-Cunilleras, E., Taylor, L.E., and Hinchcliff, K.W. (2004). Glycemic index of cracked corn, oat groats and rolled barley in horses. *J. Anim. Sci.* 82 (9): 2623–2629.

42 Schwandt, E.F., Hubbert, M.E., Thomson, D.U. et al. (2017). Flake density, roll diameter, and flake moisture all influence starch availability of steam-flaked corn. *Kansas Agric. Exp. Stn. Res. Reports* 3 (1): 1–5.

43 Vervuert, I. and Coenen, M. (2006). Factors affecting glycemic index of feeds for horses. In: *Proceedings of the 3rd European Equine Nutrition and Health Congress*, Merelbeke, Belgium, 17–18.

44 McLean, B.M.L., Hyslop, J.J., Longland, A.C. et al. (2000). Physical processing of barley and its effects on intra-caecal fermentation parameters in ponies. *Anim. Feed Sci. Technol.* 85 (1): 79–87.

45 Klendshof, C., Potter, G.D., and Lichtenwalner, R.E. (1979). Nitrogen digestion in the small intestine of horses fed crimped or micronized sorghum or oats. In: *Proceedings of the 6th Equine Nutrition and Physiology Society Symposium*, 91–94. College Station, TX: Equine Nutrition and Physiology Society.

46 Vervuert, I., Voigt, K., Hollands, T. et al. (2009). Effect of feeding increasing quantities of starch on glycaemic and insulinaemic responses in healthy horses. *Vet. J.* 182 (1): 67–72.

47 Nielsen, B.D., O'Connor-Robison, C.I., Spooner, H.S., and Shelton, J. (2010). Glycemic and insulinemic responses are affected by age of horse and method of feed processing. *J. Equine Vet. Sci.* 30 (5): 249–258.

48 Venable, E.B., Fenton, K.A., Braner, V.M. et al. (2017). Effects of feeding management on the equine cecal microbiota. *J. Equine Vet. Sci.* 49 (February): 113–121.

49 Flores, R.S., Byron, C.R., and Kline, K.H. (2011). Effect of feed processing method on average daily gain and gastric ulcer development in weanling horses. *J. Equine Vet. Sci.* 31 (3): 124–128.

50 Hintz, H., Scott, J., and Soderholm, L. (1985). Extruded feeds for horses. In: *Proceedings of the 9th Equine Nutrition and Physiology Society Symposium*, 174–176. East Lansing, MI: Equine Nutrition and Physiology Society.

51 Longhofer, S.L., Reinemeyer, C.R., and Radecki, S.V. (2008). Evaluation of the palatability of three nonsteroidal antiinflammatory top-dress formulations in horses. *Vet. Ther.* 9 (2): 122–127.

52 Francis, J.M., Thompson-Witrick, K.A., and Perry, E.B. (2021). Palatability of horse treats: comparing the preferences of horses and humans. *J. Equine Vet. Sci.* 99 (April): 103357.

53 Kennedy, M., Currier, T., Glowaky, J., and Pagan, J. (2001). The influence of fruit flavours in feed preference in thoroughbred horses. In: *Advances in Equine Nutrition II* (ed. J. Pagan and R. Geor), 145–146. Nottingham: Nottingham University Press.

54 Francis, J.M., Neander, C.R., Roeder, M.J., and Perry, E.B. (2020). The influence of topically applied oil-based palatants on eating behavior in horses. *J. Equine Vet. Sci.* 91: 102995.

55 Khelil-Arfa, H., Reigner, F., Blard, T. et al. (2021). Feed concentrate palatability in welsh ponies: acceptance and preference of flavors. *J. Equine Vet. Sci.* 102: 103619.

56 Goodwin, D., Davidson, H.P.B., and Harris, P. (2005). Selection and acceptance of flavours in concentrate diets for stabled horses. *Appl. Anim. Behav. Sci.* 95 (3–4): 223–232.

57 van den Berg, M., Giagos, V., Lee, C. et al. (2016). The influence of odour, taste and nutrients on feeding behaviour and food preferences in horses. *Appl. Anim. Behav. Sci.* 184 (November): 41–50.

58 Forbes, J.M. (1998). Dietary awareness. *Appl. Anim. Behav. Sci.* 57 (3): 287–297.

59 van den Berg, M., Giagos, V., Lee, C. et al. (2016). Acceptance of novel food by horses: the influence of food cues and nutrient composition. *Appl. Anim. Behav. Sci.* 183 (October): 59–67.

60 Freeman, D.W., Wall, D.L., Topliff, D.R. et al. (1990). Intake response of horses consuming a concentrate varying in pellet size. *Prof. Anim. Sci.* 6 (3): 10–12.

61 Venable, E.B., Bland, S., Braner, V. et al. (2016). Effect of grazing muzzles on the rate of pelleted feed intake in horses. *J. Vet. Behav.* 11 (January): 56–59.

62 Stark, C.R. and Jones, F.T. (2010). Quality assurance program in feed manufacturing. *Feedstuffs* 16: 62–67.

63 Jones, F. (1989). Feed quality control in poultry production. *Korean J. Anim. Nutr. FDST* 13 (1): 25–37.

64 Doonan, G.R., Brown, C.M., Mullaney, T.P. et al. (1989). Monensin poisoning in horses – an international incident. *Can. Vet. J. La Rev. Vet. Can.* 30 (2): 165–169.

65 Bryden, W.L. (2012). Mycotoxin contamination of the feed supply chain: implications for animal productivity and feed security. *Anim. Feed Sci. Technol.* 173 (1): 134–158.

66 Liesener, K., Curtui, V., Dietrich, R. et al. (2010). Mycotoxins in horse feed. *Mycotoxin Res.* 26 (1): 23–30.

67 Helman, R.G. and Edwards, W.C. (1997). Clinical features of blister beetle poisoning in equids: 70 cases (1983–1996). *J. Am. Vet. Med. Assoc.* 211 (8): 1018–1021.

68 Dubey, J.P., Lindsay, D.S., Saville, W.J.A. et al. (2001). A review of Sarcocystis neurona and equine protozoal myeloencephalitis (EPM). *Vet. Parasitol.* 95 (2): 89–131.

69 Francis, J.M. and Perry, E.B. (2021). The influence of packaging on palatability and shelf life stability of horse treats. *J. Equine Vet. Sci.* 98 (March): 103326.

70 Association of American Feed Control Officials (2020). Animal feed labeling guide. Champaign, IL: Association of American Feed Control Officials, Inc. https://www.aafco.org/Portals/0/SiteContent/Publications/Feed_Labeling_Guide_web_complete.pdf (accessed 2 April 2021).

71 Gille, C., Kayser, M., and Spiller, A. (2010). Target group segmentation in the horse buyers' market against the background of equestrian experience. *J. Equine Sci.* 21 (4): 67–71.

14

Dietary Supplements

Donna M. Raditic

KEY TERMS

- Feed supplements are used with other feeds to improve the nutritive balance or performance of the total feed. These may be offered free choice (salt block), fed diluted within a complete feed (chelated mineral ingredient), or fed undiluted in addition to other feeds (ration balancer).
- Animal food additives are substances not generally recognized as safe and must undergo premarket Food and Drug Administration (FDA) approval demonstrating safety and utility (selenium).
- Dosage Form Animal Health Products are, according to the National Animal Supplement Council (NASC), supplements for animals, not intended for human consumption, and recognized to mean any product intended to affect the structure or function of the animal's body other than by providing nutrition to the animal. These products include oils, tinctures, capsules, tables, liquids, soft chews and chewable limited dose products.

KEY POINTS

- The use of herbs and dietary supplements (HDS) is common and growing as owners look for inexpensive, more natural options to prevent and treat various disease states in the horse.
- Despite the low level of evidence for the use of most supplements, there is a wide range of HDS available on the market and owners believe that these were important to their horse's health and performance.
- Veterinarians must educate owners that currently there are variable degrees of regulatory scrutiny and oversight of the HDS marketed for the horse.
- Utilizing evidence-based medicine (EBM) concepts, although rigorous evidence is scarce and often inconclusive, will enable equine practitioners to answer the challenging questions from owners and give the best recommendations about the use of HDS in equine patients.

14.1 Introduction

A 2015 survey reflects the complex relationship between humans and horses. The majority of respondents were most likely to view their horses as family members (68%), companion animals (63%), performance partners (58%), and/or best friends (56%). A smaller percentage of respondents viewed their horses as an investment (22%), livestock animal (21%), or employee (8%) [1]. The use of HDS has increased dramatically with not less than 80% of people worldwide using them as part of their healthcare [2]. Therefore, it is not unexpected that in the United States about 70% of owners in 2008 were feeding one type of herb or dietary supplement to their horses [3]. Based on these statistics, equine practitioners should be prepared to address owner inquiries concerning the selection and feeding of dietary supplements.

14.2 Regulation of Supplements

The United States Congress in the Federal Food, Drug and Cosmetic Act (FFDCA) gave the FDA authority to oversee the quality of substances sold as a drug or a "food." This authority includes feed for animals because FFDCA defined food as "articles used for food or drink for man or other animals including components of such articles." Additives are "components" of food or feed (Figure 14.1).

Equine Clinical Nutrition, Second Edition. Edited by Rebecca L. Remillard.

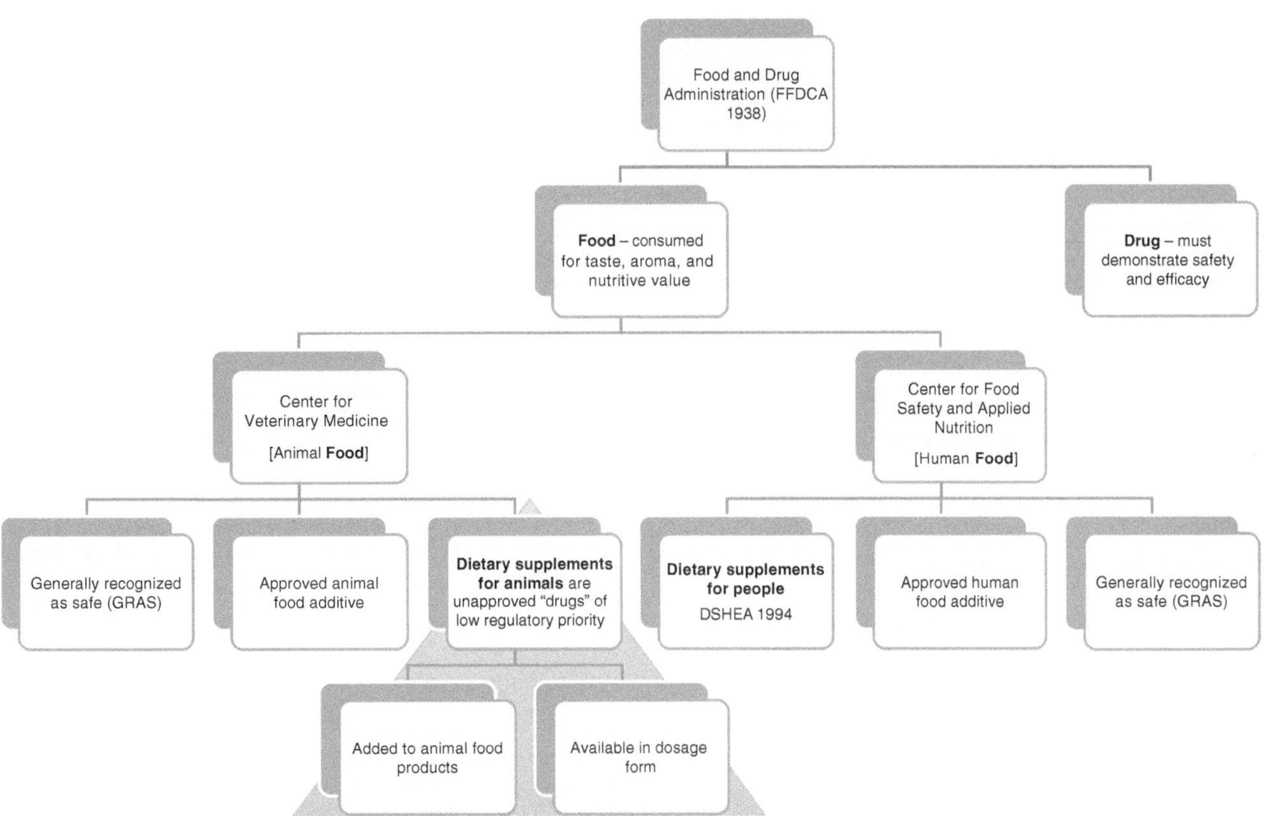

Figure 14.1 Regulation of dietary supplements: dietary supplements for animals have to meet the same regulatory requirements as those of food or food additives, and if not, then they are likely considered unapproved drugs of low regulatory priority. 'Feed additive' is not a regulatory term in the USA. 'Food' is the regulatory term for both humans and animals.

Animal food and additive regulations are the same for all animals in that there is no distinction between those producing food for humans, e.g. cattle, sheep, and poultry, and nonfood animals, e.g. companion and exotics [4]. See USA Regulatory Oversight in Chapter 15.

Dietary supplements are considered "food" under FFDCA because the 1994 Dietary Supplement and Education Health Act (DSHEA) placed dietary supplements in a distinct subcategory of human foods [5]. This subcategory allows the inclusion of substances without prior documentation of safety or utility. The DSHEA defined "dietary supplement" as a substance taken orally that contains at least one of the following: vitamins, minerals, amino acids, herbs or other plant-based compounds (botanicals), and substances, such as enzymes, organ tissues, glandular tissues and metabolites, including extracts and concentrates thereof. However, in 1996, the FDA announced that DSHEA did not apply to animals thereby leaving only two legal options for these substances: animal food additive or drug. Whether a substance is considered a food or drug depends on the intended use of the substance; therefore, labels on animal supplements are scrutinized.

Animal dietary supplements that are not on the "generally recognized as safe" (GRAS) list or FDA approved as a animal food additive are in a regulatory gray zone because these do not qualify as a food and yet have not undergone a drug approval process (Figure 14.1). At this time, for practical reasons based on the number of products and the relatively low risk of harm, dietary supplements to animals are considered "unapproved drugs" in the market. Center for Veterinary Medicine (CVM) considers dietary supplements to animals a low regulatory priority and exercises regulatory discretion when: (i) there are reasonable assurances that feeds containing these "unapproved drug" additives are safe and efficacious, and (ii) the OTC forms (tablets, powders, etc.) of these substances are not marketed as a food or a drug to animals. However, CVM does reserve the right to take action against a dietary supplement as an unapproved (adulterated) drug at any time [6].

14.3 Marketing of Supplements

14.3.1 Animal Food Additive

Typical animal food ingredients such as forages, grains, and most minerals and vitamins are GRAS sources of nutrients. Non-essential dietary substances may also be vitamins, minerals, proteins, or fatty acid feed additives intended to augment the nutritive value of the total ration and always have been regulated as a animal food additive. Commercial feeds for horses are usually formulated by nutritionists and these additives are sold through industrial channels. A feed product containing an unapproved additive is considered unsafe if the added substance is not considered GRAS and does not conform to the animal food additive regulations. For example, glucosamine, chondroitin sulfate, or a combination are found in horse feeds but neither is defined by the Association of American Feed Officials (AAFCO) nor an approved animal food additive. Glucosamine and chondroitin sulfate are perceived to be chondroprotective, yet no horse feed containing either substance has received FDA approval for such a claim. Although the feed product label may declare such substances in the product, no claim improving joint health should be found on the label [4]. This is a animal food additive violation of low regulatory priority for the CVM. Veterinarians must be able to distinguish between equine feeds that comply with the pertinent animal food regulations and those that do not. See Chapter 15 USA Feed Regulations and Safety.

14.3.2 Dosage Forms

Those substances that meet the DSHEA definition of "dietary supplements" are not added to feed products but sold in dosage forms as tablets, capsules, liquids, or powders. Such oral supplements for companion animals are mostly sold OTC direct to lay customers. In the USA, horses are not in the human food chain so considered companion animals in the context of these supplements. The labeling of OTC dietary supplements, also called animal health products, may contain claims to affect normal health, function, and structure of the body but may not claim to diagnose, cure, mitigate, treat or prevent disease. The CVM does not generally object to the marketing of oral supplements to horses provided the product conforms to the following restrictions [7]:[1]

1) There is a known need for each nutrient ingredient represented to be in the product for each animal for which the product is intended.
2) The label represents the product for use only in supplementation and not as a substitute for good daily rations.
3) The product provides a meaningful but not excessive concentration of each ingredient stated on the label.
4) The labeling should bear no disease prevention or therapeutic, including growth promotion, representations.
5) The labeling should not be otherwise false or misleading in any particular.
6) The product is neither over-potent nor under-potent nor otherwise formulated to pose a hazard to the health of the target animal.

But again, the FDA-CVM considers dietary supplements to be unapproved drugs and reserves the right to take action at any time.

Dietary supplements containing non-nutrient substances such as herbs, botanicals, and metabolites are more likely marketed as a stand-alone product sold over the counter. Such dietary supplements contain active compounds not directly related to a nutrient [5]. For example, the action of an herb supporting a body system may be based on a unique chemical compound in that herb unrelated to any nutrient or nutritional benefit. A dietary supplement is, therefore, a broad category in which some products may contain classically known nutrients (vitamins, minerals) while others may contain complex non-nutritional substances, and other products may contain both. The National Center of Complementary and Integrative Health (NCCIH) is the agency evaluating scientific research on supplements [8]. The NCCIH has adopted the DSHEA supplement definition and refers to this diverse group of products as "herbs and dietary supplements" (HDS). The NCCIH and DSHEA definitions and terms should be used in veterinary medicine; therefore, for purposes of discussion herein, these products will be called HDS or veterinary HDS. Equine practitioners must understand that HDS products for horses are being marketed without proof of effectiveness or safety as one would expect with an approved veterinary drug (Figure 14.1). As explained, the FDA considers many veterinary HDS to be unapproved drugs and in some cases, the agency may not initiate action against them unless determined to be unsafe or make drug claims.

As many veterinary HDS are not GRAS and do not undergo any FDA premarketing approval as a animal food additive or drug, veterinarians must then take on the responsibility of investigating the safety, efficacy, and manufacturing practices for products they recommend [6]. Manufacturers of veterinary HDS should be held to the same standards as drug manufacturers with FDA approved sources of raw ingredients, no contamination, proof of potency, and quality control programs that ensure accuracy in label content. Veterinarians should inquire if manufacturers participate in some oversight programs and analysis that can independently assure product quality and proper labeling such as the NASC or Consumer Testing Laboratories [9–11]. Independent oversight is warranted as analysis of equine joint health supplements reported that nine out of 23 glucosamine products failed to meet label claims and four products contained less than 30% of the amount stated on the label [12].

Companies marketing veterinary HDS should be willing to provide answers to questions regarding specific

1 FDA-CVM Compliance Policy Guide Sec. 690.100 Nutritional Supplements for Companion Animals was withdrawn 2/20/2020.

Sidebar 14.1: Questions to Ask a Company Marketing Veterinary Herbal and Dietary Supplements

Product information:

What is the evidence for the product's formulation?

What is the evidence for the clinically effective dose?

What scientific clinical studies of the product and/or the ingredients have been performed and published? Please provide citations.

Is information known, published, and available regarding any toxicities or adverse events with the product or any of its ingredients?

What is your system for receiving, investigating, and reporting any adverse events?

Are adverse events reported to a national compiling/reporting group?

Labeling:

Do labels contain the exact weight of dose/tablet/chew of all active and inactive ingredients?

Do labels have lot numbers, expiration dates, adequate directions, and appropriate warnings?

How are expiration dates determined?

Do labels state applicable warnings?

Do labels have contact information to report adverse events?

Do labels contain the name and address of the manufacturer or distributor?

Manufacturing:

Who and where is the manufacturer located?

Is it possible to visit the manufacturer?

Does the manufacturer comply with current good manufacturing practices [13]?

How do you assure the quality and handling of raw ingredients?

What quality control testing programs do you have to assure raw ingredients and final products do not contain contaminants including but not limited to heavy metals, herbicides, pesticides, microbes, foreign material, or drugs?

Is documentation of your quality control programs available to the public?

How is the consistency of ingredient content in your product assured?

Is documentation available substantiating the consistency of your product?

information on dosing and safety of their product and ingredients, labeling, and manufacturing procedures [13]. See Sidebar 14.1. The NASC, a trade organization representing many veterinary HDS manufacturers, has developed a labeling format that is decidedly different from that required by AAFCO for feed and supplements. Products labeled as per NASC guidance follow a "DSHEA-like" format, but with important differences. Examples of AAFCO feed and supplement labels vs. NASC dosage-form animal health product labels are shown in Figures 15.1–15.3, respectively. Investigating a manufacturer's product details, production and marketing is necessary to identify safe and effective equine HDS products. Using this information and sound concepts of evidence-based medicine (EBM) will enable practitioners to answer the challenging questions from owners and give the best recommendations about the use of HDS in equine patients.

14.4 Evidence-Based Medicine

The animal dietary supplement market appears to be thriving on a lack of understanding, a paucity of data, clinical trials, and efficacy, and depends on owners diagnosing their horse's medical condition and needs. Evidence-based medicine is defined as the integration of the best research, clinical expertise, and patient (client) values to make medical decisions to improve outcomes. Best research evidence is usually considered randomized controlled clinical trials (RCCT) or systematic reviews of several trials (meta-analyses). Classification systems to evaluate the quality of research evidence include published hierarchical schemes, evidence pyramids (Figure 14.2), and grading systems [14]. More often the rationale for use of a drug, therapy, or

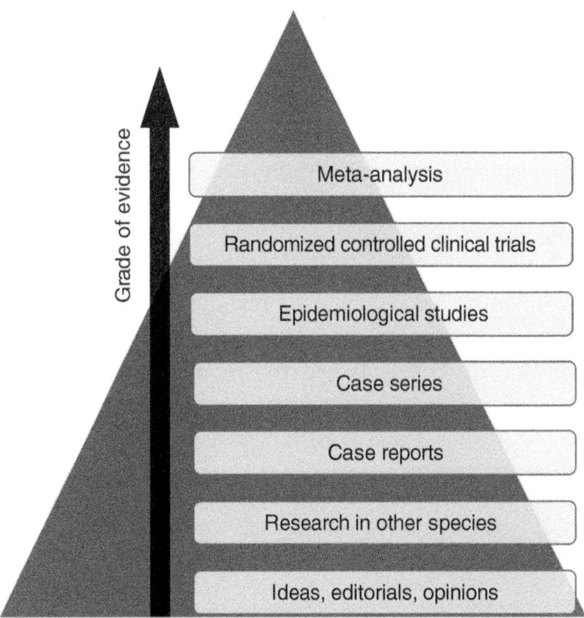

Figure 14.2 Grade of evidence: the level of evidence for the use of a supplement should be based on the number and strength of published reports. Randomized controlled clinical trials and meta-analyses provide the strongest evidence.

supplement in veterinary medicine stems from the lower grades of evidence such as extrapolations from pathophysiological principles, *in vivo* or *in vitro* studies in the same or different species rather than the higher grades of evidence-based, such as RCCTs or meta-analyses [15, 16]. Supplements used in clinical equine nutrition should be based on EBM utilizing higher grades of evidence than is presently practiced.

Utilizing EBM to make decisions about HDS requires understanding and integrating client values to include unique preferences, concerns, and expectations. The demand for HDS among horse owners, breeders, and trainers can be due to a preference for natural products over conventional pharmaceuticals. Another survey of feeding practices of horse owners in northeastern United States reported 84% feeding at least one dietary supplement. The more common supplements were chondro-protectives, electrolytes, and multivitamins. The survey noted that owners consulted multiple sources about equine nutrition, but the major source of information was reported to be the veterinarian [17]. Another descriptive study focused on owners of dressage and eventing horses in the United Kingdom reported that nearly all used supplements with only 5% of nearly 600 respondents stating they did not use supplements. The most often cited reasons for using HDS in dressage horses were "joints and mobility" and "behavior" modification, whereas "electrolytes" and "joints and mobility" were the most common reasons in eventing horses [18].

These studies and surveys highlight the importance of the human–horse bond and the increasing demand for the use of HDS in equine healthcare and treatments. Equine veterinarians are faced with multiple questions and challenges regarding the use, efficacy, and safety of HDS. Veterinarians should use EBM to answer questions and make decisions when recommending HDS, but unfortunately, there is a paucity of the higher grades of evidence regarding the use of HDS in equine healthcare. Despite the low level of evidence for most supplements, there was a wide range of HDS used, and owners perceived that these were important to their horse's health and performance. Clinically relevant research in the use of HDS in equine diseases is scarce. However, there are some relevant studies and reviews using higher grades of EBM for the use of HDS in equine musculoskeletal, gastrointestinal (GI), behavioral, respiratory, and metabolic diseases.

14.5 Musculoskeletal Diseases

Oral administration of HDS to the horse is common and perceived to be a benign treatment or prevention of osteoarthritis. A survey study noted supplements were the dietary element more commonly changed as the horse became older. Owners reported using HDS to decrease the use of drugs with adverse side effects and prevent further degradation of affected joints while expecting to restore function [19]. Supplements that have been evaluated in equine musculoskeletal diseases include chondroprotectants, omega 3 fatty acids, carnitine, creatine, antioxidants, and herbs or herbal preparations.

14.5.1 Chondro-Protectants

Chondromodulating compounds are purported to alter or slow the progression of osteoarthritis. Beneficial effects may include a positive effect on cartilage matrix synthesis and hyaluronic acid synthesis by the synovial membrane, as well as an inhibitory effect on catabolic enzymes in osteoarthritic joints. These compounds fall under two different categories. One group includes parenteral agents that are approved by the FDA, such as polysulfated glycosaminoglycan (GAG), which will have label claims of clinical effects and are considered drugs. The other group includes products that are oral supplements, such as glucosamine and chondroitin sulfate, which are not approved as drugs or acceptable for use in animal food products, and legally cannot claim any medical benefits [20].

D-Glucosamine, an amino sugar, is endogenously synthesized and is the biochemical precursor of nitrogen-containing sugars called GAG and proteoglycans. Glycosaminoglycans are major components of normal joint cartilage. Chondroitin sulfate is a form of GAG and a component of joint cartilage. The water-retaining properties enhance cartilage's function as a shock absorber and supplementation can stimulate GAG and collagen synthesis. *in vitro* studies in other species do support the concept that supplemental glucosamine-chondroitin may help rebuild cartilage, but these studies often use glucosamine-chondroitin concentrations not achieved in serum or plasma after oral administration [20].

Extensive reviews and evaluations of *in vivo/in vitro* equine cell studies of glucosamine-chondroitin in equine osteoarthritis have been published [21–23]. The evidence is conflicting on whether these oral supplements have beneficial clinical effects in equine osteoarthritis. Some of the controversy has related to study design and quality with studies criticized for being statistically underpowered, lack of blinding, inappropriate placebo control, and poorly defined inclusion and exclusion criteria. More recent studies have attempted to overcome these issues using a synovitis model and equine kinematics, but the results have been variable [24–29]. In summary, there is weak clinical evidence of the benefit of glucosamine-chondroitin in horses with osteoarthritis, but owner use is common. Rigorous randomized, controlled clinical studies to determine the role of oral glucosamine-chondroitin supplements in the management of equine osteoarthritis are needed.

14.5.2 Omega 3 Polyunsaturated Fatty Acids (n-3 PUFA)

Supplementation of omega 3 polyunsaturated fatty acids (n-3 PUFA) has been shown to have beneficial effects in many species. Studies have demonstrated beneficial effects on inflammatory status in cardiovascular, musculoskeletal, dermatological, renal, and other disease states [30]. Equine studies of omega 3 PUFA supplementation have shown similar effects on inflammation. Dietary PUFA supplementation can alter equine plasma, red blood cells, and muscle fatty acid concentrations. However, to elevate tissue concentrations of eicosapentaenoic acid (EPA) and docosapentaenoic acid (DHA), specific PUFAs, fish oil is required in the diet because there is the limited conversion of alpha-linolenic acid as from flaxseed oil to EPA and DHA in the horse [31, 32]. Direct supplementation of EPA and DHA sources has been shown to alter the inflammatory response by reducing basal tumor necrosis factor alpha (TNFα) production and increasing DHA concentration in synovial fluid [33, 34]. Studies in horses with osteoarthritis supplemented with marine sources of omega n-3 PUFAs had a decrease in inflammatory markers and an increase in stride length [35, 36]. Exercising horses supplemented with fish oil as compared with corn oil demonstrated lower heart rates and packed cell volume [37]. Feeding fish oil (11 mL/100 kg body weight (BW)) for 127 days to Thoroughbreds increased serum and red blood cell EPA and DHA concentrations, which may decrease RBC fragility in racehorses but there were no published follow-up performance studies [38]. Although the evidence for supplementing n-3 PUFA in the diet of horses is limited, consideration of studies in other species suggests n-3 PUFA supplementation may decrease the equine inflammatory state.

14.5.3 L-Carnitine

L-Carnitine plays an important role in fatty acid metabolism as a cofactor for long-chain fatty acid transport across the inner mitochondrial membrane. Carnitine availability in the exercising horse is unknown, but studies have considered supplementation to potentially increase oxidative fatty acid metabolism sparing glycogen stores. Early studies of oral carnitine supplementation demonstrated increased equine muscle carnitine concentrations, but beneficial effects on performance were not documented [37, 39]. Recent studies investigating L-carnitine supplementation on insulin sensitivity, glucose tolerance, and other metabolic parameters were unable to demonstrate benefits [40–42].

14.5.4 Creatine

Creatine or methylguanidine-acetic acid is synthesized by the horse from arginine, L-methionine, and glycine. During intense exercise, phosphocreatine is a phosphate source for the re-synthesis of ATP and supports high-energy phosphate transfers. Frequently found in human, canine, and equine supplements, creatine is marketed as an ergogenic aid for athletic performance. Early studies of creatine supplementation suggest poor oral absorption in the horse [39]. A 45-d study of creatinine supplementation at the comparatively high dose of 28 g/100 kg BW/d reported no change in athletic performance [43].

14.5.5 Antioxidants

Exercise intensity and duration, diet, age, and disease states can affect oxidative status in the horse. Herbs and dietary supplements are marketed with claims to improve oxidative status in the horse and potentially improve performance. These equine antioxidant supplements may include vitamins, minerals, enzymes, herbs, and herbal preparations. Studies using exogenous supplementation of vitamin E, vitamin C, and α-lipoic acid have shown some positive results in decreasing the effects of exercise-induced oxidative stress, but more studies are needed to determine optimal dosing [39, 44].

14.5.6 Herbal Preparations

Plant or herb extracts, preparations, or other "natural compounds" are common in equine supplements marketed to enhance performance. The primary effects of these plant or herb extracts may be due to the flavonoid content. Flavonoids are major constituents of fruits, vegetables, wine, and tea. These compounds are ketone-containing compounds that have a similar structure and may have beneficial anti-inflammatory and/or antioxidant properties [45, 46]. Some of these herbs and herbal preparations have been evaluated for their potential application in studies *in vivo* or *in vitro* in other species, but very few of these have been evaluated in a controlled manner in the horse. Randomized crossover studies have evaluated the oxidative status and inflammatory state in exercising horses fed various extracts of cranberry, orange peel, ginger, and tart cherry juice. Although some positive effects on oxidative and/or anti-inflammatory status were reported, long-term and dose–response studies using greater numbers of horses are needed [47–49].

14.6 Gastrointestinal Diseases

Horses suffer from a myriad of GI diseases that can affect their quality of life and longevity. An array of HDS to prevent and treat equine GI diseases are marketed, but again few studies support their efficacy and clinical use. Most prominent are HDS for gastric ulcer syndrome and probiotics for an array of GI diseases. Currently, probiotics are being evaluated for their effectiveness in managing GI disease states in many species. Some studies of probiotics use in the horse are presented, but the efficacy may be limited by our incomplete knowledge of the equine microbiota. See Chapter 4 The Horse: Microbiome.

14.6.1 Ulcers

The prevalence of equine gastric ulcer syndrome (EGUS) varies with breed, use, level of training, and includes equine glandular gastric disease and equine squamous gastric disease, which more specifically describe the affected portion anatomically [50]. Lesser understood and diagnosed are colonic ulcers. The GI tract of 365 horses from a variety of sources was examined in a Texas abattoir where 55% were found to have gastric ulcers and 44% had colonic ulcers. In the second group of 180 performance horses at the abattoir, 87% were shown to have gastric ulcers, while 63% exhibited colonic ulcers [51].

Treatment with pharmacological agents for ulcers is expensive and may require chronic administration; therefore, there has been increased interest in the use of HDS to treat and prevent gastric ulcers in horses. Many commercial products are available but there is little scientific data available on the efficacy of most HDS, and of those that have been studied in horses, most were tested for less than 30 days. However, in one study of 42 Thoroughbred horses in training with squamous ulceration were randomly assigned either treatment of omeprazole or a dietary supplement containing oat oil and bran, yeast, and a select few amino acids. The dietary supplement containing soluble fiber (β-glucan) was found to be equally effective to omeprazole in the treatment of squamous gastric ulcers after 3 m [52].

An intermittent feed-deprivation study evaluated a commercial sea buckthorn (*Hippophae rhamnoides*) supplement (SBT) compared with no treatment. The high flavonoid content of SBT was proposed to be a potent antioxidant that may act as a gastro-protectant. Horses were treated for four wks followed by a one wk alternating feed-deprivation period to induce or worsen existing ulcers. Gastroscopic examinations were performed, gastric juice pH was measured and gastric ulcer number and severity scores were assigned. The SBT supplement did not show efficacy in treatment or prevention of naturally occurring non-glandular ulcers in horses; however, glandular ulcer scores were significantly lower in SBT-treated horses after food deprivation [53].

Equine studies using the intermittent feed-deprivation model and crossover design have evaluated other supplements with anti-ulcer genic compounds, such as lecithin, pectins, L-glutamine, and salts of carbonic acids (SOC): sodium bicarbonate and calcium carbonates. Lecithin, a natural phospholipid, and pectins may support the hydrophobic barrier on the gastric mucosal membranes. Pectin may also protect gastric mucosal by binding bile acids while the non-essential amino acid L-glutamine is a primary fuel for rapidly dividing enterocytes [54–57].

In other species and *in vitro* studies, SOC has an antacid effect. Sodium bicarbonate-containing supplements could be a concern as there are known effects on blood pH and speculated to improve racing performance by buffering lactic acid and delaying the onset of fatigue. Total blood CO_2 concentrations are monitored in Thoroughbred racing in the United States and if the concentration exceeds 37 mmol/L, then doping is considered [56]. More research is needed to evaluate HDS in EGUS as current studies do not support their use and gastric ulcer supplements that contain sodium bicarbonate, and calcium carbonate could be problematic in performance horses.

14.6.2 Probiotics

Supplements containing probiotics are available for improving GI function, feed efficiency, and/or treatment of GI diseases in the horse.

The Food and Agriculture Organization (FAO) and the World Health Organization (WHO) define probiotics as "live microorganisms that, when administered in adequate amounts, confer a health benefit on the host" [58]. The mode of action of probiotics may include modulation of host innate and acquired immune systems, antimicrobial production, competitive inhibition of pathogens, and their bacterial toxins [59].

A limited number of research studies using probiotics in horses to improve hindgut fermentation and diet digestibility have been published. The majority of these studies used *Saccharomyces cerevisiae* (SC) with a variety of diets and demonstrated that the addition of SC improved fiber digestibility in horses offered high-starch and high-fiber diets. With high-concentrate diets, SC supplementation helped maintain cecal pH and decreased lactic acid concentration [60]. One study using lower dosing of the SC probiotic reported no differences in fiber digestibility, volatile fatty acids (VFA) concentrations, and fecal SC population [61]. Similar results were seen when horses fed low- and high-starch diets were fed a probiotic containing *Lactobacillus acidophilus* and then a mixture of *L. acidophilus, Lactobacillus casei, Bifidobacterium bifidum*, and *Enterococcus faecium*. No effect of either probiotic was noted with diet digestibility, fecal pH, and VFA concentrations [62]. Conclusions were difficult to draw from these studies as basal diets varied and the source, dosage, and strain(s) of probiotics differed.

14.6.2.1 Enterocolitis

Probiotic preparations have been evaluated in the clinical treatment of GI diseases in the horse. *Saccharomyces boulardii* was assessed in a RCCT in 14 horses with acute enterocolitis. The severity and duration of GI tract disease during hospitalization were significantly less in horses receiving *S. boulardii* as compared with horses receiving the placebo, yet no differences were seen in outcomes, duration of hospitalization, and reoccurrence of diarrhea [63]. A second RCCT, using *S. boulardii* as adjunctive treatment in 12 horses with antibiotic-induced enterocolitis reported no difference between groups for occurrence of normal feces or cessation of watery diarrhea. Again, there were no differences reported for outcomes, days to improvement, and duration of hospitalization. The investigators postulated lack of efficacy could be due to a lack of colonization by *S. boulardii* because fecal samples in some horses were negative for *S. boulardii* [64].

14.6.2.2 Neonatal Diarrhea

Neonatal diarrhea occurs in up to 60% of foals within 6 m of birth, hence studies evaluating probiotics in this group have been conducted but with variable results. A RCCT using *Lactobacillus pentosus* WE7 in neonatal foal diarrhea reported a significantly higher incidence of diarrhea and the need for further veterinary treatment in the probiotic-treated group [65]. A multi-strain probiotic was used in another RCCT in foals with the treatment group showing a statistically significant lower incidence of diarrhea and larger weight gains at one single time point. These positive effects are questionable as the diarrhea was unlikely clinically significant in this population of foals because there was little difference in the need for medical intervention between the two groups [66].

A RCCT of 72 foals using a multi-strain probiotic with four *Lactobacillus* spp. and *Bifidobacterium animalis* spp. *lactis* has been published [67]. The multi-strain probiotic had previously inhibited the growth of *Clostridium difficile* and *perfringens in vitro* [68]. The overall incidence of diarrhea, duration of diarrhea, and soft feces were not statistically significant between the treatment groups. Foals treated with the probiotic were more likely to develop diarrhea requiring veterinary interventions. The prevalence of *Clostridium perfringens* and *difficile* shedding was 55% and 11%, respectively, with no difference between treatment groups. There was no significant difference in clinical signs or *C. perfringens* and *C. difficile*-positive fecal cultures [67]. Following this study, the same probiotic was fed once a day to 38 foals and fecal samples were collected at two-wk intervals and assessed via metagenomics sequencing. There were no changes in the phylum, order, or class of fecal microbes between the probiotic-treated vs. placebo group at any age, but some significant changes in the relative abundance of families were noted. The authors concluded the four *Lactobacillus* spp. and *Bifidobacterium animalis* spp. *lactis* probiotic treatment had limited effects on the bacterial microbiota of foals and would seem to have limited potential as a therapeutic intervention [69]. Another study compared a high dose and a low dose of a probiotic containing *Bacillus cereus* var. *toyoi* to a placebo. Diarrhea occurred in 88% of the foals during the first 58 days and the probiotic at either dose did not affect the occurrence of diarrhea in foals [70].

14.6.2.3 Salmonellosis

The use of probiotics to control *Salmonella* spp. in production animals has been successful. A few studies in horses have looked at the use of probiotics on Salmonella shedding in horses. A total of 186 post colic surgery horses were enrolled in a RCCT to look at the effects of two multi-strain probiotic formulations compared with placebo for 10 days. The overall shedding rate was 21% and there were no statistical differences in postoperative diarrhea, duration of hospitalization, and medical management between the three groups [71]. A second RCCT looked at Salmonella shedding, diarrhea, and outcomes in colic cases with variable underlying diseases. No clinical differences were noted in Salmonella shedding and other clinical parameters between the probiotic and placebo treated groups [72]. Another study looked at the preventative effect of a multi-strain probiotic on Salmonella shedding in a RCCT of 130 hospitalized horses admitted without GI disease. Horses were given a probiotic or placebo upon admission and although the probiotic decreased the incidence of Salmonella shedding the results were not significantly different [73].

Although probiotics have shown promise in human and canine GI diseases, the evidence for their use to prevent and/or treat GI disease in the horse is weak and limited. In neonatal diarrhea, the use of probiotics may have some negative effects. The incomplete knowledge of the equine hindgut microbiota limits development of appropriate strains and concentrations of probiotics for improved diet utilization, treatment, and prevention of GI disease. As we gain more knowledge of the equine microbiota, this may enable the development of probiotic strains that are beneficial in the equine gut. Overall, probiotics are generally considered safe, easy to administer, and cost-effective in other species. Treatment and prevention of equine GI disease remains challenging; therefore, further research to develop effective probiotic therapeutics is warranted.

14.7 Behavior

Managing behavioral problems in horses is challenging due to their size and strength. Supplements containing the amino acid tryptophan are frequently found in supplements marketed for behavior issues in many species [74]. Early studies reported a toxic effect of oral tryptophan given at 350 or 600 mg/kg BW to adult ponies. Signs of restlessness, elevated respiratory rate, hemolysis, hemoglobinuria, and hemoglobinuria nephrosis evident at necropsy were reported [75]. A single IV administration showed no clinical abnormalities because the oral tryptophan may have led to the formation of an active toxic metabolite, possibly indole [76]. Another study evaluating IV tryptophan compared to glucose on exercise capacity confirmed the non-toxicity with parental administration [77].

A study using low oral doses of L-tryptophan (0.5 mg and 0.1 mg/kg BW) in 10 mares isolated from their herd after dosing, reported more activity and an elevated heart rate at both dosages. The study also reported no change in blood concentrations of tryptophan or serotonin, which had been previously reported in other species [78]. In a different study, 12 Thoroughbreds were administered L-tryptophan supplement at 12 mg/kg BW as used in commercial products or a placebo, and then fed roughage or concentrate and observed in an empty enclosure with an unfamiliar person or novel object in a randomized controlled crossover design. Plasma tryptophan was measured by gas chromatography and blood concentrations of tryptophan were threefold greater in the treated than in the placebo group. L-tryptophan did not affect resting heart rate after either meal but the presence of a stranger or novel object did increase heart rate regardless of treatment. No marked behavioral changes were noted in the treated group and no evidence of toxicity was noted at this dose of oral L-tryptophan. The conclusion was there was no evidence that tryptophan administered at a dose used in some commercial preparations modified the behavioral response of horses [79].

14.8 Respiratory Diseases

Respiratory diseases are a significant economic problem in working and pleasure horses. Both inflammatory airway disease (IAD) affecting horses of all ages and recurrent airway obstruction (RAO) primarily in horses over seven years of age have been described [80]. Conventional treatments using corticosteroid drugs for equine respiratory diseases can be costly and may have adverse effects. Owners may consider dietary supplements and herbs as complementary and/or data available.

A randomized crossover study compared the effects of an herbal preparation to placebo in six horses symptomatic with RAO. The herbal supplement contained garlic, white horehound, boneset, aniseed, fennel, licorice, thyme, and hyssop and was analyzed for flavonoid content via liquid chromatography. Major compounds identified were asquercetin, azaleatin, rutin, kaempferol. No statistical differences were reported in serum biochemistry, complete blood count, cytology of tracheal aspirates, ventigraph measurements, respiratory rate, and maximum intrapleural pressure [81]. A longitudinal randomized crossover study evaluated an herbal preparation compared to no treatment in nine horses with RAO. The herbal preparation was not analyzed but said to contain extracts from yellow gentian, garden sorrel, cowslip, verbena, and common elder in a tablet formulation. After two wks of treatment, a significant decrease in maximal intrapleural pressure differences in all horses was reported but there were no treatment effects on clinical signs or cytology of bronchoalveolar lavage fluid [82].

Supplements marketed for "immune support" may be used to prevent inflammatory/infectious airway diseases in horses at risk. For example, bovine colostrum (BC) is a commonly used food supplement in humans and other animals for 'immune support' and enhanced athletic performance. Studies in humans suggest BC may prevent influenza and upper respiratory disease. Bovine colostrum supplementation for four wks was evaluated in a randomized placebo-controlled study in 12 horses in race training by analyzing serum insulin-like growth factor-1 (IGF-1) concentration. Bovine colostrum has been suggested to improve performance due to its ability to increase serum IGF-1 concentration. There was reported an expected seasonal decrease in IGF-1, but there was no effect of BC supplementation as compared with placebo [83].

Omega 3 polyunsaturated fatty acids (n-3 PUFA) have known effects on the inflammatory response in humans and other species. Eight research horses and 35 client-owned horses with chronic lower airway disease were randomly assigned a pelleted, no-hay diet supplemented with 30 or 60 g of an n-3 PUFA supplement or 30 g of placebo for two months. The n-3 PUFA supplementation resulted in increased concentrations of plasma docosahexaenoic acid (DHA) as well as a statistically significant improvement in clinical signs in the n-3 PUFA treated group [84]. Feeding fish oil to Thoroughbreds did increase red blood cell EPA and DHA content which is thought to decrease RBC fragility in racehorses and may reduce pulmonary bleeding; however, there are no published studies at this time [38]. As there is extensive research in PUFA supplementation *in vitro* and *in vivo* in other species, more research is warranted to evaluate the role of n-3 PUFA supplementation in equine respiratory diseases.

Natural supplements are marketed for exercise-induced pulmonary hemorrhage or bleeding, a common respiratory disorder in racehorses. A study evaluated Yunnan Baiyao (YB) given to horses three days before an exercise challenge. No beneficial effect was reported on laboratory variables and no difference in blood loss was measured in bronchoalveolar lavage fluid [85]. YB is an herbal preparation that primarily contains *Panax pseudoginseng* and has been widely used in China as a hemostatic agent. Its active constituents are thought to be two major saponins, ginsenoside Rg1, and Rb1, which have been identified through high-performance liquid chromatography [86]. A randomized placebo-controlled study looked at the effects of YB on platelet activation and function in horses. This study reported no significant effects on any of the hemostatic variables as compared with placebo [87]. Pre-medicating with YB reduced template bleeding times in anesthetized ponies [88]. As template bleeding is an *in vivo* measurement of primary hemostasis, YB may act at endothelial or extravascular cell membrane surfaces at the site of tissue injury. Other studies support this mechanism of action for this herbal preparation and further *in vivo* and clinical treatment trials are needed.

14.9 Metabolic/Endocrine Diseases

The prevalence of equine metabolic syndrome (EMS) is unknown, but the individual components (obesity, insulin resistance, predisposition to laminitis) have been reviewed. See Chapter 28 Metabolic Syndrome. There is a large population of horses "at risk" for EMS. Owner awareness of EMS is growing and the use of HDS marketed for prevention and/or treatment has risen [89]. Herbs and dietary supplements that may improve insulin sensitivity have been evaluated in humans and laboratory animal studies. Reported mechanisms of action include anti-obesity compounds, antioxidants, compounds that slow carbohydrate absorption, insulin receptor activators, and stimulators of glucose uptake [90]. Published studies in horses include short-chain fructooligosaccharides (scFOS), which are plant constituent that slows carbohydrate absorption. Two published studies evaluated scFOS in a randomized placebo-controlled crossover design in obese or overweight horses. One study demonstrated increased insulin sensitivity in obese horses without losing bodyweight or condition, while the other reported insulin sensitivity improved with weight loss independent of the scFOS supplement [91, 92].

Herb extract studies in EMS evaluated stevia, cinnamon, and spirulina. Extracts from the stevia plant were evaluated in 8 EMS horses as compared with 7 age-matched non-EMS controls. An oral sugar test was performed using corn syrup or stevia in a random crossover design. Stevia appeared to stimulate lower glycemic and insulinemic responses when compared with corn syrup in EMS horses. Stevia extract was well tolerated and further research was indicated as stevia may be a potential candidate as a non-glycemic sugar replacer in horses with insulin dysfunction [93]. In a study of 10 mares with known low insulin sensitivity, neither cinnamon extract nor fish oil had any significant effect on insulin sensitivity, plasma insulin, and leptin concentrations [94]. In a study of *Spirulina platensis* extract, supplementation resulted in statistically significantly reduced fasting insulin, but in this 3-month study, EMS supplemented horses also had significant weight loss confounding the results [95].

Chromium, magnesium, and L-carnitine supplementation have also been evaluated in EMS. Chromium has been suggested to improve insulin sensitivity by enhancing intracellular post-insulin receptor signaling pathways. A supplement containing chromium, magnesium, and other herbs was evaluated in 12 previously laminitic obese horses in a randomized 16-wk study. The supplement did not alter morphometric measurements, blood variables, resting insulin concentrations, or insulin sensitivity [96]. L-carnitine was shown to improve glucose tolerance in one study, but the results could not be replicated in a randomized, double-blind, placebo-controlled weight reduction study in ponies [41, 42]. This review of the literature suggests herbs or herbal combinations are unlikely to be beneficial in managing EMS, but supplementation with scFOS and L-carnitine may warrant further investigation.

Case in Point

Animal Assessment

A 27-yr-old Haflinger gelding (BW 320 kg, BCS 3/9) is seen on a North Carolina farm in mid-June for increased respiratory effort and weight loss (90–100 kg) that began 3 m previously despite good spring pasture growth and receiving 0.5 kg of ration balancer pellets daily; a ration that had historically maintained the pony at BCS 6/9 for several years. Physical exam, body temperature, and heart sounds were normal but the respiratory rate was 60 breaths per minute (b/min) with significant abdominal effort. Increased lung sounds (rhonchi and wheezes) were heard dorsally but no sounds were heard ventrally due to congestion on both sides, no nasal discharge, and rarely a cough. Based on laboratory blood results, the most likely diagnosis was RAO. The owner declined bronchoalveolar lavage and radiographs but requested medical management recommendations. Deworming with ivermectin/praziquantel paste one time and a 10-d course of trimethoprim sulfadiazine powder (38 g/d once daily) was recommended for unlikely lung parasites and infection. Clenbuterol syrup (72.5 mg/mL) was prescribed at 15 mL PO q 12 hrs for 30 days and then reassess the patient. The pony was routinely housed outdoors in a 4-acre pasture with a three-sided run-in shed, so adding a fan inside the shed was recommended for the summer.

1) *What feeding recommendations should be made to regain the weight lost?*

Reassessment Visit

After 30 days of clenbuterol syrup treatments, respiratory rate taken daily in the morning averaged 35–40 b/min with mild to moderate abdominal effort, which the owner considered to be comfortable for the pony. Reluctant to reduce the dose but due to the cost of clenbuterol, the owner asked about dietary supplements.

2) *What dietary supplement could be considered as adjunctive therapy in this pony?*

See Appendix A Chapter 14

References

1 American Horse Publications (2015). 2015 AHP Equine Industry Survey sponsored by Zoetis. American Horse Publications. https://www.americanhorsepubs.org/equine-survey/2015-equine-survey/ (accessed 18 October 2018)..

2 Ekor, M. (2014). The growing use of herbal medicines: issues relating to adverse reactions and challenges in monitoring safety. *Front. Neurol.* 4 (Jan): 1–10.

3 Williams, C.A. and Lamprecht, E.D. (2008). Some commonly fed herbs and other functional foods in equine nutrition: a review. *Vet. J.* 178: 21–31.

4 National Research Council (2007). *Nutrient Requirements of Horses*. 6th Rev. Animal Nutrition Series, 1–341. Washington DC: National Academies Press.

5 U.S. Food and Drug Administration (2019). Dietary supplements. https://www.fda.gov/food/dietary-supplements (accessed 3 July 2019).

6 Dzanis, D.A. (2012). Nutraceuticals and dietary supplements. In: *Applied Veterinary Clinical Nutrition* (ed. A.J. Fascetti and S.J. Delaney), 57–67. West Sussex: Wiley.

7 Finno, C.J. (2020). Veterinary pet supplements and nutraceuticals. *Nutr. Today* 55 (2): 97–101.

8 National Institutes of Health (2019). National Center for Complementary and Integrative Health (NCCIH). https://www.nccih.nih.gov/about (accessed 3 July 2019).

9 Booth, D.M. (2004). Balancing fat and fiction of novel ingredients: definitions, regulations and evaluation. *Vet. Clin. North Am. Small Anim. Pract.* 34 (1): 7–38.

10 National Animal Supplement Council (2019). NASC live. National Animal Supplement Council. https://www.nasc.cc (accessed 3 July 2019).

11 ConsumerLab. (2019). Independent tests and reviews of vitamin, mineral, and herbal supplements. https://www.consumerlab.com (accessed 3 July 2019).

12 Oke, S., Aghazadeh-Habashi, A., Weese, J.S., and Jamali, F. (2006). Evaluation of glucosamine levels in commercial equine oral supplements for joints. *Equine Vet. J.* 38 (1): 93–95.

13 International Society for Pharmaceutical Engineering (2019). Good manufacturing practice (GMP) resources | ISPE | International Society for Pharmaceutical Engineering. https://ispe.org/initiatives/regulatory-resources/gmp (accessed 3 July 2019).

14 Burns, P.B., Rohrich, R.J., and Chung, K.C. (2011). The levels of evidence and their role in evidence-based medicine. *Plast. Reconstr. Surg.* 128 (1): 302–310.

15 Roudebush, P., Allen, T., and Novotny, B. (2010). Evidence-based clinical nutrition. In: *Small Animal Clinical Nutrition*, 5e (ed. M.S. Hand, C.D. Thatcher, R.L. Remillard, et al.), 23–30. Topeka, KS: Mark Morris Institute.

16 Rosenthal, R.C. (2004). Evidence-based medicine concepts. *Vet. Clin. North Am. Small Anim. Pract.* 34 (1): 1–6.

17 Hoffman, C.J., Costa, L.R., and Freeman, L.M. (2009). Survey of feeding practices, supplement use, and knowledge of equine nutrition among a subpopulation of horse owners in New England. *J. Equine Vet. Sci.* 29 (10): 719–726.

18 Agar, C., Gemmill, R., Hollands, T., and Freeman, S.L. (2016). The use of nutritional supplements in dressage and eventing horses. *Vet. Rec. Open* 3 (1): e000154.

19 Bushell, R. and Murray, J. (2016). A survey of senior equine management: owner practices and confidence. *Livest. Sci.* 186: 69–77.

20 Beale, B.S. (2004). Use of nutraceuticals and chondroprotectants in osteoarthritic dogs and cats. *Vet. Clin. North Am. Small Anim. Pract.* 34: 271–289.

21 Vandeweerd, J.M., Coisnon, C., Clegg, P. et al. (2012). Systematic review of efficacy of nutraceuticals to alleviate clinical signs of osteoarthritis. *J. Vet. Intern. Med.* 26 (3): 448–456.

22 Ramey, D.W., Eddington, N., Thonar, E., and Lee, M. (2002). An analysis of glucosamine and chondroitin sulfate content in oral joint supplement products. *J. Equine Vet. Sci.* 22 (3): 125–127.

23 Trumble, T.N. (2005). The use of nutraceuticals for osteoarthritis in horses. *Vet. Clin. North Am. Equine Pract.* 21 (3): 575–597.

24 Pearson, W. and Lindinger, M. (2009). Low quality of evidence for glucosamine-based nutraceuticals in equine joint disease: review of in vivo studies. *Equine Vet. J.* 41 (7): 706–712.

25 Leatherwood, J.L., Gehl, K.L., Coverdale, J.A. et al. (2016). Influence of oral glucosamine supplementation in young horses challenged with intra-articular lipopolysaccharide. *J. Anim. Sci.* 94 (8): 3294–3302.

26 Kilborne, A.H., Hussein, H., and Bertone, A.L. (2017). Effects of hyaluronan alone or in combination with chondroitin sulfate and N-acetyl-d-glucosamine on lipopolysaccharide challenge-exposed equine fibroblast-like synovial cells. *Am. J. Vet. Res.* 78 (5): 579–588.

27 van de Water, E., Oosterlinck, M., Dumoulin, M. et al. (2017). The preventive effects of two nutraceuticals on experimentally induced acute synovitis. *Equine Vet. J.* 49 (4): 532–538.

28 Higler, M.H., Brommer, H., L'Ami, J.J. et al. (2014). The effects of three-month oral supplementation with a nutraceutical and exercise on the locomotor pattern of aged horses. *Equine Vet. J.* 46 (5): 611–617.

29 Murray, R.C., Walker, V.A., Tranquille, C.A. et al. (2017). A randomized blinded crossover clinical trial to determine the effect of an oral joint supplement on equine limb kinematics, orthopedic, physiotherapy, and handler evaluation scores. *J. Equine Vet. Sci.* 50 (3): 121–128.

30 Bauer, J.E. (2011). Therapeutic use of fish oils in companion animals. *J. Am. Vet. Med. Assoc.* 239 (11): 1441–1451.

31 Hess, T.M., Rexford, J.K., Hansen, D.K. et al. (2012). Effects of two different dietary sources of long chain omega-3, highly unsaturated fatty acids on incorporation into the plasma, red blood cell, and skeletal muscle in horses. *J. Anim. Sci.* 90 (9): 3023–3031.

32 Hall, J.A., Van Saun, R.J., Tornquist, S.J. et al. (2004). Effect of type of dietary polyunsaturated fatty acid supplement (corn oil or fish oil) on immune responses in healthy horses. *J. Vet. Intern. Med.* 18 (6): 880–886.

33 Dinnetz, J.M., Furtney, S.R., Pendergraft, J.S. et al. (2013). Omega-3 fatty acid supplementation reduces basal tnfα but not toll-like receptor-stimulated tnfα in full-sized and miniature mares. *J. Equine Vet. Sci.* 33 (7): 523–529.

34 Ross-Jones, T., Hess, M.V., Rexford, J. et al. (2014). Effects of omega-3 long chain polyunsaturated fatty acid supplementation on equine synovial fluid fatty acid composition and prostaglandin E2. *J. Equine Vet. Sci.* 34 (6): 779–783.

35 Manhart, D.R., Honnas, C.M., Gibbs, P.G. et al. (2016). Markers of inflammation in arthritic horses fed omega-3 fatty acids. *Prof. Anim. Sci.* 25 (2): 155–160.

36 Woodward, A.D., Nielsen, B.D., O'Connor, C.I. et al. (2005). Dietary long chain polyunsaturated fatty acids increase plasma eicosapentaenoic acid and docosahexaenoic acid concentrations and trot stride length in horses. *Equine Comp. Exerc. Physiol.* 4 (2): 71–78.

37 O'Connor, C.I., Lawrence, L.M., St. Lawrence, A.C. et al. (2004). The effect of dietary fish oil supplementation on exercising horses. *J. Anim. Sci.* 82 (10): 2978–2984.

38 Pagan, J.D.D., Lawrence, T.L.L., and Lennox, M.A.A. (2010). Fish oil and corn oil supplementation affect red blood cell and serum EPA and docosahexaenoic acid (DHA) concentrations in Thoroughbred horses. In: *Proceedings of the 1st Nordic Feed Science Conference* Sveriges Lantbruksuniversitet, 116–118.

39 Williams, C.A. (2013). Specialized dietary supplements. In: *Equine Applied and Clinical Nutrition: Health, Welfare and PerformanceHealth, Welfare and PerformanceHealth, Welfare and Performance* (ed. R.J. Geor, P.A. Harris, and M. Coenen), 351–366. Edinburgh: Saunders Elsevier.

40 Kranenburg, L.C., Westermann, C.M., de Sain-van der Velden, M.G.M. et al. (2014). The effect of long-term oral L-carnitine administration on insulin sensitivity, glucose disposal, plasma concentrations of leptin and acylcarnitines, and urinary acylcarnitine excretion in warmblood horses. *Vet. Q.* 34 (2): 85–91.

41 Schmengler, U., Ungru, J., Boston, R. et al. (2013). Effects of l-carnitine supplementation on body weight losses and metabolic profile in obese and insulin-resistant ponies during a 14-week body weight reduction programme. *Livest. Sci.* 155 (2–3): 301–307.

42 Van Weyenberg, S., Buyse, J., and Janssens, G.P.J. (2009). Increased plasma leptin through l-carnitine supplementation is associated with an enhanced glucose tolerance in healthy ponies. *J. Anim. Physiol. Anim. Nutr. (Berl.)* 93 (2): 203–208.

43 Teixeira, F.A., Araújo, A.L., Ramalho, L.O. et al. (2016). Oral creatine supplementation on performance of quarter horses used in barrel racing. *J. Anim. Physiol. Anim. Nutr. (Berl.)* 100 (3): 513–519.

44 Williams, C.A. (2016). Horse species symposium: the effect of oxidative stress during exercise in the horse. *J. Anim. Sci.* 94 (10): 4067–4075.

45 Bitto, A., Squadrito, F., Irrera, N. et al. (2014). Flavocoxid, a nutraceutical approach to blunt inflammatory conditions. *Mediators Inflamm.* 2014: 1–8.

46 Flamini, R., Mattivi, F., De Rosso, M. et al. (2013). Advanced knowledge of three important classes of grape phenolics: anthocyanins, stilbenes and flavonols. *Int. J. Mol. Sci.* 14: 19651–19669.

47 Smarsh, D.N., Liburt, N., Streltsova, J. et al. (2010). Oxidative stress and antioxidant status in intensely exercising horses administered nutraceutical extracts. *Equine Vet. J.* 42 (38): 317–322.

48 Liburt, N.R., McKeever, K.H., Streltsova, J.M. et al. (2009). Effects of ginger and cranberry extracts on the physiological response to exercise and markers of inflammation in horses. *Comp. Exerc. Physiol.* 6 (4): 157–169.

49 Ducharme, N.G., Fortier, L.A., Kraus, M.S. et al. (2009). Effect of a tart cherry juice blend on exercise-induced muscle damage in horses. *Am. J. Vet. Res.* 70 (6): 758–763.

50 Sykes, B.W., Hewetson, M., Hepburn, R.J. et al. (2015). European College of Equine Internal Medicine Consensus Statement-equine gastric ulcer syndrome in adult horses. *J. Vet. Intern. Med.* 29 (5): 1288–1299.

51 Pellegrini, F.L. (2005). Results of a large-scale necroscopic study of equine colonic ulcers. *J. Equine Vet. Sci.* 25 (3): 113–117.

52 Kerbyson, N.C., Knottenbelt, D.K., Carslake, H.B. et al. (2016). A comparison between omeprazole and a dietary supplement for the management of squamous gastric ulceration in horses. *J. Equine Vet. Sci.* 40 (5): 94–101.

53 Huff, N.K.K., Auer, A.D.D., Garza, F. et al. (2012). Effect of sea buckthorn berries and pulp in a liquid emulsion on gastric ulcer scores and gastric juice pH in horses. *J. Vet. Intern. Med.* 26 (5): 1186–1191.

54 Sanz, M.G., Viljoen, A., Saulez, M.N. et al. (2014). Efficacy of a pectin-lecithin complex for treatment and prevention of gastric ulcers in horses. *Vet. Rec.* 175 (6): 147.

55 Hellings, I.R. and Larsen, S. (2014). ImproWin® in the treatment of gastric ulceration of the squamous mucosa in trotting racehorses. *Acta Vet. Scand.* 56 (1): 13–20.

56 Woodward, M.C., Huff, N.K., Garza, F. et al. (2014). Effect of pectin, lecithin, and antacid feed supplements (Egusin®) on gastric ulcer scores, gastric fluid pH and blood gas values in horses. *BMC Vet. Res.* 10 (1): 1–8.

57 Lindinger, M.I. and Anderson, S.C. (2014). Seventy day safety assessment of an orally ingested, l-glutamine-containing oat and yeast supplement for horses. *Regul. Toxicol. Pharmacol.* 70 (1): 304–311.

58 Binda, S., Hill, C., Johansen, E. et al. (2020). Criteria to qualify microorganisms as "probiotic" in foods and dietary supplements. *Frontiers in Microbiology* 11: 1–9.

59 Schoster, A., Weese, J.S., and Guardabassi, L. (2014). Probiotic use in horses – what is the evidence for their clinical efficacy? *J. Vet. Intern. Med.* 28 (6): 1640–1652.

60 Coverdale, J.A. (2016). Horse species symposium: cthe microbiome of the horse be altered to improve digestion. *J. Anim. Sci.* 94 (6): 2275–2281.

61 Mackenthun, E., Coenen, M., and Vervuert, I. (2013). Effects of *Saccharomyces cerevisiae* supplementation on apparent total tract digestibility of nutrients and fermentation profile in healthy horses. *J. Anim. Physiol. Anim. Nutr. (Berl.)* 97 (suppl.1): 115–120.

62 Swyers, K.L., Burk, A.O., Hartsock, T.G. et al. (2008). Effects of direct-fed microbial supplementation on digestibility and fermentation end-products in horses fed low-and high-starch concentrates. *J. Anim. Sci.* 86 (10): 2596–2608.

63 Desrochers, A.M., Dolente, B.A., Roy, M. et al. (2005). Efficacy of *Saccharomyces boulardii* for treatment of horses with acute enterocolitis. *J. Am. Vet. Med. Assoc.* 227 (6): 954–959.

64 Boyle, A.G., Magdesian, K.G., Gallop, R. et al. (2013). *Saccharomyces boulardii* viability and efficacy in horses with antimicrobial-induced diarrhoea. *Vet. Rec.* 172 (5): 128.

65 Weese, J.S. and Rousseau, J. (2005). Evaluation of *Lactobacillus pentosus* WE7 for prevention of diarrhea in neonatal foals. *J. Am. Vet. Med. Assoc.* 226 (12): 2031–2034.

66 Yuyama, T., Takai, S., Tsubaki, S. et al. (2004). Evaluation of a host-specific lactobacillus probiotic in training-horses and neonatal foals. *J. Intest. Microbiol.* 18 (2): 101–106.

67 Schoster, A., Staempfli, H.R., Abrahams, M. et al. (2015). Effect of a probiotic on prevention of diarrhea and *Clostridium difficile* and *Clostridium perfringens* shedding in foals. *J. Vet. Intern. Med.* 29 (3): 925–931.

68 Schoster, A., Kokotovic, B., Permin, A. et al. (2013). in vitro inhibition of *Clostridium difficile* and *Clostridium*

perfringens by commercial probiotic strains. *Anaerobe* 20 (Apr): 36–41.

69 Schoster, A., Guardabassi, L., Staempfli, H.R. et al. (2016). The longitudinal effect of a multi-strain probiotic on the intestinal bacterial microbiota of neonatal foals. *Equine Vet. J.* 48 (6): 689–696.

70 John, J., Roediger, K., Schroedl, W. et al. (2015). Development of intestinal microflora and occurrence of diarrhoea in suckling foals: effects of *Bacillus cereus* var. *toyoi* supplementation. *BMC Vet.* 11 (34): 1–7.

71 Parraga, M.E., Spier, S.J., Thurmond, M., and Hirsh, D. (1997). A clinical trial of probiotic administration for prevention of Salmonella shedding in the postoperative period in horses with colic. *J. Vet. Intern. Med.* 11 (1): 36–41.

72 Kim, L.M., Morley, P.S., Traub-Dargatz, J.L. et al. (2001). Factors associated with Salmonella shedding among equine colic patients at a veterinary teaching hospital. *J. Am. Vet. Med. Assoc.* 218 (5): 740–748.

73 Ward, M.P., Alinovi, C.A., Couëtil, L.L. et al. (2004). A randomized clinical trial using probiotics to prevent Salmonella fecal shedding in hospitalized horses. *J. Equine Vet. Sci.* 24 (6): 242–247.

74 Grimmett, A. and Sillence, M.N. (2005). Calmatives for the excitable horse: a review of L-tryptophan. *Vet. J.* 170 (1): 24–32.

75 Paradis, M.R., Breeze, R.G., Bayly, W.M. et al. (1991). Acute hemolytic anemia after oral administration of L-tryptophan in ponies. *Am. J. Vet. Res.* 52 (5): 742–747.

76 Paradis, M.R., Breeze, R.G., Laegreid, W.W. et al. (1991). Acute hemolytic anemia induced by oral administration of indole in ponies. *Am. J. Vet. Res.* 52 (5): 748–753.

77 Farris, J.W., Hinchcliff, K.W., McKeever, K.H. et al. (1998). Effect of tryptophan and of glucose on exercise capacity of horses. *J. Appl. Physiol.* 85 (3): 807–816.

78 Bagshaw, C.S., Ralston, S.L., and Fisher, H. (1994). Behavioral and physiological effect of orally administered tryptophan on horses subjected to acute isolation stress. *Appl. Anim. Behav. Sci.* 40 (1): 1–12.

79 Noble, G.K., Brockwell, Y.M., Munn, K.J. et al. (2008). Effects of a commercial dose of L-tryptophan on plasma tryptophan concentrations and behaviour in horses. *Equine Vet. J.* 40 (1): 51–56.

80 Couëtil, L.L., Cardwell, J.M., Gerber, V. et al. (2016). Inflammatory airway disease of horses-revised consensus statement. *J. Vet. Intern. Med.* 30 (2): 503–515.

81 Pearson, W., Charch, A., Brewer, D., and Clarke, A.F. (2007). Pilot study investigating the ability of an herbal composite to alleviate clinical signs of respiratory dysfunction in horses with recurrent airway obstruction. *Can. J. Vet. Res.* 71 (2): 145–151.

82 Anour, R., Leinker, S., and van den Hoven, R. (2005). Improvement of the lung function of horses with heaves by treatment with a botanical preparation for 14 days. *Vet. Rec.* 157 (23): 733–736.

83 Fenger, C., Tobin, T., Casey, P. et al. (2014). Bovine colostrum supplementation does not influence serum insulin-like growth factor-1 in horses in race training. *J. Equine Vet. Sci.* 34 (8): 1025–1027.

84 Nogradi, N., Couetil, L.L., Messick, J. et al. (2015). Omega-3 fatty acid supplementation provides an additional benefit to a low-dust diet in the management of horses with chronic lower airway inflammatory disease. *J. Vet. Intern. Med.* 29 (1): 299–306.

85 Epp, T., McDonough, P., Padilla, D. et al. (2005). The effect of herbal supplementation on the severity of exercise-induced pulmonary haemorrhage. *Equine Comp. Exerc. Physiol.* 2 (1): 17–25.

86 Liu, X.X., Wang, L., Chen, X.Q. et al. (2008). Simultaneous quantification of both triterpenoid and steroidal saponins in various Yunnan Baiyao preparations using HPLC-UV and HPLC-MS. *J. Sep. Sci.* 31 (22): 3834–3846.

87 Ness, S.L., Frye, A.H., Divers, T.J. et al. (2017). Randomized placebo-controlled study of the effects of Yunnan baiyao on hemostasis in horses. *Am. J. Vet. Res.* 78 (8): 969–976.

88 Graham, L., Farnsworth, K., and Cary, J. (2002). The effect of Yunnan Baiyao on the template bleeding time and activated clotting time in healthy halothane anesthetized ponies under halothane anesthesia. *J. Vet. Emerg. Crit. Care* 12 (4): 279.

89 Morgan, R., Keen, J., and McGowan, C. (2015). Equine metabolic syndrome. *Vet. Rec.* 177 (7): 173–179.

90 Tinworth, K.D., Harris, P.A., Sillence, M.N., and Noble, G.K. (2010). Potential treatments for insulin resistance in the horse: a comparative multi-species review. *Vet. J.* 186: 282–291.

91 Respondek, F., Myers, K., Smith, T.L. et al. (2011). Dietary supplementation with short-chain fructo-oligosaccharides improves insulin sensitivity in obese horses. *J. Anim. Sci.* 89 (1): 77–83.

92 McGowan, C.M., Dugdale, A.H., Pinchbeck, G.L., and Argo, C.M.G. (2013). Dietary restriction in combination with a nutraceutical supplement for the management of equine metabolic syndrome in horses. *Vet. J.* 196 (2): 153–159.

93 Elzinga, S.E., Rohleder, B., Schanbacher, B. et al. (2017). Metabolic and inflammatory responses to the common sweetener stevioside and a glycemic challenge in horses with equine metabolic syndrome. *Domest. Anim. Endocrinol.* 60 (Jul): 1–8.

94 Earl, L.R., Thompson, D.L., and Mitcham, P.B. (2012). Factors affecting the glucose response to insulin injection in mares: epinephrine, short- and long-term prior feed intake, cinnamon extract, and omega-3 fatty acid supplementation. *J. Equine Vet. Sci.* 32 (1): 15–21.

95 Nawrocka, D., Kornicka, K., Śmieszek, A., and Marycz, K. (2017). Spirulina platensis improves mitochondrial function impaired by elevated oxidative stress in adipose-derived mesenchymal stromal cells (ASCs) and intestinal epithelial cells (IECs), and enhances insulin sensitivity in equine metabolic syndrome (EMS) horse. *Mar. Drugs* 15 (8): 237–265.

96 Chameroy, K.A., Frank, N., Elliott, S.B., and Boston, R.C. (2011). Effects of a supplement containing chromium and magnesium on morphometric measurements, resting glucose, insulin concentrations and insulin sensitivity in laminitic obese horses. *Equine Vet. J.* 43 (4): 494–499.

15

USA Feed Regulations and Safety

David A. Dzanis

KEY TERMS

- Animal food (feed) is any article that is provided to the animal in orally consumable form for its taste, aroma, or nutritive value.
- Labeling includes not only the label directly affixed to the feed bag or container, but also any information related to the product that is found in brochures, shelf talkers, etc. or on websites, but depending on the jurisdiction may not necessarily include advertisements.
- Adulteration means that the feed contains a contaminant, is made with a substance that is not approved for such use, is not manufactured under acceptable conditions, or is otherwise unfit for consumption.
- Misbranding refers to false or misleading information associated with a product in labeling, or the failure for the label to bear mandatory information in a prescribed format.
- Generally Recognized As Safe ("GRAS") is a regulatory term referring to a substance added to feed that in the broad judgment of qualified experts has been adequately shown to be safe under the conditions of its intended use.
- A food additive is a substance intentionally added (directly or indirectly) to an animal food that is not GRAS or otherwise sanctioned for use in feed.

KEY POINTS

- Feed is food, and irrespective of intended species, it is a violation for a feed to be adulterated or misbranded.
- There is no Food and Drug Administration (FDA) premarket approval process for animal feeds, although many state laws require registration of products and/or licensure of companies as a condition of distribution within that jurisdiction.
- The distributor of the product is responsible for ensuring the product is safe, wholesome, and properly labeled.
- Marketing claims (aka romance copy), the catchy phrases, attributes, or pictures on the label or in labeling to market the product, are not mandatory under the law but are subject to oversight under general false and misleading principles if not expressly addressed by regulation or policy.
- The US equine feed industry enjoys a long history of providing safe and suitable products, however, incidents of feed-borne illness can occur, and the timely reporting of a suspected problem with a feed not only may aid in the diagnosis of a clinical case but also may help curtail a larger outbreak.
- The equine practitioner is not expected to be an expert on horse feed regulations, but a working knowledge of the fundamentals is expected and can prove helpful.

15.1 Introduction

A well-rounded understanding of the science of equine nutrition and the art of feeding horses demands an appreciation for the regulatory requirements that commercial feed products must meet. It behooves the equine practitioner to know how to read the feed or supplement label to best offer advice on the suitability and proper use of a given product to the horse owner. See Sidebar 15.1. Further, it may become the veterinarian's role to deal directly with regulators in reporting suspect adulterated or misbranded products, so a working knowledge of how that is done is necessary for the practitioner, helpful to the horse owner, and beneficial to the industry.

Equine Clinical Nutrition, Second Edition. Edited by Rebecca L. Remillard.

Sidebar 15.1: Horse Owner's Views

A 2015 survey illustrated that horse owners were most likely to view their horses as family members (68%), companion animals (63%), performance partners (58%), and/or best friends (56%). However AAFCO has defined "pet" as limited to dogs and cats. It also has defined "specialty pet" to refer to other species commonly kept in households, such as ornamental fish, birds (non-poultry), reptiles, and small mammals, but again, the definition does not pertain horses of any size. Therefore, veterinarians need to be mindful that regardless of how the horse owner views their horse(s), from a food/feed regulatory standpoint, horses are not considered "pets" and that regulations for horse foods vs. dog and cat foods are different [1–3].

15.2 USA Regulatory Oversight

Commercial feeds for horses, including complete feeds, concentrates, supplements, treats, and the components of these types of products, are regulated at two levels in the United States [4]. At the federal level, the FDA has primary jurisdiction over all animal feeds in interstate commerce, including products imported into the United States. Secondly, many states also exercise authority over horse feeds distributed within their respective borders.

15.2.1 Food and Drug Administration Authority

The authority of the FDA to regulate animal feeds comes from the Federal Food, Drug, and Cosmetic Act of 1938 (FFDCA), in which "food" is defined in part as "food or drink for man or other animals." Regulations promulgated under this Act appear in Title 21 of the Code of Federal Regulations (aka "21 CFR"). Those applying to foods and drugs for animals, including equine feeds, are found in 21 CFR Parts 500–599 [5]. Facilities involved in the manufacturing and handling of feeds must register with FDA under the Bioterrorism Act of 2002. Importers must give FDA notice of all shipments into the United States before arrival at the port of entry. As a practical matter, the regulations in 21 CFR may differ between animal feeds vs. foods for human consumption. Still, feed is food, and irrespective of intended species, it is a violation of the Act for a feed to be adulterated or misbranded.

15.2.1.1 Adulteration

Adulteration includes contamination of the feed with a substance that may render the feed injurious to health, a failure on the part of the manufacturer to follow current Good Manufacturing Practices (cGMPs), a lack of a nutrient normally expected or professed to be in that feed, or inclusion of an ingredient not deemed suitable for that use, i.e. one that is not GRAS or approved as a food additive.

15.2.1.2 Misbranding

Misbranding may occur when information about the product on the label and any materials associated with the product available at the point of sale (store) or website (aka, labeling) does not conform to regulatory requirements. For example, if the label is missing required information such as product weight or manufacturer information, or if the labeling bears false or misleading information or makes a "drug claim," the product could be deemed misbranded.

There is no premarket approval process for foods at the federal level unless it is a "food additive." The FDA does not require registration of a feed product or preapproval of a label before distribution. More importantly, veterinarians and horse owners must understand that a manufacturer does not have to prove the safety and utility of a feed item to FDA before distribution. Rather, the onus is on the distributor of the product to ensure that what is being marketed is safe, wholesome, and properly labeled.

15.2.2 State Authority

Beyond FDA oversight, the majority of states also enforce animal feed regulations under their versions of laws akin to FFDCA, which most often does require product registration, company licensure, or both to distribute an equine feed within its jurisdiction. This most often requires the manufacturer or other distributor to submit labels and other information, with a fee, to the state feed control official, and products found not to comply with applicable law can be denied registration and the ability to be legally distributed in that state.

Regulations can be different in each state, so not surprisingly, compliance can sometimes prove cumbersome for products distributed in multiple states or when sold nationwide. It is often logistically infeasible for a manufacturer to have different labels for different states; therefore, the label on a widely distributed product must comply with every applicable state's feed regulations because the denial of registration in one state usually has much broader consequences. Fortunately, approximately two-thirds of states have adopted, in whole or in part, a version of the Association of American Feed Control Officials (AAFCO) Model Bills and Regulations.

AAFCO is a non-governmental body whose members must be government officials who are involved in animal feed regulation, such as state and territorial feed control officials, employees from the FDA, and a few representatives from foreign countries (presently, Canada and Costa Rica are members of AAFCO). Among its many functions is the establishment and maintenance of model laws and regulations that constitute a consensus among its members as to how feed should be regulated, and which are published annually in the AAFCO Official Publication [1]. The models are intended to facilitate minimally restrictive interstate commerce by the encouragement of uniform interpretation and enforcement among the individual states. They cover many aspects not addressed in FDA regulations. Importantly, they have no authority in and of themselves, i.e. technically, a company does not have to comply with AAFCO rules per se. However, many states incorporate the AAFCO models by reference or copy much of the language into their laws and regulations, at which time they become enforceable at the state level. Also, while AAFCO does not and cannot dictate how a state feed control official chooses to interpret and enforce its regulations, in the case where a discrepancy between the state's and AAFCO's regulations exists, to avoid unnecessary hindrance in interstate trade a state may opt to defer to AAFCO's interpretation. Notwithstanding the lack of any direct effect of the AAFCO Models on the regulation of feed, they are effectively the national standard. Thus, it is very prudent for manufacturers to comply with AAFCO requirements for their products to be broadly distributed within the United States.

Commodities such as hay, unmixed whole seeds e.g. bulk whole oats, and some individual chemical compounds are not included in the AAFCO definition of "commercial feed." Depending on the state, they are often exempt from state registration and labeling requirements although labeling, if any, would still need to meet FDA regulations. For example, typically there is no label on bales of hay and in most states, there is no requirement for the hay to be registered or the seller to be licensed with the state feed control official. Buying forage locally or from a national distributor comes with very limited or no information as commonly found on bags of commercial horse feed. Average nutrient analyses for forages and individual grains have been published; nevertheless, neither federal nor state regulations dictate that a given feed item must conform to these published "textbook" average nutrient profiles [6, 7]. However, these feed items are still "food" under the law, hence the FDA and states still have the authority to take appropriate enforcement action in the case of adulteration or misbranding. Information written about a hay product at the feed store or on the web, e.g. on a blackboard or price sheet, identifying the type of hay and/or any other information offered about the hay is "labeling" under the law.

15.3 Basic Label Requirements

Mandatory label information under FDA regulations is codified in 21 CFR 501 [5]. These cover basic requirements, such as a statement of identity, net contents, the name and address of the manufacturer or distributor, and a declaration of ingredients. They do not address many other aspects of proper horse feed labeling, such as nutrient content and directions for use. However, the AAFCO Model Regulations help cover these gaps [1]. The regulations in those states that have not adopted the AAFCO Models usually address these same aspects.

An example of a compliant horse feed label bearing the mandatory information from both an FDA and AAFCO perspective is shown in Figure 15.1. Historically, this information was all contained on a single tag sewn to a plain or minimally marked feed bag. While many bagged feeds may still bear a tag, the information may also be printed directly on the bag to allow for a more stylistic presentation to the purchaser. For feed items normally sold in smaller quantities, such as supplements and treats, there often is not a tag (or even a bag), but regardless, the mandatory information must still appear on the label of the container as seen by the purchaser at the time of sale. Some of the mandatory information must appear on the label's principal display panel (PDP), the panel most likely to be displayed to the purchaser at the time of sale. Other mandatory information must appear on the information panel, defined by FDA regulations as the panel immediately to the right of the PDP, if it does not already appear on the PDP. For much of the information required by AAFCO, but not FDA, the exact placement is left to the manufacturer's discretion [2].

15.3.1 Brand/Product Name

The product name, and brand name, if applicable, will generally be at the top of the tag, or if no tag, somewhere on the PDP. A product name may be fanciful with no direct indication as to contents or purpose, but if it bears any description as to intended purpose, the contents must be suitable for that use. The product name cannot be derived from one or more ingredient names unless all ingredients are part of the product name, with some exceptions.

YOUR 12% TEXTURED HORSE FEED

For maintenance of mature horses

Guaranteed Analysis

Crude Protein (min)	12.0%
Crude Fat (min)	3.0%
Crude Fiber (max)	12.0%
Acid Detergent Fiber (max)	23%
Neutral Detergent Fiber (max)	18%
Calcium (min)	1.0%
Calcium (max)	1.5%
Phosphorus (min)	1.0%
Copper (min)	20 ppm
Selenium (min)	0.20 ppm
Zinc (min)	40 ppm
Vitamin A (min)	2000 IU/lb.

Ingredient Statement

Grain Products, Plant Protein Products, Processed Grain By-Products, Molasses Products, Roughage Products, Vitamin A Supplement, Vitamin D_3 Supplement, Vitamin E Supplement, Vitamin B_{12} Supplement, Riboflavin Supplement, Folic Acid, Biotin, Thiamine Mononitrate, Calcium Carbonate, Salt, Dicalcium Phosphate, Manganous Oxide, Ferrous Sulfate, Copper Sulfate, Magnesium Oxide, Zinc Oxide, Ethylenediamine Dihydroiodide, Cobalt Carbonate, Potassium Chloride, Sodium Selenite.

Feeding Directions:

Feed ½ to 1 lb. of feed per 100 lb. of bodyweight for the maintenance of mature horses. Feed good quality hay at the rate of 1 to 2 lb. per 100 lb. of bodyweight daily. Provide fresh, clean water at all times.

Important: Feed hay along with this ration, as per directions.

Manufactured By:
YOUR NAME FEEDS
City, State Zip

NET Wt.: 50 lb. (22.67 kg)

Figure 15.1 Example of a tag for a horse feed in compliance with AAFCO Model Regulations. *Source:* Courtesy of AAFCO [1].

Unless expressly noted otherwise, a percentage value in the product name, e.g. "14% Horse Feed," is understood to refer to protein content.

15.3.2 Statement of Identity/Purpose Statement

Federal regulations require a "statement of identity," i.e. a succinct description of the contents in common terms on the PDP. For single-ingredient products, such as "rolled oats," that verbiage may be sufficient as both the product name and statement of identity. In the case of a fanciful product name, e.g. "Betty's Bites," something like "treats for horses" would suffice as the statement of identity.

AAFCO also requires a "purpose statement" on the PDP, which identifies the species and class for which the feed is intended. Established classes for horses under AAFCO regulations include growing, maintenance, broodmare, and performance, although manufacturers have some liberty as to the exact terminology used. The label may be exempt from the need to identify species and class in the case of single-ingredient feeds, e.g. corn, or those products intended for the further manufacture of feeds. Otherwise, the statement on the label may appear as something like "performance horse feed" or "vitamin supplement for foals."

15.3.3 Guaranteed Analysis

Although nutrient content is not addressed in FDA regulations, AAFCO has established mandatory guarantees to appear on the labels of all animal feeds to allow the purchaser to evaluate the nutritional value of the product. The specific guarantees mandated for a given feed depends on the intended species, as determined to be critical nutritional indicators for that species by a panel of experts from academia and industry. For most horse feeds, AAFCO requires minimum percentage guarantees for crude protein and crude fat. Also, maximum percentage guarantees for crude fiber, and more recently, acid detergent fiber and neutral detergent fiber are required (Figure 15.1). Further, minimum and maximum guarantees for calcium (%), and minimum guarantees for phosphorus (%), zinc (parts per million, or ppm), and selenium (ppm) must be declared. Guarantees for minimum copper (ppm) and vitamin A (IU/lb) content are needed if those substances have been added to the product formulation. Unlike pet foods, a maximum moisture (%) guarantee is not required on horse feed labels.

Additional guarantees may be added voluntarily, or in the case where a specific nutrient content claim is made, as needed to support the claim and otherwise inform the purchaser of the product's contents, in units as stipulated in the regulations. For example, a claim "high in iron" on a complete feed label requires an additional guarantee for minimum iron (ppm) content. Claims for probiotic activity require a guarantee for minimum viable microbiologic content in terms of colony-forming units (CFUs) per pound or per gram,[1] depending on how the product is fed, for the named organism(s), e.g. *Saccharomyces cerevisiae* minimum 3.5 billion CFU/lb. A product represented to be a vitamin or mineral supplement must provide guarantees for every added vitamin and/or mineral in the product as evidenced by their inclusion in the ingredient list. However, for vitamin and mineral supplements, the guarantees optionally can be expressed in terms of units consistent with the feeding directions, e.g. Zinc (min) 10 mg per tablespoon vs. 500 ppm

Some equine products may be exempt from the requirement for certain guarantees. In cases where the feed is not intended to provide, nor does it provide appreciable amounts of protein, fat, or fiber, e.g. a vitamin supplement in a starch-based carrier, these guarantees do not have to appear on the label. On the other hand, an oil intended as a fatty acid supplement would not have to bear protein or fiber guarantees, but would still have to declare minimum percentage crude fat and guarantees for the minimum content of any specifically claimed fatty acids.

A recent amendment to the AAFCO Model Regulations has defined the requirements for a livestock "treat," which is an item fed occasionally for purposes of enjoyment or training, not necessarily for its nutritive value. Under the new rule, the label of a horse feed prominently identified as a "snack" or "treat" on the PDP needs only declare crude protein, crude fat, and crude fiber guarantees. The exception would be that additional guarantees still would be needed to support any nutrient content claims for the treat, e.g. "Betty's Bites with calcium" would require a minimum and maximum guarantee for calcium (%) on the label.

15.3.4 Ingredient Declaration

Under both FDA and AAFCO regulations, each ingredient in the horse feed product must be declared on the information panel, if not already on the PDP by its "common or usual" name in descending order of predominance by weight in the formulation. Some ingredients are universally understood by the purchaser as "common food," e.g. barley, apples, so that no official definition or other sanction by a regulatory body is required. For some others, names are established via the Food Additive Petition or GRAS Notice processes as administered by FDA. See Section 15.6.2.

For many if not most ingredients, though, the common or usual names and characteristic qualities of feedstuff are established via the AAFCO Feed Ingredient Definition process. Another important function of AAFCO involves establishing definitions for many of the common or usual ingredients that have been further processed or fractioned, such as "oat hulls" or "corn gluten meal." This naming is especially important for feed ingredients that may be recognized by different names in different regions of the country. However, nutrient and processing specifications often established in the definition of an ingredient

1 The amount of viable microorganisms per serving is also acceptable and permitted only as supplemental information, and not in lieu of per lb or g.

also help ensure that the ingredient is consistent in nature and composition wherever it is sold. For example, “dried plain beet pulp” must be the same ingredient and meet the same specifications whether it is purchased in Maine or California. From a legal perspective, some of these AAFCO-defined ingredients may not be formally approved as food additives or deemed to be GRAS, which is required by the strict interpretation of FFDCA. In other words, the AAFCO definition process is “informal” from the regulatory perspective. However, FDA works closely with AAFCO in the definition process, and under a Memorandum of Understanding between the two bodies, FDA reviews data demonstrating safety and utility for a new ingredient before a definition can be published in the AAFCO Official Publication [1]. As a practical matter, then, AAFCO-defined ingredients are universally acceptable to all US regulatory bodies.

One exception to the rule that applies to horse and other livestock feeds, but not pet foods, is the use of “collective terms” in the ingredient statement. Manufacturers often may need to replace key ingredients in a formulation based on availability, season, price, or to correct for nutrient variability. However, to avoid the need for frequent and potentially expensive label changes with each variation in the formula, a term such as “grain products” or “forage products” may be substituted for the actual ingredient name in the label declaration. For each category of collective terms, the applicable ingredients are listed in the AAFCO Official Publication. Also, the use of a collective term requires that all ingredients within that category in the formulation be included under that term, and the term appears in order of predominance based on the combined weights of all applicable ingredients. In other words, “dehulled soybean meal” cannot appear as a separate ingredient on a label that also declares “plant protein products.”

There is also an exemption from a declaration of ingredients identified as “incidental additives” (21 CFR 501.100). These include a processing aid or other technical additive that may be used in manufacturing, but is removed, destroyed, or otherwise present in insignificant quantities in the finished product where it no longer serves any function. This may also include an ingredient in the product only by the fact that it is a component of another ingredient, where again, it is present in insignificant amounts and no longer serves a functional role in the finished feed. A good example of this is a carrier, such as a starch or oil, that is used in vitamin or mineral premixes to help with the handling of the premix during the manufacture of the feed, but whose contribution to the nutrient content of the finished feed is negligible. On the other hand, an antioxidant preservative added to a fat source to retard degradation may be expected to retain significant function in the finished feed as well, in which case, it is not exempt and must be disclosed on the final label, for example, “cottonseed oil (preserved with BHA).”

15.3.5 Directions for Use/Precautions

Under AAFCO regulations, directions on the feed or supplement label must be sufficient to allow for safe and suitable use by a person with no special knowledge as to the purpose and use of the feed and include cautionary information as may be required elsewhere in the regulations. Statements of microbial or enzyme content, such as “This product contains viable, naturally occurring microorganisms” or “Contains protease to hydrolyze proteins” are mandatory for products containing claims for probiotic or enzyme activity, respectively. Special directions for feeds containing approved drugs, i.e. medicated feeds, non-protein nitrogen sources, or raw milk-based ingredients are also required by the regulations, but rarely if ever apply to horse feed labels.

15.3.6 Name and Address of the Guarantor

The name of the party responsible for registering the product for distribution of the feed, the “guarantor,” in AAFCO-speak, must appear on the information panel of the label, if not already on the PDP. When the named party is not the actual manufacturer, i.e. it does not own or directly control the feed facility, words such as “manufactured for” or “distributed by” must accompany the name. Also required on the label are the city, state, and postal (ZIP) code of the named responsible party. Further, unless the physical street address, not a post office box, of the principal place of business of that party, is publicly available, e.g. in a local telephone directory or on the company’s website, the physical address must appear on the label. This is to allow regulators to visit the company unannounced in the case of an emergency.

15.3.7 Net Contents

An accurate declaration of a quantity of content is deemed critical information for the purchaser to assess value, e.g. cost per pound, and to compare between products. For this reason, both FDA and AAFCO regulations require a net content statement, most often in terms of net weight, the weight of product without packaging, but it can be in terms of volume (fluid ounces/milliliters) for liquid products, and on rare occasions for horse products, by numerical count, e.g. “XX tablets.” Under FDA rules, this statement must appear on the bottom 30% of the PDP (or feed tag, if present) in lines generally parallel to the base. Further, it must be of sufficient contrast and boldness, separated from all other text, and of sufficient size relative to the area of the PDP to be easily identified and read by the purchaser. Use of terms that may serve to mislead the purchaser as to the quantity, e.g. "jumbo quarts," is prohibited. Regulations promulgated by the Federal Trade Commission (FTC) under the Fair Packaging and Labeling Act, yet to be codified by FDA, is for the declaration to be provided in terms of both avoirdupois (pound/ounce or gallon/quart/fluid ounce) and their equivalent units in the metric system.

15.3.8 Country of Origin Declaration

Under regulations promulgated by US Customs and Border Protection but subject to enforcement by FDA and state feed control officials, the labels of all imported products must bear a country of origin statement, such as "Made in Canada" or "Product of Mexico." This needs to be at least the same type size and reasonably juxtaposed with the guarantor's name and address. Domestically manufactured products that are materially transformed in the United States are not required to declare a country of origin regardless of the origin of their ingredients.

15.3.9 Expiration Dates and Identifying Codes

There is no provision in FDA or AAFCO regulations that requires an expiration date, "best by" date, or similar indicator of usability or freshness on the horse feed label. Similarly, there is nothing in the regulations mandating the identification of the specific production batch, lot code, or other markings that would serve the same purpose. However, it is generally prudent for the manufacturer to include such markings, not only for the benefit of the purchaser but also for practical reasons.

In response to a complaint or as a matter of routine surveillance, feed control officials often obtain samples of products from the retail market to conduct their analyses. Products on the market must be found to meet their guarantees or be subject to enforcement action as an adulterated feed. Without an expiration date on the label, the company has no viable defense when a violation is detected. Also, some sort of indicator of the production batch that a particular bag of product comes from can be very important in case of a recall. Without some way of distinguishing one batch from another, all products on the market can be subject to the same enforcement action, i.e. a massive vs. strategic recall of products. The size and placement of these markings are left to the discretion of the manufacturer.

Bar codes, QR codes, etc. that may appear on the label to facilitate the purchase of the product at retail are not subject to regulatory oversight. Rather, the manufacturers obtain their codes through private parties and place them on the label at their discretion. However, a state may opt to use the bar code number, if any, as a means of product identification for registration purposes.

15.4 Labeling Claims

When in the past the label consisted only of the tag sewn onto a plain feed bag, there was often no room to add more than the basic mandatory information. Today, marketing claims on the packaging ("romance copy") that extol the benefits of the product, the ingredients or nutrient content, or other qualities of the feed abound, sometimes surpassing the amount of mandatory information appearing on the label. More expansive or elaborate marketing claims are often made on websites or other labeling. Only a few regulations address specific labeling claims. However, as per the general provisions of the law, all claims and other statements on the labeling must be truthful and not misleading to the purchaser.

15.4.1 Carbohydrate-Related Claims

One claim recently allowed on livestock feed labels is a carbohydrate-related claim, e.g. "low carbs" or "less dietary starch." Historically, AAFCO policy discouraged these types of claims, primarily because there were no effective means to directly measure carbohydrate content per se. Under AAFCO Model Regulations, a nutrient content claim most often requires a stated guarantee to support it, so as interpreted by most states, if you cannot make a guarantee, you cannot make the claim. However, validation of analytical methods for specific carbohydrate fractions has allowed that to be more feasible.

As a result, carbohydrate-related claims are now allowed on horse and other livestock feed labels, but only if additional guarantees for both maximum percentages of "sugars" and "dietary starch" appear on the label. Both guarantees must be made regardless of the nature of the claim. Any carbohydrate-related claim for a forage-containing product must include a maximum percentage "fructans" guarantee as well. All three guarantees are subject to verification by defined and validated analytical methods. Importantly, AAFCO makes no judgments as to how low is "low," e.g. hypothetically, a molasses-based horse treat could claim to be "low in sugars" provided the guarantees for sugars and dietary starch were added to the label. So, the horse owner and veterinarian must assess the merits of the carbohydrate-related claim in light of the stated guarantees and evaluate the appropriateness of those concentrations for the individual animal.

15.4.2 "Natural" Claims

AAFCO also has established guidelines for "natural" claims. When pertaining to a product as a whole, all ingredients in the product must be of natural origin (plant, animal, or mined sources). Certain processing of the feed or its ingredients are allowed, e.g. physical processing, heat processing, fermentation, enzymolysis, but any ingredient or component that is derived by chemically synthetic means would invalidate the claim. However, an exception is made in the case of added trace nutrients, such as vitamins, minerals, or amino acids. In that case, though, the presence of these chemically synthetic components must be disclaimed in association with the "natural" claim, e.g. "natural with added vitamins." While such a disclaimer is suitable for a complete feed or treat, it is not allowed for products that are in fact predominately formulated with synthetic trace nutrients, such as a vitamin or mineral supplement.

The term "natural" as defined by AAFCO does not address other reasonable interpretations of the word, such as whether the ingredients are "non-GMO" or are normally a part of the animal's diet in nature. In essence, it only means the product does not contain artificial preservatives, flavors, or colors. These synthetic ingredients are not harmful, provided that they have been deemed acceptable for that purpose and are used in accordance with the regulation or definition. Some preservatives, such as mixed tocopherols extracted from wheat germ oil or other plant sources, are considered natural but may not be as effective in preventing fat degradation as some synthetic antioxidants [8]. Oxidized fats may impact palatability and affect the degree of oxidative stress in the animal. Still, the "naturalness" of a product may be a driving factor in the purchasing decision, so to the extent feasible, the veterinarian can advise the purchaser of perceived benefit vs. potential risks.

15.4.3 "Made in USA" Claims

As mentioned above, labels of domestically manufactured products do not have to bear country of origin declarations. However, if a manufacturer chooses for marketing purposes to add a "made in USA" statement, include depictions of the American flag, or make a claim of similar implication as to the product's origin, it becomes subject to FTC guidance. Under FTC, a product whose label bears the claim must not only be physically produced in the United States, but "all or virtually all" ingredients must be of US origin as well.

Some states will ask companies for documentation to substantiate compliance with this guidance. The FTC does not define what "virtually all" means, except to say products bearing the claim must be of "negligible foreign content," so it is left to the state regulator's discretion as to how much is too much. Many ingredients that may be in a horse feed, especially vitamins, amino acids, and other trace nutrient ingredients simply are not available from US manufacturers, but those are typically used in small amounts. However, other ingredients that may be in a horse feed may or may not be of US origin, e.g. legumes, grains, or in the case of tropical fruits, vegetables, tapioca, or palm oil are unlikely produced in the United States. Thus, products containing these types of ingredients may be required to further qualify the claim, such as "Made in the USA with ___ from ___" or "Made in the USA with ingredients from around the world."

15.4.4 Drug Claims

Perhaps the claims of greatest concern to regulators are "drug claims." Under FFDCA, a drug is an article intended for the diagnosis, cure, treatment, prevention, or mitigation of disease, or one intended to affect the structure or function of the body in a manner beyond classical nutritional precepts. "Intent" is an important factor in the determination of drug status. In fact, intent can be established by means beyond what is on the label or labeling. For example, although FDA defers primary authority to FTC in matters relating to advertising vs. labeling, in the case of a drug claim, the advertising, and even verbal statements by a salesperson can be used as evidence of intent. Any expressed or implied claim to affect an animal in this manner can make the product a "drug" by definition, regardless of the actual composition of the product. Further, because the product was not approved as a drug for this use by submission of data to support safety and efficacy to FDA, the food becomes an "adulterated drug" under FDA law. Bottom line, drug claims cannot be made on the label or other materials, websites, or advertisements or the company faces the risk of enforcement action.

A perfectly acceptable feed ingredient, such as calcium carbonate, may be safely added to feed as a nutritional substance. A claim to "help support healthy bone growth and development in foals" is within the realm of acceptable food claims, as that is the recognized function of calcium in the ration. However, a promise to "cure bone deformations" is a drug claim. Similarly, garlic may be added to a horse feed for flavor or aroma, but claims relating to any effect on the structure or function of the animal are objectionable. Details on how FDA views product labels bearing drug claims can be found at https://www.fda.gov/media/69982/download

15.5 Special Products

15.5.1 Supplements

Supplements are a unique category of feeds, and not all "supplements" are subject to the same regulatory oversight. Many nutrient supplements, such as vitamin, mineral, or fatty acid products, are regulated as animal feed and subject to the same FDA and AAFCO regulations as any other feed. There are some label provisions particular to supplements in the guaranteed analysis in terms of expressed units allowed, but otherwise, these should be labeled in accordance with all applicable federal and state regulations. All ingredients must be sanctioned for use in feed, and any drug claims on labels or elsewhere are strictly prohibited. In other words, all components in the label ingredient list must be AAFCO-defined, or otherwise acceptable for use in feeds for the intended species, e.g. ingredients allowed in a supplement for cattle or pets may not necessarily be allowed in products intended for horses.

Nutritional supplement products have been on the market for many decades. However, the passage of the Dietary Supplement Health and Education Act of 1994 (DSHEA) fundamentally changed the country's perception of what constitutes a "dietary supplement." In addition to vitamins, minerals, etc. DSHEA also allows herbs and botanicals, metabolites, and many other substances that normally would not be allowed in food in conventional form (or if allowed, not for the stated purpose) to be used in products in dietary supplement form. Further, the Act provides for supplement claims not routinely tolerated on food labels including an effect on the structure or function of the body apart from its purely nutritive value. This resulted in an explosive expansion of the supplement industry, providing a much broader range of products to the consumer. These supplements are still legally "foods" and not "drugs" under the law, and therefore came to the market without the same degree of regulatory scrutiny as drugs. Hence, demonstration of safety and efficacy as normally expected for a drug is often lacking for many of these supplements. Although FDA concluded authoritatively in 1996 that DSHEA was neither intended by Congress nor applied to supplements for species other than humans, the animal supplement industry, initially for pets, and now horses, has seen dramatic growth. This caused a considerable regulatory conundrum because many animal supplement products were simply not compliant with the existing feed requirements; either because they contained unapproved ingredients or professed objectionable claims.

A workable albeit tenuous solution to this dilemma was reached with the formation of the National Animal Supplement Council (NASC), a non-profit trade association representing many manufacturers of horse and pet supplements, aka "dosage-form animal health products" (www.nasc.cc). The NASC developed product quality standards, a process for auditing of members, and an adverse event reporting system that in negotiation with FDA and AAFCO alleviated many concerns of regulators. The NASC also established a label format that is decidedly distinct from that for FDA/AAFCO-labeled products. Rather, labels following NASC guidance are more closely akin to those allowed under DSHEA for dietary supplements for human consumption. So, the "guaranteed analysis," has been replaced by a "Product Facts Box" stating levels of "active ingredients," both nutritional and non-nutritional components, in the product. Also, ingredients in NASC-labeled products are not declared in order of predominance but rather the "inactive ingredients" are declared separately and in lower predominance to the active components. While disease treatment/prevention claims are not allowed by NASC, structure/function claims not allowed on a feed label are permitted, i.e. attributes pertaining to effects on the body beyond nutritional merits. Examples of typical information panels on labels for FDA/AAFCO-compliant products vs. NASC-labeled products are shown in Figures 15.2 and 15.3.

NASC-labeled supplements generally escape the scrutiny of state feed control officials because they are not identified as "food." They are subject to oversight by FDA as "unapproved drugs of low regulatory priority" and may need to be registered in the few states that have "animal remedy" laws. Otherwise, the veterinarian must remain aware that supplements of this type have not been evaluated for safety and effectiveness by a regulatory body. See Chapter 14 Dietary Supplements.

15.5.2 Medicated Feeds/Veterinary-Directed Feeds

A medicated feed is a feed containing a drug intended for specific therapeutic or production purposes. The drug must be approved by FDA, and in addition to other requirements to demonstrate safety and efficacy, be shown to remain potent and available to the animal in a feed matrix. Facilities producing medicated feeds are subject to additional FDA and state oversight to ensure proper cGMPs are followed and the drug is properly and uniformly mixed. Feeds must be properly identified with the term "medicated," the name and concentration of the drug, its intended use, and any cautionary statements as determined to be necessary for safe use. While medicated feeds are very common in feeds for other livestock and poultry, only one drug for use in medicated feeds for horses (pyrantyl palmitate) is approved.

While veterinary-directed (aka, "therapeutic") foods for dogs or cats are much more common in the market, such

Melanie's Happy Hoof Co.

Vitamin & Mineral Supplement for Adult Horses and Ponies

Apple Flavor

Ingredients

Dicalcium Phosphate, Tapioca Starch, Dried Apple Pomace, Magnesium Oxide, Zinc Amino Acid Complex, Thiamine Mononitrate, Caramel (color), Silicon Dioxide, Vitamin A Palmitate, Copper Proteinate, dl-Alpha Tocopherol Acetate. Riboflavin, Citric Acid (preservative), Cholecalciferol, Vitamin B_{12} Supplement.

Guaranteed Analysis

Calcium (min)..15%
Calcium (max)..18%
Phosphorus (min)...............................13.5%
Magnesium (min).................................1.2%
Copper (min)..................................45 ppm
Zinc (min).......................................210 ppm
Thiamine (Vitamin B_1)(min)..........150 mg/lb
Riboflavin (Vitamin B_2)(min)...........70 mg/lb
Vitamin B_{12} (min)..........................15 mcg/lb
Vitamin A (min)...........................6500 IU/lb
Vitamin D_3 (min)............................479 IU/lb
Vitamin E (min).............................260 IU/lb

Feeding Directions

Top dress or mix in a small amount of sweet feed. One scoop (enclosed) = 60 g

Body weight (lbs)	Scoops/day
Less than 500	1/2
500	1
750	2
1000	3
Greater than 1000	4

Contact Us!

Distributed by Melanie's Happy Hoof Co., San Angeles,.CA 90298
Toll free: 800-555-4959
www.melanieshappyhoof.com

See Best Before date on bottom of container

Figure 15.2 Example of the information panel on a label for a nutritional supplement in conformance with AAFCO Model Regulations.

feed products for the intended use of affecting specific medical conditions of horses have been available as well. These are not medicated feeds and do not contain drugs or unapproved food additives, but rather are formulated to exert an effect on a disease or condition by manipulation of common feedstuffs to alter nutrient profiles, e.g. minimizing the non-structural carbohydrate content for the management of insulin dysregulation. Such products may be construed as "unapproved drugs" under the law because these feeds are expressly intended for the treatment or prevention of disease and, hence, potentially subject to enforcement action as an adulterated product. Admittedly, enforcement of the law for these sorts of products has been lacking, and in seeing the potential value of these products on the market, FDA has historically exercised enforcement discretion and not taken strong action to date.

Although it does not directly impact equine products, FDA has developed guidance for veterinary-directed foods for dogs and cats to identify under which conditions it is less likely to initiate an enforcement action. Recently, AAFCO has developed very similar guidance. Theoretically, these conditions can be reasonably applied to similarly intended horse feeds. Briefly, they include:

- The product is made available only through veterinarians or on the order of a veterinarian. While not a "prescription" in the legal sense of the term, it encourages the use of products where a valid veterinarian–client–patient relationship has been established.
- Promotional materials available to the veterinarian may include a discussion of its therapeutic intent and provide the rationale for that distinction. However, all materials intended for the animal owner, in electronic form or

Melanie's Happy Hoof Co.

HEALTHY JOINT SUPPORT FOR HORSES

Product Facts

ACTIVE INGREDIENTS PER OUNCE:

Glucosamine HCl (shellfish)	1500 mg
Chondroitin Sulfate (poultry)	800 mg
Proprietary Herbal Blend (Ginger Root, Boswellia, Turmeric)	250 mg
Ascorbic Acid (Vitamin C)	100 mg
Manganese (manganese amino acid complex)	15 mg

INACTIVE INGREDIENTS:
Artificial apple flavor, beet molasses, BHA and BHT (preservatives), dehydrated alfalfa meal, oat hulls, propionic acid (preservative) and silicon dioxide

CAUTIONS:
Safe use in pregnant animals or animals intended for breeding has not been proven.
If lameness worsens, discontinue use and contact your veterinarian.
Administer during or after the animal has eaten to reduce incidence of gastrointestinal upset.

FOR USE IN HORSES ONLY.
RECOMMENDED TO SUPPORT HEALTHY JOINT FUNCTION.
DIRECTIONS FOR USE:
Enclosed scoop holds 1 ounce.
Give 2 scoops morning and night for initial loading dose (3-4 weeks).
For maintenance, give 1 scoop daily (based on an 1000 lb adult horse).

WARNINGS:
For animal use only.
Keep out of the reach of children and animals. In case of accidental overdose, contact a health professional immediately.
This product should not be given to animals intended for human consumption.

QUESTIONS?

Distributed by: Melanie's Happy Hoof Co., San Angeles, CA 90298

Call us at 1-800-555-4959 or visit www.melanieshappyhoof.com

Lot #: *Best before:*

Figure 15.3 Example of the information panel on a label for a "dosage form animal health product" following NASC guidance. *Source:* Dzanis [4] with permission of Elsevier.

print, and including the label of the product itself, would not bear any indications of therapeutic use or other drug claims. This discourages diagnoses and treatment by the owner without veterinary supervision.

- The product would not be marketed as an alternative to approved new animal drugs.
- The product would contain only acceptable feed ingredients, and would not contain a drug or unapproved food additive.
- The product would be otherwise compliant with all regulatory requirements for animal feed, and the labeling would not be false or misleading in any other respect.

It is anticipated that the establishment of this guidance will allow for stronger enforcement capabilities concerning dog and cat foods, in that once the legitimate players comply, it will be easier for regulators to move against those that refuse to conform to these conditions of distribution. Importantly, though, this regulatory guidance was neither intended nor does it directly apply to equine products. Still, equine practitioners may wish to consider these basic tenets when evaluating the suitability of horse feeds of this nature. In any respect, it is crucial to note that data to support the safety and utility of therapeutic feed products are not typically reviewed by FDA before marketing. Thus, the equine veterinarian should closely evaluate the available information and the rationale for use before recommending a given product to the horse owner.

15.6 Feed Safety

15.6.1 Regulatory Oversight

The safety of feeds as it pertains to both animal and human health has always been a high priority to regulators. In the past, however, most enforcement efforts were reactionary, i.e. steps were taken only after an incident occurred. The Food Safety Modernization Act of 2012 (FSMA) fundamentally changes that mode of conduct.

In the regulations promulgated under FSMA (21 CFR 507), feed facilities must follow cGMPs for animal food production. These take into consideration the wide diversity of production types, e.g. a mining operation producing a mineral supplement would be held to different standards than a grain storage facility, a feed mill, or the manufacturer of a vitamin premix. Still, all must adhere to a set of appropriate standards, and failure to follow cGMPs can be used as de facto evidence of adulteration. For example, failure to follow proper sanitation steps could cause the product to be deeded adulterated, regardless of lack of direct evidence of contamination, e.g. product analysis for pathogenic bacteria.

Equine feed companies are also mandated to prepare a written food safety plan, which includes the performance of a hazard analysis. This is to identify known or reasonably foreseeable biological, chemical, and physical hazards, be they naturally occurring, unintentionally introduced, or intentionally introduced for economic or another gain. The establishment and implementation of risk-based preventive controls, e.g. specified processing or sanitation steps, must adequately address any identified hazards. Where the hazard may stem from raw materials, a supply-chain program must be instituted. Facilities are obligated to dutifully monitor and verify the effectiveness of these measures and make corrections to the plan as indicated. Finally, a written recall plan is also required under the regulations.

Another key component to feed safety is the "Reportable Food Registry." This was implemented far before FSMA as an outcome of the Food and Drug Administration Amendments Act of 2007 (FDAAA) and was done in part after hearings by the US Congress on the melamine contamination incident in dog foods earlier that year. With some exceptions, it applies to all food and feed manufacturers. As a result, horse feed companies now must electronically report to FDA on any incident of contamination when there is a reasonable probability of serious adverse health consequences within 24 hours of discovery.

15.6.2 Ingredient Approval

Many ingredients intended for use in horse feed are "common foods" or allowed via the AAFCO Feed Ingredient Definition process. For those substances that may impose potentially higher safety risks, a more formal procedure may be required prior to acceptance. A Food Additive Petition requires submission to the FDA of data and other information to substantiate the safety and utility of a substance for use in feed. Petitioners submit information on the nature and composition of the substance, demonstration of its functionality at proposed use levels, and adequate safety studies (including target animal feeding trials) to prove that the substance is safe when incorporated in feeds as intended. Upon review of the data and concurrence by the FDA as to its suitability, a regulation is codified in 21 CFR 573 to define the substance name, specifications, and any limitations or restrictions on use. This means of approving an ingredient is often reserved for those substances that may pose unique safety concerns when not properly used. A good example of an approved food additive common in horse feeds is the various selenium compounds (21 CFR 573.920) [5].

While FDA regulations do allow for a substance to be deemed GRAS by virtue of its history of safe use before the passage of the Food Additive Amendments Act of 1958, that option is largely inapplicable today. To be shown as GRAS by scientific procedures, the quantity and quality of data needed to support safety must be comparable to that required in a Food Additive Petition, with the additional caveat that it is primarily derived from information available to the public, e.g. as in the peer-reviewed scientific literature. Usually, a panel of experts with sufficient knowledge and training in the evaluation of the safety of food ingredients is convened to make the determination. Technically, a sponsor of a proposed GRAS substance does not have to inform FDA of its inclusion in a product. However, at this time, many states will not accept an "independent conclusion of GRAS" as an adequate demonstration of safety, so for practical purposes, many will submit to FDA what is called a "GRAS Notice." FDA does not reach its own conclusion of GRAS for that substance but will provide the sponsor with a "no questions" letter, in other words, more of a tacit rather than formal approval. The findings of FDA are not published in 21 CFR but do appear in a list on FDA's website (https://www.fda.gov/animal-veterinary/generally-recognized-safe-gras-notification-program/current-animal-food-gras-notices-inventory) and the AAFCO Official Publication.

15.6.3 Nutritional Suitability

AAFCO regulations require that a feed be nutritionally appropriate for its intended species and class when fed as directed. However, unlike dog and cat foods, horse feeds do not have to meet an expressly identified nutritional standard, e.g. be formulated to meet the AAFCO Dog or Cat Food Nutrient Profiles or successfully pass an AAFCO-specified feeding trial. Further, horse feed manufacturers do not have to identify the means of substantiation of nutritional suitability on the label at all. If requested by a state feed control official, a company may have to file an "Affidavit of Suitability." This is a legally binding document in which the guarantor attests to its knowledge of the nutritional composition of the product and the scientific basis by which nutritional suitability was substantiated. For horse products in the USA, the *Nutrient Requirements of Horses* is most commonly cited as the source of supporting scientific evidence [6].

15.7 Enforcement

There is a great deal of cooperative effort between FDA and state feed control officials, both individually and through interaction within AAFCO. For example, in contemplation of an enforcement action, FDA may provide scientific and regulatory expertise to the state feed control official to facilitate its efforts. On the other hand, the states may have the ability to move faster or more effectively against a violative product compared with FDA. Many states also have agreements with FDA to conduct facility inspections and/or product sampling and analysis on behalf of the FDA as part of a routine surveillance program.

Unlike most states, FDA cannot deny product registration as an enforcement tool. Also, FDA lacks the authority to fine companies for violations of the FFDCA. However, there are other options at its disposal to help impose compliance. For one, it can initiate a "seizure" against the violative product. This involves the physical detainment of the product and filing of a legal suit against the product rather than the manufacturer or distributor per se, e.g. "*The United States vs. 5000 bags of horse feed*." Unless the manufacturer or owner of the detained product can satisfy the FDA demands for remedy, e.g. relabeling or reconditioning the 5000 bags of horse feed, the product is typically destroyed.

As a consequence, such an action can have a severe economic impact on the owner of the horse feed. However, when indicated, other enforcement options are available. For more egregious or repeated offenses, FDA may also seek an injunction against the company, legally barring it from certain practices. Other possible actions include suspension of the manufacturers' food facility registration, refusal of entry for imported goods, and in some cases, criminal prosecution of the principals of the company.

Although FSMA does grant FDA mandatory recall authority, most recalls are "voluntary," be they initiated by the company or by FDA. Depending on the violation, FDA assesses the risk to human and animal health and assigns the class and depth of the recall. While the company does the bulk of the work in retrieving products, FDA oversees all aspects of a recall to help ensure that the violative product is swiftly removed from the market.

With respect to state enforcement options, most feed control officials do have the authority to impose product registration and/or company licensure requirements before distribution in that state. While labels are typically submitted to the state as part of this process, a state may look at all labeling, such as the company's website, and in some states, the advertising in its determination of compliance. As such, a quick and effective means of addressing labeling or other violations is at their disposal. Upon denial of registration/licensure, a feed product may not be entered into distribution unless and until it is brought into compliance as directed. Technically, that action only restricts movement in that state, and the company could still be free to distribute products into other states. However, because states frequently interact between themselves and FDA on these types of matters, one initial complaint can quickly grow to dozens. Also, it is usually impractical for companies to hold inventories of different labels for different jurisdictions, or for distributors to effectively prevent the product from moving into isolated states while still selling in neighboring jurisdictions. The product that is denied registration but is found in distribution anyway may be subject to a "stop sale." This state action is essentially the same as a seizure action by FDA. Depending on the state, it may also have the authority to file an injunction, impose criminal penalties, or issue fines for noncompliance.

15.8 Reporting Problems with Horse Feed Products

Contamination of a horse feed product, whether physical, chemical, or microbiologic in origin, can lead to serious health consequences. Also, formulation errors or even improper labeling can result in adverse events. While the US equine feed industry enjoys a long history of providing safe and suitable products, incidents of feed-borne illness can occur. For example, if a feed mill fails to practice proper production sequencing and equipment clean-out procedures, residues of a drug commonly used in cattle feed such as monensin can be carried over into a horse feed with disastrous results. Timely reporting of a suspected problem with a feed not only may be of assistance in the diagnosis of a clinical case but also may help curtail a larger outbreak.

It is not uncommon for horse owners to implicate the feed as the cause of an acute onset of illness. However, since signs of a feed-borne disease are often non-specific, it is prudent to diligently rule out other potential causes of sudden illness as a matter of course. Still, the possibility of adverse effects stemming from feed contamination or improper formulation must remain on the differential diagnosis list until ruled out or when the definitive cause is determined.

Before filing a complaint, a veterinarian who suspects a case of feed-borne illness needs to collect as much information related to the product in question as feasible (Table 15.1). A record of the dietary history of a sick animal is always prudent and may become important if a pattern emerges or a notice of a recall is announced at a later date. Pertinent information includes details about the feed and its labeling, as well as clinical observations of the animal. Collection of feed samples for laboratory analysis may be indicated. Proper handling of the sample as legal evidence and in accordance with the protocols of the FDA, state, or other suitable diagnostic laboratory may be critical if there is a possibility of a lawsuit at a later date [9]. A thorough description of clinical findings may give clues to the testing facility as to which contaminants are likely and hence which analyses to conduct.

Details on how veterinarians and the public-at-large can file a complaint regarding an FDA-regulated product, including an equine feed or supplement, can be found at: Reporting Problems with Horse or other Livestock Feed/Food (https://www.fda.gov/animal-veterinary/report-problem/reporting-problems-horse-or-other-livestock-feedfood). To facilitate the receipt of complaints online, FDA has instituted an electronic reporting portal (Table 15.2). Alternatively, the Consumer Complaint Coordinator at the nearest FDA District Office can be contacted directly. The link in Table 15.2 provides the appropriate telephone number to call organized by state, although more than one state may be handled by a given District Office. Also, the product manufacturer or distributor should be contacted promptly any time a feed is suspected to be contaminated, as the company may be able to recognize an emerging pattern if multiple complaints regarding a product are received. Such notification should be done

Table 15.1 Helpful information in reporting horse feed complaints.

Source	Information to obtain
Feed	Type of feed (e.g. forage, mixed feed, supplement)
	Where purchased (store name and street address)
	Date of purchase
	Appearance (e.g. mold, off odor, foreign material)
	Results of diagnostic testing (e.g. microbial, mycotoxin, chemical), if any
Label	Brand, product, and variety name
	Manufacturer's or distributor's name and address
	Package size
	Batch identification (e.g. lot code, best by date, any other markings)
Animal	Number of animals affected
	Signalment and previous health history
	Quantity of feed consumed
	Onset and progression of signs relative to the time of consumption
	Other foods, treats, supplements, medications involved
	Results of diagnostic testing, if any
	Tentative or confirmed diagnosis

Table 15.2 Reporting suspected problems with horse feed products.

To whom	How to contact
FDA	FDA Safety Reporting Portal
	https://www.safetyreporting.hhs.gov/SRP2/en/Home.aspx?sid=25143bf1-c475-4980-9e17-f39aa5b1f430
	Consumer Complaint Coordinator
	https://www.fda.gov/consumer-complaint-coordinators
Feed company	Company website or "800" telephone number on the label
State feed control official	AAFCO state directory
	https://www.aafco.org/Regulatory/State-Information

in addition to, not instead of, direct reporting to FDA, even though reports of serious problems to the company should initiate its investigation and possible reporting to FDA through the Reportable Food Registry. In any case, but especially for locally made products, notification of the state feed control official (varies, but usually in the state department of agriculture) is also prudent. The link in the table brings up a map, so one need only click on the appropriate state to call up the correct contact information.

15.9 Summary

The regulation of horse feed products in the United States is complex. The equine practitioner is not expected to be an expert in the field, but a working knowledge of the fundamentals can prove helpful. Especially for those veterinarians contemplating the introduction of equine feeds or supplements into the market, further knowledge of the regulatory requirements are instrumental to success.

References

1 Association of American Feed Control Officials (2021). *Official Publication AAFCO*. Champaign, IL: Association of American Feed Control Officials, Inc. https://www.aafco.org (accessed 2 February 2021).

2 Association of American Feed Control Officials (2020). *Animal Feed Labeling Guide*. Champaign, IL: Association of American Feed Control Officials, Inc. https://www.aafco.org/Portals/0/SiteContent/Publications/Feed_Labeling_Guide_web_complete.pdf (accessed 2 April 2021).

3 American Horse Publications (2015). 2015 AHP Equine Industry Survey sponsored by Zoetis. American Horse Publications. https://www.americanhorsepubs.org/equine-survey/2015-equine-survey/ (accessed 18 October 2018).

4 Dzanis, D. (2018). Veterinary products. In: *An Overview of FDA Regulated Products* (ed. E. Pacifici and S. Bain), 181–198. London: Elsevier.

5 United States Congress. Title 21. (2020). Food and Drugs; Subchapter E – Animal, Drugs, Feeds and Related Products, §500–599. In: Electronic Code of Federal Regulations. Washington DC. https://www.ecfr.gov/cgi-bin/text-idx?SID=c8787638238163005 68cc1852626d0bc&mc=true&tpl=/ecfrbrowse/Title21/21cfrv6_02.tpl#0 (accessed 2 April 2021).

6 National Research Council (2007). *Nutrient Requirements of Horses*. 6th Rev. Animal Nutrition Series, 1–341. Washington, DC: National Academies Press.

7 National Research Council (1982). *United States-Canadian Tables of Feed Composition*. 3rd Rev. Nutritional Data for United States and Canadian Feeds, 1–148. Washington, DC: National Academies Press.

8 Gross, K., Bollinger, R., Thawnghmung, P., and Collings, G.F. (1994). Effect of 3 different preservative systems on the stability of extruded dog food subjected to ambient and high temperature storage. *J. Nutr.* 124 (Supp 12): 2638S–2642S.

9 Miller, E.P. and Cullor, J.S. (2000). Food safety. In: *Small Animal Clinical Nutrition*, 4e (eds. M.S. Hand, C.D. Thatcher, R.L. Remillard, et al.), 183–198. Topeka, KS: Mark Morris Institute.

Section III

Feeding Management

Healthy Horses

16

Feeding and Drinking Behaviors

Katherine A. Houpt and Rebecca L. Remillard

KEY TERMS

- Herbaceous plants are mainly made up of cellulose with no persistent woody stem above ground (graminoids, forbs).
- Graminoids are grass-like plants (orchardgrass, fescue, timothy).
- Forbs are flowering, broad-leafed plants (clovers).
- Browse refers to shoots, twigs, leaves of trees, and shrubs.
- Concentrates refer to grain and/or supplement mixes used to improve the nutritive balance of the total ration, fed either separately or mixed into a complete feed product.
- Chaff is the dry, scaly protective casing of cereal grain seeds (hulls) or finely chopped straw.
- Patch grazing is the close and repeated grazing of some areas (or individual plants) while nearby areas (or plants) are left ungrazed creating uneven growth and nutritional value across the pasture.

KEY POINTS

- Grazing as a group is called social facilitation with some individuals watching for predators while others eat or rest.
- Mature horses on pasture with ample forage, no other feed, during mild weather will spend from 40 to 60% of the time grazing.
- Feeding behaviors of stabled horses can be very different or similar to that of grazing free-range horses depending on the amount of hay available to the confined horse.

16.1 Introduction

Horses are kept in three general types of management systems: (i) on pasture, (ii) pasture during the day and stabled at night, or (iii) confined to a stall for the majority of the time with a few hours in a grassless paddock. Based on behavioral studies of the Przewalski horses in Mongolia, feeding behaviors have not been changed by domestication [1]. Appetite and feed intake in horses are thought to be ultimately controlled by the central nervous system in the modulation of overall energy balance (intake vs. expenditure) through hormonal, neuronal, and macronutrient signals [2]. Hormones such as ghrelin and leptin have been studied in horses on a limited basis and are thought to act similarly as in other mammalian species [3, 4]. A specific nutrient-seeking appetite, as found across many species, including the horse, exists for only energy, salt, and water. Like other species, horses do not seek out certain non-food substances (dirt, feces, wood) due to specific micronutrient (mineral or vitamin) deficiencies. It has been shown that palatability responses are associated with specific macro-nutrients (protein > hydrolyzed carbohydrate > lipid-rich diets) and those nutrient associations related to digestion and absorption can be learned in five days [5]. Understanding the feeding and drinking behaviors are important considerations in the management of horses to optimize nutritional intake and foster their physical, social, and psychological well-being.

16.2 Feeding Behaviors

Horses have been observed in a variety of environments from the south of France to the Canadian plains, and from the Bronx Zoo to the Mongolian Steppes. Remarkably, their behavior is similar in the different environments. Grazing

Equine Clinical Nutrition, Second Edition. Edited by Rebecca L. Remillard.

consists of grasping a tuft of grass with the prehensile upper lip, tearing it off with the incisors (prehending), and then using the molars to masticate (chew). Prehending bites are different from chewing bites. The grazing horse prehends about 25 bites/min and chews at a rate of 30–50 bites/min for 8–12 h/d. The usual pattern is to take two to five bites in one place and then to walk a step or more and then take another few bites.[1] The number of bites per stop decreases and the number of steps increases as the pasture grass decreases in quantity and nutritional quality.

Horses prefer not to eat alone, presumably because grazing requires lowering their head, which increases their vulnerability to predators. Ponies eating from mangers spent more time eating when they could see one another than when a board obscured their view [6]. Similarly, feeding a pair of horses eating from a trough with a removable barrier, the dominant horse spent more time eating than the subordinate one when there was no barrier between the horses; however, when a solid barrier was placed in the trough to obstruct their view of each other, the dominant horse spent less time eating [7]. Grazing as a group, allowing some to be eating, while, one or more horses may be watching for predators, is an example of social facilitation [8].

When feeding horses as a group, a social hierarchy will become readily apparent, particularly when feed or water is limited. Incidence of dominance, biting, and kicking can be minimized by providing ample headroom at the feeding station(s) for all horses in the group to feed contentedly. Monitoring for losses in body weight (BW) and condition of the more submissive horses within the group will indicate a possible problem with access to the feeder. The use of several feeding stations with sufficient space between feeders may be necessary to discourage a dominant horse from controlling more than one station at a time.

Horses defecate and urinate frequently while eating, and the majority of the time do so in or near their feeding area, contaminating feed on the ground and increasing feed waste. Horses spend about 70% of their day eating and prefer to eat off the ground. When all hay offered was initially placed in a feed bunk, the horses pulled the hay out of the bunk and spent 59% of their eating time eating from the ground vs. 41% from the bunk. Horses will frequently (25 times/h) raise their head to view the surroundings when forced to consume hay from a blinding feed bunk, likely to better see oncoming dominant horses and/or predators [6].

[1] The idea that horses keep moving is the basis for "Paradise Paddocks" in which the horse must walk from one resource such as water, hay, salt, a rolling pit, to another. Jackson, J. (2016). Paddock Paradise: A Guide to Natural Horse Boarding. Revised. 122. James Jackson Publishing.

16.2.1 Time Management

Mature horses, tame or feral, on pasture with ample forage, and no other feed, during mild weather reportedly spend from 40% to 60% of a 24-hr period grazing [9–12]. On the lush pastures of northern Virginia, Przewalski horses spent 46% of 24-hrs grazing [13]. In the arid and overgrazed Steppes of Mongolia, Przewalski horses spent 46% of the daylight hours grazing [1]. Horses also spend 9% of their time walking, more on poor pasture or if alone. They spend 5–10% of their time, primarily three to four hrs before dawn, lying down, with 25–30% of this time in lateral recumbency.

Foals do not have to eat initially as they receive their nutrient needs suckling their dam, but gradually they graze more and suckle less [11]. A one-d-old foal spends 6–9% of the time grazing, increasing to 20–30% by eight wks of age and 40–50% by 21 wks of age [9, 10, 14]. Foals graze when their mares graze and likely learn which species of plant to ingest. Yearlings' grazing time is similar to that of an adult.

Eating behaviors do not change when horses are confined to a paddock or stall if offered free-choice hay. When individually confined to a pen, the adult horse reportedly spent 57% of the time eating hay and 10% lying down [15]. Individually stalled horses fed hay ad libitum spent 73% of daylight hours eating when they could see other horses and 60% when they could not [6]. Ponies fed ad libitum hay in a box stall spent 76% of their time eating, and draft mares tethered in single straight stalls spent from 32% to 58% of their time eating hay (Figure 16.1) [16].

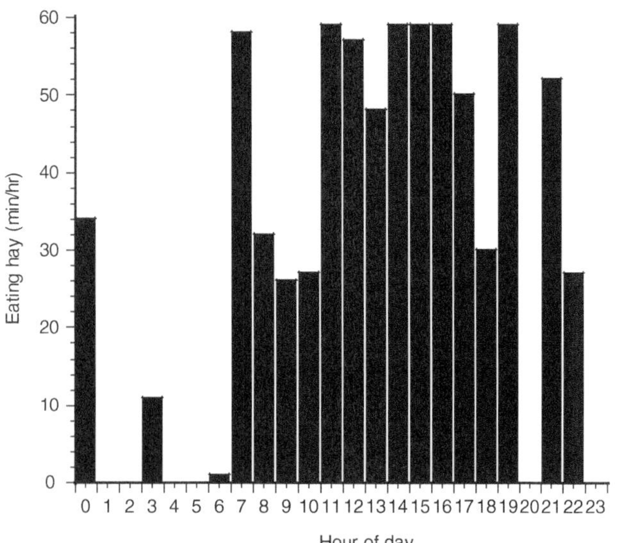

Figure 16.1 Time of day spent eating ad libitum hay by one pregnant draft mare tethered in a straight stall. *Source:* Data from Houpt et al. [16].

16.2.1.1 Time of Day and Feeding

The normal pattern is to graze continuously for several hours, and to rest for longer or shorter periods, depending on weather conditions and distance to be traveled for water and sufficient forage. The time devoted to grazing decreases with severe weather (hot or cold) and the presence of pests such as biting flies. A common pattern is for almost all horses in a herd to graze first thing in the morning with rest periods mid-morning and mid-afternoon. A study of the Assateague ponies reported 54% of the 10 overnight hours was spent grazing [17]. The nadir of grazing was at 2 a.m. when horses were likely to be lying down. Nighttime grazing also increased as day length shortened, which served to keep grazing time and, therefore, food intake, constant [18]. During the warmer (15–30 °C) parts of the day, the Mongolian Przewalski horses moved to cooler no forage elevations to avoid the flies [19]. Domesticated horses will also spend hours in cooler darker protected areas (trees, run-in sheds) not eating to avoid biting flies, but then graze at night to sufficiently maintain BW when pasture is adequate.

16.2.2 Pastured Horse Feeding Behaviors

Horses are selective grazers and do not simply feed on plants that are in the greatest abundance in their range. Until preferred forages are depleted, horses will eat only a few of the many species available. Wild horses in the Douglas Mountain areas of Colorado ate mostly needlegrass (*Stipa* spp.), wheatgrass (*Agropyron* spp.), and brome (*Bromus* spp.). In southern New Mexico, free-roaming horses chose Russian thistle (*Salsola kali tenuifolia*) and jungrass (*Koeleria cristata*), especially in the winter and spring, whereas during summer and fall, they chose dropseed (*Prosopis juliflora*). Stage of growth, as well as availability, determine the seasonal difference in preference as younger immature plants within a plant species are preferred. In Alberta, Canada, free-ranging feral horses ate grasses, especially hairy wild rye (*Elymus innovatus*), tall fescue (*Festuca* spp.), and sedge (*Carex* spp.) despite having more than 24 other species of grasses and browse available. The crude protein content of the feral horse diet varies between 4% in the winter and 16% in spring as acid detergent fiber varies from 30% to 55% [20]. Horses do learn to avoid foods that make them ill (food aversion) by associating the taste with the illness. However, this type of learned aversion in horses only occurs if the latency time, i.e. between consumption and illness, is 30 min or less. Hence horses are susceptible to chronic plant poisonings (*Senecio* plants) [21]. See Chapter 12 Toxic Plants.

The plants preferred by horses vary seasonally. For example, in the Mediterranean climate of the Camargue, France, horses consume graminoids in the marshy areas, moving to the less preferred long grasses in the winter. On Shackleford Island, off the eastern United States, the ponies eat primarily sea oats, smooth cordgrass, and centipede grass in the summer and fall, but eat a more varied diet in the winter, including more forbs. Similarly, meadow and shrubland are the vegetation types grazed by feral horses in the Great Basin of Nevada, but food preferences and nutritional needs have to be weighed against the dangers of predators, cold in winter and the irritation of insects and heat in the summer. Grasses are chosen in preference to forbs or browse but as the grass dies off in winter, feral horses eat a higher percentage of browse [22]. Australian horses consume a range of non-pasture grasses and frequently demonstrate bark-chewing behavior while at pasture [23]. Horses kept in pastures or paddock with trees will routinely eat the bark at the root collar or trunk, and if the bark is lost completely around the trunk, i.e. girdling or ring-barking, the tree will die.

Horses consume about 80 g dry matter (DM)/min when grazing or 100–200 g DM/kg $BW^{0.75}$/d [24, 25]. There have been several studies of the plants that ponies and horses choose to eat on pasture. The New Forest Ponies of England eat eight different species of plants but avoid the poisonous *Senecio* plants [26]. When given access to strips of pure strands of 29 species of grass, horses and ponies preferred timothy, white (not red) clover, and perennial ryegrass. When preferred grasses are overgrazed, the distribution of species in the pasture will change and less preferred plants will dominate. See Sidebar 16.1. Horses also avoid fecal, contaminated grass areas, and more mature, more fibrous tall grasses [22].

Most pastures contain several different types of forage, e.g. the average central Kentucky horse pasture is reported to contain about 50% bluegrass, 30% tall fescue, and 20% orchardgrass with the highest nutrient content in spring and fall growth. Soil quality and conditions are not homogeneous, which also results in varied plant growth and nutritive value across a pasture. Herbivores navigate between the available quantity of digestible DM and energy content in the tall/mature grasses vs. higher concentrations of digestible protein in the short/young grasses. See Sidebar 16.2. Digestible protein was the best predictor of the horses' choice of grass. When digestible protein was not limiting, i.e. protein content was adequate across the different stages of plant growth as in spring, the horses selected patches where food was ingested faster (tall/mature plants). However, when protein was limited, horses maximized their protein intake rate by feeding on the short/immature grasses [19].

Sidebar 16.1: Pasture Management and Horse Preferences

The key to obtaining the highest feeding value from pasture is to graze forages while they are in the young growing stages of development, uniformly across the pasture, and not allow horses to overgraze young plants. See Chapter 11 Forages. As forages mature, their palatability and utilizable nutrient content decreases, and horses will instead overgraze more palatable young plants such that they may not be able to recover. Weeds will increase in the overgrazed areas while areas of mature forage, not eaten, continue to grow and become contaminated with feces. The manure then also contributes to uneven grazing because: (i) most mature horses avoid grazing fecal contaminated areas, and (ii) plants, fertilized by manure, grow and mature rapidly and will remain ungrazed. The net effect is a pasture with weeds and unpalatable mature grass. Preventing uneven or a patched pasture involves either harvesting the pasture for hay at the appropriate time, or using rotational grazing that forces horses to eat less palatable plants within a small area before being moved to the next section. To correct an uneven pasture, remove horses, mow the overmature forage close to the ground, kill or mow the weeds, scatter the manure piles with a harrow, fertilize and lime as needed per a soil test, and keep horses off the pasture until plant growth can sustain rotational grazing, which is usually a height of 3–6 in (10–15 cm) depending on the grass species.

Sidebar 16.2: The Herbivore Dilemma

For any pasture grass species, immature growing plants are relatively more nutritious and palatable than mature versions of the same plant; however, immature plants are smaller, contain more water, and provide less total food DM for the same area. For example, digestible energy and protein content in fescue and orchardgrass pastures were more than adequate in the spring; however, both nutrients in both types of grass were below mature horse requirements by winter [27]. The quandary for grazing herbivores is balancing the intake of forage digestible energy and protein over the energy expended to travel distances across the pasture or plains. Tall mature grasses can be ingested more efficiently than short immature plants but mature plants have lower energy and protein digestibility coefficients because of the higher fiber content, i.e. taller plants have more fiber (lignin) to remain upright than shorter plants. Immature grass plants are highly digestible, contain more protein, sugar, less fiber, but DM intake rates are limited compared with the tall grasses for the same area.

16.2.3 Stabled Horse Feeding Behaviors

The feeding time of stalled horses can be largely different or very similar to the grazing time of free-range horses depending on the amount of hay available to the animal [28]. There are methods of minimizing wasted hay and slowing the rate of hay ingestion by stabled horses, such as hanging hay in small (2.5 cm) holed nets at a height between shoulder and head. Using more than one hay net can significantly slow hay consumption, e.g. horses consumed 1 kg of hay in 39 min from a single hay net, 67 min/kg hay from a double-layered hay net, and 78 min/kg hay from a triple-layered hay net [29]. Horses offered, during separate weeks, either free-choice hay or a pelleted nutritionally complete ration, spent 62% of their time eating hay but only 10% of the time eating pellets. The remaining time was spent standing or foraging through the bedding (Figure 16.2) [30]. Stabled horses spent 8.5–12 h/d in

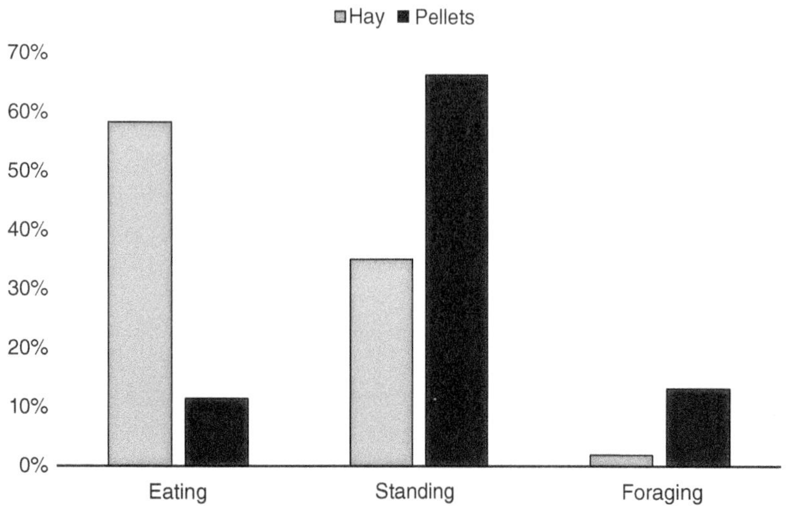

Figure 16.2 Average time spent eating, standing, and foraging within the stall/d by horses (n = 8) fed long-stem hay ad libitum vs. meal-fed pelleted complete ration. *Source:* Adapted from Elia et al. [30].

foraging-related behaviors, e.g. investigating or ingesting wood-shavings and/or feces [31]. Horses bedded on straw, spent 8% of the time eating the straw, whereas horses bedded on wood shaving spent 1% of the time eating the shavings [32]. Additionally, the lack of access to long-stem hay has been associated with behavioral stereotypes, e.g. cribbing, wood chewing, and weaving associated with confined horses [33].

Typically, stalled horses are fed two meals/d, each of which may be consumed in as little as 30 min to four hrs depending on the feed form provided. Extruded forms are eaten more slowly than pellets of the same grain mixture; however, sweet feed intake by horses has been measured at 140–190 g/min (~1/3 lb/min). Mixing the concentrate with chaff, straw, or sawdust will slow the rate of consumption [34]. Horses have preferences for whole grains as measured by single and two-bucket feeding tests (sweet feed > oats > corn > wheat > barley > rye > soybean) (Figure 13.4) and the composition of a grain mix can affect palatability [35–37]. Additionally, there are an array of palatants used in manufactured feed to encourage consumption of concentrates and supplements. See Chapter 13 Manufactured Feeds.

There are significant physiologic changes that occur with feeding large meals, i.e. plasma volume decreases, plasma glucose, and thyroid hormones increase. The meal pattern and physiologic changes associated with feeding are in sharp contrast to the nearly continuous infusion of high-fiber feed that occurs in grazing animals. Changes in circulating blood volume and regional blood flow may account for the digestive disturbances (colic) frequently afflicting stabled horses [22, 38].

16.2.4 Food and Water Intake

Food intake is related to water intake as the lack of one leads to less ingestion of the other. When the water intake of pregnant mares was restricted, they ate less hay, and when ponies were deprived of hay, they drank less water [39, 40]. The amount of water consumed depends on the amount of food consumed and does not vary with the frequency of feeding. Ponies fed one large meal of pellets/d drank the same amount as ponies fed six small meals/d [41]. However, horses fed meals have been observed to commonly drink within two hrs of eating hay [10, 25, 42, 43].

On a lush pasture, horses acquire much of their water needs from grass. When horses were moved from pasture to a stall, they drank 6 L/100 kg BW/d, whereas on pasture, they consumed 2 L/100 kg BW/d [44]. In some environments and some years in many environments, there will be droughts. During a drought, the horses must apportion their time so that they get both water and food. During a severe Australian drought, a herd of feral horses drank at the one remaining water hole every two and half days, walked 12 hrs (15 km) to the remaining grass, ate for a day or two, and then returned to the water [45].

16.2.5 Pica

Pica is the eating of substances with little or no nutritional value, such as dirt, soil, clay, wood, bedding, hair, and feces, which has been observed in horses of all ages, breeds, and genders. Although mineral or vitamin imbalances are often cited as the cause of pica, this is rarely the reason. Nutritionists have found that across most domestic species, including horses, a true and specific appetite exists for only three nutrients: energy, salt, and water. Horses, like other species, do not demonstrate nutrient deficiencies or toxicities as a desire to eat non-food substances, i.e. specific nutrient-seeking behaviors, to rectify dietary imbalances [46, 47].

16.3 Drinking Behavior

Evolutionarily, watering sites were relatively dangerous places with both prey and predator species present at the same time, therefore short periods at water sources favored survival. Additionally, lowering the head, below the horizon, to drink was a vulnerable position for a prey species to maintain. Drinking during daylight in a wide-open place with an unobstructed 360° view of the horizon was less dangerous than in the dark. The less time spent in a defenseless position, i.e. head at ground level, in a perilous place was a survival advantage.

Horses have small stomachs with a limited capacity to take in water at one time and have developed a pattern of effectively consuming water in short bouts, often in less than 30 seconds (sec). The swallow is biphasic with one long draw followed by sips. Some horses may first splash across the top of the water to clear floating debris and scum, and then ingest water by immersing nearly closed lips just below the water surface, some use the tongue to filter out large debris and, with a sucking action, pull the water into the mouth (Figure 16.3) [25, 48]. When water needs increase, water consumption increases mainly as a result of increased frequency of drinking episodes rather than an increased duration of drinking. Leading a horse to water more often, instead of spending more time at the water source, may increase water intake.

Daily patterns of drinking for domesticated horses are dependent on availability, palatability, source, and feeding schedule. The horse, like all animals, consumes more water than needed if palatable water is readily available. See

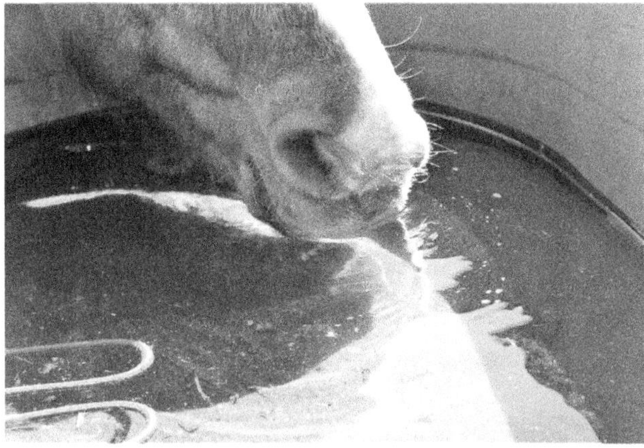

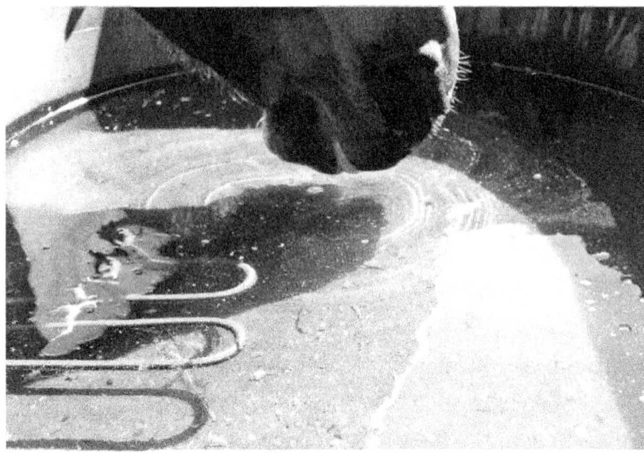

Figure 16.3 Ingesting water through nearly closed lips just below the water surface (top). Some use the tongue between the lips to filter out large debris (bottom).

Water Quality in Chapter 5. The amount of water consumed, however, will decrease to just meet the need if water is not readily accessible or unpalatable. There is a direct correlation between drinking frequency and ambient temperature, with a large increase in frequency at temperatures above 85 °F (30 °C). For example, at ambient temperatures of 85–95 °F (32–35 °C), pastured lactating mares with water readily available drank once every 1.8 hrs whereas, at 40–50 °F (5–10 °C), the same mares drank only once every 3.0 hrs [10].

Present-day, feral bands of horses have been observed to visit water sources early and late during daylight but leave the source soon after drinking. Free-roaming horses several miles from the nearest water source, reportedly return to drink once a day or as little as every other day. Przewalski horses have reportedly drunk as seldom as every two or three days [48]. The ability to tolerate days without drinking is in part due to the large intestine in horses that acts as a reservoir during times of water deprivation [49].

References

1 King, S.R.B. (2002). Home range and habitat use of free-ranging Przewalski horses at Hustai National Park, Mongolia. *Appl. Anim. Behav. Sci.* 78 (2): 103–113.

2 Schwartz, M.W., Woods, S.C., Porte, D. et al. (2000). Central nervous system control of food intake. *Nature* 404 (6778): 661–671.

3 Geor, R.J. (2013). Endocrine and metabolic physiology. In: *Equine Applied and Clinical Nutrition: Health, Welfare and Performance* (ed. R.J. Geor, P.A. Harris, and M. Coenen), 33–63. Edinburgh: Saunders Elsevier.

4 Geor, R.J. and Harris, P.A. (2013). Obesity. In: *Equine Applied and Clinical Nutrition: Health, Welfare and Performance* (ed. R.J. Geor, P.A. Harris, and M. Coenen), 487–502. Edinburgh: Saunders Elsevier.

5 Redgate, S.E., Cooper, J.J., Hall, S. et al. (2014). Dietary experience modifies horses' feeding behavior and selection

patterns of three macronutrient rich diets. *J. Anim. Sci.* 92 (4): 1524–1530.

6 Sweeting, M.P., Houpt, C.E., and Houpt, K.A. (1985). Social facilitation of feeding and time budgets in stabled ponies. *J. Anim. Sci.* 60 (2): 369–374.

7 Holmes, L.N., Song, G.K., and Price, E.O. (1987). Head partitions facilitate feeding by subordinate horses in the presence of dominant pen-mates. *Appl. Anim. Behav. Sci.* 19 (1): 179–182.

8 Houpt, K.A. and Houpt, T.R. (1988). Social and illumination preferences of mares. *J. Anim. Sci.* 66 (9): 2159–2164.

9 Beaver, B. (1983). A day in the life of a horse. *Vet. Med.* 78 (2): 227–228.

10 Crowell-Davis, S.L., Houpt, K.A., and Carnevale, J. (1985). Feeding and drinking behavior of mares and foals with free access to pasture and water. *J. Anim. Sci.* 60 (4): 883–889.

11 Duncan, P. (1980). Time-budgets of Camargue horses II. Time-budgets of adult horses and weaned sub-adults. *Behaviour* 72 (1, 2): 26–48.

12 Berger, J. (1986). *Wild Horses of the Great Basin: Social Competition and Population Size*, 326. Chicago, IL: The University of Chicago Press.

13 Boyd, L.E., Carbonaro, D.A., and Houpt, K.A. (1988). The 24-hour time budget of Przewalski horses. *Appl. Anim. Behav. Sci.* 21 (1): 5–17.

14 Kusunose, R., Hatakeyama, H., Ichikawa, F. et al. (1986). Behavioral studies on yearling horses in field environments 2. Effects of the group size on the behavior of horses. *Bull. Equine Res. Inst.* 1986 (23): 1–6.

15 Kiley-Worthington, M. (1997). *The Behaviour of Horses: in Relation to Management and Training*, 265. London: J. A. Allen.

16 Houpt, K., Houpt, T.R., Johnson, J.L. et al. (2001). The effect of exercise deprivation on the behaviour and physiology of straight stall confined pregnant mares. *Anim. Welf.* 10 (3): 257–267.

17 Keiper, R.R. and Keenan, M.A. (1980). Nocturnal activity patterns of feral ponies. *J. Mammal.* 61 (1): 116–118.

18 Houpt, K.A., O'Connell, M.F., Houpt, T.A., and Carbonaro, D.A. (1986). Night-time behavior of stabled and pastured peri-parturient ponies. *Appl. Anim. Behav. Sci.* 15 (2): 103–111.

19 Edouard, N., Duncan, P., Dumont, B. et al. (2010). Foraging in a heterogeneous environment: an experimental study of the trade-off between intake rate and diet quality. *Appl. Anim. Behav. Sci.* 126 (1, 2): 27–36.

20 McInnis, M.L. and Vavra, M. (1987). Dietary relationships among feral horses, cattle, and pronghorn in southeastern Oregon. *J. Range Manag.* 40: 60–66.

21 Houpt, K.A., Zahorik, D.M., and Swartzman-Andert, J.A. (1990). Taste aversion learning in horses. *J. Anim. Sci.* 68 (8): 2340–2344.

22 Houpt, K.A. (1990). Ingestive behavior. *Vet. Clin. North Am. Equine Pract.* 6 (2): 319–337.

23 van den Berg, M., Brown, W.Y., Lee, C., and Hinch, G.N. (2015). Browse-related behaviors of pastured horses in Australia: a survey. *J. Vet. Behav.* 10 (1): 48–53.

24 Pratt-Phillips, S.E., Stuska, S., Beveridge, H.L., and Yoder, M. (2011). Nutritional quality of forages consumed by feral horses: the horses of Shackleford banks. *J. Equine Vet. Sci.* 31 (11): 640–644.

25 National Research Council (2007). *Nutrient Requirements of Horses*. 6th Rev. Animal Nutrition Series, 1–341. Washington, DC: National Academies Press.

26 Tyler, S.J. (1972). The behaviour and social organization of the new forest ponies. *Anim. Behav. Monogr.* 5 (Jan): 87–196.

27 Moffitt, D.L., Meacham, T., Fontenot, J., et al. (1987). Seasonal differences in apparent digestibilities of fescue and orchardgrass/clover pastures in horses. In: *Proceedings of the 10th Equine Nutrition and Physiology Society Symposium*, 79–85. Fort Collins, CO: Equine Nutrition and Physiology Society.

28 Houpt, K.A. (2006). Mastication and feeding in horses. In: *Feeding in Domestic Vertebrates: From Structure to Behaviour* (ed. V.L. Bels), 195–209. CABI Publishing.

29 Ellis, A.D., Redgate, S., Zinchenko, S. et al. (2015). The effect of presenting forage in multi-layered haynets and at multiple sites on night time budgets of stabled horses. *Appl. Anim. Behav. Sci.* 171 (Oct): 108–116.

30 Elia, J.B., Erb, H.N., and Houpt, K.A. (2010). Motivation for hay: effects of a pelleted diet on behavior and physiology of horses. *Physiol. Behav.* 101 (5): 623–627.

31 Ellis, A.D. (2010). Biological basis of behaviour and feed intake in horses. In: *The Impact of Nutrition on the Health and Welfare of Horses. EAAP 128* (ed. A.D. Ellis, A. Longland, M. Coenen, and N. Miraglia), 53–74. Wageningen: Wageningen Academic Publishers.

32 Greening, L., Shenton, V., Wilcockson, K., and Swanson, J. (2013). Investigating duration of nocturnal ingestive and sleep behaviors of horses bedded on straw versus shavings. *J. Vet. Behav.* 8 (2): 82–86.

33 McGreevy, P.D., Cripps, P.J., French, N.P. et al. (1995). Management factors associated with stereotypic and redirected behaviour in the thoroughbred horse. *Equine Vet. J.* 27 (2): 86–91.

34 Hintz, H.F., Schryver, H.F., Mallette, J., and Houpt, K. (1989). Factors affecting rate of grain intake by horses. *Equine Pract.* 11 (4): 35–42.

35 Houpt, K.A. (1983). Taste preferences in horses. *Equine Pract.* 5 (4): 22–26.

36 van den Berg, M., Giagos, V., Lee, C. et al. (2016). The influence of odour, taste and nutrients on feeding behaviour and food preferences in horses. *Appl. Anim. Behav. Sci.* 184 (Nov): 41–50.
37 Hintz, H.F. (1980). Feed preferences for horses, In: *Proceedings of Cornell Nutrition Conference for Feed Mfg*, Ithaca, NY, 113–116.
38 Youket, R.J., Carnevale, J.M., Houpt, K.A., and Houpt, T.R. (1985). Humoral, hormonal and behavioral correlates of feeding in ponies: the effects of meal frequency. *J. Anim. Sci.* 61 (5): 1103–1110.
39 Houpt, K.A., Eggleston, A., Kunkle, K., and Houpt, T.R. (2000). Effect of water restriction on equine behaviour and physiology. *Equine Vet. J.* 32 (4): 341–344.
40 Norris, M.L., Houpt, K.A., and Houpt, T.R. (2013). Effect of food availability on the physiological responses to water deprivation in ponies. *J. Equine Vet. Sci.* 33 (4): 250–256.
41 Houpt, K.A., Perry, P.J., Hintz, H.F., and Houpt, T.R. (1988). Effect of meal frequency on fluid balance and behavior of ponies. *Physiol. Behav.* 42 (5): 401–407.
42 Pagan, J.D. and Harris, P.A. (1999). The effects of timing and amount of forage and grain on exercise response in thoroughbred horses. *Equine Vet. J.* 31 (S30): 451–457.
43 Jansson, A. and Dahlborn, K. (1999). Effects of feeding frequency and voluntary salt intake on fluid and electrolyte regulation in athletic horses. *J. Appl. Phys.* 86 (5): 1610–1616.
44 Williams, S., Horner, J., Orton, E. et al. (2015). Water intake, faecal output and intestinal motility in horses moved from pasture to a stabled management regime with controlled exercise. *Equine Vet. J.* 47 (1): 96–100.
45 Hampson, B.A., De Laat, M.A., Millis, P.C., and Pollitt, C.C. (2010). Distances travelled by feral horses in "outback" Australia. *Equine Vet. J.* 42 (Suppl. 38): 582–586.
46 Kentucky Equine Research Staff (2012). Pica: the peculiar palate. *EquiNews* https://ker.com/equinews/pica-peculiar-palate (accessed 14 June 2021).
47 Barnes, J.C. (2005). Effect of block and loose forms on ad libitum mineral consumption in equine. M.S. Thesis. Texas A&M University. https://www.proquest.com/openview/8116eb94c34f7feaa9a6d5aa5493f7a5/1?pq-origsite=gscholar&cbl=18750&diss=y (accessed 14 June 2021).
48 Waring GH. Ingestive Behavior: Drinking. In: Horse Behavior. 2nd ed. Norwich, NY: Noyes Publications; 2003. p. 136–8.
49 Sneddon, J.C.C. and Argenzio, R.A.A. (1998). Feeding strategy and water homeostasis in equids: the role of the hind gut. *J. Arid. Environ.* 38 (3): 493–509.

17

Feeding Adult and Senior Horses

Géraldine Blanchard and Nettie R. Liburt

KEY TERMS

- A concentrate feed is a combination of ingredients used to improve the nutritive balance of the total ration, intended to be further diluted and mixed to produce supplement, complementary, or complete feed [1].
  - Energy concentrates may contain small grains and/or fat.
  - Mineral concentrates (supplements) are concentrated refined forms of macrominerals and/or trace minerals.
  - Vitamin concentrates (supplements) are concentrated synthetic forms of vitamins.
  - Protein concentrates contain high-quality proteins and/or specific amino acids.
- Complementary feeds come in a variety of forms, including pellets, extruded nuggets, and/or a coarse mix of grains (textured), concentrates, and fat/oil, providing calories, protein, minerals, and/or vitamins to be fed in addition to forage.
- Ration balancer is generally recognized as a palatable, pelleted meal or block feed containing minerals and vitamins; it may also contain amino acids and/or energy concentrates to provide nutrients lacking in specific forage types (grass vs. legume).
- Complete feed is a nutritionally adequate fiber-enriched (≥12%) product formulated to be fed as the sole ration and capable of maintaining life/production without additional substances, other than water [1].

KEY POINTS

- Forage is the foundation of the ration. A forage intake of at least 1% BW daily is recommended (>10 lbs for 1000 lb horse).
- Maintenance horses are open (not pregnant, not lactating) mares and geldings >5-yr-old, not in active work or training or performance. Many adult horses do not work regularly or have been retired from performance activities and are kept as companion animals.
- Some aged horses, in the last third of their expected life span, can and do still work and are in regular use.
- Aging is an irreversible, progressive, time-dependent decline of overall body functions as a result of genetic and environmental factors.
- Aging is not a disease but rather a process on a continuum where the rate of age-related changes is unique to the individual horse.

17.1 Introduction

The horse, as a domesticated species originally used as a means of travel and working the land, has progressively become a companion animal, similar to the dog and cat, in affluent Western societies. In a 2007 survey from almost 50 thousand USA households, 38% of horse owners considered their horses to be family members, and 56% considered them to be a pet or companion. Similarly, 47% of respondents in the Netherlands indicated that horses were like a "partner or child" to them [2, 3]. In Australian and UK surveys of horses ≥15 yrs, approximately 60% of the horses were used for leisure riding, whereas 30–40% of the horses were retired or kept as a pasture pet [4].

Equine Clinical Nutrition, Second Edition. Edited by Rebecca L. Remillard.

The nutritional needs of adult horses are dependent on a myriad of factors, that is, genetics, activity level, health status, and environment/housing, each of which needs to be taken into consideration when designing an appropriate diet. Two horses living in the same environment may likely have different sets of nutritional needs, thus one ration for the barn or farm is unlikely to be appropriate for all adult horses. There is no specific age at which a horse is considered "senior," as the course of aging is influenced by both inborn genetic programs and environmental factors. However, by age 20 yrs, there are typically physiological changes associated with the aging process that may or may not be outwardly noticeable by the caretaker. Thus, it is critical to consider a horse's individual needs when designing a proper diet. When nutritional or diet-related problems arise, a systematic iterative review of the horse, the ration, and the feeding method is recommended. See Appendix C Nutrition Competencies of Equine Veterinarians.

17.2 Animal Assessment

Horses in the physiological state of maintenance, requiring daily energy intake sufficient to maintain current body weight (BW) and body condition score (BCS), are open (not pregnant, not lactating) mares and geldings (castrated stallions) more than 5 years old, not in regular active work or training or performance. Horses, having only maintenance nutritional needs, owned as pets, or for light recreational activities, comprise the majority of the total captive equine USA population. Given the BW of horses at maintenance ranges from 200 to 900 kg, the recommended daily nutrient intakes are presented in Table 17.1 per 100 kg of mature BW, regardless of age, as there are some indications that the macronutrient requirements do not vary with age [5–7]. See Appendix E Average Body Weight and Height of Horses.

Table 17.1 Recommended daily nutrient intakes for mature horses at maintenance per 100 kg of body weight regardless of age.

Nutrient		Adult maintenance		
		Temperament or voluntary activity		
	Units	Minimum	Average	Elevated
Digestible energy	Mcal	3.04	3.34[a]	3.64
Crude protein	g	108	126	144
Lysine	g	4.6	5.4	6.2
Calcium	g	4.0	4.0	4.0
Phosphorus	g	2.8	2.8	2.8
Magnesium	g	1.5	1.5	1.5
Potassium	g	5.0	5.0	5.0
Sodium	g	2.0	2.0	2.0
Chloride	g	8.0	8.0	8.0
Sulfur	g	3.0	3.0	3.0
Copper	mg	20	20	20
Iron	mg	80	80	80
Manganese	mg	80	80	80
Zinc	mg	80	80	80
Cobalt	mg	0.1	0.1	0.1
Iodine	mg	0.7	0.7	0.7
Selenium	mg	0.2	0.2	0.2
Vitamin A	KIU	3	3	3
Vitamin D	IU	660	660	660
Vitamin E	IU	100	100	100
Thiamine	mg	6	6	6
Riboflavin	mg	4	4	4

[a] For example, a 650 kg adult horse with average temperament would require $3.34 \times 6.5 = 21.71$ Mcal DE/d.

Source: Adapted from NRC [5]; Table 16-3 using nutrients required for a 500 kg mature horse with BCS 4–6/9 consuming 2% BW.

17.2.1 Body Condition Score

Horses should be fed to maintain a BCS of 4/9 (moderately thin) to 6/9 (moderately fleshy); however, both over and under ideal weights are prevalent problems in adult horses [8, 9]. See Body Condition Scoring in Chapter 2. An adult non-working horse (5 to 20-yr-old) kept as a companion animal, that is, a pet, if improperly fed grain concentrates, or allowed unlimited access to pastures, is likely to be overweight or obese (BCS >6/9). There is substantial evidence that being overweight/obese is deleterious. Of the comorbidities associated with obesity, insulin resistance may be of most importance to the adult horse [10–12]. See Chapter 28 Metabolic Syndrome. Conversely, for horses with an orthopedic condition, musculoskeletal injury, or other conditions limiting mobility, a BCS of 4/9 is recommended for comfort.

In horses ≥15-yr-old, 28% of owners reported weight loss (BCS <3/9) as an important health issue and was the second most common reason for euthanasia [4, 13]. Therefore, routine physical assessments are recommended for the adult maintenance horse based on history, activity level, and feeding management. The assessment frequency is case-dependent in that an active 10-yr-old mare with a history of having an ideal BW and BCS for years may need only be assessed twice a year, whereas a 20-yr-old mare with an elevated temperament and history of poor dental care and feed intake may need to be assessed monthly until stabilized. See Chapter 2 Nutritional Assessment of the Horse and Chapter 23 Weight Management.

17.2.2 Temperament

Within the realm of mature, non-working horses, there is a recognition that there is a range of natural instinctive behaviors that affect energy requirements, for example, voluntary activity, alertness, and reactionary movements. Body mass explains 95% of the variation in the resting energy requirement observed across all mammalian species; however, within a species, the variation due to body mass is small (20%) [14]. Within a species, individual personality differences may explain the variation in resting energy required for weight maintenance [15].

Similarly, different personalities of horses may explain the variation in the energy required to maintain BW in the absence of work, growth, or reproduction. The basis for these behaviors affecting digestible energy for maintenance (DE_m) is that activity, exploration, alertness, and reactions cost energy to perform. As a result, there are different daily energy intakes based on the adult horse's temperament, lifestyle, or extent of voluntary activity [5]. The maintenance energy need for horses that are sedentary, docile, often confined to a small area (stalled), have a non-reactive temperament, or have low voluntary activity even in a large area, often termed easy keepers or left-brained, is considered to have a minimal DE_m (3.04 Mcal/100 kg BW) (Table 17.1). The DE_m for horses with an attentive but calm temperament and moderate voluntary activity relative to that of a sedentary horse is considered to be average (3.34 Mcal/100 kg BW). Whereas horses most reactive, with an alert nervous temperament and high levels of voluntary activity, regardless of the area available, often termed hard keepers or right-brained, have an elevated DE_m (3.64 Mcal/100 kg BW).

17.2.3 Environment

Climate, seasonal and daily weather, that is, temperature, humidity, wind, and exposure to sun, rain, snow, and ice directly increase the DE_m requirement of horses. Housing or the availability of shelter, shade, and ponds can mitigate that rise in energy requirement. Consistently providing access to dry feed (with particular attention to forage), clean water, and salt supplements requires attention to feeding management protocols as each is affected by adverse weather conditions (heat, cold, wind, mud, rain, snow, ice and combinations). See Cold Weather Care and Hot Weather Care in Chapter 6.

17.2.4 Aging

The point in time at which aging begins, as a process, is still debated among biodemographers, that is, before birth, after birth vs. after puberty; however, most agree that aging begins after the natural longevity of a species, which is 40–50 yrs in humans [16, 17]. The essential life span of horses has not been suggested. Chronological age refers to the number of years the horse has lived. Expected longevity in horses however is 30 yrs with some reported to live into their 40s or even longer [18, 19]. In 2015, approximately 11.5% of horses in the USA were over the age of 20 yrs, compared to 7.4% in 1998, which has been accredited to improvements in preventative health care, disease diagnostics, and the willingness of owners to provide for a horse in later years [20]. The average age of death in feral horses was reported to be 7–8 yrs in the Nevada Great Basin Desert [21]. Death at a younger age in feral, relative to domesticated, horses due to injury, starvation, dehydration, disease, and predation is understandable. However, Assateague ponies die of natural causes at about 20 yrs of age, and a few sold at auction as foals maintained as domesticated horses have lived longer than 30 yrs [22]. Although horses tend to be retired and cared for well past 20 yrs of age, horses over 16.5 yrs of age are less likely to be purchased [18].

There is no specific age at which a horse is considered "old" or a "senior" because there is considerable variation between individuals in the physiologic changes of aging, although 20 yrs is the common chronological benchmark and may be the natural longevity of horses [23–26]. A 20-yr-old horse is approximately equivalent to a 60-yr-old person having completed 65–70% of their expected natural life span. As witnessed in other species with a large range in mature BW, for example, canines, smaller individuals may live longer than larger cohorts in that pony breeds are significantly overrepresented in the ≥30-yrs-of-age group [25]. The gastrointestinal (colic), musculoskeletal (lameness), and respiratory tract problems were most frequently reported within a population of ≥20-yr-old horses [25, 26], whereas conditions commonly attributed to the cause of death in ≥20-yr-old horses were colic (13.4%), cancer (13.2%), neurologic conditions (12.1%), and chronic weight loss (11.7%) [20]. The most common (26.6%) cause of death was cited as "other," an unspecified condition but attributable to being of old age.

Feeding horses over a lifetime requires the understanding that aging is not a disease but rather a process on a continuum. The rate of age-related changes is unique to the individual horse based on genetics and environment, that is, stochastic factors. Aging is the progressive loss of redundant tissues and metabolic processes, that is, loss of capacity to withstand an insult or injury, which then increases the susceptibility of the animal to disease and risk of death [27]. For large complex biological organisms, such as mammals, the rate of aging is different not only within the organs and tissues of an individual but also between animals exposed to the same environment [27]. Therefore, horses, as they age like other species, become more susceptible, or less resistant, to immunological challenges, and have decreased tissue function but these changes are not a disease process as such. Aging, as the loss of capacity, is not linear with time as individuals experiencing severe illness or trauma early in life may outwardly recover but have a loss of capacity, or decreased resiliency, to deal with future insults. An animal surviving an injury or disease process may not have the same reserve capacity as a healthy herd mate. Recognition and understanding of aging may warrant nutritional or dietary modifications based on medical history and the clinical expression of age-related changes, and should not necessarily be related to a specific year of age. See Sidebar 17.1.

There are naturally occurring physical characteristics commonly related to increasing age in horses (Table 17.2). Common outward signs of aging, which for most horses become increasingly noticeable after 20 yrs of age, include: graying of the hair, particularly around the eyes, temples, and nostrils; increased sinking of the hollows above the eyes; a swayback, increased prominence of the backbone and poll; sometimes drooping of the lower lip; and changes in the teeth showing wear. There is a reduced ability to regulate body temperature outside of the thermoneutral zone (TNZ) and during exercise with aging [41]. Muscles and joints lose

Sidebar 17.1: Aging is a Loss of Resilience, and not a Disease

Aging is understood as a progressive time-dependent decline of overall body functions occurring in every individual and cannot be considered a disease. Considering aging as a disease implies the condition can be reversed with treatment or prevented, which is not true [16]. Biological aging begins after the natural or essential life span, for example, mutations in mitochondrial DNA (mtDNA) are known to occur in people after their fourth decade [27]. Aging at the cellular level is the progressive accumulation of molecular damage caused by: (i) ROS formed as a result of external factors (UV rays, chemical agents) and internal sources involving oxygen and metals; (ii) nutritional metabolites, such as amino acid modifications, misincorporation and misfolding of proteins, lipid peroxidation, and advanced glycation end products from carbohydrates, and (iii) spontaneous errors in nuclear and mtDNA, such as mutations, base modifications or deletions, and the miscoding of RNA [28].

ROS damage to mitochondrial proteins, lipids, and DNA leads to the loss of function, decreased energy production, and the subsequent clinical expression of aging [29]. The number of skeletal muscle mitochondria is decreased in sarcopenia with the loss of strength, decreased metabolic rate, and aerobic capacity [30]. Peroxidation within the lipid membrane of cells alters membrane fluidity, permeability, and function. Damage to mtDNA may have greater implications than damaged proteins and lipids because mitochondria propagate as cells divide and therefore errors persist and may be amplified.

Repair to damaged cellular proteins, nucleic acids, and lipid macromolecules occurs through biological maintenance and repair systems (MRSs), that is, antioxidant nutrients handling of free radicals, or repair of nuclear and mtDNA damage. [16]. Therefore, the survival of an organism depends on the balance between the occurrence of cellular damage and a functioning MRS. Damage to MRS itself leads to increased cellular dysfunctions, reduced tolerance to stress and diseases, and ultimately, death [31]. Decreased functioning of the MRS to control cellular damage and remodel leads to increased vulnerability and increased probabilities of age-related diseases. An organism's resiliency to withstand external and internal sources of cellular damage, therefore, depends on the MRS, which in turn depends on dietary sources of energy and, at the very least, essential nutrients (amino acids, minerals, and vitamins). The current thinking of gerontologists is that aging is not a disease, but a condition that allows for the emergence of one or more diseases.

Table 17.2 Major changes observed in the older horse and practical consequences.

Changes in the aging horse		Practical dietary considerations
Teeth and dentition	Erosion and irregularities of the dental arcade [32]	Provide wet/cooked foods and easily chewable foods; avoid whole and hard grains
Digestive tract	Decreased microbial diversity [33] Specific parasitism [34]	Offer easily digestible foods (cooked starch, flakes rather than whole grains), maintain the intake of fiber, salt, minerals, and water-soluble vitamins. Adopt deworming program
Hair coat	More frequent dry hair and dermatitis, and white hairs	Provide supplemental fat high in essential fatty acids (e.g. oil), vitamins, and trace minerals. Favor forages at the expense of cereals. Supply with biotin if hoof horn is impaired
Respiratory system	Chronic emphysema, chronic obstructive pulmonary disease	Avoid dusty foods, wet or soak forage, and higher energy concentrate. House outdoors if possible
Muscle mass	Loss of muscle mass	Supply of easily digestible, high-quality proteins and review dietary amino acid profile. Maintain light regular physical activity
Musculoskeletal system	Osteoarthritis, weakness, lameness, increased risk of laminitis	Feed for the optimal desired weight, not the actual weight if overweight or underweight. Maintain light regular physical activity
Endocrine system	pituitary pars intermedia dysfunction, weight loss, insulin dysregulation, laminitis, increased susceptibility to infections [35]	Decrease sugar and starch intake. Soak and prioritize forage + oil energy sources, split concentrates feedings into several meals/d. Supply of vitamins and trace minerals
Immune function	Increased sensitivity to infections, decreased acquired immune response [36–38]	Feed high-quality proteins, vitamins, trace elements, and prebiotics
Reproduction	Poor reproductive efficiency [39]; Pathology more frequent (uterine artery rupture and hemorrhages) [40]	Monitor BCS and feed intake, and adjust as needed for 4/9–5/9 BCS. Increased frequency of medical examines

elasticity with age requiring a longer warm-up period before working. Exercise capacity decreases, recovery time increases, and there is a natural change in the endocrine system, some of which can be mitigated by maintaining a light training program [41–44]. For some horses, maintaining weight and/or muscle tone requires specific dietary modifications, e.g. increased caloric density and/or higher quality protein. Recent research has also suggested a decrease in microbial diversity in the hindgut with aging [33].

Despite clear outward signs of aging, some well-cared-for horses over 20, and even 25, yrs of age continue to be actively ridden and worked, and both mares and stallions can reproduce [18, 41, 45]. Although their physical performance ability has slowed, many are ideal starter horses. Old horses, particularly those still working or at least in regular use, are truly wonderful creatures, and will patiently educate the inexperienced person. This, and the attachment people develop for them through the years, makes many older horses one of the most valued in many stables, ranches, and farms.

17.2.4.1 Dentition

Healthy teeth are important for chewing and grinding food. Horses normally have a "full mouth" of permanent teeth, 12 incisors, 12 premolars, and 12 molars by the age of 5 yrs. Male horses may also have 4 additional canine teeth in the interdental space that are rarely present in mares. See Figure 3.2. Horses evolved with hypsodont teeth, meaning the teeth continue to erupt from the gum after forming in the jaw. See Sidebar 1.4.

Teeth wear naturally from daily chewing of forages, but if wear is abnormal, hooks, points, oral ulcers, and tongue lesions may arise. The prevalence of dental abnormalities in adult equines has been reported to be 10–80%, depending on the population studied [46–48]. Signs a horse is having difficulty chewing food include quidding of forage, that is, hay falls out of the mouth in the shape of a ball or rod, halitosis, feed packing in cheeks, long pieces (>3.7 mm) of fiber in the manure, weight loss, and history of choke [49, 50]. Correction of dental abnormalities, however, may not improve digestion and absorption of nutrients, body condition, or weight in horses that were in good body condition before the procedure was performed, regardless of the type of ration fed [47, 51, 52].

Regular dental examinations throughout a horse's lifetime can help minimize problems associated with aging teeth. It is recommended that examination and correction of dental abnormalities should be done annually. Horses with severe dental abnormalities (missing incisors, molars, premolars, wave mouth, severe malocclusions) can maintain good body condition if fed a balanced ration using feeds and delivered in a manner appropriate for their specific limitations. See Case in Point in Chapter 3.

17.2.4.2 Digestion and Absorption

It may have been a long-held belief that as horses age, diets needed to be more heavily fortified to make up for losses in digestive efficiency; however, the digestibility of macronutrients in three different rations fed to healthy >15-yr-old vs. <15-yr-old horses was not different [53, 54]. Healthy senior horses may not experience declines in digestibility with aging, but those with medical or physical conditions are at risk for impaired nutrient absorption. A soft, water-soaked ration that meets all nutritional requirements without having to chew is helpful when mastication and swallowing have been compromised. Horses with chronic parasite problems may have decreased digestion and absorption of nutrients due to scarred intestinal tissue [5]. Horses with compromised liver function may have difficulty synthesizing a sufficient supply of vitamin C and endogenous proteins, and declining kidney function may impair the elimination of nitrogen. For these reasons, regular veterinary examinations are essential for detecting changes to health as the horse ages, and helpful dietary and nutritional changes can be implemented before weight loss and poor BCS are clinically apparent.

17.3 Ration Assessment

Ration digestible energy (DE) concentrations of 1.5–1.8 Mcal DE/kg dry matter (DM) are suitable for adult horses intended to maintain a BW and BCS (4/9–6/9) (Table 17.3). Adult non-working mares and geldings should be provided a complete and balanced ration, meeting the energy and nutrient requirements fed within 1.5–2.0% BW dry matter intake (DMI).

17.3.1 Feeds

17.3.1.1 Forage

Forage (pasture or hay) should provide the preponderance (>60%) of the adult horse ration. Forage quality is assessed objectively using laboratory nutrient analyses, and subjectively through the assessment of smell, color, feel, and physical contents. See Ration Analysis and Subjective Assessments in Chapter 10. The forage offered must be palatable to the horse to ensure an adequate DMI [57]. The forage digestible dry matter (DDM) and energy density (Mcal/kg DM) must be sufficient to meet the estimated daily energy requirement (DER) within an edible volume of feed (DMI). DDM and voluntary DMI are inversely related to the forage acid detergent fiber (%ADF) and neutral detergent fiber (%NDF), respectively. As ADF and NDF increase in the forage DM, the voluntary DMI and DM digestibility decrease, and the nutritional value of the forage decreases. Forages with less than 45% ADF and 65% NDF are recommended for adult horses unless weight loss is desirable. Forage with relative feeding values (RFVs) of 85–115 is recommended for adult horses at maintenance [5, 55]. See Relative Feed Value in Chapter 10. In cases where the available forage energy density is insufficient to meet the horse's nutrient requirement within the voluntary DMI, an energy concentrate can be fed to provide the difference between the animal requirement and that provided by forage alone [58].

Horses evolved consuming small amounts of forage frequently, and therefore forage should be fed at a rate no less than 1% of ideal BW on a DM basis [5]. Most forage types, grass or legume, as pasture or hay provide sufficient energy, protein, calcium, phosphorus, and essential fatty acids for the adult horse at maintenance (Table 17.3). Legumes are generally higher in energy, protein, and calcium content compared to grass species. Examples of common grass varieties, as hay or pasture, are timothy, bromegrass, orchard grass, canary grass, Bermuda grass, ryegrass, fescue, and teff, whereas the most common legume hay fed to horses is alfalfa. See Chapter 11 Forages. It is not common to graze an all-legume pasture, but most (42%) of the hay harvested in the USA is alfalfa or an alfalfa–grass mixture.[1] Mixtures of hay that are predominately legume are known as "mixed mainly legume" (MML), whereas mixtures comprising mostly grass are known as "mixed mainly grass" (MMG). The nutritional content of the mixture will reflect the relative proportions of each forage type, that is, MML will typically have a higher protein and calcium content compared with MMG.

Within a species of forage, the single most important factor affecting forage quality is the stage of growth (maturity) at the time of harvest as hay or pasture. Poor-quality forages of low nutritional value RFV <85 are of limited benefit to the horse [59]. Most horses will generally consume more legume than grass hay if offered both, even if the legume hay is of lower quality [60]. For equal-quality grass hays, preference based on consumption in descending order was: timothy > bromegrass, canary grass, and orchard grass > fescue and Bermuda grass. Bahiagrass appears to be

1 US Dept. of Agriculture stats. https://quickstats.nass.usda.gov/ results/ 2AD59A92-C025-30B6-A573-01141AC51636 (accessed 20 May 2022)

Table 17.3 Comparison of major nutrient concentrations between forage averages and rations for adult horses at maintenance. [5, 55, 56].

Horse to Forage Comparison	Digestible energy	Protein	Calcium	Phosphorus	DMI	RFV
	Dry matter basis				% BW	
Temperament:	Mcal/kg	%	%	%		
Minimum	1.52	5.40	0.20	0.14	2.0	85–115
Average	1.67	6.30	0.20	0.14	2.0	
Elevated	1.82	7.20	0.20	0.14	2.0	
Forages:						
Legume						
Pasture: vegetative	2.71	26.5	1.31	0.37	3.6[a]	197[b]
Hay: immature	2.62	20.5	1.56	0.31	3.3	171
Hay: mid-mature	2.43	20.8	1.37	0.30	2.8	136
Hay: mature	2.21	17.8	1.22	0.28	2.4	106
Grass						
Pasture: vegetative	2.39	26.5	0.56	0.44	2.6	141
Hay: immature	2.36	18.0	0.72	0.34	2.4	121
Hay: mid-mature	2.18	13.3	0.66	0.29	2.1	97
Hay: mature	2.04	10.8	0.47	0.26	1.7	76

[a] Forage %DMI = 120/%NDF.
[b] Forage relative feeding value = %DDM × %DMI × 0.775, where %DDM = 88.9 − (0.779 × %ADF).
Source: Adapted from NRC [5]; Table 16-3 using nutrients required for a 500 kg mature horse BCS 4–6/9. Forage data from Table 16-6.

the least palatable of hays, is of low nutritional value to horses, and is not recommended [61]. Within the same grass or legume hay, the amount consumed was directly related to hay quality [60]. Although feeding adequate to good-quality hay is recommended, if the only feed available is weathered, nutritionally deficient hay with a low leaf-to-stem ratio with (non-toxic) weeds, feeding *ad libitum*, is an option because horses will sort through the bale and eat the better portions. However difficult the situation, moldy or dusty hay should not be fed, instead, an alternative solution using a bagged, pelleted, chopped, or cubed commercial forage is recommended.

The appearance, feel, and smell of hay are the most common and practical means of determining the presence of mold, dust, weeds, and other undesirable foreign materials such as metal, plastic, or trash. Mold may grow on hay at moisture concentrations of 15% or more which can occur when the hay has not dried sufficiently before baling [62]. The hay will smell musty, contain black areas that feel damp and warm, and may have a plume of white-talcum-like powder (fungal spores) when moved. Molds commonly found in hay include *Alternaria*, *Aspergillus*, *Cladosporium*, *Fusarium*, *Mucor*, *Penicillium*, and *Rhizopus* [63]. These molds produce spores that cause respiratory problems in horses and indicate the possible presence of a mycotoxin. If uncertain, hay may be tested for mold and quantitated. Safe upper limits of mold, bacteria, and yeast in hay have been suggested depending on the species [64]. Moldy hay causes recurrent airway obstruction, a chronic, inducible, inflammatory lung disease, in mature horses [65, 66]. Such hay will likely be refused by the horse reducing DMI and nutrient intakes, and, eventually, weight loss.

Most commonly square baled hay (40–80 lb; approximately \$0.25/lb) is fed to horses because the size is convenient to handle, store, and feed out as flakes. Hay sold as a compressed flaked bale (50–55 lb; approximately \$0.60/lb) has been compacted, bagged, banded, or shrink-wrapped, and may have a guaranteed analysis. Large round baled hay (600–1000 lb; approximately \$0.06/lb)[2] is used in feeding a large number of horses; however, proper equipment is needed to move the bales, and large storage areas and covered feeders are needed to keep the hay contained and to control spoilage [56]. Alternative forms of forage can fill an important need in the equine diet under various circumstances. Alternative forms include cubed, chopped, or pelleted hay, beet pulp, and much less so in the USA, silage, and haylage.

Hay cubes are typically (2 × 2 in.) made of coarsely chopped grass, legume, or mixed hay, and sold in bags with

2 Relative cost of the various forms of hay Jan 2023. Small shrink-wrapped compressed bales cost about 10 x/lb than large round baled hay.

nutrient composition guarantees [56]. Hay cubes are easy to store, handle, and minimize wastage. The cubes are usually hard and horses with normal dentition learn to chew, and not to gulp, the cubes. Chopped hay has been mechanically cut to 1-in. lengths and compressed into a bag with nutrient composition guarantees. A variety of forage types (grass, alfalfa, or a mix) are available and can be mixed with a grain concentrate that allows for easy adjustment of the forage to concentrate ratio when needed without changing the feedstuffs. Pelleted hay is available in a variety of pellet sizes and forage types; however, the fine grind and small particle size within the pellet increases the rate of digesta passage, does not provide adequate satiety, and horses consume more total feed when fed a pelleted forage [56]. Feeding pellets can be a portion of the forage ration, should not be the sole form of forage, and feeding at least 1% BW in long-stem hay is recommended.

Beet pulp (approximately $0.60/lb) is a secondary or by-product of the sugar beet industry and is the dried fibrous material that remains after most of the sugar has been removed. Beet pulp is a >65% digestible fiber (27% ADF, 45% NDF, RFV 140) source and an excellent source of volatile fatty acid energy (2.33 Mcal DE/kg DM). For these reasons, beet pulp is a good addition to a forage ration for a horse needing to gain weight or a higher DE concentration to maintain BW. Beet pulp lacks vitamins, is high in calcium, and is low in other minerals, so the ration will likely require a mineral–vitamin supplement to be nutritionally balanced.

Forage as cubes, chopped or pelleted hays (approximately $0.40/lb), or beet pulp can provide a consistent and convenient source of forage for horses while traveling, or as an adjunct to poor-quality pasture or long-stem hay. For older horses with poor dentition, forage alternatives provide a variety of convenient options when soaking in water before feeding is necessary. The nutrient balance of a forage-based ration should be checked and perfected with mineral, vitamin, and protein supplementation if needed.

17.3.1.2 Complementary Feeds

Concentrates are a feed product used to improve the nutritive balance of the total ration. The proper amount to feed initially could be based on a ration formulation or commercial manufacturer's recommendations and then adjusted as necessary to maintain a proper body condition for that individual horse.

Energy concentrates, containing small grains, that is, corn, oats, and barley, are a concentrated form of energy and low in fiber compared with forages. Mineral concentrates (supplements) contain macrominerals and/or trace minerals, whereas vitamin concentrates (supplements) contain fat and water-soluble vitamins to be used as needed to complement the forage portion of the ration. "Straight" grains, such as corn, oats, barley, and wheat, are excellent energy sources for horses, but do not have a full complement of vitamins and minerals, and many have more phosphorus than calcium, that is, creating an inverse calcium to phosphorus ratio. Combinations of two or more concentrates may be needed to complete the nutrient profile of the forage ration. Low intakes of forage with high intakes of concentrate increase the risk of colic, gastric ulcers, behavioral issues, and hindgut acidosis. The concentrates added to the ration should be reverse-engineered to meet the horse's daily nutrient requirements based on the analysis of the forage.

Ration balancer products are palatable commercially pelleted combinations of nutrients designed to complement a forage ration. Some contain high-quality protein sources providing essential amino acids, while others contain only minerals and vitamins. See Sidebar 17.2. Such products do not have one universal nutrient profile, although most contain some minerals and vitamins. Products marketed as a "ration balancer" generally contain 1-3 Mcal DE/kg and typically are low in sugar, starch, and fat. These products should be selected based on the forage type (grass vs. legume) used in the ration. Many adult horses at maintenance, light work, or low temperaments survive well on pasture with no supplemental energy concentrates. However, the nutritional value of pasture changes by the season and with forage type and species. Harvested hay stored under proper conditions can maintain sufficient energy, protein, and mineral content for 2–3 yrs; however, vitamins are lost within weeks of storage. For these reasons, it is recommended that mature horses be provided, at least, a commercial source of trace minerals and vitamins A and E consistently year-round. For working and reproducing horses, forage alone may not provide sufficient calories, protein, vitamins, and minerals to meet daily needs;

Sidebar 17.2: Comparison of 3 Ration Balancer Products

There is not one nutrient profile for products called "ration balancers," although most contain some macrominerals and microminerals and vitamins. For example, product A contains more protein and calories than products B or C. Product B, high in phosphorus, low in calcium (inverse Ca:P ratio), is designed to be fed with legume forages inherently high in calcium such as alfalfa. Product C with a balanced Ca:P ratio is intended to be fed with grass forages. A ration balancer product should be selected specifically to balance the forage and fed based on a ration formulation or at the manufacturer's recommended dose. Feeding less may result in deficiencies and feeding more may result in excessive intakes and increase cost.

Ration balancer product comparison[a]		**Product A**[b]	**Product B**[c]	**Product C**[e]
Supplement marketing descriptor		**Vitamins and minerals (*with protein*)**	**Vitamins and minerals to be fed w/alfalfa**	**Vitamins and minerals to be fed w/grass**
Recommended feeding rate for 454 kg BW		1.0–1.5 lb	3 oz	3 oz
Cost/d for 454 kg BW		$0.80–1.20	$0.25	$0.25
Macronutrients:	Units		as fed	
Crude protein	%	30	11	11
Crude fat	%	3	6*	11*
Crude fiber	%	5	9.5	11.5
Acid detergent fiber	%	7	11*	14*
Neutral detergent fiber	%	13	15*	16*
Non-structural CHO	%	9.8	8*	8.7*
Caloric density	Mcal/kg	2.78	1.51*	1.63*
Amino acids:				
Lysine	%	2.0	1.0	1.1
Methionine	%	0.62	1.3	1.3
Threonine	%	1.35		
Tryptophan	%	0.44		
Leucine	%	2.25		
Macrominerals:				
Calcium	%	4	1.1*	6.05*
Phosphorus	%	1.5	6.9*	2.98*
Ca:P		3:1	0.2:1	2:1
Magnesium	%	2.4	2.9	2.9
Salt (NaCl)	%	1.5	2.8	2.8
Microminerals:				
Selenium	ppm	3.4	12	12
Zinc	ppm	1000	4400	4400
Manganese	ppm	575	1818	1818
Cobalt	ppm	2.1	18	18
Copper	ppm	300	1349	1349
Iodine	ppm		23	23
Iron	ppm	500	1170*	1221*
Vitamins:				
Vitamin A	IU/lb	36 000	80 000	80 000
Vitamin D3	IU/lb	6000	13 334	13 334
Vitamin E	IU/lb	1000	2666	2666
Thiamine	mg/lb	42	1067	1067
Riboflavin	mg/lb	16	853	853

[a]Data from label or web site.
[b]Triple Crown Balancer. http://triplecrownfeed.com. (accessed 26 July 2021). First ingredient: soybean provides protein and essential amino acids.
[c]Select Alfalfa. http://selectthebest.com. (accessed 26 July 2021). First ingredients: ammonium phosphate and rice bran provide phosphorus for Ca:P ratio.
[d]Select Grass. http://selectthebest.com. (accessed 26 July 2021). Second and third ingredients: alfalfa meal and calcium carbonate provide calcium for Ca>P.
*Data based on laboratory analysis Aug 2021. Blanks are missing data and should not be assumed to be zero.

therefore, an appropriate energy–mineral–vitamin ration balancer with a high-quality protein source, for example, soybean, should be fed.

Complementary feed products sold as "senior" feeds combine grains, micronutrient concentrates, and a high-quality protein source, for example, soybean providing 12–16% protein, and oils providing 4–7% fat for older horses. The grains are ground or cooked to improve small intestinal starch digestion for low BW horses with dental disease. Many senior feed products intended as the sole source of feed contain >12% crude fiber with a recommended feeding rate of 2.0% BW divided into 4 meals/d [49].

17.3.2 Key Nutrients

17.3.2.1 Water

At all times, adequate quantities of good-quality palatable water should be readily available. Whether the horse drinks before or after feeding does not affect feed digestibility, but consuming water does affect feed intake. Horses deprived of water will reduce feed intake, and horses deprived of feed will reduce water intake. The average daily water requirement of healthy adult horses is approximately 5 L/100 kg BW/d of which 85% is from drinking water [67]. The importance of checking the functionality of automatic waterers or refilling two 5-gallon water buckets at least twice a day per horse cannot be understated as important. See Chapter 5 Water.

17.3.2.2 Energy

The energy cost of first and foremost maintaining body tissues and function is the maintenance energy requirement (MER). For a horse at maintenance (not growing, working, or reproducing), the MER equals the DER (Table 17.1). The best indicators of energy balance in the body are BW, BCS, and trends over time. Initial estimates of the DER for mature horses, when a diet and weight history are unavailable, is likely 3.04–3.64 Mcal DE/100 kg BW depending upon temperament. The BW and BCS should be assessed at reasonable intervals and, per the iterative process, repeated at regular intervals particularly if changes to the feed or feeding protocol were made to address a problem. Most adult horses derive DE from the fermentation of the forage fiber content. Forage has very little fat and, although the concentrations of sugar and starch are variable across forages, there is relatively less in forage than in grains.

17.3.2.2.1 Fat

Fats are sources of energy, essential fatty acids, and carriers of fat-soluble vitamins. Dietary fats, often using oil, are used to increase the energy density of equine rations. Increasing dietary fat concentration increases ration energy density, which in turn decreases the amount of feed needed to meet DER. Ration caloric density is increased for athletic performance, milk production, reproductive efficiency, growth, and to maintain or increase BW during hot humid weather. Adding fat to the ration of maintenance adult horses is rarely needed. However, adding fat in the form of vegetable oil can substantially increase the caloric density of a ration with a minimal increase in food volume for aged low BCS horses. One cup (224 g/d) provides approximately 2.0 Mcal DE which would be a 12% increase in caloric intake for an adult 454 kg horse. The addition of 1–2 cups of oil to the ration must be titrated over several weeks to avoid steatorrhea.

Both linoleic acid (LA; 18:2 n-6) and α-linolenic acid (ALA; 18:3 n-3) are essential fatty acids in mammals. Although ponies fed diets containing 0.03% linoleic acid for 7 m showed no ill effects, a dietary minimum of 0.5% DM has been suggested, which is relatively easy to meet with ≤1% fat in the ration [5]. The forage portion of the ration of horses provides primarily ALA. There are no dietary omega-3 fatty acid recommendations, but dietary fatty acid content does affect circulating and cellular fatty acid profiles in horses [68]. Oils are used to increase the fat content of feeds and generally contain no biologically useful vitamins or minerals, but dietary fat is necessary for the intestinal absorption of vitamins A, D, E, and K. Fat is calorically dense (9 kcal/g), but does not elicit an insulin response and is therefore used to increase caloric intake in carbohydrate-sensitive animals. See Chapter 27 Endocrine System Disorders.

17.3.2.3 Protein

Estimate of the maintenance crude protein (CP) requirement for adult non-working horses is 1.08–1.44 g CP/100 kg BW/d depending on DER (Table 17.1) on the assumption that more active horses have more lean mass to support. Lysine is considered the first limiting amino acid and is recommended at 4.3% of CP. Other amino acids considered essential are arginine, histidine, isoleucine, leucine, methionine, phenylalanine, threonine, tryptophan, and valine, but sufficient information to make a quantitative dietary recommendation is lacking [5]. Ration balancer products for adult horses will often include lysine and methionine, a sulfur-containing amino acid, providing a small margin of safety in the face of unknown requirements (Table 17.2). Alternatively, the products will contain high-quality proteins such as soybean or alfalfa meal to provide essential amino acids, albeit quantitatively the requirements are not known.

17.3.2.4 Macrominerals

Forage is the major source of macrominerals in the ration. The dietary intake of calcium (Ca), phosphorus (P), magnesium, potassium, sodium, chloride, and sulfur is based on the BW of the adult horse regardless of temperament and age (Table 17.1). The Ca:P ratio should be between 1.2:1 and 3:1. If P intake exceeds Ca intake, Ca absorption will be impaired, resulting in skeletal abnormalities. Grains (oats and barley) and grain by-products (wheat bran) have reversed Ca:P ratios. Legume forages typically contain more Ca than P (10:1), whereas most grass forages have a moderate Ca:P ratio of ≤2:1; therefore, laboratory mineral analysis of the forage, particularly for MML and MMG forages, is warranted to ensure proper calcium to phosphorus balance in the total ration.

17.3.2.5 Antioxidants

Antioxidant nutrients are typically listed as Vitamins A, E, C, and beta-carotene, and trace minerals selenium, iron, copper, zinc, and manganese. Endogenously synthesized antioxidants require dietary precursors. For example, coenzyme Q is a unique lipid-soluble antioxidant involved in mitochondrial oxidative phosphorylation (energy production) requiring phenylalanine, manganese, and vitamins (B_5, B_6) for endogenous synthesis [29]. Interest in these nutrients stems from the increased understanding that free radical events may be involved in many disease processes. The aging process has been recognized as the progressive decreased ability to mitigate and repair oxidative damage to cellular macromolecules. Free radicals and reactive oxygen species (ROS) damage DNA, proteins, and polyunsaturated phospholipids, which results in disruption of membrane architecture and cell function.

Historically, the daily recommended intake of vitamins and trace minerals is based on preventing clinical deficiencies. Recommendations were determined from feeding studies in which zero or low concentrations of the nutrient produced a gross clinical sign of deficiency, for example, night blindness and Vitamin A, or a biochemical parameter, for example, erythrocyte stability and Vitamin E. In the same study, a higher concentration that resulted in a "normal" animal or at least no evidence of the same clinical sign of deficiency or the point at which blood concentrations plateaued, then determined the dietary recommendation. The recommendation was appropriately increased when feed digestibility or availability of the nutrient was known. In the case of horses, the daily nutrient intake of some vitamins and trace minerals has been extrapolated from studies conducted in other species, and for most B vitamins, given the large bowel microbiome, requirements have understandably been difficult to determine.

There are no specific guidelines or dietary recommendations for the class of nutrients functioning as antioxidants and anti-aging nutrients. Optimal concentrations of nutrients known to be essential to mitigating free-radical-mediated injury have not been determined. The client's attitudes toward the use of micronutrients to optimize disease prevention currently outpace our knowledge of effective dosages or daily intakes. See Chapter 14 Dietary Supplements.

17.3.2.5.1 Trace Minerals

The dietary intake of copper, iron, manganese, zinc, cobalt, iodine, and selenium is based on the BW of the adult horse regardless of temperament and age (Table 17.1). Additionally, the balance between trace minerals is important to maintain, as minerals do compete for intestinal absorption. A Ca:Zn ratio should not exceed 100:1, and the Zn and Cu should not exceed a 35:1 ratio in the total diet [5].

17.3.2.5.2 Vitamins A and E

The dietary intake of vitamins A, D, E, thiamine, and riboflavin is based on the BW of the adult horse regardless of temperament and age (Table 17.1). Horses consuming fresh forage (pasture) of moderate quality unlikely need a vitamin concentrate; however, those maintained on preserved forage (hay) should receive a supplement fortified by vitamins A and E. It is commonly said that horses maintained on a forage-only (hay or pasture) ration would likely benefit from consistently consuming a vitamin ration balancer considering the natural variation in pasture and forage quality.

17.4 Feeding Management

Adult horses should be maintained with a BCS of 4/9–6/9 and preferably fed moderate to good-quality forage as pasture or hay, with water and salt (NaCl) available *ad libitum*. For idle or occasionally ridden horses, a white or trace mineralized salt (block or loose), specific for horses, should be available *ad libitum*, preferably under cover from weather, and monitored. White salt should be offered if a commercial feed or ration balancer contains trace minerals. The suggested feeding recommendations apply only to mature horses in moderate body condition.

Forage quality should be sufficiently palatable and digestible (<42% ADF; <60% NDF; RFV of 85–115) such that the horse will meet requirements consuming 1.5–2.0% BW DMI (Tables 10.3 and 17.3) [5, 55]. The forage must have adequate concentrations of energy, protein, calcium, and phosphorus (Table 17.3). Mature horses fed fresh forages will likely require a trace mineral source, whereas feeding hays with comparable RFV may require a trace mineral–vitamin supplementation fed at 0.1% BW to complete the ration. If lower-quality forages or those with DE <1.5 Mcal/kg, or CP <6–8% DM are fed, a complementary feed or ration balancer providing calories and/or protein with minerals and vitamins will be needed. See Sidebar 17.3.

Sidebar 17.3: Calculating Daily Feeding Recommendations for an Adult Horse at Maintenance

Animal Assessment

- 550 kg (BCS 5/9) 25-yr-old Quarter Horse gelding elevated temperament trail ridden maybe for 2 hrs/month, i.e. non-working.
- DMI for an adult horse at maintenance 2.0% BW (Table 17.3).
- Gelding's daily DE_m requirement: 3.64 Mcal/100 kg BW × 5.5 = 20.0 Mcal DE (Table 17.1).
- Forage recommendations for adult horses are RFVs of 85–115 and 1.82 Mcal DE/kg DM (Table 17.3). ADF <42%, NDF <60% is recommended for adult horses (Table 10.3).

Ration Assessment

Hay available at the boarding stable is a mixed mainly legume (MML) forage with 90% DM. The smell and texture of the hay are sufficiently palatable for the gelding to consume 2% BW. On a DM basis, the forage had textbook values of:

International Feed Number (IFN)	DE	CP	Ca	P	ADF	NDF	Cu	Zn
#	Mcal/kg	%	%	%	%	%	ppm	ppm
1-02-277	2.35	19.1	1.17	0.30	35.4	47.2	9.0	24

- Calculate forage RFV values:
  - %DDM = 88.9 − (0.779 × %ADF) = 61%.
  - %DMI = 120/%NDF = 2.5% BW.
  - RFV = %DDM × %DMI × 0.775 = 120 good-quality (Table 10.3).
  - Forage quality is adequate compared with that recommended for mature horses at maintenance.
- Calculate daily forage intake required to meet the horse's DE on DM and as fed (AF) basis:
  - Horse requires 20 Mcal DE/2.35 Mcal DE/kg DM = 8.5 kg forage DM/0.9 = 9.5 kg forage AF.
  - Check DMI: 8.5 kg hay DM intake/550 kg BW = 1.5% BW.
- Compare forage crude protein (CP), calcium (Ca), and phosphorus (P) concentrations with recommendations (Table 17.3):
  - Recommended CP is 7.2%; forage contains 19.1% CP.
  - Recommended Ca is 0.20%; forage contains 1.17% Ca.
  - Recommended P is 0.14% P; forage contains 0.30% P with Ca:P ratio = 3.9:1.
  - If 9.5 kg AF of hay is consumed daily, the CP, Ca, and P needs should be met.
- If the horse consumed 8.5 kg DM hay daily, compare copper (Cu) and zinc (Zn) intakes with recommendations (Table 17.1):
  - Cu: intake is 76.5 mg [8.5 kg forage DM/d x 9 mg/kg] whereas 110 mg Cu is required [20 mg x 5.5].
  - Zn: intake is 204 mg whereas 440 is required.
  - Copper and zinc needs will not be met consuming this hay.

Feeding Management Recommendations

The nutrient composition of the hay, based on textbook values, exceeds the gelding's requirements for energy, protein, calcium, and phosphorus. Specific instructions:

- Laboratory assay the hay for DE, ADF, NDF, and re-assess feeding plan based on client's hay laboratory analysis.
- Feed 9–10 kg hay AF/d and monitor BW and BCS monthly.
- Feed trace mineral–vitamin ration balancer to meet micronutrient requirements with sufficient phosphorus to correct Ca:P ratio to about 1.5:1.
- Lysine intake should be checked. The book value is 0.72% DM.
- Offer water and salt *ad libitum*.

Feeding intake, BCS, and BW must be monitored to maintain mature horses in ideal BW and condition. The amount of hay to maintain a moderate BCS weight should be initially calculated, and the horse assessed as activity levels, weather, and hay source change. The intake of pasture is difficult to determine; therefore, assessing BW and BCS 4–6 times a year as the pasture changes is warranted.

17.4.1 Maintenance of Weight and Condition

17.4.1.1 BCS >6/9

An adult non-working horse (5 to 20-yr-old) kept as a companion animal is more likely to be overweight or obese (BCS >6/9), frequently attributable to a misunderstanding of the horse's true dietary needs. Often maintenance horses are fed unnecessary grain concentrates, and/or allowed unlimited access to pastures with little to no imposed exercise. Hence, the weight gain and high BCS are due to excess caloric intake relative to energy expenditure, although genetics is a strong underlying factor. The comorbidities associated with obesity are orthopedic (laminitis and osteoarthritis), endocrine, and metabolic disorders (insulin dysregulation, dyslipidemia, equine metabolic syndrome), heat and exercise intolerance, and colic associated with pedunculated lipomas [11, 69]. The ideal situation is to prevent weight gain with regular BW and BCS animal assessments and close monitoring of feeds and feeding management. Weight loss programs are successful with assistance from a qualified equine nutritionist and veterinarian [10–12]. See Feeding for Weight Loss in Chapter 23.

17.4.1.2 BCS <4/9

A common problem for senior horses is the maintenance of weight or condition. Underweight horses in the UK >15-yr-old were reported to have a higher mortality risk compared to animals with a higher BCS [70]. In a survey of owners, loss of weight and condition, arthritis, and dental care topped their concerns for their aged horses [71]. Reasons for the lack of condition are varied, but are often linked to an underlying clinical disease process. Clinical conditions most commonly seen in older horses are neoplasia (pituitary pars intermedia dysfunction and thyroid tumors), increased incidence of colic and dental abnormalities, a decreased function in the aortic valve and respiratory system, decreased immunocompetence and increased incidence of bacterial and viral infections, increased risk of tendon and ligament damage due to changes in the collagen structure, and there are several age-related changes seen in the brain of horses [72]. Older horses have a more difficult time regulating body temperature during exercise [41]. Extreme heat or cold demands more energy reserves to compensate. Pain from old injuries, arthritis, or other causes potentially limits ease of movement, leading to a decrease in overall muscle tone. Strategically managing these conditions to relieve pain may increase the horse's comfort, ease of movement, and provide a better quality of life. See Chapter 22 Pain and Discomfort Behaviors.

Maintaining BW and condition requires maintaining feed intake, as there is no recovery from disease or injury without dietary inputs of energy, protein, and micronutrients. Ration reformulations with appropriate changes are often needed to meet nutritional needs within a consumable amount of feed. If an older horse is losing BW and BCS, it must first be determined whether the horse is or is not consuming sufficient calories. Determining the cause of weight loss is of paramount concern. Consuming insufficient calories intuitively leads to weight loss; however, consuming an adequate amount of feed and calories in the face of weight loss redirects the investigation. A review of the feeding protocol is important to assess because the appropriate feeds fed incorrectly can result in weight loss. See Sidebar 17.4.

A veterinary examination is required to determine the root cause of the poor feed intake or poor feed utilization when the ration and method of feeding are appropriate. Medical and dietary history, physical examination including the oral cavity, reviewing laboratory biochemical data, and time spent observing horse behaviors during feeding are helpful in the investigation. The horse's interest in, or lack of, eating, ability to prehend, masticate, and swallow feed are necessary observations in addition to a physical examination. See Oral Cavity in Chapter 3.

Stress may contribute to weight loss, and a horse low in the pecking order may have a more difficult time acquiring sufficient feed in group-fed horses. Feeding underweight older horses separately, with herd mates nearby, may result in increased food consumption and will aid in monitoring progress. Providing feed and water from a raised position, for example, shoulder level or from a fence rail, instead of ground level, may be easier for older horses with osteoarthritis in the forelimbs or neck [49]. An underweight horse may need more total feed, a calorically dense feed, or both to stop loss of condition and regain weight. If pasture is unavailable, high-quality hay or chopped forage should be considered. Forage in the vegetative stage (fresh or dried) is softer, easier to chew, and has a higher digestibility coefficient. If a better forage is not available or does not provide sufficient calories, or weight loss is due to poor dentition, a complete, high-fat extruded product is an option. Adding fat to the diet is the most effective method of increasing caloric intake without increasing feed volume, and adding vegetable oil avoids high intakes of starch and sugar which may exacerbate the age-related decline in insulin sensitivity. See Feeding for Weight Gain in Chapter 23.

Sidebar 17.4: A case of unexplained weight loss and the importance of a diet history according to Robert M Miller, DVM.[a]

A young woman called me because her horse was losing weight despite eating everything offered.

Animal Assessment

I went to her home and examined a middle-aged mare that was almost 200 lb underweight. She was only used for light trail riding 2–4 times/wk. My examination revealed no abnormalities except for her early emaciation.

Ration Assessment

I asked the client what she fed. "A huge flake of hay two times/d and some carrots," the owner replied. I was puzzled and examined her hay. It was excellent. I took a blood sample for a complete blood count, and a fresh stool sample to check for parasites. Both were normal.

Dietary Recommendations:
I suggested adding a couple of pounds of grain to her ration daily and said that I would return in 2 wks to recheck the mare.

Follow-up:
Two weeks later I returned to find that she had not regained any weight. I asked if she cleaned up all her food. "Well, no," the owner replied. "She eats all of the grain and the carrots, but only eats half the hay. I have to clean up all the hay she will not eat."

It was 3:30 p.m., a bit early to feed, but I asked her to feed while I watched. She obediently fed a large flake of very nice hay, a coffee can full of grain, and then dragged out a huge washtub full of carrots. The mare went promptly to the carrot tub. "Do you feed this many carrots *every* day?" I asked amazed. She said, "No, I do it twice a day. She loves carrots."

Problem solved! I told her to continue the hay and grain, but to limit the mare to two carrots, twice a day.

Outcome:
She called me a month later. "She's getting fat! Should I quit the grain?" Take home message: Palatability can lead us into making feeding mistakes.

[a] Dr. Robert M Miller is an equine behaviorist and veterinarian, and was an early adopter of natural horsemanship. His cartoons, done under his initials RMM, have been published in veterinary and horse magazines around the world. He has authored scientific papers and magazine articles for veterinary and equine publications, has published four books and six videos on equine behavior, health, and horsemanship.

Case in Point

The owner asks for a consult because a friend recently cautioned about overweight older horses being insulin-resistant, so the owner asks: "Is my horse fat and how much hay should I be feeding him per day?"

Animal Assessment

An 18-yr-old Quarter Horse gelding, BW 500 kg BCS 5/9, minimum temperament, used occasionally giving pony rides walked in hand at children's parties (2 hrs of walking/month), is maintained in a 1 ac dry lot with a run-in shed. No abnormalities were noted on physical examination, and there were no current medical concerns.

Ration Assessment

Water and a white salt block were available *ad libitum*. The horse is offered 1/2 (60 lb) bale/d of fescue/orchard grass-mixed hay but does not finish all of it. Based on laboratory analysis, the cool-season grass hay with 90% DM contains the following nutrients on a DM basis:

DE	CP	Ca	P	Lysine	ADF	NDF
Mcal/kg	%	%	%	%	%	%
2.1	8.8	0.31	0.29	0.35	37.8	58.7

1) *Calculate relative feed value (RFV) and determine the nutritional quality of the forage.*
2) *Based on the calculated DE_m requirement, how much hay (lb as fed) should this horse consume daily?*
3) *Does feeding an adequate amount of this hay/d meet the horse's protein, calcium, and phosphorus requirements?*
4) *The owner asks: "Is my horse fat and how much hay should I be feeding him per day?" What are your nutritional recommendations?*

See Appendix A Chapter 17.

References

1 Association of American Feed Control Officials (2021). *Official Publication AAFCO*. Champaign, IL: Association of American Feed Control Officials, Inc. www.aafco.org.

2 Veterinary Economics Division (2007). *U.S. Pet Ownership & Demographics Sourcebook*. Schaumburg, IL: American Veterinary Medical Association.

3 Visser, E.K. and Van Wijk-Jansen, E.E.C. (2012). Diversity in horse enthusiasts with respect to horse welfare: an explorative study. *J. Vet. Behav. Clin. Appl. Res.* 7 (5): 295–304.

4 McGowan, C.M. and Ireland, J.L. (2016). Welfare, quality of life, and euthanasia of aged horses. *Vet. Clin. North Am. Equine Pract.* 32 (2): 355–367.

5 National Research Council (2007). *Nutrient Requirements of Horses*. 6th Rev. Animal Nutrition Series, 1–341. Washington D.C.: National Academies Press.

6 Siciliano, P.D. (2002). Nutrition and feeding of the geriatric horse. *Vet. Clin. North Am. Equine Pract.* 18 (3): 491–508.

7 Wagner, A.L., Urschel, K.L., Betancourt, A. et al. (2013). Effects of advanced age on whole-body protein synthesis and skeletal muscle mechanistic target of rapamycin signaling in horses. *Am. J. Vet. Res.* 74 (11): 1433–1442.

8 Henneke, D.R., Potter, G.D., Kreider, J.L., and Yeates, B.F. (1983). Relationship between condition score, physical measurements and body fat percentage in mares. *Equine Vet. J.* 15 (4): 371–372.

9 Mottet, R., Onan, G., and Hiney, K. (2009). Revisiting the Henneke body condition scoring system: 25 years later. *J. Equine Vet. Sci.* 29 (5): 417–418.

10 Johnson, P.J., Wiedmeyer, C.E., Messer, N.T., and Ganjam, V.K. (2009). Medical implications of obesity in horses – lessons for human obesity. *J. Diabetes Sci. Technol.* 3 (1): 163–174.

11 Frank, N., Geor, R.J., Bailey, S.R. et al. (2010). Equine metabolic syndrome. *J. Vet. Intern. Med.* 24 (3): 467–475.

12 Geor, R.J. (2013). Endocrine and metabolic physiology. In: *Equine Applied and Clinical Nutrition: Health, Welfare and Performance* (ed. R.J. Geor, P.A. Harris, and M. Coenen), 33–63. Edinburgh: Saunders Elsevier.

13 McGowan, T.W., Pinchbeck, G., Phillips, C.J.C. et al. (2010). A survey of aged horses in Queensland, Australia. Part 2: clinical signs and owners' perceptions of health and welfare. *Aust. Vet. J.* 88 (12): 465–471.

14 Careau, V., Thomas, D., Humphries, M.M., and Réale, D. (2008). Energy metabolism and animal personality. *Oikos* 117 (5): 641–653.

15 Brinkmann, L., Gerken, M., Hambly, C. et al. (2014). Saving energy during hard times: energetic adaptations of Shetland pony mares. *J. Exp. Biol.* 217 (24): 4320–4327.

16 Rattan, S.I.S. (2014). Aging is not a disease: implications for intervention. *Aging Dis.* 5 (3): 196.

17 Rattan, S.I.S. (2018). Biogerontology: research status, challenges and opportunities. *Acta Biomed.* 89 (2): 291–301.

18 Brosnahan, M.M. and Paradis, M.R. (2003). Assessment of clinical characteristics, management practices, and activities of geriatric horses. *J. Am. Vet. Med. Assoc.* 223 (1): 99–103.

19 Ireland, J.L., McGowan, C.M., Clegg, P.D. et al. (2012). A survey of health care and disease in geriatric horses aged 30 years or older. *Vet. J.* 192 (1): 57–64.

20 United States Department of Agriculture (2015). Baseline reference of equine health and management in the United States. Fort Collins, CO. https://www.aphis.usda.gov/animal_health/nahms/equine/downloads/equine15/Eq2015_Rept1.pdf (accessed 28 December 2021).

21 Waring, G.H. (2003). Ecological influences on reproduction and social behavior: influences on reproductive success. In: *Horse Behavior*, 2e, 320–323. Norwich, NY: Noyes Publications.

22 Keiper, R.R. (1985). Population dynamics. In: *The Assateague Ponies*, 84. Atglen, PA: Schiffer Publishing.

23 Ralston, S., Nockels, C., and Squires, E.L. (1988). Differences in diagnostic test results and hematologic data between aged and young horses. *Am. J. Vet. Res.* 49 (8): 1387–1392.

24 Satue, K., Blanco, O., and Munoz, A. (2009). AGE-related differences in the hematological profile of Andalusian broodmares of Carthusian strain. *Vet. Med. (Praha)* 54 (4): 175–182.

25 Brosnahan, M.M. and Paradis, D.M.R. (2003). Demographic and clinical characteristics of geriatric horses: 467 cases (1989–1999). *J. Am. Vet. Med. Assoc.* 223 (1): 93–98.

26 Silva, A.G. and Furr, M.O. (2013). Diagnoses, clinical pathology findings, and treatment outcome of geriatric horses: 345 cases (2006–2010). *J. Am. Vet. Med. Assoc.* 243 (12): 1762–1768.

27 Figueiredo, P.A., Mota, M.P., Appell, H.J., and Duarte, J.A. (2008). The role of mitochondria in aging of skeletal muscle. *Biogerontology* 9 (2): 67–84.

28 Rattan, S.I.S. (2008). Increased molecular damage and heterogeneity as the basis of aging. *Biol. Chem.* 389 (3): 267–272.

29 Lenaz, G., D'Aurelio, M., Merlo Pich, M. et al. (2000). Mitochondrial bioenergetics in aging. *Biochim. Biophys. Acta, Bioenerg.* 1459 (2, 3): 397–404.

30 Bua, E.A., McKiernan, S.H., Wanagat, J. et al. (2002). Mitochondrial abnormalities are more frequent in muscles undergoing sarcopenia. *J. Appl. Phys.* 92 (6): 2617–2624.

31 Rattan, S.I.S. (2006). Theories of biological aging: genes, proteins, and free radicals. *Free Radical Res.* 40 (12): 1230–1238.

32 Lowder, M.Q. and Mueller, P.O. (1998). Dental disease in geriatric horses. *Vet. Clin. North Am. Equine Pract.* 14 (2): 365–380.

33 Dougal, K., De La Fuente, G., Harris, P.A. et al. (2014). Characterisation of the faecal bacterial community in adult and elderly horses fed a high fibre, high oil or high starch diet using 454 pyrosequencing. *PLoS One* 9 (2): e87424.

34 Bucknell, D.G., Gasser, R.B., and Beveridge, I. (1995). The prevalence and epidemiology of gastrointestinal parasites of horses in Victoria, Australia. *Int. J. Parasitol.* 25 (6): 711–724.

35 Dickinson, C.E. and Lori, D.N. (2002). Diagnostic workup for weight loss in the geriatric horse. *Vet. Clin. North Am. Equine Pract.* 18 (3): 523–531.

36 Fermaglich, D.H. and Horohov, D.W. (2002). The effect of aging on immune responses. *Vet. Clin. North Am. Equine Pract.* 18 (3): 621–630.

37 Goto, H., Yamamoto, Y., Ohta, C. et al. (1993). Antibody responses of Japanese horses to influenza viruses in the past few years. *J. Vet. Med. Sci.* 55 (1): 33–37.

38 Horohov, D.W., Dimock, A., Guirnalda, P. et al. (1999). Effect of exercise on the immune response of young and old horses. *Am. J. Vet. Res.* 60 (5): 643–647.

39 Madill, S. (2002). Reproductive considerations: mare and stallion. *Vet. Clin. North Am. Equine Pract.* 18 (3): 591–619.

40 Paradis, M.R. (2002). Demographics of health and disease in the geriatric horse. *Vet. Clin. North Am. Equine Pract.* 18 (3): 391–401.

41 McKeever, K.H., Eaton, T.L., Geiser, S. et al. (2010). Age related decreases in thermoregulation and cardiovascular function in horses. *Equine Vet. J.* 42 (Suppl. 38): 220–227.

42 Betros, C.L., McKeever, K.H., Kearns, C.F., and Malinowski, K. (2002). Effects of ageing and training on maximal heart rate and VO_2 max. *Equine Vet. J.* 34 (S34): 100–105.

43 Malinowski, K., Shock, E.J., Rochelle, P. et al. (2006). Plasma β-endorphin, cortisol and immune responses to acute exercise are altered by age and exercise training in horses. *Equine Vet. J.* 38 (Suppl. 36): 267–273.

44 Liburt, N.R., McKeever, K.H., Malinowski, K. et al. (2013). Response of the hypothalamic-pituitary-adrenal axis to stimulation tests before and after exercise training in old and young Standardbred mares. *J. Anim. Sci.* 91 (11): 5208–5219.

45 Ireland, J.L., Clegg, P.D., Mcgowan, C.M. et al. (2011). A cross-sectional study of geriatric horses in the United Kingdom. Part 2: health care and disease. *Equine Vet. J.* 43 (1): 37–44.
46 Rucker, B.A. (2002). Diseases of the oral cavity and soft palate. In: *Manual of Equine Gastroenterology* (ed. T. Mair, T. Divers, and N.G. Ducharme), 69–77. London: Saunders Elsevier.
47 Carmalt, J.L., Townsend, H.G.G., Janzen, E.D., and Cymbaluk, N.E. (2004). Effect of dental floating on weight gain, body condition score, feed digestibility, and fecal particle size in pregnant mares. *J. Am. Vet. Med. Assoc.* 225 (12): 1889–1893.
48 Nicholls, V.M. and Townsend, N. (2016). Dental disease in aged horses and its management. *Vet. Clin. North Am. Equine Pract.* 32 (2): 215–227.
49 Jarvis, N.G. (2009). Nutrition of the aged horse. *Vet. Clin. North Am. Equine Pract.* 25 (1): 155–166.
50 Easley, K.J. (2003). Dental and oral examination. In: *Equine Dentistry* (ed. G. Baker and J. Easley), 107–126. Philadelphia: W.B. Saunders.
51 Ralston, S.L., Foster, D.L., Divers, T., and Hintz, H.F. (2001). Effect of dental correction on feed digestibility in horses. *Equine Vet. J.* 33 (4): 390–393.
52 Carmalt, J.L. and Allen, A. (2008). The relationship between cheek tooth occlusal morphology, apparent digestibility, and ingesta particle size reduction in horses. *J. Am. Vet. Med. Assoc.* 233 (3): 452–455.
53 Ralston, S.L., Malinowski, K., Christensen, R, and Breuer, L. (2000). Apparent digestion of hay/grain rations in aged horses – revisited. In: *Proceedings 2000 Equine Nutrition Conference for Feed Manufacturers* (ed. Kentucky Equine Research Inc.), 193–195.
54 Elzinga, S., Nielsen, B.D., Schott, H.C. et al. (2014). Comparison of nutrient digestibility between adult and aged horses. *J. Equine Vet. Sci.* 34 (10): 1164–1169.
55 Swinker, A.M. (2014). Hay quality for different classes of horses. Pennsylvania State Extension Service. https://extension.psu.edu/hay-quality-for-different-classes-of-horses (accessed 2 July 2021).
56 Russell, M.A. and Johnson, K.D. (2007). *Selecting Quality Hay for Horses.* West Lafayette, IN: Department of Agriculture Cooperative Extension Service. https://www.agry.purdue.edu/ext/forages/publications/id-190.htm (accessed 5 July 2021).
57 van den Berg, M., Giagos, V., Lee, C. et al. (2016). The influence of odour, taste and nutrients on feeding behaviour and food preferences in horses. *Appl. Anim. Behav. Sci.* 184 (Nov): 41–50.
58 Geor, R., Harris, P.A., and Coenen, M. (2013). Nutritional requirements, recommendations and example diets. In: *Equine Applied and Clinical Nutrition Health, Welfare and Performance* (ed. R. Geor, P.A. Harris, and M. Coenen), 639–643. Edinburgh: Saunders Elsevier.
59 Redfearn, D.D., Freeman, D.W., and Hiney, K. (2017). *Forage for Horses*. Stillwater, OK: Oklahoma Cooperative Extension Service ANSI-3980. https://shareok.org/bitstream/handle/11244/49954/oksd_ansi_3980_2013-08.pdf?sequence=1 (accessed 11 July 2021).
60 Fonnesbeck, P., Lydman, R., Vander Noot, G., and Symons, L. (1967). Digestibility of the proximate nutrients of forage by horses. *J. Anim. Sci.* 26 (5): 1039–1045.
61 Lieb, S., Ott, E., and French, E. (1993). Digestible nutrients and voluntary intake of rhizomes peanut, alfalfa, bermudagrass and bahiagrass by equine. In: *Proceedings of the 13th Equine Nutrition and Physiology Society Symposium*, 98–99. Gainsville, FL: Equine Nutrition and Physiology Society.
62 Martinson, K., Coblentz, W., and Sheaffer, C. (2011). The effect of harvest moisture and bale wrapping on forage quality, temperature, and mold in orchardgrass hay. *J. Equine Vet. Sci.* 31 (12): 711–716.
63 Undersander, D., Hall, M, Leep, R. et al. Moldy hay for horses. Madison, WI: University of Wisconsin Extension. https://fyi.extension.wisc.edu/forage/moldy-hay-for-horses (accessed 25 July 2021).
64 Kamphues, J. (2013). Feed hygiene and related disorders in horses. In: *Equine Applied and Clinical Nutrition Health, Welfare and Performance* (ed. R.J. Geor, P.A. Harris, and M. Coenen), 367–380. Edinburgh: Saunders Elsevier.
65 Beeler-Marfisi, J., Clark, M.E., Wen, X. et al. (2010). Experimental induction of recurrent airway obstruction with inhaled fungal spores, lipopolysaccharide, and silica microspheres in horses. *Am. J. Vet. Res.* 71 (6): 682–689.
66 Clarke, A.F. and Madelin, T. (1987). Technique for assessing respiratory health hazards from hay and other source materials. *Equine Vet. J.* 19 (5): 442–447.
67 Schott, H.C. (2011). Water homeostasis and diabetes insipidus in horses. *Vet. Clin. North Am. Equine Pract.* 27 (1): 175–195.
68 Pagan, J.D.D., Lawrence, T.L.L., and Lennox, M.A.A. (2010). Fish oil and corn oil supplementation affect red blood cell and serum eicosapentaenoic acid (EPA) and docosahexaenoic acid (DHA) concentrations in Thoroughbred horses. In: *Proceedings of the 1st Nordic Feed Science Conference Sveriges Lantbruksuniversitet*, 116–118.
69 Geor, R.J. and Harris, P.A. (2013). Obesity. In: *Equine Applied and Clinical Nutrition: Health, Welfare and Performance* (ed. R.J. Geor, P.A. Harris and M. Coenen), 487–502. Edinburgh: Saunders Elsevier.
70 Ireland, J.L., Clegg, P.D., McGowan, C.M. et al. (2011). Factors associated with mortality of geriatric horses in the United Kingdom. *Prev. Vet. Med.* 101 (3): 204–218.
71 McGowan, C. (2011). Welfare of aged horses. *Animals* 1 (4): 366–376.
72 Ralston, S. and Harris, P. (2013). Nutritional considerations for aged horses. In: *Equine Applied and Clinical Nutrition: Health, Welfare and Performance* (ed. R.J. Geor, P.A. Harris and M. Coenen), 289–303. Edinburgh: Saunders Elsevier.

18

Feeding Athletes and Working Horses

Shannon Pratt-Phillips and Jenna Kutzner Mulligan

KEY POINTS

- Horses performing imposed exercise require additional energy and some nutrients proportional to the increased metabolism required to accomplish the work as measured by time and intensity. Quantifying the duration of work is possible; however, characterizing the intensity is less precise.
- Energy-concentrated feeds should be fed at as low a level as possible with forage making up the major portion of the diet regardless of discipline.
- Glycogen muscle loading in horses does not appear to be possible due to a limited rate of muscle replenishment.

18.1 Introduction

Athletic and working horses have specific nutritional needs to support a variety of work efforts. It would be difficult to feed to the exact nutrient requirements for each day's work, and therefore the work effort is generally considered for a week. The nutrient requirements, above maintenance needs, are influenced primarily by the duration, intensity, and frequency of the workouts (hrs or days/wk). The work performed by horses has been divided into light, moderate, heavy, or very heavy work classifications based on mean heart rate (HR) (Table 18.1) [1]. Light working horses are those used primarily for recreation or low-level riding/training 1 to 3 hrs/wk at a walk or trot for the majority of the time. Moderate work refers to those horses involved in a regular riding program and ranch work, and competition horses working between 3 to 5 hrs/wk at a walk or trot 85% of the time with 5% skill work. Examples of skill work are dressage, jumping, racing, sprinting, cutting, reining, or working cattle. Heavy work includes horses at high levels of competition with more demanding skills, such as rodeo events, show jumping, and low-level eventing horses, and those in early race training working 4 to 5 hrs/wk at higher intensities of cantering, galloping, and skill work. Very heavy work refers to those working at the highest skill levels and intensities as required for national and international racing, show jumping, and eventing competitions. The intensity of work is related to the speed, number/height of obstacles, the weight pulled or carried (rider and tack), and performing in extended or collected gaits. Work effort will also be affected by the footing and terrain traveled, the fitness of the horse, and environmental temperatures.

Performing work requires endogenous energy. There are three general types of physical exertion based upon the endogenous source of energy required by performing horses. Endurance activities generally of 2 hrs or more of low-intensity exertion utilize aerobic energy metabolism for long-distance races, competitive trail rides, and ranch, draft, show, and lesson work. Sprint (0.25 mile or less) activities of a minute or less at near 100% maximum exertion use anaerobic energy production as in Quarter Horse racing, barrel racing, rodeo events, and draft pulling contests. Middle-distance (0.5–2 miles) activities of several minutes at an average of 75–95% of maximum-intensity exertion utilize aerobic and anaerobic energy metabolism together as in Thoroughbred and Standardbred trotter racing, whereas polo, cutting, and show jumping will require both sources at different moments. In summary, the specific nutritional needs of working horses are dependent on

Equine Clinical Nutrition, Second Edition. Edited by Rebecca L. Remillard.

Table 18.1 Work descriptors and examples of workload.

Work descriptor	Approximate work rate	Heart rate (beats/min)	Examples of work[a]
Maintenance (average)	At rest	30–40	None or off-season
Light work	1–3 hrs/wk 40% walk, 50% trot, 10% canter	80	Recreational trail riding Occasional low-level shows
Moderate work	3–5 hrs/wk 30% walk, 55% trot, 10% canter with 5% skill work	90	Competitive trail riding Regular shows with skills School horses Ranch work Western pleasure show Racing (barrel)
Heavy work	4–5 hrs/wk 20% walk, 50% trot, 15% canter with 5% skill work	110	Regular shows with skills Ranch work Polo/rodeo competitions Eventing (low to medium level) Racing (flat track)
Very heavy/intense work	1 hr/wk of speed work to 6–12 hrs/wk of slow work	110–150	Racing: endurance, steeplechase Elite show Jumping Eventing (high level)

[a] Examples of skill work are dressage, jumping, racing, sprinting, cutting, reining, working cattle, etc. Eventing is an equestrian triathlon where a horse/rider pair competes in three disciplines: dressage, cross-country, and show jumping over 1–4 d. Racing (ridden or harnessed) is on straight or oval flat track. Steeplechase is flat track racing with jumps.

a myriad of factors each of which is to be taken into consideration when designing an appropriate ration and feeding program. When nutritional or diet-related problems arise, a systematic iterative review of the horse, the ration, and the feeding method is recommended. See Appendix C Nutrition Competencies of Equine Veterinarians.

18.2 Animal Assessment

Working horses are open mares, geldings, and stallions requiring daily energy intake sufficient to maintain current body weight (BW) and body condition score (BCS). Those horses in training under 5 yrs of age are in the late stages of growth, whereas horses 5 yrs and older have fully matured. Given the mature BW ranges from 200 to 900 kg in horses, the recommended daily nutrient intakes are presented in Table 18.2 per 100 kg of mature BW for adult horses and Table 18.3 for 18-mo-old (long yearlings) and 2-yr-old horses. [2].

18.2.1 Body Condition Score

Working horses, regardless of sport or type of work, should be fed to maintain a BCS of 4/9 (moderately thin) to 6/9 (moderately fleshy) [3, 4]. Young horses in high-intensity level training programs are likely to be underweight (BCS <4/9). In feeding relatively high-grain/low-forage rations to meet the daily energy requirement (DER) of maintenance, growth plus training, or maintenance plus work, there is an increased risk of gastric ulcers and colic [5, 6]. Therefore, routine physical assessments are recommended for working horses based on history, work expenditures, and feeding management. The assessment frequency is case-dependent in that a 6-yr-old Quarter Horse mare with a history of having an ideal BW and BCS through years of competitive trail riding may need only be assessed at the start and mid-point of the show season. Whereas a 3-yr-old Thoroughbred mare with an elevated temperament and history of poor appetite in flat track racing training 3 to 5 hrs/wk may need be assessed monthly until stabilized. See Chapter 2 Nutritional Assessment of the Horse.

18.2.2 Skeletal Muscle Energy Metabolism

Skeletal muscle is made of bundles of muscle fibers that are elongated cells that have multiple nuclei and mitochondria and store both fat (as triglyceride [TG]) and glucose (as glycogen). The key proteins within muscle fibers are the contractile proteins, actin, and myosin, which are supported by troponin and tropomyosin. These actin and myosin filaments are arranged across the length of the muscle fiber in units called sarcomeres. Upon stimulation from the nervous system, an action potential travels down t-tubules within the muscle cell and triggers the release of

Table 18.2 Recommended daily nutrient intakes for mature horses at work per 100 kg of body weight regardless of age.

Nutrient		Level of work				
	Units	Maintenance average[a]	Light	Moderate	Heavy	Very heavy
Digestible energy	Mcal	3.34	4.00[b]	4.66	5.32	6.90
Crude protein	g	126.0	139.8	153.6	172.4	200.8
Lysine	g	5.4	6.0	6.6	7.4	8.6
Calcium	g	4.0	6.0	7.0	8.0	8.0
Phosphorus	g	2.8	3.6	4.2	5.8	5.8
Magnesium	g	1.5	1.9	2.3	3.0	3.0
Potassium	g	5.0	5.7	6.4	7.8	10.6
Sodium	g	2.0	2.8	3.6	5.1	8.2
Chloride	g	8.0	9.3	10.7	13.3	18.6
Sulfur	g	3.0	3.0	3.4	3.8	3.8
Copper	mg	20	20.0	22.5	25.0	25.0
Iron	mg	80	80	90	100	100
Manganese	mg	80	80	90	100	100
Zinc	mg	80	80	90	100	100
Cobalt	mg	0.10	0.10	0.12	0.12	0.12
Iodine	mg	0.70	0.70	0.80	0.88	0.88
Selenium	mg	0.20	0.20	0.23	0.25	0.25
Vitamin A	KIU	3.0	4.5	4.5	4.5	4.5
Vitamin D	IU	660	660	660	660	660
Vitamin E	IU	100	160	180	200	200
Thiamin	mg	6.0	6.0	9.3	12.5	12.5
Riboflavin	mg	4.0	4.0	4.5	5.0	5.0

[a] Average temperament. Average DE_m = 3.34 Mcal/100 kg BW/d [2].
[b] For example, a 525kg adult horse in light work would require 4.00 × 5.25 = 21.0 Mcal DE/d.
Source: Adapted from NRC [2]; Table 16-3 using nutrients required for a 500kg mature horse with BCS 4-6/9 consuming 2.5% BW for very heavy and heavy exercise, 2.25% BW for moderate exercise and 2% BW for light exercise and maintenance.

calcium from the sarcoplasmic reticulum. Calcium binds to troponin and causes a conformational change in tropomyosin that exposes binding sites on actin. The head structure myosin is energized, and can now bind to actin. This results in a "power stroke" wherein myosin and actin slide over each other toward the center of the sarcomere, thus shortening the muscle fiber length. For the myosin to release actin and the muscle to relax, adenosine triphosphate (ATP) binds to myosin, and ATP is then hydrolyzed to adenosine diphosphate (ADP) and phosphate, thus recharging the myosin head. For muscular work to continue, ATP supply to the muscle must meet the demands of the contraction. There is some ATP stored within the muscle and available for that first second or two of work but quickly depleted. ATP must be replenished rapidly through two high-energy phosphate reactions catalyzed by creatine kinase and myokinase to have continuous muscular contractions. Creatine phosphate stores in the muscle can supply one high-energy phosphate to ADP creating ATP and creatine. In addition, two units of ADP catalyzed by myokinase donate high-energy phosphate to produce ATP. These stores are also depleted quickly and the body must rely on further metabolism of energy substrates, that is, carbohydrates, fats, and, to some lesser degree, proteins to continue producing ATP.

Dietary carbohydrates (CHO), primarily the non-structural carbohydrates of sugar and starch, are used to replenish liver or muscle glycogen serving as energy substrates for continued muscular contraction. Insulin facilitates glucose uptake to the sarcolemma by recruitment of the glucose transporter type 4 (GLUT4) protein. Complex carbohydrates, structural fibers, are fermented in the large intestine to

Table 18.3 Recommended daily nutrient intakes for young horses in training per 100 kg of expected mature body weight.

Nutrient		Growth (month of age)					
	Units	18 with light exercise	18 with moderate exercise	24 with light exercise	24 with moderate exercise	24 with heavy exercise	24 with Very heavy exercise
Digestible energy	Mcal	4.42[a]	5.00	4.36	4.96	5.94	6.50
Crude protein	g	170.6	181.2	165.8	177.6	193.8	218.2
Lysine	g	7.3	7.8	7.1	7.6	8.3	9.4
Calcium	g	7.4	7.4	7.3	7.3	7.3	7.3
Phosphorus	g	4.1	4.1	4.1	4.1	4.1	4.1
Magnesium	g	1.2	1.2	1.3	1.3	1.3	1.3
Potassium	g	4.0	4.0	4.4	4.4	4.4	4.4
Sodium	g	1.6	1.6	1.8	1.8	1.8	1.8
Chloride	g	6.4	6.4	7.1	7.1	7.1	7.1
Sulfur	g	2.9	2.9	3.2	3.2	3.2	3.2
Copper	mg	19	19	21	21	21	21
Iron	mg	97	97	107	107	107	107
Manganese	mg	78	78	86	86	86	86
Zinc	mg	78	78	86	86	86	86
Cobalt	mg	0.1	0.1	0.1	0.1	0.1	0.1
Iodine	mg	0.7	0.7	0.8	0.8	0.8	0.8
Selenium	mg	0.2	0.2	0.2	0.2	0.2	0.2
Vitamin A	KIU	3.48	3.48	3.86	3.86	3.86	3.86
Vitamin D	IU	1232	1232	1176	1176	1176	1176
Vitamin E	IU	155.0	155.0	171.6	171.6	171.6	171.6
Thiamin	mg	5.82	5.82	6.44	6.44	6.44	6.44
Riboflavin	mg	3.88	3.88	4.30	4.30	4.30	4.30

[a] For example, an 18-mo-old, average tempered horse in light work with a mature BW estimated at 550 kg would require 4.42 × 5.5 = 24.3 Mcal DE/d.
Source: Adapted from NRC [2]; Table 16-3 using nutrients required for a 500kg mature horse with BCS 4–6/9 consuming 2.5% BW.

produce volatile fatty acids (acetate, propionate, and butyrate). While most butyrate is used by the enterocytes, acetate can be used by the muscle for energy production or can be converted to fat for storage. Propionate is largely glucogenic and the resulting glucose is stored or used. Fats are digested into free fatty acids, which can be available in the blood, and/or stored primarily in the adipose tissue, but also muscle and liver. Proteins are digested to amino acids, which are used primarily for body protein synthesis, but when fed in excess of need, the carbon skeleton is metabolized for energy after deamination. The process of deamination requires water and energy and produces ammonia. The cell toxic ammonia is converted to urea and excreted by the kidneys also requiring water. For this reason, athletic horse rations should not contain excessive crude protein (CP) (>15%) because dietary protein used as a source of energy requires the additional metabolic work of the liver and kidneys to handle the nitrogen and draws on body water resources. Of the potential energy stored in dietary protein, only 60–65% is available for metabolic work compared with 80–90% from CHO and fat, respectively.

Following digestion, energetic substrates consumed beyond that required for maintenance will be stored for later use, for example, exercise. In the postprandial state, it has been estimated that a 500-kg horse has approximately 40 kg adipose tissue and 1.4–2.8 kg muscle triglycerides that could be metabolized to 385 Mcal (42 kg × 9.15 Mcal/kg), whereas muscle glycogen (3.2–4.0 kg) and liver glycogen (0.09–0.22 kg) would provide only 15 Mcal (3.7 × 4.15 Mcal/kg) [7–10]. Therefore, energy stored as body fat is by far the largest reserve for the horse and potentially can provide 25 times more megacalories than body stores of CHO. Protein is not stored in the body as an energetic substrate. During exercise, the body primarily relies on blood glucose concentrations from dietary carbohydrates and/or gluconeogenesis from the hepatic glycogen, and fats, as free fatty acids or acetate derived from the last meal, adipose tissue, or stored muscle triglycerides. The contribution of each endogenous substrate type (fat vs. CHO) and source (blood glucose vs. muscle glycogen vs. muscle triglyceride) depends largely on the timing, intensity, and duration of the exercise. Amino acids do not contribute, typically <5%, to energy production, except during extensive prolonged exercise when muscle mass is catabolized to release amino acids for deamination and energy.

18.2.2.1 Anaerobic Metabolism

At the start of exercise, that is, a burst from the starting gate, residual ATP, ATP from creatine phosphate, and the myokinase reaction will be the major sources of energy, but these are depleted quickly. In this early phase of muscle work and during very intense exercise, the demand for ATP is high; however, oxygen delivery is initially limited. Glucose from muscle glycogen is metabolized through the process of glycolysis in the absence of oxygen, that is, anaerobic metabolism. Glycolysis proceeds very rapidly to produce ATP and nicotinamide adenine dinucleotide (NADH), a carrier of high-energy electrons, from NAD^+ and pyruvate. For glycolysis to continue, NAD^+ is replenished. Anaerobic metabolism readily converts NADH back to NAD^+ with the conversion of pyruvate to lactate. Lactate concentrations can increase in muscle and, subsequently, in blood and potentially contribute to fatigue.

18.2.2.2 Aerobic Metabolism

During continued exercise with oxygen available, pyruvate from glycolysis is converted to acetyl coenzyme A and enters the tricarboxylic acid (TCA) cycle. The TCA cycle requires oxygen and a continuous influx of two carbon units to continue producing ATP, NADH, and flavin adenine dinucleotide ($FADH_2$). Fatty acids, acetate, and amino acid carbon skeletons can be converted to acetyl-co A for entry into the Krebs cycle. Both NADH and $FADH_2$ donate electrons to the electron transport chain producing an electrical gradient that also produces ATP, and regenerates NAD^+ using oxygen as the final electron acceptor to produce water. Therefore, while glucose and glycogen can produce energy via anaerobic metabolism, aerobic metabolism can use glucose or glycogen and fat sources, and to a lesser degree amino acids, for energy production.

The various energy substrates are metabolized through glycolysis, the TCA cycle, electron transport chain, and oxidative phosphorylation. As a result, cells produce and store ATP, consume oxygen, and exhale carbon dioxide as a by-product. Aerobic metabolism of one glucose unit produces 32 ATPs, whereas anaerobic glycolysis of one glucose unit produces 2 ATPs. Fats metabolized during oxidative phosphorylation generate a high yield of ATP depending on the carbon length, for example, 129 ATP from the oxidation of palmitic acid. Amino acids yield much lower quantities of ATP if catabolized for energy, again depending on the length of the carbon skeletal.

It is possible to determine which substrate(s) are providing energy using indirect calorimetry, which is a method of estimating energy expenditure from respiratory gases. The respiratory exchange ratio (RER) is the ratio between the volume of CO_2 exhaled and the volume of O_2 consumed. This value closely matches the respiratory quotient (RQ) which is the proportion of CO_2 volume generated to the O_2 volume consumption at cellular concentrations. Therefore, the RER is more easily and commonly measured and serves as an estimate of RQ. The oxidation of CHO results in an RER of 1.0, whereas the oxidation of fat results in an RER closer to 0.7. Tracers that label and quantify carbohydrate and fat oxidation rates can also be used. Muscle biopsies can estimate energetic substrate use by estimating muscle glycogen and intramuscular triglyceride concentrations.

Exercise intensity has the greatest effect on substrate use in that as the intensity of the exercise increases, a greater portion of energy production will come from the metabolism of local glycogen stores, and decreasing amounts from body fat. At lower intensities of exercise, there is a greater proportion of energy production from the metabolism of fat, and less from endogenous CHO. This shift from one substrate to the other is often referred to as the crossover concept. However, it should be noticed that at any point in time, both CHO and fats can be used for energy production. It is also recognized that as exercise duration continues resembling more endurance, less sprint type of exercises, the intensity of the exercise is lowered, and there is a greater contribution of energy production from fat.

More specifically, at rest and during a low-intensity type of exercise, a majority of the ATP will be produced through fat oxidation. As the intensity of the exercise increases through the 30–50% VO_2 max range, fat oxidation increases peaking at 55–65% VO_2 max in humans [11]. As exercise intensity increases above 65% VO_2 max, the relative contribution of fat to oxidation decreases. Carbohydrate oxidation is relatively low during low-intensity exercise (30–40% of total energy expenditure), but increases with exercise intensity to nearly 100% of energy expenditure. Muscle glycogen accounted for approximately 30% of the total energy expenditure at 30% VO_2 max [12]. This increased to 65% of total energy expenditure at 60% VO_2 max. Blood glucose contribution was about 10%, and amino acid metabolism was negligible at both work levels [13]. Thus, at lower intensities of work, fat oxidation accounts for a larger percentage of relative energy expenditure (approximately 55%)

compared to higher intensities (approximately 25%). The shift in metabolism type and substrate can be attributed to many factors, including hormones and energy status, as well as breed and individual variations, dietary influence, and training.

In feeding to maintain an adequate energy supply for exercise, the very large body stores of fat, relative to glycogen, produce ATP more slowly and less CO_2, a major determinant of respiratory rate. Carbohydrate stores as muscle glycogen are limited and, although immediately available, produce less energy and more CO_2. During high-intensity exercise, when muscle glycogen is used primarily, the exercise duration is typically short but not exhausted. For example, Thoroughbred and Standardbred horses racing a distance of 0.5–1.25 miles will deplete 20–35% of available muscle glycogen [14, 15]. Cross-country eventers may deplete glycogen stores to 60%, though glycogen is likely not the limiting factor [16]. Whereas, during low-intensity endurance exercise (50–100-mile ride), there was significant glycogen depletion (50–75%) despite a slower rate of use [17, 18]. During prolonged exercise, hypoglycemia and fatigue are associated with depleted muscle glycogen [17, 19]. Muscle protein catabolism may also support gluconeogenesis during this type of exercise, and increased alanine concentrations have been observed in horses following endurance exercise [20]. Although a supply of fatty acids may be available during low-intensity exercise, carbohydrates (or amino acid skeletons) are still required for the TCA cycle to continue. A common phrase in human exercise physiology is "fat burns in a carbohydrate flame," but runners can "hit the wall" when glycogen has been depleted.

It has been shown that reduced glycogen stores can negatively affect exercise bouts and impair performance [21–23]. In sports when a horse might be asked to compete on consecutive days, it is important to replenish glycogen stores quickly. In humans, the replenishment of glycogen following exercise is rapid and depends on the supply of glucose to the muscle. Human athletes consume carbohydrates as starch/sugar at 1 g/kg BW immediately after glycogen depleting exercise and then every 2 hrs for a total of 6 hrs to maximize glycogen resynthesis [24]. In horses, however, glycogen replenishment following exercise is rate-limited and much slower than other species. Starch consumption (15 Mcal) following glycogen-depleting exercise resulted in minimal net muscle glycogen replenishment (52% of resting concentrations) 24 hrs post exercise [25]. Nasogastric administration of glucose (3 g/kg BW over 6 hrs) following glycogen-depleting exercise only replenished glycogen to 56% pre-exercise concentration, while even intravenous glucose administration (3 g/kg BW over 6 hrs) replenished glycogen faster but only reached 75% of pre-exercise concentrations [26]. Glycogen synthase is activated by insulin, substrate availability, and perhaps low glycogen concentrations. In humans and rodents, insulin sensitivity is high following exercise, promoting glycogen synthesis. Relative to other species, horses appear to be comparatively insulin resistant and do not have significant increases in insulin sensitivity after exercise [27, 28]. Regardless, it is still of interest to hasten the recovery of muscle glycogen following exercise in preparation for the next event. While protein or fat supplementation appears to have little impact on glycogen synthesis, the provision of acetate along with electrolytes and fluids may be beneficial [29]. Acetate may be helpful as a readily available energy source for the horse and may spare glucose for glycogen synthesis [30, 31].

18.2.2.3 Skeletal Muscle Fiber Types

Within a muscle, there are differences among the types of fibers, and different muscle groups may have different proportions of different fiber types. Further, some horse breeds have more or less of a specific type of muscle fiber. Muscle fibers can be categorized differently based on functional capacity or the structures within them. From a functional standpoint, muscle fibers can be classified as either slow-twitch or fast-twitch, based on the speed at which the fibers contract. Slow-twitch muscle fibers (Type I) contract slowly and resist fatigue, are also highly oxidative, produce ATP via aerobic metabolism, and are important for endurance exercise. These types of fibers are also found in higher concentrations in breeds known for endurance abilities, for example, Arabians. In horses, the fast-twitch muscle fibers are categorized as Type IIA or Type IIX. Type IIA fibers found in high concentrations in horses are considered fast-twitch high/low oxidative that use anaerobic and aerobic ATP pathways [32]. Type IIX muscle fibers are fast-twitch, low oxidative/high glycolytic which preferentially use anaerobic metabolism to produce ATP and are associated with speed and power. Quarter Horses and Thoroughbreds, known for their bursts of speed, have higher concentrations of Type II fibers. With exercise training, there is some adaptability of muscle types to shift toward oxidative vs. glycolytic, depending on the training program [33]. At rest, horses rely on Type I fibers to generate muscle force in postural muscles. As a horse might begin to exercise, additional muscle fibers are recruited, depending on the type of exercise. As the intensity of an exercise increases, Type II fibers are recruited. Therefore, whole-body substrate utilization depends on both substrate availability and the muscle fiber types contracting. In summary, muscles use ATP for contraction, and ATP must be regenerated for exercise to continue. Athletes must consume sufficient quantities of dietary energetic substrates to endogenous fuels and reserves are available for muscular work.

18.2.3 Temperament

Within the realm of mature, working horses, there is a recognition that there is a range of natural instinctive behaviors that affect energy requirements, for example, voluntary activity, alertness, and reactionary movements. Between horses, individual personality differences may explain the variation in digestible energy (DE) required for BW maintenance [34]. The basis for these behaviors affecting digestible energy for maintenance (DEm) is that activity including stable vices, alertness, and reactions cost energy to perform. There are therefore different daily energy intakes based on the maintenance horse's temperament, lifestyle, or extent of voluntary activity [6]. The DE_m for average horses with an attentive but calm temperament is 3.34 Mcal/100 kg BW, while the DE_m for horses most reactive, with an alert nervous temperament and high levels of voluntary activity, regardless of the area available, is elevated to 3.64 Mcal/100 kg BW. It is not clear at this time whether an average or elevated maintenance DE_m is fitting for working horses [2]. Most likely, the average DE_m closely approximates the energy required for some horses, while the elevated DE_m is appropriate for others. It is important to note that dietary energy intake must first satisfy DE_m before additional functions may be performed, for example, work. Loss of BW and condition are clinical signs of insufficient DE intake for maintenance when working.

18.2.4 Environment

Specific to the water and mineral requirements of working horses, environmental temperature and humidity are major factors to be considered. About 75–80% of the energy used in the body is given off as heat. Energy utilization and, therefore, heat production are greatly increased during exercise. Even at light exercise (a trot, canter, or lope at 9–11 mph), heat production increases 10–20 times that produced at rest, and during a sprint, heat production increases 40–60 times over resting. Without the dissipation of heat produced, at a sprint, body temperature would increase 1.2 °F/min or to a life-threatening level above 106 °F within 4–6 min [35]. The evaporative cooling of sweat accounts for about 55–60% of heat dissipation, whereas evaporative cooling from the respiratory tract accounts for about 25% of the heat dissipated by the horse. The remaining 15–20% of heat dissipation is primarily by convection if the ambient temperature is less than body temperature. Heat production is greater and heat losses are decreased for a similar amount of exercise in physically unfit versus fit horses, and heat loss is further impaired in overweight horses and those with a winter coat.

Sweating results in the loss of not only water but also sodium, chloride, potassium, and lesser amounts of calcium and magnesium, and if excessive, will result in a significant body deficit of these electrolytes. Since the concentration of sodium, potassium, and chloride in the sweat is higher than plasma, excessive sweating decreases body concentrations. Dehydration and electrolyte imbalances contribute to exercise fatigue. In contrast to many nutrients, there are no body stores of water or electrolytes other than those carried in the gastrointestinal (GI) tract. Any excess quantities of electrolytes consumed are absorbed and rapidly excreted in the urine. Thus, body water and electrolyte deficits cannot be prevented by administration before there is a deficit; however, severe deficits can be prevented by the use of replacement solutions offered regularly throughout the workout or event.

18.3 Ration Assessment

Ration DE concentrations of 2–3 Mcal DE/kg dry matter (DM) are suitable for growing in training, whereas 2–2.8 Mcal DE/kg DM are recommended for mature working horses with BCS of 4/9–6/9. All horses should be provided a complete and balanced ration, meeting the energy and nutrient requirements within 2.0–2.5% BW dry matter intake (DMI) depending on the age and DER. Rations, predominately forage, with relative feeding values (RFV) greater than 95 are suggested for working mature horses, but greater than 115 RFV is recommended for growing horses in training [36–38] (Table 18.4).

18.3.1 Feeds

18.3.1.1 Forages

Forage (pasture or hay) should provide the preponderance (>60%) of the working horse ration. Forage quality is assessed through objective nutrient analyses and subjective measures, that is, smell, color, feel, and physical contents. See Ration Analysis and Subjective Assessments in Chapter 10. The forage offered must be palatable, that is, in odor and texture, to the horse to ensure an adequate DMI [40]. The forage digestible dry matter (DDM) and energy density (Mcal/kg DM) must be sufficient to meet the estimated DER within an edible volume of feed (DMI). DM digestibility and voluntary DMI are inversely related to the forage acid detergent fiber (%ADF) and neutral detergent fiber (%NDF), respectively. As ADF and NDF increase in the forage DM, the voluntary DMI and DM digestibility decrease, and the nutritional value of the forage decreases. See Relative Feed Value in Chapter 10.

Table 18.4 Comparison of major nutrient concentrations between forage averages and ration recommendations for working horses [37, 39].

Horse to Forage Comparison	Digestible energy	Protein	Calcium	Phosphorus	DMI	RFV
	Dry matter basis				% BW	
Growth + work:	Mcal/kg	%	%	%		115–150
18 mos old						
Light	2.28	8.8	0.38	0.21	2.5	
Moderate	2.58	9.4	0.38	0.21	2.5	
24 mos old						
Light	2.03	7.7	0.30	0.19	2.5	
Moderate	2.31	8.3	0.30	0.19	2.5	
Heavy	2.38	9.0	0.30	0.19	2.5	
Very heavy	3.03	10.2	0.30	0.19	2.5	
Adult + work:						>95
Light	2.00	7.0	0.30	0.18	2.0	
Moderate	2.07	7.0	0.31	0.19	2.25	
Heavy	2.13	7.0	0.32	0.23	2.5	
Very heavy	2.76	8.0	0.32	0.23	2.5	
Forages:						
Legume						
Pasture: vegetative	2.71	26.5	1.31	0.37	3.6[a]	197[b]
Hay: immature	2.62	20.5	1.56	0.31	3.3	171
Hay: mid-mature	2.43	20.8	1.37	0.30	2.8	136
Hay: mature	2.21	17.8	1.22	0.28	2.4	106
Grass						
Pasture: vegetative	2.39	26.5	0.56	0.44	2.6	141
Hay: immature	2.36	18.0	0.72	0.34	2.4	121
Hay: mid-mature	2.18	13.3	0.66	0.29	2.1	97
Hay: mature	2.04	10.8	0.47	0.26	1.7	76

[a] Forage %DMI = 120/NDF%.
[b] Forage relative feeding value = %DDM × %DMI × 0.775; where %DDM = 88.9 − (0.779 × ADF%).
Source: Adapted from NRC [2]; Table 16-3 using nutrients required for a 500 kg mature horse BCS 4–6/9. Forage data from Table 16-6.

Horses foraging on pasture have many advantages: natural social interactions, voluntary exercise with a reduction in incidences of gastric ulcers, colic, stereotypical behaviors, and orthopedic diseases, and forage is a nutritious feed [38]. For example, a well-managed pasture of cool-season grasses can provide 22–28 Mcal DE/d to horses grazing at 2.0–2.5% DMI which is the daily DE required by a 500-kg horse performing moderate to heavy work [38, 41]. However, the nutritional value of a pasture is dependent on management (fertilization, grazing pattern, etc.), plant species, access time, seasons, and weather, and therefore can be variable. Additionally, time at pasture is reduced by training and travel schedules. Legume or mixed mainly legume (MML) hay (RFV >95, >2.0 Mcal/kg DM) can also provide a 500-kg horse at moderate to heavy work with sufficient DE. Hay providing the preponderance (>75%) of the working horse ration will require a mineral–vitamin supplement to be nutritionally complete.

18.3.1.2 Complementary Feeds

In those instances when forage cannot meet the energy needs, regardless of reason, concentrated energy products (grain/fat mixtures) are fed to provide the difference between the animal requirement and that provided by forage alone [34, 42]. See Chapter 13 Manufactured Feeds. Commercial performance feeds provide energy, in the form of carbohydrates, fiber and fat, protein, minerals, and vitamins. These products are usually sold as bagged pelleted or textured (sweet feeds) with a minimum guaranteed analysis and ingredient list. See Basic Label Requirements in Chapter 15. The proper amount to feed is initially suggested by the manufacturer or that determined by a ration formulator, but then as little as necessary is fed to maintain a proper body condition for that individual horse.

18.3.2 Key Nutrients

For frequent or prolonged physical activity, such as training for and competing in athletic events, the nutrients needed, in their order of importance, are (i) water, (ii) body salts or electrolytes, and (iii) energy. A horse can use essentially all available body fat stores and up to one-half of body protein, whereas a loss of 15% of body water is fatal. Electrolytes are lost with the water from the body. In some performances, large quantities of water and electrolytes are lost during physical exertion to dissipate the heat produced in the production and utilization of energy necessary for physical activity.

18.3.2.1 Water

Water is the most important nutrient comprising roughly 65% of an adult horse's mass, and 85% is acquired by drinking water [43–45]. The normal voluntary daily water intake of horses is dependent on factors including body heat produced, environmental temperature and humidity, rate of exercise, and food composition. Thirst is influenced by plasma osmolality, which is affected by diet composition and feed DM consumption [44, 46–48]. The average daily water intake of healthy adult horses is approximately 54–64 mL/kg BW/d [45]. Water losses primarily, up to 55% of total daily water loss, occur through defecation and urination, with the remainder of water lost via sweating and respiration [49]. Losses through sweating and respiration are greatly impacted by temperature, humidity, and work [43, 50, 51].

The increase in water requirement for athletic horses is largely to replace the sweat losses that occur with exercise. Muscle contraction is inefficient, using only some of the potential energy for work, and the remaining energy being released as heat. Most body heat is dissipated from the horse via sweat, and horses can sweat up to 10 L/hr of exercise. Further, increases in feed intake and the likely decreased access to fresh pasture in place of dried hay result in increased drinking of water. Fresh, clean water should be made available to all horses at all times. It is an error not to offer water to hot horses. Supplying cool water continuously helps horses dissipate body heat via convection. Hydration status should be monitored during workouts and as part of the recovery protocol.

18.3.2.2 Energy

Total DE requirements for work include that required for maintenance (DE_m), and that needed for work (DE_w), plus DE for growth (DE_g) if the horse has not yet reached maturity. Energy requirement for work is ultimately based on calories consumed at various intensities of work, as DE_w increases with increasing intensity, for example, speed (Table 18.5). Suggested DE for horses performing various levels of work were calculated based on studies that measured oxygen consumed at different intensities of exercise, extrapolated to weekly averages, and then divided into four workout groups: light, moderate, heavy, and intense (Table 18.2) [2]. These values are based on the 3.34 Mcal/100 kg BW DE_m plus 20%, 40%, and 60% for light, moderate, and heavy work, respectively. However, at the most intense level, very heavy work, the DERs are based on the "elevated" maintenance metabolic rate (DE_m 3.63 Mcal/100 kg BW) plus 90% above maintenance due to a typically higher lean body condition and the more active temperament of these horses. Energy requirements are more than double (3.34–6.9 Mcal DE/100 kg BW) from a horse at maintenance to a horse in very heavy work. It should be noted that these values are estimates, and body condition should be monitored to ensure calorie intake is sufficient to maintain BW and condition.

18.3.2.2.1 Carbohydrates

Dietary sources of energy are fat (9 kcal/g), carbohydrate (4 kcal/g), and protein (4 kcal/g); however, in the equine ration, carbohydrates predominate. Starch and sugars in grain and molasses, respectively, in concentrate feeds may

Table 18.5 Gait speeds and approximate energy expenditures needed above maintenance [52, 53].

Gait	Speed	DE above DE_m
	Miles/hr	Mcal/hr/100 kg BW[a]
Slow walk	2.1	0.17
Fast walk	3.5	0.25
Slow trot	7.5	0.65
Medium trot	9.3	0.95
Fast trot/slow canter	11.2	1.37
Medium canter	13.0	1.9
Gallop[b]	18–37[c]	2.0+

[a] Total weight of horse, rider, and tack. For example, a mature Paint mare BW 549 kg (w/o rider and tack) exercised at a medium speed trot for 15 min in-hand would expend 1.3 Mcal.
[b] Sprinting at a full gallop is generally for less than 1 min in most races and training sessions. Race distances are 0.25 mile for Quarter Horses, 1.0 mile for Standardbreds, and 1.0–1.5 mile for Thoroughbreds.
[c] Average speed of Kentucky Derby winners.

comprise 40–60% of the ration providing DE. The energy from these sources is converted to glucose and either used immediately by tissues or stored in the liver or muscle as glycogen for later use. Glycogen is readily converted back to blood glucose for energy relative to volatile fatty acids from fiber fermentation and body fat. Muscle glycogen, used in anaerobic energy production, and hence dietary starch and sugar are primary energy sources for short fast sprint activities at near 100% maximum exertion as in Quarter Horse racing, barrel racing, rodeo events, and draft pulling contests.

18.3.2.2.2 Fat

Oils are primarily used to increase the fat content and energy density of equine rations. Dietary fats are concentrated sources of energy, carriers of fat-soluble vitamins, and sources of essential fatty acids. Increasing dietary fat concentration increases ration caloric density which in turn decreases the amount of feed needed to meet DER because fats provide 2.25 times (9 vs. 4 kcal/g) more utilizable energy than an equal weight of carbohydrate or protein. Ration caloric density is increased for athletic performance, growth, and to maintain or increase BW during hot humid weather. Specific to athletic performance, mobilizing body fat, compared with glycogen stores, decreases the heat load and increases the energy available for physical activity [54]. Additionally, high-fat diets have been shown to enhance both aerobic and anaerobic performance activities and to delay fatigue [55, 56]. A high-fat diet (15% DM) appeared to be better than either a high-starch (40% DM) or a high-protein (25% DM) diet for both high-speed and moderate-speed exercises. At high speed, muscle glycogen use and plasma lactate concentration were both substantially lower than when the horses were consuming the high-starch, low-fat (3% DM) diet [57]. A crude fat content of at least 6% DM is recommended in the complementary products fed to performance horses [34].

Both linoleic acid (LA; 18:2 n-6) and α-linolenic acid (ALA; 18:3 n-3) are essential fatty acids in horses. A dietary minimum of 0.5% DM has been suggested which is relatively easy to meet with ≤1% fat in the ration, whereas the forage portion of the ration provides primarily ALA [2]. There are no dietary omega-3 fatty acid recommendations, but dietary fatty acid content does affect circulating and cellular fatty acid profiles in horses [58].

18.3.2.3 Protein

With exercise, muscle hypertrophy is an increase in size and not an increase in the number of muscle fibers. Work is the major stimulus for muscle growth, and protein synthesis increases after a bout of exercise [59]. Exercise stress and damage to the muscle from heavy work activate satellite cells [60]. These satellite cells can divide and multiply and will fuse with existing muscle fibers, to increase muscle size. Numerous hormones promote muscle growth, such as insulin-like growth and fibroblast growth factors, growth hormone, and testosterone. Insulin can also promote muscle growth by activating protein synthesis and facilitating glucose uptake into cells. Therefore, while the major factor stimulating muscle synthesis is exercise, the diet must provide sufficient amino acids to support muscle growth as well as sufficient energy [61]. A common misconception is that feeding amino acids alone will improve back musculature, for example, "topline supplements." However, without the exercise stimulus in those muscle groups, there is no muscle hypertrophy regardless of the increased protein or amino acid intake. There is no storage form of amino acids in the body. Dietary amino acids consumed are either used for endogenous protein or tissue synthesis immediately, or the amino acids are deaminated and the carbon skeleton is converted to glucose or fat. Overfeeding protein will not increase tissue protein synthesis, but does ultimately increase blood urea followed by increased urination to excrete the excessive nitrogen. Hence, high-protein diets may be detrimental to athletic horses by altering water balance [62, 63].

Dietary protein concentrations for athletes are higher than maintenance primarily for increased tissue synthesis and repair, and not as an energy source. Nitrogen is also lost in sweat in the protein latherin, the soapy substance secreted with sweat. Therefore, protein intakes for working horses must support muscle hypertrophy, repair, replenish lost nitrogen in addition to maintenance of cell membranes, enzymes, hormones, immune function, and carrier/transport functions. Dietary CP concentration increases as workload increases (Tables 18.2–18.4). Several studies have demonstrated either no benefit or detrimental effects of high-protein diets, and, therefore, 10–16% DM is recommended to adequately meet, but not greatly exceed, the protein requirement [64–67]. The CP content of at least 11–13% is recommended in the non-forage portion fed to performance horses [34].

Many commercial horse feeds designed for athletes contain high-quality protein sources, for example, soybean meal, and/or added amino acids to ensure adequate intake. Lysine is the first limiting amino acid, and hence dietary concentrations have been recommended in a performance horse ration that increase with greater levels of work. Threonine is likely the second limiting amino acid for horses, though a dietary recommendation has not been established [68, 69]. Leucine has been shown to increase satellite cell activity in rats when accompanied by appropriate exercise training and is commonly supplemented to working horses; however, a dietary recommendation has not been established [70].

18.3.2.4 Macrominerals

Calcium (Ca), phosphorus (P), and magnesium (Mg) are major constituents of bone, and the recommended dietary concentrations in athletic horse rations increase with the level of exercise to support bone remodeling (Table 18.2) [71]. Bone remodeling occurs in response to the forces applied to the bone proportional to the exercise intensity and frequency. Feeding additional calcium without an exercise stimulus, with or without phosphorus, does not increase bone density. It is important to ensure adequate absolute intakes of both Ca and P, first separately, and then that the Ca:P ratio is within 1.5:1 to 2:1. The macromineral recommendations for young growing horses in training are the same as those for growth (Table 18.3) [2]. Rations high in cereal grains, for example, oats or barley, to increase energy intake, are likely to have low concentrations of Ca and high in phosphorus. High-forage rations may also be relatively high in oxalate which reduces calcium absorption.

The electrolytes, sodium (Na), chloride (Cl), and potassium (K), are an important group of macrominerals that are lost in significant quantities in sweat, which occurs at all levels of work even when sweat is not visible, and during transportation in hot temperatures. Requirements of Na, Cl, and K almost double from maintenance in intense exercise, though might be higher in hot temperatures. Sodium concentrations are typically low in forages and cereal grains, while potassium intake is typically sufficient with the consumption of forages. All athletic horses should be fed salt (NaCl) in addition to that in commercial feeds, which are typically low, and may need further electrolyte supplementation under more extreme circumstances, that is, endurance racing in high ambient temperatures and humidity.

18.3.2.5 Trace Minerals

The stressors of exercise on bones likely increase the need for copper and zinc to maintain bone integrity (Tables 18.2 and 18.3). Iron is an important component of hemoglobin, the oxygen-carrying protein in red blood cells. Iron absorption from the digestive tract is well regulated and is stored in the liver. There is no excretory mechanism for iron and sweat content is minor. Therefore, iron deficiency is typically only seen in horses with gastric ulcers or exercise-induced pulmonary hemorrhaging where iron is lost from the body. Iron supplements to increase hemoglobin stores and enhance the oxygen-carrying capacity of the blood do not appear to be effective [72]. Iron concentrations in most forages are relatively high (200–400 ppm DM) and iron in commercial feeds is common, and therefore intake is typically adequate, as iron requirements increase little with increasing exercise demands [2]. Cobalt is a required cofactor of vitamin B_{12} (cobalamin) which is essential for red blood cell synthesis. In some species, cobalt supplementation is associated with an increase in erythropoietin and red blood cell production. However, research in horses shows that cobalt administration does not affect red blood cell volume or performance [73]. Selenium is a required cofactor of the glutathione peroxidase system that intercepts pro-oxidants and buffers the reactive oxygen species produced during exercise. Although no benefit against muscle damage or improved antioxidant defense was found in horses fed 0.25 or 0.75 mg of Se/100 kg BW, often more Se is supplemented than recommended [1, 2, 74].

18.3.2.6 Vitamins

The B vitamins and vitamin K are produced in sufficient quantities by the GI microbes to meet the needs of idle adult horses; however, the recommended dietary concentrations of thiamin and riboflavin increase with work effort (Tables 18.2 and 18.3) [2]. Many B vitamins are required in intermediary metabolism and energy production, and therefore would be needed at a higher rate in a working horse with a higher metabolic rate. Predominantly, thiamin, riboflavin, and niacin are essential to the workings of the TCA cycle (Krebs cycle) and energy ATP production. Intravenous thiamin administration was shown to improve glucose metabolism in exercising horses [75]. B vitamins are relatively inexpensive ingredients with no known upper toxic limit, and hence often a component of commercial feeds and supplements [1].

Vitamin E, as α-tocopherol, functions as an antioxidant endogenously and recommended intakes increase with exercise level. Contractions cause oxidative damage to muscle cells and vitamin E works as an antioxidant to help restore muscle integrity. As a preservative, delta and gamma forms of vitamin E scavenge free radicals and are often added to higher-fat diets of exercising horses to help prevent lipid peroxidation. Vitamin C (ascorbic acid) is an antioxidant that is normally produced in the liver and is not considered a dietary essential nutrient. Vitamin C restores the activity of vitamin E, and when supplemented together, blood vitamin E concentrations are higher than vitamin E fed alone [76]. Beta-carotene, in addition to its function as a precursor to vitamin A, also functions as an antioxidant. Sport horses are commonly supplemented with multivitamins, though caution should be taken as excessive vitamin E intake may reduce beta-carotene status [1, 77].

18.4 Feeding Management

Working adult and young horses should be maintained with a BCS of 4/9–6/9. The working horse should be fed a ration containing good- to high-quality forage as pasture or hay, with water and salt (NaCl) as white or trace mineralized salt (block or loose), specific for horses, should be available *ad libitum*, preferably under cover from weather and consumption monitoring. For idle or occasionally ridden horses, white salt should be offered if a commercial feed or ration balancer contains trace minerals. Feeding intake, BCS, and BW must be monitored to maintain working horses in ideal BW and condition. The amount of feed to maintain a moderate BCS weight should be initially calculated, and the horse assessed as activity levels, weather, and forage source change. The intake of pasture is difficult to determine, but assessing BW and BCS regularly as the pasture changes is warranted. The suggested feeding recommendations apply only to horses in moderate body condition.

Most athletic horses meet the nutritional requirements of work by increasing feed intake within 3.0% BW [2, 38]. This is particularly important for athletic horses where speed and power influence performance that is negatively impacted by the weight of the GI tract. Most maintenance horses consume 2% BW when offered forages free choice. Athletic horses can easily increase DMI to 2.5% BW. As forage quality decreases and fiber increases, DMI maximums are reached before the horse can meet macronutrient needs. When nutrient requirements exceed the maximum forage DMI, a portion of the ration must become more concentrated in calories, protein, and most all other nutrients. Complementary feeds, cereal grains, and commercial sweet or textured feeds with higher DE densities (>3.0 Mcal/kg DM) must replace some portion of the forage in the ration. A predominantly forage ration consumed at 2–2.25% BW is adequate for most idle or light working horses; however, as energy requirements increase with the workload, athletic horses have increased proportions of non-forage feeds in their diets. At an extreme, the concentration portion may exceed the forage portion, that is, a 30:70 concentrate to forage ratio. Feeding energy-concentrated feeds decreases the volume and weight of feed consumed, for example, a commercial performance feed may contain 4.5 Mcal DE_g vs. grass hay with 1.9 Mcal DE per kg feed. The challenge in feeding athletic horses is to balance the higher nutritional needs, principally energy, with recognized safe feeding practices, that is, high-fiber/low-grain rations. Some horses in high levels of work need large amounts (>1% BW) of grain mixes daily. In such cases, it is recommended that horses be fed their total daily ration divided into four or more meals/d. Feeding small meals and slowing down feeding rate through the use of objects placed in a horse's feed tub can hasten the blood glucose and insulin response to each meal [78, 79].

Bowel ballast weight refers to the weight of the feed in the horse's digestive tract and is significantly increased with forage intake. Reducing forage (<60%) intake is detrimental to equine health, but in some instances, limiting feed intake before exercise may have some advantages. In sports where power and speed are tested, a leaner BCS may also be desirable. One BCS represents 16–20 kg BW, and keeping some horses in leaner condition (4/9 vs. 5/9) might be advantageous over a more conditioned horse (BCS >5/9). The feed should never be withheld from horses, so a balance between maintaining enough forage (fiber) in the GI tract for health but avoiding ballast weight must be attained. Limiting feed intake before high-intensity exercise may have advantages in terms of substrate selection during exercise. Horses that were fasted maintained higher blood glucose concentrations during high-intensity exercise than those horses fed corn before exercise [80]. This is likely due to the additive effects of insulin and exercise driving glucose from the bloodstream and into muscle. Insulin also inhibits lipolysis decreasing the concentrations of free fatty acids in the blood. Similarly, feeding forage before exercise was not detrimental to substrate utilization and performance [81]. Further, meal feeding before exercise results in hemodynamic changes shifting fluids to the digestive tract. Ponies fed before exercise had higher heart rates and cardiac outputs during the exercise than unfed horses [82]. Because forage is so important for GI health, it is recommended that athletic horses be fed good-quality or better (RFV >115) forages in smaller meals when approaching an intense bout of exercise [83].

There is some evidence that the source of dietary energy can influence the fuel substrate used during high-intensity exercises, that is, flat track racing, polo, and eventing. Fat adaptation can shift fuel use away from carbohydrates, thus sparing muscle glycogen in high-intensity work [55]. Diets high in forages have been shown to increase acetate and fatty acid availability during exercise which produced lower lactate concentrations in racing Standardbreds [84]. Whereas feeding corn (high starch) to horses before high-intensity exercises resulted in increased carbohydrate oxidation during the workout [85]. However, horses performing at high levels of work intensity, that is, Quarter Horse races and rodeo work (cutting, reining, and barrel racing), rely on muscle glycogen, and dietary simple carbohydrates should be sufficient to maintain adequate glycogen stores.

During lower-intensity and endurance exercises, fat is the primary source of fuel. In some cases, glycogen can become limiting, for example, endurance rides >50 mi (80 km), which contributes to fatigue. Horses should be offered forages as much as possible, as large bowel fermentation of forages provides a longer-term energy source from volatile fatty acids [30, 31, 83]. Horses fed a higher fat diet also had an increase in fat oxidation during low-intensity exercise, thus sparing glucose and glycogen [86]. During lower intensity types of exercise, for example, dressage, show hunters and western pleasure horses benefit from having more calories from fat and fiber compared to starch and sugar.

Some feeds high in starch and sugar, for example corn, are said to cause some horses to be "hot" or "high", or overly spirited. The best physiological explanation would be that some horses are more sensitive to fluctuations in blood glucose after consuming high non-structural carbohydrate meals rather than an attribute of corn. By contrast, some trainers complain of horses being less reluctant to exercise at the desired intensity, that is, lazy. Unfortunately, no nutrient or substance can be fed or administered (legally) to increase the desire to run faster or jump higher. The administration of a sweet meal may momentarily raise blood glucose concentrations, but these are often short-lived. In some situations, a horse may struggle to exercise adequately because of undiagnosed pain, psychological barriers, or excessive weight which not only increases workload but contributes to heat stress.

In summary, athletic horses should consume good- to high-quality forage rations, supplemented with nutrient-concentrated feed products only as needed based on meeting nutrient requirements, and not based on marketing. Horses that work at high intensities should be fed before (>8 hrs) and after exercise to optimize muscle glycogen concentrations. Immediately prior (<4 hrs) to competitive events, horses should receive small amounts of forages (0.5% BW).

18.4.1 Growing Athlete

To have as much forage in the ration as possible, growing horses in heavy training may require excellent-quality forage to meet energy requirements. Forage quality should be sufficiently palatable and digestible (<30% ADF, <40% NDF, RFV >124) such that 18 to 24-mo-old horses will meet energy requirements. The forage must have adequate concentrations of energy, protein, calcium, and phosphorus to meet needs within 2.5% BW DMI (Tables 10.3 and 18.4). Feeding young equine athletes will likely require a complementary feed, although the better the forage quality, the less will be needed, that is, forage to grain ratio is higher using better-quality forages. Feeding a ration with CP 8–12% is recommended [2, 36–38]. If lower RFV forages are fed, greater quantities of a complementary growth product for calories and/or protein will be needed, in addition to mineral–vitamin supplements, and the total ration will have a lower forage to grain ratio.

18.4.2 Mature Athlete

Forage quality for fully grown mature horses should be sufficiently palatable and digestible (<40% ADF, <50% NDF, RFV >95) such that the horse will meet energy requirements. The forage must have adequate concentrations of energy, protein, calcium, and phosphorus to meet needs consuming 2-2.5% BW DMI (Tables 10.3 and 18.4). Feeding equine athletes in very heavy training may require excellent-quality forage to meet energy requirements with as much forage in the ration as possible. Feeding forage with RFV >95 is recommended with 7 to 11 % CP [2, 36–38]. If lower RFV forages are fed, a complementary performance feed for calories will be needed, in addition to mineral–vitamin supplements, and the ration will have a lower forage to grain ratio. See Sidebar 18.1.

Sidebar 18.1: Calculating Daily Feeding Recommendations for a Mature Horse at Light Work

Animal Assessment

- A 550 kg (BCS 5/9) 15-yr-old Quarter Horse gelding trail ridden (walk/trot) 2–3 hrs/wk in Florida year-round; considered light work (Table 18.1).
- DMI is 2.0% BW (Table 18.4).
- Gelding's daily DE requirement: 4.00 Mcal/100 kg BW × 5.5 = 22.0 Mcal DE/d (Table 18.2).
- Forage recommendations for adult horses in light work are RFVs of 95–150 and 2.0 Mcal DE/kg DM (Table 18.4). ADF <45% and NDF <65% is recommended for adult horses (Table 10.3).

Ration Assessment

Hay available is a MML forage with 90% DM. The smell and texture of the hay are sufficiently palatable for the gelding to consume 2% BW. On a DM basis, the forage had estimated textbook values of:

IFN	DE	CP	Ca	P	ADF	NDF	Na	Cl	K
#	Mcal/kg				%				
1-02-277	2.35	19.1	1.17	0.30	35.4	47.2	0.08	0.43	2.34

- Calculate DDM, DMI, and RFV values:
  - %DDM = 88.9 − (0.779 × %ADF) = 61%.
  - %DMI = 120/%NDF = 2.5% BW.
  - RFV = %DDM × %DMI × 0.775 = 120 good-quality (Table 10.3).
  - Forage quality matches that recommended for a working adult horse.
- Calculate daily forage intake required to meet the horse's DE on DM and as fed (AF) basis:
  - Horse requires 22 Mcal DE/2.35 Mcal DE/kg DM = 9.4 kg forage DM/0.9 = 10.4 kg forage AF.
  - Check DMI: 9.4 kg forage DM intake/550 kg BW = 1.7% BW.

- Compare forage crude protein (CP), calcium (Ca), and phosphorus (P) concentrations with recommendations (Table 18.4).
  - Recommended [CP] is 7.0%; forage contains 19.1% CP.
  - Recommended [Ca] is 0.30%; forage contains 1.17% Ca.
  - Recommended [P] is 0.18% P; forage contains 0.30% P with Ca:P ratio = 3.9:1.
  - If a sufficient quantity of hay is consumed, the CP, Ca, and P needs should be met.
- If the horse consumed 9.4 kg DM hay daily, compare sodium (Na), chloride (Cl) and potassium (K) intake and daily recommendations (Table 18.2):
  - Na: intake is 7.5 g Na/d [9.4 kg forage DM/d × 0.08%] whereas 15 g Na is required [2.8 g/d × 5.5].
  - Cl: intake is 40 g Cl/d whereas 51 g Cl is required.
  - K: intake is 220 g K/d whereas 31 g K is required.
  - Na and Cl needs will not be met, K need is met.

Feeding Management Recommendations

The nutrient composition of the hay, based on textbook values, exceeds the gelding's requirements for energy, protein, calcium, and phosphorus. Specific instructions:

- Laboratory assay the hay for DE, ADF, and NDF, and re-assess feeding plan based on client's hay data.
- Feed 10 to 11 kg hay AF/d which is 1.7% BW [9.4 kg DM/550 kg] and monitor BW and BCS monthly.
- Feed 1 tbsp white table salt (NaCl)/d [15 g Na required minus 7.5 g Na forage = 7.5 g deficit/39% Na in salt = 19 g salt/d] (Table 18.6).
- Feed trace mineral–vitamin ration balancer to meet micronutrient requirements.
- Lysine intake should be checked. The book value is 0.72% DM which is adequate.
- Offer water and salt block *ad libitum*.

18.4.3 Feeding Management Based on Workload

18.4.3.1 Feeding Horses for Infrequent Light Exercise

Horses that are ridden occasionally (30–180 min/wk) at a walk or slow trot on the flat ground such as pleasure trail riding or in an arena often do well fed a moderate- to good-quality forage (pasture or hay) at quantities that maintain a BCS 4/9–5/9. The DE intake for maintenance adult horses doing occasional light exercise is 3.34 Mcal/100 kg BW/d based on average temperament (Table 18.2) to 3.64 Mcal/100 kg BW/d for elevated temperament [2]. On feeding a moderate- to good-quality hay (RFV >86), these horses will likely require a mineral–vitamin supplement, that is, low-calorie, low-fat, ration balancer, fed at 0.1% BW with no special feeding before, during, or after the ride [34]. Ensure the minimum sodium requirement is met (5 g NaCl/100 kg BW/d), and that water and salt (white or trace mineral) are available *ad libitum*. See Chapter 17 Feeding Adult and Senior Horses.

Table 18.6 Daily sodium requirements of horses at different workloads and the amount of NaCl required to meet sodium requirement [2, 87].

Level of work	Sodium per 100 kg BW[a] (g)	NaCl per 100 kg BW (g)	White table salt per 100 kg BW[b]	White table salt for a 500-kg horse (tbsp)
Maintenance	2.0	5	1 tsp	1.5
Light work	2.8	7	1.25 tsp	2
Moderate work	3.6	9	2 tsp	2.5
Heavy work	5.1	13	2.25 tsp	3.5
Very heavy work	8.2	21	1.25 tbsp	6

[a] This does not account for sodium needs with excessive sweat losses due to high environmental temperatures and humidity. Weight lost during exercise × 3.1 g Na/kg BW approximates an individual horse's Na requirement on a given day.

[b] Rounded up using 6 g/teaspoon (tsp) or 18 g/tablespoon (tbsp) of white table salt. https://fdc.nal.usda.gov/fdc-app.html#/food-details/173468/measures.

18.4.3.2 Feeding Horses for Frequent Light Exercise and Low-Intensity Events

Horses exercised (45–60 min; 4–5 d/wk) at a walk (40%), trot (50%), and canter (10%) and involved in recreational trail riding and occasional low-level competitions are considered to be in a light exercise routine (Table 18.1). The DE intake for horses in light exercise is 4.0 Mcal/100 kg BW/d (Table 18.2) [2]. The competitions are low-intensity types of events, such as dressage, western pleasure, timed trail riding with obstacles, and show ring hunters, which require athleticism and a focused and engaged disposition. Many horses perform well and maintain BCS on moderate- to good-quality forage (RFV >86) ration (pasture or hay) with a mineral–vitamin ration balancer. Depending on the frequency of shows, traveling, and extent of activities, a forage ration with a complementing feed (4–6% fat, 11–13% protein with minerals and vitamins) fed at 0.3–0.5% BW may be required to maintain BCS 4/9–6/9 [34]. On event days, portions of the daily ration containing grains should be fed

4 or more hrs before a competition to ensure blood glucose concentrations have stabilized [81]. Feeding a low non-structural carbohydrate ration in multiple meals/d will minimize fluctuations in blood glucose concentrations which may help maintain an even temperament and responsiveness in those horses reactive to high blood glucose concentrations. Adding fat in the form of vegetable oil to maintain optimal BCS is rarely needed, but an option if needed periodically, that is, during the show season vs. the off-season. Fish oils may also be fed to improve skin and hair coat when a show quality shine is desirable. Ensure the minimum sodium requirement is met (5 g NaCl/100 kg BW/d) recognizing more will be needed proportional to work and sweat production (Table 18.6). Water and white salt, or trace mineral salt if no complementing feed is used, should be available *ad libitum* or offered frequently.

18.4.3.3 Feeding Horses for Moderate Exercise and Mid-Intensity Events

Horses worked (45–60 min; 4–5 d/wk) at a walk (30%), trot (55%), or canter (10%) on the flat ground involved in low-level skilled competitions (dressage, eventing, etc.), school horses, western speed events (roping, cutting, and reining), western pleasure are considered to be doing moderate work. The DE intake for horses in moderate exercise is 4.66 Mcal/100 kg BW/d (Table 18.2) [2]. These horses will likely require a complementary feed (8–10% fat, 11–13% protein with minerals and vitamins) fed at 0.5–0.8% BW in addition to a good-quality forage (RFV >100) (pasture or hay) to maintain BCS 4/9–6/9 during certain times of the year, that is, show season or work schedules [34]. Ensure the minimum sodium requirement is met (5 g NaCl/100 kg BW/d) daily recognizing more will be needed proportional to work and sweat production [87]. Water and white salt should be available *ad libitum* or offered frequently.

18.4.3.4 Feeding Horses for Heavy Exercise and High-Intensity Sports and Events

Horses worked (60 min; 4–6 d/wk) at a walk (20%), trot (50%), canter (15%), and 15% specialized training as in flat track racing, polo, eventing, and rodeo skill work are considered to be in heavy work routines (Table 18.1). The DE intake for horses in heavy exercise is 5.32 Mcal/100 kg BW/d (Table 18.2) [2]. Horses may be frequently traveling to participate in high-intensity sports such as cross-country racing, Grand Prix level jumping, low- to mid-level 3-d eventing, high levels of dressage, polo, and endurance riding. These horses need large reserves of muscle and hepatic glycogen to fuel such activities and do require dietary energy (sugar, starch) beyond that supplied by forage. These horses also benefit from fat in their diets to provide sufficient calories and potentially decrease lactic acid production. A complementary feed (10–14% fat, 13–15% protein with minerals and vitamins) should be fed at 0.8–1.0% BW in addition to a good- to high-quality forage (RFV >100) (pasture or hay) to maintain BCS 4/9–6/9 [34]. The grain portion of the ration concentrate should be fed in several meals/d (<300 g starch/100 kg BW/meal) and at least 4–6 hrs before an event [88, 89]. These horses also tend to have a high occurrence of gastric ulcers; therefore, long-stem good- to high-quality grass forage should predominate the ration (1.5–2.0% BW). On event days, feeding limited amounts of grass or mixed mainly grass (MMG) (<30% alfalfa) in the hours before an event is advised to minimize bowel ballast, and not feeding excessive protein and calcium before an event is recommended [88]. Ensure the minimum sodium requirement is met (5 g NaCl/100 kg BW/d) recognizing more will be needed proportional to work and sweat production (Table 18.6). Water and white salt should be available *ad libitum* or offered frequently.

18.4.3.5 Feeding Horses for Very Heavy Exercise and Endurance Events

Horses performing very heavy workloads are exercised (4–6 d/wk) at galloping or sprinting speeds for <10 min/d or 1–2 hrs of skill or endurance work. These horses perform in elite 3-d eventing, high-goal polo, steeplechase, and 50–100 mile endurance races (Table 18.1) [2, 34]. The DE intake for horses in very heavy exercise is 6.9 Mcal/100 kg BW/d (Table 18.2) [2]. Feeding high- to excellent-quality forage (RFV >125) is required to maximize energy intake from fiber sources (volatile fatty acids), improve DMI intake as horses will consume more of a higher RFV hay than the more mature lower RFV hays, and lower the risk of GI disturbances. It is challenging, if not impossible, to meet the daily DE requirement of such horses if feed intake (DMI) is <2% BW [89]. To meet the daily DE requirement of these horses requires feeding a complementary feed (8–10% fat, 13–15% protein with minerals and vitamins) fed at 1.2–1.5% in forage (pasture or hay) to maintain BCS 4/9–6/9 BW [34]. BCS of 4/9–4.5/9 has been suggested for endurance horses [88]. Ensure the minimum sodium requirement is met (5 g NaCl/100 kg BW/d) recognizing more will be needed proportional to work and sweat production (Table 18.6). Water and white salt should be available *ad libitum* or offered frequently.

In general, higher fat concentrates are not recommended for sprinting activities because anaerobic activities utilize glycogen stores. Carbohydrate loading the muscle before an event, as used by human marathon runners, is of little value in horses due to a slow rate of replenishment after depletion [90]. In horses, 2–3 d may be required to fully replenish muscle glycogen stores after exertional

Sidebar 18.2: Endurance Events

Endurance racing is a timed event using a pre-marked, pre-measured trail over natural terrain consisting of distances between 20 and 100 miles in 1 d. The total race distance can be longer when held over multiple days. The sport is overseen by the International Federation for Equestrian Sports (Fédération Équestre Internationale, FEI). Horses are checked by qualified veterinarians at regular intervals before, during, and after the ride, and will be disqualified for showing clinical signs of lameness or metabolic abnormalities, i.e., heat stress, dehydration, electrolyte disorders, synchronous diaphragmatic flutter, rhabdomyolysis. Historically, championship races were won at relatively low speeds (5–6 mph); however, average race speeds have increased over the years, and winners of international races are now averaging 12–18 mph [52].[a] Local events run for pleasure and low-level competitions are more commonly completed at 5–8 mph which is a slow trot for most breeds (Arabians, Stock, and Warmbloods).

The terrain, horse's and rider's athleticism, confidence, and experience generally dictate the speed over the course. Most horses canter or gallop on flat terrain, but walk or trot during up or downhill sections. To cover tens of miles of trail in a day over varying terrain, managing the horse's energy reserves is important. Performance during endurance exercise is dependent on the supply of endogenous stores of energy substrates: muscle and liver glycogen, intramuscular triglycerides (TGs), adipose, and dietary glucose and fatty acids supplied during rest stops. The adipose stores (40 kg) in a 454-kg horse far outweigh total muscle and hepatic glycogen and TGs (3–5 kg) stores [52]. Monitoring heart rate (HR) and adjusting the gait and speed accordingly to keep the horse in aerobic energy metabolism (HR 80–150 bpm) using body fat, rather than anaerobic energy metabolism (HR 160–220 bpm) using glycogen, are important factors in completing the course. Anaerobic depletion of liver and muscle energy stores, dehydration, and electrolyte imbalances are thought to be the primary factors contributing to fatigue during long distances.

a The U.S. Pony Express in operation between 1860 and 1861 carried mail and newspapers 1966 miles between Missouri and California in 10 days. Riders covered 75–100 miles as fast as possible using 5–8 horses during their shift. Morgans and Thoroughbreds were preferred on eastern end, while Mustangs were preferred on the western end of the route. http://nationalponyexpress.org.

depletion. Flat track sprinters may only run one race every few days and have time for repletion between races. However, horses that may compete in more than one event/d, for example, Standardbred racers, or over multiple days, for example, show jumpers and 3-d eventers, are repeatedly diminishing glycogen stores faster than the rate of replenishment. Feeding a high-starch diet risks gastric ulcers, colic, and laminitis, which are more detrimental than exertional fatigue. The current recommendation is to continue feeding a high-forage ration, with the appropriate type and quantity of concentrate fed in 4+ meals/d, ample water, and salt replacement [90]. On event days, consider reducing forage intake before an event to decrease bowel weight and not feeding grain within 3 hrs of an event to avoid: (i) decrease in plasma volume as the fluid shifts to GI lumen, (ii) postprandial hyperglycemia and hyperinsulinemia, and (iii) insulin suppression of fatty acid oxidation [82, 91].

Horses that participate in endurance types of events that last for several hours strive to have glycogen reserves maximized before and throughout the event. See Sidebar 18.2. This will require feeding (and watering) horses at all rest stops a mix of highly palatable forages and concentrates to encourage consumption. Forage fermentation in the hindgut will provide a steady supply of volatile fatty acids for energy and carbohydrate concentrates to replenish liver and muscle glycogen stores. On event days, feed a mix of concentrates, chopped hay, and water at rest stops based on the individual palatability choices of each horse. Watering with electrolytes will replenish body sodium, chloride, and potassium concentrations. Electrolyte loading 2–3 d before a ride is unlikely useful; however, feeding 70 g of 3:1 NaCl/KCl in a concentrate meal 2 hrs before the ride may be of benefit. There are no specific feeding recommendations during race rest stops, and at best a variety of highly palatable feedstuffs (alfalfa, cereal grains, wheat bran, and stabilized rice bran) and water should be offered. Feeding recommendations after the ride include both plain and 0.9% NaCl water, free-choice forage, providing electrolyte supplements with potassium 24 hrs post race, and then routine feeding of concentrates [52].

18.4.4 Feed and Water During Transport

Another important consideration for feeding athletic horses is travel. Horses travel internationally more than any other animal species and account for >50% of USA[1] total live animal exports. One reason is that for many species the trip is one-way; however, most horses make many trips to and from states and other countries. Horses travel to compete, for training and breeding, and for recreational activities all year-round in many instances for days at a time, hence feed and watering require a preplanned

1 USDA Animal and Plant Health Inspection Service. https://www.aphis.usda.gov/aphis/maps/animal-health/horse-protection.

strategy. Horses may voluntarily drink water once or twice daily, or as little as every other day; however, would not voluntarily fast for more than 3–4 hrs. See Drinking Behavior in Chapter 16. Transporting horses by road, rail, or air is physically and psychologically demanding which may result in decreased feed and water intake. There are individual horse differences in coping with transportation stressors and the ability to recover. It has been suggested that a horse's temperament and ability to handle transport and competition stressors be taken into consideration in sport horse breeding decisions [69].

Traveling in a moving container is physically tiring and requires constant muscular work to remain balanced during unforeseen acceleration/deceleration, ascending/descending, and turns. Horses are not in a relaxed position while traveling in a trailer, although some horses learn to lean against a wall or divider that helps maintain balance [92]. The horse in motion does not maintain the normal body posture with 60% BW on the forelegs, but rather all legs are splayed out directly under the body with head raised. It is also possible that some horses experience motion sickness while moving in a confined space with a limited view [93]. There are also variables related to road conditions, terrain, trailer features, and driver technique that can add or minimize stressors. Additionally, horses are naturally claustrophobic, would not enter a dark enclosed or novel space with limited options for escape, and so instinctively avoid confinement having evolved on open plains where fleeing has been a successful defense. Hence, restricted movement with a limited view of the horizon and solidarity in a trailer, that is, a metal cave, with unfamiliar outside noises, are stressors even when the trailer is not moving. Traveling with a herd mate is helpful however; traveling with a dominant horse, with no options to move off, could be more stressful. Horses are less willing to feed and drink in stressful situations, as their instinct to escape and avoid danger can override the desire to eat or drink. Understandably then transportation has been associated with elevated heart rates, increased blood glucose concentrations, plasma cortisol, and muscle-related enzymes aspartate transaminase and creatine kinase [94, 95].

Therefore, transporting horses is physically and psychologically stressful, and a disrupted feeding schedule can be associated with fatigue and illness which hinders well-being and performance. Transportation has been associated with illnesses such as gastric ulcers, colitis, diarrhea, laminitis, transit tetany, choke, and clinical signs referable to the respiratory tract (cough and mucus discharge) [94, 95]. The performance of transport-experienced horses over relatively short distances does not appear to be affected by travel, whereas longer trips or less travel-experienced horses are likely to exhibit signs of stress. Many horses compete on the same day as trailering to the event which may impact energy substrate availability given increased cortisol concentrations increase free fatty acid and blood glucose concentration [96]. The change in the environment, food, and water does negatively impact some competitors. It is recommended that horses arrive at a destination at least 4 hrs before an event [97]. Many horses also suffer from transport stress, even when transported several days before an event. Horses transported by road for 6 hrs, with food and water offered, lost an average of 2.5% BW which was not recovered until the third day after transport [98]. Weight loss was related to the distance traveled and was attributed to decreased feed and water intake, increased energy requirement, and sweat losses [99]. Prior proper training and familiarity with trailer loading, unloading, movement and maintaining a regular feeding schedule while traveling will reduce anxiety and associated health risks.

Research data are lacking, but anecdotal reports of horses refusing feed and/or water following transport are common. Decreasing the overall transport stress begins with using low-pressure trailer training techniques at home and acclimating the horse to feedstuffs and water to be used on the road weeks before traveling. To decrease the stress of travel to competitions, ideally owners should attempt to bring the same hay and feed, for example, if needed to feed cubes or pellets while traveling to save space and convenience, and introduce the feedstuff into the feeding protocol at home several weeks before departure. In some instances, it may not be possible to bring a sufficient quantity of feed for the entire trip. Then feeding commercially available hay products at home weeks before travel, for example, bagged hay bales or cubes, from a reputed manufacturer with a wide distribution area should diminish the variation in forage between "home" and the venue. In some instances, particularly for international travel, owners are not allowed to bring hay and other feeds and the horses must adapt suddenly to new feeds available at the competition venue. Owners and managers at horse show venues should ensure the feeds available for athletes are of very high quality and hence highly palatable [70].

Water will also taste different at venues, which might affect water intake. Some horses do well after adapting to water flavoring agents that can be added to tubs and buckets first at home and then at the venue to masks new smells and tastes. Drinking water and maintaining hydration can be a logistical problem while traveling, and even a travel-experienced horse, with no previous issue, may refuse to drink at a new venue. Treated (chlorine, fluoride) water from municipal sources may not be accepted by horses accustomed to drinking well, pond, or stream waters. One option is to transport water from the home source to be used only if needed or to mix with the new water source 50/50 for a few days. Another option is to flavor (apple, cider vinegar, flavored drink mix) the home water and train the horse to drink from buckets weeks before travel and then use the same flavoring and buckets at the new venue. Ensuring an adequate daily salt (NaCl) intake (5 g [1 tsp]/100 kg BW) mixed into the textured feed is a relatively simple method of maintaining adequate blood sodium concentrations and the desire to drink [2].

Short trips (<500 miles) are unlikely to be associated with transport-related diseases, dehydration, and fatigue, or result in reduced feed intake [95]. Ranch, rodeo, companion, and performance horses can be and are commonly transported (5–8 hrs/d with overnight stops for longer trips) with relatively few problems. Healthy horses transported with periodic access to water became severely fatigued (closed eyes, lower head carriage, less social interaction, and less responsive to stimuli) after a 28-hr drive [100]. A reasonable schedule for working, companion, and performance horses is a 20–30-min rest stop every 3–5 hrs of travel allowing horses to stand still, although restricted, with a wide view at a comfortable temperature appears to be adequate and frequently coincides with fuel stops. It is neither necessary nor recommended to unload horses from the trailer during short rest stops. Offering a forage feed (0.2–0.5% BW) and water is advisable, although rarely will a horse drink in the trailer unless accustomed to doing so. Forage in the form of cubes, pellets, or a hanging hay net of long-stem hay offered during short rest stops can easily be removed before resuming the drive. Having water or feeds available to the horse while traveling is not necessary, as horses rarely consume feed while in motion, with distractions, or in unfamiliar surroundings [101].

Minimizing stress and respiratory illness favors feed consumption. Air quality in the trailer is an important factor to monitor. Opening vents and screened windows, avoiding exhaust fumes (NO_2 and CO), and minimizing flying debris, dust, and ammonia (NH_3) within the trailer decrease the risk of respiratory illness. Careful trip planning using major roadways and highways and avoiding traffic delays and congestion will minimize exhaust fumes and temperatures rising within a still trailer. Covering hay bales, for example, using hay bags, stored in the horse compartment, and using pelleted forms of bedding, rather than shavings, minimize airborne particles. Removing manure and urine-soaked bedding when possible improves air quality within the trailer because airflow recirculates rear to the front along the floor in most trailers [95]. Increasing the rest time and cleaning the interior of the vehicle during rest stops have been shown to reduce transportation stress and respiratory insults [102]. Quick-release head restraints should allow the horse to move into a safe and comfortable position while in motion and to lower their head which aids draining of the respiratory tract. An interesting observation is that horses, facing either toward or away from the direction of travel, exhibited less stress when allowed to raise and lower their heads, and horses that were not crosstied during transport had lower cortisol, glucose, and white blood cell counts than those crosstied in the same vehicle [94].

18.4.5 Feeding Management for Specific Conditions

Major diet-related conditions of performance horses are dehydration, gastric ulceration, respiratory diseases, and joint health. Feeding management recommendations for these conditions include the use of specific feeds, supplements, and feeding methods. See Evidence-based Medicine in Chapter 14 and Labeling Claims in Chapter 15.

18.4.5.1 Hydration

Electrolytes are a class of minerals that are integral to the function of many organ systems, including but not limited to muscles, heart, digestion, nervous system, and kidneys. Sodium, chloride, potassium, calcium, and magnesium are electrolytes with the first three of major concerns in working horses. Further, electrolyte balance is intertwined with hydration status, so disruptions in either electrolytes or hydration can lead to fatigue, muscle twitching, heart arrhythmias, respiratory distress, abnormal GI tract motility, poor performance, and abnormal thermoregulation [103]. Electrolyte imbalances can be created by exercise primarily because even well-trained horses experience significant sweat losses during exercise, which is related to workload and ambient temperatures, with electrolytes and water lost through sweat. One study found that over a 4-d training period, horses in moderate work lost an average of 6 kg of sweat/500 kg BW, while very heavy exercise resulted in an average loss of 7.8 kg of sweat/500 kg BW [104]. Horse sweat contains 2.5–3.0 g Na/L, 4.3–5.0 g Cl/L, and 1.2–1.6 g K/L [52].

Multiple studies have shown the significant imbalances in electrolytes and hydration that occur as a result of exercise in non-supplemented horses, putting the health and performance of horses at risk, and particularly when exercise bouts are repeated day-to-day, since imbalances carry over if not corrected [104–109]. Horses adapted to high-intensity exercise over multiple days, if not supplemented, will experience electrolyte derangements, and often stray farther from normal each day with back-to-back or week-to-week competitions [110]. In endurance sports particularly, electrolyte imbalances have been correlated with a higher chance of not completing the race successfully [111].

Sodium is naturally low (<0.1%) in forages and horses are unlikely to meet sodium needs by diet alone, and since electrolytes are lost at higher concentrations in sweat, electrolytes in some form should be supplemented to horses [2]. Commercial equine feeds may supply some concentration of electrolytes, though often intakes are too low to meet the daily needs of working animals. Horses at maintenance and cool temperatures can meet their daily sodium requirement by consuming 5 g NaCl/100 kg BW which can be met with 1 tsp/100 kg BW/d of white salt (39% Na) (Table 18.2) [2]. This can be in the form of white table salt or commercial electrolyte blends top-dressed to feeds, electrolyte supplements intended to be added to water, or through salt block access. Of note, salt blocks are less efficient in stimulating voluntary intake of sufficient salt to meet daily needs and drinking, thus top-dressing salt/electrolyte supplements to feed or offering electrolytes in water is typically better suited to ensure adequate intake during training and performance periods [112].

The athletic horse is particularly in need of daily electrolyte supplementation to match their workloads (Table 18.6), as needs increase as workload increases and/or the environmental temperature and humidity increase [2]. Horses in moderate exercise or hot climates will need to receive high concentrations and additional electrolytes in their supplement, that is, Na, Cl, K plus Ca, and Mg, to match ratios lost in sweat. These horses may require a daily intake of commercially formulated, palatable top-dressed supplements that can be dosed for BW and workload to ensure the electrolyte needs are met. It has been shown that horses in very heavy exercise, when maintained on a balanced electrolyte supplement for weeks leading up to increased exercise levels, can maintain electrolyte balance [104]. However, for some training or environmental conditions, typical daily supplementation may not be sufficient. It is possible with particularly intense exercise, on consecutive days of exercise, or endurance riding, additional dosing of electrolytes may be needed during and/or after competition to quickly and efficiently replace lost electrolytes and to help maintain hydration [105]. In these cases, a syringe/paste version of electrolytes given during or immediately after exercise may be the easiest and most efficient way to ensure rapid intake of electrolytes and prevent an imbalance from escalating and creating organ system dysfunction.

Increased quantities of salt or electrolytes ingested each day may reduce the palatability of water or feed and limit voluntary intake. For horses that decline to eat salty flavors at the dosing needed to prevent electrolyte imbalances, commercial electrolyte blends have been formulated to reduce palatability problems. Options such as added flavors, sweeteners, or micro-encapsulated electrolytes may entice the horse to ingest the needed dose of electrolytes. Whenever offering electrolytes added to water, an additional non-electrolyte water source should always be accessible as well. This is to ensure that if the horse refuses the electrolyte water, another water source is still available. Insulin-resistant horses requiring a low sugar/starch diet may not tolerate a sweetened electrolyte blend. Horses with gastric ulcers may experience pain when salt contacts the ulcerated tissues in the stomach, and typical electrolyte supplementation can exacerbate gastric ulcers [113]. These horses may develop a feed avoidance to salty tastes. In this case, micro-encapsulated electrolytes, that is, coated with a thin layer of oil, might be needed, as the coating helps reduce detectable flavors and physically prevents contact between the electrolytes and the ulcerated tissues.

Electrolyte and hydration imbalances are related to exercise, as sweating also leads to water loss, though not at the same rate as electrolyte loss, which alters relative electrolyte and water concentrations in the blood. Once an imbalance is created, both electrolyte and water needs must be addressed, but correcting one impacts the other. For humans and horses, with exercise and subsequent sweat loss, water and electrolytes are lost in sweat. For humans, losing either water or electrolytes creates hormonal and neural stimuli to drink, that is, there is a redundant stimulus to drink more water. The loss of body water in horses does not create strong thirst signals, which was likely an evolutionary advantage allowing for watering once or every other day. See Drinking Behavior in Chapter 16. The thirst drive is controlled by plasma osmolality. Administering or feeding electrolytes that increase plasma osmolality will drive horses to voluntarily increase water consumption at the same time, whereas providing only plain water to a horse with electrolyte imbalances will lower plasma osmolality, lowering electrolyte concentrations further and reducing the stimulus to voluntarily drink [107]. Voluntary water intake was increased for 4 hrs post administration of electrolytes [114]. Hence, providing the horse unlimited access to clean water simultaneously after administering supplemental electrolytes is important. So, "you can lead a horse to water, but you cannot make them drink"—unless electrolytes are replenished first.

Salt supplementation to some extent is warranted in horses year-round, regardless of competition or training season, but working horses may need additional intakes and additional electrolytes (Ca, K, Mg) whenever exercised and/or sweating heavily. Ideally, providing additional and diverse electrolyte supplementation should begin weeks before changes in exercise or sweating to prevent imbalances. If an imbalance is created, special attention should be given to replenishing electrolytes through palatable, easy-to-dose methods and providing unlimited access to water to reduce the escalation of electrolyte and hydration imbalances.

18.4.5.2 Equine Gastric Ulceration Syndrome

Gastric ulcers are a common concern of horse owners, and the greater the level of training and competition, the greater the risk is considered for gastric ulcer development and hindrance for equine performance and comfort. See Ulcers in Chapter 26. The majority of recommended management practices to reduce gastric ulcer formation in competition horses are related to the amount of feed provided and timing of feed access. While many of these recommendations would be beneficial to most horses in modern housing, difficulties are created when trying to provide enough feed to meet the energy demands of competition and feeding around boarding facility limitations, training schedules, travel, and competition timetables. As it is accepted that gastric ulcer formation is considered multifactorial, enacting as many management practices as possible to help reduce the incidence of ulcers may be needed, and yet may still prove insufficient to fully prevent gastric ulcer formation for some horses.

The quantity of long-stem forage recommended to reduce gastric ulcer incidence is 1–1.5% DM BW/d and a maximum of 0.5% BW/d concentrate (grains, pellets, textured feeds) [115]. Research on access to pasture and forage species has shown variable impacts on ulcer rates, but the amount of long-stem forage versus concentrate/d is accepted as correlated with gastric health [116–119]. More than the type of forage, consistent access to forage is likely the key to aiding gastric health, as consuming long-stem forage forces more chewing, which stimulates more saliva production and saliva is a natural buffer for the stomach [120]. Further, long-stem forage consumption prolongs the time taken to consume feed, leading to longer periods with feed physically within the stomach and acting as a buffer [121–123]. Thus, providing access to long-stem forage consistently, including while traveling, at shows, between training bouts, and as part of regular daily management, should be part of the management plan to reduce gastric ulcer formation [124]. The use of hay nets or slow feeders can help prolong horses' intake time and reduce labor associated with providing consistent access to hay.

To meet the energy and nutrient needs of the competition horse, likely some form of concentrate feeding will be needed to help maintain body condition and physiological demands. As such, most competition horses will be given additional meals each day of grains, processed feeds, supplements, or ration balancers, and timing these meals can also help reduce their impact on gastric ulcer formation. When giving concentrate meals, providing the concentrate in small frequent meals throughout the day can help reduce gastric risk, as going from 2 to 3 meals/d decreases ulcer risk by almost 20% [125]. Further, timing the meals to be fed less than 6 hrs apart also reduces ulcer risk, likely as this correlates with more frequent feedings of smaller amounts [126]. When developing a feeding schedule around training or competition, care should be taken to ensure the horse is given access to forage, maintain consistency in concentrate meal feeding to avoid prolonged "empty" stomach, and have some substrate in the stomach going into exercise to help act as a buffer. Neither very large meals nor the absence of meals before exercise is recommended during exercise, as intra-abdominal pressure leads to a smaller stomach volume with a lower pH, increasing vulnerable gastric tissue exposure to damaging acids [127].

Horses should have consistent access to clean water at a desirable temperature in their daily housing, when traveling, at competitions, and between exercise bouts, as limited water access is also associated with gastric ulcer formation, likely related to the direct buffering capacity of water in the short term and the reduction in saliva and mucus production during dehydration in the long term [126]. The administration of salt or electrolytes should be done conscientiously in horses with gastric ulcers, as direct contact between salt and ulcerated stomach tissues can induce immediate gastric pain that can lead to food avoidance, and repeated administration of hypertonic electrolytes has been shown to increase both number and severity of gastric ulcers [113]. Horses with gastric ulcers benefit from either delivering electrolytes dissolved in a water solution or utilizing micro-encapsulated electrolytes where the salts are coated with a protective layer to reduce contact between salts and ulcerated tissues. Providing unlimited access to clean water is a core component of gastric health, but this is especially important if supplying electrolytes, as electrolyte intake will stimulate additional water intake [126].

Training factors are also of concern when attempting to reduce gastric ulcer risk [128]. Whenever starting a horse for training, increasing intensity level of exercise, or training for a new discipline, more focus on reducing gastric ulcer risks should be employed, as simply starting new training programs has been associated with gastric ulcer development [129], though the intensity of the training, teaching techniques, and individual horse's demeanor would likely impact the gastric ulcer formation risk level. Exercise intensity is considered a major factor in gastric ulcer risk, as the incidence rate in racehorses and endurance horses is common, likely due to a combination of high stress and GI impacts during exercise, typically less access to long-stem forage, or long periods without feed or water during training/competition bouts combined with relatively high volumes of concentrate meals to maintain BW [124, 129–131]. The cause-and-effect relationship between stressful stimuli and gastric ulcers is not fully established. It is reasonable that the connection between stress and gastric ulcer formation exists, as the neural and hormonal responses to stress shift physiological resources away from the GI tract and toward the peripheral tissues. This shift results in reduced blood flow to the stomach, decreased stomach volume, limited saliva and mucus production, slowing of GI transit rate, and changes in digestive reflexes, all of which can increase the exposure of sensitive gastric tissues to low pH solutions [127, 132, 133]. Cribbing and wind sucking have also been shown to be correlated with gastric ulcers, and though again the cause or effect relationship is not clear, attempts should be made to suppress such behaviors for the gastric-ulcer-prone horse [134].

For horses at risk for gastric ulcers, low-starch feeds and supplements may be helpful, particularly when large volumes of feed are needed to maintain weight. Specifically, a goal of no more than 2 g starch/kg BW/d with less than 1 g starch/kg BW/meal has been recommended [126]. This is related to the fermentation of the starch in the stomach, resulting in volatile fatty acid formation, which is correlated with a higher gastric ulcer risk and the presence of aerobic bacteria in mesenteric lymph nodes and liver [122, 135]. The use of oil for weight gain instead of additional starch intake can be gastroprotective, as significant calorie intake can be achieved with small volumes of oil. While some research has shown that oil itself results in decreased gastric acid secretion and thus may protect against gastric irritation, other research has not shown such benefits [136, 137]. Evidence exists for the use of feeds and supplements with natural or chemical buffers to offer an immediate short-term buffering of low gastric pH. Alfalfa comprises proteins that naturally buffer the stomach acid and calcium that moderates gastric secretions, and can be fed as a long-stem forage [6, 138]. Chemical buffers such as magnesium hydrochloride, magnesium hydroxide, aluminum hydroxide, and calcium carbonate are common components of gastric health supplements for their buffering capacity, although the duration of their effectiveness in the gastric environment is short [139, 140].

Due to the often chronic and widespread tissue damage associated with gastric ulcers, supplementing anti-oxidants is reasonable to aid healing and support future tissue integrity, such as vitamin C, vitamin E, selenium, zinc, thioredoxin, glutamine, glycine, or naturally anti-oxidant-rich compounds such as sea buckthorn, fenugreek, or grape components [141–144]. Specific to the gastric environment, ingredients that stimulate mucus production can offer protection for damaged gastric tissues, or ingredients that provide a physical coating over ulcerated tissues help reduce acid exposure to the damaged gastric wall. As such, ingredients such as apple pectin and lecithin, Aloe vera, beta-glucan, hyaluronan, licorice root, marshmallow root, and slippery elm bark are included in gastric support supplements for mucogenic or gel-like properties that physically coat the gastric wall [145–152]. Probiotics may be included in gastric health supplements, as the typically diverse microbial population of the equine gastric mucosa is reduced during ulceration [153]. Due to the naturally anti-microbial environment of the stomach, colonizing probiotics may be limited and more research is needed to determine the feeding rates and beneficial microbial species.

Likely a combination of buffering gastric pH, increasing stomach mucus, supporting gastric tissue integrity, and emulsifying is probably the best approach. Various supplements show promise, with most having a wide range of ingredients, although beneficial effects may take longer than veterinary grade treatments [149, 154–159]. For acute or higher-grade ulcers, a combination of management with veterinary treatments, such as omeprazole and sucralfate, and gastric supplements with efficacy could be utilized to support more inclusive or prolonged relief for the horse [160]. Long-term use of omeprazole is associated with unwanted metabolic side effects, and both omeprazole and sucralfate are relatively expensive treatments, particularly when dealing with chronic gastric ulcers [161, 162].

18.4.5.3 Respiratory Disease

Respiratory problems in equine athletes can stem from a wide variety of causes, such as stabling conditions with long-term confinement for an injury, related to weather or transportation, particles in the air from debris burning or pollution, contaminated or dusty feed, specific respiratory viruses, bacteria, and internal parasites, allergies or immune system disorders, and diseases such as inflammatory airway disease (IAD), asthma, chronic obstructive pulmonary disease (COPD), and recurrent airway obstruction (RAO) also known as heaves. Many of these are correlated with training and/or the competition season either directly or indirectly, as spring allergies often coincide with the start of the show year, the risk of exposure to diseases is more likely when horses gather at competitions. Stress levels are generally higher with advancing levels of competition which may compromise the immune system. Additionally, the rigors of exercise are associated specifically with high respiratory demands and the risk of respiratory tissue injury. Most equine athletes experience a variety of respiratory offenses that can overwhelm the tract and lead to impaired breathing, gas exchange, and ultimately decreased athletic function.

Respiratory diseases can present in a variety of clinical signs such as nasal discharge of mucus or blood, repeated or excessive snorting, cough, blowing, wheezing, lack of air movement despite active attempts to inhale, chronically flared nostrils, increased respiratory rate, and changes in respiratory muscle tone [163]. Probably the least appreciated is that a cough is abnormal in horses and an indicator of a respiratory problem. Horses with IAD often only present with a cough at the onset of exercise. These horses could benefit from management changes, respiratory supplements, and/or veterinary treatment that could ease discomfort, facilitate breathing, and improve athleticism. Preventing, diagnosing, and treating the disease early are often key to reducing the risk of permanent changes in the respiratory tract and preventing secondary diseases from developing. General management practices that benefit all horses but especially athletes with respiratory problems should be aimed at reducing inhalation of hazardous particles, including dust, ammonia, allergens, pollution, and mold. For horses with respiratory disease, management practices such as using pelleted low-dust/low-odor shavings, lightly wetting down shavings, removing urine and feces frequently from stalls, aggressively treating mold, increased ventilation, or outdoor housing should be followed.

Feeding management of horses with respiratory disease requires the use of high-quality, palatable feed as appetite and intake may be diminished with reduced ability to smell and difficulty breathing while eating. Reduced feed intake plus the increased physiological effort and energy to breathe may lead to weight loss, reduced capacity of the immune system, and further reduced tissue strength in the respiratory tract. Ensuring access to clean water and monitoring hydration daily are important, as water is a major component of mucus and dehydration can lead to viscous mucus that may accumulate within the tract. Electrolyte intake can help increase water intake if needed. Other recommendations are (i) adding water or oil to dusty feeds when feeding concentrates or supplements reduces inhalation of small particles, (ii) feeding hay from the ground instead of elevated feeders, and (iii) reducing hay dust by shaking out small particles, soaking the hay before feeding, or using commercial hay steamers to reduce both dust and microbial presence. Steaming hay can be particularly helpful for respiratory allergies, as research has shown steaming can reduce particles, bacteria, and mold by 99% when a high-quality commercial steamer is used. On the other hand, soaking hay or retail steaming methods at home can be helpful to reduce physical contaminants, but if not properly executed, these less controllable practices may increase microbial contamination [164, 165].

A complementary route of protecting the equine respiratory tract has been postulated by feeding supplements that target respiratory tract health, reduce airway inflammation, and/or suppress allergic responses. Antioxidants such as vitamin E and selenium can offer a level of respiratory tissue protection against damage, help develop respiratory tissue integrity, and aid the process of tissue repair [166–168]. Key minerals such as copper, zinc, and manganese can facilitate the development of respiratory tract tissues, provide immune system support, and are associated with beneficial effects in respiratory diseases in people. As respiratory tract inflammation is a common factor in horses with IAD, asthma, chronic COPD, and RAO/heaves, adding anti-inflammatory components to the diet may help alleviate respiratory symptoms associated with reduced airflow or changes in inflammation at the alveolar level [163]. Although methylsulfonylmethane (MSM) may provide respiratory support through anti-inflammatory effects in people and rats, research specific to horses has not been published. However, omega-3 fatty acids eicosapentaenoic acid (EPA) and docosahexaenoic acid (DHA) have demonstrated anti-inflammatory effects in the respiratory symptoms of horses, likely a combination of helping ease airflow through the tract, reducing allergic responses, and/or suppressing inflammatory markers in bronchoalveolar tissues [169, 170].

18.4.5.4 Joint Disease

Horses in work experience high levels of multidirectional strain on joint tissues, with added stressors related to conformation, breed characteristics, level of fitness, stage of growth, aging, immune function, housing, diet, tack fit, rider effect, and even temperament. The health and function of joints are a complex compilation of the working loads for cartilage, ligaments, tendons, synovial fluid, bones, and the muscles that generate motion. While damage (strain or injury) to any one of these tissues can affect the total joint mobility and comfort of the horse, the associated inflammation subsequently generated is a major factor in joint health and function, leading to both acute and long-term joint issues.

Cartilage is a highly specialized tissue that promotes the smooth, frictionless movement between the bones during locomotion. Cartilaginous chondrocytes produce a matrix of structural collagen and proteoglycans composed of proteins and sugars with shock-absorbing properties. Cartilage tissue undergoes a continuous cycle of turnover necessary for a healthy joint. Damage to the cartilage of any type induces inflammation, and mediators, such as interleukins, interfere with cartilage turnover. Specifically, inflammation causes accelerated cartilage breakdown and decreased cartilage production. Therefore, chronic inflammation causes degradation and ossification of cartilage, impairment of synovial fluid function, and permanent joint disease [171]. Cartilage, tendons, and ligaments have a very limited or negligible ability to repair once the damage has taken place, due to the nature of the tissues' components [172]. Some success in the repair has been achieved with blood-derived and stem cell therapies of late, but is an expensive, time-consuming, and often very involved treatment plan for all but the exceptional performance horse [173]. Thus, the best plan is to prevent or minimize progressive joint damage. This includes a comprehensive initiative for preventing joint damage through conscientious training programs, regular hoof and shoeing care, attention to footing and bedding composition, diet formulation for appropriate body condition and demands of the sport, and observing closely for indicators of pain, stiffness, or changes in joint appearance and function and treating such issues early in their development.

An overall balanced ration with proper protein, mineral, vitamin, water, and energy concentrations influences both the growth and maintenance of the equine athlete's skeleton [2]. Providing the equine athlete with sufficient dietary intake of required nutrients to perform the requirements of the sport helps reduce the risk of joint damage due to incoordination, weakness, fatigue, mineral imbalances, or altered immune response. In particular to joint tissues, sufficient protein is required for tissue integrity and fluids; sufficient intake and balanced ratios of calcium, phosphorus, and magnesium are needed to develop and maintain healthy skeletal tissues; sufficient intake and ratios of manganese, zinc, and copper support connective tissue development; and sufficient sulfur and vitamin C aid collagen formation [2]. Other dietary components that support healthy joint function include omega-3 fatty acids EPA and DHA. Typical equine commercial feeds are relatively high in omega-6 fatty acids; thus, specifically supplying sources of omega-3 helps support lesser inflammatory pathways and modulate the immune response, possibly joint inflammation, and subsequent joint damage [169, 174]. Supra-nutritional intakes of antioxidants (vitamin A, vitamin C, vitamin E, selenium, zinc, copper, manganese, beta-carotene, lutein, lycopene, alpha-lipoic acid) theoretically may protect against free-radical damage associated with chronic joint inflammation and development of osteoarthritis [175].

Feeding the athletic horse to meet and maintain an appropriate weight helps maintain joint health. Overweight horses have additional strain placed on connective tissues, added pressure within joint cavities, require more effort to accomplish training tasks, and overall increased risk of joint damage. Conversely, a horse with low muscle mass or low adipose stores may have difficulty executing maneuvers or having the endurance required for training and competition, increasing the risk of joint injury due to imprecision of movements. Thus, ensuring a horse is in proper body condition for their sport and without excess weight helps protect joints from damage during exercise.

Joint supplements are among the most popular equine nutritional products, available in oral and injectable forms, and contain a wide range of ingredients; however, evidence of efficacy for most commercially available products is lacking. Supplements that alleviate inflammation and help protect joint tissues from further damage are indicated for the horse in a high level of training or competition with an increased risk of joint injury or those with joint damage. Many oral joint supplements recommend a loading dose period of a few weeks to reach reportedly effective concentrations within the joint. For horses with a higher risk of joint damage or with known joint disease, remaining on an inclusive joint supplement throughout the year, regardless of training or show schedule, might better promote joint health and minimize the inflammatory response to an acute injury.

Common oral ingredients include glucosamine (HCl or sulfate), chondroitin sulfate, MSM, and hyaluronic acid (HA), while some products may also contain EPA and DHA, collagen peptides, herbal ingredients, antioxidants, vitamins, and minerals (Table 18.7). The preventive administration of some nutraceuticals was found to have anti-inflammatory effects similar to meloxicam using a synovitis model in healthy horses [180]. The reportedly higher efficacy or response rate noted with supplement blends may be due to a multifaceted approach

Table 18.7 Joint supplement ingredients and a proposed method of action in horses.

Ingredient	Proposed method of action
Glucosamine	Chondroprotective, component of cartilage [176]
Chondroitin sulfate	Chondroprotective, component of cartilage, increases synovial fluid [176]
Methylsulfonylmethane	Anti-inflammatory, anti-oxidant, source of organic sulfur [177]
Hyaluronic acid	Anti-inflammatory, component of synovial fluid [178]
Omega-3 fatty acids: α-linolenic acid, eicosapentaenoic acid, docosahexaenoic acid	Immune system modulators, anti-inflammatory [169, 174]
Collagen peptides	chondroprotective, component of various connective tissues [179]
Rosehip extract	Anti-inflammatory, anti-oxidant (source of vitamin C and lycopene) [180]
Devil's claw	Anti-inflammatory, pain reduction [181]

to reducing inflammation, the root cause of joint swelling, pain, stiffness, and arthritic changes in joint tissues [171]. See Sidebar 18.3. Overall the evidence to date is conflicting on whether these oral supplements have beneficial clinical effects in equine joint health. Some of the controversies are related to study design as in statistically underpowered, lack of blinding, inappropriate placebo control, and poorly defined inclusion/exclusion criteria. In summary, there is some clinical evidence suggesting a benefit to horses with joint damage and osteoarthritis; however, rigorous randomized, controlled clinical studies are needed.

Sidebar 18.3: Effectiveness of Supplement Blends

- A supplement comprising glucosamine and chondroitin fed to veteran horses had no effect at wk 4, but by wk 8, horses had increased elbow, stifle, and hind fetlock range of motion, and increased stride length and stride duration [181].
- A proprietary blend of glucosamine and chondroitin showed steady improvements in pain control, range of motion, lameness score, and flexion scores over 56 d and continued to have beneficial results throughout the rest of the 24-wk trial [182].
- Horses fed a commercial blend of glucosamine HCl, chondroitin sulfate, MSM, vitamin C, and marine omega-3 fatty acids had lower lameness grades, improved joint flexion, and improved range of motion and muscle tone, and earned higher movement scores after 21 d of supplementation [183].
- Supplemental fatty acids given alone have been shown to increase synovial fluid concentrations of conjugated LA in 28 d, and effectively reduced cartilage degradation and increased cartilage regeneration [184].
- Supplemental oils given in a proprietary anti-oxidant and anti-inflammatory blend (mushrooms, yeast, melon concentrate, flaxseeds, fish oil, and enzymes) produced positive results in 23 d with evidence of decreased markers of skeletal muscle injury and decreased joint damage indicators [185].

The more rapid onset of positive effects could be due to the greater breadth of active ingredients, dosing rate, and/or synergistic interactions between ingredients. Thus, it may be of benefit to choose a joint supplement with a wider range of ingredients to support a synergistic approach to joint health.

Case in Point

The owner asks for a consult because, at the last competition, a friend suggested "StrongHeart" supplement which is a mineral–vitamin pellet with a recommended feeding rate of 1–2 lb/1000 lb horse/d. The owner asks, "The supplement is expensive ($1–2/d), but is this a good idea, and, if so, how much to feed per day?"

Animal Assessment

A 9-yr-old Morgan gelding, BW 1200 lb, BCS 3/9, average temperament, used in competitive trail rides (walk/trot/canter) requiring about 5 hrs/wk of low-level obstacle skill work training. The horse is maintained in a 3 ac poorly managed pasture/dry lot with a run-in shed. Horse has an excellent appetite. Water is available *ad libitum*. The horse is offered 1/4 bale (80 lb bale) of MMG hay/d.

Ration Assessment

A hay-only ration is fed. Water is accessible using an automatic waterer and a white salt block is always available. No concentrate or complementary feed is fed. Based on laboratory analysis, the MMG hay (94% DM) contains the following nutrients on a DM basis:

DE	CP	Ca	P	Lysine	ADF	NDF	Cu	Zn
Mcal/kg				%			ppm	ppm
2.3	13.3	0.8	0.31	0.6	31.5	49.6	9.0	25

1) *Calculate relative feed value (RFV) and determine nutritional quality of the forag*
2) *Based on the calculated DE requirement, how much hay (lb as fed)/d should be offered to this horse?*
3) *Based on nutrient concentrations* (Table 18.4), *could this hay meet the ration protein (CP), calcium (Ca), and phosphorus (P) recommendations for this horse?*
4) *Does feeding an adequate amount of this hay/d meet the horse's lysine, copper (Cu), and zinc (Zn) requirements?* (Table 18.2).
5) *Does feeding the suggested vitamin–mineral ration balancer with copper (100 ppm) and zinc (850 ppm) at the suggested 1 lb/d dose fulfill the Cu and Zn requirements?*
6) *The owner asks, "Is this a good idea and how much to feed/d?" What is your nutritional recommendation?*

See Appendix A Chapter 18.

References

1 Burk, A.O. and Williams, C.A. (2008). Feeding management practices and supplement use in top-level event horses. *Comp. Exerc. Physiol.* 5 (2): 85–93.

2 National Research Council (2007). *Nutrient Requirements of Horses*. 6th Rev. Animal Nutrition Series, 1–341. Washington, DC: National Academies Press.

3 Henneke, D.R., Potter, G.D., Kreider, J.L., and Yeates, B.F. (1983). Relationship between condition score, physical measurements and body fat percentage in mares. *Equine Vet. J.* 15 (4): 371–372.

4 Mottet, R., Onan, G., and Hiney, K. (2009). Revisiting the Henneke body condition scoring system: 25 years later. *J. Equine Vet. Sci.* 29 (5): 417–418.

5 Durham, A.E. (2009). The role of nutrition in colic. *Vet. Clin. North Am. Equine Pract.* 25 (1): 67–78.

6 Nadeau, J.A., Andrews, F.M., Mathew, A.G. et al. (2000). Evaluation of diet as a cause of gastric ulcers in horses. *Am. J. Vet. Res.* 61 (7): 784–790.

7 McMiken, D.F. (1983). An energetic basis of equine performance. *Equine Vet. J.* 15 (2): 123–133.

8 Snow, D.H. and Vogel, C. (1987). *Equine Fitness: The Care and Training of the Athletic Horse*, 271. London: David & Charles.

9 Harris, P. (1997). Energy sources and requirements of the exercising horse. *Annu. Rev. Nutr.* 17 (1): 185–210.

10 Pagan, J. (2006). Energy and the performance horse. In: *Tennessee Nutrition Conference*, 1–6. Knoxville, TN: University of Tennessee.

11 Achten, J., Gleeson, M., and Jeukendrup, A.E. (2002). Determination of the exercise intensity that elicits maximal fat oxidation. *Med. Sci. Sports Exerc.* 34 (1): 92–97.

12 Geor, R.J., Hinchcliff, K.W., and Sams, R.A. (2000). β-adrenergic blockade augments glucose utilization in horses during graded exercise. *J. Appl. Phys.* 89 (3): 1086–1098.

13 Prince, A., Geor, R., Harris, P. et al. (2002). Comparison of the metabolic responses of trained Arabians and Thoroughbreds during high- and low-intensity exercise. *Equine Vet. J.* 34 (S34): 95–99.

14 Lindholm, A., Bjerneld, H., and Saltin, B. (1974). Glycogen depletion pattern in muscle fibres of trotting horses. *Acta Physiol. Scand.* 90 (2): 475–484.

15 Harris, R.C., Marlin, D.J., and Snow, D.H. (1987). Metabolic response to maximal exercise of 800 and 2,000 m in the Thoroughbred horse. *J. Appl. Phys.* 63 (1): 12–19.

16 Hodgson, D.R., Rose, R.J., Allen, J.R., and Dimauro, J. (1985). Glycogen depletion patterns in horses competing in day 2 of a three day event. *Cornell Vet.* 75 (2): 366–374.

17 Snow, D.H., Baxter, P., and Rose, R.J. (1981). Muscle fibre composition and glycogen depletion in horses competing in an endurance ride. *Vet. Rec.* 108 (17): 374–378.

18 Snow, D.H., Kerr, M.G., Nimmo, M.A., and Abbott, E.M. (1982). Alterations in blood, sweat, urine and muscle composition during prolonged exercise in the horse. *Vet. Rec.* 110 (16): 377–384.

19 Coyle, E.F. and Coggan, A.R. (1984). Effectiveness of carbohydrate feeding in delaying fatigue during prolonged exercise. *Sport Med.* 1 (6): 446–458.

20 Trottier, N.L., Nielsen, B.D., Lang, K.J. et al. (2002). Equine endurance exercise alters serum branched-chain amino acid and alanine concentrations. *Equine Vet. J.* 34 (34): 168–172.

21 Snow, D.H. and Harris, R.C. (1991). Effects of daily exercise on muscle glycogen in the Thoroughbred racehorse. *Equine Exerc. Physiol.* 3: 299–304.

22 Lacombe, V.A., Hinchcliff, K.W., Geor, R.J., and Baskin, C.R. (2001). Muscle glycogen depletion and subsequent replenishment affect anaerobic capacity of horses. *J. Appl. Phys.* 91 (4): 1782–1790.

23 Lacombe, V.A., Hinchcliff, K.W., and Taylor, L.E. (2003). Interactions of substrate availability, exercise performance, and nutrition with muscle glycogen metabolism in horses. *J. Am. Vet. Med. Assoc.* 223 (11): 1576–1585.

24 Ivy, J.L. (1998). Glycogen resynthesis after exercise: effect of carbohydrate intake. *Int. J. Sports Med.* 19 (Suppl. 2): S142–S145.

25 Jose-Cunilleras, E., Hinchcliff, K.W., Lacombe, V.A. et al. (2006). Ingestion of starch-rich meals after exercise increases glucose kinetics but fails to enhance muscle glycogen replenishment in horses. *Vet. J.* 171 (3): 468–477.

26 Geor, R.J., Larsen, L., Waterfall, H.L. et al. (2006). Route of carbohydrate administration affects early post exercise muscle glycogen storage in horses. *Equine Vet. J.* 36 (Suppl): 590–595.

27 Jeffcott, L.B., Field, J.R., McLean, J.G., and O'Dea, K. (1986). Glucose tolerance and insulin sensitivity in ponies and Standardbred horses. *Equine Vet. J.* 18 (2): 97–101.

28 Pratt, S.E., Geor, R.J., Spriet, L.L., and McCutcheon, L.J. (2007). Time course of insulin sensitivity and skeletal muscle glycogen synthase activity after a single bout of exercise in horses. *J. Appl. Phys.* 103 (3): 1063–1069.

29 Waller, A.P. and Lindinger, M.I. (2010). Nutritional aspects of post exercise skeletal muscle glycogen synthesis in horses: a comparative review. *Equine Vet. J.* 42 (3): 274–281.

30 Pethick, D.W., Rose, R.J., Bryden, W.L., and Gooden, J.M. (1993). Nutrient utilisation by the hindlimb of Thoroughbred horses at rest. *Equine Vet. J.* 25 (1): 41–44.

31 Pratt, S.E., Lawrence, L.M., Warren, L.K., and Powell, D.M. (2005). The effect of exercise on the clearance of infused acetate in the horse. *J. Equine Vet. Sci.* 25 (6): 266–271.

32 Kawai, M., Minami, Y., Sayama, Y., Kuwano, A., Hiraga, A., and Miyata, H. (2009). Muscle fiber population and biochemical properties of whole body muscles in thoroughbred horses. *Anat Rec.* 292 (10): 1663–9.

33 Gondim, F.J., and Modolo, L. V. (2005). Campos GER, Salgado I. Neuronal nitric oxide synthase is heterogeneously distributed in equine myofibers and highly expressed in endurance trained horses. *Can J Vet Res.* 69 (1): 46–52.

34 Duren, S.E., and Cubitt, T. (2020). How to select a concentrate for performance horses. In: *Proceedings of the 66th Annual Convention of the American Association Equine Practitioners*. Virtual, 50–54. American Association of Equine Practitioners (AAEP).

35 Carlson, G.P. (1983). Thermoregulation and fluid balance in the exercising horse. In: *Equine Exercise Physiology* (ed. D. Snow, S. Persson and R. Rose), 291–309. Cambridge: Granta Editions.

36 National Research Council (1989). *Nutrient Requirements of Horses*. 5th Rev. Animal Nutrition Series, 1–100. Washington, DC: National Academies Press.

37 Swinker, A.M. (2014). Hay quality for different classes of horses. Pennsylvania State Extension Service. https://extension.psu.edu/hay-quality-for-different-classes-of-horses (accessed 2 July 2021).

38 Martinson K. (2020). How to select forages for equine athletes. In: *Proceedings of the 66th Annual Convention of the American Association of Equine Practitioners*, 44–45. Virtual: American Association of Equine Practitioners (AAEP).

39 Russell, M.A. and Johnson, K.D. (2007). Selecting quality hay for horses. West Lafayette, IN: Department of Agriculture Cooperative Extension Service. https://www.agry.purdue.edu/ext/forages/publications/id-190.htm (accessed 5 July 2021).

40 van den Berg, M., Giagos, V., Lee, C. et al. (2016). The influence of odour, taste and nutrients on feeding behaviour and food preferences in horses. *Appl. Anim. Behav. Sci.* 184 (Nov): 41–50.

41 DeBoer, M.L., Sheaffer, C.C., Grev, A.M. et al. (2017). Yield, nutritive value, and preference of annual warm-season grasses grazed by horses. *Agron. J.* 109 (5): 2136–2148.

42 Geor, R., Harris, P.A., and Coenen, M. (2013). Nutritional requirements, recommendations and example diets. In: *Equine Applied and Clinical Nutrition Health, Welfare and Performance* (ed. R. Geor, P.A. Harris, and M. Coenen), 639–643. Edinburgh: Saunders Elsevier.

43 Lindinger, M.I., McKeen, G., and Ecker, G.L. (2004). Time course and magnitude of changes in total body water, extracellular fluid volume, intracellular fluid volume and plasma volume during submaximal exercise and recovery in horses. *Equine Comp. Exerc. Physiol.* 1 (2): 131–139.

44 Cymbaluk, N.F. (2013). Water. In: *Equine Applied and Clinical Nutrition: Health, Welfare and Performance* (ed. R.J. Geor, P.A. Harris and M. Coenen), 80–95. Edinburgh: Saunders Elsevier.

45 Schott, H.C. (2011). Water homeostasis and diabetes insipidus in horses. *Vet. Clin. North Am. Equine Pract.* 27 (1): 175–195.

46 Houpt, K.A., Eggleston, A., Kunkle, K., and Houpt, T.R. (2000). Effect of water restriction on equine behaviour and physiology. *Equine Vet. J.* 32 (4): 341–344.

47 Lester, G.D., Merritt, A.M., Kuck, H.V., and Burrow, J.A. (2013). Systemic, renal, and colonic effects of intravenous and enteral rehydration in horses. *J. Vet. Intern. Med.* 27 (3): 554–566.

48 Norris, M.L., Houpt, K.A., and Houpt, T.R. (2013). Effect of food availability on the physiological responses to water deprivation in ponies. *J. Equine Vet. Sci.* 33 (4): 250–256.

49 Gerber, V., Schott, H.C., and Robinson, N.E. (2011). Owner assessment in judging the efficacy of airway disease treatment. *Equine Vet. J.* 43 (2): 153–158.

50 Fielding, C.L. (2015). Potassium homeostasis and derangements. In: *Equine Fluid Therapy* (ed. C.L. Fielding and K.G. Magdesian), 27–44. John Wiley & Sons, Inc.

51 Naylor, J.R., Bayly, W.M., Gollnick, P.D. et al. (1993). Effects of dehydration on thermoregulatory responses of horses during low-intensity exercise. *J. Appl. Phys.* 75 (2): 994–1001.

52 Harris, P.A. and Schott, H.C. (2013). Nutritional management of elite endurance horses. In: *Equine Applied and Clinical Nutrition: Health, Welfare and Performance* (ed. R.J. Geor, P.A. Harris, and M. Coenen), 272–288. Edinburgh: Saunders Elsevier.

53 Pagan, J.D., Hintz, H.F., and Equine energetics. II. (1986). Energy expenditure in horses during submaximal exercise. *J. Anim. Sci.* 63 (3): 822–830.

54 Scott, B.D., Potter, G.D., Greene, L.W. et al. (1993). Efficacy of a fat supplemented diet to reduce thermal stress in exercising Thoroughbred horses. In: *Proceedings of the 13th Equine Nutrition and Physiology Society Symposium*, 66–71. Gainesville, FL: Equine Nutrition and Physiology Society.

55 Oldham, S.L., Potter, G.D., Evans, J.W. et al. (1990). Storage and mobilization of muscle glycogen in exercising horses fed a fat-supplemented diet. *J. Equine Vet. Sci.* 10 (5): 353–359.

56 Hambleton, P.L., Slade, L.M., Hamar, D.W. et al. (1980). Dietary fat and exercise conditioning effect on metabolic parameters in the horse. *J. Anim. Sci.* 51 (6): 1330–1339.

57 Pagan, J.D., Essén-Gustavsson, B., Lindholm, A., and Thorton, J. (1987). The effect of dietary energy source on blood metabolites in Standardbred horses during exercise. In: *Proceedings of the 10th Equine Nutrition and Physiology*

Society Symposium, 425–430. Fort Collins, CO: Equine Nutrition and Physiology Society.

58 Pagan, J.D.D., Lawrence, T.L.L., and Lennox, M.A.A. (2010). Fish oil and corn oil supplementation affect red blood cell and serum eicosapentaenoic acid (EPA) and docosahexaenoic acid (DHA) concentrations in Thoroughbred horses. In: *Proceedings of the 1st Nordic Feed Science Conference Sveriges Lantbruksuniversitet*, 116–118.

59 Rasmussen, B.B. and Phillips, S.M. (2003). Contractile and nutritional regulation of human muscle growth. *Exerc. Sport Sci. Rev.* 31 (3): 127–131.

60 Charge, S.B.P. and Rudnicki, M.A. (2004). Cellular and molecular regulation of muscle regeneration. *Physiol. Rev.* 84 (1): 209–238.

61 Graham-Thiers, P.M. and Kronfeld, D.S. (2005). Amino acid supplementation improves muscle mass in aged and young horses. *J. Anim. Sci.* 83 (12): 2783–2788.

62 Meyer, H. (1987). Nutrition of the equine athlete. In: *International Conference on Equine Exercise Physiology* (ed. J.R. Gillespie and N.E. Robinson), 644–673. Davis, CA: ICEEP Publications.

63 Miller-Graber, P.A., Lawrence, L.M., Foreman, J.H. et al. (1991). Dietary protein level and energy metabolism during treadmill exercise in horses. *J. Nutr.* 121 (9): 1462–1469.

64 Frank, N., Meacham, T.N., and Fontenot, J.P. (1987). Effect of feeding two levels of protein on performance and nutrition of exercising horses. In: *Proceedings of the 10th Equine Nutrition and Physiology Society Symposium*, 579–583. Fort Collins, CO: Equine Nutrition and Physiology Society.

65 Smith, R.R., Rumsey, G.L., and Scott, M.L. (1978). Heat increment associated with dietary protein, fat, carbohydrate and complete diets in salmonids comparative energetic efficiency. *J. Nutr.* 108 (6): 1025–1032.

66 Miller, P.A. and Lawrence, L.A.M. (1988). The effect of dietary protein level on exercising horses. *J. Anim. Sci.* 66 (9): 2185–2192.

67 Pagan, J.D., Essen-Gustavasson, B., Lindholm, A., and Thorton, J. (1987). The effect of energy source on exercise performance in Standardbred horses. In: *International Conference on Equine Exercise Physiology* (ed. J.R. Gillespie and N. Robinson), 686–700. Davis, CA: ICEEP Publications.

68 Mok, C.H., Levesque, C.L., and Urschel, K.L. (2018). Using the indicator amino acid oxidation technique to study threonine requirements in horses receiving a predominantly forage diet. *J. Anim. Physiol. Anim. Nutr. (Berl).* 102 (5): 1366–1381.

69 Mok, C.H. and Urschel, K.L. (2020). Amino acid requirements in horses. *Asian-Australas. J. Anim. Sci.* 33 (5): 679.

70 Lim, C.H., Gil, J.H., Quan, H. et al. (2018). Effect of 8-week leucine supplementation and resistance exercise training on muscle hypertrophy and satellite cell activation in rats. *Phys. Rep.* 6 (12): 1–12.

71 Gray, J., Harris, P., and Snow, D.H. (1988). Preliminary investigations into the calcium and magnesium status of the horse. In: *Animal Clinical Biochemistry* (ed. D. Blackmore), 307–317. Cambridge, MA: Cambridge University Press.

72 Loch, W.E., Brockschmidt, L., and Harmon, H. (1984). Effect of supplemental iron, live *Saccharomyces cerevisiae* yeast and exercise on hemoglobin and packed cell volume of the blood of horses. *J. Equine Vet. Sci.* 4 (3): 125–127.

73 McKeever, K.H., Malinowski, K., Fenger, C.K. et al. (2020). Evaluation of cobalt as a performance enhancing drug (PED) in racehorses. *Comp. Exerc. Physiol.* 16 (4): 243–252.

74 White, S.H. and Warren, L.K. (2017). Submaximal exercise training, more than dietary selenium supplementation, improves antioxidant status and ameliorates exercise-induced oxidative damage to skeletal muscle in young equine athletes. *J. Anim. Sci.* 95 (2): 657–670.

75 Laus, F., Faillace, V., Tesei, B. et al. (2017). Effect of thiamine pyrophosphate (bicarbossilasi®) administration on the exercising horse metabolism. *Isr. J. Vet. Med.* 72 (2): 15–21.

76 Williams, C.A., Kronfeld, D.S., Hess, T.M. et al. (2004). Antioxidant supplementation and subsequent oxidative stress of horses during an 80-km endurance race. *J. Anim. Sci.* 82 (2): 588–594.

77 Williams, C.A. and Carlucci, S.A. (2006). Oral vitamin E supplementation on oxidative stress, vitamin and antioxidant status in intensely exercised horses. *Equine Vet. J.* 38 (Suppl. 36): 617–621.

78 Pratt-Phillips, S., Kutzner-Mulligan, J., Marvin, R. et al. (2014). The effect of feeding two or three meals per day of either low or high nonstructural carbohydrate concentrates on postprandial glucose and insulin concentrations in horses. *J. Equine Vet. Sci.* 34 (11): 1251–1256.

79 Kutzner-Mulligan, J., Eisemann, J., Siciliano, P. et al. (2013). The effect of different feed delivery methods on time to consume feed and the resulting changes in postprandial metabolite concentrations in horses. *J. Anim. Sci.* 91 (8): 3772–3779.

80 Lawrence, L., Soderholm, L.V., Roberts, A. et al. (1993). Feeding status affects glucose metabolism in exercising horses. *J. Nutr.* 123 (12): 2152–2157.

81 Pagan, J.D. and Harris, P.A. (1999). The effects of timing and amount of forage and grain on exercise response in Thoroughbred horses. *Equine Vet. J.* 31 (S30): 451–457.

82 Duren, S.E. (1998). The gut during exercise. *Aust. Equine Vet.* 61 (1): 10–16.

83 Robyn, J., Plancke, L., Boshuizen, B. et al. (2017). Substrate use in horses during exercise – the "fasted" compared to the postprandial state. *Vlaams Diergeneeskd. Tijdschr.* 86 (5): 275–284.

84 Jansson, A. and Lindberg, J.E. (2012). A forage-only diet alters the metabolic response of horses in training. *Animal* 6 (12): 1939–1946.

85 Jose-Cunilleras, E., Taylor, L.E., and Hinchcliff, K.W. (2004). Glycemic index of cracked corn, oat groats and rolled barley in horses. *J. Anim. Sci.* 82 (9): 2623–2629.

86 Pagan, J.D., Geor, R.J., Harris, P.A. et al. (2002). Effects of fat adaptation on glucose kinetics and substrate oxidation during low-intensity exercise. *Equine Vet. J.* 34 (Suppl): 33–38.

87 Coenen, M. (2005). Exercise and stress: impact on adaptive processes involving water and electrolytes. *Livest. Prod. Sci.* 92 (2): 131–145.

88 Harris, P. (2009). Feeding management of elite endurance horses. *Vet. Clin. North Am. Equine Pract.* 25 (1): 137–153.

89 Lawrence, L. (2008). Nutrient needs of performance horses. *Rev. Bras. Zootec.* 37: 206–210.

90 Geor, R.J. (2013). Endocrine and metabolic physiology. In: *Equine Applied and Clinical Nutrition: Health, Welfare and Performance* (ed. R.J. Geor, P.A. Harris, and M. Coenen), 33–63. Edinburgh: Saunders Elsevier.

91 Jose-Cunilleras, E., Hinchcliff, K.W., Sams, R.A. et al. (2002). Glycemic index of a meal fed before exercise alters substrate use and glucose flux in exercising horses. *J. Appl. Phys.* 92 (1): 117–128.

92 Roberts, T.D. (1990). Staying upright in a moving trailer. *Equine Athl.* 3 (3): 1–8.

93 Santurtun, E. and Phillips, C.J.C. (2015). The impact of vehicle motion during transport on animal welfare. *Res. Vet. Sci.* 100 (June): 303–308.

94 Waran, N.K., Leadon, D., and Friend, T. (2002). The effects of transportation on the welfare of horses. In: *The Welfare of Horses* (ed. N.K. Waran), 125–150. London: Kluwer Academic Publishers.

95 Stull C. (2013). Transporting horses by road and air recommendations for reducing the stress. In: *Center for Equine Health: Horse Report. School of Veterinary Medicine*, 1–13. Davis, CA: University of California.

96 Connysson, M., Muhonen, S., and Jansson, A. (2017). Road transport and diet affect metabolic response to exercise in horses. *J. Anim. Sci.* 95 (11): 4869–4879.

97 Tateo, A., Padalino, B., Boccaccio, M. et al. (2012). Transport stress in horses: effects of two different distances. *J. Vet. Behav.* 7 (1): 33–42.

98 Waran, N.K. (1993). The behaviour of horses during and after transport by road. *Equine Vet. Educ.* 5 (3): 129–132.

99 Foss, M.A. and Lindner, A. (1996). Effects of trailer transportation duration on body weight and biochemical variables of horses. *Pferdeheilkunde* 12: 435–437.

100 Friend, T.H. (2000). Dehydration, stress, and water consumption of horses during long-distance commercial transport. *J. Anim. Sci.* 78 (10): 2568–2580.

101 Waran, N.K. and Cuddeford, D. (1995). Effects of loading and transport on the heart rate and behaviour of horses. *Appl. Anim. Behav. Sci.* 43 (2): 71–81.

102 Oikawa, M., Hobo, S., Oyamada, T., and Yoshikawa, H. (2005). Effects of orientation, intermittent rest and vehicle cleaning during transport on development of transport-related respiratory disease in horses. *J. Comp. Pathol.* 132 (2, 3): 153–168.

103 Lindinger, M.I. (2005). Determinants of surface membrane and transverse-tubular excitability in skeletal muscle: implications for high-intensity exercise. *Equine Comp. Exerc. Physiol.* 2 (4): 209–217.

104 Hoyt, J.K., Potter, G.D., Greene, L.W. et al. (1995). Electrolyte balance in exercising horses fed a control and a fat-supplemented diet. *J. Equine Vet. Sci.* 15 (10): 429–435.

105 Düsterdieck, K.F., Schott, H.C., Eberhart, S.W. et al. (1999). Electrolyte and glycerol supplementation improve water intake by horses performing a simulated 60 km endurance ride. *Equine Vet. J.* 31 (S30): 418–424.

106 Hyyppä, S., Saastamoinen, M., and Pösö, A.R. (1996). Restoration of water and electrolyte balance in horses after repeated exercise in hot and humid conditions. *Equine Vet. J.* 28 (S22): 108–112.

107 Kronfeld, D.S. (2001). Body fluids and exercise: replacement strategies. *J. Equine Vet. Sci.* 21 (8): 368–375.

108 Robert, C., Goachet, A.G., Fraipont, A. et al. (2010). Hydration and electrolyte balance in horses during an endurance season. *Equine Vet. J.* 42 (Suppl. 38): 98–104.

109 McConaghy, F.F., Hodgson, D.R., Evans, D.L., and Rose, R.J. (1995). Equine sweat composition: effects of adrenaline infusion, exercise and training. *Equine Vet. J.* 27 (S20): 158–164.

110 Assenza, A., Bergero, D., Congiu, F. et al. (2014). Evaluation of serum electrolytes and blood lactate concentration during repeated maximal exercise in horse. *J. Equine Vet. Sci.* 34 (10): 1175–1180.

111 Muñoz, A., Riber, C., Trigo, P. et al. (2010). Dehydration, electrolyte imbalances and renin-angiotensin-aldosterone-vasopressin axis in successful and unsuccessful endurance horses. *Equine Vet. J.* 42 (S38): 83–90.

112 Gordon, M. and Jerina, M. (2013). Water intake in horses fed supplemental salt compared to free-choice access to salt blocks. *J. Equine Vet. Sci.* 33 (5): 348–349.

113 Holbrook, T.C., Simmons, R.D., Payton, M.E., and MacAllister, C.G. (2005). Effect of repeated oral administration of hypertonic electrolyte solution on equine gastric mucosa. *Equine Vet. J.* 37 (6): 501–504.

114 Pagan, J., Waldridge, B., and Lange, J. (2013). Dextrose does not affect rate of absorption or retention of electrolytes in idle Thoroughbreds. *J. Equine Vet. Sci.* 33 (5): 349–350.

115 Videla, R. and Andrews, F. (2009). New perspectives in equine gastric ulcer syndrome. *Vet. Clin. North Am. Equine Pract.* 25 (2): 283–301.

116 Bell, R.J.W., Kingston, J.K., Mogg, T.D., and Perkins, N.R. (2007). The prevalence of gastric ulceration in racehorses in New Zealand. *N.Z. Vet. J.* 55 (1): 13–18.

117 Husted, L., Sanchez, L.C., Olsen, S.N. et al. (2008). Effect of paddock vs. stall housing on 24 hour gastric pH within the proximal and ventral equine stomach. *Equine Vet. J.* 40 (4): 337–341.

118 Le Jeune, S., Nieto, J., Dechant, J., and Snyder, J. (2009). Prevalence of gastric ulcers in Thoroughbred broodmares in pasture: a preliminary report. *Vet. J.* 181 (3): 251–255.

119 Lester, G.D., Robinson, I., and Secombe, C. (2008). *Risk Factors for Gastric Ulceration in Thoroughbred Racehorses*, 1–42. Rural Industries Research and Development Corporation, Australian Government.

120 Alexander, F. (1966). A study of parotid salivation in the horse. *J. Phys.* 184 (3): 646–656.

121 Meyer, H., Ahlswede, L., and Reinhardt, H. (1975). Duration of feeding, frequency of chewing and physical form of the feed for horses. *Dtsch. Tierarztl. Wochenschrift.* 82: 54–58.

122 Nadeau, J.A., Andrews, F.M., Patton, C.S. et al. (2003). Effects of hydrochloric, acetic, butyric, and propionic acids on pathogenesis of ulcers in the nonglandular portion of the stomach of horses. *Am. J. Vet. Res.* 64 (4): 404–412.

123 Brøkner, C., Nørgaard, P., and Hansen, H.H. (2008). Effect of feed type and essential oil product on equine chewing activity. *J. Anim. Physiol. Anim. Nutr. (Berl).* 92 (6): 621–630.

124 Murray, M.J. and Eichorn, E.S. (1996). Effects of intermittent feed deprivation, intermittent feed deprivation with ranitidine administration, and stall confinement with ad libitum access to hay on gastric ulceration in horses. *Am. J. Vet. Res.* 57 (11): 1599–1603.

125 Feige, K., Furst, A., and Eser, M. (2002). Effects of housing, feeding, and use on equine health with emphasis on respiratory and gastrointestinal disease. *Schweiz. Arch. Tierheilkd.* 144 (7): 348–355.

126 Luthersson, N., Nielsen, K.H., Harris, P. et al. (2009). Risk factors associated with equine gastric ulceration syndrome (EGUS) in 201 horses in Denmark. *Equine Vet. J.* 41 (7): 625–630.

127 Lorenzo-Figueras, M. and Merritt, A.M. (2002). Effects of exercise on gastric volume and pH in the proximal portion of the stomach of horses. *Am. J. Vet. Res.* 63 (11): 1481–1487.

128 Malmkvist, J., Poulsen, J.M., Luthersson, N. et al. (2012). Behaviour and stress responses in horses with gastric ulceration. *Appl. Anim. Behav. Sci.* 142 (3, 4): 160–167.

129 Vatistas, N.J., Sifferman, R.L., Holste, J. et al. (1999). Induction and maintenance of gastric ulceration in horses in simulated race training. *Equine Vet. J.* 31 (S29): 40–44.

130 Dionne, R.M., Vrins, A., Doucet, M.Y., and Pare, J. (2003). Gastric ulcers in Standardbred racehorses: prevalence, lesion description, and risk factors. *J. Vet. Intern. Med.* 17 (2): 218–222.

131 Nieto, J.E., Snyder, J.R., Beldomenico, P. et al. (2004). Prevalence of gastric ulcers in endurance horses – a preliminary report. *Vet. J.* 167 (1): 33–37.

132 Furr, M., Taylor, L., and Kronfeld, D. (1994). The effects of exercise training on serum gastrin responses in the horse. *Cornell Vet.* 84 (1): 41–45.

133 Lester, G.D. (2004). Gastrointestinal diseases of performance horses. In: *Equine Sports Medicine and Surgery: Basic and Clinical Sciences of the Equine Athlete* (ed. A. Kaneps, K. Hinchcliff, and R. Geor), 1037–1048. Saunders.

134 Nicol, C.J., Davidson, H.P.D., Harris, P.A. et al. (2002). Study of crib-biting and gastric inflammation and ulceration in young horses. *Vet. Rec.* 151 (22): 658–662.

135 Raspa, F., Colombino, E., Capucchio, M. et al. (2021). Effects of feeding managements on microbial contamination of mesenteric lymph nodes and liver and on intestinal histo-morphology in horses. In: *Proceedings 25th Congress of the European College of Veterinary and Comparative Nutrition*, 93. Vila Real, Portugal: European College of Veterinary and Comparative Nutrition.

136 Cargile, J.L., Burrow, J.A., Kim, I. et al. (2004). Effect of dietary corn oil supplementation on equine gastric fluid acid, sodium, and prostaglandin E 2 content before and during pentagastrin infusion. *J. Vet. Intern. Med.* 18 (4): 545–549.

137 Frank, N., Andrews, F.M., Elliott, S.B., and Lew, J. (2005). Effects of dietary oils on the development of gastric ulcers in mares. *Am. J. Vet. Res.* 66 (11): 2006–2011.

138 Lybbert T, Gibbs P, Cohen N, et al. (2007). Feeding alfalfa hay to exercising horses reduces the severity of gastric squamous mucosal ulceration. In: *Proceedings of the 53rd Annual Convention of the American Association of Equine Practitioners*, 525–526. Orlando, FL: American Association of Equine Practitioners (AAEP).

139 Clark, C.K., Merritt, A.M., Burrow, J.A., and Steible, C.K. (1996). Effect of aluminum hydroxide/magnesium hydroxide antacid and bismuth subsalicylate on gastric pH in horses. *J. Am. Vet. Med. Assoc.* 208 (10): 1687–1691.

140 Murray, M.J. and Grodinsky, C. (1992). The effects of famotidine, ranitidine and magnesium hydroxide/aluminium hydroxide on gastric fluid pH in adult horses. *Equine Vet. J.* 24 (S11): 52–55.

141 Shawaf, T., El-Deeb, W., and Elgioushy M. (2020). The contribution of specific and nonspecific biomarkers in diagnosis of equine gastric ulcer syndrome (EGUS) under field condition. *J. Equine Vet. Sci.* 84 (1): 102853.

142 Huff, N.K.K., Auer, A.D.D., Garza, F. et al. (2012). Effect of sea buckthorn berries and pulp in a liquid emulsion on gastric ulcer scores and gastric juice pH in horses. *J. Vet. Intern. Med.* 26 (5): 1186–1191.

143 Loftin, P., Woodward, M., Bidot, W.A. et al. (2012). Evaluating replacement of supplemental inorganic minerals with Zinpro performance minerals on equine gastric ulcers. *J. Vet. Intern. Med.* 26: 737–738.

144 Zavoshti, F.R. and Andrews, F.M. (2017). Therapeutics for equine gastric ulcer syndrome. *Vet. Clin. North Am. Equine Pract.* 33 (1): 141–162.

145 Köller, G., Recknagel, S., Spallek, A. et al. (2010). Magenschleimkonzentration und intragastraler pH-Wert adulter Pferde während der Nahrungskarenz und nach oraler Applikation von Pronutrin®. *Pferdeheilkunde* 26: 186–190.

146 Venner, M., Lauffs, S., and Deegen, E. (1999). Treatment of gastric lesions in horses with pectin-lecithin complex. *Equine Vet. J.* 31 (S29): 91–96.

147 Bush, J., Van Den Boom, R., and Franklin, S. (2018). Comparison of *Aloe vera* and omeprazole in the treatment of equine gastric ulcer syndrome. *Equine Vet. J.* 50 (1): 34–40.

148 Chen, H., Nie, Q., Xie, M. et al. (2019). Protective effects of β-glucan isolated from highland barley on ethanol-induced gastric damage in rats and its benefits to mice gut conditions. *Food Res. Int.* 122 (Aug): 157–166.

149 Slovis, N. (2017). Polysaccharide treatment reduces gastric ulceration in active horses. *J. Equine Vet. Sci.* 50 (3): 116–120.

150 Elghandour, M.M.M.Y., Reddy, P.R.K., Salem, A.Z.M. et al. (2018). Plant bioactives and extracts as feed additives in horse nutrition. *J. Equine Vet. Sci.* 69 (Oct): 66–77.

151 Zaghlool, S.S., Shehata, B.A., Abo-Seif, A.A., and Abd El-Latif, H.A. (2015). Protective effects of ginger and marshmallow extracts on indomethacin-induced peptic ulcer in rats. *J. Nat. Sci. Biol. Med.* 6 (2): 421.

152 McCullough, R.W. (2013). Expedited management of ulcer, colic and diarrhea in 209 horses: an open-labeled observational study of a potency-enhanced sucralfate-like elm phyto-saccharide. *J. Vet. Med. Anim. Heal.* 5 (2): 32–40.

153 Al Jassim, R., McGowan, T., Andrews, F., and McGowan, C. (2008). *Gastric Ulceration in Horses the Role of Bacteria and Lactic Acid.* Rural Industries Research and Development Corporation, Australian Government.

154 Andrews FM, Camacho P, Gaymon G, et al. (2014). Effect of a supplement on non-glandular gastric ulcer scores and gastric juice pH. In: *Proceedings of the 60th Annual Convention of the American Association of Equine Practitioners*, 189–190. Salt Lake City, UT: American Association of Equine Practitioners (AAEP).

155 Bonelli, F., Busechian, S., Meucci, V. et al. (2016). pHyloGASTRO in the treatment of equine gastric ulcer lesions. *J. Equine Vet. Sci.* 46 (11): 69–72.

156 Kerbyson, N.C., Knottenbelt, D.K., Carslake, H.B. et al. (2016). A comparison between omeprazole and a dietary supplement for the management of squamous gastric ulceration in horses. *J. Equine Vet. Sci.* 40 (5): 94–101.

157 Stucchi, L., Zucca, E., Serra, A. et al. (2017). Efficacy of the administration of a natural feed supplement in the management of equine gastric ulcer syndrome in 7 sport horses: a field trial. *Am. J. Anim. Vet. Sci.* 12 (3): 104–110.

158 Sykes, B.W., Sykes, K.M., and Hallowell, G.D. (2014). Efficacy of a combination of Apolectol®, live yeast (CNCM I-1077) and magnesium hydroxide in the management of equine gastric ulcer syndrome in Thoroughbred racehorses: a randomised, blinded, placebo controlled clinical trial. *J. Equine Vet. Sci.* 34: 1274–1278.

159 Woodward, M.C., Huff, N.K., Garza, F. et al. (2014). Effect of pectin, lecithin, and antacid feed supplements (Egusin®) on gastric ulcer scores, gastric fluid pH and blood gas values in horses. *BMC Vet. Res.* 10 (1): 1–8.

160 Andrews, F.M., Camacho-Luna, P., Loftin, P.G. et al. (2015). Effect of a pelleted supplement fed during and after omeprazole treatment on nonglandular gastric ulcer scores and gastric juice pH in horses. *Equine Vet. Educ.* 28 (4): 196–202.

161 Mélo, S.K.M., Santiago, T.A., de Lima, D.T. et al. (2014). A proton-pump inhibitor modifies the concentration of digestion biomarkers in healthy horses. *J. Equine Vet. Sci.* 34 (11, 12): 1318–1323.

162 Pagan, J.D., Petroski-Rose, L., Mann, A., and Hauss, A. (2020). Omeprazole reduces calcium digestibility in Thoroughbred horses. *J. Equine Vet. Sci.* 86: 102851.

163 Loving, N. (2016). Respiratory Problems. https://aaep.org/horsehealth/respiratory-problems (accessed 2 September 2021).

164 Moore-Colyer, M.J.S., Taylor, J.L.E., and James, R. (2016). The effect of steaming and soaking on the respirable particle, bacteria, mould, and nutrient content in hay for horses. *J. Equine Vet. Sci.* 39 (4): 62–68.

165 Humer, E., Hollmann, M., Stögmüller, G., and Zebeli, Q. (2019). Steaming conditions enhance hygienic quality of the compromised equine hay with minimal losses of nonfiber carbohydrates. *J. Equine Vet. Sci.* 74 (3): 28–35.

166 Avellini, L., Chiaradia, E., and Gaiti, A. (1999). Effect of exercise training, selenium and vitamin E on some free radical scavengers in horses (*Equus caballus*). *Comp. Biochem. Physiol. Part B Biochem. Mol. Biol.* 123 (2): 147–154.

167 Brummer, M., Hayes, S., Dawson, K.A., and Lawrence, L.M. (2013). Interrelationships among selenium status, antioxidant capacity and oxidative stress in the horse. *J. Equine Vet. Sci.* 5 (33): 332.

168 Velázquez-Cantón, E., de la Cruz-Rodríguez, N., Zarco, L. et al. (2018). Effect of selenium and vitamin E supplementation on lactate, cortisol, and malondialdehyde in horses undergoing moderate exercise in a polluted environment. *J. Equine Vet. Sci.* 69 (10): 136–144.

169 Hall, J.A., Van Saun, R.J., and Wander, R.C. (2004). Dietary (n-3) fatty acids from menhaden fish oil alter plasma fatty acids and leukotriene B synthesis in healthy horses. *J. Vet. Intern. Med.* 18 (6): 871–879.

170 Nogradi, N., Couetil, L.L., Messick, J. et al. (2015). Omega-3 fatty acid supplementation provides an additional benefit to a low-dust diet in the management of horses with chronic lower airway inflammatory disease. *J. Vet. Intern. Med.* 29 (1): 299–306.

171 Tew, W.P. and Hotchkiss, R.N. (1981). Synovial fluid analysis and equine joint disorders. *J. Equine Vet. Sci.* 1 (5): 163–170.

172 Bertone, A.L., Bramlage, L.R., McIlwraith, C.W., and Malemud, C.L. (2005). Comparison of proteoglycan and collagen in articular cartilage of horses with naturally developing osteochondrosis and healing osteochondral fragments of experimentally induced fractures. *Am. J. Vet. Res.* 66 (11): 1881–1890.

173 Monteiro, S.O., Bettencourt, E.V., and Lepage, O.M. (2015). Biologic strategies for intra-articular treatment and cartilage repair. *J. Equine Vet. Sci.* 35 (3): 175–190.

174 McCann, M.E., Moore, J.N., Carrick, J.B., and Barton, M.H. (2000). Effect of intravenous infusion of omega-3 and omega-6 lipid emulsions on equine monocyte fatty acid composition and inflammatory mediator production in vitro. *Shock* 14 (2): 222–228.

175 Dimock, A.N., Siciliano, P.D., and McIlwraith, C.W. (2000). Evidence supporting an increased presence of reactive oxygen species in the diseased equine joint. *Equine Vet. J.* 32 (5): 439–443.

176 Neil, K.M., Caron, J.P., and Orth, M.W. (2005). The role of glucosamine and chondroitin sulfate in treatment for and prevention of osteoarthritis in animals. *J. Am. Vet. Med. Assoc.* 226 (7): 1079–1088.

177 Marañón, G., Muñoz-Escassi, B., Manley, W. et al. (2008). The effect of methyl sulphonyl methane supplementation on biomarkers of oxidative stress in sport horses following jumping exercise. *Acta Vet. Scand.* 50 (1): 1–9.

178 Williams, V.S. (2007). Intraarticular hyaluronic acid supplementation in the horse: the role of molecular weight. *J. Equine Vet. Sci.* 27 (7): 298–303.

179 Dobenecker, B., Reese, S., Jahn, W. et al. (2018). Specific bioactive collagen peptides (PETAGILE®) as supplement for horses with osteoarthritis: a two-centred study. *J. Anim. Physiol. Anim. Nutr. (Berl).* 102 (Suppl. 1): 16–23.

180 Winther, K., Kharazmi, A., Hansen, A.S.V., and Falk-Rønne, J. (2010). A randomised placebo controlled double blind study on the effect of subspecies of rose hip (*Rosa canina*) on the immune system, working capacity and behaviour of horses. In: *The Impact of Nutrition on the Health and Welfare of Horses*. EAAP Volume 128 (ed. A. Ellis, A. Longland, M. Coenen, and N. Miraglia), 283–287. Wageningen: Wageningen Academic Publishers.

181 Torfs, S., Delesalle, C., Vanschandevijl, K. et al. (2008). Anti-inflammatory phytotherapeutics: a valuable alternative to NSAID treatment in horses? *Vlaams Diergeneeskd. Tijdschr.* 78: 161–170.

182 van de Water, E., Oosterlinck, M., Dumoulin, M. et al. (2017). The preventive effects of two nutraceuticals on experimentally induced acute synovitis. *Equine Vet. J.* 49 (4): 532–538.

183 Forsyth, R.K., Brigden, C.V., and Northrop, A.J. (2006). Double blind investigation of the effects of oral supplementation of combined glucosamine hydrochloride (GHCL) and chondroitin sulphate (CS) on stride characteristics of veteran horses. *Equine Vet. J.* 36 (Suppl): 622–625.

184 Montgomery, M. (2011). Evaluation of the safety and efficacy of the dietary supplement Actistatin® on established glucosamine and chondroitin therapy in the horse. *Int. J. Appl. Res. Vet. Med.* 9 (2): 101.

185 Murray, R.C., Walker, V.A., Tranquille, C.A. et al. (2017). A randomized blinded crossover clinical trial to determine the effect of an oral joint supplement on equine limb kinematics, orthopedic, physiotherapy, and handler evaluation scores. *J. Equine Vet. Sci.* 50 (3): 121–128.

186 Bradbery, A.N., Coverdale, J.A., Vernon, K.L. et al. (2018). Evaluation of conjugated linoleic acid supplementation on markers of joint inflammation and cartilage metabolism in young horses challenged with lipopolysaccharide. *J. Anim. Sci.* 96 (2): 579–590.

187 Lindinger, M.I., MacNicol, J.M., Karrow, N., and Pearson, W. (2017). Effects of a novel dietary supplement on indices of muscle injury and articular GAG release in horses. *J. Equine Vet. Sci.* 48 (1): 52–60.

19

Feeding Stallions

Stewart K. Morgan and Megan Shepherd

KEY POINTS

- Breeding stallions are optimally maintained between body condition score (BCS) of 4 and 6/9.
- Nutritional requirements of breeding stallions range between adult maintenance and work.
- Nutritional requirements of stallions are also influenced by temperament and work level.
- The ration of stallions should be nutritionally complete and balanced according to current recommendations year-round.
- There are no studies with high grades of evidence to suggest that specialized nutritional supplements improve semen quality or stallion performance.

19.1 Introduction

The proportion of intact male horses (stallions and colts) is assumed to be ≤10% of the total captive equine population given horses are most commonly owned for recreational or performance activities. Male horses are usually castrated (gelded) at a young age to prevent undesirable behavioral traits, prevent the perpetuation of genetic defects, and reduce the population of unwanted horses [1, 2]. Mature stallions are retained for breeding with the more desirable mares, breeding up to 200 in a season [3–5]. The percentage of stallions that breed more than 120 mares per season has increased since the late 1980s [4]. Athletic performance, before and following sexual maturity, is a key factor in selecting stallions for breeding [6, 7]. Successful sires may also be significant sources of revenue as some owners receive more than $100 000 USD in stud fees. Inherited traits, responsiveness to training, husbandry, and nutrition contribute to a stallion's performance in competition and subsequent economic value. Proper nutritional management of stallions involves routine physical evaluations, at key points throughout the year, that is, before, during, and after the breeding season, to ensure the stallion is healthy and maintaining adequate body weight (BW) and BCS. When nutritional or diet-related problems arise, a systematic iterative review of the stallion, the ration, and the feeding method is recommended. See Appendix C Nutrition Competencies of Equine Veterinarians.

19.2 Animal Assessment

Given the BW for horses ranges from 200 to 900 kg, the recommended daily nutrient intakes for non-breeding and breeding stallions are presented in Table 19.1 per 100 kg of mature BW [8]. Stallions do vary in age, temperament, voluntary activity, imposed exercise (riding, driving, training), and service frequency (number of mares or collections/wk). Therefore, the nutritional requirement and feeding management should be reviewed at least twice a year to accommodate individual stallion needs.

19.2.1 Body Condition Score

Stallions should be fed to maintain a BCS of 4/9 (moderately thin) to 6/9 (moderately fleshy) [9, 10]. Live-cover breeding is seasonal, for example, February to May in North America. Stallions may gain BW and BCS during the non-breeding times and/or may lose BW and BCS during the breeding season. Therefore, routine physical assessments should be tailored to the breeding schedule, activity level, and individual horse history. The assessment frequency is case-dependent in that an inactive stallion that remains at target weight and BCS may need only be assessed twice a year, whereas an active stallion with a recent history of losing weight and decreased appetite should be assessed weekly. See Chapter 2 Nutritional Assessment of the Horse.

Equine Clinical Nutrition, Second Edition. Edited by Rebecca L. Remillard.

Table 19.1 Recommended daily nutrient intakes for mature stallions per 100 kg of body weight regardless of age.

Nutrient		Stallion	
	Units	Non-breeding	Breeding
Digestible energy	Mcal	3.64[a]	4.36
Crude protein	g	144	158
Lysine	g	6.2	6.8
Calcium	g	4.0	6.0
Phosphorus	g	2.8	3.6
Magnesium	g	1.5	1.9
Potassium	g	5.0	5.7
Sodium	g	2.0	2.8
Chloride	g	8.0	9.3
Sulfur	g	3.0	3.0
Copper	mg	20	20
Iron	mg	80	80
Manganese	mg	80	80
Zinc	mg	80	80
Cobalt	mg	0.1	0.1
Iodine	mg	0.7	0.7
Selenium	mg	0.2	0.2
Vitamin A	KIU	3	4.5
Vitamin D	IU	660	660
Vitamin E	IU	100	160
Thiamin	mg	6	6
Riboflavin	mg	4	4

[a] For example, a 560 kg non-breeding, average tempered stallion would require 3.64 × 5.6 = 20.38 Mcal DE/d.
Source: Adapted from NRC [8]; Table 16-3 using nutrients required for a 500 kg mature horse with BCS 4–6/9 consuming 2% BW.

19.2.2 Breeding Soundness

Assessing a stallion's true fertility is difficult, as true fertility is the product of the stallion and the mare [11]. Thus, the observed fertility of a stallion is significantly impacted by mare fertility [11–13]. Factors that may impact a stallion's observed fertility include the number of mares the stallion is bred to, the number of times the stallion is allowed to breed a mare (or number of artificial inseminations), and age [14, 15].

Stallions must be physiologically sound to breed efficiently, and generally achieve reproductive maturity by approximately 4–5 years of age, based on hormonal and physical changes [16, 17]. Spermatozoa first appear in stallion ejaculate at 11–15 m of age, and stallions may be put into breeding service as young as 2–3 years of age. However, spermatozoa production, but not fertility of the spermatozoa produced, is generally lower in 2-year-old and 3-year-old stallions than in older horses, and is lower in 2-year-olds than in 3-year-olds [18]. However, there are large individual differences, and, therefore, fertility evaluations should be done to determine how the stallion and the semen should be used to obtain maximum reproductive efficiency. Regardless of semen quality, young horses should be used sparingly, as overuse may lead to poor breeding behavior. Although the percentage of live foals born per breeding decreases as mature mares' age increases, the age of the mature breeding stallion appears to not affect the live foal percentage. This is based on all registered Thoroughbred horses bred in North America (NA) during two breeding seasons in which live foal percentage averaged 58.1% [19].

Breeding soundness examinations help assess a stallion for reproductive fitness. Briefly, stallion breeding soundness examinations involve performing a physical examination to assess the animal's general health, comparing the animal's sperm and semen quality to those generally accepted as being satisfactory, checking the stallion for infectious diseases that may negatively impact fertility, and assessing libido [20, 21]. Musculoskeletal soundness also plays a role in breeding soundness. Poor breeding performance in the stallion has been associated with poor libido, and difficulty in mounting, thrusting, and ejaculatory dysfunction [15, 22].

Testicular size and sperm output, but not motility, are significantly affected by the time of year. Total scrotal width, seminal volume, and the number of sperm per ejaculation increased 20%, 40%, and 50%, respectively, from mid-winter to late spring/early summer. Since the number of spermatozoa per ejaculate is the most important seminal characteristic related to fertility, with the possible exception of motility, semen obtained early in the breeding season is only about half as good as that obtained during peak physiological breeding season [23]. Seasons do not affect the percentage of progressively motile spermatozoa or their chemical characteristics, however, because fewer spermatozoa are produced, and the sex drive is lower from fall to spring, fewer mares can be bred during this time. Plasma testosterone, total androgen concentrations, and libido in the stallion are lowest in the winter and highest in the spring. As with mares, artificial light beginning an hour before sunset to increase total light to 16 hrs daily beginning 2–3 m before the desired breeding season will increase the stallion's fertility in terms of spermatozoa per ejaculate and libido.

19.3 Ration Assessment

The energy requirement of non-breeding and breeding stallions is similar to horses at elevated maintenance and those doing light work, respectively. Ration digestible energy (DE) concentrations of 1.8–2.2 Mcal DE/kg dry matter (DM) are suitable for non-breeding and breeding stallions depending on activity. Stallions should be provided a complete and balanced ration, meeting the energy and nutrient requirements, fed within the limits of dry matter intake (DMI) which is 1.5–2.0% BW.

19.3.1 Feeds

Given the seasonality of breeding, the feeding management of these horses may vary throughout the year. Therefore, general guidelines must be fine-tuned for the individual stallion as needed throughout the year and their lifetime.

Forage (pasture or hay) should provide the preponderance of the stallion ration. Forage quality is assessed through objective nutrient analyses and subjective measures, that is, smell, color, feel, and physical contents. See Ration Analysis and Subjective Assessments in Chapter 10. The forage offered must be palatable in odor and texture, to the stallion to ensure an adequate DMI [24]. The forage digestible dry matter (DDM) and energy density (Mcal/kg DM) must be sufficient to meet the estimated daily energy requirement (DER) within an edible volume of feed (DMI). DM digestibility and voluntary DMI are inversely related to the forage acid detergent fiber (%ADF) and neutral detergent fiber (%NDF), respectively. As ADF and NDF increase in the forage DM, the voluntary DMI and DM digestibility decrease, and the nutritional value of the forage decreases. Forages with relative feeding values (RFVs) of 86–124 are recommended for stallions (Table 19.2) [8, 25, 26]. See Relative Feed Value in Chapter 10.

In cases where the available forage energy density is insufficient to meet the stallion's nutrient requirement within the voluntary DMI, an energy concentrate can be fed to provide the difference between the animal requirement and that provided by forage alone [26]. The proper amount to feed initially could be based on a ration formulation or commercial manufacturer's recommendations and then adjusted as necessary to maintain a moderate body condition for that individual stallion. For stallions that have an orthopedic disease or other conditions limiting mobility, a BCS of 3/9–4/9 has been recommended for "breeding comfort" [15]. There is no evidence that being overweight is advantageous to an adult reproducing stallion; however, there is

Table 19.2 Comparison of major nutrient concentrations between forage averages and ration recommendations for stallions [25].

Horse to Forage Comparison	Digestible energy	Protein	Calcium	Phosphorus	DMI	RFV
	Dry matter basis				% BW	
Stallion:	Mcal/kg	%	%	%		
Non-breeding	1.8	7.2	0.2	0.1	1.5–2.0	86–100
Breeding	2.2	7.9	0.3	0.2	1.5–2.0	86–124
Forages:						
Legume						
Pasture: vegetative	2.71	26.5	1.31	0.37	3.6[a]	197[b]
Hay: immature	2.62	20.5	1.56	0.31	3.3	171
Hay: mid-mature	2.43	20.8	1.37	0.30	2.8	136
Hay: mature	2.21	17.8	1.22	0.28	2.4	106
Grass						
Pasture: vegetative	2.39	26.5	0.56	0.44	2.6	141
Hay: immature	2.36	18	0.72	0.34	2.4	121
Hay: mid-mature	2.18	13.3	0.66	0.29	2.1	97
Hay: mature	2.04	10.8	0.47	0.26	1.7	76

[a] Forage %DMI = 120/%NDF.
[b] Forage relative feeding value = %DDM × %DMI × 0.775; where %DDM = 88.9 − (0.779 × %ADF).
Source: Adapted from NRC [8]; Table 16-3 using nutrients required for a 500 kg mature horse BCS 4–6/9. Forage data from Table 16-6.

substantial evidence that being overweight is deleterious. Of the comorbidities associated with obesity in horses, osteoarthritis may be of most importance to the stallion [27–32].

19.3.2 Key Nutrients

There is a paucity of direct evidence suggesting that a stallion's reproductive performance is significantly impacted by dietary management or that stallions have significantly different nutrient requirements than geldings or non-breeding mares. Undernutrition early in life can later negatively affect reproduction in mature animals, for example, during growth, both energy and nutrient deficiencies can delay the onset of sexual maturity and impair the development of reproductive organs [33]. Thus, an individual adult stallion's nutrient requirements are largely determined by the environment, voluntary physical activity, and daily energy expenditure [34, 35]. The National Research Council (NRC) and the French Institut National de la Recherche Agronomique (INRA) provide nutritional recommendations for stallions [8, 36, 37].

19.3.2.1 Water

Voluntary water intake may be affected by factors including food intake, diet composition, exercise, physiologic status, and temperature. Water is the most important but often forgotten nutrient. For convenience, many stallions meet their water requirement using automatic waterers which should be cleaned and checked daily to ensure proper function. Monitoring daily water intake is not possible with automatic water unless the waterer is metered. Noting a problem or change in the stallion's intake is more likely with buckets that need to be filled several times daily [38]. In general, however, the daily maintenance water requirement of the average adult horse fed a dry diet is approximately 5 L/100 kg BW or 5% of BW [8]. Although there is no evidence that breeding stallions have water requirements that differ from those of geldings or mares, it is prudent to ensure that stallions have ready access to a source of clean drinking water at all times [8].

19.3.2.2 Energy

The energy cost of work added to the energy cost of first and foremost maintenance energy requirement determines the total DER for a stallion (Table 19.1). Breeding does not require an increase in any nutrient except for energy and the increase needed for the act of breeding itself is small. However, the increased physical activity associated with breeding, such as pacing and apprehension, in addition to temperament, housing (stalled vs. pasture), and imposed activity (performance, training), may substantially increase dietary energy needs. Mature inactive stallions with a quiet temperament and low levels of voluntary activity likely have a DER similar to the mature horse at maintenance; whereas a very active stallion during the breeding season may have an energy requirement approximating light to moderate work [26].

A study of 33 Thoroughbred stallions on a Central Kentucky breeding farm during one season, covering 70–90 mares/month, consumed an average of 4.4 Mcal DE/100 kg BW daily [35]. Yet during this period, the weight of the stallions decreased about 2%. All of these stallions were kept in box stalls, allowed access to pasture for about 3 hrs/d, and fed a concentrate and alfalfa hay twice daily. Although BCS was not reported in this study and feed intake was estimated, BW changes were documented and the energy requirement was estimated to be 20% above average maintenance horse needs [8, 26].

The NRC estimates that digestible energy for maintenance (DEm) of adult horses with elevated levels of voluntary activity or with nervous temperaments is 3.6 Mcal DE/100 kg BW, and some adult stallions are included in that group [8]. The INRA provides methods for estimating the DER of both breeding and non-breeding stallions during the breeding season and provides housing allowances (box stall vs. paddock or free roaming in pens), activity, and breeding intensity (light, moderate, or intense). The INRA estimates that DER for sexually quiescent adult draft stallions is 5% greater than for adult draft geldings, while the DER for non-breeding adult stallions of sport and racing breeds (light horses) is 15–20% greater than those of light horse geldings [36].

In summary, the best indicators of energy balance in the body are BW, BCS, and changes, if any. Initial estimates of the DER for a stallion, when a diet and weight history are unavailable, are likely 3.6–4.4 Mcal DE/100 kg BW/d depending upon activity and season. The BW and BCS should be assessed at reasonable intervals and, per the iterative process, repeated more often when changes to the feed or feeding protocol were made to address a problem.

19.3.2.2.1 Fatty Acids

Fats are sources of energy, carriers of fat-soluble vitamins, and sources of essential fatty acids, which are precursors of prostaglandins. While linoleic acid (LA; 18:2 n-6) and α-linolenic acid (ALA; 18:3 n-3) are essential fatty acids, there is only an intake recommendation for linoleic (0.5% DM). Horses fed a forage-based diet will consume primarily ALA [39, 40]. Although there are no dietary omega-3 fatty acid recommendations, the long-chain omega-3 polyunsaturated fatty acid (PUFA) docosahexaenoic acid (DHA; 22:6 n-3) is the major PUFA composition of sperm [41–44]. Although dietary fatty acid content does affect circulating and cellular fatty acid profiles, there is insufficient evidence to suggest that dietary supplementation with omega-3 fatty acids will have a significant positive impact on stallion sperm [40, 45, 46].

19.3.2.3 Protein

Adequate intake of dietary protein is essential for the synthesis and maintenance of proteins, cells, tissues, and hormones. Both the INRA and NRC suggest that the dietary protein requirement for non-breeding stallions is greater than that of geldings or non-breeding mares of the same BW [8, 36]. This is presumably based upon the assumption that stallions are more active or need greater dietary protein to maintain greater muscle mass. Although testosterone is anabolic and promotes skeletal muscle development, there is insufficient experimental data to suggest substantial anabolism as a consequence of either exogenous or endogenous androgens [47, 48]. The NRC estimates the maintenance crude protein (CP) requirement for a non-breeding stallion is 1.44 g CP/kg BW/d. For breeding stallions, the NRC assumes a 10% increase in protein requirements relative to the non-breeding stallion (1.6 g CP/kg BW/d). The only specific amino acid recommendation is lysine at 4.3% of CP. The INRA also assumes that horse digestible crude protein (Matières Azotées Digestibles Cheval [MADC]) requirement, for non-breeding stallions, is higher than those for geldings and non-breeding mares. Like the NRC, the INRA assumes that a stallion's protein requirement is increased by that level of reproductive activity (light, medium, or heavy), although there is no empirical evidence that this is the case.

19.3.2.4 Macrominerals

Forage is the major source of macrominerals in the ration. The dietary intake of calcium, phosphorus, magnesium, potassium, sodium, chloride, and sulfur is based on the BW of the adult horse for non-breeding stallions and slightly higher for working stallions (Table 19.1). The Ca:P ratio should be between 1.2:1 and 2:1. Legume forages contain more Ca than P (Ca:P = 10:1), whereas most grass forages have a moderate Ca:P ratio of <2:1; therefore, laboratory mineral analysis of the forage, particularly for mixed forages, is warranted to ensure proper calcium to phosphorus balance in the total ration.

19.3.2.5 Antioxidants

The high concentration of long-chain PUFAs in the plasma membranes of spermatozoa increases the susceptibility of spermatozoa to lipid peroxidation and the formation of reactive oxygen species (ROS). Although involved in normal sperm function and capacitance, ROS can also cause DNA fragmentation in sperm and reduce sperm motility [49]. Cryopreserved spermatozoa, in particular, are negatively impacted by ROS. Meeting recommended intakes of antioxidant nutrients, such as Vitamin C, Vitamin E, selenium, and zinc, is thus important in reducing the negative effects of ROS on sperm. Vitamin C and E supplements are reported fed to enhance the stallion's reproductive performance or ability; however, there is insufficient evidence that administering a stallion supplemental dietary antioxidants increases fresh semen quality [50, 51].

19.3.2.5.1 Selenium

Selenium is an essential micronutrient that functions as a component of proteins (selenoproteins) and as an antioxidant [52–60]. Selenium also plays an essential role in testicular development and spermatogenesis [43]. Testes have a greater concentration of selenium than most organs and retain normal selenium concentrations, even under conditions of moderate selenium deficiency [61–63]. For the breeding stallion, selenium is of particular importance in reducing oxidative damage to spermatozoa [41, 43, 49, 64, 65].

Spermatozoa are particularly susceptible to oxidative damage as a consequence of high concentrations of PUFAs in their cellular membranes. Selenium deficiency is associated with poor sperm production and quality presumably as a consequence of oxidative damage [66]. Sperm motility defects have been reported in selenium-deficient animals [64, 66, 67]. *In vitro* studies suggest that reductions in stallion sperm motility that occur as a consequence of oxidative stress may be abrogated by glutathione peroxidase and catalase (ferroprotein) [49]. Fragmentation of the equine sperm DNA is also abrogated by reduced glutathione and catalase [65]. The NRC recommended selenium intake for breeding and non-breeding stallions of 0.1 mg/kg DM [8]. While a maximum tolerable concentration of selenium of 5 mg/kg DM has been suggested, based upon interspecies extrapolation, a "more advisable upper limit" of 2 mg selenium/kg ration DM is appropriate [68].

19.3.2.5.2 Zinc

Zinc is essential for normal testicular development, serum testosterone, and spermatogenesis [43, 69]. While there appears to be a paucity of research detailing the specific effects of zinc on stallion reproduction, feeding the maintenance requirement of 40 mg/ration kg DM is prudent [8].

19.3.2.5.3 Ascorbic Acid

Vitamin C has been given to treat impaired fertility or to enhance the fertility of mares and stallions, and there have been anecdotal reports, without confirmatory data: (i) feeding 1 g of vitamin C/horse/d may help get hard-to-breed mares to conceive, and (ii) a stallion that had reduced semen motility was successfully treated by giving ascorbic acid. However, giving 10 g of ascorbic acid/horse/d orally for 70 d to five stallions who had less than 25% spermatozoal progressive motility did not increase motility, although it did increase their plasma ascorbic acid concentrations 40–140% and decreased spermatozoal tail abnormalities 20–58% [70]. There is insufficient evidence to suggest a dietary requirement of vitamin C for horses of any life stage. If feeding a vitamin C supplement is desired, or to ensure that the stallion's diet contains a sufficient amount of all vitamins for optimum health and reproductive ability, feeding excessive vitamin C is unlikely to be harmful.

19.3.2.5.4 Vitamin E

Vitamin E, like selenium, has essential functions as a cellular antioxidant. Vitamin E plays a critical role in preventing lipid peroxidation in cellular membranes. The cellular membranes of mammalian spermatozoa are rich in PUFAs and are particularly susceptible to oxidative damage. The major PUFA in mammalian sperm is DHA, which constitutes >60% of sperm cell membranes [43]. Oxidative damage to spermatozoa cellular membranes increases the membrane's permeability to both intra- and extra-cellular ions, impairing the membrane potentials that are critical to normal sperm motility, and thus hindering fertilization.

A vitamin E deficiency is known to impair reproduction in both males and females of many species of animals. The impairments include early embryonic death, abortion, retained placenta, and degenerative changes in the testes. However, these effects have never been reported in horses, and there is no substantial evidence to indicate that vitamin E supplementation helps resolve reproductive problems in horses. Numerous studies have failed to confirm any benefit of vitamin E supplementation on the reproductive performance or libido in stallions. While there is no clear evidence that vitamin E supplementation above maintenance (100 IU/100 kg BW) is necessary for reproduction, there is a recommended dietary intake of 160 IU/100 kg BW for breeding stallions which corresponds to the recommended dietary intake for horses undergoing light exercise [8].

19.4 Feeding Management

Stallions should be maintained with a BCS of 4–6/9 and preferably fed moderate to good quality forage as pasture or hay, and water and salt should be available to all stallions *ad libitum*. The suggested feeding recommendations apply only to stallions in moderate body condition.

Forage quality should be sufficiently palatable and digestible (<40% ADF; <53% NDF, RFV 86–124) such that the breeding stallion will meet requirements consuming 1.5–2.0% BW DMI (Tables 10.3 and 19.2) [8, 25]. The forage must have adequate concentrations of energy, protein, calcium, and phosphorus. Stallions fed fresh forages will likely require a trace mineral source, whereas feeding hays with comparable energy and protein content may require a trace mineral–vitamin supplementation fed at 0.1–0.3% BW to complete the ration. If dry forages with DE <1.8 Mcal/kg, or CP <7–8% DM are fed, a complementary feed or ration balancer providing calories and/or protein with minerals and vitamins will be needed. For breeding stallions, a concentrate with 3.5 Mcal/kg DM fed at 0.5% BW divided into two or three feedings daily may be needed to provide sufficient calories [26]. If activity level and energy expenditure are high while turned out to pasture, turn out in a smaller area, less time turned out, turn out separate from mares, or turn out with a gelding companion may help to reduce activity. See Sidebar 19.1.

Sidebar 19.1: Calculating Daily Feeding Recommendations for a Breeding Stallion

Animal Assessment

- 600 kg (BCS 4/9) 5-yr-old Hanoverian stallion average temperament covering 6–8 mares/wk.
- DMI for a breeding stallion is 1.5–2.0% BW (Table 19.2).
- Stallion's daily DE requirement: 4.36 Mcal/100 kg BW × 6 = 26.2 Mcal DE (Table 19.1).
- Forage recommendations for breeding stallions are RFVs of 86–124 and 2.2 Mcal DE/kg DM (Table 19.2). ADF <42% and NDF <60% is recommended for stallions (Table 10.3).

Ration Assessment

- The farm has several tons of mature MMG hay with 92% DM. The smell and texture of the hay are sufficiently palatable for the stallion to consume 2% BW, but of questionable nutritional quality based on plant maturity. The forage was analyzed and reported on a DM basis to be:

International Feed Number (IFN)	DE	CP	ADF	NDF
#	Mcal/kg	%	%	%
1-02-280	2.08	13.3	42.1	62.5

- Calculate forage DDM, DMI, and RFV values:
  - %DDM = 88.9 − (0.779 × %ADF) = 56%.
  - %DMI = 120/%NDF = 1.9% BW.
  - RFV = %DDM × %DMI × 0.775 = 82 fair-quality (Table 10.3).
  - Forage quality is marginally adequate compared with that recommended for stallions.
- Calculate daily forage intake required to meet the stallion's DE on DM and as fed (AF) basis:
  - Stallion requires 26.2 Mcal DE/2.08 Mcal DE/kg DM = 12.5 kg forage DM/0.92 = 13.7 kg forage AF.
  - Check DMI: 12.5 kg hay DM intake/600 kg BW = 2.1% BW.

- If the horse consumed 12.5 kg hay DM daily, compare crude protein (CP) intake with daily recommendations (Table 19.1):
  - Consumption is 1663 g CP [12.5 kg forage DM × 13.3%].
  - 948 g CP is recommended [158 g × 6].
  - The stallion's protein need will be met eating 13–14 kg AF of this forage per day, however, lysine intake should be checked.

Feeding Management Recommendations

The nutrient composition of the hay, based on laboratory tests, is of fair-quality and marginally low in DE (2.08 Mcal vs. horse recommendation of 2.2 Mcal DE/kg DM), but adequate in protein for the stallion. DE requirement could be met if the stallion consumed 12.5 kg forage DM (2.1% BW) which is plausible. The low quality and marginal caloric density may result in loss of weight and condition if the stallion's actual DE requirement is higher than calculated, and/or if DMI does not increase >2% BW of which is unknown at this point. Specific recommendations:

- Monitor daily feed intake and assess BW and BCS every 2 wks during breeding season.
- If BW should decrease >5%, consider:
  - Feeding higher quality forage: RFV >100 with ≥2.2 Mcal DE/kg DM.
  - Adding an energy concentrate (3.5 Mcal DE/kg DM) to the ration fed at 0.5% BW, initially, and re-assess.
  - Take measures to reduce breeding activity level.
- Feed mineral–vitamin ration balancing supplement to ensure adequate micronutrient intakes per manufacturer's feeding recommendations usually at 0.1–0.3% BW.
- Offer water and salt block *ad libitum*.

During the breeding season, the appetite may be reduced in some stallions, and/or activity level may increase, both resulting in weight loss. If BW and BCS decrease during the breeding season due to an observed decrease in feed intake, offering highly palatable feeds, an energy concentrate mix, or allowing access to green pasture grasses may be needed. Turning the stallion out on green grass pasture for a few hours daily may improve appetite; however, the nutritional content of pastures routinely changes over weeks to months, and, therefore, pasture grass quality and energy intake must be monitored. See Chapter 11 Forages. If BW and BCS decrease despite adequate or increased feed intake (approximately 2% BW) with an observed increased activity level, the energy density of the ration must be increased (>2.2 Mcal DE/kg DM) (Table 19.2), and/or energy expenditure must be decreased.

Feeding intake, BCS, and BW must be monitored throughout the breeding season to maintain stallions in ideal BW and condition. If a stallion is known historically to lose weight during the breeding season, then it may be necessary to have that animal at or above BCS 6/9 at the start of the season [26]. Conversely, the amount and/or energy density of the complementing feed should be reduced if BCS increases above 6/9.

Case in Point

A 20-year-old Arabian stallion presented to the veterinary teaching hospital for poor libido and reluctance to mount during the prior breeding season. The stallion had previously been used competitively in endurance rides, but was currently turned out for exercise 1 h daily, and housed in a stall the remainder of the time.

Animal Assessment

On examination, the stallion weighed 523 kg and had evidence of reduced muscle mass in both hind limbs. Palpation of the stallion's thoracic vertebrae elicited pain. The horse was reluctant to make sharp turns and showed evidence of back pain during lunging. Radiographs revealed overriding dorsal spinous processes ("kissing spines"). The attending clinician recommended a combination of shockwave therapy, light exercise, and referred the patient to the nutrition service for weight-loss feeding recommendations. The stallion was overweight (BCS 7/9). Controlled weight loss was recommended to minimize mechanical load on the painful thoracic vertebrae, reduce the subclinical inflammatory state associated with increased body fat, and provide a better quality of life as the animal aged. Ideal BW was estimated between 455 and 477 kg corresponding to BCS 4/9–5/9. The plan was to reassess the horse's pain level and mobility at a lower BW and BCS, and continue weight loss if needed.

Ration Assessment

Based on dietary history, the nutrition service calculated the stallion was consuming approximately 21.4 Mcal DE/d.

1) *What is the recommended DE for a non-breeding stallion weighing 455 kg?* (Table 19.1).
2) *What dietary and management recommendations should be made for this stallion?*
3) The stallion achieved a BW of 466 kg (BCS 5/9) in 6 mos. *What was the %BW loss/wk?*

See Appendix A Chapter 19.

References

1 American Association of Equine Practitioners (2021). Castration: from stallion to gelding. https://aaep.org/horsehealth/castration-stallion-gelding (accessed 22 June 2021).

2 American Association of Equine Practitioners (2009). Genetic defects. https://aaep.org/guidelines/aaep-ethical-and-professional-guidelines/aaep-position-statements/aaep-statement-genetic-defects-2009 (accessed 22 June 2021).

3 Campbell, M.L.H. and Sandøe, P. (2015). Welfare in horse breeding. *Vet. Rec.* 176 (17): 436–440.

4 Turner, R.M. and McDonnell, S.M. (2007). Mounting expectations for Thoroughbred stallions. *J. Am. Vet. Med. Assoc.* 230 (10): 1458–1460.

5 Umphenour, N.W., McCarthy, P., and Blanchard, T.C. (2011). Management of stallions in natural service programs. In: *Equine Reproduction* (ed. A.O. McKinnon, E.L. Squires, W.E. Vaala, and D.D. Varner), 1208–1227. Oxford: Wiley.

6 Rosenberg, J.L., Cavinder, C.A., Love, C.C. et al. (2013). Effects of strenuous exercise on stallion sperm quality. *Prof. Anim. Sci.* 29 (5): 482–489.

7 Thorén Hellsten, E., Viklund, Å., Koenen, E.P.C. et al. (2006). Review of genetic parameters estimated at stallion and young horse performance tests and their correlations with later results in dressage and show-jumping competition. *Livest. Sci.* 103 (1, 2): 1–12.

8 National Research Council (2007). *Nutrient Requirements of Horses*. 6th Rev. Animal Nutrition Series, 1–341. Washington, DC: National Academies Press.

9 Henneke, D.R., Potter, G.D., Kreider, J.L., and Yeates, B.F. (1983). Relationship between condition score, physical measurements and body fat percentage in mares. *Equine Vet. J.* 15 (4): 371–372.

10 Mottet, R., Onan, G., and Hiney, K. (2009). Revisiting the Henneke body condition scoring system: 25 years later. *J. Equine Vet. Sci.* 29 (5): 417–418.

11 Amann, R.P. (2006). The fertility dilemma: perception vs. actuality. *Equine Vet. Educ.* 18 (3): 159–164.

12 Blanchard, T., Thompson, J., Brinsko, S. et al. (2010). Sources of variation in fertility of Thoroughbred stallions. *Anim. Reprod. Sci.* 121 (1, 2): 128–129.

13 Blanchard, T.L., Thompson, J.A., Brinsko, S.P. et al. (2010). Some factors associated with fertility of Thoroughbred stallions. *J. Equine Vet. Sci.* 30 (8): 407–418.

14 Blanchard, T.L., Varner, D.D., Love, C.C. et al. (2012). Management options for the aged breeding stallion with declining testicular function. *J. Equine Vet. Sci.* 32 (8): 430–435.

15 McDonnell, S.M. (2005). Techniques for extending the breeding career of aging and disabled stallions. *Clin. Tech. Equine Pract.* 4 (3): 269–276.

16 Johnson, L., Varner, D.D., and Thompson, J.D.L. (1991). Effect of age and season on the establishment of spermatogenesis in the horse. *J. Reprod. Fertil. Suppl.* 44 (Jan): 87.

17 Davies-Morel, M.C.G. (2008). Stallion management. In: *Equine Reproductive Physiology, Breeding and Stud Management*, 3e, 225–236. Cambridge, MA; Wallingford: CABI.

18 Sigler, D.H. and Kiracofe, G.H. (1988). Seminal characteristics of two- and three-year-old quarter horse stallions. *J. Equine Vet. Sci.* 8 (2): 160–164.

19 McDowell, K.J., Powell, D.G., and Baker, C.B. (1992). Effect of book size and age of mare and stallion on foaling rates in Thoroughbred horses. *J. Equine Vet. Sci.* 12 (6): 364–367.

20 Kenney, R.M., Hurtgen, J.P., and Pierson, R.H. (1983). Clinical fertility evaluation of the stallion. *J. Soc. Theriogenology* 9: 7–62.

21 Turner, R.M. (2005). Current techniques for evaluation of stallion fertility. *Clin. Tech. Equine Pract.* 4 (3): 257–268.

22 Martin, B.B. and McDonnell, S.M. (2003). Lameness in breeding stallions and broodmares. In: *Equine Lameness* (ed. M. Ross), 1077–1084. Philadelphia, PA: Saunders.

23 Pickett, B.W., Voss, J.L., Bowen, R.A. et al. (1988). Seminal characteristics and total scrotal width (TSW) of normal and abnormal stallions. In: *Proceedings of the 34th Annual Convention of the American Association of Equine Practitioners*, 487–518. San Diego, CA: American Association of Equine Practitioners (AAEP).

24 van den Berg, M., Giagos, V., Lee, C. et al. (2016). The influence of odour, taste and nutrients on feeding behaviour and food preferences in horses. *Appl. Anim. Behav. Sci.* 184 (Nov): 41–50.

25 Swinker, A.M. (2014). Hay quality for different classes of horses. Pennsylvania State Extension Service. https://extension.psu.edu/hay-quality-for-different-classes-of-horses (accessed 2 July 2021).

26 Lawrence, L.M. (2013). Feeding stallions and broodmares. In: *Equine Applied and Clinical Nutrition: Health, Welfare and Performance* (ed. R.J. Geor, P.A. Harris, and M. Coenen), 231–242. Edinburgh: Saunders Elsevier.

27 Johnson, P.J., Wiedmeyer, C.E., Messer, N.T., and Ganjam, V.K. (2009). Medical implications of obesity in horses – lessons for human obesity. *J. Diabetes Sci. Technol.* 3 (1): 163–174.

28 Frank, N., Geor, R.J., Bailey, S.R. et al. (2010). Equine metabolic syndrome. *J. Vet. Intern. Med.* 24 (3): 467–475.

29 Garcia-Seco, E., Wilson, D.A., Kramer, J. et al. (2005). Prevalence and risk factors associated with outcome of surgical removal of pedunculated lipomas in horses: 102 cases (1987-2002). *J. Am. Vet. Med. Assoc.* 226 (9): 1529–1537.

30 Harris, P. (2009). Feeding management of elite endurance horses. *Vet. Clin. North Am. Equine Pract.* 25 (1): 137–153.

31 Geor, R.J. and Harris, P.A. (2013). Obesity. In: *Equine Applied and Clinical Nutrition: Health, Welfare and Performance* (ed. R.J. Geor, P.A. Harris, and M. Coenen), 487–502. Edinburgh: Saunders Elsevier.

32 Schlueter, A.E. and Orth, M.W. (2004). Equine osteoarthritis: a brief review of the disease and its causes. *Equine Comp. Exerc. Physiol.* 1 (4): 221–231.

33 Brown, B.W. (1994). A review of nutritional influences on reproduction in boars, bulls and rams. *Reprod. Nutr. Dev.* 34 (2): 89–114.

34 Mantovani, R. and Bailoni, L. (2011). Energy and protein allowances and requirements in stallions during the breeding season, comparing different nutritional systems. *J. Anim. Sci.* 89 (7): 2113–2122.

35 Siciliano, P., Wood, C., Lawrence, L., and Duren, S. (1993). Utilization of a field study to evaluate the digestible energy requirements of breeding stallions. In: *Proceedings of the 13th Equine Nutrition and Physiology Society Symposium*, 293–298. Gainesville, FL: Equine Nutrition and Physiology Society.

36 Institut National de la Recherche Agronomique (2015). *Equine Nutrition: INRA Nutrition Requirements, Recommended Allowances and Feed Tables*, 1e (ed. W. Martin-Rosset), 691. Wageningen: Wageningen Academic Publishers.

37 Martin-Rosset, W., Vermorel, M., Doreau, M. et al. (1994). The French horse feed evaluation systems and recommended allowances for energy and protein. *Livest. Prod. Sci.* 40 (1): 37–56.

38 Freeman, D.W. (2001). An overview of stallion breeding management. ANSI -3922, Stillwater, OK. https://shareok.org/bitstream/handle/11244/49914/oksd_ansi_3922_2001-09.pdf?sequence=1 (accessed 22 June 2021).

39 Glasser, F., Doreau, M., Maxin, G., and Baumont, R. (2013). Fat and fatty acid content and composition of forages: a meta-analysis. *Anim. Feed Sci. Technol.* 185 (1, 2): 19–34.

40 Warren, L.K. and Vineyard, K.R. (2013). Fat and fatty acids. In: *Equine Applied and Clinical Nutrition: Health, Welfare and Performance* (ed. R.J. Geor, P.A. Harris, and M. Coenen), 136–155. Edinburgh: Saunders Elsevier.

41 Macías García, B., González Fernández, L., Ortega Ferrusola, C. et al. (2011). Membrane lipids of the stallion spermatozoon in relation to sperm quality and susceptibility to lipid peroxidation. *Reprod. Domest. Anim.* 46 (1): 141–148.

42 Freitas, M.L., Bouéres, C.S., Pignataro, T.A. et al. (2016). Quality of fresh, cooled, and frozen semen from stallions supplemented with antioxidants and fatty acids. *J. Equine Vet. Sci.* 46 (Nov): 1–6.

43 Cheah, Y. and Yang, W. (2011). Functions of essential nutrition for high quality spermatogenesis. *Adv. Biosci. Biotechnol.* 2 (4): 182.

44 de Arruda, R.P., da Silva, D.F., Alonso, M.A. et al. (2010). Nutraceuticals in reproduction of bulls and stallions. *Rev. Bras. Zootec.* 39 (Suppl): 393–400.

45 King, S.S., AbuGhazaleh, A.A., Webel, S.K., and Jones, K.L. (2008). Circulating fatty acid profiles in response to three levels of dietary omega-3 fatty acid supplementation in horses1. *J. Anim. Sci.* 86 (5): 1114–1123.

46 O'Connor, C.I., Lawrence, L.M., and Hayes, S.H. (2007). Dietary fish oil supplementation affects serum fatty acid concentrations in horses. *J. Anim. Sci.* 85 (9): 2183–2189.

47 Fajt, V.R. and McCook, C. (2008). An evidence-based analysis of anabolic steroids as therapeutic agents in horses. *Equine Vet. Educ.* 20 (10): 542–544.

48 Soma, L.R., Uboh, C.E., Guan, F. et al. (2007). Pharmacokinetics of boldenone and stanozolol and the results of quantification of anabolic and androgenic steroids in race horses and nonrace horses. *J. Vet. Pharmacol. Ther.* 30 (2): 101–108.

49 Baumber, J., Ball, B.A., Gravance, C.G. et al. (2000). The effect of reactive oxygen species on equine sperm motility, viability, acrosomal integrity, mitochondrial membrane potential, and membrane lipid peroxidation. *J. Androl.* 21 (6): 895–902.

50 Deichsel, K., Palm, F., Koblischke, P. et al. (2008). Effect of a dietary antioxidant supplementation on semen quality in pony stallions. *Theriogenology* 69 (8): 940–945.

51 Contri, A., De Amicis, I., Molinari, A. et al. (2011). Effect of dietary antioxidant supplementation on fresh semen quality in stallion. *Theriogenology* 75 (7): 1319–1326.

52 Streeter, R.M., Divers, T.J., Mittel, L. et al. (2012). Selenium deficiency associations with gender, breed, serum vitamin E and creatine kinase, clinical signs and diagnoses in horses of different age groups: a retrospective examination 1996-2011. *Equine Vet. J.* 44 (Dec): 31–35.

53 Ludvikova, E., Jahn, P., Pavlata, L., and Vyskocil, M. (2005). Selenium and vitamin E status correlated with myopathies of horses reared in farms in the Czech Republic. *Acta Vet. Brno.* 74 (3): 377–384.

54 Secombe, C.J. and Lester, G.D. (2012). The role of diet in the prevention and management of several equine diseases. *Anim. Feed Sci. Technol.* 173 (1, 2): 86–101.

55 Brummer, M., Hayes, S., Dawson, K.A., and Lawrence, L.M. (2013). Measures of antioxidant status of the horse in response to selenium depletion and repletion. *J. Anim. Sci.* 91 (5): 2158–2168.

56 Calamari, L., Capelli, P., Ferrari, A., and Bertin, G. (2007). Glutathione peroxidase responses in mature horses following the withdrawal of an organic selenium supplement. *Ital. J. Anim. Sci.* 6 (Suppl 1): 275–277.

57 Montgomery, J.B., Wichtel, J.J., Wichtel, M.G. et al. (2012). The effects of selenium source on measures of selenium status of mares and selenium status and immune function of their foals. *J. Equine Vet. Sci.* 32 (6): 352–359.

58 Richardson, S.M., Siciliano, P.D., Engle, T.E. et al. (2006). Effect of selenium supplementation and source on the selenium status of horses. *J. Anim. Sci.* 84 (7): 1742–1748.

59 Calamari, L., Ferrari, A., and Bertin, G. (2009). Effect of selenium source and dose on selenium status of mature horses. *J. Anim. Sci.* 87 (1): 167–178.

60 Ullrey, D.E. (1987). Biochemical and physiological indicators of selenium status in animals. *J. Anim. Sci.* 65 (6): 1712.

61 Schomburg, L. and Schweizer, U. (2009). Hierarchical regulation of selenoprotein expression and sex-specific effects of selenium. *Biochim. Biophys. Acta* 1790 (11): 1453–1462.

62 Schomburg, L. (2016). Sex-specific differences in biological effects and metabolism of selenium. In: *Selenium: Its Molecular Biology and Role in Human Health* (ed. D.L. Hatfield, U. Schweizer, P.A. Tsuji, and V.N. Gladyshev), 377–388. Cham: Springer International Publishing.

63 Sunde, R.A. and Raines, A.M. (2011). Selenium regulation of the selenoprotein and nonselenoprotein transcriptomes in rodents. *Adv. Nutr.* 2 (2): 138–150.

64 Foresta, C., Flohé, L., Garolla, A. et al. (2002). Male fertility is linked to the selenoprotein phospholipid hydroperoxide glutathione peroxidase. *Biol. Reprod.* 67 (3): 967–971.

65 Baumber, J., Ball, B.A., Linfor, J.J., and Meyers, S.A. (2003). Reactive oxygen species and cryopreservation promote DNA fragmentation in equine spermatozoa. *J. Androl.* 24 (4): 621–628.

66 Beckett, G.J. and Arthur, J.R. (2005). Selenium and endocrine systems. *J. Endocrinol.* 184 (3): 455–465.

67 Surai, P.F. and Fisinin, V.I. (2016). Selenium in livestock and other domestic animals. In: *Selenium: Its Molecular Biology and Role in Human Health* (ed. D.L. Hatfield, U. Schweizer, P.A. Tsuji, and V.N. Gladyshev), 595–606. Cham: Springer International Publishing.

68 National Research Council (2005). *Mineral Tolerance of Animals*. 2nd Rev., 1–496. Washington, DC: National Academies Press.

69 Omu, A.E., Al-Azemi, M.K., Al-Maghrebi, M. et al. (2015). Molecular basis for the effects of zinc deficiency on spermatogenesis: an experimental study in the Sprague-Dawley rat model. *Indian J. Urol.* 31 (1): 57–64.

70 Ralston, S.L., Barbacini, S., Squires, E.L., and Nockels, C.F. (1988). Ascorbic acid supplementation in stallions. *J. Equine Vet. Sci.* 8 (4): 290–293.

20

Feeding Broodmares

Stewart K. Morgan and Megan Shepherd

KEY TERMS

- Colostrogenesis is the prepartum transfer of immunoglobulins from the maternal circulation into mammary secretions.
- Open mares are not pregnant, whereas gravid mares are pregnant.
- Feed digestibility is the percent of a feed nutrient (energy, protein, mineral) digested and absorbed by the animal depending on the form of the feed, ingredients and nutrient interactions.
- Feed efficiency conversion is the quantity of feed dry matter, calories or protein consumed per unit of weight gained during growth or milk produced.

KEY POINTS

- Mares are seasonally polyestrous breeders when daylight hours are increasing, regardless of hemisphere, which coincides with forage availability.
- Broodmares are optimally maintained between body condition score (BCS) 4 and 6/9 throughout the reproductive cycle.
- Early gestational nutrient requirements are the same as maintenance mares.
- Nutritional requirements increase about 20% by late gestation but increase by 90% in early lactation over maintenance mares.
- Reproductive efficiency is directly related to BCS in broodmares.

20.1 Introduction

The nutritional goals for the mare are to maximize fertility, fetal development, and milk production, and prevent disease, reduced fertility, and poor fetal development. Mare reproductive capacity is affected by breed, age, season, nutrition, and body condition [1–8]. Mares are classified as maiden (never bred), barren (never pregnant), open (not pregnant), pregnant or in foal, or lactating. Maiden, barren, and open mares are fed as adult non-pregnant, non-lactating maintenance horses [9]. When feeding the broodmare, three physiological states are considered: maintenance, gestation, and lactation. Nutrient requirements of the late gestating and lactating broodmare are greater than those for maintenance plus requirements involved in placental, uterine, and fetal growth, mammary development, colostrogenesis, and lactation.

The broodmare plays a substantial role in determining foal birth weight, rate of growth, and metabolism [10–12]. Experiments in which pony embryos are transferred into a draft horse or Thoroughbred mares ("small into large") resulted in increased birthweights, rates of growth, and changes in markers of energy homeostasis, adrenocortical function, and cardiovascular function in foals relative to control pregnant ponies with pony embryos [11]. Opposite effects are noted in embryo transfer experiments in which Thoroughbred or Saddlebred embryos are transferred into pony mares ("large into small"). Many of the changes noted in these embryo transfer experiments impact the foal until adulthood. While the exact cause(s) of these changes is not entirely understood, the conclusion is that mares play a role in determining foal rate of growth, metabolism, and hormonal activity. Proper nutritional management of mares involves routine physical evaluations at key points

Equine Clinical Nutrition, Second Edition. Edited by Rebecca L. Remillard.

throughout the year such as pre-breeding, late gestation, peak lactation, and weaning to ensure the mare is healthy and maintaining adequate body weight (BW) and body condition score (BCS). When nutritional or diet-related problems arise, a systematic iterative review of the mare, the ration, and the feeding method is recommended. See Appendix C Nutrition Competencies of Equine Veterinarians.

20.2 Animal Assessment

Given the mature BW for horses range from 200 to 900 kg, the recommended daily nutrient intakes for gestating (Table 20.1) and lactating (Table 20.2) mares are presented per 100 kg of mature mare BW [9]. Feeding the broodmare should be seen as feeding on a continuum through three distinct life stages, that is, maintenance, gestation, and then lactation. The gestational period in horses is on average 340 d, but varies from 310 to 370, and is influenced by the month of foaling, for example, longer for foals born in the spring vs. summer [6, 13, 14]. Historically, the gestational period has been divided into early (≤8 mos) and late (months 9 to 11) [9]. Presently, the nutritional requirements for gestation have been divided into early (months 0 to 4), mid (months 5 to 8), and late (months 9 to 11) [9]. Expected weight gain during gestation is 12–16% of initial BW due to an increase in reproductive (fetal, uterine, and placental) tissues. The onset of lactation signals pending parturition producing colostrum for the first 12–24 hrs. The lactation cycle is divided into early (month 1 & 2) and late (months 3 to 6). Milk produced peaks in about 60 days post parturition and then declines until weaning. Weaning generally occurs at 10 m of age in feral or free-roaming horses, but at 4–6 m of age in the horse industry [15–19].

Table 20.1 Recommended daily nutrient intakes for gestating mares per 100 kg of mature body weight.[a]

Nutrient		**Gestation (month)**							
	Units	**<5**	**5**	**6**	**7**	**8**	**9**	**10**	**11**
Digestible energy	Mcal	3.34[b]	3.42	3.48	3.58	3.7	3.84	4.04	4.28
Crude protein	g	126	137	141	146	152	159	168	179
Lysine	g	5.4	5.9	6.1	6.3	6.5	6.9	7.2	7.7
Calcium	g	4.0	4.0	4.0	5.6	5.6	7.2	7.2	7.2
Phosphorus	g	2.8	2.8	2.8	4.0	4.0	5.3	5.3	5.3
Magnesium	g	1.5	1.5	1.5	1.5	1.5	1.5	1.5	1.5
Potassium	g	5.0	5.0	5.0	5.0	5.0	5.2	5.2	5.2
Sodium	g	2.0	2.0	2.0	2.0	2.0	2.2	2.2	2.2
Chloride	g	8.0	8.0	8.0	8.0	8.0	8.2	8.2	8.2
Sulfur	g	3.0	3.0	3.0	3.0	3.0	3.0	3.0	3.0
Copper	mg	20	20	20	20	20	25	25	25
Iron	mg	80	80	80	80	80	100	100	100
Manganese	mg	80	80	80	80	80	80	80	80
Zinc	mg	80	80	80	80	80	80	80	80
Cobalt	mg	0.1	0.1	0.1	0.1	0.1	0.1	0.1	0.1
Iodine	mg	0.7	0.7	0.7	0.9	0.9	0.8	0.8	0.8
Selenium	mg	0.2	0.2	0.2	0.2	0.2	0.2	0.2	0.2
Vitamin A	KIU	6	6	6	6	6	6	6	6
Vitamin D	IU	660	660	660	660	660	660	660	660
Vitamin E	IU	160	160	160	160	160	160	160	160
Thiamin	mg	6	6	6	6	6	6	6	6
Riboflavin	mg	4	4	4	4	4	4	4	4

[a] Calculated based on pre-pregnancy weight.
[b] For example, a 435 kg average tempered mare less than 5 mos pregnant would require 3.34×4.35 = 14.53 Mcal DE/d.
Source: Adapted from NRC [9]; Table 16-3 using nutrients required for a 500 kg mature horse with BCS 4–6/9 consuming 2% BW.

Table 20.2 Recommended daily nutrient intakes for lactating mares per 100 kg of mature body weight.

Nutrient		Lactation (month)					
	Units	1	2	3	4	5	6
Digestible energy	Mcal	6.34[a]	6.34	6.12	5.88	5.66	5.44
Crude protein	g	307	306	293.6	279.6	266	253
Lysine	g	17.0	16.9	16.1	15.1	14.2	13.4
Calcium	g	11.8	11.8	11.2	8.3	7.9	7.5
Phosphorus	g	7.7	7.6	7.2	5.2	4.9	4.6
Magnesium	g	2.2	2.2	2.2	2.1	2.0	1.7
Potassium	g	9.6	9.5	9.2	7.2	7.0	6.7
Sodium	g	2.6	2.6	2.5	2.4	2.3	2.3
Chloride	g	9.1	9.1	9.1	9.1	9.1	9.1
Sulfur	g	3.8	3.8	3.8	3.8	3.8	3.8
Copper	mg	25	25	25	25	25	25
Iron	mg	125	125	125	125	125	125
Manganese	mg	100	100	100	100	100	100
Zinc	mg	100	100	100	100	100	100
Cobalt	mg	0.12	0.12	0.12	0.12	0.12	0.12
Iodine	mg	0.88	0.88	0.88	0.88	0.88	0.88
Selenium	mg	0.25	0.25	0.25	0.25	0.25	0.25
Vitamin A	KIU	6	6	6	6	6	6
Vitamin D	IU	660	660	660	660	660	660
Vitamin E	IU	200	200	200	200	200	200
Thiamin	mg	7.5	7.5	7.5	7.5	7.5	7.5
Riboflavin	mg	5	5	5	5	5	5

[a] For example, a 435 kg average tempered mare in the first month of lactation would require 6.34×4.35 = 27.6 Mcal DE/d.
Source: Adapted from NRC [9]; Table 16-3 using nutrients required for a 500 kg mature horse with BCS 4–6/9 consuming 2.5% BW.

The digestible energy (DE) required (Mcal/100 kg BW) increases steadily (130%) through gestation to foaling. There is a 150% increase at the start of lactation that then steadily declines to weaning (Figure 20.1). Similarly, crude protein (CP) (g/100 kg BW) increases steadily (140%) through gestation with a 170% increase at the start of lactation. The calcium (Ca) and phosphorus (P) needs also increase proportionately (180%) through gestation due to increases in fetal and reproductive tissues. At parturition, however, the calcium requirement increases (165%) disproportionately to the phosphorus increases (145%) likely related to the composition of milk (0.12% Ca and 0.075% P) in the first month of lactation [9]. Milk production (kg/d) changes between parturition and weaning, peaking in month 2, and is affected by breed, age, and nutrition of the mare. For practical purposes, milk yield can be estimated for light breeds at 3% BW wks 1–12 and 2% BW wks 13–24, or 4% and 3% BW for ponies, respectively [20].

20.2.1 Body Condition Score

The BCS of reproducing mares should be 5/9 (moderate) to 6/9 (moderately fleshy) [4, 21]. The mare's BCS is indicative of a prior energy intake and has a significant impact on reproductive performance [4, 6–8, 22]. The BW will change as the mare cycles through an early gestation (equal to maintenance), late gestation, and then lactation. However, BW measurements do not differentiate between mare and reproductive tissues. BCS estimates subcutaneous body fat,

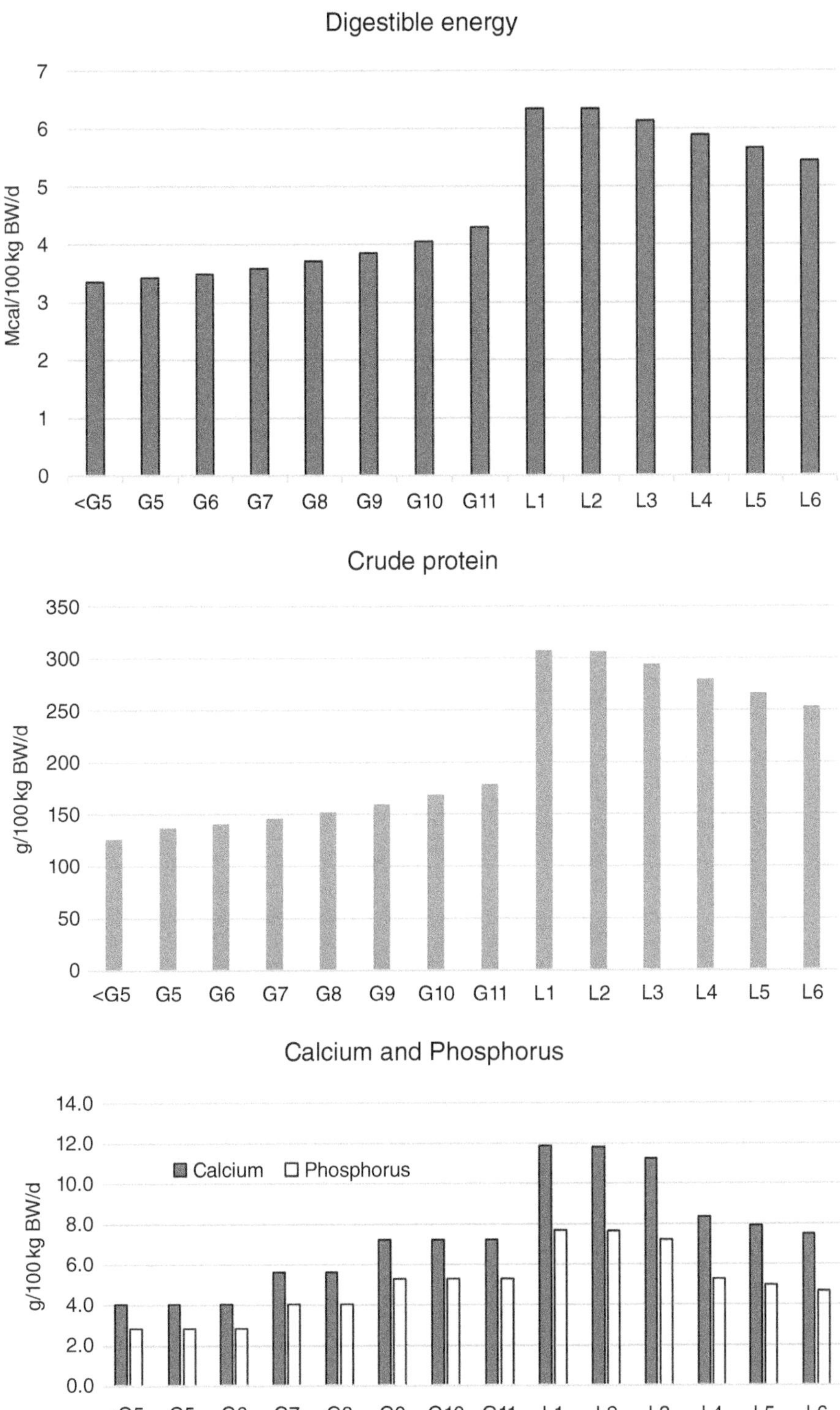

Figure 20.1 Digestible energy, protein, calcium, and phosphorus requirements per 100 kg BW increase steadily above maintenance (<G5) through the second half of gestation (G5 to G11), increase markedly with the onset of lactation (L1), and then decline each month to weaning (L2 to L6). *Source:* Adapted from NRC [9].

and taken together with BW, provides an assessment of energy balance.

In general, when horse owners error, they typically overfeed relative to actual energy need during gestation and underfeed during lactation. Mares are likely to be overfed, gain weight and BCS before breeding and during early gestation but then lose BW and BCS during lactation due to underfeeding. Therefore, regular physical assessments of the mare, including BW and BCS, throughout the reproductive cycle, are recommended. Body condition scoring must include palpation. For example, late pregnant mares with a winter coat require deliberate palpation of ribs, tail head, spine, etc., as a simple visual assessment will be inaccurate. The assessment frequency is case-dependent. For example, a 2nd mo gestating 8-yr-old mare with a history of maintaining an ideal BW and BCS may need only be assessed every month before parturition, whereas a 2nd mo first time lactating 4-yr-old mare may need to be assessed weekly. See Chapter 2 Nutritional Assessment of the Horse.

Energy deficiency, and subsequent weight loss, can negatively impact reproductive performance in the mare as in other species, and the broodmare's BCS and changes influence both broodmare fertility and the suckling foal's growth rate [4, 6, 23–27]. Having a BCS of <5/9 may negatively affect the brain–hypothalamic–pituitary axis and has been associated with a prolonged anovulatory period, more cycles to conceive, and lower conception rates in mares [2, 9]. Mares at a BCS ≤4/9 have a longer interval to first seasonal ovulation, to first postpartum ovulation, and between first and second postpartum ovulations than mares at a BCS ≥5/9 [4, 8, 28]. Furthermore, mares fed to maintain a BCS of <4/9 (both before and after parturition) had significantly reduced pregnancy rates over three estrus cycles [4]. Mares that are below an ideal BCS or that have evidence of muscle wasting should not be bred until the condition has been corrected.

Historically, feeding broodmares to maintain a BCS≥6/9 from conception through lactation was recommended. While the negative effects of low BCS on mare reproduction have been described, the role of excessive BW on broodmare reproductive performance is less clear [4, 20, 28–30]. Increasing body condition at conception has favorable results on mare fertility, and mares overweight during gestation appear to lose less body fat through lactation [6, 23]. Overweight mares (BCS 6/9–7/9) appear to ovulate similarly to mares of ideal BCS; however, overconditioned (BCS>7/9) is associated with reduced reproductive performance and non-seasonal cycling in the mare [2, 4, 6, 28, 29, 31, 32]. Additionally, obesity is a risk factor for metabolic alterations in the horse. These alterations have a direct impact on mares' ovaries and oocytes, although the effects of these impacts are still not characterized. Obesity should be avoided nevertheless as fat mass is associated with equine metabolic syndrome (increased adiposity, insulin resistance, laminitis, etc.), hypertriglyceridemia, and increased markers of inflammation [31, 33, 34]. Excessive BW appears to neither increase the risk for dystocia in the mare nor negatively impact foaling rates [35].

While obesity should be avoided in broodmares at all times due to the overall negative impacts on health, intentional weight loss to correct BW is less than ideal in the gestating or lactating mare, or at the time of active breeding, because metabolic processes of losing weight negatively affect fertility. The negative effect of weight loss upon fertility may be due to the effects of adipose-tissue-derived fatty acids on hormones [6]. Negative energy balance during lactation can reduce rebreeding conception rates and induce endogenous tissue catabolism to support milk production [4, 36]. Therefore, controlled feeding for weight loss should occur months before breeding.

20.3 Ration Assessment

Ration energy concentrations of 1.5–2.0 Mcal DE/kg dry matter (DM) are suitable for maiden, barren, and open mares and those in the first 8 mos of gestation, 2.0 Mcal DE/kg DM is recommended for gestating mares between 9 and 10 mos, and 2.2 Mcal DE/kg DM is suggested for month 11 of gestation (Table 20.3). Ration energy density recommended for mares in the first 3 mos of lactation is 2.5 Mcal DE/kg DM, but lower (2.3 DE/kg DM) for the last 3 mos [9]. Mares should be provided a complete and balanced ration, meeting the energy and nutrient requirements, fed within the limits of their dry matter intake (DMI) as a % BW (Table 20.3).

20.3.1 Feeds

20.3.1.1 Forage

Forage should be the foundation of the ration, as many legumes and grasses, as pasture or hay, can provide the mare's major nutrient needs. Additionally, feeding forage is an important factor for foal health. Maintaining normal blood glucose concentrations and insulin sensitivity in the mare is thought to be beneficial for foal health and growth [10, 12, 38, 39]. Consumption of forage reduces fluctuations in blood glucose and insulin relative to meal feeding an energy concentrate.

Assessment of forage quality is important in feeding broodmares properly and utilizes both objective nutrient analyses and subjective assessments (smell, color, feel, and physical contents). See Ration Analysis and Subjective Assessments in Chapter 10. The forage offered must be palatable in odor and texture, to the horse to ensure an adequate DMI [40]. The forage digestible dry matter (DDM) and energy density (Mcal/kg DM) must be sufficient to

Table 20.3 Comparison of major nutrient concentrations between forage averages and ration recommendations for broodmares. [37].

Horse to Forage Comparison	Digestible energy	Protein	Calcium	Phosphorus	DMI	RFV
	Dry matter basis				% BW	
Reproductive Stage:	Mcal/kg	%	%	%		
Gestation <9 mos	1.5–2.0	6–8	0.20	0.15	1.5–2.0	85–115
9 mos	2.00	8.0	0.36	0.26		>120
10 mos	2.02	8.4	0.36	0.26		
11 mos	2.14	8.9	0.36	0.26		
Lactation						
1–3 mos	2.51	12.1	0.46	0.32	2.0–3.0	>120
4–6 mos	2.26	10.6	0.30	0.20	2.0–2.5	>100
Forages:						
Legume						
Pasture: vegetative	2.71	26.5	1.31	0.37	3.6[a]	197[b]
Hay: immature	2.62	20.5	1.56	0.31	3.3	171
Hay: mid-mature	2.43	20.8	1.37	0.30	2.8	136
Hay: mature	2.21	17.8	1.22	0.28	2.4	106
Grass						
Pasture: vegetative	2.39	26.5	0.56	0.44	2.6	141
Hay: immature	2.36	18.0	0.72	0.34	2.4	121
Hay: mid-mature	2.18	13.3	0.66	0.29	2.1	97
Hay: mature	2.04	10.8	0.47	0.26	1.7	76

[a] Forage %DMI = 120/%NDF.
[b] Forage relative feeding value = %DDM × %DMI × 0.775; where %DDM = 88.9 − (0.779×%ADF).
Source: Adapted from NRC [9]; Table 16-3 using nutrients required for a 500-kg mature horse BCS 4–6/9. Forage data from Table 16-6.

meet the estimated daily energy requirement (DER) within an edible volume of feed (DMI). DM digestibility and voluntary DMI are inversely related to the forage acid detergent fiber (%ADF) and neutral detergent fiber (%NDF), respectively. Forages should have relative feeding values (RFV) of 85–115 for early-mid gestation and >120 for late gestation through peak lactation (Table 20.3) [37]. See Relative Feed Value in Chapter 10. A concentrate will be required if a better quality forage is not available. As nutritional requirements increase through gestation to peak lactation, ensuring a digestible forage is foremost to meeting those nutritional demands.

In cases where the available forage energy density is insufficient to meet the mare's nutrient requirement within the voluntary DMI, common in late gestation and lactation periods, a concentrate or complementary feed should be fed to provide the difference between the animal's requirement and that provided by forage alone [36]. Throughout most of the reproductive cycle, most forage types can meet the mare's protein requirement (8–13% DM); however, when mature hays or poor-quality pastures do not meet the mare's requirement, higher-protein forage legumes (alfalfa, clover, lespedeza) can be incorporated into the ration (Table 20.3). Trace minerals commonly insufficient in forages must be supplied using a low-sodium trace mineral supplement or ration balancer pellet. Ideally, the forage quality and nutrient profile are determined first, and then concentrates and supplements are added to complement the nutrient profile of the forage to meet the mare's energy, protein, and micronutrient needs. See Chapter 13 Manufactured Feeds.

20.3.1.2 Complementary Feeds

Complementary feeds or concentrates include grain mixtures and life-stage commercial feeds. Many commercial concentrates also provide minerals and vitamins, in addition to calories and protein. Therefore, concentrates are needed when forage alone does not meet the mare's energy, protein, or other essential nutrient requirements. While mares in 1–8 m of gestation do not necessarily need concentrates in the ration as they may be able to consume enough energy and protein from the forage, concentrates are often needed in mos 9–11 of gestation and during lactation when the mare's energy and other essential nutrient requirements have substantially increased over maintenance [36]. However, there are reports of successful reproductive programs where the mares never receive concentrates [41, 42].

Concentrate feeding is associated with reduced microbial diversity in the hindgut, increased risk for colic, and reduced insulin sensitivity [43–45]. Concentrate feeding also negatively influences voluntary forage intake during late gestation and lactation [39, 41]. An observational study reported that mares fed concentrates during gestation were more likely to produce foals that will develop osteochondrosis, compared to mares that were not fed concentrates likely due to a relatively increased growth rate in foals [46]. See Chapter 21 Feeding Growing Horses.

Feeding straight commodity grains (barley, corn, oats, or a mix thereof) should be done with caution because grains are higher in phosphorus than calcium. It is, therefore, possible to create an inverse calcium:phosphorus (Ca:P) ratio in the total ration. Cereal grains lack sufficient trace minerals (copper, iron, manganese, zinc, cobalt, iodine, and selenium) and vitamins A & E as needed (Tables 20.1 and 20.2). Feeding a ration balancer with trace minerals, vitamins, and a Ca:P ratio that has been adjusted to match the forage, resulting in a total ration ratio of 1:1 to 1.5:1, is advisable. When feeding concentrates, particularly high-starch concentrates, for example, corn grain contains approximately 70% starch, dividing the total daily amount into more frequent small meals should help to reduce the risk of glucose peaks and changes to the hindgut microbiome [43]. Feeding large meals decreases transit time through the foregut, and digestible nutrients are carried to the hindgut before digestion and absorption are completed. Highly digestible carbohydrates are then fermented in the hindgut. Currently, the recommendation is to limit starch and sugar intake to <200 g/100 kg BW/d and to adjust the number of daily meals such that each is ≤100 g/100 kg BW [47]. If concentrates are needed by some mares or only during certain reproductive stages, then mares should be grouped such that feeding concentrates can be targeted to those individuals.

20.3.2 Key Nutrients

The importance of appropriate maternal nutrition during gestation has gained a greater appreciation in the last two decades. In the first 150 days of gestation, mares at optimal BCS may be managed as mares at maintenance because fetal growth is slow; however, nutritional needs of the mare begin to increase in the second trimester (mos 6–8) even though most of the fetal growth occurs during the third trimester [9, 36]. Lactation is comparatively a nutritionally demanding life stage for the mare. The efficiency of feed DE conversion to milk DE has been estimated at 60% for horses whereas feed CP to milk CP is 35–40% [9].

20.3.2.1 Water

Water is the most important nutrient and comprises roughly 65% of an adult horse's mass [48–50]. In the horse, as in other mammals, water is supplied via drinking, moisture in feed, and through water derived from metabolic processes (metabolic water). The normal voluntary daily water intake of horses is dependent on factors including heat, humidity, exercise, and food composition. Thirst is influenced by plasma osmolality, which is affected by diet composition and feed consumption [49, 51–54]. The average daily water intake of healthy adult horses is approximately 54–64 mL/kg BW/d [50, 54] of which 85% is provided by drinking water [50]. While the water requirements for the pregnant broodmare do not appear to be that different from those of the open mare, milk is a substantial route for water loss in the lactating mare [55].

Mare's milk is approximately 90% water and the average daily milk yield for mares in early lactation has been estimated to be 3% BW [9, 56, 57]. The water requirements of lactating mares maintained in a thermoneutral environment are approximately 37–74% above maintenance requirements [9, 58]. In the horse, there is a positive correlation between food and free water intake [52, 53, 59]. Thus, horses deprived of free water reduce their intake of food, and horses deprived of food have reduced voluntary water intake. Unlimited access to water is therefore important in allowing the lactating broodmare to meet her dry matter intake of feed. To compensate for the feed intake that occurs during lactation (2–3% DMI), water intake is predicted to increase by 50–75% [9]. Properly functioning automatic waterers, or checking water buckets 3–4 times daily, are essential for meeting lactating mare's water requirement. See Chapter 5 Water.

20.3.2.2 Energy

The DE requirement in the first 5 mos of gestation is equivalent to open mares (average 3.34 Mcal/100 kg BW). Monitoring of BW and BCS will help determine when the gravid mare's energy requirement is no longer similar to maintenance. Increases in BW begin mid-gestation due to placental, uterine, and fetal weight and continue linearly until foaling. The caloric value of these tissues was determined and used to estimate the increasing DE requirement from mid (3.42 Mcal/100 kg BW) to late gestation (4.28 Mcal/100 kg BW) [9]. The energy cost of growing a fetus added to the energy cost of first and foremost of maintenance determines the total daily energy requirement (DER) for a gestating mare (Table 20.1).

Milk production begins days before parturition and increases for the first 60 days, and then declines and ceases at weaning. Therefore, DE requirement increases again from 4.28 to 6.34 Mcal/100 kg BW within days of foaling (Figure 20.1). Mare's milk contains 6% lactose, less than 2% fat, and has a caloric value of 500–600 kcal/kg as fed. The energy content of milk times the yield (kg/d) approximates the additional DE required for milk production. The energy cost of milk production added to the energy cost of first and foremost of maintenance determines the total DER for a lactating mare (Table 20.2).

20.3.2.2.1 Fat

Fats are sources of energy, carriers of fat-soluble vitamins, and sources of essential fatty acids. Dietary fats (oils) are used to increase the energy density of equine rations. Increasing dietary fat concentration increases ration energy density, which in turn decreases the amount of feed needed to meet DER. Ration caloric density is increased for milk production and reproductive efficiency. Both linoleic acid (LA; 18:2 n-6) and α-linolenic acid (ALA; 18:3 n-3) are essential fatty acids in mammals. A dietary minimum of 0.5% DM has been suggested for linoleic acid, which is relatively easy to meet with <1% fat in the ration while the forage portion of the ration provides ALA [9]. There are no dietary omega-3 fatty acid recommendations.

20.3.2.3 Protein

The pregnant mare, from conception to 4th mo of gestation, has protein requirements equal to those of average maintenance mares [9]. For the pregnant mare ≥5 mos gestation through parturition, the protein requirement is estimated by calculating the sum of the protein needed for mare maintenance plus the average daily fetal protein gain (130 g CP/d for horses; 45 g CP/d for the pony). As fetal growth progresses, the protein requirement increases (Figure 20.1). This calculation assumes that lysine comprises ≥4.3% of the dietary CP, a mare dietary protein digestibility coefficient of 80%, and a 50% feed conversion efficiency by the fetus [9]. The dietary CP concentration of the mare's ration DM must therefore increase accordingly from 5th m to parturition (Table 20.3) [9, 60, 61].

Arginine is considered an essential amino acid in the horse. In the horse and other mammals, arginine functions in the urea cycle, protein synthesis, nitric oxide synthesis, polyamine synthesis, and proline, glutamate, and creatine synthesis [62]. Nitric oxide functions as a vasodilator and helps in the regulation of placental blood flow. Deficiencies in both nitric oxide and polyamines are implicated in intrauterine growth retardation (IUGR). Arginine is involved in postpartum maternal health, and characterizing the requirement of the reproducing broodmare horse is an area of active study [63, 64].

The lactating mare must consume sufficient protein to maintain body mass plus that required in milk. Milk contains 2% protein and lysine comprises about 8% of the milk protein [36, 65]. These factors determine the lactating mare requirements over and above maintenance protein and lysine needs which change throughout the lactating cycle with milk yield. Mare protein requirement is highest in month 1 and 2 when milk production is highest and then declines as milk yield declines (Figure 20.1 and Table 20.2).

20.3.2.4 Macrominerals

In late gestation (mos 9–11), the dietary calcium, phosphorus, and sodium (Na) requirements of the mare are increased over that of the mare during earlier periods of pregnancy. The increased requirement during late pregnancy is a consequence of maintaining fetal tissues and continued fetal growth. The calculated mare requirement of macrominerals in late gestation is based on that sufficient to maintain mare tissues and function, plus fetal maintenance and growth using estimated dietary (50% Ca, 35% P, and 80% Na) absorption rates [9]. With the onset of lactation, the dietary calcium and phosphorus concentrations must increase to meet the demands of milk production (Figure 20.1). Sodium requirements increase with the increased water consumption associated with lactation [9, 49, 54, 66]. Given milk macromineral concentration and dietary absorption rates, the daily intakes of macrominerals have been estimated [9].

20.3.2.5 Trace Minerals

The maternal ration directly influences fetal trace mineral stores, that is, hepatic copper (Cu), iodine (I), and selenium (Se) which are essential for pre-weaning growth because milk is generally a poor source of trace minerals. Copper is a key nutrient in the prevention of nutrition-related developmental orthopedic disease in foals, in that those with low Cu liver concentrations had worsening osteochondrosis scores from 5 to 11 m of age compared with foals with higher liver Cu concentrations [67].

Broodmares with iodine deficiency may give birth to foals with congenital hypothyroidism associated with two syndromes: congenital hypothyroidism and dysmaturity syndrome (CHD), and congenital hyperthyroidism with goiter (CHG). CHD is a disease with a poor prognosis, with most foals dying or being euthanized within days of birth [68]. CHG has a guarded prognosis for the ability of the horse to later perform an intended function. Dietary factors affecting bioavailability include excessive nitrates in the feed, insufficient dietary selenium, or ingestion of goitrogenic plants, such as brassicas [69–71]. The dietary iodine concentration for mares gestation mos ≥9 is 0.4 mg I/kg DM on the increased dietary iodine intake recommended for humans [9]. For all other equine life stages, a dietary intake of 0.35 mg I/kg DM is recommended with a maximum tolerable concentration of 5 mg I/kg DM [72].

Selenium deficiency, characterized by serum concentrations <65 ng/mL, is associated with an increased risk of white muscle disease, and a mare's Se status determines that of the foal [9, 73–76]. In late gestation, Se is transferred transplacentally from the broodmare to the foal [73–79]. Postpartum, Se is transferred from the mare to the newborn foal in the first few hours after birth through colostrum, while negligible Se is imparted thereafter through milk [74, 79]. The recommended dietary selenium for broodmares (0.1 mg/kg DM) is the same as that for other life stages [79]. Assessing serum Se concentrations to be adequate (180–240 ng/mL) in broodmares before breeding is prudent. Selenium supplementation in deficient broodmares in late gestation (≤2 m before parturition) was not sufficient to normalize mare or foal plasma Se concentrations before parturition [79]. Both inorganic and organic (typically selenomethionine from selenized yeast[1]) forms fed at 0.3 mg/kg DM improved blood selenium with glutathione activity plateauing 154 d later.

Assessing mare status before breeding, even in regions not deficient in selenium, is prudent because Se bioavailability is dependent on numerous soil factors and plant species [73, 80, 81]. Correcting for Se deficiency in broodmares feeding a diet with 0.3 mg Se/kg DM, rather than 0.1 mg/kg DM, is advisable. There is evidence that, in the horse, as in other species, organic forms may be more effective than inorganic Se sources at increasing blood concentrations in the neonate via placental and colostral transfer [77, 79]. Organic Se (selenomethionine) may also improve foal Se reserves, within muscles and other tissues, serving as reserves before weaning in selenium-deficient regions [79].

20.3.2.6 Vitamins

Fresh forage (pasture) generally supplies adequate vitamins A and E to the broodmare, whereas hay content depends on the quality and storage conditions. Laboratory analysis of vitamins is not done routinely due to sampling errors and cost. Regardless of the type of forage, hay, or pasture, if the forage contains a significant recognizable green color and constitutes the majority of the horse's ration, likely the beta-carotene and alpha-tocopherol intake will be adequate. Although carotenes are a yellow-orange pigment, the green color present in forage gives a rough approximation of the beta-carotene and alpha-tocopherol concentrations. Ensuring broodmares vitamins A and E intake during gestation and lactation is important, as both are primarily transferred to foals through colostrum, and to a lesser extent milk.

20.3.2.6.1 Vitamin A

Carotenes are destroyed gradually by light and heat; even with optimum harvesting, the carotene concentration in sun-cured forage or hay is lower than in green forage. Carotenes are destroyed gradually by light, heat, and moisture, thus their concentration in conserved forages (hay and silage) can be unpredictable. See Table 9.2. Horse tissue stores of vitamin A were depleted within 2 m when fed hay with no access to pasture [82]. Broodmares with limited access to growing pasture or green hay require vitamin A supplied as part of the concentrate or a vitamin supplement. Vitamin A requirement increases at parturition, at least partially due to the presence of high concentrations of vitamin A and β-carotene in mare colostrum [83]. Vitamin A required for reproduction and lactation is suggested to be at least two times the amount required for maintenance, that is, 6 KIU/100 kg BW (Tables 20.1 and 20.2); hence, feeds containing 3000–4500 IU/kg DM are more appropriate for reproduction [9]. Colostrum contains concentrations of vitamin A (approximately 235 IU/mL) which then stabilize to 7–25 IU/mL in the first 48 hrs of lactation providing a relatively stable intake until the foal is weaned [83]. Provided the mare's vitamin A status is adequate, milk is sufficient to meet the foal's requirements until they begin eating fresh forages.

20.3.2.6.2 Vitamin E

Fresh forages have the highest concentration of vitamin E (100–600 IU/kg DM), hays at 15–60 IU/kg DM, and grains at the lowest concentration (5–80 IU/kg DM) [9, 84]. The vitamin E content of forages decreases with plant maturity, that is, 70–90% from early growth to maturity in grasses and 35–65% in alfalfa from bud to post-flowering. The vitamin E recommendation during gestation is 160 IU/100 kg BW, while the vitamin E requirement for lactation is 200 IU/100 kg BW [9]. The colostrum of mares fed a diet meeting the recommended vitamin E intake had concentrations of α-tocopherol approximately fivefold that of milk at day 21 postpartum [83].

20.4 Feeding Management

Forage quality must be sufficiently palatable and digestible such that the mare will meet requirements voluntarily which varies from 1.4–5.4% BW depending on the environment, for example, housing, weather, and psychological

1 Approximately 50–70% of yeast selenium is in the form of selenomethionine, while 10–15% of yeast selenium is in the form of selenocysteine, which has poor bioavailability [77].

factors, such as temperament and herd status. Water and salt should be available to all mares *ad libitum*.

A trace mineral–vitamin concentrate or ration balancer, composed of calories, protein, vitamins, or minerals, is added as needed to complement the forage nutrient profile in meeting the broodmare's nutrient requirements. Fresh forage (pasture) can be a good source of energy and essential nutrients, that is, protein, calcium, phosphorus, and is a better source of vitamins A and E compared to hays. Feeding fresh forages will likely require trace mineral supplementation, whereas feeding hays will likely require trace mineral–vitamin supplementation to complete the ration. If lower-quality forages or low-caloric-density (Mcal DE/kg) rations with % CP less than recommended are to be fed, a ration balancer with grain for calories and/or protein will be needed in addition to the trace mineral–vitamin concentrate.

Open and early gestation mares can easily overconsume calories relative to requirements, gaining excessive weight, when fed a high-quality forage (RFV >120) free choice, for example, allowing mares to graze *ad libitum* on legume or grass pasture in the vegetative state. Therefore, feeding specific quantities of hay or limiting time on pastures and monitoring BCS are employed to avoid excessive weight gain in these life stages. Conversely, a forage of lower quality offered even *ad libitum* to a lactating mare may limit feed intake before meeting the DE requirement resulting in weight loss and poor condition, for example, feeding mature grass hay (RFV < 100) to the lactating mare (Table 20.3).

20.4.1 Gestation

Suggested feeding recommendations for gestation apply only to broodmares in moderate body condition BCS 5 to 6/9. Gestating mares will consume (1.5–2.0% BW) to attain and maintain body fat stores during pregnancy for utilization late in gestation and lactation [85]. Mares in <9 mos gestation are fed moderate-quality forage (<42% ADF, <60% NDF, RFV >86) (Table 10.3). Late gestation (mos 9–11) mares are fed a high-quality forage (<35% ADF, <46% NDF, RFV>120) (Table 10.3) and a concentrate at 0.1% BW for the third-trimester fetal growth and in preparation for transition to the lactation ration. If lower-quality forages or those with DE < 2.1 Mcal/kg or CP < 9% DM are fed, a complementary feed or ration balancer providing calories and/or protein with minerals and vitamins fed at 0.3–0.5% BW, divided into 2 or 3 feedings daily, may be required [86].

Body condition scoring of mares should be assessed in the fall and, if not 4 to 6/9, then feeding to correct before spring breeding because BCS influences reproductive efficiency [36]. Increasing DE intake to achieve a BCS 5 to 6/9 by mid-gestation is recommended in gravid mares with a low score. Practically, this could be accomplished by feeding 110% of the DE requirement for the estimated ideal BW (BCS 5/9). Energy excess in late gestation will promote mare weight gain, but not fetal, and will not affect foaling [35]. For the obese broodmare (BCS ≥8/9), prescribed weight loss should ideally have been implemented before breeding. See Feeding for Weight Loss in Chapter 23. Severe underfeeding energy may prolong gestation due to the effects of negative energy balance on prostaglandin concentrations and glucose homeostasis [87, 88]. Although not ideal, controlled weight loss for the mare is possible by feeding at her ideal BW, rather than current BW through gestation and lactation. See Case in Point.

20.4.1.1 Fescue Toxicity

Tall fescue (*Festuca arundinacea*) is a dominant forage across the USA and is an important forage to consider when feeding broodmares, particularly in late gestation. Fescue toxicosis occurs when a broodmare consumes tall fescue infected with the symbiotic endophyte fungus *Neotyphodium coenophialum* (formerly *Acremonium coenophialum*), which is concentrated in seed heads and stems. The toxic agents within the fungus are believed to be ergot alkaloids [89]. Fungal toxins reduce progesterone, prolactin, and estrogen concentrations in both mares and cows. Detection of *N. coenophialum* requires staining for the endophyte within the seed or stem. The concentration of ergot alkaloids increases as the fescue plant matures, and a toxic concentration of the ergot alkaloid ergovaline is considered to be >200 ppb [89–91].

Sequelae of fescue toxicosis include abortion, prolonged gestation, agalactia, and thickened placentas [90]. In affected broodmares, foals grow larger *in utero* past their due date, and with thicken placentas, dystocia is common. Udder development and signs of impending parturition may not occur. Affected mares tend to gain less weight during pregnancy and may be in poorer BCS than those not consuming infected fescue. Management and prevention of fescue toxicosis involve preventing animals from consuming infected hay or pastures. Feeding hay that is cut at an early stage, that is, before seed head formation, also prevents toxicity. Removing mares from infected fescue 60–90 d prior to parturition is recommended. Alternatives to this include grazing/feeding a tall-fescue-mixed pasture/hay, that is, legume mix or mixed grass, and mowing to remove the seed heads. Growing horses may also be negatively impacted by the consumption of endophyte-infected tall fescue [92]. See Chapter 21 Feeding Growing Horses.

20.4.2 Lactation

Suggested feeding recommendations for lactation apply only to broodmares in moderate body condition BCS 5 to 6/9 (Table 20.2). Serum parathyroid hormone increases 3 days before parturition signaling lactation [93]. The mare's nutrient requirements increase >50% with the onset of lactation and feed intake will increase accordingly; however, the transition from the gestation to lactation ration should be gradual to lower the risk of digestive disturbances, as there are increased risks of diarrhea, colic, and laminitis when changing the forage or concentrate portion of the ration in horses [44, 94, 95]. The DMI for mares in early and late lactation is 2.0–3.0% and 2.0–2.5% BW, respectively [9, 36]. Depending on the forage RFV, starch, and sugar content of the lactation ration relative to the gestation ration, the transition should occur over 1 wk for relatively small differences whereas 2 wks or more are suggested for large differences. The greater the proportion of high RFV forage in the gestation ration, the less grain concentrate is needed, and less time is needed for the transition to the lactation ration. A general guideline is to replace 25% of the old ration DM with a new ration DM every 4–6 days and monitor for GI changes and laminitis. See Sidebar 26.1.

20.4.2.1 Early Lactation (mos 1–3)

A high-quality forage (<35% ADF, <46% NDF, RFV >120) (Table 10.3) should dominate the lactating mare ration, as energy restriction of the mare during lactation has negative effects on mare body condition, milk production, and subsequent foal growth [4]. If lower-quality forages or those with DE < 2.5 Mcal/kg or CP < 12.0% DM are fed, a complementary feed or ration balancer providing calories and/or protein with minerals and vitamins fed at 0.5–1.0% BW divided into 2 or 3 feedings daily may be required [86].

The forage to grain concentrate ratio of a mare's ration, particularly fiber and starch, influences the macronutrient composition of the mare's milk. High starch rations (low forage) result in higher concentrations of lactose and higher milk yields, while high fiber rations (low concentrate) result in higher milk fat concentrations and lower milk yields. Due to the higher caloric density of fat, the total daily energy consumed by the foal on a mare consuming a high forage ration may not be different from a foal on a mare fed a high starch ration. The fat content and fatty acid profile of the lactating ration positively and directly influence the milk fat content and fatty acid profile [96, 97].

Water requirements are highest for the lactating mare with the production of 3–4% of BW in milk/d, that is, 9–14 L (2–4 gal) of milk from a 500-kg BW mare, of which 90% is water. Increased consumption of water without access to salt results in hyponatremia [59, 66]. Mild hyponatremia is not typically associated with clinical signs; however, severe hyponatremia is associated with neurologic abnormalities including dysphagia, seizures, coma, and death [66]. Given there is a salt appetite, that is, hyponatremia promotes salt intake, lactating mares should have unlimited access to potable water and sodium chloride (salt block).

20.4.2.2 Late Lactation (mos 4–6)

Milk production declines to 2% BW/d by month 5 of lactation [9], and compared to early lactation, the mare in late lactation has relatively lower requirements for energy and nutrients. A good-quality forage (<40% ADF, <53% NDF, RFV >100) (Table 10.3) should still dominate the mare's ration. If lower-quality forages or those with DE < 2.3 Mcal/kg or CP < 11.0% DM are fed, a complementary feed or ration balancer providing calories and/or protein with minerals and vitamins fed at 0.5–0.75% BW divided into 2 or 3 feedings daily will be needed. The amount of concentrate fed should decrease in the weeks prior to weaning, as feeding energy concentrates slows the decline in milk production. See Sidebar 20.1.

Mares usually have fewer psychological problems at weaning time than do foals; however, some mares will also experience a high degree of stress. Five to seven days before weaning, decrease the forage fed to that of the mare and discontinue feeding the grain concentrate. The reduced energy intake will decrease milk production and help prevent excessive udder pressure and discomfort once the foal has been removed. The udder should become soft and pliable within a week of weaning. The mare, post weaning, in good condition (BCS 4 to 5/9) may be fed as an open mare. However, if the mare has a poor BCS (<4/9), feeding sufficient forage and restarting an energy concentrate to increase BW and improve BCS at this time are advised. Feeding more DE will enhance the mare's reproductive efficiency, chances of rebreeding, and replenishing energy stores for the next pregnancy–lactation cycle.

20.4.3 BCS for Reproductive Efficiency

Mares should have a BCS of 5 to 6/9 at foaling. The first estrus after foaling will occur in 45% of mares by d 9, 93% by d 15, and 97% by d 20 postpartum [98]. If successfully bred during the foal heat, the mare will be gravid while lactating. Early gestation nutritional requirements are the same as maintenance; however, monitoring of BCS through to weaning is necessary for proper feeding management

Sidebar 20.1: Calculating Daily Feeding Recommendations for a Lactating Broodmare

Animal Assessment

- A 650-kg (BCS 5/9) 6-yr-old Trakehner broodmare in fifteenth wk of lactation. The owner wants to put the mare (and foal) out on pasture (no hay ration). Compare the nutrient recommendations for the mare during the remaining months of lactation with a pasture based ration.
- DMI for a late-lactating mare is 2.0–2.5% BW (Table 20.3).
- Mare's daily DE requirement month 4 of lactation: 5.88 Mcal DE/100 kg BW × 6.5 = 38.2 Mcal DE (Table 20.2).
- Forage recommendations for lactating mares are RFV >100 and 2.26 Mcal DE/kg DM (Table 20.3). ADF <35% and NDF <46% is recommended for lactating horses (Table 10.3).

Ration Assessment

- Forage available on the farm is a cool-season grass pasture in the vegetative state. The grass is highly palatable, the pasture is well managed, and the horse would likely consume 2.5% BW. The pasture grass had 20% DM and dry matter book values of:

International feed number (IFN)	DE	CP	Lysine	ADF	NDF	Ca	P
#	Mcal/kg	%	%	%	%	%	%
2-02-260	2.39	26.5	0.92	25.0	45.8	0.56	0.44

- Calculate forage DDM, DMI, and RFV values:
  - %DDM = 88.9 − (0.779 × %ADF) = 69.4%.
  - %DMI = 120/%NDF = 2.6% BW.
  - RFV = %DDM × %DMI × 0.775 = 140 high-quality (Table 10.3).
  - Forage quality is adequate compared with that recommended for late lactating mares.
- Calculate daily forage intake required to meet the mare's DE on DM and as fed (AF) basis:
  - Horse requires 38.2 Mcal DE/2.39 Mcal DE/kg DM = 16 kg forage DM/0.2 = 80 kg (175 lb) fresh forage.
  - Check DMI: 16 kg pasture DM/650 kg BW = 2.46% BW.
- Compare forage crude protein (CP), calcium (Ca), and phosphorus (P) concentrations with recommendations (Table 20.3).
  - Recommended [CP] is 10.6%; forage contains 26.5% CP.
  - Recommended [Calcium] is 0.30%; forage contains 0.56% Ca.
  - Recommended [Phosphorus] is 0.20% P; forage contains 0.44% P with Ca:P ratio = 1.3:1.
  - If sufficient quantity of fresh pasture is consumed, the CP, Ca, and P needs should be met.

Feeding Management Recommendations

In summary, the pasture available on the farm based on textbook values is adequate in DE, CP, calcium, and phosphorus for a mos 4–6 lactating mare, and requirements should be met within her voluntary DMI (2.0–2.5% BW). Specific instructions:

- The mare should be able to consume 2.5% BW in forage DM if allowed sufficient time on pasture and if ample growth and acreage are available.
- The mare must be able to consume 80 kg of fresh pasture grass/d to meet her DE requirement, but it is not possible to directly quantify forage intake on pasture; therefore, monitoring mare and foal BW and BCS every 2 wks is advisable.
  - The mare is post-peak lactation and nutritional requirements will decrease from this point to weaning.
  - Similarly, cool-season pasture nutrient profiles will decrease as grass plants mature.
- Monitoring for BW and BCS changes is recommended for reproduction efficiency if rebreeding.
- Feed mineral ration balancer supplement per manufacturer's feeding recommendations (0.1–0.3% BW). Vitamin intake on the fresh green forge (pasture) is likely adequate.
- Lysine intake was also checked and found to be adequate.
- Offer water and salt *ad libitum*.

after weaning. Mares with BCS 5 to 6/9 have higher conception rates and require fewer cycles to conceive.

20.4.3.1 BCS <5/9

Assessment of BCS in open mares should be done at least 3 m before the breeding, and if less than 5/9, adjustments to increase energy intake should be made to the feeding program to improve the BCS prior to breeding season. Feeding a good-quality (>2.0 Mcal/kg DM, RFV >100) forage, usually, legume–grass mixed hay or pasture with a trace mineral–vitamin concentrate will improve poor BCS in most mares over 4–8 mos. Improving BCS is more easily accomplished during the mild weather of late summer and fall. With the onset of cold weather or as the time to rebreeding shortens, higher energy concentrates will be needed to correct the BCS.

Increasing BCS 1 point in maintenance horses requires a BW gain of 16–20 kg and each kg of gain requires about 18–24 Mcal DE [9]. A mare may consume 0.5% BW of appropriately fortified concentrate daily, and, therefore, improving the BCS by 1 point in 500 kg BW gravid late lactating mare will require feeding 2–3 kg/d of an energy concentrate (3–3.5 Mcal DE/kg DM) for 1–2 mos.

20.4.3.2 BCS >6/9

Reproductive efficiency in mares with BCS >7/9 is not reduced [36]. Obese broodmares are at risk of developing hyperlipidemia during periods of negative energy balance. Late gestation and early lactation are periods of high metabolic demand, with a higher risk of negative energy balance if dietary intake should become insufficient due to anorexia, malnutrition, stress, pain, or disease. These periods of peak fetal development and increased use of adipose tissue for milk production are associated with changes in mare insulin sensitivity and serum triglyceride concentration, and free fatty acids are released into circulation [99–102]. Hyperlipidemias are a form of dyslipidemia characterized by elevated serum triglycerides occurring almost exclusively in older, obese, pregnant, or lactating mares of pony and miniature horse breeds. See Hyperlipemia in Chapter 27. If the mare is overweight, feeding a less energy dense forage (1.0–1.5 Mcal/kg DM, RFV 80–100) and a trace mineral–vitamin concentrate to reduce BW and BCS before rebreeding is advisable. In general, a recommended rate of weight loss is 0.5–1 BCS point/month, for example, a BCS 8/9 mare would require 3–6 mos of weight loss to reach BCS 5/9.

Case in Point

An 11-yr-old paint mare 10.5 mos pregnant presents to the nutrition service in early July. The owner is concerned about the mare's weight due to a chronic forelimb lameness. The veterinarian and owner request a weight management ration appropriate for gestation.

Animal Assessment

A BW history was not available. The current walk-on scale BW was 638 kg. The mare's BW was adjusted 10% for a fetus. Starting mare BW was estimated at 574 kg (BCS 7/9). Ideally, for managing the mare's lameness, goal BCS would be 4/9. However, given the mare is in late gestation, the goal BCS is set at 5/9 and the estimated target BW was set at 535 kg.

Ration Assessment

Diet history from February to May, the mare was on a spring pasture. As pasture declined, the mare was fed 6–9 lb alfalfa hay, offered fescue hay *ad libitum*, a handful of a mare-specific concentrate, and a mineral–vitamin concentrate daily. In June, the owner confined the mare to a dry lot, offered 5 lb of fescue hay (2.2 Mcal DE/kg or 1.0 Mcal DE/lb AF) twice daily with water *ad libitum* from buckets. The veterinarian was concerned that feeding 10 Mcal/d met neither energy nor nutrient requirements for late gestation and that an accelerated weight loss in late gestation would pose health problems for both the mare and foal, yet current BW was uncomfortable for the mare due to chronic lameness.

Nutritional Recommendations

Although not ideal to induce weight loss during late gestation, a ration was formulated to meet the recommended energy and nutrient requirements for an 11 month pregnant mare at her ideal BW.

1) What is the recommended DE for an 11 month pregnant mare at BW of 535 kg (Table 20.1) and how much fescue hay should be fed per day?

The mare foaled in August and a ration for early lactation was requested. According to the owner, the mare weighed 565 kg using a weight tape, appeared thinner but still overweight. The ration was reformulated using the same hay and supplement to meet the lactation recommendations.

2) What is the recommended DE for a mare during the first month of lactation at BW of 535 kg? (Table 20.2).

In January, the owner reported that the mare and foal were doing well and a weight tape indicated the mare weighed 540 kg, losing 34 kg over the 6 month period. No BCS was available.

3) What was the %BW loss/wk overall?

See Appendix A Chapter 20.

References

1 Guillaume, D., Salazar-Ortiz, J., and Martin-Rosset, W. (2006). Effects of nutrition level in mares' ovarian activity and in equines' puberty. In: *Nutrition and Feeding of the Broodmare. AEEP #120* (ed. N. Miraglia and W. Martin-Rosset), 315–339. Wageningen: Wageningen Academic Publishers.

2 Henneke, D.R., Potter, G.D., Kreider, J.L., and Yeates, B.F. (1983). Relationship between condition score, physical measurements and body fat percentage in mares. *Equine Vet. J.* 15 (4): 371–372.

3 Donadeu, F.X. and Pedersen, H.G. (2008). Follicle development in mares. *Reprod. Domest. Anim.* 43 (Suppl 2): 224–231.

4 Henneke, D.R., Potter, G.D., and Kreider, J.L. (1984). Body condition during pregnancy and lactation and reproductive efficiency of mares. *Theriogenology* 21 (6): 897–909.

5 Davies-Morel, M.C.G., Newcombe, J.R., and Hayward, K. (2010). Factors affecting pre-ovulatory follicle diameter in the mare: the effect of mare age, season and presence of other ovulatory follicles (multiple ovulation). *Theriogenology* 74 (7): 1241–1247.

6 Fradinho, M.J., Correia, M.J., Gracio, V. et al. (2014). Effects of body condition and leptin on the reproductive performance of Lusitano mares on extensive systems. *Theriogenology* 81 (9): 1214–1222.

7 Smith, S., Marr, C.M., Dunnett, C., and Menzies-Gow, N.J. (2016). The effect of mare obesity and endocrine function on foal birthweight in Thoroughbreds. *Equine Vet. J.* 49 (4): 461–466.

8 Vecchi, I., Sabbioni, A., Bigliardi, E. et al. (2010). Relationship between body fat and body condition score and their effects on estrous cycles of the Standardbred maiden mare. *Vet. Res. Commun.* 34 (Suppl.1): 41–45.

9 National Research Council (2007). *Nutrient Requirements of Horses.* 6th Rev. Animal Nutrition Series, 1–341. Washington, DC: National Academies Press.

10 Peugnet, P., Robles, M., Mendoza, L. et al. (2015). Effects of moderate amounts of barley in late pregnancy on growth, glucose metabolism and osteoarticular status of pre-weaning horses. *PLoS One* 10 (4): e0122596.

11 Peugnet, P., Robles, M., Wimel, L. et al. (2016). Management of the pregnant mare and long-term consequences on the offspring. *Theriogenology* 86 (1): 99–109.

12 Robles, M., Gautier, C., Mendoza, L. et al. (2017). Maternal nutrition during pregnancy affects testicular and bone development, glucose metabolism and response to overnutrition in weaned horses up to two years. *PLoS One* 12 (1): e0169295.

13 Heidler, B., Aurich, J.E., Pohl, W., and Aurich, C. (2004). Body weight of mares and foals, estrous cycles and plasma glucose concentration in lactating and non-lactating Lipizzaner mares. *Theriogenology* 61 (5): 883–893.

14 Bos, H. and van der Mey, G.J.W. (1980). Length of gestation periods of horses and ponies belonging to different breeds. *Livest. Prod. Sci.* 7 (2): 181–187.

15 Duncan, P., Harvey, P.H., and Wells, S.M. (1984). On lactation and associated behaviour in a natural herd of horses. *Anim. Behav.* 32 (1): 255–263.

16 Waran, N.K., Clarke, N., and Farnworth, M. (2008). The effects of weaning on the domestic horse (*Equus caballus*). *Appl. Anim. Behav. Sci.* 110 (1): 42–57.

17 Stoneham, S.J., Morresey, P., and Ousey, J. (2017). Nutritional management and practical feeding of the orphan foal. *Equine Vet. Educ.* 29 (3): 165–173.

18 Apter, R.C. and Householder, D.D. (1996). Weaning and weaning management of foals: a review and some recommendations. *J. Equine Vet. Sci.* 16 (10): 428–435.

19 Gibbs, P.G. and Cohen, N.D. (2001). Early management of race-bred weanlings and yearlings on farms. *J. Equine Vet. Sci.* 21 (6): 279–283.

20 Kubiak, J.R., Crawford, B.H., Squires, E.L. et al. (1987). The influence of energy intake and percentage of body fat on the reproductive performance of nonpregnant mares. *Theriogenology* 28 (5): 587–598.

21 Mottet, R., Onan, G., and Hiney, K. (2009). Revisiting the Henneke body condition scoring system: 25 years later. *J. Equine Vet. Sci.* 29 (5): 417–418.

22 Morley, S.A. and Murray, J. (2014). Effects of body condition score on the reproductive physiology of the broodmare: a review. *J. Equine Vet. Sci.* 34 (7): 842–853.

23 Newcombe, J.R. and Wilson, M.C. (2005). Age, body weight, and pregnancy loss. *J. Equine Vet. Sci.* 25 (5): 188–194.

24 Roche, J.R., Friggens, N.C., Kay, J.K. et al. (2009). Invited review: body condition score and its association with dairy cow productivity, health, and welfare. *J. Dairy Sci.* 92 (12): 5769–5801.

25 Johnson, C.A. (2008). Pregnancy management in the bitch. *Theriogenology* 70 (9): 1412–1417.

26 Martin, B., Golden, E., Carlson, O.D. et al. (2008). Caloric restriction: impact upon pituitary function and reproduction. *Ageing Res. Rev.* 7 (3): 209–224.

27 Cline, J. (2012). Cattery management and nutrition of the queen and her offspring. In: *Management of Pregnant and Neonatal Dogs, Cats, and Exotic Pets* (ed. C. Lopate), 15–24. Wiley.

28 Kubiak, J.R., Evans, J.W., Potter, G.D. et al. (1989). Postpartum reproductive performance in the multiparous mare fed to obesity. *Theriogenology* 32 (1): 27–36.

29 Cavinder, C.A., Vogelsang, M.M., Gibbs, P.G. et al. (2009). Variances in reproductive efficiency of mares in fat and moderate body conditions following parturition. *Prof. Anim. Sci.* 25 (3): 250–255.

30 Waller, C.A., Thompson, D.L., Cartmill, J.A. et al. (2006). Reproduction in high body condition mares with high versus low leptin concentrations. *Theriogenology* 66 (4): 923–928.

31 Sessions-Bresnahan, D.R. and Carnevale, E.M. (2014). The effect of equine metabolic syndrome on the ovarian follicular environment. *J. Anim. Sci.* 92 (4): 1485–1494.

32 Vick, M.M., Adams, A.A., Murphy, B.A. et al. (2007). Relationships among inflammatory cytokines, obesity, and insulin sensitivity in the horse. *J. Anim. Sci.* 85 (5): 1144–1155.

33 Sessions-Bresnahan, D.R., Schauer, K.L., Heuberger, A.L., and Carnevale, E.M. (2016). Effect of obesity on the preovulatory follicle and lipid fingerprint of equine Oocytes1. *Biol. Reprod.* 94 (1): 1–15.

34 Frank, N., Geor, R.J., Bailey, S.R. et al. (2010). Equine metabolic syndrome. *J. Vet. Intern. Med.* 24 (3): 467–475.

35 Kubiak, J.R., Evans, J.W., Potter, G.D. et al. (1988). Parturition in the multiparous mare fed to obesity. *J. Equine Vet. Sci.* 8 (2): 135–140.

36 Lawrence, L.M. (2013). Feeding stallions and broodmares. In: *Equine Applied and Clinical Nutrition: Health, Welfare and Performance* (ed. R.J. Geor, P.A. Harris, and M. Coenen), 231–242. Edinburgh: Saunders Elsevier.

37 Swinker, A.M. (2014). Hay quality for different classes of horse. Pennsylvania State Extension Service. https://extension.psu.edu/hay-quality-for-different-classes-of-horses (accessed 2 July 2021).

38 Rodiek, A.V. and Stull, C.L. (2007). Glycemic index of ten common horse feeds. *J. Equine Vet. Sci.* 27 (5): 205–211.

39 Winsco, K.N., Coverdale, J.A., Wickersham, T.A. et al. (2013). Influence of maternal plane of nutrition on mares and their foals: determination of mare performance and voluntary dry matter intake during late pregnancy using a dual-marker system. *J. Anim. Sci.* 91 (9): 4208–4215.

40 van den Berg, M., Giagos, V., Lee, C. et al. (2016). The influence of odour, taste and nutrients on feeding behaviour and food preferences in horses. *Appl. Anim. Behav. Sci.* 184 (Nov): 41–50.

41 Collas, C., Fleurance, G., Cabaret, J. et al. (2014). How does the suppression of energy supplementation affect herbage intake, performance and parasitism in lactating saddle mares? *Animal* 8 (8): 1290–1297.

42 Lepeule, J., Bareille, N., Robert, C. et al. (2013). Association of growth, feeding practices and exercise conditions with the severity of the osteoarticular status of limbs in French foals. *Vet. J.* 197 (1): 65–71.

43 Julliand, V. and Grimm, P. (2017). The impact of diet on the hindgut microbiome. *J. Equine Vet. Sci.* 52 (5): 23–28.

44 Tinker, M.K., White, N.A., Lessard, P. et al. (1997). Prospective study of equine colic risk factors. *Equine Vet. J.* 29 (6): 454–458.

45 Hoffman, R.M., Boston, R.C., Stefanovski, D. et al. (2003). Obesity and diet affect glucose dynamics and insulin sensitivity in Thoroughbred geldings. *J. Anim. Sci.* 81 (9): 2333–2342.

46 Vander Heyden, L., Lejeune, J.P., Caudron, I. et al. (2013). Association of breeding conditions with prevalence of osteochondrosis in foals. *Vet. Rec.* 172 (3): 68.

47 Harris, P. and Shepherd, M. (2021). What would be good for all veterinarians to know about equine nutrition. *Vet. Clin. North Am. Equine Pract.* 37 (1): 1–20.

48 Lindinger, M.I., McKeen, G., and Ecker, G.L. (2004). Time course and magnitude of changes in total body water, extracellular fluid volume, intracellular fluid volume and plasma volume during submaximal exercise and recovery in horses. *Equine Comp. Exerc. Physiol.* 1 (2): 131–139.

49 Cymbaluk, N.F. (2013). Water. In: *Equine Applied and Clinical Nutrition: Health, Welfare and Performance* (ed. R.J. Geor, P.A. Harris, and M. Coenen), 80–95. Edinburgh: Saunders Elsevier.

50 Schott, H.C. (2011). Water homeostasis and diabetes insipidus in horses. *Vet. Clin. North Am. Equine Pract.* 27 (1): 175–195.

51 Houpt, K.A., Eggleston, A., Kunkle, K., and Houpt, T.R. (2000). Effect of water restriction on equine behaviour and physiology. *Equine Vet. J.* 32 (4): 341–344.

52 Lester, G.D., Merritt, A.M., Kuck, H.V., and Burrow, J.A. (2013). Systemic, renal, and colonic effects of intravenous and enteral rehydration in horses. *J. Vet. Intern. Med.* 27 (3): 554–566.

53 Norris, M.L., Houpt, K.A., and Houpt, T.R. (2013). Effect of food availability on the physiological responses to water deprivation in ponies. *J. Equine Vet. Sci.* 33 (4): 250–256.

54 Fielding, C.L. (2015). Potassium homeostasis and derangements. In: *Equine Fluid Therapy* (ed. C.L. Fielding and K.G. Magdesian), 27–44. Wiley.

55 Magdesian, K.G. (2015). Maintenance fluid therapy in horses. In: *Equine Fluid Therapy* (ed. C.L. Fielding and K.G. Magdesian), 175–189. Wiley.

56 Doreau, M. and Boulot, S. (1989). Recent knowledge on mare milk production: a review. *Livest. Prod. Sci.* 22 (3): 213–235.

57 Centoducati, P., Maggiolino, A., De Palo, P., and Tateo, A. (2012). Application of Wood's model to lactation curve of Italian heavy draft horse mares. *J. Dairy Sci.* 95 (10): 5770–5775.

58 Groenendyk, S., English, P.B., and Abetz, I. (1988). External balance of water and electrolytes in the horse. *Equine Vet. J.* 20 (3): 189–193.

59 Lopes, M.A., White, N.A. 2nd, Donaldson, L. et al. (2004). Effects of enteral and intravenous fluid therapy, magnesium sulfate, and sodium sulfate on colonic contents and feces in horses. *Am. J. Vet. Res.* 65 (5): 695–704.

60 van Niekerk, F.E. and van Niekerk, C.H. (1997). The effect of dietary protein on reproduction in the mare. I. the composition and evaluation of the digestibility of dietary protein from different sources. *J. S. Afr. Vet. Assoc.* 68 (3): 78–80.

61 van Niekerk, F.E. and van Niekerk, C.H. (1998). The effect of dietary protein on reproduction in the mare. VII. Embryonic development, early embryonic death, foetal losses and their relationship with serum progestagen. *J. S. Afr. Vet. Assoc.* 69 (4): 150–155.

62 Wu, G. and Morris, S.M. (1998). Arginine metabolism: nitric oxide and beyond. *Biochem. J.* 336 (Pt 1): 1–17.

63 Kelley, D.E., Warren, L.K., and Mortensen, C.J. (2013). Oral L-arginine supplementation impacts several reproductive parameters during the postpartum period in mares. *Anim. Reprod. Sci.* 138 (3–4): 233–240.

64 Mesa, A.M., Warren, L.K., Sheehan, J.M. et al. (2015). L-arginine supplementation 0.5% of diet during the last 90 days of gestation and 14 days postpartum reduced uterine fluid accumulation in the broodmare. *Anim. Reprod. Sci.* 159 (Aug): 46–51.

65 Wickens, C.L., Ku, P.K., and Trottier, N.L. (2002). An ideal protein for the lactating mare. *J. Anim. Sci.* 80 (Suppl 1 Abstr 620): 155.

66 Fielding, C.L. (2015). Sodium and water homeostasis and derangements. In: *Equine Fluid Therapy* (ed. C.L. Fielding and K.G. Magdesian), 11–26. Wiley.

67 Van Weeren, P.R., Knaap, J., and Firth, E.C. (2003). Influence of liver copper status of mare and newborn foal on the development of osteochondrotic lesions. *Equine Vet. J.* 35 (1): 67–71.

68 Koikkalainen, K., Knuuttila, A., Karikoski, N. et al. (2014). Congenital hypothyroidism and dysmaturity syndrome in foals: first reported cases in Europe: congenital hypothyroidism and dysmaturity syndrome in foals. *Equine Vet. Educ.* 26 (4): 181–189.

69 Hotz, C.S., Fitzpatrick, D.W., Trick, K.D., and L'Abbé, M.R. (1997). Dietary iodine and selenium interact to affect thyroid hormone metabolism of rats. *J. Nutr.* 127 (6): 1214–1218.

70 Rotruck, J., Pope, A., Ganther, H. et al. (1973). Selenium: biochemical role as a component of glutathione peroxidase. *Science* 179 (Feb): 588–590.

71 Contempre, B., Denef, J.F., Dumont, J.E., and Many, M.C. (1993). Selenium deficiency aggravates the necrotizing effects of a high iodide dose in iodine deficient rats. *Endocrinology* 132 (4): 1866–1868.

72 National Research Council (2005). *Mineral Tolerance of Animals*. 2nd Rev., 1–496. Washington, DC: National Academies Press.

73 Delesalle, C., de Bruijn, M., Wilmink, S. et al. (2017). White muscle disease in foals: focus on selenium soil content. A case series. *BMC Vet. Res.* 13 (1): 121.

74 Lee, J., McAllister, E., and Scholz, R. (1995). Assessment of selenium status in mares and foals under practical management conditions. *J. Equine Vet. Sci.* 15 (5): 240–245.

75 Thorson, J.F., Karren, B.J., Bauer, M.L. et al. (2010). Effect of selenium supplementation and plane of nutrition on mares and their foals: foaling data. *J. Anim. Sci.* 88 (3): 982–990.

76 Karren, B.J., Thorson, J.F., Cavinder, C.A. et al. (2010). Effect of selenium supplementation and plane of nutrition on mares and their foals: selenium concentrations and glutathione peroxidase. *J. Anim. Sci.* 88 (3): 991–997.

77 Surai, P.F. and Fisinin, V.I. (2016). Selenium in livestock and other domestic animals. In: *Selenium: Its Molecular Biology and Role in Human Health* (ed. D.L. Hatfield, U. Schweizer, P.A. Tsuji, and V.N. Gladyshev), 595–606. Cham: Springer International Publishing.

78 Secombe, C.J. and Lester, G.D. (2012). The role of diet in the prevention and management of several equine diseases. *Anim. Feed Sci. Technol.* 173 (1–2): 86–101.

79 Montgomery, J.B., Wichtel, J.J., Wichtel, M.G. et al. (2012). The effects of selenium source on measures of selenium status of mares and selenium status and immune function of their foals. *J. Equine Vet. Sci.* 32 (6): 352–359.

80 Gissel-Nielsen, G., Gupta, U.C., Lamand, M., and Westermarck, T. (1984). Selenium in soils and plants and its importance in livestock and human nutrition. *Adv. Agron.* 37 (Jan): 397–460.

81 Gupta, U.C. and Gupta, S.C. (2000). Selenium in soils and crops, its deficiencies in livestock and humans: implications for management. *Commun. Soil Sci. Plant Anal.* 31 (11–14): 1791–1807.

82 Greiwe Crandell, K.M., Kronfeld, D.S., Gay, L.A., and Sklan, D. (1995). Seasonal vitamin A depletion in grazing horses is assessed better by the relative dose response test than by serum retinol concentration. *J. Nutr.* 125 (10): 2711–2716.

83 Schweigert, F.J. and Gottwald, C. (1999). Effect of parturition on levels of vitamins A and E and of B-carotene in plasma and milk of mares. *Equine Vet. J.* 31 (4): 319–323.

84 National Research Council (1982). *United States-Canadian Tables of Feed Composition*. 3rd Rev. Nutritional Data for United States and Canadian Feeds, 1–148. Washington, DC: National Academies Press.

85 Powell, D., Lawrence, L.M., Parrett, D.F. et al. (1989). Body composition changes in broodmares. In: *Proceedings of the 11th Equine Nutrition and Physiology Society Symposium*, 91–94. Stillwater, OK: Equine Nutrition and Physiology Society.

86 Geor, R., Harris, P.A., and Coenen, M. (2013). Nutritional requirements, recommendations and example diets. In: *Equine Applied and Clinical Nutrition Health, Welfare and Performance* (ed. R. Geor, P.A. Harris, and M. Coenen), 639–643. Edinburgh: Saunders Elsevier.

87 Silver, M. and Fowden, A.L. (1982). Uterine prostaglandin F metabolite production in relation to glucose availability in late pregnancy and a possible influence of diet on time of delivery in the mare. *J. Reprod. Fertil.* 32 (Jan Suppl): 511–519.

88 George, L.A., Staniar, W.B., Treiber, K.H. et al. (2009). Insulin sensitivity and glucose dynamics during pre-weaning foal development and in response to maternal diet composition. *Domest. Anim. Endocrinol.* 37 (1): 23–29.

89 Aiken, G.E. and Strickland, J.R. (2013). Forages and pastures symposium: managing the tall fescue-fungal endophyte symbiosis for optimum forage-animal production. *J. Anim. Sci.* 91 (5): 2369–2378.

90 Blodgett, D.J. (2001). Fescue toxicosis. *Vet. Clin. North Am. Equine Pract.* 17 (3): 567–577.

91 Osweiler, G.D. (2016). Fescue poisoning. In: *The Merck Veterinary Manual*, 11e (ed. S.E. Aiello, M.A. Moses, and D.G. Allen). Kenilworth, NJ: Merck & Co., Inc.

92 Aiken, G.E., Bransby, D.I., and McCall, C.A. (1993). Growth of yearling horses compared to steers on high-and low-endophyte infected tall fescue. *J. Equine Vet. Sci.* 13 (1): 26–28.

93 Martin, K.L., Hoffman, R.M., Kronfeld, D.S. et al. (1996). Calcium decreases and parathyroid hormone increases in serum of periparturient mares. *J. Anim. Sci.* 74 (4): 834–839.

94 Cohen, N.D., Gibbs, P.G., and Woods, A.M. (1999). Dietary and other management factors associated with equine colic. *J. Am. Vet. Med. Assoc.* 215 (1): 53–60.

95 Hillyer, M.H., Taylor, F.G.R., Proudman, C.J. et al. (2002). Case control study to identify risk factors for simple colonic obstruction and distension colic in horses. *Equine Vet. J.* 34 (5): 455–463.

96 Hoffman, R.M., Kronfeld, D.S., Herbein, J.H. et al. (1998). Dietary carbohydrates and fat influence milk composition and fatty acid profile of Mare's milk. *J. Nutr.* 128 (12): 2708S–2711S.

97 Kronfeld, D.S., Holland, J.L., Rich, G.A. et al. (2004). Fat digestibility in *Equus caballus* follows increasing first-order kinetics. *J. Anim. Sci.* 82 (6): 1773–1780.

98 Loy, R.G. (1980). Characteristics of postpartum reproduction in mares. *Vet. Clin. North Am. Large Anim. Pract.* 2 (2): 345–360.

99 McKenzie, H.C. (2011). Equine hyperlipidemias. *Vet. Clin. North Am. Equine Pract.* 27 (1): 59–72.

100 Watson, T.D.G., Burns, L., Packard, C.J., and Shepherd, J. (1993). Effects of pregnancy and lactation on plasma lipid and lipoprotein concentrations, lipoprotein composition and post-heparin lipase activities in Shetland pony mares. *J. Reprod. Fertil.* 97 (2): 563–568.

101 Burden, F.A., Du, T.N., Hazell-Smith, E., and Trawford, A.F. (2011). Hyperlipemia in a population of aged donkeys: description, prevalence, and potential risk factors. *J. Vet. Intern. Med.* 25 (6): 1420–1425.

102 Hammond, A. (2004). Management of equine hyperlipaemia. *In Pract.* 26 (10): 548–552.

21

Feeding Growing Horses

Stewart K. Morgan and Megan Shepherd

KEY POINTS

- Mares are seasonal "long-day" breeders with an 11 m gestation period; therefore, foal growth is seasonal as well, and forage accessibility varies by region and pasture management.
- Horses are a precocial species and foals are relatively mature and mobile from the moment of birth.
- Feeding young growing horses requires a balanced diet that contains all of the essential nutrients, in adequate quantities and correct proportion to each other.

21.1 Introduction

Although a continuum, the first 2 years of growth in horses is linear and can be divided into 5 periods based on the source of nutrients (diet and season) and physiological differences in the pattern of growth [1]. The neonate or newborn (0–2 mos) undergoes an incredibly complex array of changes in which the source of nutrition must change from the passive intake via the umbilical cord and placenta to standing, finding, and sucking mare's milk, and relies on milk quality for the majority of energy and nutrients. The suckling foal (2–6 mos) is still nursing; however, milk quality and quantity are decreasing as foal growth is increasing through summer. The weanling (6–12 mos) has completed their transition from milk to forage, often in the form of hay, and concentrates through the fall and winter. A yearling (12–24 mos) consumes forage, possibly in the form of spring and summer pasture, and a feed. Two- to five-year-olds are growing at a slower rate and might be in training or an imposed exercise program. When nutritional or diet-related problems arise, a systematic iterative review of the growing horse, the ration, and the feeding method is recommended. See Appendix C Nutrition Competencies of Equine Veterinarians.

21.2 Animal Assessment

The body weight (BW) for growing horses ranges from 20 to 900 kg between birth and maturity (Table 21.1). The recommended daily nutrient intakes are presented (Table 21.2) per 100 kg of expected mature, not current, weight. The growth pattern of horses is such that the most rapid rate of growth occurs *in utero* during late gestation; however, post-parturition growth rate resembles a sine wave notably mirroring seasons (day length and temperature) and forage availability (Figure 21.1) [3]. In general, growth rates are highest in the youngest, and therefore malnutrition before weaning is likely to result in abnormalities more rapidly and likely more detrimental than after weaning, highlighting the importance of broodmare nutrition and milk composition. See Chapter 20 Feeding Broodmares.

In 2015, 5.8% of foals died in the first 30 d following birth; 3.3% in the first 2 d, and the other 2.5% between 3 and 30 d. For foals <1 yr of age, conditions commonly attributed to causing death were injury, wounds, or trauma (27.8% of deaths); digestive problems other than colic, such as diarrhea (17.8%); respiratory problems (15.4%); and failure to get milk or colostrum (13.2%) [5].

Equine Clinical Nutrition, Second Edition. Edited by Rebecca L. Remillard.

Table 21.1 Growth rate of young horses from birth to maturity as a percent of mature size.[a]

Age	Light horse breeds[b]		Pony breeds[c]	Draft breeds[d]
(mos)	Weight (%)	Height[e] (%)	Weight (%)	Weight (%)
Birth	8–11	61–64	7.5–8.5	
1	17–20	67–70	15–17	
3	30–33	76–79	28–31	
6	44–47	83–86	41–45	34–38
9	55–58	87–90	51–59	
12	63–67	90–92	66–75	52–55
18	78–85	94–96	84–86	69–73
24	87–92	96–98	95	75–80
30	91–96	97–99		
36	94–99	98–100		90
48	98–99	99–100		
60	100	100		

[a] See Appendix E. Average Body Weight and Height of horses.
[b] Thoroughbreds, Quarter Horse, and Arabians.
[c] Shetland and Welsh crosses with mature weight 175–182 kg.
[d] Percherons are on the high end; Belgians are on the low end.
[e] Height at withers is less variable and less affected by conditions than weight.

21.2.1 Growth

Neonates weigh approximately 10% of adult weight at birth and achieve nearly 30 and 45% of adult BW by 3 and 6 m, respectively, consuming mare's milk [1, 2, 6]. By 1 yr of age, the young horse will weigh nearly 65% of adult BW, long yearling (≥18 mos) will be about 80% whereas 2-yr-old horses generally will be 90% of adult BW. Skeletal growth, represented by gains in wither height, will achieve maturity by

Table 21.2 Recommended daily nutrient intakes for growing horses per 100 kg expected mature body weight.

Nutrient	Units	Age (mos) 4	6	12	18	24
Digestible energy	Mcal	2.66[a]	3.10	3.76	3.84	3.74
Crude protein	g	134	135	169	160	154
Lysine	g	5.8	5.8	7.3	6.9	6.6
Calcium	g	7.8	7.7	7.5	7.4	7.3
Phosphorus	g	4.3	4.3	4.2	4.1	4.1
Magnesium	g	0.7	0.8	1.1	1.2	1.3
Potassium	g	2.2	2.6	3.5	4.0	4.4
Sodium	g	0.8	1.0	1.4	1.6	1.8
Chloride	g	3.1	4.0	5.3	6.4	7.1
Sulfur	g	1.3	1.6	2.4	2.9	3.2
Copper	mg	8	11	16	19	21
Iron	mg	42	54	80	97	107
Manganese	mg	34	43	64	78	86
Zinc	mg	34	43	64	78	86
Cobalt	mg	0.0	0.1	0.1	0.1	0.1
Iodine	mg	0.3	0.4	0.6	0.7	0.8
Selenium	mg	0.1	0.1	0.2	0.2	0.2
Vitamin A	KIU	1.5	1.9	2.9	3.5	3.9
Vitamin D	IU	748	959	1118	1232	1176
Vitamin E	IU	67	86	128	155	172
Thiamin	mg	2.52	3.24	4.82	5.82	6.44
Riboflavin	mg	1.68	2.16	3.22	3.88	4.30

[a] For example, a 4-month-old foal with a mature BW estimated at 550 kg would require 2.66 × 5.5 = 14.63 Mcal DE/d.
Source: Adapted from NRC [2]; Table 16-3 using nutrients required for a growing horse with a mature BW of 500 kg BCS 4–6/9 consuming 2.5% BW.

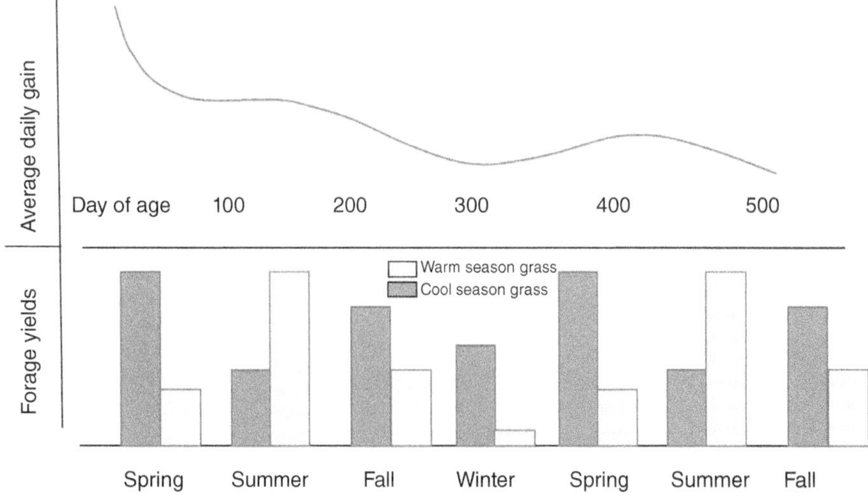

Figure 21.1 Average daily gain of growing horses relative to forage yields through the seasons. *Source:* Adapted from Staniar [3] and Mowrey and Pond [4].

3 yrs of age, but final mature BW may not occur until 5 yrs of age (Table 21.1).

A foal's rate of growth is dependent on foal genetics (breed) and outside factors such as epigenetics and nutrition. Average daily gain (ADG) of a 500-kg mature horse is highest for nursing foals (1 kg/d) and decreases to 0.7, 0.6, 0.5, and 0.2 kg/d for 6-, 9-, 12-, and 24-mo-old horses, respectively (Figure 21.1) [1, 3]. A slower growth rate decreases the need for energy and nutrients but also masks nutrient deficiencies, and if slowed sufficiently, mature body size will be reduced. Foals display catch-up growth after periods of malnutrition; however, catch-up growth is successful when malnutrition spans over a relatively short period, i.e. a few weeks. A fast growth rate does not influence adult stature, but does increase the risk of developmental orthopedic diseases (DOD). This risk is reduced after 1 yr of age because skeletal growth rate, using wither height rather than BW, has slowed considerably (Table 21.1). For example, 100% of the cannon bone's length and 90% of the circumference are reached by 1 yr of age. Bone mineral content and strength also increase during growth. Although bone mineral content peaks between 3 and 4 yrs of age, most of the increase occurs during the first year of life [7].

21.2.2 Body Condition Score

Although the 9-point body condition score (BCS) scale was not developed using foals, it is still helpful in identifying foals that are under- or over-conditioned [8]. Ideal BCS for adult horses ranges from 4/9 (moderately thin) to 6/9 (moderately fleshy) and is likely ideal for the foal [9, 10]. As in other species, promoting a lean body condition may promote longevity and reduce the risk of DOD [11]. Tracking serial foal BW, height, and BCS over time is critical for monitoring the rate and quality of growth. Ideally, growth will be steady from birth to maturity across different seasons and environments through the first 2 yrs, avoiding severe growth depressions or spurts. The assessment frequency is case-dependent in that a 3-yr-old with an ideal BW and BCS may need only be assessed four times a year, whereas a 6-mo-old weanling with a high ADG and early signs of DOD should be assessed weekly. See Chapter 2 Nutritional Assessment of the Horse.

21.3 Ration Assessment

The gastrointestinal tract (GIT) is relatively smaller and the liver larger in foals, with each constituting 3.5% of BW at birth and similar to adults by 6 m of age [12]. The foal has an undeveloped large intestine at birth. Intestinal tract length increases rapidly in the fetus and foal, from mid-gestation to 1 yr of age, and changes little thereafter [13]. Small intestine length increases rapidly during the first month of life, while large intestine length increases when forage consumption begins. Feeding the growing horse must take into consideration the GIT physiology and the changes through the first year of life.

Mares' milk contains 10% dry matter (DM) and 5–6 Mcal digestible energy (DE)/kg DM. Solid feed ration DE concentrations of 3.2, 2.9, and 2.3 Mcal DE/kg DM are recommended for 4-, 6-, and 12-mo-old horses, respectively, whereas 2.0–1.7 DE/kg DM are suggested for 18- and 24-mo-old horses, respectively [2]. Growing horses should be provided a complete and balanced ration, meeting the energy and nutrient requirements, fed within the limits of their voluntary dry matter intake (DMI) as a %BW (Table 21.4). Solid feeds (e.g., forage, manufactured feed, etc.) should be introduced before weaning to allow the nursing foal to adjust. Although foals begin consuming forages within days of birth, the feeding program should progressively increase the proportion of forages in the ration through to maturity. Ideally, the forage quality and nutrient profile are determined first, and then manufactured feeds are added to complement the nutrient profile of the forage to meet the growing horse's energy, protein, and micronutrient needs. See Chapter 13 Manufactured Feeds.

21.3.1 Feeds

21.3.1.1 Milk

The first milk consumed, within 1–6 hrs of birth, is colostrum, which provides a concentrated form of immunoglobulins, nutrients, and water to support the newborn. Colostrum is produced by the selective secretion of circulating immunoglobulins (Ig) into the udder during the last month of gestation, with most of the Ig secreted during the last 2 wks. The mare's colostrum contains three major types of immunoglobulins: IgG, 1gM, and IgA, which normally at foaling are present at concentrations of approximately 4000–10 000, 500–1500, and 50–200 mg/dL, respectively [15]. The nutrient content of colostrum is primarily protein (19%) due to immunoglobulins, low fat (0.7%), and 5% lactose with macrominerals and microminerals.

By day 2, the foal is sucking mare's milk containing 500–600 kcal DE/kg, 2–3% protein, 0.3% lysine, 1.5–2.0% fat and 6% lactose with 1200 ppm Ca, 725 ppm P (as fed), macrominerals (magnesium, potassium, sodium, sulfur), and trace minerals (copper, zinc, selenium, manganese, iron, and cobalt) for the first 4 wks [2]. Although difficult to directly measure, foals may consume 15–25% of the BW in milk/d in the first wk [1]. The greatest increase in intestinal length after birth is in the small intestine from 1 to 4 wks postpartum in response to milk consumption which corresponds to the period of most rapid growth in the foal [16]. Assessing the nutritional adequacy of the milk must be done based on observing normal suckling times and frequency, increase in foal BW and condition, and observing the mare's udder and behaviors toward the foal.

21.3.1.2 Complementary Feeds

As the small intestinal enzyme lactase decreases and sucrose and maltase activity increase, the foal will transition to solid feeds with other sources of carbohydrates [17]. Concentrates fed to growing horses often contain soybean, corn, oats, and barley, providing approximately 3.0 Mcal DE/kg DM, 15% crude protein (CP) with macrominerals and trace minerals, and vitamins A and E. After 2 m of age, the amount of milk produced by most mares has declined and may no longer meet the foal's nutritional needs, thus a concentrate specifically formulated for nursing foals may be needed. As the energy and nutrient requirements of weanlings cannot be met feeding forage alone in the fall and winter, concentrates are also fed at 1.5–3.0% BW. Yearlings in spring may also require an energy concentrate (1–2% BW) if an adequate forage is not available. The nutritional requirement of 18 to 24-mo-old horses may be met by feeding a legume forage; however, if, in training, additional calories may be provided with a concentrate fed at 1–1.5% BW (Table 21.3 and Figure 21.1) [2]. The proper amount to feed initially could be based on a ration formulation or commercial manufacturer's recommendations and then adjusted as necessary to maintain a proper body condition for that individual horse.

21.3.1.3 Forage

Foals graze very little at less than 30 d of age, but as they mature, the time spent foraging increases from 20% to almost 50% of the day between 1 and 5 m of age. By 10 m, weanlings spend 60% of their time grazing [17]. The greatest change in hindgut length segments occurs between 1 and 6 m of age as foals increase their foraging activity. The development of a functional large bowel is important in the dietary transition from milk and grain (soluble carbohydrates) to the structural carbohydrates of forage [16].

The forage offered must be palatable to weanlings, yearlings, and older, to ensure an adequate DMI [20]. The forage digestible dry matter (DDM) and energy density (Mcal/kg DM) must be sufficiently high to meet the estimated daily energy requirement (DER) of the growing horse within an edible volume of feed (DMI). Forage quality is assessed through objective nutrient analyses and subjective measures (smell, color, feel, and physical contents). See Ration Analysis and Subjective Assessments in Chapter 10. DM digestibility and voluntary DMI are inversely related to the forage acid detergent fiber (%ADF) and neutral detergent fiber (%NDF), respectively. As ADF and NDF increase in the forage DM, the voluntary DMI and DM digestibility decrease, and the nutritional value of the forage decreases. Initially, high-quality forages with relative feeding values (RFV of >120) are fed to weanlings; good-quality forages (RFV >100) are fed to yearlings (12 to 18 mos old), and moderate-quality forages (RFV 85–100) are fed to 2 to 5-yr-old horses (Table 21.4) [14]. See Relative Feed Value in Chapter 10. In cases where the available forage energy density and protein are insufficient to meet the growing horse's nutrient requirement within the voluntary DMI, a concentrate or complementary feed should provide the difference between the animal requirement and that provided by forage alone [21].

The legumes, of which alfalfa and the clovers are the most common, are higher in protein, vitamins, and some minerals (calcium and magnesium) than are the grasses. Immature forages are higher in protein, vitamins, and minerals on a DM basis relative to more mature forages. The seasonality of foal growth generally matches the nutrient

Table 21.3 Approximate feed dry matter intakes and forage to concentrate ratios for growing horses.

	Weanlings		Yearlings		Long Yearlings		> 2-yr-olds	
Age (months)	(4–12)		(12–18)		(18–24)		(24–36)	
	Average daily gain				Training			
	Moderate	High	Moderate	High	No	Yes	No	Yes
Dry Matter Intake (% BW)	2.0%	3.5%	2.0%	3.0%	2%	2.5%	1.8%	2.5%
Dry matter ratio								
Forage (minimum)	30		40		55	50	65	50
Concentrate	70		60		45	50	35	50

Source: Adapted from NRC [19]; Tables 5-2A and 5-4, and Geor et al. [18].

Table 21.4 Comparison of major nutrient concentrations between forage averages and ration recommendations for growing horses [14].

Horse to Forage Comparison	Digestible energy	Protein	Lysine	Calcium	Phosphorus	DMI	RFV
	Dry matter basis					% BW	
Age:	Mcal/kg	%	%	%	%		
Weanling: 4 mos	3.17	15.9	0.7	0.93	0.52	2.0–3.5	>120
Weanling: 6 mos	2.87	12.5	0.5	0.71	0.40	2.0–3.5	>120
Yearling: 12 mos	2.34	10.5	0.5	0.47	0.26	2.0–3.0	>100
Long yearling: 18 mos	1.98	8.3	0.4	0.38	0.21	2.0–2.5	>100
2 yr old	1.74	7.2	0.3	0.34	0.19	1.8–2.5	85–100
Forages:							
Legume							
Pasture: vegetative	2.71	26.5	1.37	1.31	0.37	3.6[a]	198[b]
Hay: immature	2.62	20.5	1.05	1.56	0.31	3.3	171
Hay: mid-mature	2.43	20.8	1.06	1.37	0.30	2.8	136
Hay: mature	2.21	17.8	0.89	1.22	0.28	2.4	106
Grass							
Pasture: vegetative	2.39	26.5	0.92	0.56	0.44	2.6	141
Hay: immature	2.36	18	0.63	0.72	0.34	2.4	121
Hay: mid-mature	2.18	13.3	0.46	0.66	0.29	2.1	97
Hay: mature	2.04	10.8	0.38	0.47	0.26	1.7	76

[a] Forage %DMI =120/%NDF.
[b] Forage relative feeding value = %DDM × %DMI × 0.775; where %DDM = 88.9 − (0.779 × %ADF).
Source: Adapted from NRC [2]; Table 16-3 using nutrients required for a 500 kg mature horse BCS 4-6/9. Forage data from Table 16-6.

availability of grassland forages in North America (Figure 21.1). Forage consumption by nursing foals, raised by mares on spring pastures, is initially minimal. However, as the large bowel and microbiome develop, summer (warm-season grasses) forages are consumed in increasingly greater quantities. Weanlings with access to cool-season grass pasture have an average ADG of approximately 1.0 kg/d depositing body fat in preparation for winter. Growth (ADG) through the winter is typically slowed (0.5 kg/d) when pasture forage is unavailable, but the reappearance of grasses in the spring provides energy and nutrients for a higher (approximately 1.0 kg/d) ADG (Figure 21.1).

21.3.2 Key Nutrients

While all nutrients are important during growth, those of greatest concern are involved with healthy musculoskeletal development. Nutrients of concern for musculoskeletal development include energy (deficit, excess), protein (deficiency), calcium (absolute or relative deficiency), phosphorus (relative excess), copper (deficiency), and zinc (deficiency). The requirement for energy and nutrients expressed as a concentration in ration DM is highest in the youngest (Table 21.4) because younger animals have lower BWs but higher ADG than older animals. See Ration Assessment in Chapter 10.

21.3.2.1 Water

Foals, like other young animals, have greater total body water content than adults [22, 23]. The body water content of the neonatal foal ranges from 71% to 83% of BW at birth and declines to approximately 60–70% body water in adulthood. Furthermore, for the first 8 wks of life, foals also have reduced urinary concentrating ability, compared to adult horses [23–25]. This reduced ability to concentrate urine indicates that water availability is of particular importance to the foal. Milk consumption by foals generally meets their daily water requirement [26–28]. Foals on pasture that are actively nursing generally do not consume water, even when freely available [26]. However, foals should have access to unlimited free-choice potable water throughout growth. While clinical evidence of dehydration is not as obvious in the foal as in the adult horse, signs of dehydration may include loss of skin turgor (skin tenting when raised), dry mucous membranes, and reduced corneal moisture [23].

21.3.2.2 Energy

Foal DER is the sum of that required for tissue maintenance plus that needed to increase tissue mass measured as growth (Table 21.1). Energy is the first limiting nutrient, for example, the growth rate is lower in an energy-deficient ration with adequate concentrations of all other essential nutrients. DE requirements are also inversely associated with environmental temperature, particularly with low temperatures. Foals have a lower critical temperature (LCT) depending on age ranging from 20 °C for 1-wk-old neonates to 0 °C for yearlings. The DE intake for the foal should be increased by 1.3% daily for each degree Celsius the environmental temperature is below the LCT [29, 30]. Conversely, excess energy, fueling a high growth rate (high ADG), increases the risk of orthopedic disease in foals [31]. The impact of excess energy in DOD is likely due to an imbalance of protein and minerals relative to the growth rate.

21.3.2.2.1 Fat

Fats are sources of energy, carriers of fat-soluble vitamins, and sources of essential fatty acids. Both linoleic acid (LA; 18:2 n-6) and α-linolenic acid (ALA; 18:3 n-3) are essential fatty acids in mammals. Dietary fats (oils) are used to increase the energy density of equine rations. Increasing dietary fat concentration increases ration energy density which in turn decreases the amount of feed needed to meet DER. Ration caloric density is highest for growth (2–3 Mcal/kg DM), and accomplished using oils (Table 13.4) and oilseeds (Table 13.2). A dietary minimum of 0.5% DM has been suggested for linoleic acid which is relatively easy to meet with <1% fat in the ration while the forage portion of the ration provides ALA [2]. There are no dietary omega-3 fatty acid recommendations for growing horses. See Dietary Fatty Acids in Chapter 6.

21.3.2.3 Protein

The protein requirements for foals less than 4 mos old have not been defined, and are assumed to be met largely by mare's milk [2]. For horses older than 4 m, the protein requirement for growth is calculated using the "elevated" crude protein requirement for a horse at maintenance (1.44 g CP/kg BW), the quantity of protein required for a given ADG, and an estimate of dietary protein efficiency which declines with age. The efficiency in which dietary protein is converted to tissue protein is highest (50%) for 4 to 6-mo-old foals and declines to 30% for yearlings and older. The quantity of dietary protein required by growing horses, as similar to other species, is also dependent on the essential amino acid profile, referred to as the quality of the protein source [32]. See Protein Quality in Chapter 7.

The amino acid requirement has been assumed to be similar to that of skeletal muscle and mare's milk which are similar [2, 33]. Lysine and threonine are thought to be limiting amino acids for growth; however, to date, recommendations on other amino acids (arginine, histidine, isoleucine, leucine, methionine, phenylalanine, and valine) are lacking to establish an accurate recommendation. Lysine is the first limiting amino acid in growth, essential for normal tissue accretion and daily gain in the growing horse [34–36]. Threonine has been suggested as the second-limiting amino acid for yearlings given threonine added to lysine adequate rations increased muscle gain [37, 38]. Dietary threonine (0.47–0.50% DM) and lysine (0.55–0.62% DDB) for weanlings have been suggested as sufficient, and synthetic forms of both have been utilized by horses [38, 39]. The lysine requirement for growth is calculated as 4.3% of the CP requirement [2].

21.3.2.4 Macrominerals

Ensuring adequate calcium (Ca) and phosphorus (P) intake is critical for musculoskeletal development. Ninety-nine percent of total body calcium and 81% total phosphorous are found within the bone of the growing horse [40]. The proportion of calcium should be greater than that of phosphorus in the diet, for example, Ca:P should be 1:1 to 3:1. Feeding a diet with a Ca:P ratio below 1:1, where P > Ca, leads to impaired calcium absorption and may lead to nutritional secondary hyperparathyroidism. Phosphorus can also interfere with trace mineral availability [41]. Deficiencies or excesses in dietary calcium or phosphorus intake may be associated with DOD [42–45]. The requirement for Ca and P during growth is calculated based on that needed for maintenance of current BW plus that for growth. The recommendation for dietary calcium during growth is based on an estimated dietary calcium absorption efficiency of 50%, that required by skeletal growth, and endogenous losses of calcium [2].

21.3.2.5 Trace Minerals

21.3.2.5.1 Copper

Copper (Cu) is an essential micronutrient in the synthesis and maintenance of connective tissue and metalloenzyme lysyl oxidase activity, an enzyme involved in cross-linking the extracellular matrix proteins collagen and elastin [46, 47]. Copper is also essential in cellular metabolism, superoxide dismutase activity, hematopoiesis, pigmentation because tyrosinase is a copper metalloenzyme, and neurotransmitter synthesis. Multiple studies have reported an association between low copper intake and DOD in foals such as physitis and osteochondrosis, specifically osteochondritis dissecans (OCD) [43, 48]. Dietary Cu intake has been increasingly recognized as chondroprotective for horses at risk for OCD [42, 43, 49, 50]. Foals born with higher hepatic Cu concentrations showed greater resolution of OCD lesions at 11 m of age than those with lower hepatic copper concentrations [49]. Milk is a poor source of copper, and, therefore, fetal hepatic copper stores are dependent on the mare's intake during gestation. There is a relationship between Cu and zinc such that zinc poisoning of pasture or water exposed to smelter efflux has been associated with osteochondrotic lesions [51, 52]. Dietary Zn to Cu ratio of 4:1 to 5:1 has been recommended [2, 53, 54].

21.3.2.5.2 *Iodine*

Iodine is a nutrient with essential functions in thyroid hormone synthesis. Thyroid hormones are essential regulators of metabolism and are thus of particular importance during growth. Milk is a poor source of iodine and fetal iodine stores are dependent on the mare's ration during gestation.

Broodmares with iodine deficiency may give birth to foals with congenital hypothyroidism associated with two syndromes: congenital hypothyroidism and dysmaturity syndrome, and congenital hyperthyroidism with goiter [55–57]. See Iodine in Chapter 8 and Trace Minerals in Chapter 20.

21.3.2.5.3 *Selenium*

Selenium (Se) functions as an antioxidant and prevents lipid peroxidation. Foals initially obtain Se from the dam transplacentally, and then through colostrum and milk [58]. Selenium deficiency is most common in regions with low concentrations of soil selenium [59]. White muscle disease (WMD) is nutritional muscular dystrophy that is associated with lipid peroxidation of muscle, giving the muscle a chalky white appearance (Figure 8.4). Most (82%) cases of WMD occur in horses younger than 4 yrs, with the majority in foals younger than weaning age [45, 60]. Foals at risk for WMD are those born to dams fed a selenium-deficient diet, that is, low soil Se and no dietary Se supplementation. The lipid peroxidation seen in WMD is believed to occur as a consequence of elevated free radical damage in the myocytes. The condition has a high (30–45%) mortality rate in affected horses [60].

White muscle disease can occur as an acute or subacute (or skeletal) condition. The acute form of WMD is associated with the highest mortality [60, 61]. Foals may be stillborn, alive but affected at birth, or appear normal at birth but develop symptoms later. These symptoms may include a listless appearance, stiffness, weakness, a stilted hopping gait in the rear legs, and muscle pain. The tongue may be affected, resulting in difficulty with nursing and swallowing which may result in aspiration pneumonia.

Serum activities of creatine phosphokinase (CPK) and aspartate transferase (AST) may be above 5000 and 500 IU/L, respectively. The increase in CPK and AST activities may occur before clinical signs. Myoglobin that is lost from damaged muscles is excreted in the urine, giving urine a pink to coffee-colored appearance. Both the skeletal and myocardial muscles may be affected. Young foals exhibit more myocardial, diaphragmatic, and respiratory muscle involvement. These foals develop respiration difficulties, pulmonary edema, heart failure, and frequently die within a few hours to 2 days after the onset of clinical symptoms. Older foals may become recumbent and have a normal temperature, increased heart and respiratory rate, excess salivation, painful subcutaneous swellings under the mane, and desquamation of tongue epithelium. Muscular exertion may initiate the onset of symptoms. Other conditions, including infectious diseases (tetanus and botulism) and cardiac toxins (monensin and oleander) may mimic WMD.

Foal selenium status can be determined using Se concentration or glutathione peroxidase activity in plasma or whole blood. Treatment of WMD involves exercise restriction, to minimize oxidative stress and further muscle trauma, and repeated administration of intramuscular selenium (0.06 mg/kg BW) [62]. Vitamin E and selenium behave synergistically, as both function as antioxidants. In most species studied, clinical signs of a deficiency of either vitamin E or selenium can be at least partially rectified by supplementing the diet with the other. While selenium is considered essential for thyroid hormone synthesis, there is no evidence suggesting that selenium deficiency in the foal negatively impacts thyroid hormone production.

21.3.2.6 Vitamins

Vitamin E, like selenium, functions as an antioxidant and prevents lipid peroxidation. Vitamin E deficiency has been associated with the development of neuroaxonal dystrophy/equine degenerative myeloencephalopathy (NAD/EDM) and equine motor neuron disease (EMND) [63–66]. NAD/EDM is a chronic progressive neurodegenerative disease that is associated with lipid peroxidation and axonal degeneration in the brain stem and spinal cord of horses <1 yr old. Foals at risk for NAD/EDM are those that have a genetic predisposition to developing the disorder and are born to vitamin-E-deficient dams [63, 65, 67, 68]. See Muscle Disorders in Chapter 25. Plasma or serum α-tocopherol concentrations are used to determine vitamin E status; <1.5 μg/mL indicates a deficit, 1.5–2 μg/mL are considered marginal, and >2 μg/mL are indicative of an adequate vitamin E status [67].

21.4 Feeding Management

21.4.1 Neonate

21.4.1.1 Feeding Behavior

Over 80% of mares foal between evening and dawn, and most foals will stand within 15–180 min following birth, an inherent protection mechanism of a prey species. This time to stand averages about 60–70 min for colts and 40–55 min for fillies. The time is not affected by birth weight, although tends to be faster for pony breeds. Within 3–9 min after standing, most foals, although unsteady and uncoordinated, search for the mare's udder. The foal should be allowed to find the udder unassisted, as this helps imprinting and recognition of each other. Most foals will have nursed twice within 2.5 hrs from birth. Both successful nursing and the passing of fetal-formed feces, meconium, usually occur at 1–2 hrs of age, but may take place up to 6 hrs. About 5% of foals need help nursing, and about 2% need help passing meconium. The foal's difficult task of lying down will generally be accomplished shortly following nursing, although some foals will sleep while standing, and may fall while in a deep sleep [69]. If on pasture with the dam, newborn foals spend 6–9% of the time grazing [26]. As a precocial species, by the end of the first day of life, the foal will be self-grooming, urinating, defecating, galloping, and grazing. Foals are orphaned for a variety of reasons, such as loss of the dam, rejection, or inadequate milk production by the mare. In a 2015 USDA report, 3.3% of foals die within the first 2 d of life and 13.2% of all deaths in foals under 1 yr of age was attributed to failure to get milk or colostrum [5]. See Sidebar 21.1.

Sidebar 21.1: Feeding Milk Replacer to Orphans

For orphans, the best solution for foals younger than 4 mos of age is grafting the orphan onto another lactating mare for psychological reasons, or hand-feeding milk from a different mare. However, feeding the orphan milk replacer may be most practical. Due to nutrient differences in milk across species, an equine-specific milk replacer from a familiar, reputable manufacturer is advised. Check the manufacturer's feeding and reconstituting instructions, as a liquid with 11% w/w total solids (110 g powder/1000 g water) is desirable to mimic mare's milk. More water added delivers lower quantities of nutrients. Less water added creates higher concentrations of total solids which may cause diarrhea, gas, and pain.

Begin feeding milk at 10% BW on an as-fed basis daily, and gradually increase to 20–25% BW by 10 d of age. Daily milk consumed should be divided into multiple small meals; every 2–4 hrs during the first 2 wks of age, reducing to every 6 hrs between 2–4 wks of age, then to every 8 hrs after 1 m of age. Teaching the foal to drink from a bucket with a nipple requires less direct involvement. Introducing milk replacer pellets in the first wk of age and transitioning the orphan to milk replacer pellets early will further simplify management. Once the foal's milk replacer pellet consumption is 1–2% BW DMI, introduce a suckling foal growth concentrate (labeled for suckling foals, not weanlings) into the daily feedings and gradually transition the foal off the milk replacer pellets. Discontinue liquid milk replacer once the foal's solid feed consumption is about 2–3% BW DMI.

21.4.1.2 Colostrum

Immediately following the parturition, within the first 12 hrs of life, the first nutrients that the neonate receives are in the form of colostrum. The early consumption of colostrum also contributes to the circulatory volume in the newborn [27]. Colostrum is a thick, sticky, yellow-white protein-rich fluid produced by the mare's udder that provides passive delivery of maternal antibodies [70–74]. The mare's placenta does not transfer immunoglobulins to the fetus; hence, the foal, for the first 4 m of life, is reliant on the passive transfer of mare immunoglobulins via colostrum for immune protection [73, 75, 76]. Within the first 12 hrs of birth, the foal's small intestinal mucosa is permeable to the immunoglobulin macromolecules, after which the mucosa no longer allows the passage of immunoglobulin and the mare ceases to produce colostrum [77]. Generally, consumption of 1–2 L of colostrum within 12 hrs following birth is considered an adequate intake, although ingestion of colostrum is difficult to assess directly. Milking the mare's udder for a sample to verify the production of thick sticky fluid and observing the foal suckling within hours of birth are suggestive of colostrum intake. If in doubt, detectable concentrations of immunoglobulins are present within 6 hrs of birth in nursing foals [77]. See Sidebar 21.2. In addition to immunoglobulins, colostrum also contains vitamins, minerals, free amino acids, and other proteins, such as bactericidal lysozyme, hormones, growth factors, cytokines, and bile salt-activated lipase [16, 71, 74, 78].

Sidebar 21.2: Failure of Passive Transfer

Failure of passive transfer (FPT) is the failure of the foal to consume an adequate volume of colostrum or ingestion of poor-quality (low immunoglobulin [IgG]) colostrum. FPT is a risk factor for septicemia, the most common cause of neonatal foal mortality [79, 80]. Factors that reduce/inhibit adequate colostrum intake by the foal include difficult foaling, mare or foal orthopedic problems, mare rejection of foal, injuries to the foal's tongue, premature birth, poor mare udder conformation, and twin foals [80, 81]. In addition, unsanitary environmental conditions and month of birth can negatively influence colostrum intake [76].

Foals born late in the season may be less vigorous due to environmental conditions or receive less rigorous attention than foals born early in the season [80]. Adequacy of passive transfer is generally determined by assessing serum immunoglobulin concentrations in the foal at 12 hrs postpartum [78, 79, 82, 83]. Serum IgG >800 mg/dL is considered adequate, 400–800 mg/dL is considered partial, and <400 mg/dL indicates complete FPT. If FPT or partial FPT is detected (or suspected) in a foal <12-hrs-old, administration of colostrum through a nasogastric tube or bottle should be completed. In the foal >12-hrs-old, intravenous administration of plasma from an adult horse and placing the foal into a sanitary environment with a low risk of exposure to environmental pathogens are recommended [78, 79, 83]

21.4.1.3 Milk

The nutrient content of milk produced by the well-fed healthy mare is assumed to sufficiently meet the foal's macronutrient needs for the first 8 wks of life. The mare's milk does contain trace minerals; however, during the early suckling period, the foal depends on milk and hepatic stores to meet daily requirements [2, 84]. Mare's milk does contain fatty acids, arachidonic acid (ARA), and docosahexaenoic acid (DHA), which are essential for proper neural development [27, 72–74, 85, 86]. Breed-related differences do not appear in the composition of mare's milk [72, 74].

In the first week of lactation, there is a decrease in energy density, amino acid content, and protein content of mare's milk, relative to colostrum content on day 1 [72, 74]. The energy density and protein content of the mare's milk gradually decrease through the first month of lactation, and then remains relatively stable until weaning [27]. Most foals begin nibbling on the mare's forage and the grain mix, if present, within a few days of birth, and generally feeding at the same time as the dam [24]. In this early phase of growth, foals are merely imitating the dam feeding behaviors, deriving little nutritional sustenance from but learning about solid feeds and initiating the physiologic changes to come in the GIT.

21.4.2 Suckling Foal

Nutrient requirements for foals <4 mos of age have not been well defined but as such extrapolated from the composition of mare's milk which is assumed to approximate the maintenance and growth requirements of nursing foals [2, 70, 87]. Foal milk intake is greatest in early lactation and then declines until weaning. Suckling foals consume about 25% BW daily in milk as fed at day 11 which decreases to 18% BW by day 39 postpartum [27, 70]. For the first several weeks, most foals will nurse for 0.5–2 min 18–24 times/d and lie down laterally to sleep for 15–30 min 20–25 times/d. By one month old, foals are nursing 3 times/hr which decreases to one (1 min) bout of nursing/hr by 4 mos of age [2, 26, 88]. The amount of solid feed eaten is inversely associated with the amount of milk consumed. The foal will spend progressively more time consuming solid feed, for example, 23% by 8 wks of age which increases to 40–50% by 21 wks of age [26]. Concurrently, after 2 mos, the quantity of the milk produced by the mare is declining. Therefore, by 2 mos of age, foals are fed a specifically formulated concentrate, called a creep feed, to meet the growing nursing foal's needs as the mare's milk production wanes.

21.4.2.1 Creep Feeding

Creep feeding is the term used to describe the method of intentionally feeding only the foal(s) while still with the mare(s) (Figure 21.2 [top]). The intentional introduction of a creep feed is beneficial not only in ensuring that the nursing foal's nutritional needs are met as mare milk quantity declines, but also to ensure that the weanling is accustomed to eating a grain mix separate from the mare [89]. Creep feeding may also be financially beneficial. Creep-fed foals had 10% greater ADG, lost less weight post weaning, and had better overall general assessment scores than those foals not creep-fed [90, 91]. Given BW and height are positively associated with the sale price, the post-weaning price for creep-fed foals was also significantly greater than for foals not creep-fed [90, 92].

There are numerous types of physical barriers used to provide feed to a foal(s) only and not the dam(s). The mares routinely fed in a stall can be tied and a separate feeder provided to the foal. Alternatively, a feed box or bucket with bars across the top placed close enough together to prevent the mare from inserting her muzzle into the box but far enough apart to allow the foal to eat from the box may also be used as a creep feeder. Another option is to place a barrier across the stall such that the foal can walk under a bar or board, about 54 in. high for light breeds, to eat creep feed placed in a corner but the mare cannot pass under the barrier. If mare and foal are on pasture, creep-feeding sheds are placed in a location attractive to foals which are close to where mares are fed with good drainage, water, salt, and shade. The creep feeders must be sturdy and safe and with openings wide enough and high enough to allow the foal to enter and exit safely while preventing mare entrance. Feeders should be large enough to accommodate the necessary number of foals and covered to keep the feed dry (Figure 21.2 [bottom]).

Generally, the growth concentrate should be offered at a rate of 0.25–0.5 kg per 100 kg foal BW, but should be tailored to the foal's BCS and growth rate. The macronutrient profile of the creep feed may also reduce the stress of weaning as a higher fat and fiber concentrate was associated with less stress in foals undergoing weaning compared to foals fed a high starch and sugar concentrate [93]. For foals with access to excellent-quality fresh forage, pasture RFV >140, an energy mineral ration balancer may be the only commercial feed needed.

On an as-fed basis, creep feeds should provide ≥16% crude protein, 0.7% lysine, 0.8–0.9% calcium, 0.5–0.6% phosphorus, ≥6% crude fiber, and ≤3% crude fat to ensure the foal can meet their recommended intakes of these

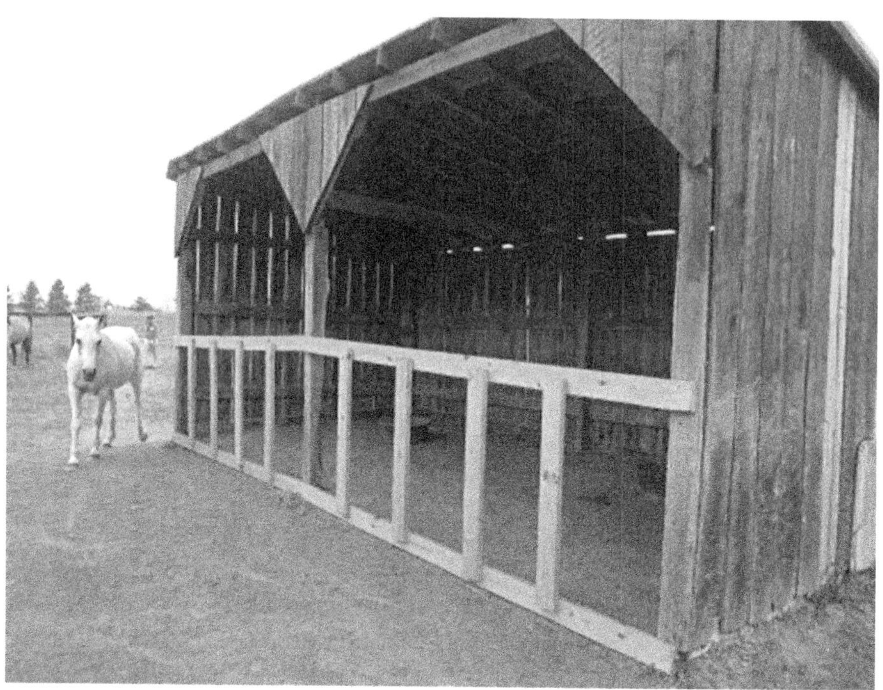

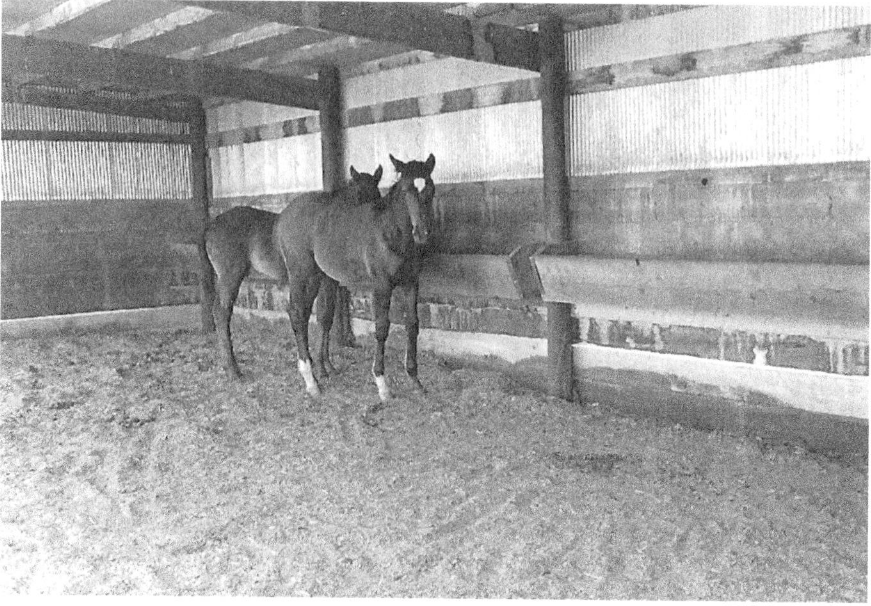

Figure 21.2 A creep-feeder shed (top) with openings wide and high enough to allow foals to access inside rubber feeding pans while preventing mares from entering the shed (*Source:* open access https://doi.org/10.1111/j.2042-3306.2011.00522.x). Inside creep-feeder shed (bottom) providing ample space with sturdy feed troughs.

nutrients [70]. Creep feeds are formulated to provide essential nutrients based on a foal's anticipated ADG. A foal with higher than anticipated ADG requires a creep feed properly formulated with nutrients balanced to the energy density of the product. Conversely, creep feed with an improper balance between non-energy nutrients and caloric density will have nutrient deficiencies. See Case in Point in Chapter 25.

21.4.2.2 Weaning

Weaning is a stressful event and foals are prone to injury; nearly one-third of deaths in foals were attributed to injury, wounds, or trauma [5]. Weaning-induced stress increases plasma cortisol concentration and decreases cell-mediated immune response in foals for up to 40 hrs and mares for 24–36 hrs following separation [94]. These physiological effects decrease food intake and growth rate and increase susceptibility to infectious diseases, gastric ulcers, and the risk of self-induced injury. Depending on the degree of stress and sickness, foals may take several weeks to recover and restart gaining BW. To decrease these risks, in addition to creep feeding, procedures should be utilized to minimize weaning stress.

There are many methods for weaning foals. These methods are the least stressful and most successful when the foal remains in a safe and familiar place. One method referred to as the pasture or interval weaning method removes one or two of the mares with the oldest foals from the herd, leaving their foals with the other familiar mares and foals. The mares should be removed quickly, quietly, and completely, preferably when the foals are occupied somewhere else, to reduce the disturbance to the herd. The mares should be removed to an area completely out of sight and hearing of the herd.

Another method separates the foal from the dam where foals can see, hear, smell, and touch their mothers through a fence, but cannot nurse. Foals physically separated but near the dam for 7 days before complete separation had lower plasma cortisol responses at 2 and 9 days following weaning, and had higher feed intakes in wk 1 of weaning than did foals completely weaned abruptly [95]. This corroborates behavioral observations in which abruptly weaned foals exhibit more emotional stress, increased vocalizations, and activity than gradually weaned foals [96]. Thus, it appears that gradual weaning is preferable to total and abrupt weaning. Although by the second wk after weaning there was no difference in feed intake between foals weaned gradually or abruptly, the major benefit of minimizing weaning stress is reduced risk of injury and disease susceptibility [95].

21.4.2.3 Forages and Concentrates

A range of ration forage to concentrate intakes based on ADG for growing horses is available (Table 21.3); however, forage should be the foundation of the feeding program, and should increase as a portion of the ration as the young horse matures. Forage quality fed to young horses should be sufficiently palatable and digestible to meet a portion of the protein, calcium, and phosphorus requirements within the forage DMI range of the growing horse (Table 21.3). The concentrate portion should complement the forage to meet the requirements which will change as the animal matures and as forage contribution and quality change throughout the year. A growth concentrate is often required initially. Preserved forages are generally lower in fat-soluble vitamins than fresh forages (pasture), hence a concentrate with vitamins will be needed when feeding hay. A general recommendation is to feed the lowest quantity of concentrate divided into 2–3 feedings as needed to complement the forage and balance the ration. All young horses should be provided water and salt *ad libitum*.

Fescue toxicosis in growing horses may be negatively impacted by the consumption of endophyte-infected tall fescue [97]. Tall fescue is infected with the symbiotic endophyte fungus *Neotyphodium coenophialum*, which produces toxic ergot alkaloids [98]. There is evidence that yearlings fed and maintained on a pasture containing ≥80% endophyte-infected tall fescue have significantly lower ADG when compared to young horses maintained on a pasture containing ≤25% endophyte-infected tall fescue [97]. However, yearlings fed a ration containing concentrate and endophyte-infected hay, designing for rapid growth, ADG similar to yearling-fed concentrate and endophyte-free tall fescue [99]. Given that the effects of endophyte-infected tall fescue fed to growing horses have not been determined, feeding infected fescue should be done with caution if ADG is an important parameter [92].

21.4.3 Weanling

Weaning generally occurs at approximately 10 mos of age in feral or free-roaming horses, but at approximately 4–6 mos of age in today's horse industry [100–104]. Weaning is considered stressful and gradually weaning the foal is generally considered most humane and less traumatic than abrupt separation from the dam [90, 103]. Weanlings should be fed to maintain a BCS of 4–5/9 and to achieve a moderate rate of growth (144 g weight gain/100 kg mature BW/d) appropriate for the age and mature BW [2]. Excessive rates of growth, excessive dietary energy intake, and high BCSs have been associated with DOD [44, 105]. The effect of excess energy on DOD risk is likely compounded when key nutrients are not in balance [106, 107].

Forage of high-quality (<35% ADF, <46% NDF, RFV > 120) should be sufficiently palatable and digestible to provide DE and protein to weanlings within 0.5–1.0% BW (Tables 10.3, 21.3, 21.4) [2, 18]. A general recommendation is to feed a growth concentrate at a rate of 1.5–3.0% of current BW divided into 2–3 daily feedings [18]. Ideally, the concentrate should be fed individually; however, for large operations, group feeding is more practical. Energy sources, regardless of quantity, may influence growth. Quarter Horse weanlings fed a concentrate with 52% nonstructural carbohydrates (NSC) DM had higher postprandial glycemic and insulinemic responses and altered growth hormone secretion compared to weanlings fed an 11% NSC DM [108].

21.4.4 Yearling

As the horse grows and the large bowel adaptions to fiber utilization proceed, greater daily quantities of forage should be consumed. Yearlings should be fed to maintain a BCS of 4–5/9 and to achieve a moderate rate of growth (90 g weight gain/100 kg mature BW/d) appropriate for the age and mature BW [2]. Forage of good-quality (<40% ADF, <53% NDF, RFV > 100) should be sufficiently palatable and digestible to provide DE and protein to yearlings at approximately 1% BW (Tables 10.3, 21.3, 21.4) [2]. A general recommendation is to feed a growth concentrate, at a rate of 1.25–2% of current BW divided into 2–3 daily feedings if forage alone is not adequate. See Sidebar 21.3.

21.4.5 Two- to Five-Year-Olds

Two- to five-year-old horses have achieved more than 90% of their mature size. These horses will have a slower rate of growth (36 g weight gain/100 kg mature BW/d) and should have a BCS of 4–5/9 [2]. Forage of moderate-quality (<42% ADF, <60% NDF, RFV 85–100) should be sufficiently palatable and digestible to provide DE and protein within approximately 2.0% BW (Tables 10.3, 21.3, 21.4) [2]. Feeding a legume or grass pasture or immature hay with more than 2 Mcal/kg DM will likely meet the DE, protein and macro mineral recommendations for 2-yr-old horses, whereas feeding a grass pasture or mature hay will likely meet the DE, protein and macro mineral recommendations of 4 to 5-yr-old horses (Table 21.4). A ration balancer providing trace minerals will be needed when pasture is available, however, trace mineral and vitamin A and E supplementation will be needed if there is no access to fresh forage. As the horse approaches maturity, DMI should resemble adult maintenance; however, a higher calorically dense rations (Mcal/kg DM) will be required for imposed exercise or performance training. See Chapter 18 Feeding Athletes and Working Horses.

Sidebar 21.3: Calculating Daily Feeding Recommendations for a Yearling

Animal Assessment

- 355 kg (BCS 4/9) 12-mo-old Thoroughbred colt. Estimated adult BW 545 kg (Table 21.1 and Appendix E).
- DMI for yearlings is 2-3% BW (Table 21.3):
  - Use 2.5% as a starting point, 355 kg x 0.025 = 9 kg feed DM/d with forage to concentrate ratio of 40:60.
- Yearling's daily DE requirement: 3.76 Mcal/100 kg BW × 5.45 = 20.5 Mcal (Table 21.2).
- Forage recommendations for yearlings are RFV >100 and 2.34 Mcal DE/kg DM (Table 21.4). ADF <40% and NDF <53% NDF is recommended for yearlings (Table 10.3).

Ration Assessment

- The best available forage with 20%DM on the farm is a cool-season grass pasture in late spring. The pasture should is highly palatable and the yearling should willingly consume ~1%BW of the pasture forage. On a DM basis, the pasture had estimated textbook values of:

IFN	DE	CP	Lysine	ADF	NDF	Ca	P
#	Mcal/kg	%	%	%	%	%	%
2-02-260	2.39	26.5	0.92	25.0	45.8	0.56	0.44

- Calculated digestible dry matter (DDM), DMI and RFV values:
  - %DDM = 88.9 − (0.779 × %ADF) = 69.4%
  - %DMI = 120/%NDF = 2.6% BW.
  - RFV = %DDM × %DMI × 0.775 = 140 high-quality (Table 10.3).
  - Forage quality is adequate compared with that recommended for yearlings.
- Calculate daily forage intake required to meet the yearling's DE on DM and as fed (AF) basis.
  - Yearling requires 20.5 Mcal/2.39 Mcal DE/kg DM = 8.6 kg forage DM/0.20 = 43 kg (95 lb) pasture forage AF.
  - Check DMI: 8.6 kg forage DM intake/355 kg BW = 2.4% BW.
- Compare forage crude protein (CP), lysine, calcium (Ca), and phosphorus (P) concentrations with recommendations (Table 21.4)

- Recommended [CP] is 10.5%, pasture contains 26.5% CP.
- Recommended [lysine] is 0.5%, pasture contains 0.92% lysine.
- Recommended [Ca] is 0.47%, pasture contains 0.56% Ca.
- Recommended [P] is 0.26% P, pasture contains 0.44 P with Ca:P ratio = 1.3:1.
- If a sufficient quantity of pasture forage is consumed, the CP, lysine, Ca and P needs should be met.

Feeding Management Recommendations

In summary, the pasture grass fulfills the yearling's requirements for CP, lysine, Ca and P, and likely vitamins, within the yearling's voluntary DMI (2-3% BW). Specific instructions:

- The yearling should be able to consume sufficient forage DM if allowed sufficient time on pasture and if ample growth and acreage are available.
- The yearling must be able to consume 43 kg of fresh pasture grass/d to meet his DE requirement, but it is not possible to directly quantify forage intake on pasture; therefore, monitoring yearling's BW and BCS every 2 wks is advisable.
- The cool-season pasture nutrient profiles will decrease as grass plants mature. An energy concentrate may be added if the colt cannot meet daily DE requirement for steady growth on pasture alone.
- Feed mineral ration balancer supplement per manufacturer's feeding recommendations (0.1–0.3% BW). Vitamin intake on the fresh green pasture is likely adequate.
- Offer water and salt block *ad libitum*.

Case in Point

Animal Assessment

In late October, a client asks for a consult on how to feed a 175-kg (BCS 4/9) 6-mo-old Connemara filly she bought at an auction. She has experience feeding horses, but not weanlings. After examining the filly, there are no apparent physical problems. Initial feeding recommendations should be conservative given there is no dietary history:

- An estimated adult BW of 400 kg is based on breed (Appendix E).
- The 6-mo-old pony is 45% of adult weight (Table 21.1).
- DMI is approximately 2–3.5% BW/d (Table 21.4).
- Minimum forage to concentrate to ratio of 30:70 for weanlings (Table 21.3).

1) *What are the filly's daily DE requirement and feed DM intake using 3% DMI?* (Table 21.2).
2) *Using a 30:70 forage to concentrate ratio, what is the approximate weight of forage DM and concentrate DM recommended for this filly?*

Ration Assessment

The best available fresh forage on the farm was the fall growth of a cool-season grass pasture, predominately fescue. The pasture is palatable to the adult horses, and the filly should be able to consume a portion of her DMI. On a DM basis, the pasture last year had the following laboratory analysis:

DE	CP	Lysine	ADF	NDF
Mcal/kg	%	%	%	%
2.2	15.0	0.57	34.4	59.8

3) *Can the pasture be used as forage for the filly?*
4) *How much DE will the filly derive consuming a minimum of 1% BW as pasture? And then how many Mcal of DE from the concentrate will be needed to meet daily DE requirement?*
5) *What does the caloric density of the concentrate need to be to meet the filly's DE requirement?*
6) *The pasture consumed at 1% of BW will not provide sufficient protein, calcium, or phosphorus for the filly. What are your feeding recommendations?*

See Appendix A Chapter 21

References

1 Staniar, W.B. (2013). Feeding the growing horse. In: *Equine Applied and Clinical Nutrition Health, Welfare and Performance* (ed. R.J. Geor, P.A. Harris, and M. Coenen), 243–260. Edinburgh: Saunders Elsevier.

2 National Research Council (2007). *Nutrient Requirements of Horses*. 6th Rev. Animal Nutrition Series, 1–341. Washington, DC: National Academies Press.

3 Staniar, W.B. (2002). Growth and the somatotropic axis in young Thoroughbreds. MS thesis. Virginia Polytechnic Institute and State University. https://vtechworks.lib.vt.edu/handle/10919/26273 (accessed 7 September 2021).
4 Mowrey, R.A. and Pond, K.R. (2008). *Managing Pastures to Feed your Horses*. Raleigh: North Carolina Cooperative Extension Service. https://content.ces.ncsu.edu/managing-pastures-to-feed-your-horse (accessed 19 July 2021).
5 United States Department of Agriculture (2015). *Baseline Reference of Equine Health and Management in the United States*. Fort Collins, CO. https://www.aphis.usda.gov/animal_health/nahms/equine/downloads/equine15/Eq2015_Rept1.pdf (accessed 28 Dec 2021).
6 Martin-Rosset, W. (2005). Growth and development in the equine. In: *The Growing Horse Nutrition and Prevention of Growth Disorders. EAAP #114* (ed. V. Julliand and W. Martin-Rosset), 15–50. Wageningen Academic Publishers.
7 Lawrence, L.A. and Ott, E.A. (1985). The use of non-invasive techniques to predict bone mineral content and strength in the horse. In: *Proceedings of the 9th Equine Nutrition and Physiology Society Symposium*, 110. East Lansing, MI: Equine Nutrition and Physiology Society.
8 Pagan, J.D. (2005). Nutrition of the growing horse: feeding management to reduce DOD. In: *Applied Equine Nutrition: Equine Nutrition Conference (ENUCO)* (ed. A. Lindner), 127–138. Wageningen Academic Publishers.
9 Henneke, D.R., Potter, G.D., Kreider, J.L., and Yeates, B.F. (1983). Relationship between condition score, physical measurements and body fat percentage in mares. *Equine Vet. J.* 15 (4): 371–372.
10 Mottet, R., Onan, G., and Hiney, K. (2009). Revisiting the Henneke body condition scoring system: 25 years later. *J. Equine Vet. Sci.* 29 (5): 417–418.
11 Kealy, R.D., Lawler, D.F., Ballam, J.M. et al. (2002). Effects of diet restriction on life span and age-related changes in dogs. *J. Am. Vet. Med. Assoc.* 220 (9): 1315–1320.
12 Meyer, H., Coenen, M., and Stadermann, B. (1993). The influence of size on the weight of the gastrointestinal tract and the liver of horses and ponies. In: *Proceedings of 13th Equine Nutrition and Physiology Society Symposium*, 18–23. Gainesville, FL: Equine Nutrition and Physiology Society.
13 Smyth, G.B. (1988). Effects of age, sex, and post mortem interval on intestinal lengths of horses during development. *Equine Vet. J.* 20 (2): 104–108.
14 Swinker, A.M. (2014). Hay quality for different classes of horses. Pennsylvania State Extension Service. https://extension.psu.edu/hay-quality-for-different-classes-of-horses (accessed 2 July 2021).
15 Kohn, C.W., Knight, D., Hueston, W. et al. (1989). Colostral and serum IgG, IgA, and IgM concentrations in Standardbred mares and their foals at parturition. *J. Am. Vet. Med. Assoc.* 195 (1): 64–68.
16 Lawrence, L.A. and Lawrence, T.J. (2009). Development of the equine gastrointestinal tract. In: *Advances in Equine Nutrition* IV (ed. J.D. Pagan), 173–183. Nottingham: Nottingham University Press.
17 Boy, V. and Duncan, P. (1979). Time-budgets of camargue horses I. Developmental changes in the time-budgets of foals. *Behaviour* 71 (3–4): 187–201.
18 Geor, R., Harris, P.A., and Coenen, M. (2013). Nutritional requirements, recommendations and example diets. In: *Equine Applied and Clinical Nutrition Health, Welfare and Performance* (ed. R. Geor, P.A. Harris, and M. Coenen), 639–643. Edinburgh: Saunders Elsevier.
19 National Research Council (1989). *Nutrient Requirements of Horses*. 5th Rev. Animal Nutrition Series, 1–100. Washington, DC: National Academies Press.
20 van den Berg, M., Giagos, V., Lee, C. et al. (2016). The influence of odour, taste and nutrients on feeding behaviour and food preferences in horses. *Appl. Anim. Behav. Sci.* 184 (November): 41–50.
21 Lawrence, L.M. (2013). Feeding stallions and broodmares. In: *Equine Applied and Clinical Nutrition: Health, Welfare and Performance* (ed. R.J. Geor, P.A. Harris, and M. Coenen), 231–242. Edinburgh: Saunders Elsevier.
22 Schoeller, D.A. (1989). Changes in total body water with age. *Am. J. Clin. Nutr.* 50 (5): 1175–1176.
23 Magdesian, K.G. (2015). Fluid therapy for neonatal foals. In: *Equine Fluid Therapy* (ed. C.L. Fielding and K.G. Magdesian), 279–298. Wiley.
24 Brewer, B.D., Clement, S.F., Lotz, W.S., and Gronwall, R. (1991). Renal clearance, urinary excretion of endogenous substances, and urinary diagnostic indices in healthy neonatal foals. *J. Vet. Intern. Med.* 5 (1): 28–33.
25 Edwards, D.J., Brownlow, M.A., and Hutchins, D.R. (1990). Indices of renal function: values in eight normal foals from birth to 56 days. *Aust. Vet. J.* 67 (7): 251–254.
26 Crowell-Davis, S.L., Houpt, K.A., and Carnevale, J. (1985). Feeding and drinking behavior of mares and foals with free access to pasture and water. *J. Anim. Sci.* 60 (4): 883–889.
27 Oftedal, O.T., Hintz, H.F., and Schryver, H.F. (1983). Lactation in the horse: milk composition and intake by foals. *J. Nutr.* 113 (10): 2096.
28 Martin, R.G., McMeniman, N.P., and Dowsett, K.F. (1992). Milk and water intakes of foals sucking grazing mares. *Equine Vet. J.* 24 (4): 295–299.

29 Cymbaluk, N.F. (1994). Thermoregulation of horses in cold, winter weather: a review. *Livest. Prod. Sci.* 40 (1): 65–71.

30 Cymbaluk, N.F. (1990). Cold housing effects on growth and nutrient demand of young horses. *J. Anim. Sci.* 68 (10): 3152–3162.

31 Lepeule, J., Bareille, N., Robert, C. et al. (2013). Association of growth, feeding practices and exercise conditions with the severity of the osteoarticular status of limbs in French foals. *Vet. J.* 197 (1): 65.

32 Saastamoinen, M.T. and Koskinen, E. (1993). Effect of fast vs. moderate growth rate related to nutrient intake on developmental orthopaedic disease in the horse. *Anim. Sci.* 56 (1): 135–144.

33 Franco, D., Crecente, S., Vázquez, J.A. et al. (2013). Effect of cross-breeding and amount of finishing diet on growth parameters, carcass and meat composition of foals slaughtered at 15 months of age. *Meat Sci.* 93 (3): 547–556.

34 Ott, E.A., Asquith, R.L., and Feaster, J.P. (1981). Lysine supplementation of diets for yearling horses. *J. Anim. Sci.* 53 (6): 1496–1503.

35 Ahtila, L. and Saastamoinen, M. (2005). Effect of nutrition on the growth curve of weanling foals. In: *The Growing Horse Nutrition and Prevention of Growth Disorders. EAAP #114* (ed. V. Julliand and W. Martin-Rosset), 79–80. Wageningen Academic Publishers.

36 Ott, E.A., Asquith, R.L., Feaster, J.P., and Martin, F.G. (1979). Influence of protein level and quality on the growth and development of yearling foals. *J. Anim. Sci.* 49 (3): 620–628.

37 Graham, P.M., Ott, E.A., Brendemuhl, J.H., and TenBroeck, S.H. (1994). The effect of supplemental lysine and threonine on growth and development of yearling horses. *J. Anim. Sci.* 72 (2): 380–386.

38 Staniar, W.B., Kronfeld, D.S., Wilson, J.A. et al. (2001). Growth of thoroughbreds fed a low-protein supplement fortified with lysine and threonine. *J. Anim. Sci.* 79 (8): 2143.

39 Saastamoinen, M.T. (1996). Protein, amino acid and energy requirements of weanling foals and yearlings. *Pferdeheilkunde* 12 (3): 297–302.

40 Grace, N.D., Pearce, S.G., Firth, E.C., and Fennessy, P.F. (1999). Content and distribution of macro-and micro-elements in the body of pasture-fed young horses. *Aust. Vet. J.* 77 (3): 172–176.

41 Schryver, H.F., Hintz, H.F., and Craig, P.H. (1971). Calcium metabolism in ponies fed a high phosphorus diet. *J. Nutr.* 101 (2): 259–264.

42 van Weeren, P.R. and Jeffcott, L.B. (2013). Problems and pointers in osteochondrosis: twenty years on. *Vet. J.* 197 (1): 96–102.

43 van Weeren, P.R. and Olstad, K. (2016). Pathogenesis of osteochondrosis dissecans: how does this translate to management of the clinical case? *Equine Vet. Educ.* 28 (3): 155–166.

44 van Weeren, P.R. (2006). Etiology, diagnosis, and treatment of OC(D). *Clin. Technol. Equine Pract.* 5 (4): 248–258.

45 Secombe, C.J. and Lester, G.D. (2012). The role of diet in the prevention and management of several equine diseases. *Anim. Feed Sci. Technol.* 173 (1–2): 86–101.

46 Smith-Mungo, L.I. and Kagan, H.M. (1998). Lysyl oxidase: properties, regulation and multiple functions in biology. *Matrix Biol.* 16 (7): 387–398.

47 Rucker, R.B., Kosonen, T., Clegg, M.S. et al. (1998). Copper, lysyl oxidase, and extracellular matrix protein cross-linking. *Am. J. Clin. Nutr.* 67 (5): 996S–1002S.

48 Coskun, A., Ozdemir, O., Erol, M., and Kirbiyik, H. (2016). The relationship of copper concentrations in feed and plasma to developmental orthopedic disease in foals. *Vet. Arh.* 86 (3): 287–294.

49 Van Weeren, P.R., Knaap, J., and Firth, E.C. (2003). Influence of liver copper status of mare and newborn foal on the development of osteochondrotic lesions. *Equine Vet. J.* 35 (1): 67–71.

50 Gee, E.K., Firth, E.C., Morel, P.C.H. et al. (2005). Articular/epiphyseal osteochondrosis in Thoroughbred foals at 5 months of age: influences of growth of the foal and prenatal copper supplementation of the dam. *N. Z. Vet. J.* 53 (6): 448–456.

51 Gunson, D.E., Kowalczyk, D.F., Shoop, C.R., and Ramberg, J.C.F. (1982). Environmental zinc and cadmium pollution associated with generalized osteochondrosis, osteoporosis, and nephrocalcinosis in horses. *J. Am. Vet. Med. Assoc.* 180: 295–299.

52 Messer, N.T. (1981). Tibiotarsal effusion associated with chronic zinc intoxication in three horses. *J. Am. Vet. Med. Assoc.* 178 (3): 294–297.

53 Coger, L.S., Hintz, H.F., Schryver, H.F., and Lowe, J.E. (1987). The effect of high zinc intake on copper metabolism and bone development in growing horses. In: *Proceedings of the 10th Equine Nutrition and Physiology Society Symposium*, 173. Fort Collins, CO: Equine Nutrition and Physiology Society.

54 Hintz, H.F. (1996). Mineral requirements of growing horses. *Pferdeheilkunde* 12 (3): 303–306.

55 Allen, A.L. (2014). Congenital hypothyroidism in horses: looking back and looking ahead. *Equine Vet. Educ.* 26 (4): 190–193.

56 Koikkalainen, K., Knuuttila, A., Karikoski, N. et al. (2014). Congenital hypothyroidism and dysmaturity syndrome in foals: first reported cases in Europe: congenital hypothyroidism and dysmaturity syndrome in foals. *Equine Vet. Educ.* 26 (4): 181–189.

57 Coleman, M.C. and Whitfield-Cargile, C. (2017). Orthopedic conditions of the premature and dysmature foal. *Vet. Clin. North Am. Equine Pract.* 33 (2): 289–297.

58 Montgomery, J.B., Wichtel, J.J., Wichtel, M.G. et al. (2012). The effects of selenium source on measures of selenium status of mares and selenium status and immune function of their foals. *J. Equine Vet. Sci.* 32 (6): 352–359.

59 Jones, G.D., Droz, B., Greve, P. et al. (2017). Selenium deficiency risk predicted to increase under future climate change. *Proc. Natl. Acad. Sci.* 114 (11): 2848–2853.

60 Delesalle, C., de Bruijn, M., Wilmink, S. et al. (2017). White muscle disease in foals: focus on selenium soil content. A case series. *BMC Vet. Res.* 13 (1): 121.

61 Valberg, S.J. (2017). Muscular system. In: *Nutritional Management of Equine Diseases and Special Cases* (ed. B.M. Waldridge), 51–72. Ames, IA: Wiley Blackwell.

62 Johnson, A.L., Divers, T.J., and de Lahunta, A. (2014). Nervous system. In: *Equine Emergencies Treatment and Procedures*, 4e (ed. J.A. Orsini and T.J. Divers), 339–378. St. Louis: Elsevier.

63 Finno, C.J., Miller, A.D., Sisó, S. et al. (2016). Concurrent equine degenerative myeloencephalopathy and equine motor neuron disease in three young horses. *J. Vet. Intern. Med.* 30 (4): 1344–1350.

64 Divers, T.J. (2005). Equine motor neuron disease. *J. Equine Vet. Sci.* 25 (5): 238.

65 Mayhew, I.G., Brown, C.M., Stowe, H.D. et al. (1987). Equine degenerative myeloencephalopathy: a vitamin E deficiency that may be familial. *J. Vet. Intern. Med.* 1 (1): 45–50.

66 Finno, C.J., Estell, K.E., Katzman, S. et al. (2015). Blood and cerebrospinal fluid α-tocopherol and selenium concentrations in neonatal foals with neuroaxonal dystrophy. *J. Vet. Intern. Med.* 29 (6): 1667–1675.

67 Finno, C.J. and Valberg, S.J. (2012). A comparative review of vitamin E and associated equine disorders. *J. Vet. Intern. Med.* 26 (6): 1251–1266.

68 Rech, R. and Barros, C. (2015). Neurologic diseases in horses. *Vet. Clin. North Am. Equine Pract.* 31 (2): 281–306.

69 Waring, G.H. (1982). Onset of behavior patterns in the newborn foal. *Equine Pract.* 4 (5): 28–34.

70 Becvarova, I. and Buechner-Maxwell, V. (2012). Feeding the foal for immediate and long-term health. *Equine Vet. J.* 44 (February): 149–156.

71 Venig, J.C. and Fink-Gremmels, J. (2012). Intestinal barrier function in neonatal foals: options for improvement. *Vet. J.* 193 (1): 32–37.

72 Csapó, J., Stefler, J., Martin, T.G. et al. (1995). Composition of mares' colostrum and milk. Fat content, fatty acid composition and vitamin content. *Int. Dairy J.* 5 (4): 393–402.

73 Pecka, E., DobrzaŃSki, Z., Zachwieja, A. et al. (2012). Studies of composition and major protein level in milk and colostrum of mares. *Anim. Sci. J.* 83 (2): 162–168.

74 Csapó-Kiss, Z., Stefler, J., Martin, T.G. et al. (1995). Composition of mares' colostrum and milk. Protein content, amino acid composition and contents of macro and micro-elements. *Int. Dairy J.* 5 (4): 403–415.

75 Sanchez, L.C. (2005). Equine neonatal sepsis. *Vet. Clin. North Am. Equine Pract.* 21 (2): 273–293.

76 Davis, E. (2012). Maintaining health in foals: the role of colostrum constituents. *Vet. Rec.* 170 (2): 49–50.

77 Jeffcott, L.B. (1974). Studies on passive immunity in the foal. *J. Comp. Pathol.* 84 (1): 93–101.

78 Giguère, S. and Polkes, A.C. (2005). Immunologic disorders in neonatal foals. *Vet. Clin. North Am. Equine Pract.* 21 (2): 241–272.

79 Crisman, M.V. and Scarratt, W.K. (2008). Immunodeficiency disorders in horses. *Vet. Clin. North Am. Equine Pract.* 24 (2): 299–310.

80 Raidal, S.L. (1996). The incidence and consequences of failure of passive transfer of immunity on a thoroughbred breeding farm. *Aust. Vet. J.* 73 (6): 201–206.

81 Pemberton, D.H., Thomas, K.W., and Terry, M.J. (1980). Hypogammaglobulinaemia in foals: prevalence on Victorian studs and simple methods for detection and correction in the field. *Aust. Vet. J.* 56 (10): 469–473.

82 Hofsaess, F.R. (2001). Time of antibody absorption in neonatal foals. *J. Equine Vet. Sci.* 21 (4): 158–159.

83 Sellon, D.C. (2000). Secondary immunodeficiencies of horses. *Vet. Clin. North Am. Equine Pract.* 16 (1): 117–130.

84 Anderson, R.R. (1992). Comparison of trace elements in milk of four species. *J. Dairy Sci.* 75 (11): 3050–3055.

85 Caroprese, M., Albenzio, M., Marino, R. et al. (2007). Behavior, milk yield, and Milk composition of machine- and hand-milked Murgese mares. *J. Dairy Sci.* 90 (6): 2773–2777.

86 Pikul, J. and Wójtowski, J. (2008). Fat and cholesterol content and fatty acid composition of mares' colostrums and milk during five lactation months. *Livest. Sci.* 113 (2): 285–290.

87 Schryver, H.F., Oftedal, O.T., Williams, J. et al. (1986). Lactation in the horse: the mineral composition of mare milk. *J. Nutr.* 116 (11): 2142.

88 Carson, K. and Wood-Gush, D.G.M. (1983). Behaviour of Thoroughbred foals during nursing. *Equine Vet. J.* 15 (3): 257–262.

89 Lawrence, L. (2009). Assessing energy balance. In: *Advances in Equine Nutrition IV* (ed. J.D. Pagan), 43–50. Nottingham: Nottingham University Press.

90 Coleman, R.J., Mathison, G.W., and Burwash, L. (1999). Growth and condition at weaning of extensively managed creep-fed foals. *J. Equine Vet. Sci.* 19 (1): 45–50.

91 Pagan, J., Jackson, S., and DeGregorio, R. (1993). The effect of early weaning on growth and development in Thoroughbred foals. In: *Proceedings of the 13th Equine*

Nutrition and Physiology Society Symposium, 76–79. Gainsville, FL: Equine Nutrition and Physiology Society.

92 Pagan, J., Koch, A., and Caddel, S. (2009). Size matters at the sales. In: *Advances in Equine Nutrition IV* (ed. J. Pagan), 221–222. Nottingham: Nottingham University Press.

93 Nicol, C.J., Badnell-Waters, A.J., Bice, R. et al. (2005). The effects of diet and weaning method on the behaviour of young horses. *Appl. Anim. Behav. Sci.* 95 (3): 205–221.

94 Malinowski, K., Hallquist, N.A., Helyar, L. et al. (1990). Effect of different separation protocols between mares and foals on plasma cortisol and cell-mediated immune response. *J. Equine Vet. Sci.* 10 (5): 363–368.

95 McCall, C.A., Potter, G.D., Kreider, J.L., and Jenkins, W.L. (1987). Physiological responses in foals weaned by abrupt or gradual methods. *J. Equine Vet. Sci.* 7 (6): 368–374.

96 McCall, C.A., Potter, G.D., and Kreider, J.L. (1985). Locomotor, vocal and other behavioral responses to varying methods of weaning foals. *Appl. Anim. Behav. Sci.* 14 (1): 27–35.

97 Aiken, G.E., Bransby, D.I., and McCall, C.A. (1993). Growth of yearling horses compared to steers on high-and low-endophyte infected tall fescue. *J. Equine Vet. Sci.* 13 (1): 26–28.

98 Aiken, G.E. and Strickland, J.R. (2013). Forages and pastures symposium: managing the tall fescue-fungal endophyte symbiosis for optimum forage-animal production. *J. Anim. Sci.* 91 (5): 2369–2378.

99 Pendergraft, J., Arns, M.J., and Brazle, F.K. (1993). Tall fescue utilization by exercised – yearling horses. *J. Equine Vet. Sci.* 13 (10): 548–552.

100 Duncan, P., Harvey, P.H., and Wells, S.M. (1984). On lactation and associated behaviour in a natural herd of horses. *Anim. Behav.* 32 (1): 255–263.

101 Waran, N.K., Clarke, N., and Farnworth, M. (2008). The effects of weaning on the domestic horse (*Equus caballus*). *Appl. Anim. Behav. Sci.* 110 (1): 42–57.

102 Stoneham, S.J., Morresey, P., and Ousey, J. (2017). Nutritional management and practical feeding of the orphan foal. *Equine Vet. Educ.* 29 (3): 165–173.

103 Apter, R.C. and Householder, D.D. (1996). Weaning and weaning management of foals: a review and some recommendations. *J. Equine Vet. Sci.* 16 (10): 428–435.

104 Gibbs, P.G. and Cohen, N.D. (2001). Early management of race-bred weanlings and yearlings on farms. *J. Equine Vet. Sci.* 21 (6): 279–283.

105 Savage, C.J., McCarthy, R.N., and Jeffcott, L.B. (1993). Effects of dietary energy and protein on induction of dyschondroplasia in foals. *Equine Vet. J.* 25 (S16): 74–79.

106 Donabédian, M., Fleurance, G., Perona, G. et al. (2006). Effect of fast vs. moderate growth rate related to nutrient intake on developmental orthopaedic disease in the horse. *Anim. Res.* 55 (5): 471–486.

107 Valette, J.P., Paragon, B.M., Blanchard, G. et al. (2005). The growing horse nutrition and prevention of growth disorders. In: *The Growing Horse Nutrition and Prevention of Growth Disorders. EAAP #114* (ed. V. Julliand and W. Martin-Rosset), 291–301. Wageningen Academic Publishers.

108 Gray, S.M., Bartell, P.A., and Staniar, W.B. (2013). High glycemic and insulinemic responses to meals affect plasma growth hormone secretory characteristics in Quarter Horse weanlings. *Domest. Anim. Endocrinol.* 44 (4): 165–175.

Clinical Nutrition

22

Pain and Discomfort Behaviors

Katherine A. Houpt

KEY TERMS

- Anorexia is a loss of appetite.
- Anhedonia is the loss of interest in pleasant activities.
- Optimism is the speed or willingness to perform a task.
- Stereotypies or "vices" are spontaneous, repetitive, compulsive, topographically invariant response patterns commonly observed in captive or domestic animals.

KEY POINTS

- Display, or lack, of natural behaviors (grooming, thermoregulatory, foraging, resting, sleeping, and playing) can be used to assess animal welfare.
- Behaviors provide valuable insight into a horse's subjective state and are a good indicator of welfare.
- As a survival mechanism, horses often suppress signs of pain in the presence of predators, including humans.
- The horse values safety and comfort before food, hence horses in pain, afraid, distressed, or diseased may be partially or fully anorexic.
- Horses, like other species, are less able to cope with physical and psychological challenges when they experience discomfort, pain, depression, or distress.
- The recognition of pain remains a major barrier to animals being managed appropriately.
- For horses to thrive, caretakers must be able to recognize discomfort and pain, fear and distress, and accommodate their natural behaviors.

22.1 Introduction

When humans domesticated the horse, keeping them in artificial housing (box stalls), feeding a diet (low forage) different from their physiologic design, and using them for our pleasure and profit, we then become responsible for their welfare. Most healthy horses under our care are free of thirst and hunger, but we do cause them fear, distress, injury, and pain, and some are not free to express many of their natural behaviors such as living in a grazing group. As clinically observed, horses in pain, those in fear or distress, and those with a disease may not consume a sufficient amount of food, and some become anorectic. One can assess animal welfare using the Five Freedoms that are attributes compiled by a group of scientists and ethicists initially in response to public outcry over "factory" farming [1]. See Sidebar 22.1. Within the framework of the Five Freedoms, the objective is to improve early recognition of discomfort and pain, fear and distress, and to accommodate the horse's natural behaviors as an antecedent to promoting appetite and ingestion of proper nutrition [2].

22.2 Assessments of Discomfort, Pain, Depression, and Distress

22.2.1 Physical Assessments

Horses are highly perceptive of surroundings, instinctually reactive, and will suppress signs of pain or injury in the presence of predators, including humans. Caretakers must

Equine Clinical Nutrition, Second Edition. Edited by Rebecca L. Remillard.

Sidebar 22.1: The Five Freedoms [1, 2]

Freedom from thirst, hunger, and malnutrition
Freedom from thermal and physical discomfort
Freedom from pain, injury, and disease
Freedom from fear and distress
Freedom to express normal behaviors

Table 22.1 The facial muscles of the horse.

Action	Muscle
Inner brow raiser	Levator anguli oculi medialis
Eye closure and blink	Orbicularis oculi and levator palpebrae superioris
Half blink	Orbicularis oculi
Upper lid raiser	Levator palpebrae
Upper lip raiser	Levator labii superioris and transverse nasii
Lip corner puller	Zygomatic major
Sharp lip puller	Levator labii superioris alaeque
Nostril lift	Levator annulioris fascialis
Lower lip depressor	Depressor labii inferioris
Chin raiser	Mentalis
Lip pucker	Orbicularis oris and incisvii labii
Upper lip curl	Levator labii superioris and transverse nasi
Lip presser	Orbicularis oris
Lips part	Depressor labii or relaxation of the mentais or orbicularis oris
Jaw drop	Masseter, temporal, and internal pterygoid relaxed
Mouth stretch	Ptergoids and digastric

Source: Data from Wathan et al. [4].

be able to read the sometimes subtle body language of a horse in pain or distress. The ideal pain scoring system should be linear, weighted, sensitive to pain type, breed, and species-specific, and easy to interpret [3].

22.2.1.1 Facial Appearance

Many muscles supply the horse's face. Contraction or relaxation of these muscles provides clues as to the level of discomfort and pain (Table 22.1 and Figure 22.1). The Facial Action Coding System is a method of identifying facial expressions based on the underlying musculature and movement [4]. The Horse Grimace Scale (HGS) is a facial-expression-based pain coding system using six Facial Action Units, each independently coded using a three-point scale (Figure 22.2) [5]. For example, signs of pain in a horse while ridden are detected using the HGS (Figure 22.3) [6].

22.2.1.2 Posture

The number and severity of aversive past experiences may cause a horse to be depressed and withdrawn. States of depression or withdrawal are characterized by a stationary, flat-necked posture, i.e. the nape, neck, and back are held at the same height with no angle difference between them (Figure 22.4). The horse stands motionless with wide open, unblinking eyes with a fixed gaze and backward-pointing ears. Longer times to interact with a novel object are reflective of higher levels of anxiety or neophobia. Anhedonia is a key indicator of depression. When horses had access to novel flavored (cherry, banana, and apple) sugar blocks, horses spending the most time withdrawn consumed less sugar, i.e. loss of interest in pleasant activities [7]. Moving stabled horses onto pasture induced the expression of natural behaviors; however, for several days initially, the horses were withdrawn due to the change in environment and social conditions [9]. Conversely, the occurrence of stereotypies and maintaining the withdrawn posture increased during the first five days of returning pastured horses to confinement.

22.2.1.3 Heart Rate

A heart rate increase is the best indicator of pain in a resting horse. However, heart rate variability (HRV) describes the antagonistic influences of both the sympathetic and vagal branches of the autonomic nervous system on the sinus node of the heart. A decrease in HRV indicates a shift toward sympathetic dominance, i.e. a stress response, while increased values indicate parasympathetic dominance or a resting state [10].

22.2.2 Behavioral Assessments

There are different kinds of pain, so there are different horse responses. Sharp sudden pain will usually cause the horse to move or run off. For example, an insect bite may cause the horse to stomp, bite at the source of pain, or even gallop off. Head pain can cause head shaking, snorting, or restlessness. Jaw or mouth pain can result in difficulty eating, drooling saliva, or chewing on one side only. Tail swishing may be to ward off flies or other horses; however, tail lashing is indicative of agitation. Pawing has several associations as it may occur with foaling or colic pain, a learned behavior linked with meals, or an undesirable behavior (vice) with no obvious function. A horse pawing may be wanting to go forward as an escape or to join another horse. Pawing serves to expose grass under snow or to uncover water in a hole.

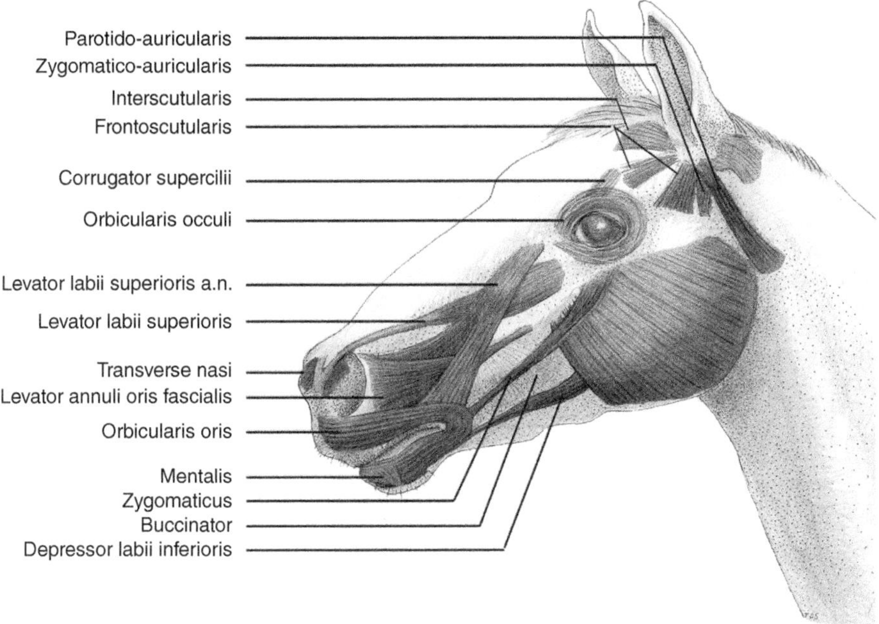

Figure 22.1 Facial muscles of the horse. *Source:* Wathan et al. [4].

22.2.2.1 Stereotypic Behaviors

The relationship between oral stereotypic behaviors (cribbing, wind sucking) and endorphins has been investigated with no clear association [11]. Opioid receptor density in the midbrains of crib-biting horses was significantly ($p < 0.001$) higher compared to control animals giving support to a hereditary component to stereotypic behavior [12]. Feed type (textured, sweet, grain vs. low forage) and timing have also been thought related to endorphin release and oral vices. A greater number of oral stereotypical behaviors were noted in horses fed concentrate at 1.0% BW vs. those fed 0.5% BW, and conversely, more events occurred in horses fed 0.5% BW hay vs. those fed at 0.9–1.5% BW; however, ration carbohydrate and fiber details were lacking [13].

22.2.2.2 Cognitive Bias

Cognitive bias is based on the premise that subjects in a negative affective state will form more undesirable judgments about ambiguous stimuli than subjects in a positive affective state. It is usually measured by rewarding a horse for going to a feed tub on the right but never for going to the tub on the left. When offered a tub in the middle, the optimistic horse approaches it quickly, whereas the pessimistic horse approaches slowly, if at all. The speed at which the horse approaches the tub is used as the measure of optimism. Horses kept on pasture before the test were more optimistic than those confined to stalls [14].

22.2.2.3 Time Budget Analysis

Healthy, stress-free horses exhibit highly repetitive daily routines which, if quantified, can provide an objective and unambiguous evidence-based assessment. A systematic review of the literature (12 papers) reported 24-hr time budgets of 10–66.6% eating, 8.1–66% resting, and 0.015–19.1% moving which varied due to age, environment, and access to feed and water. Domesticated horses' time budget became more similar to semiferal horses when restraints of food and space were not limiting [15].

22.3 Freedom from Thirst, Hunger, and Malnutrition

Previous chapters on nutrients (water, energy, protein, minerals, and vitamins) and those on forages, manufactured feeds, and supplements are ultimately dedicated to the prevention of thirst, hunger, and malnutrition in horses. Equids in our care should have access to a complete and balanced diet (feed and water) based on their physiological needs to achieve and maintain full health and vigor [2]. Horses in pain, discomfort, or malaise may require specialized nutrient profiled rations. Those with oral injuries may require different physical forms of the feed, and horses with limited mobility due to trauma or pain may require specialized methods of feeding. See

Stiffly backward ears

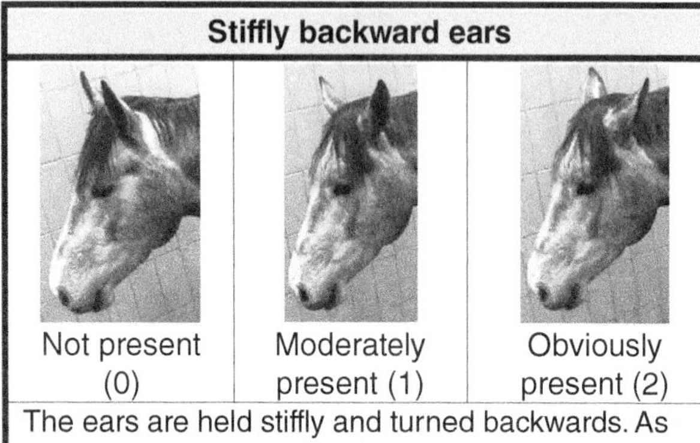

The ears are held stiffly and turned backwards. As a result, the space between the ears may appear wider relative to baseline.

Orbital tightening

Not present (0) | Moderately present (1) | Obviously present (2)

The eyelid is partially or completely closed. Any eyelid closure that reduces the eye size by more than half should be coded as "obviously present" or "2".

Tension above the eye area

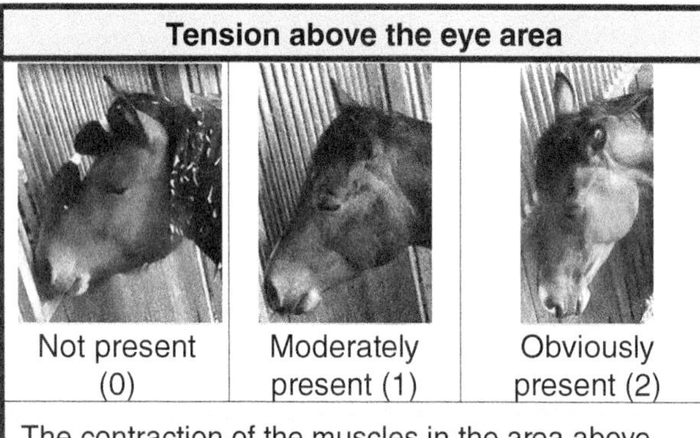

The contraction of the muscles in the area above the eye causes the increased visibility of the underlying bone surfaces. If temporal crest bone is clearly visible should be coded as "obviously present" or "2".

Prominent strained chewing muscles

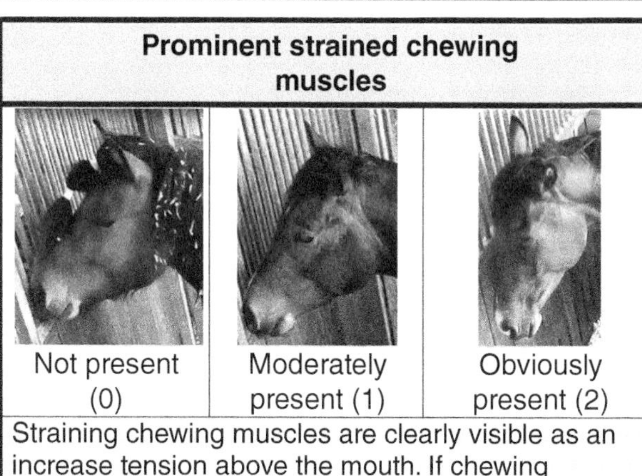

Straining chewing muscles are clearly visible as an increase tension above the mouth. If chewing muscles are clearly prominent and recognizable the score should be coded as "obviously present" or "2".

Mouth strained and pronounced chin

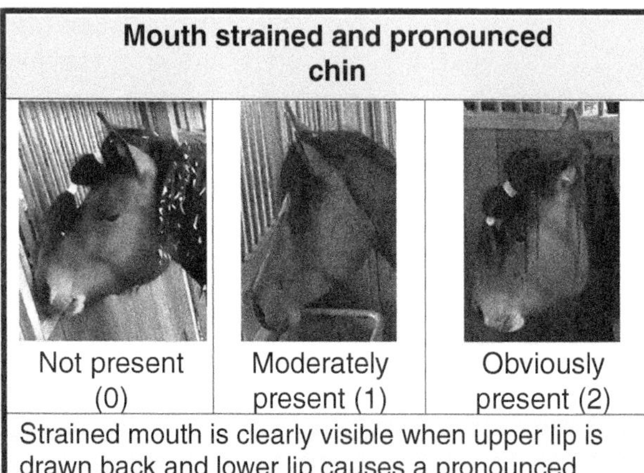

Strained mouth is clearly visible when upper lip is drawn back and lower lip causes a pronounced "chin".

Strained nostrils and flattening of the profile

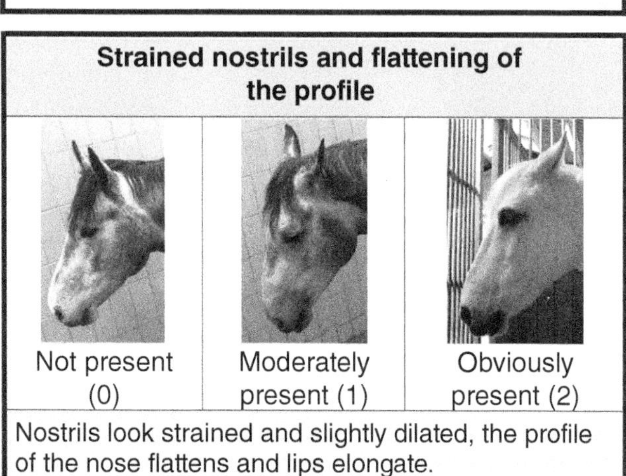

Nostrils look strained and slightly dilated, the profile of the nose flattens and lips elongate.

Figure 22.2 The Horse Grimace Scale with six facial action units scored: not present (score 0), moderately present (score 1) or obviously present (score 2). *Source:* Dalla Costa et al. [5].

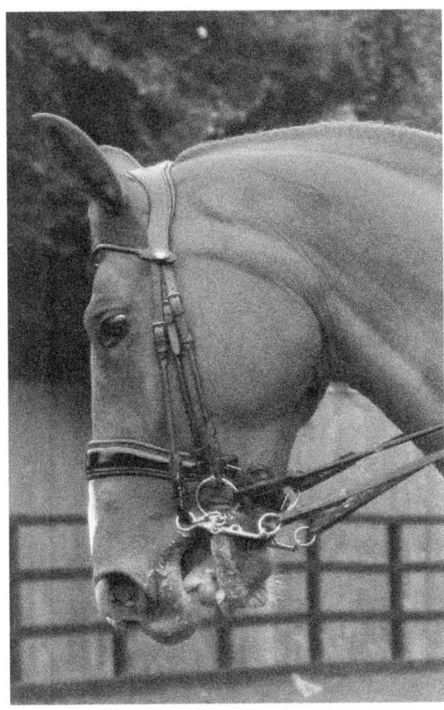

Figure 22.3 Facial signs of pain in a horse: left eye has an intense stare (pain score [PS] 2), tension in the muscles above the eye (PS 1), left ear rotated outward (PS 1), mouth is wide open exposing teeth and tongue (PS 3), left nostril flared with angular sides and a wrinkle below the nostril (PS 1), and lower muzzle is tense (PS 1) [6]. *Source:* Photo courtesy of Sue Dyson.

Chapter 2 Nutritional Assessment of the Horse and Assisted Feeding in Chapter 24.

22.4 Freedom from Thermal and Physical Discomfort

22.4.1 Shelter

Horses should always have shelter available so that they can escape wind and rain in cold weather, and the sun and heat in hot weather. Horses can behaviorally thermoregulate and can even be taught to signal for a blanket or to have the blanket removed [16, 17]. Horses may require changes in the energy density of their feed to accommodate environmental extremes. See Chapter 6 Energy.

22.4.2 The Twitch

One can make use of the horse's tactile sense or more likely pain receptors, using the twitch – a wooden handle with a loop of rope or chain attached. When the chain around the horse's upper lip is twisted, endorphins are released and temporary analgesia is produced for 15 min or less. The same can often be accomplished using one hand gasped tightly around the upper lip with a slight twist.The horse is behaviorally and physiologically calm based on a lower heart rate and higher vagal tone. This method can be used, if needed, to restrain a horse for mildly frightening short procedures, such as ear clipping, vaccination, or blood draws [18].

22.5 Freedom from Pain, Injury, and Disease

As caretakers, horse owners are responsible for the prevention of injury and disease. Veterinarians are responsible for basic care and preventive recommendations, efficient diagnosis of a problem, recommending therapies, and the administration of some treatments. There are many medications to help reduce pain in horses ranging from nonsteroidal anti-inflammatory drugs, e.g. phenylbutazone, alpha-2-agonists, i.e. detomidine, and opiates. Local anesthesia can be used for pain relief and should be used as soon as possible to prevent suffering and further injuries.

Medicating feed, although common, may cause discomfort if the horse is nauseated by the medication and will learn to avoid that food. Using a method of conditioned taste aversion and pairing, the drug suspected to cause nausea first with a novel flavor, i.e. raspberry, and then feeding the flavor without the drug will separate the possible side effect of the drug from the feed. If the drug causes nausea, the horse will not eat the flavored feed or will consume less vs. feed alone in a two-bucket test [19].

22.5.1 Neurological Diseases

Several diseases cause neurological deficits and subsequently decreased feed consumption. The American Association of Equine Practitioners has vaccination guidelines for tetanus, rabies, encephalitis (Eastern, Western, and West Nile virus), and Lyme disease [20, 21]. Although these forms of encephalitis have a high mortality rate, and euthanasia is electable, those surviving will require nutritional support. See Assisted Feeding in Chapter 24.

22.5.2 Lameness and Back Pain

Pain is the most common cause of lameness. Diagnosing lameness requires clinical experience and is an art of veterinary medicine. Currently, observers are asked to grade lameness on a visual analog scale where one end indicates "sound" and four indicates nonweight bearing or immobile (Table 22.2) [23]. However, the use of a Ridden Horse Pain Ethogram may also be a valuable tool in helping veterinarians to recognize musculoskeletal pain, when overt lameness has not been recognized [24, 25]. Less commonly

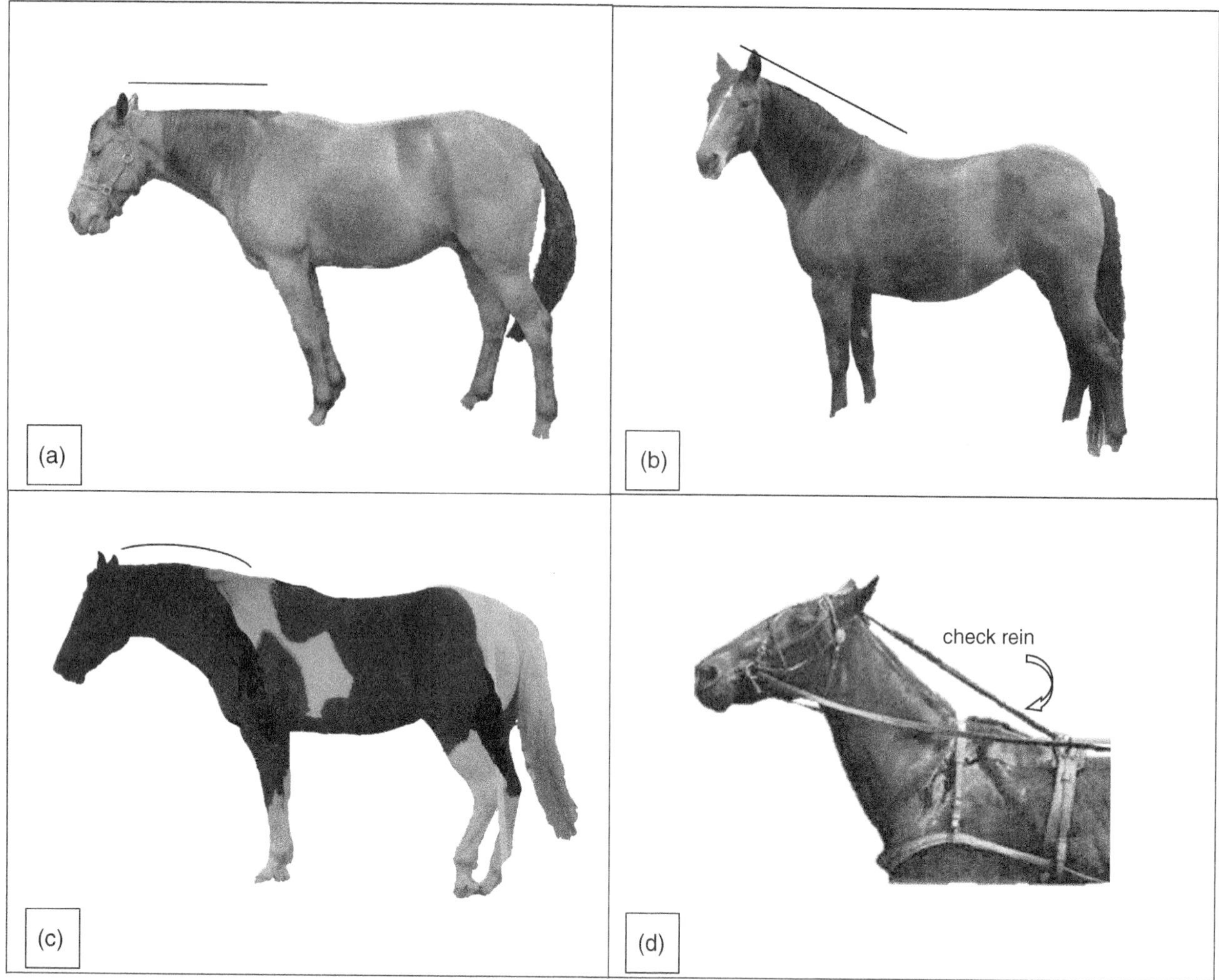

Figure 22.4 The head and neck posture of a withdrawn horse (a) compared with a focused stance (b) and standing at ease (c) (note: cocked hind limb) vs. dorsal flexion held by overuse of check rein (d). *Source:* Fureix et al. [7] and Roberts [8].

Table 22.2 Modified Obel score for detecting lameness.

Grade	Description
Normal	Sound
1	No gait abnormalities at a walk or trot. At rest, the horse exhibited foot lifting. The horse exhibited a normal gait at a walk. The trot showed a shortened stride and showed even head and neck lifting for each foot.
2	The walk was stilted but showed no abnormal head or neck lifting. The trot showed obvious lameness with uneven head and neck lifting. A forefoot could be lifted off the ground easily.
3	The lameness was obvious at a walk and trot. The horse resisted attempts to have a forefoot lifted and was reluctant to move.
4	The horse experienced difficulty bearing weight at rest or was very reluctant to move.

Source: Data from Menzies-Gow et al. [22].

recognized is back pain but must be included when assessing "bad" acting horses. Those with back pain may show signs of discomfort such as tail lashing, tooth grinding, reluctance to lie down, inappetence, resentment of grooming or saddling, or problems under saddle such as sinking when mounted, bolting, rearing, bucking, and refusal to move forward. Back pain is especially difficult to assess in an animal too large to be radiographed successfully; however, temperament may be a cue. Fifty-nine lesson horses, mostly French Saddlebred geldings, were investigated for aggression toward humans and examined by a licensed chiropractor for lesions of the spinal column. Horses severely affected by vertebral problems (33 of 43 horses, $p < 0.001$) were prone to react aggressively toward humans, and the percentage of affected vertebrae was negatively correlated ($rs = -0.31$, $p = 0.02$) with the number of positive reactions during behavioral testing, i.e. the more pain, the fewer positive responses from the horse [26].

22.5.3 Colic

Gastrointestinal distress is one of the most common causes of pain in horses and the number one cause of death. Some colics will resolve on their own, some need conservative treatment, and some require major surgery and may result in euthanasia. The ability to recognize the signs of colic early is very important both to reduce pain and suffering and to begin treatment before the situation worsens. The first sign of colic is anorexia. Horses spend the majority of their time (~60%) eating ad libitum hay; therefore, a horse not eating hay while herd mates are eating is a good reason to investigate further. The next sign is restlessness and turning to look at the belly or Flehmen (lip curl). The horse may kick at the abdomen in an apparent effort to dislodge the pain. Finally, the horse will throw himself down and roll. This rolling can be differentiated from comfort rolling because the colicing horse will not whole body shake after rising. Often a colicing horse will walk a few paces and then go down again, and unattended, this sequence may be repeated for hours. The advent of closed-circuit TV cameras in barns enables owners to observe their horses anytime. As most episodes of colic occur at night, the problem may be caught on camera and treated earlier in the course of the event.

Behavioral observations indicative of pain in horses post colic surgery can be based on (i) posture; to be consistent with other chapters. (ii) response to food; and (iii) interactive behavior. Postural behaviors indicative of abdominal pain are ears held back and head held below the level of the withers, restlessness, or no movement with arched back and tucked up belly. The response to food can be strong, mild, or nonexistent. Interactive behavior is the expected response to a human, whereas the response of a postsurgical patient may be limited to looking at the observer, moving away, or no movement. A postabdominal surgery pain assessment scale has been described [27].

22.6 Freedom from Fear and Distress

No matter the discipline, e.g. a weight-pulling Belgian, a racing thoroughbred, or an endurance-ridden Arabian, a horse can be overworked physically and mentally. The physical and psychological stress of excessive training, abusive equipment, improper environment, and inappropriate ration can create fear, depression, chronic distress, and subsequently decrease appetite. In most sports, horses bleeding from the tongue, lips, or flanks from bits and spurs are eliminated from competitions; however, training sessions are not monitored.

22.6.1 Training Techniques and Equipment

Check (bearing or overcheck) reins run from the horse's bit, over the front of the face, between the ears, down the neck, and connect to the harness designed to keep the horse's head up, hyperextended in some cases. Check reins were fashionable in the nineteenth century (Figure 22.4) and were recognized as a welfare issue in the classic story Black Beauty by Anna Sewell. We may no longer misuse check reins, but there are still items of equipment that produce pain and discomfort in this century.

A clear indication of the horse's preference, between two riding styles, was demonstrated by 15 horses given the choice to choose the direction of travel within a maze. After being conditioned, horses learned that in one direction they were ridden hyperflexed at the poll (Rollkur) vs. the other direction where they were ridden with normal poll flexion [28]. Fourteen horses chose ($p < 0.05$) the direction where the normal flexion riding style was used. Horses more often showed behavioral signs of discomfort, such as tail-swishing, head-tossing, or attempted bucks ($p < 0.05$) during the hyperflexed ride. The Rollkur riding style is more often associated with dressage but is used in other disciplines. The extreme curb or leverage bits with long shanks, to amplify rein pressure several fold depending on the length of the shank, is used in some western-style events to get hyperflexion at the poll. Rollkur was banned in 2013 by the International Federation for Equestrian Sports (FEI).

There are several issues involving tails that produce discomfort or pain. Tails can be altered by breaking the tail so it can be set to produce an artificially elevated tail. The tail can be denervated to make a nervous western pleasure horse appear calmer or ginger in the anus can be used to encourage a high tail posture in Arabians and American Saddlebreds. The tail set harnesses used on American Saddlebreds may be uncomfortable. Tails of Clydesdales, among other breeds, can be docked which deprives the animal of protection from insects.

Other practices, in addition to equipment, may produce pain. Caustic substances are applied to the pasterns of Tennessee Walking horses to stimulate the horses to raise their forelegs high. This process is called soring and is outlawed in the United States, but the law is not enforced. Whipping horses is painful, but jockeys will whip their mounts during the final moments of a race. In some countries, the type of whip, when it can be used, and the area of the horse that can be struck is regulated in racing so that only the horses in contention for the first three places can be whipped. In developing countries, horses or donkeys may have an ill-fitting harness that produces skin sores. Even the sight of saddles can increase cortisol concentrations in horses used for trail rides. Horses are less stressed when ridden by a novice than by an experienced rider. There were no significant differences in the mean number of stress-related behaviors in horses when ridden by recreational riders, physically handicapped riders, psychologically handicapped riders, or special education children [29, 30].

22.6.2 Endurance Rides

The abuses of horses on endurance rides, especially competitive rides with prize money, have led to frequent veterinary checks to remove horses before they become seriously lame, dehydrated, or simply fatigued. Exhaustion is accompanied by dehydration, electrolyte imbalance, and glycogen depletion. See Chapter 18 Feeding Athletes and Working Horses. It is optimal to have three veterinary checks on a 50-mile ride. In order to pass the vet check, after resting for a few minutes, the horse must have a pulse <64 beats/min, trot soundly for 250 ft and have normal abdominal sounds on auscultation. Endurance riding is the only equine sport that involves veterinarians in deciding the horse's "fitness to continue."

22.6.3 Dressage

Dressage horses are particularly prone to tendonitis and suspensory desmitis as a result of tendon and ligament fatigue. The length of daily training sessions is often longer than other disciplines. Exhaustion is indicated when the horse's sides are heaving, nostrils flaring, and flanks lathered after a performance or warm-up. Dressage horses are often confined to a stall and then are overworked at "warm-up" to calm them before the training session. The extent of confinement may lead to the development of stereotypic behaviors in dressage horses vs. other disciplines [9]. However, a hereditary component has been suggested because certain thoroughbred bloodlines are more likely to exhibit stereotypies [31].

22.6.4 Hunter Jumpers

Hunter jumpers may also be confined for long periods with no turnout. Additionally, there are a variety of methods used to encourage the horse to jump higher, from rapping or poling, i.e. striking the horse in the belly with the rail just before the jump, using electric wire on the jumps, whips, or spurs. A recent trend has been to apply caustic substances to the lower legs to encourage the horse to pick up their feet, similar to the "soring" of Tennessee Walkers.

22.6.5 Reining and Cutting Horses

Reining is a popular sport in which the horse must spin repeatedly and execute a sliding stop from a full gallop followed by a rollback, i.e. a 180° turn followed by a lope. Other maneuvers include spinning and flying lead changes on command. A major welfare issue is the training method called "fencing" in which a young horse is galloped toward a fence to teach him to stop suddenly. Other issues are the use of inhumane bits to stop the horse and the subsequent orthopedic consequences of repetitive high-velocity halts and turns.

22.6.6 Rodeo Horses

There has been much public concern about the welfare of bucking horses which the Professional Rodeo Cowboys Association has taken pains to address. Spurs used by riders must be blunted, and the flank strap used to encourage bucking is lined with sheepskin or neoprene and has a quick-release mechanism used to provide relief as soon as a ride is complete. In general, bucking horses are valuable animals, bred for this purpose, and owners are unlikely to hurt them [32].

22.6.7 Racehorses

The issue with racehorses that garner most public attention is fractures or other "breakdowns" on the track. There have been many studies investigating track surface (s) as it relates to injuries, and results from these investigations have led to safer surfaces. A larger, less obvious problem is racing horses that are too old or too lame to be humanely raced, but who, with sufficient medication and other treatments, can pass prerace veterinary examinations. Some racetracks pay enough prize money to make placing sixth profitable. Standardbred racehorses often paw or dig in their stalls, not usually before meals but rather in the afternoon following training, and paw less on Sundays, the only day not worked. Standardbreds have been known to dig a hole in the stall area, then place the hind limbs in the hole to take the pressure off the forelimbs. In this case, pawing and standing in the hole may be a sign of seeking relief from discomfort [33].

22.6.8 Carriage Horses

In developing countries, where horsepower is commonly used, horses, donkeys, and mules may be asked to pull loads that are much too heavy or to work long hours with neither food nor water. In many large cities, carriage rides are offered for a romantic and quiet experience. In the United States, carriage horses have been the target of welfare groups and this has resulted in restricting the number of hours a horse can work and to avoid the hottest part of the day, provision of bigger stalls, and more veterinary examinations. Carriage horses that have worked many hours for a few days may present with rhabdomyolysis. Trauma from automobiles is also a common injury.

22.7 Freedom to Express Normal Behaviors

The environment we provide must ensure the horse can adequately exhibit natural comforting behaviors and avoid mental suffering.

22.7.1 Rolling, Scratching, and Mutual Grooming

Horses roll as a comfort behavior. They can scratch their back in places they cannot reach with hoof or teeth, and often roll after being ridden or bathed. For their comfort, a horse should have access to a safe place to roll in soft dirt or bedding without restraints, e.g. harnesses and saddles. The area must be large enough for the horse to roll and get itself upright again. In a stall, a horse can cast itself (unable to rise again) because they are too close to a wall. When a horse arises after rolling, a partial or whole body shake to remove debris is normal and indicates the roll was a comfort behavior. Rolling is particularly common when a horse has colic pain but then is unlikely to shake after rising. Horses should be provided a place to safely scratch other body areas (chest and rump) and allowed mutual grooming among herd mates.

22.7.2 Biting Insects

Insect bites are very irritating to horses and the sound of buzzing insects associated with a painful bite can cause horses to stop grazing and gallop to shelter. They avoid them by moving to areas with fewer insects such as grassless areas or patches of snow or even into water. In confined domestic conditions (stalls, paddocks, and small pastures), they cannot move away from the insects, and therefore other measures (insect control and deterrents) must be used and comfort measures (fans, cool, dark shelters, fly masks, and repellents) should be provided [34]. Horses should not be tethered to prevent head shaking or have tails shortened to prevent swishing which wards off insects.

22.7.3 Herd Bound

After millions of years, the horse, as a prey species, has learned well that there is safety in numbers because horses, vulnerable to predators, have limited defenses, i.e. early detection, flight, and, when cornered, biting, rearing, and kicking. As herd animals, horses do not prefer to be alone, although some do learn to live as such. For example, a single horse living in a paddock spent more time eating, and less time walking, when there were other horses in an adjacent paddock than when no horses were within sight [35]. The stress hormone, cortisol, is reliably increased in horses separated from herd mates likely because that individual has lost the protection of the herd and social facilitation. A herd of horses was found to have synchronized behaviors 81% of the time which allowed some horses to perform more vulnerable tasks, i.e. lying down, sleeping, grazing, or drinking, while others watched for predators, i.e. social facilitation [36]. Horses in a group act out natural behaviors of exploration, social interaction, play, and grooming to fulfill psychological needs [14]. This strong, innate, survival instinct to remain in a herd and the undeniable need to be with other horses (at least by sight) must be addressed in the housing management of horses in our care [9].

References

1 Brambell F.W.R. (1967). *Report of the Technical Committee to Enquire into the Welfare of Animals Kept Under Intensive Livestock Systems*. London, UK; Her Majesty's Stationery Office; 1967. Cmnd. 2836. 1–85. London: HMSO.

2 Webster, J. (2016). Animal welfare: freedoms, dominions and "A life worth living". *Animals* 6 (6): 35–40.

3 Ashley, F.H., Waterman-Pearson, A.E., and Whay, H.R. (2005). Behavioural assessment of pain in horses and donkeys: application to clinical practice and future studies. *Equine Vet. J.* 37 (6): 565–575.

4 Wathan, J., Burrows, A.M., Waller, B.M., and McComb, K. (2015). The equine facial action coding system. *PLoS One* 10 (8): e0131738.

5 Dalla Costa, E., Minero, M., Lebelt, D. et al. (2014). Development of the horse grimace scale (HGS) as a pain assessment tool in horses undergoing routine castration. *PLoS One* 9 (3): e92281.

6 Mullard, J., Berger, J.M., Ellis, A.D., and Dyson, S. (2017). Development of an ethogram to describe facial expressions in ridden horses (FEReq). *J. Vet. Behav.* 18 (Mar): 7–12.

7 Fureix, C., Beaulieu, C., Argaud, S. et al. (2015). Investigating anhedonia in a non-conventional species: do some riding horses *Equus caballus* display symptoms of depression? *Appl. Anim. Behav. Sci.* 162 (Jan): 26–36.

8 Roberts, I.P. (1905). Education and care of roadsters and other light horses: harness. In: *The Horse*, 2e, 286. New York: The MacMillan Company.

9 Ruet, A., Arnould, C., Levray, J. et al. (2020). Effects of a temporary period on pasture on the welfare state of horses housed in individual boxes. *Appl. Anim. Behav. Sci.* 228 (Jul): 105027.

10 von Borell, E., Langbein, J., Després, G. et al. (2007). Heart rate variability as a measure of autonomic regulation of cardiac activity for assessing stress and welfare in farm animals – a review. *Physiol. Behav.* 92 (3): 293–316.

11 Pell, S.M. and McGreevy, P.D. (1999). A study of cortisol and beta-endorphin levels in stereotypic and normal thoroughbreds. *Appl. Anim. Behav. Sci.* 64 (2): 81–90.

12 Hemmings, A., Parker, M.O., Hale, C., and McBride, S.D. (2018). Causal and functional interpretation of mu- and delta-opioid receptor profiles in mesoaccumbens and nigrostriatal pathways of an oral stereotypy phenotype. *Behav. Brain Res.* 353 (Nov): 108–113.

13 Hanis, F., Chung, E.L.T., Kamalludin, M.H., and Idrus, Z. (2020). The influence of stable management and feeding practices on the abnormal behaviors among stabled horses in Malaysia. *J. Equine Vet. Sci.* 94 (11): 103230.

14 Löckener, S., Reese, S., Erhard, M., and Wöhr, A.C. (2016). Pasturing in herds after housing in horseboxes induces a positive cognitive bias in horses. *J. Vet. Behav.* 11 (Jan): 50–55.

15 Auer, U., Kelemen, Z., Engl, V., and Jenner, F. (2021). Activity time budgets – a potential tool to monitor equine welfare? *Animals* 11 (3): 850.

16 Houpt, K.A. (1991). Animal behavior and animal welfare. *J. Am. Vet. Med. Assoc.* 198 (8): 1355–1360.

17 Mejdell, C.M., Buvik, T., Jørgensen, G.H.M., and Bøe, K.E. (2016). Horses can learn to use symbols to communicate their preferences. *Appl. Anim. Behav. Sci.* 184 (Nov): 66–73.

18 Flakoll, B., Ali, A.B., and Saab, C.Y. (2017). Twitching in veterinary procedures: how does this technique subdue horses? *J. Vet. Behav.* 18 (Mar): 23–28.

19 Houpt, K.A., Zahorik, D.M., and Swartzman-Andert, J.A. (1990). Taste aversion learning in horses. *J. Anim. Sci.* 68 (8): 2340–2344.

20 American Association of Equine Practitioners. Vaccination guidelines. https://aaep.org/guidelines/vaccination-guidelines (accessed 15 April 2021).

21 The Center for Food Security and Public Health (2008). *Mosquito Control Measures in Animal Shelter Settings*. The Center for Food Security and Public Health. https://www.cfsph.iastate.edu.

22 Menzies-Gow, N.J., Stevens, K.B., Sepulveda, M.F. et al. (2010). Repeatability and reproducibility of the Obel grading system for equine laminitis. *Vet. Rec.* 167 (2): 52–55.

23 Baxter, G.M. (2011). Assessment of the lame horse. In: *Manual of Equine Lameness*, 83–148. Ames, IA: Wiley Blackwell.

24 Dyson, S. (2022). The ridden horse pain ethogram. *Equine Vet Educ.* 34(7): 372–80.

25 Dyson, S. Ellis, A.D. (2022). Application of a Ridden Horse Pain Ethogram to horses competing at 5-star three-day-events: Comparison with performance. *Equine Vet Educ.* 34(6): 306–15.

26 Fureix, C., Menguy, H., and Hausberger, M. (2010). Partners with bad temper: reject or cure? A study of chronic pain and aggression in horses. *PLoS One* 5 (8): e12434.

27 Graubner, C., Gerber, V., Doherr, M., and Spadavecchia, C. (2011). Clinical application and reliability of a post abdominal surgery pain assessment scale (PASPAS) in horses. *Vet. J.* 188 (2): 178–183.

28 von Borstel, U.U., Duncan, I.J.H., Shoveller, A.K. et al. (2009). Impact of riding in a coercively obtained Rollkur posture on welfare and fear of performance horses. *Appl. Anim. Behav. Sci.* 116 (2): 228–236.

29 Kaiser, L., Heleski, C.R., Siegford, J., and Smith, K.A. (2006). Stress-related behaviors among horses used in a therapeutic riding program. *J. Am. Vet. Med. Assoc.* 228 (1): 39–45.

30 McKinney, C., Mueller, M.K., and Frank, N. (2015). Effects of therapeutic riding on measures of stress in horses. *J. Equine Vet. Sci.* 35 (11): 922–928.

31 Vecchiotti, G.G. and Galanti, R. (1986). Evidence of heredity of cribbing, weaving and stall-walking in thoroughbred horses. *Livest. Prod. Sci.* 14 (1): 91–95.

32 Corey, D. (2011). Welfare issues in the rodeo horse. In: *Equine Welfare* (ed. C.W. McIlwraith and B.E. Rollin), 275–301. London: Blackwell Wiley.

33 Butler, C.L. and Houpt, K.A. (2014). Pawing by Standardbred racehorses: frequency and patterns. *J. Equine Sci.* 25 (3): 57–59.

34 The Center for Food Security and Public Health (2008). *Fly Control Measures in Animal Shelter Settings*. The Center for Food Security and Public Health. https://www.cfsph.iastate.edu.

35 Houpt, K.A. and Houpt, T.R. (1988). Social and illumination preferences of mares. *J. Anim. Sci.* 66 (9): 2159–2164.

36 Rifá, H. (1990). Social facilitation in the horse (*Equus caballus*). *Appl. Anim. Behav. Sci.* 25 (1): 167–176.

23

Weight Management

Shannon P. Phillips and Rebecca L. Remillard

KEY TERMS

- Lean body mass refers to muscle mass within the context of weight management.
- Fat-free mass includes internal organs, bone, muscle, water, blood, and connective tissue and is calculated as total body weight (BW) minus total fat mass.
- Drylot is a fenced grassless area of variable size.
- Non-structural carbohydrates (NSC) are simple sugars, starch, and fructans contained within the plant cells.
- Start BW is weight at the beginning of a weight management program.
- Goal BW is estimated BW at condition score (BCS) 4–6/9 depending on life stage and performance.

KEY POINTS

- Obesity is a chronic, low-grade inflammation affecting many body systems.
- A forage analysis is helpful as hay should be the foundation of the weight loss diet, and is the starting point of ration balancing.
- A successful weight loss program involves a nutritionally complete calorie-restricted ration, a restricted feed intake, an exercise plan, owner compliance, and monitoring.
- When weight loss is necessary for a horse with concurrent disease, i.e. orthopedic, endocrine, metabolic, or heat/exercise intolerance, close supervision by a veterinarian is recommended and precautions are needed.
- A successful weight gain program involves a balanced high-energy ration, an appropriate feeding method, a modified exercise plan, owner compliance, and monitoring.

23.1 The Healthy Weight as a Concept

Weight management is an important aspect of the overall health management of horses. The concept of a "healthy" BW and BCS is important to understand and then apply appropriately to each case as there is not a one-size-fits-all depiction, e.g. the BW and BCS desirable for a broodmare is not the same as that for an elite endurance horse. Additionally, feral horses do not maintain a constant weight as might be expected of a domesticated horse. There is a physiologically fluctuation of body condition in free-ranging horses that occurs over the year. The flux in BW and BCS depends on feed quality, water, and the environment, i.e. weather and seasonal effects. There is seasonal variation in the quality of pasture grasses, and concurrently, there are seasonal energy needs by gestating and lactating mares and stallions in protecting the herd [1]. The net effect of feed quality vs. energy need will be revealed in the BCS of the horses, and these changes throughout the year for wild horses are acceptable.

It has been well recognized in all species that chronically underweight individuals have an increased risk of mortality when concurrently confronted with trauma or illness at a time when food intake is limited. Animals with less than optimal body fat (BF) stores are at a distinct disadvantage should either decrease food intake or increase energy need, or when both occur simultaneously. When endogenous fat stores have been depleted, the body begins to catabolize muscle. Time to muscle catabolism is directly related to BF stores, and the daily energy deficit, i.e. the difference between intake and expenditure [2]. Death

Equine Clinical Nutrition, Second Edition. Edited by Rebecca L. Remillard.

occurs when there is greater than 25–30% loss of body protein that compromises cardiac and pulmonary muscle strength. Hence time to death during an energy deficit is firstly related to BF stores, and a "healthy" weight carries adequate BF stores to survive times of low or no food intake and disease. A lean horse with a BCS 3 to 4/9 may have more difficulty recovering from an illness or injury compared with a BCS 5 to 6/9 horse. While a thin horse (BCS < 3) may not have adequate energetic reserves to independently forage, and is at a greater risk of general malnutrition and death.

Conversely, excess BF is not better when considering a "healthy" weight for horses. Body fat has been traditionally thought of as an inert tissue of stored energy; however, adipocytes are now known to produce and secrete numerous cytokines and pro-inflammatory peptides [3–5]. Across different mammals, i.e. mice, rats, cats, dogs, primates, and people, numerous diseases have been associated with obesity and/or exacerbated by excess BF [6, 7]. The multisystem effects of obesity are linked to an imbalance between homeostatic and pro-inflammatory immune responses [8, 9]. Chronic systemic inflammation of obesity is a key component in the pathogenesis of insulin resistance [10]. Insulin dysregulation previously documented in other species and people has now been recognized in obese horses [11]. Hyperinsulinemia in horses is a risk factor for the life-limiting disease laminitis, and, therefore, efforts to develop obesity prevention and weight loss strategies are of immediate interest to veterinarians [12, 13].

If excess energy intake occurs over a prolonged period, most of the surplus is stored in the body as fat. Some of the excess energy is given off as heat and used for increased physical activity. Increased body heat production is used by many animal species, including people, to compensate for excess dietary energy intake; however, the horse is unique in compensating by increasing physical activity [14]. These horses may show increased anxiety, increased voluntary exercise when outside, and/or stereotypic behaviors that burn calories. Research in horses is ongoing to determine the individual factors that affect metabolism and energy requirements that may contribute to high vs. low BF stores.

In most species studied, feeding to maintain a lean body type is advantageous to overall health. The well-recognized Nestlé Purina's Life Span Study showed that dogs fed 25% less food than littermates over their lifespan had a 6/9 vs. 8/9 BCS and lived 18–24 m longer with a later onset of the same chronic conditions [15]. Other than in people and non-human primates, there are no lifetime studies in mammals larger than the dog to date [16, 17]. Therefore, the consequences of high BW due to high BF content for horses must be extrapolated from other species. However, in every species studied to date, excessively high BF has negative health consequences and shortens the potential life span. A long lifespan is a desirable trait for companion animals, and as the horse is increasingly considered a companion, horses living well in old age is becoming important to owners.

Most horses should be kept at a BCS between 4 and 6 on the Henneke 9-scale where a score of 5 is the median, while 3 indicates inadequate, and 7 or greater indicates excess energy intake [18]. See Chapter 2 Nutritional Assessment of the Horse. Veterinarians should consistently assess BW and BCS during physical examinations using one of the recognized BCS systems and relay to the caretaker in a two-way, active dialogue any potential problems [18–20]. Horse owners should be taught and encouraged to regularly assess BW and BCS using weight tapes properly and consistently positioned if calibrated weight scales are not available. Calibrated tapes and various weight equations using height and length are inexpensive and useful for monitoring BW. A consistent method should be applied, e.g. same person, tape and position, time relative to feeding, etc. However, such measures are less accurate at extreme BWs, in pregnant mares, growing foals, and well-muscled, fit horses. Practitioners should remain current on the advantages and disadvantages of the various methodologies by which to manage BW, i.e. in the proper use of grazing muzzles or restricting time out at pasture [21, 22]. Additionally, feeding low-calorie forages does require the supplementation of specific ration balancers to ensure a balanced intake of essential nutrients.

23.1.1 Reproductive Efficiency

The Henneke work describing body condition scoring in horses was used to show that mares of higher BCS, i.e. "over-conditioned," and those receiving higher planes of nutrition that created a positive energy balance and weight gain had better reproductive efficiency traits, as measured by faster foal heat and higher rates of conception than leaner counterparts [23]. See Chapter 20 Feeding Broodmares.

23.1.2 Performance

The welfare issues related to underconditioned horses are readily recognized by owners, whereas the health-related issues of overconditioning are rarely appreciated. Unfortunately, in events, such as halter classes or some hunter divisions, horses with more condition are often rewarded, which may be contributing to owner misperception of the ideal BCS.

Obesity in horses is associated with several negative performance consequences such as heat and exercise intolerance. The ideal BCS for a performance horse is not established, but, intuitively, excessive weight as BF would be a handicap, as well as an additional load on joints and limbs. In racehorses, the performance was related to fat-free mass while %BF was negatively correlated with race time [24]. A noticeable effect of excess BF in the horse is decreased physical activity and increased sweating with exercise. These effects are due primarily to a decreased ability to transfer heat to the air and cool the body due to excessive subcutaneous fat cover. Without cooling, 20 min of moderate exercise, i.e. trotting at 8.5–11 mph produces sufficient heat to cause hyperthermia-induced fatigue and even death [25]. Conversely, endurance horses with BCS ranging from 1.5 to 5.5/9 in a 160 km race illustrated that BCS had a significant effect on race completion rate. Horse performance improved at BCS greater than 3/9 while rider weight did not affect the outcome of the race [26].

Respiratory difficulties also contribute to decreased physical activity and performance in the overweight horse, as is known to occur in other species. The major respiratory complications of obesity are increased work of breathing, respiratory muscle inefficiency, and diminished respiratory compliance [27]. Obesity increases respiratory difficulties because excess body mass increases oxygen demand, but decreases the ability to expand the lungs during inhalation. The additional fat mass against the chest wall increases respiratory effort, reduces respiratory compliance and efficiency, and may lead to alveolar hypoventilation and exercise intolerance.

Similarly, excessive weight even in minimal work puts an added load on joints and limbs, which over a lifespan can be detrimental. Overweight and obese dogs have an increased prevalence of traumatic and degenerative orthopedic disease with greater severity of osteoarthritis at a younger age compared with those maintained at an ideal BCS [15, 28]. Similar correlations have been established in horses between BCS, activity level, and inflammatory biomarkers in the intercarpal joint [29]. See Chapter 18 Feeding Athletes and Working Horses.

23.1.3 Establishing Daily Digestible Energy Intake

Energy, measured in calories, is derived from the digestion and metabolism of dietary carbohydrates, fats, the carbon skeleton remaining after the deamination of proteins, and volatile (or short chain) fatty acids. In North America (NA), digestible energy (DE) is typically used to describe a horse's energy requirement and the available energy from food, i.e. feed gross energy minus the fecal energy. Most of Europe and abroad use the net energy system based on the ability of a feed to provide energy after metabolic losses, i.e. fecal, urine, gases, and heat. See Figure 6.1.

As in other species, people, dogs, and cats, despite having similar body weight, size and composition, two horses may require different energy intakes to maintain BW due to innate differences in metabolism. Variation in expected energy intake required to maintain optimal BW has been well documented in people, dogs, and cats, and the same should be expected for horses. Daily digestible energy recommendations have been suggested for horses at maintenance (DE_m) with "minimum", "average", and "elevated" energy need as a result of individual variation related to metabolic rate, environment or lifestyle, temperament, and voluntary activity [30]. See Chapter 17 Feeding Adult and Senior Horses.

- Minimum DE_m = 3.04 Mcal/100 kg BW/d
- Average DE_m = 3.34 Mcal/100 kg BW/d
- Elevated DE_m = 3.64 Mcal/100 kg BW/d

The minimum DE_m equation is a mean determined from horses and ponies that were confined to stalls during feeding trials to estimate DE intake. The minimum equation is an estimated DE_m for sedentary, docile, non-reactive temperament horses such as older or disabled horses maintained in stalls or small areas, or for those horses with low voluntary activity regardless of the space provided and should be used for overweight and obese (BCS $\geq$ 7/9) horses. The average DE_m is an estimate for horses with some turn out to pasture or a large drylot or those with a moderately reactive temperament or moderate voluntary activity in large areas, e.g. a performance horse during the off-season. The elevated DE_m is an estimate for horses, such as stallions or young animals, with relatively high reactive temperaments and/or high voluntary activity regardless of area size, e.g. physically active within a stall, drylot, or pasture. The elevated DE_m equation is not intended to include the energy needed for gestation, lactation, performance, or recovery, but should be used for BCS 3 to 4/9 horses in need of weight gain.

At face value, the equations suggest the DE required by an individual horse might be +/− 10% from the calculated average DE_m due to biological variations. However, the variation may be more than 10% based on data collected in other species. The generic equation for estimating daily energy requirement (DER) in an individual dog or cat can be as much as +/− 50% off the group mean. An individual dog's or cat's DER, and the amount of food needed to maintain a constant optimal BW, even under similar environmental conditions and confined to cages or runs, varied threefold [31]. Therefore, the calculated DE_m intake must be considered an estimate or starting point, and individual animal monitoring with feed adjustments is needed to achieve and maintain the desirable BCS given the magnitude of individual horse-to-horse variation has not been determined [30]. Conversely, the actual DE_m requirement of any horse may be reversely calculated but only when the animal maintains a relatively constant BW and ideal BCS over time. When the daily feed intake is quantified and the DE of each feed is determined, using laboratory analysis, the total DE intake can be calculated, and will be the DE_m requirement of that horse when BW has been constant.

Energy is the easiest nutrient class to visualize in the horse when there is an excessive or insufficient intake. While DE values of feeds are not readily available to most horse owners, it is relatively easy for an owner to feed for energy balance. Using BCS, a scale, or measuring tapes regularly, owners can ensure the horse at an ideal BCS is not gaining or losing weight. If a horse is chronically losing weight, the feed total or caloric density needs to be increased, whereas, less feed or a lower caloric density should be fed if the horse is chronically gaining weight. The regularity of assessing weight, i.e. weekly or monthly, should be as warranted by the individual case. There will be relatively small, i.e. 5–10% fluctuations in weight due to hydration, gastrointestinal tract (GIT) fill, eliminations, and the method of assessing BW. However, the detection of a trend, e.g. a consistent plus 8–10% change every 30 days, is an indication to reassess the animal, the feed, and the feeding method. See Appendix C Nutrition Competencies of Equine Veterinarians.

Horses that tend to gain weight easily such as ponies and miniature horses, several gaited breeds, Andalusians, and some warmbloods are said to be "easy keepers." These horses may have a lower than average maintenance energy requirement, in part due to a genetic predisposition that may have been an evolutionary advantage at one time. Using the minimum DE_m equation would be advisable for these horses until the individual horse had a trend of losing weight. For horses considered "hard keepers," such as Arabians or Thoroughbreds, the elevated DE_m equation may be used until the individual horse chronically gained weight. For all other breeds not characterized as easy or hard keepers, using the average DE_m equation may be used until the individual horse chronically gains or loses weight. The suggested daily DE for minimum, average and elevated needs are in 10% increments and thus provide only a guideline. When the BW trend is increasing over several weeks to months, the recommendation to decrease DE intake by 10–15% would be a reasonable first recommendation. Likewise, when the BW trend is decreasing over time, advising an increase in DE intake by 10–15% would be warranted. Whenever changing the daily DE intake to attain ideal BCS, subsequent regular, e.g. monthly, monitoring is required.

To further define the energy requirements at maintenance, studies feeding horses fed at different DE intakes for weight gain, then regressing to zero gain, estimated that for every 1 Mcal of DE consumed above maintenance need, 513 kcal was retained as fat, i.e. 51% efficiency [32]. Adipose tissue is 10–15% water and 85–90% fat, and the fat would provide approximately 9 Mcal/kg, therefore, one kg BF (1 kg × 85–90% fat × 9 Mcal/kg) is equivalent to 7.65–8.1 Mcal/kg. Given 1 kg of fat averages 7.88 Mcal, feeding about 15 Mcal of DE (7.88/0.51) above energy requirements would result in a gain of 1 kg BF. More recent work in 35 Quarter horses determined that an average of 24 Mcal above maintenance resulted in 1 kg of weight gain; although across all horses, the range was 11–34 Mcal/kg weight gain [33]. From a different perspective, horses fed nearly 197% of DE_m requirement gained 86 kg BW, 67 kg as fat, over 28 d, which increased BCS by 2 units (6 to 8/9) [34]. In summary, useful energy intake to BW estimates are:

- Metabolism of 1 kg of BF provides approximately 7.88 Mcal.
- 15 Mcal DE intake above maintenance will result in 1 kg of BF gain [32].
- 24 Mcal DE intake above maintenance will result in 1 kg of BW gain [33].
- 1 Mcal of DE intake above maintenance will result in 0.5 Mcal stored as fat [32].
- Each BSC unit above 5/9 is approximately a 5% BW gain as BF [34].

Obtaining a diet history can be invaluable in estimating current daily DE intake and, therefore, the source of excess calories responsible for the weight gain. The caloric intake of horse treats, now appearing on the market, cannot be underestimated as treats can be a substantial source of calories. See Sidebar 23.1. Treats may contain 300–400 kcal/100 g with instructions to feed 1–2 lb/d to a 500 kg horse. Treat-feeding instructions may add 1–4 Mcal/d, which is a 6–25% increase in daily DE intake for a 500 kg horse. Most horse treat products advertise "no sugar added," but this should not be mistaken for a sugar-free or even a low-sugar product. See Marketing Concepts in Chapter 13.

23.2 Feeding for Weight Loss

23.2.1 Animal Assessment

To maintain a constant BW and BCS, calorie intake must equal caloric expenditure. Therefore, horses with high BCS have DE intake greater than energy expenditure, and both aspects need to be investigated to determine the reasons for the weight gain before attempting to induce weight loss.

Most often, the DE consumption of overweight or obese horses has been chronically excessive relative to

Sidebar 23.1: Calorie Intake of Treats

Feeding treats, according to product directions when available, to horses with low or average DE_m requirements increases daily calorie intake substantially, which is often unappreciated by the owner:

- Example 1. Treat A (92 kcal/treat) marketed for horses suggests feeding 3 or 4 treats per 200 kg horse BW/d. A 400 kg horse with an average DE_m of 13.3 Mcal/d fed 8 treats/d (8 × 92 = 736 kcal/d) would be an additional 5.5% of DE_m (0.736/13.3 × 100) and likely not a significant source of calories.
- Example 2. Treat B (3.5 kcal/g) marketed for horses suggests feeding 1–2 lb/d to a 500 kg horse. Feeding 2 lb is 3.18 Mcal (908 g × 3.5). For a 500 kg horse with an average DE_m of 16.7 Mcal/d, feeding 2 lb of Treat B daily would be an additional 19% of DE_m (3.18/16.7 × 100), which is a significant source of calories.

expenditure due to simple overfeeding. Other complicating factors are age, genetics, housing, management, and secondary diseases. A complete physical examination and minimal laboratory database, i.e. complete cell count and serum biochemistry profile, should be assessed before initiating a weight loss plan. It is important to understand conditions commonly associated with obesity, such as orthopedic, endocrine, and metabolic disorders, as well as heat or exercise intolerances [7]. Rarely is a high BCS or weight gain due to a decrease in metabolic rate, i.e. hypothyroidism. It must be said that primary hypothyroidism is exceedingly rare in adult horses even when thyroid hormone concentrations are borderline or low. If the weight gain is relatively recent, i.e. weeks or months, most likely there has been a change in the animal, feeds, feeding method, and/or management factors (Table 23.1).

As in people, dogs, and cats, weight loss in horses is a challenge. Also similarly, many fads and tricks are promoted to enhance weight loss. However, the best tried and true method across species is creating a negative energy balance, i.e. the horse expends more calories than consumed. There are two ways to produce a daily energy deficit: decrease energy intake or increase expenditure, e.g. exercise or work, but the use of both together is more effective. A successful weight loss program involves a nutritionally complete calorie-restricted ration, an appropriate feeding method, an exercise plan, owner compliance, and monitoring. When weight loss is necessary for a horse with concurrent disease, i.e. orthopedic, endocrine, metabolic, GIT, or heat/exercise intolerance, close supervision by a veterinarian is recommended and additional precautions are needed [7].

Table 23.1 Factors affecting body weight and condition.

Factors to consider when a horse has unintended	Weight gain	Weight loss
Animal:		
Change in DE_m requirement	x	x
Pain (dental, GI, orthopedic)		x
Injury		x
Parasitism		x
Feed:		
Change in caloric density	x	x
Change in form or texture		x
Change in taste or smell		x
Contamination or spoilage		x
Feeding method:		
Incorrect food dosing	x	x
Change in feeding routine	x	x
Change in herd dynamics	x	x
Environmental limitation		x
Management:		
Change in feeding personnel	x	x
Change in feeding logistics	x	x
Limited water access		x
Change in an exercise program	x	x

A BCS between 4 and 6 on the Henneke scale [1–9] is thought to be healthy in horses, while those over 7 are said to be "over-conditioned" with more than 20% BW as BF [20]. In dogs and cats, % BF terminology was adapted from people and was presented as linear with BCS, i.e. a BCS 7/9 with 30% BF are "overweight," BCS 8/9 with 35% BF are "obese" and BCS 9/9 with 40% fat are "morbidly obese" [35, 36]. However, in horses, the Henneke scale was not originally intended to estimate BF and the association between BCS and BF fat appears to be nonlinear above 6/9 [20]. Therefore, estimating %BF, fat tissue weight to be lost, and time to reaching goal BW cannot be accurately predicted, only estimated, in horses using the BCS scale.

Body fat to be lost can be estimated using the current BW minus ideal BW. Ideal BW can be estimated using breed skeletal length and height measurements that do not change with %BF. See Tables 2.2 and 2.3. Given the difference between starting and ideal BW is primarily BF and each kilogram averages 7.88 Mcal, the calorie content of the weight difference can be estimated, e.g. 100 kg overweight × 7.88 Mcal/kg = 788 Mcal less must be fed over time to reduce BW by 100 kg. The total caloric value of the excess BF divided by the daily caloric deficit will approximate the time required to achieve the ideal BW, e.g. 788 Mcal excess divided by the daily caloric deficit of 3 Mcal/d = 263 days to lose 100 kg of BF.

23.2.2 Ration Assessment

Any plan will involve strategies for caloric restriction, and wherever possible, increased calorie expenditure. Obtaining a ration history detailing the forage, concentrate, and treat intakes to estimate the average daily DE intake and the exercise routine in the prior weeks to months will provide a valuable reference point from which to develop a weight loss feeding program. Dietary calorie restriction may be based on feeding some percent less than the current DE intake or feeding that required at the desired BW [37].

23.2.2.1 Feeds

The success of a weight loss ration begins with a low ration energy density. Most often rations containing 1.7–2.0 Mcal DE/kg dry matter (DM) composed primarily of forage are used. The ration should be nutritionally complete, i.e. include all of the nutrients recommended for an adult horse but restricted in DE calories. Most weight loss rations will require supplementation of vitamins, minerals, and possibly protein to meet recommended nutrient intakes for the start BW, and should have palatable water and white salt available at all times.

23.2.2.1.1 Forage

A forage analysis or estimated book value is necessary as hay should be the foundation of the weight loss ration, and is the starting point of ration balancing. Fair-quality forages (43–45% acid detergent fiber (ADF), 61–65% neutral detergent fiber (NDF), RFV 75–87) are appropriate for weight loss [7]. Grass forages are generally lower in energy, protein, and calcium content compared with those containing legumes. Examples of common grass varieties, as hay or pasture, are cool-season timothy, bromegrass, orchardgrass, canarygrass ryegrass, and fescue, or warm-season Bermudagrass and Teff.

Hay Whenever possible, feeding a lower DE hay is preferable to feeding a lower dry matter intake (DMI) of higher DE hay. For example, keeping DMI the same, feeding 7 kg of 2.0 Mcal DE/kg hay will provide the horse with 14 Mcal/d compared with 7 kg of 1.7 Mcal DE/kg hay providing 11.9 Mcal/d is a 15% reduction in calorie intake without changing DMI. Feeding lower quality hays with a lower DE, higher %NDF, and %ADF, could also be an advantage in reducing undesirable behaviors. For example, an owner could offer a higher quantity of a higher fiber (lower RFV) hay, which should increase chewing time, increase saliva production, lower the risk of ulcers, and occupy the horse longer in foraging behaviors. Teff hay fed free choice facilitated weight loss in horses due to lower palatability coupled with a low energy density, which resulted in low DE intake relative to other hay types [38]. It should be noted that Teff hay has higher nitrate concentrations, and while horses are more tolerant of nitrates than other livestock, soaking Teff hay for one hr decreased the nitrate concentrations [39].

Pasture Similar to feral and wild horses, domesticated horses turned out 24-hr/d graze 45% of the time (10–12 hrs) predominantly before dawn and after dusk. Similarly, inactive adult maintenance horses can meet their DE requirements within 8–10 hrs of grazing a fescue pasture. [40, 41]. Confined ponies turned out onto pasture spent a greater portion of the time grazing, consuming 4.9%BW, in some type of compensatory type of behavior [42]. When forage growth is not limiting, horses may have DMI near 3.2% BW/d and will become overweight and obese on palatable pasture [43].

Therefore, pasture should not be the main source of feed intake for overweight horses for several reasons. First, pasture grass may be more energy-dense than hay, i.e. cool-season grass pasture (2.4 Mcal DE/kg) vs. the same grass as mature hay (2.0 Mcal DE/kg), and may have higher concentrations of NSC than dried forages [30, 44]. Second, monitoring and regulating intake at pasture is difficult. Several studies have aimed to quantify DMI for a horse at pasture 24-hr/d; however, determining intake when horses are only out for shorter periods is more difficult [45]. Uncontrolled pasture access is counterproductive because a goal of weight loss is to limit DE intake. However, many owners do not have drylot facilities that preclude the use of pasture. For these reasons, some studies have investigated means of limiting pasture intake, either through the use of a grazing muzzle, reducing the size and time at pasture, and/or using different management practices, such as mowing before allowing horses out to graze or seeding different pasture grasses to affect calorie and NSC intake. Teff grass pasture consistently had lower DE, crude protein and NSC, and higher NDF and ADF fiber compared with alfalfa and cool-seasoned grasses [46].

Grazing muzzles have been used successfully to decrease pasture intake in horses and ponies but some owners have a negative perception of using muzzles, and therefore, it is important to ensure grazing muzzles are used correctly [22, 47]. The use of a grazing muzzle decreased forage consumed by 30% compared with no grazing muzzle on alternating days in the same horses [48]. DMI restrictions of 77–83% were found when ponies wore muzzles but, when turned out to pasture with no muzzle, ponies consumed more than 0.8% BW in the 3-hr period [49–51]. Many horses learn to remove muzzles, or can learn to strategically place the muzzle on grass that allows a higher than expected intake.

Pasture intake by horses can also be limited by time and space. Restricting the time a horse spends on pasture can decrease the feed consumed, but then drylot or stall facilities are needed with additional forage to prevent boredom and maintain healthy gut function. The DMI rate can be high initially when allowed access to pasture limited by time/d [40, 52]. Strip or rotational grazing can reduce grass intake and help with weight maintenance but may reduce activity although not seen in all studies [53, 54]. Horses restricted to grazing cells estimated to provide 80% of the DE requirements for 7 d lost significant amounts of weight but also exhibited decreased activity as determined by heart rate monitors and GPS-quantified distance traveled [55]. Some horses may initially graze heavily on the new sections of grass, which might increase the risk of laminitis under certain conditions. While limiting horses to specific pasture cells was an effective strategy for weight loss, and can promote uniform pasture grazing, the practice is labor-intensive in managing fences and grass yields to avoid overgrazing and weeds. In summary, maintaining the horse in a drylot or paddock with ad libitum water and salt, and adequate shelter may be preferable at some facilities.

23.2.2.1.2 Complementary Feeds

For overweight horses on a weight loss program, an all forage ration of pasture or hay will not provide sufficient vitamins and minerals to meet daily needs; therefore, it is advisable to feed a low-calorie/fat ration balancer at start BW. Recommended nutrient intakes increase with BW; therefore, feeding the non-energy vitamins and minerals at start BW will be greater than that recommended at the lower goal BW, and provide a margin of safety given none are near known toxic intakes. A low-calorie (1.5 Mcal DE/kg) pelleted equine ration balancing product containing vitamins and minerals plus an excellent protein source, such as soybean meal for essential amino acids, fed at 0.1–0.3% of start BW, or according to the manufacturer's feeding instructions, should complement a fair-quality forage to nutritionally complete the ration.

23.2.2.2 Key Nutrient is Digestible Energy

Ideally, lean body mass should be preserved, and BF mass should be decreased during weight loss. Dogs and cats at ideal BW in thermoneutral environments spend about 70% of the daily energy intake to maintain lean body mass [56]. Therefore, feeding horses a caloric intake equal to 70% of the DE required at ideal BW would be a reasonable initial recommendation. However, restricting Shetland ponies to a DE intake equal to 70% of the ideal BW requirement did achieve a weight loss rate of 0.6% BW/wk initially. DE had to be further restricted to 50% of ideal BW for 8 wks and then further restricted to 35% of ideal BW for 4 wks to achieve an overall loss of 1% BW/wk over a 17-wk trial. Changes in lean body mass or muscle were not assessed and likely metabolic rate declined in response to decreasing food intake [57]. Without an exercise plan, the resting metabolic rate normally down regulates with DE restrictions, and further caloric restrictions are then required for continued weight loss.

There are several means by which a limited daily DE intake may be calculated: (i) feed a lower percentage of DMI at start or goal BW, or (ii) feed a lower percentage of the minimum DE_m equation at starting or goal BW (Table 23.2). Ponies fed a chaff-based complete diet at 1% of start BW for 12 wks, which equated to 67% of DE_m at obese weight, lost on average 11% of the original weight. Of the weight lost, 45% was due to decreases in BF as measured by total body water using deuterium oxide. Heart girth circumference, belly girth circumference, rump width, and subcutaneous fat depth at the rib-eye area decreased, and, interestingly, play behavior increased [59]. Similarly, increased voluntary activity and social behavior have been noted in dogs and cats with as little as 5% weight loss.

It should be emphasized that there can be significant variation between horses in DE_m required to maintain BW. An obese horse may be found in a group of non-obese horses of similar breeds, workload, and feeding regimes. Feed DM and DE intakes were determined to be similar in a group of geldings of similar breed and age but ranged in BCS from overweight (BCS $\geq$ 7/9) or moderate (BCS 4 to 5/9) while living in the same pasture for several years [28]. Additionally, there can be substantial variation between overweight horses when placed on the same dietary restriction. In 12 overweight horses and ponies restricted to a DMI of 1.25% BW, considerable animal differences in weight loss were noted. When sources of the variable response were analyzed, 65% of the variation was attributed to the individual animal response to weight loss, whereas, diet and initial animal assessments were independent [60]. Based on successful weight loss programs in dogs and cats, the strategy of restricting DE based on the calculated current DE intake for the individual overweight horse may also be effective. If individual animal variation overshadows a standard DMI or DE_m restrictions based on current BW, determining first the current DE intake than maintains the obese weight, from the diet history, and then applying a percent (90%) restriction of current DE intake would likely be successful.

23.2.3 Feeding Management

Owners, managers, caretakers, available facilities, and resources, i.e. time and finances will most likely need to be amended to implement a weight loss plan. Successful weight loss protocols feed a nutritionally complete low-calorie ration at a reduced DMI. Small frequent meals are recommended in weight loss programs for most other species, and horses having feed available 20–24 hrs/d is the

Table 23.2 Comparison of different weight loss protocols, theoretically, for the same horse fed the same grass hay ration using minimum DE_m. [30, 34, 59]

Weight loss programs comparisons[a]	Current protocol 2.2% DMI		2% DMI at start BW	2% DMI at goal BW	2% DMI at goal BW + Ex	90% DE_m at start BW	90% DE_m at goal BW	100% DE_m at goal BW + Ex
Protocol #	0	1	2	3	4	5	6	7
Consuming hay	MML	Grass hay						
Daily DE intake (Mcal/d)	25.56	20.91	19.01	15.84	15.84	14.45	12.04	13.38
DMI (kg/d)	11.62	11.62	10.56	8.80[b]	8.80	8.03	6.69[c]	7.43
Exercise (Mcal/d)[d]	0	0	0	0	1.22	0	0	1.22
DE deficit (Mcal/d)	0	4.65	6.55	9.72	15.54	6.46	8.87	12.26
Wks to goal BW	0	21	15	10	7	15	11	8
Weight loss rate (% BW/wk)[e]	0	0.8%	1.1%	1.6%	2.6%	1.1%	1.5%	2.1%

[a] Based on BW 528 kg BCS 8/9 adult horse fed MML hay (2.2 Mcal/kg DM) has a goal weight of 440 kg BCS 5/9 fed grass hay (1.8 Mcal/kg DM). Minimal DE_m starting BW = 16.0 Mcal/d, minimum DE_m at goal BW = 13.4 Mcal/d. Total fat to be lost is 88 kg fat × 7.88 Mcal/kg fat = 693 Mcal deficit. Total Mcal deficit /daily Mcal deficit = d to goal BW. %BW wt loss rate = [88 kg/528 kg]/wks to goal BW × 100. Exercise = 528 kg × 6.5 kcal/kg/hr slow trot for 30 min (Table 18.5) × 5 d/wk / 7 d/wk = 1.22 Mcal/d.
[b] 1.66% DMI at start BW.
[c] 1.26% DMI at start BW.
[d] Slow trot (0.65 Mcal/100 kg BW) for 30 minutes 5x wk (Table 18.5).
[e] Actual rates of weight loss will likely be 0.5–1.0 %BW lost/wk [7].
Source: Based on NRC [30]; Carter et al. [34]; Pagan and Hintz [58].

norm. A weight loss program in horses should provide feed frequently (4–6 meals/d) in amounts that still limit the total daily DE intake. All hay and supplement meals should be fed by weight and not volume, e.g. a scoop of rocks does not weigh the same as a scoop of cotton balls.

To determine a reasonable estimate of a limiting DMI, the current hay intake based on diet history and feed analysis should be determined first to ensure a lower DE will be fed at the start of the weight loss program. If the horse has been allowed ad libitum hay, most consume 2–2.25% BW/d. A reasonable recommendation is to reduce feed intake to 1.2–1.5% BW/d, if current DMI is greater than 1.5%, and assess BW weekly for 6–8 wks. Reduce feed DMI further to 1% BW if needed. Horses should not be fed <1% BW unless under veterinary supervision due to potential negative consequences. The DMI quantity is less than actual "as fed" instructions. Most hays and pelleted feeds contain about 10% water and providing feeding recommendations in "as fed" quantities (DMI/0.9) for horse owners is advisable.

With the use of a weight tape or scale, owners can track BW weekly and can adjust the diet accordingly by weighing the feed. Although feeding a coarse but palatable long-stem hay during a weight loss program is preferred, it can be difficult to accurately weigh flaked long-stem hay. Owners estimating hay weight for a meal based on square bale or average flake weight is not sufficiently accurate to adjust feed intake by 10%. Placing the hay in a 1-inch^2 mesh net and weighing the bundle using a pull-type or digital hanging spring scale with ½ lb or kg increments will be reasonably accurate and consistent (Figure 23.1). Hay can be removed through the mesh openings to obtain the correct amount of hay to be fed (Figure 23.2). If giving treats is an important bonding behavior for the owner, calories from treats must be counted in the total DE intake and the specific treat and daily allotment must be prescribed and agreed upon by the owner. See Sidebar 23.1.

Muzzles alone are rarely successful in controlling BW but are a useful tool as part of a larger weight management program. Careful monitoring of a horse's behavior in the pasture, and monitoring of BW and BCS, will determine if a muzzle is effective at restricting weight gain or conducive to weight loss. Monitoring for potential issues includes rubbing, altered social interactions and increased wearing of the teeth [50]. Miniature horses muzzled for 24 hrs showed no apparent physiological stress, weight gain was prevented, and more time was spent foraging [61, 62]. The National Equine Welfare Council[1] provides Grazing Muzzle Guidance on the proper fitting and adaption of

1 National Equine Welfare Council https://newc.co.uk.

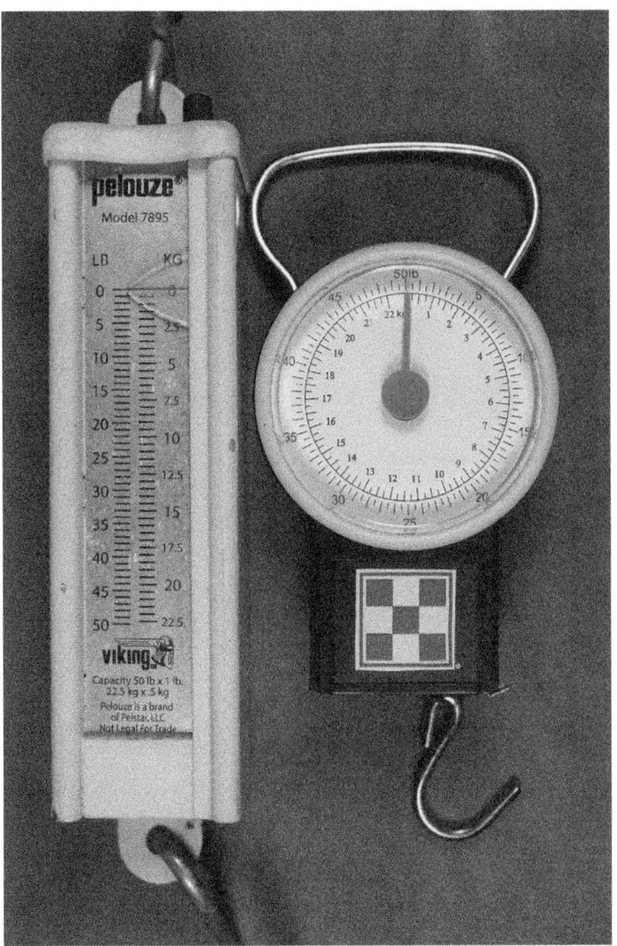

Figure 23.1 Examples of pull-down hanging feed scales.

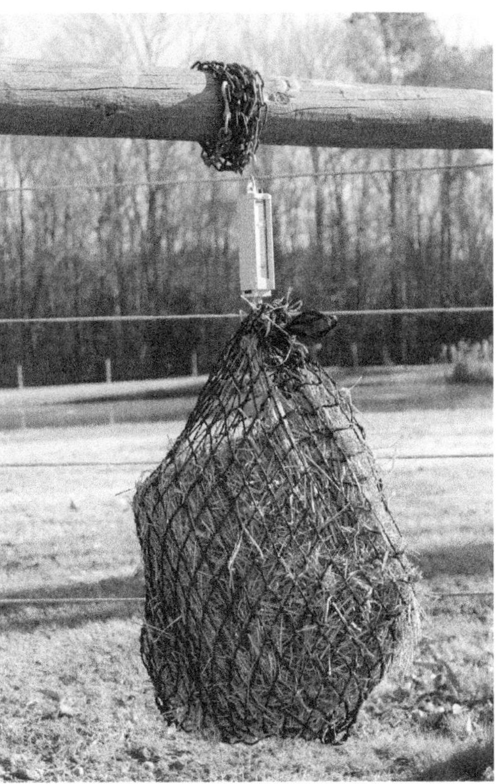

Figure 23.2 Weighing long-stem hay using a net and pull-down hanging scale.

muzzles. The guidance recommends muzzles not be worn for more than 10–12 hrs/d and ensures the consumption of water is not hindered. See Sidebar 23.2.

23.2.3.1 Fads and Supplements

As with people, there are numerous fads and supplements marketed to promote weight loss in horses. See Evidence-based Medicine in Chapter 14. The so-called "low carb" diets are misleading – as "carbs" would include structural carbohydrates such as fiber, without which there is a likely increase in the risk of digestive disturbances. There are also numerous claims that supplements containing magnesium can improve insulin sensitivity. However, most equine diets have more than adequate concentrations of magnesium, nor is there any scientific data to suggest that additional magnesium promotes weight loss. Thyroid medication, e.g. Thyro-L, provides thyroid hormone for hypothyroid horses. Research has shown that supplementation of Thyro-L, containing levothyroxine sodium, in euthyroid healthy horses

Sidebar 23.2: Quick Notes for Weight Loss

- Determine or estimate current DE intake using a diet history.
- Obtain forage nutrient profile and balance non-energy nutrients for start BW.
- Feed lower energy density forage to allow maximum weight loss with the most forage provided.
- Initially feed DMI at 1.5% BW if lower than the current rate.
- Provide forage in slow feeders such as hay nets with 1.25 x 1.25 inch (or 1 x 1 in) mesh openings.
- Select for low NSC intake when insulin dysregulation has been diagnosed or suspected; soak hay that has more than 12% NSC DM.
- Increase exercise when possible; hand walking may be sufficient. Eliminate or minimize the routine use of blankets on the horse.
- Monitor BW, neck, girth and belly circumference every 2 wks, and BCS monthly (Table 2.2).
- Aim for 1% BW loss/wk on average.
- Decrease DMI further to 1.25% BW, if needed.
- If needed, decrease feed intake further (1.2–1% BW) with veterinary monitoring.
- Be patient as weight loss requires weeks to months to accomplish.

decreases BW and improves insulin sensitivity [63]. However, this is a prescription drug and federal law restricts the use of this product by or on the order of a licensed veterinarian.

23.2.3.2 Exercise

Creating an energy deficit as a result of decreased DE intake and increased exercise has many advantages over maintaining an idle horse fed a reduced DE intake. However, in the case of weight gain as a result of inactivity due to lameness, a dietary restriction may be the only option. Exercise in conjunction with reduced caloric intake has been shown in other species to be beneficial for weight reduction for several reasons:

1) Increases daily energy expenditure over the idle horse.
2) Prevents the down regulation of resting metabolic rate, due to decreasing thyroid hormone concentrations that would otherwise occur when caloric intake is reduced [64].
3) Moderate exercise has been known to reduce appetite.
4) Prevention of bone mineral and muscle losses that occur when caloric intake is reduced in the idle horse.

Few studies have examined the various types of exercises specifically for weight loss in horses, although exercise in addition to the restricted diet provided enhanced health benefits over restricted DE intake alone [65, 66]. There was significant weight loss in horses that were placed on energy intake restriction to 80% of estimated DE requirements for start BW by using either dietary restriction or an exercise protocol to burn 20% of estimated DE requirements [67]. While both groups lost similar amounts of weight and BCS, exercised horses had significant improvements in insulin and glucose metabolism. The horse should lose BF with exercise training, build muscle, improve glucose metabolism, and heat tolerance. An additional benefit to exercising during weight loss is that as muscle mass increases, resting metabolic rate also increases.

Exercise intensity is defined by the amount of energy required to perform a physical activity per unit of time. Aerobic exercise, i.e. using oxygen-dependent energy reactions, with a RQ between 0.7 and 1.0 is catabolizing fat tissue for calories [68]. Hence, low-intensity exercise such as fast walk (0.25 Mcal/100 kg BW/hr) to a medium trot (0.95 Mcal/100 kg BW/h) or combinations several times a week is preferred during a weight loss program. See Table 18.5. The DE expenditure of an exercise session is directly related to the weight of the horse, time, and speed. For example, a 615 kg BCS 7/9 mature Paint mare performing a fast walk (3.5 mph) for 60 min would expend approximately 1.54 Mcal (Table 18.5) [59]. The same 615 kg horse requires 18.7 Mcal DE /d, [6.15 × 3.04] hence fast walking for 1 hr/d would equate to 8.2% (1.54/18.7) of her idling horse DE daily requirement [30]. Exercise programs must start slowly for short periods (20–30 min/session) but regularly (2–3 sessions/wk) to be effective, and should progress in frequency, duration, and increase in intensity as respiratory and cardiovascular responses to exercise improve for continued weight loss [7]. If the exercise protocol intensity increased to a medium trot (9 mph) for 45 min, then the same 615 kg horse would expend 4.4 Mcal equal to 23% of the idle horse DE requirements [59, 67]. Exercise is an effective weight loss tool in addition to decreased caloric intake (Table 23.2).

23.2.3.3 Owner Compliance

In controlled research studies where feed is weighed daily and horses are carefully monitored, calorie restriction and/or exercise have been shown to be effective at achieving weight loss in horses. It is important to consider that across species, adherence to dietary restrictions and exercise protocols[2] is key to having favorable results [63, 69, 70]. Owners who strictly followed weight loss protocols for 24 overweight horses by removing the horse from pasture, used a grazing muzzle, or weighed feed daily to restrict intake, achieved significantly greater weight loss than less compliant owners [71]. While owners should be taught how to assess BCS, scores are regularly lower than that of a trained individual, and hence objective measurements, i.e. BW, girth, and belly circumference are likely the more accurate home-monitoring tool [72]. Photos taken monthly consistently can be an excellent way to document weight loss progress and motivate owners.

23.2.3.4 Risks

Simple feed and calorie intake restrictions are not without risks. Horses restricted to 1.25% BW lost weight, but high fecal dry matter (DM) output was reported. This was attributed to the consumption of the wood shaving bedding by at least 5 of the 12 horses [73]. Limited forage intake is also attributed to the development of stereotypic disorders in horses [74]. Abnormal behavior increased in racehorses when forage intake was less than 6.8 kg/d which is 1.5–1.7% BW in horses weighing between 400 and 450 kg. Providing environmental enrichment is recommended with intake below 1.5% BW [75]. To avoid boredom in horses undergoing weight loss, it is generally recommended that forage is offered:

- divided into 4–6 meals/d.
- in a 1x1 inch mesh hay net[3] which has been shown to double the eating time compared with those eating the same amount of hay without a net [76, 77].

---

2 Exercise 3–5x/wk in the same round pen or arena can become mind-numbing for both horse and rider. Consider a diversity of exercise patterns with purpose such as the Parelli Freestyle or Finesse Patterns (www.parelli.com).

3 For example: https://haychix.com/collections/square-bale.

- using single or doubled hay nets. Tripled nets may promote frustration.
- in multiple nets in different places within range.

Another potential consequence of restricting forage intake is the risk of gastric ulcers. Horses continually produce and secrete acid into the stomach, and continuous forage consumption helps to buffer these acids, both through the bicarbonate-rich saliva secreted with the chewing of forages, and the fibrous mat that can help protect the upper lining of the stomach from acid. Withdrawing feed from horses for 12 and then 24 hrs is the protocol used to induce gastric ulcers before testing the efficacy of different ulcer treatments [78]. Feeding multiple meals/d and/or slow feeding of forage is advisable to reduce the risk of ulcers. See Ulcers in Chapter 26.

Hyperlipemia or fatty liver syndrome is a metabolic disease most commonly associated with weight loss in overweight female miniature horses, donkeys, and ponies, particularly those that are insulin resistant [79, 80]. Sudden dietary restriction to achieve negative energy balance, with stress and increased cortisol concentrations causes rapid BF breakdown from the adipose tissue. The liver normally converts fatty acids from BF to very-low-density lipoproteins (VLDL) and then secretes the VLDL into the plasma for peripheral tissue uptake. When hepatic production of VLDL exceeds peripheral tissue uptake, high plasma concentrations result, which in turn cause liver and kidney saturation. This may become a life-threatening disease due to multi-organ dysfunction and failure. At-risk animals should be carefully monitored for hyperlipidemia when placed on calorie-restricted diets. See Hyperlipemia in Chapter 27.

23.2.3.5 Monitoring

Monitoring, initially every 2 wks then every 4 wks, is essential to a successful weight loss plan to ensure the prescribed feeding instruction is effective and to motivate the owner if needed. Caretakers often benefit from support, e.g. regular discussions with a veterinary technician, client groups overseen by a veterinary practice, or consultations with a clinical nutritionist [71]. Reviewing the feeds and feeding method is key to preventing and uncovering discrepancies during setbacks. There are three critical time points to recheck: (i) in the first 1–2 wks to ensure the plan has been implemented and to catch early any questions or unexpected problems; (ii) at the end of the program to oversee the transition from weight loss to maintenance feeding instructions, and (iii) any time during the program when weight loss is not occurring or there has been a logistical change, i.e. feed, people, housing, or a change to feeding instructions is needed [56].

Weight loss can safely occur at 1% BW/wk but on average will likely be 0.5–1.0% BW/wk [7]. The rate of weight loss should be calculated excluding the first week as weight loss at that time is most likely due to reduced gut fill. Changes in BW, heart girth and belly circumference will be noted sooner than changes in BCS and crest neck score [7, 58, 60, 81]. If no change in heart girth or belly circumference has occurred within 4–6 wks, BW should be assessed using a calibrated weigh scale. A review of the feed and feeding recommendations is advisable and consider decreasing DE intake by 10–15%, or if possible, increasing exercise by 10%. Reviewing the feeds and feeding method with the person responsible for delivering the feed is necessary to find inconsistencies between the feeding instructions and the ration offered to the horse.

23.3 Feeding for Weight Gain

23.3.1 Animal Assessment

To maintain a constant BW and BCS, calorie intake must equal caloric expenditure. Therefore, healthy horses with low BW and BCS (3–4/9) have an insufficient DE intake relative to energy expenditure, and both aspects need to be investigated to determine the reasons before attempting to induce weight gain.

A complete physical examination and minimal laboratory data, i.e. complete cell count and serum biochemistry profile, should be assessed before initiating a weight gain plan. On-site observation of the feeding routine and the horse's eating behavior may also provide valuable insight as to the origin of the poor BCS. The provision of a nutritionally adequate and palatable ration to a horse reluctant to eat is suggestive of underlying disease or pain [82]. It is important to rule out conditions commonly associated with low BCS, such as oral/dental, orthopedic, endocrine, organ, and metabolic disorders. Decreased voluntary feed intake is most commonly related to underlying disease and the medical condition must be addressed before or simultaneously while attempting weight gain. Healthy horses that are underweight and underconditioned (BCS 3–4/9), not related to a concurrent medical condition or a welfare problem involving neglect or abuse, should require only additional calories or less exercise/work to achieve or regain the desired BCS. For malnourished starved horses BCS < 3/9, see Chapter 24 Refeeding and Assisted Feeding.

Estimating the average daily DE intake and detailing the exercise or work routine in the weeks to months before loss of BW and BCS will provide a valuable reference point. Energy expenditure higher than the average DE_m may occur in animals with a higher than average resting energy metabolism due to innate metabolic and temperament differences, or counterproductive behaviors such as stall walking or weaving. Those animals with elevated innate DE_m requirements referred to as "hard keepers" may require greater DE intake permanently and the elevated DE_m equation is recommended as a starting point. Increasing the daily DE intake temporarily to correct a low BCS may be sufficient. For example, in broodmares with a low BCS and conception rate, a manager may increase DE intake to improve the conception rate [23]. A successful weight gain program involves a balanced high-energy ration, an appropriate feeding method, a modified exercise plan, owner compliance, and monitoring.

23.3.2 Ration Assessment

Low BCS (3–4/9) horse with a good to excellent appetite indicates an insufficient DE intake more likely due to ration or feeding management issues (Table 23.1). Obtaining a ration history detailing the forage and concentrate intakes to estimate the average daily DE intake in the weeks to months before loss of BW and BCS will provide a valuable reference point. Evaluating the appearance, feel, and smell of the forage and complementary feeds is a practical means of determining the presence of mold, dust, and weeds, which may be limiting intake, or undesirable foreign materials, such as metal or glass, which may have caused oral trauma [83, 84].

23.3.2.1 Feeds

The ration designed for weight gain contains >2 Mcal DE/kg DM and micronutrients to be nutritionally complete and balanced.

23.3.2.1.1 Forage

A generally safe method of increasing calorie intake is to increase the forage offered to the horse. Most horses offered ad libitum hay consume 2-2.25% DMI. Forage is high in fiber and typically lower in sugars than cereal grains, and there is a lower risk of digestive disorders when increasing more the same forage as compared with changing the feed type. Offering more forage may decrease innate behaviors such as stall walking or weaving that increased DE expenditure. Increased forage intake may occur with increased time at pasture, improving the quality of the pasture, increased amounts and frequency of hay offered, increased forage quality (>2.0 Mcal DE/kg DM, RFV > 100). Typically, increasing long-stem forage is desirable, but processed forages, such as haylage or hay cubes, may also improve intake. Other high-fiber concentrate feeds such as beet pulp without molasses (2.8 Mcal DE/kg DM) or rice bran (3.35 Mcal DE/kg DM) will effectively increase the caloric density of the ration while keeping sugar intake relatively low.

23.3.2.1.2 Complementary Feeds

Increasing quantities of cereal grains and commercial concentrate feeds minimally increases the caloric density of the ration but effectively increase caloric intake. Adding cereal grains will also increase the starch and sugar intake, which may exacerbate metabolic disorders, e.g. insulin dysregulation unrelated to obesity. Higher rates of concentrate intake are also associated with an increased risk of colic and gastric ulcers. For these reasons, it is generally advised to not feed more than 1 kg of cereal grain concentrates (1g starch/kg BW) at one meal and when additional calories are to be provided in the form of grain concentrates, the horse should be fed additional small meals/d rather than more concentrate at 1 or 2 meals/d. See Figure 26.2.

There is an upper limit to the amount of high-fiber feeds and cereal grains a horse can consume. Once this has been maximized, fat sources may be introduced into the diet to increase DE intake. Corn or canola oil is an excellent source of calories, palatable, economical, and safe, although messy to feed at higher intakes. One 8 vol-oz "cup" (244 g) of oil has ~2 Mcal DE and most horses can generally tolerate two cups/d if gradually introduced over 7–14 days [85]. When maximum absorption from the GIT has been exceeded, owners report "shiny stools," which is steatorrhea, and then the amount of oil fed should be titrated down until manure appears normal. There are several palatable high-fat commercial supplements, some of which might be cost-prohibitive when high intakes are needed. There is a 99% fat dry supplement powder easier to feed than liquid oil, and there are 30% fat pellcted supplements with vitamins and minerals.[4,5]

If there is an interest in feeding more calories using omega-3 (n3) oils with alpha-linolenic acid (ALA), flaxseed or flax oil (aka linseed oil) with 50% ALA is a reasonable option although more expensive than corn or canola oil with less than 10% ALA. The conversion rate of dietary ALA to eicosapentaenoic acid (EPA) or docosahexaenoic acid (DHA), by the liver in the horse is not known but is known to be less than 10% in other species including people. The optimal n3 : n6 ratio is not known for any species; however, having both in the ration is thought to be beneficial. Feeding marine-derived with EPA and DHA are known to be more effective at dampening the inflammatory response as precursors of cellular membranes and local cytokines than plant-based ALA. Feeding marine-derived oil with 35% DHA and EPA would have to be advantageous for reasons other than merely increasing

4 Cool Calories https://www.mannapro.com/equine/nutritional-supplements/cool-calories-100.
5 Amplify https://www.purinamills.com/horse-feed/products/detail/purina-amplify-high-fat-horse-supplement.

energy intakes, such as dampening the immune response in inflammatory airway disease or osteoarthritis to justify the increased cost.[6] Some horses may have palatability issues when fed marine-based oil due to the odor; however, starting with small amounts mixed with the grain in a large wide-mouth feeding pan or on a mat on the ground might be necessary to reduce odor and improve acceptability.

23.3.2.2 Key Nutrient is Digestible Energy

Increased calories consumed results in BW gain in healthy horses, which may be accomplished by increasing total feed consumed and, when DMI has been maximized, increasing caloric density of the ration (Mcal DE/kg DM). Carbohydrates, regardless of structure, have a caloric density of 3.5 Mcal DE/kg, and feeding more increases caloric intake but not the caloric density of the ration. Fat or oils have 8.5 Mcal DE/kg, and therefore the addition of fat effectively increases the caloric density of the ration while minimally increasing feed volume. Concurrently, intakes of protein, minerals, and vitamins are needed for tissue synthesis and accrual of muscle, bone, and viscera, proportional to the increase in BW. For example, increasing calorie intake without a proportional intake of essential amino acids may result in BF accumulation in place of lean muscle mass. Non-energy nutrients must be provided in the ration proportional to the caloric density such that no nutrient is limiting the synthesis of new body tissues resulting in a net weight gain. For example, 37 g protein/Mcal DE is recommended for adult maintenance horses, however, 45 g protein/Mcal DE is recommended for growing yearlings.

23.3.3 Feeding Management

The amount of additional daily calories required to gain weight depends on the amount of weight gain desired, the timeline, and is influenced by individual horse factors, such as metabolic rate and temperament, and external factors, such as housing or environment. It is generally recommended that the amount fed be increased gradually to prevent acute laminitis, diarrhea, colic, or other digestive tract disturbances. Although, no changes in heart or respiratory rate, rectal temperature, signs of laminitis or GIT disturbances occurred in 20 mature healthy low BCS (3.9/9) horses, when, without any feed adjustment period, were allowed free access to one of two complete diets [86]. Both diets provided 3.12 Mcal DE/kg, 13% crude protein containing either 14% crude fiber and no added fat or 18% crude fiber with 5% added fat. The horses consumed 2.8% BW, gained 1 kg/d, and BCS increased to 6/9 in 45 days. There was no difference in animal response to either diet fed ad libitum.

There are a few published studies to suggest successful weight gain protocols in horses. Thirteen Arabian or Arab-cross geldings ranging in age from 8 to 20 yrs gained 2 BCS units fed approximately 1.9 times DE_m requirements in 30 wks [34]. Likewise, in 35 Quarter horses, average age 5.3 yrs, 462 kg BW, and 4.5/9 BCS were fed 1.5, 1.6, and 1.7 times DE_m gained 8, 24, and 22 kg, respectively in 42 days, although there was substantial variation between horses [33]. Similarly, 10 Shetland ponies and 9 warmblood horses fed 2 times the estimated DE_m requirement for 2 yrs gained approximately 130% and 117% of initial BW, respectively, primarily in the first year [87]. Data from the few but varied studies suggest feeding 1.5–2 times DE_m at start BW results in 0.2–0.5 kg/d weight gain.

Based on these weight gain studies, a reasonable first recommendation for a low BCS horse to gain BW would be to increase current DE intake by 1.5 using a 2–3 Mcal/kg DM nutritionally complete and balanced ration divided into 4–6 meals/d. The DE intake may be increased in a stepwise fashion to 2 times DE_m should the rate of weight gain be inadequate. A diet of legume or mixed grass-legume hay (2.2–2.6 Mcal/kg DM) may be offered ad libitum with high-fiber concentrates. If forage intake is limiting calorie intake, increasing the caloric density of the high-fiber concentrate with the addition of a fat supplement may be necessary. Water and salt should be available ad libitum. See Sidebar 23.3.

Sidebar 23.3: Quick Notes for Weight Gain

- Determine or estimate current DE intake using a diet history.
- Obtain forage nutrient profile and balance non-energy nutrients for goal BW.
- Feed higher energy density forage, if possible.
- Increase feed intake, e.g. offering forage ad libitum.
- Add fat (oil) as a concentrated source of calories up to 1 mL fat/kg BW/d.
- Carefully increase the starch intake from a concentrate ensuring <2g starch/kg BW/d, <1g starch/kg BW/meal and <0.5% BW cereal grain concentrate/d. See Chapter 26 Digestive System Disorders.
- Increased protein intake does not increase weight or muscle gain in the absence of exercise.
- Monitor BW, neck, girth and belly circumference every 2 wks, and BCS monthly (Table 2.2).
- Be patient as weight gain may require weeks to months to accomplish.

6 EO-3 https://ker.com/hoof-coat/eo-3. See Case in Point in Chapter 14.

23.3.3.1 Supplements

Most supplements promoting weight gain contain fat, generally between 30% and 60%, plus additional perceived favorable ingredients, such as vitamins, minerals, pro-and prebiotics, yeast cultures, protein, and particular fatty acid types. Rigorous evidence is scarce and often inconclusive regarding the addition of ingredients other than fat in promoting weight gain. In healthy underweight horses, the addition of fat alone is often sufficient to increase BW.

23.3.3.2 Exercise

For weight gain, in a performance horse that is frequently exercised, it may be necessary to reduce the daily or weekly workouts until BW and condition have improved. Discontinuance of training or the exercise program is rarely necessary. It should be noted that in some cases, there is a difference in the desired tissue type to be gained. To avoid the horse from appearing thin, i.e. improving BCS, the goal is to increase subcutaneous fat coverage. However, owners and trainers of many disciplines want to increase the muscle groups that run along a horse's spine, referred to as "top line." The topline includes the muscle groups that are along the vertebral column from the base of the neck, along the back and loin, and over the top of the hip to the tail head. It is well recognized that adequate protein intake is required for muscular development; however, increasing dietary protein intake greater than the amino acid requirements does not drive muscle development alone. Muscle stimulation, i.e. exercise, is required for muscle cell hypertrophy and hyperplasia. Most muscle development in mature animals is the result of muscle cell hypertrophy. Lysine, methionine, leucine, and threonine are essential amino acids for the horse. Leucine has been shown to upregulate some pathways in muscle protein synthesis and hypertrophy. A diet balanced using sources of seed meals or legumes will provide sufficient quantities of these amino acids in support of muscle development during exercise.

23.3.3.3 Owner Compliance

Owners generally demonstrate better compliance in weight gain vs. weight loss programs. The issue is more likely owners overfeeding or adding weight "boosting or building" supplements touted for "hard keepers." It is sufficiently effective for horse owners to feed based on a %BW rather than total calorie intake. With the use of a weight tape or scale, owners can track BW weekly and can adjust the diet accordingly by weighing the feed (Figure 23.2).

23.3.3.4 Monitoring

A calculated DE intake is only an estimate or starting point, and individual animal monitoring is essential, with feed adjustments as needed, to achieve and maintain the desirable BCS. As with monitoring during a weight loss program, there are three critical time points to recheck [56]: (i) in the first 1–2 wks to ensure the plan has been implemented and to catch early any questions or unexpected problems; (ii) at the end of the program to oversee the transition from gaining to maintaining weight, and (iii) any time during the program when weight gain is not occurring or a change in the feeding plan is required due to a logistical change. Although the Henneke BCS scoring estimating %BF is not linear but logarithmic for BCS >7/9, it was considered useful in estimating the BF content in horses and ponies BCS <7/9 [20]. Monitoring BW every 2 wks and BCS monthly, and adjusting the feeding recommendations based on the individual horse's response is often successful in improving BCS in healthy underweight horses.

Case in Point

In March, an owner presents an 8-yr-old Quarter horse gelding, BW 540 kg, BCS 7/9 that has gained weight over the winter months while stall-resting for a left hind ligament injury. The horse was regularly trained and performed in several rodeo events until an injury last October. The owner did not change the feeding regime while the horse was stall-resting because she did not want the horse to lose his "condition". The horse has been maintained in a stall (12′ × 12′), within a heated barn, with access to an outdoor fenced drylot area (12′ × 24′) for 2 hrs/d. An ultrasound recheck of the left hind leg is scheduled for next week, and if approved, exercise will be restarted using an increasingly progressive protocol in time for performing next summer. The owner had been advised by the radiologist at the previous recheck visit that it would be in the horse's best interest to lose weight before returning to competition.

Animal Assessment

Physical examination was unremarkable and routine complete blood count and serum biochemistry tests were all within normal limits. There was no evidence of lameness. This patient's ideal BW, using anatomical measurements, was estimated at 460 kg; therefore, the horse is 17% overweight.

1) *How to begin a weight loss program?*

Ration Assessment

The horse is fed *ad libitum* legume-grass hay and 4 scoops a textured feed designed for performance horses divided into two feedings/d. Water and a salt block are readily available. Owner had nearly 2 tons of hay stored indoors that was of good to high-quality, free of weeds, mold, dust, and insects, and still had an aromatic pleasant smell. Most of the alfalfa leaves were missing but the grass leaves and seed heads were readily visible. Hay analysis was not available but a book value of 2.07 Mcal DE/kg DM was used. The concentrate fed is a sweet feed mixed with an extruded pellet called Super Performance Horse Feed. The DE information is not on the label but the owner called customer service to learn the product contains 1625 kcal DE/lb or 3.58 Mcal DE/kg as fed. The owner feeds 4 scoops/d and the weight of 1 scoop was determined to be 1 lb or 454g.

2) *What is the daily DE intake from the concentrate?*
3) *Assume ad libitum consumption is 2.1% BW, what is the daily DE intake from the hay?*
4) *What is the total DE intake per day?*

Dietary Recommendations

5) *How would you summarize the current total DE intake compared with DE intake recommended for the ideal BW?*
6) *What are your initial feeding recommendations for weight loss, expected rate of weight loss, and timeline to optimal BW? There are 7 plausible weight loss protocols in Table 27.2.*

See Appendix A Chapter 23.

References

1 Brabender, K., Zimmermann, W., and Hampson, B. (2016). Seasonal changes in body condition of Przewalski's horses in a seminatural habitat. *J. Equine Vet. Sci.* 42 (7): 73–76.

2 Engelking, L.R. (2011). Starvation. In: *Textbook of Veterinary Physiological Chemistry*, 2e, 412–432. Amsterdam: Elsevier.

3 Trayhurn, P. (2006). Inflammation in obesity: down to the fat? *Compend. Contin. Educ. Pract. Vet.* 28 (4): 33–36.

4 Gayet, C., Bailhache, E., Dumon, H. et al. (2004). Insulin resistance and changes in plasma concentration of TNFα, IGF1, and NEFA in dogs during weight gain and obesity. *J. Anim. Physiol. Anim. Nutr.* 157–165.

5 Miller, C., Bartges, J., Cornelius, L. et al. (1998). Tumor necrosis factor-α levels in adipose tissue of lean and obese cats. *J. Nutr.* 128 (Suppl): 2751S–2752S.

6 Laflamme, D.P. (2006). Understanding and managing obesity in dogs and cats. *Vet. Clin. North Am. Small Anim. Pract.* 36: 1283–1295.

7 Geor, R.J. and Harris, P.A. (2013). Obesity. In: *Equine Applied and Clinical Nutrition: Health, Welfare and Performance* (ed. R.J. Geor, P.A. Harris, and M. Coenen), 487–502. Edinburgh: Saunders Elsevier.

8 Lumeng, C.N. and Saltiel, A.R. (2011). Inflammatory links between obesity and metabolic disease. *J. Clin. Invest.* 121 (6): 2111–2117.

9 Vick, M.M., Adams, A.A., Murphy, B.A. et al. (2007). Relationships among inflammatory cytokines, obesity, and insulin sensitivity in the horse. *J. Anim. Sci.* 85 (5): 1144–1155.

10 de Luca, C. and Olefsky, J.M. (2008). Inflammation and insulin resistance. *Fed. Eur. Biochem. Soc.* 582 (1): 97–105.

11 de Laat, M.A., McGree, J.M., and Sillence, M.N. (2016). Equine hyperinsulinemia: investigation of the enteroinsular axis during insulin dysregulation. *Am. J. Physiol. Metab.* 310 (1): E61–E72.

12 Geor, R.J. (2008). Metabolic predispositions to laminitis in horses and ponies: obesity, insulin resistance, and metabolic syndromes. *J. Equine Vet. Sci.* 28 (12): 753–759.

13 de Laat, M.A., McGowan, C.M., Sillence, M.N., and Pollitt, C.C. (2010). Hyperinsulinemic laminitis. *Vet. Clin. North Am. Equine Pract.* 26 (2): 257–264.

14 Houpt, K.A. (1982). Feeding problems. *Equine Pract.* 4 (7): 17–20.

15 Kealy, R.D., Lawler, D.F., Ballam, J.M. et al. (2002). Effects of diet restriction on life span and age-related changes in dogs. *J. Am. Vet. Med. Assoc.* 220 (9): 1315–1320.

16 Omodei, D. and Fontana, L. (2011). Calorie restriction and prevention of age-associated chronic disease. *FEBS Lett.* 585 (11): 1537–1542.

17 Kitahara, C.M., Flint, A.J., Berrington de Gonzalez, A. et al. (2014). Association between class III obesity (BMI of 40–59 kg/m^2) and mortality: a pooled analysis of 20 prospective studies. *PLoS Med.* 11 (7): e1001673.

18 Henneke, D.R., Potter, G.D., Kreider, J.L., and Yeates, B.F. (1983). Relationship between condition score, physical measurements and body fat percentage in mares. *Equine Vet. J.* 15 (4): 371–372.

19 Kienzle, E. and Schramme, S.C. (2004). Body condition scoring and prediction of body weight in adult warm blooded horses. *Pferdeheilkd Equine Med.* 20 (6): 517–524.

20 Dugdale, A.H.A., Grove-White, D., Curtis, G.C. et al. (2012). Body condition scoring as a predictor of body fat in horses and ponies. *Vet. J.* 194 (2): 173–178.

21 Ince, J.C., Longland, A.C., Moore-Colyer, M. et al. (2005). A pilot study to estimate the intake of grass by ponies with restricted access to pasture. In: *Proceedings of the British Society of Animal Science*, 109. Cambridge University Press.

22 Longland, A.C., Barfoot, C., and Harris, P.A. (2016). Effects of grazing muzzles on intakes of dry matter and water-soluble carbohydrates by ponies grazing spring, summer, and autumn swards, as well as autumn swards of different heights. *J. Equine Vet. Sci.* 40: 26–33.

23 Henneke, D.R., Potter, G.D., and Kreider, J.L. (1984). Body condition during pregnancy and lactation and reproductive efficiency of mares. *Theriogenology* 21 (6): 897–909.

24 Kearns, C.F., McKeever, K.H., Kumagai, K. et al. (2002). Fat-free mass is related to one-mile race performance in elite standardbred horses. *Vet. J.* 163 (3): 260–266.

25 Schott, H., Hodgson, D., Naylor, J., and Bayly, W. (1990). Thermoregulation and heat exhaustion in the exercising horse. In: *Proceedings of the 36th Annual Convention of the American Association of Equine Practitioners*, 505–513. Lexington, KY: American Association of Equine Practitioners (AAEP).

26 Garlinghouse, S.E. and Burrill, M.J. (1999). Relationship of body condition score to completion rate during 160km endurance races. *Equine Vet. J.* 31 (S30): 591–595.

27 Parameswaran, K., Todd, D.C., and Soth, M. (2006). Altered respiratory physiology in obesity. *Can. Respir. J.* 13 (4): 203–210.

28 Edney, A.T. and Smith, P.M. (1986). Study of obesity in dogs visiting veterinary practices in the United Kingdom. *Vet. Rec.* 118 (14): 391–396.

29 Pearson, W., Wood, K., Stanley, S., and MacNicol, J. (2018). Exploring relationships between body condition score, body fat, activity level and inflammatory biomarkers. *J. Anim. Physiol. Anim. Nutr. (Berl).* 102 (4): 1062–1068.

30 National Research Council (1978). *Nutrient Requirements of Horses*. 4th Rev. Animal Nutrition Series, 1–33. Washington, DC: National Academies Press.

31 Gross, K.L., Yamka, R.M., Khoo, C. et al. (2010). Macronutrients. In: *Small Animal Clinical Nutrition*, 5e (ed. M.S. Hand, C.D. Thatcher, R.L. Remillard, et al.), 49–105. Topeka,: Mark Morris Institute.

32 Pagan, J.D. and Hintz, H.F. (1986). Equine energetics. I. Relationship between body weight and energy requirements in horses. *J. Anim. Sci.* 63 (3): 815–821.

33 Gill, J.C., Lloyd, K.E., Bowman, M. et al. (2017). Relationships among digestible energy intake, body weight, and body condition in mature idle horses. *J. Equine Vet. Sci.* 54 (7): 32–36.

34 Carter, R.A., McCutcheon, L.J., George, L.A. et al. (2009). Effects of diet-induced weight gain on insulin sensitivity and plasma hormone and lipid concentrations in horses. *Am. J. Vet. Res.* 70 (10): 1250–1258.

35 Laflamme, D. (1997). Development and validation of a body condition score system for dogs. *Canine Pract.* 22 (4): 10–15.

36 Laflamme, D.P. (1997). Development and validation of a body condition score system for cats: a clinical tool. *Feline Pract.* 25: 13–18.

37 Shepherd, M., Harris, P., and Martinson, K.L. (2021). Nutritional considerations when dealing with an obese adult equine. *Vet. Clin. North Am. Equine Pract.* 37 (1): 111–137.

38 Askins, M.J., Palkovic, A.G., Leppo, K.A. et al. (2017). Effect of feeding teff hay on dry matter intake, digestible energy intake and resting insulin/glucose concentrations in horses. *J. Equine Vet. Sci.* 52 (5): 45.

39 Hansen, T.L., Fowler, A.L., Strasinger, L.A. et al. (2016). Effect of soaking on nitrate concentrations in teff Hay. *J. Equine Vet. Sci.* 45 (10): 53–57.

40 Dowler, L.E., Siciliano, P.D., Pratt-Phillips, S.E., and Poore, M. (2012). Determination of pasture dry matter intake rates in different seasons and their application in grazing management. *J. Equine Vet. Sci.* 32 (2): 85–92.

41 King, S., Jones, K., Schwarm, M., and Oberhaus, E.L. (2013). Daily horse behavior patterns depend on management. *J. Equine Vet. Sci.* 33 (5): 365–366.

42 Longland, A.C., Ince, J., and Harris, P.A. (2011). Estimation of pasture intake by ponies from liveweight change during six weeks at pasture. *J. Equine Vet. Sci.* 5 (31): 275–276.

43 Sharpe, P. and Kenny, L. (2019). Grazing behavior, feed intake, and feed choices. In: *Horse Pasture Management* (ed. P. Sharpe), 121–140. London, UK: Elsevier Science.

44 Equi-Analytical Laboratories Services (2020). Common Feed Profiles. http://equi-analytical.com/common-feed-profiles (accessed 28 February 2019).

45 Dowler, L.E. and Siciliano, P.D. (2009). Prediction of hourly pasture dry matter intake in horses. *J. Equine Vet. Sci.* 29 (5): 354–355.

46 DeBoer, M.L., Hathaway, M.R., Kuhle, K.J. et al. (2018). Glucose and insulin response of horses grazing alfalfa, perennial cool-season grass, and teff across seasons. *J. Equine Vet. Sci.* 68 (9): 33–38.

47 Cameron, A., Harris, P., Longland, A. et al. (2021). UK horse carers' experiences of restricting grazing when aiming to prevent health issues in their horses. *J. Equine Vet. Sci.* 104: 103685.

48 Glunk, E.C., Sheaffer, C.C., Hathaway, M.R., and Martinson, K.L. (2014). Interaction of grazing muzzle use and grass species on forage intake of horses. *J. Equine Vet. Sci.* 34 (7): 930–933.

49 Longland, A.C., Barfoot, C., and Harris, P.A. (2012). The effect of wearing a grazing muzzle vs. not wearing a grazing muzzle on intakes of spring, summer and autumn pastures by ponies. In: *Forages and Grazing in Horse Nutrition* (ed. M. Saastamoinen, M.J. Fradinho,

A.S. Santos, and N. Miraglia), 185–186. Wageningen: Wageningen Academic Publishers.

50 Longland, A.C., Barfoot, C., and Harris, P.A. (2016). Efficacy of wearing grazing muzzles for 10 hours per day on controlling bodyweight in pastured ponies. *J. Equine Vet. Sci.* 45 (Oct): 22–27.

51 Pollard, D., Wylie, C.E., Verheyen, K.L.P., and Newton, J.R. (2019). Identification of modifiable factors associated with owner-reported equine laminitis in Britain using a web-based cohort study approach. *BMC Vet. Res.* 15 (1): 1–12.

52 Glunk, E.C., Pratt-Phillips, S.E., and Siciliano, P.D. (2013). Effect of restricted pasture access on pasture dry matter intake rate, dietary energy intake, and fecal pH in horses. *J. Equine Vet. Sci.* 33 (6): 421–426.

53 Maisonpierre, I.N., Sutton, M.A., Harris, P. et al. (2019). Accelerometer activity tracking in horses and the effect of pasture management on time budget. *Equine Vet. J.* 51 (6): 840–845.

54 Cameron, A., Longland, A., Pfau, T. et al. (2021). The effect of strip grazing on physical activity and behaviour in ponies. *J. Equine Vet. Sci.* 110: 103745.

55 Gill, J.C., Pratt-Phillips, S.E., and Siciliano, P.D. (2017). The effect of time- and space-restricted grazing on body weight, body condition score, resting insulin concentration, and activity in grazing horses. *J. Equine Vet. Sci.* 52 (5): 87–88.

56 Toll, P., Yamka, R., Schoenherr, W., and Hand, M. (2010). Obesity. In: *Small Animal Clinical Nutrition*, 5e (ed. M.S. Hand, C.D. Thatcher, R.L. Remillard, et al.), 501–542. Topeka, KS: Mark Morris Institute.

57 Van Weyenberg, S., Hesta, M., Buyse, J., and Janssens, G.P.J. (2008). The effect of weight loss by energy restriction on metabolic profile and glucose tolerance in ponies. *J. Anim. Physiol. Anim. Nutr. (Berl).* 92 (5): 538–545.

58 Pagan, J.D. and Hintz, H.F. (1986). Equine energetics. II. Energy expenditure in horses during submaximal exercise. *J. Anim. Sci.* 63 (3): 822–830.

59 Dugdale, A.H.A., Curtis, G.C., Cripps, P. et al. (2010). Effect of dietary restriction on body condition, composition and welfare of overweight and obese pony mares. *Equine Vet. J.* 42 (7): 600–610.

60 Argo, C.M., Curtis, G.C., Grove-White, D. et al. (2012). Weight loss resistance: a further consideration for the nutritional management of obese Equidae. *Vet. J.* 194 (2): 179–188.

61 Davis, K.M., Iwaniuk, M.E., Dennis, R.L. et al. (2020). Effects of grazing muzzles on behavior, voluntary exercise, and physiological stress of miniature horses housed in a herd. *Appl Anim. Behav. Sci.* 232 (Nov): 105108.

62 Davis, K.M., Iwaniuk, M.E., Dennis, R.L. et al. (2020). Effects of grazing muzzles on behavior and physiological stress of individually housed grazing miniature horses. *Appl. Anim. Behav. Sci.* 231 (Oct): 105067.

63 Porsani, M.Y.H., Teixeira, F.A., Amaral, A.R. et al. (2020). Factors associated with failure of dog's weight loss programmes. *Vet. Med. Sci.* 6 (3): 299–305.

64 Engelking, L.R. (2015). Starvation (the intermediate phase). In: *Textbook of Veterinary Physiological Chemistry*, 3e, 476–481. Amsterdam: Elsevier.

65 Bamford, N.J., Potter, S.J., Baskerville, C.L. et al. (2019). Influence of dietary restriction and low-intensity exercise on weight loss and insulin sensitivity in obese equids. *J. Vet. Intern. Med.* 33 (1): 280–286.

66 Moore, J.L., Siciliano, P.D., and Pratt-Phillips, S.E. (2019). Effects of exercise on voluntary intake, morphometric measurements, and oral sugar test response in horses on ad libitum forage. *Comp. Exerc. Physiol.* 15 (3): 209–218.

67 Moore, J.L., Siciliano, P.D., and Pratt-Phillips, S.E. (2019). Effects of diet versus exercise on morphometric measurements, blood hormone concentrations, and oral sugar test response in obese horses. *J. Equine Vet. Sci.* 78 (7): 38–45.

68 Engelking, L.R. (ed.) (2015). Exercise (VO2 max and RQ). In: *Textbook of Veterinary Physiological Chemistry*, 3e, 493–497. Amsterdam: Elsevier.

69 Annunziato, R.A., Timko, C.A., Crerand, C.E. et al. (2009). A randomized trial examining differential meal replacement adherence in a weight loss maintenance program after one-year follow-up. *Eat. Behav.* 10 (3): 176–183.

70 German, A.J. (2016). Weight management in obese pets: the tailoring concept and how it can improve results. *Acta Vet. Scand.* 58 (1): 3–9.

71 Gill, J.C., Pratt-Phillips, S.E., Mansmann, R., and Siciliano, P.D. (2016). Weight loss management in client-owned horses. *J. Equine Vet. Sci.* 39 (4): 80–89.

72 Potter, J.S., Bamford, J.N., Harris, A.P. et al. (2016). Prevalence of obesity and owners' perceptions of body condition in pleasure horses and ponies in South-Eastern Australia. *Aust. Vet. J.* 94 (11): 427–432.

73 Curtis, G.C., Barfoot, C.F., Dugdale, A.H. et al. (2011). Voluntary ingestion of wood shavings by obese horses under dietary restriction. *Br. J. Nutr.* 106 (S1): S178–S182.

74 McGreevy, P.D., Cripps, P.J., French, N.P. et al. (1995). Management factors associated with stereotypic and redirected behaviour in the thoroughbred horse. *Equine Vet. J.* 27 (2): 86–91.

75 Harris, P.A., Ellis, A.D., Fradinho, M.J. et al. (2017). Review: feeding conserved forage to horses: recent advances and recommendations. *Animal* 11 (6): 958–967.

76 Glunk, E.C., Hathaway, M.R., Weber, W.J. et al. (2014). The effect of hay net design on rate of forage consumption when feeding adult horses. *J. Equine Vet. Sci.* 34 (8): 986–991.

77 Rochais, C., Henry, S., and Hausberger, M. (2018). "Hay-bags" and "slow feeders": testing their impact on horse behaviour and welfare. *Appl. Anim. Behav. Sci.* 198 (1): 52–59.

78 Murray, M.J. and Eichorn, E.S. (1996). Effects of intermittent feed deprivation, intermittent feed deprivation with ranitidine administration, and stall confinement with ad libitum access to hay on gastric ulceration in horses. *Am. J. Vet. Res.* 57 (11): 1599–1603.

79 McKenzie, H.C. (2011). Equine hyperlipidemias. *Vet. Clin. North Am. Equine Pract.* 27 (1): 59–72.

80 Durham, A. (2013). Hyperlipemia. In: *Equine Applied and Clinical Nutrition: Health, Welfare and Performance* (ed. R.J. Geor, P.A. Harris and M. Coenen), 512–520. Philadelphia, PA: Saunders, Elsevier.

81 Rendle, D., McGregor Argo, C., Bowen, M. et al. (2018). Equine obesity: current perspectives. *UK-Vet. Equine* 2 (5): 1–19.

82 Kronfeld, D.S. (1993). Starvation and malnutrition of horses: recognition and treatment. *J. Equine Vet. Sci.* 13 (5): 298–304.

83 Rocateli, A. and Zhang, H. (2017). Evaluating hay quality based on sight, smell and feel - hay judging. Oklahoma Cooperative Extension Service PSS-2588. Stillwater, OK. http://osufacts.okstate.edu (accessed 28 June 2021).

84 Kamphues, J. (2013). Feed hygiene and related disorders in horses. In: *Equine Applied and Clinical Nutrition Health, Welfare and Performance* (ed. R.J. Geor, P.A. Harris and M. Coenen), 367–380. Edinburgh: Saunders Elsevier.

85 Kronfeld, D.S., Holland, J.L., Rich, G.A. et al. (2004). Fat digestibility in Equus caballus follows increasing first-order kinetics. *J. Anim. Sci.* 82 (6): 1773–1780.

86 Heusner, G.L. (1993). Ad libitum feeding of mature horses to achieve rapid weight gain. In: *Proceedings of the 13th Equine Nutrition and Physiology Society Symposium*, 86–87. Gainsville, FL: Equine Nutrition and Physiology Society.

87 Blaue, D., Schedlbauer, C., Starzonek, J. et al. (2019). Effects of body weight gain on insulin and lipid metabolism in equines. *Domest. Anim. Endocrinol.* 68 (Jul): 111–118.

24

Refeeding and Assisted Feeding of Horses

Meri Stratton-Phelps and Rebecca L. Remillard

KEY TERMS

- Anorexia is the complete loss of appetite or lack of desire for food; usually occurs secondary to a primary disease.
- Hyporexia is decreased appetite and feed intake.
- Admixtures are commercially available multi-chambered bags containing standard concentrations of dextrose, amino acids, and lipid solutions.

KEY POINTS

- Veterinarians play a key role in helping identify diseases that alter the weight and body condition score of a horse and should be consulted when weight loss is diagnosed.
- Malnutrition is defined as any disorder of inadequate, excessive, or unbalanced nutrient intake.
- Basal energy rate (BMR) for mammals is 70 (kg BW)$^{0.75}$ kcal/d.
- Resting energy rate (RER) for stalled horses is (21.28 (kg BW) + 975) kcal/d or 75% minimal DE_m.
- Minimum maintenance energy requirement (min DE_m) of adult horses is 3.04 Mcal/100 kg BW.

24.1 Introduction

Nutrition is a medical therapy, and basic rules should be followed regarding indications, contraindications, the timing of initiation of therapy, dose adaptation for different nutrients, and patient monitoring [1]. At any age, horses with inadequate nutrient intake become malnourished. The major consequences of malnutrition are decreased immunocompetence, decreased tissue synthesis and repair, and altered intermediary metabolism [2, 3]. Horses with a low body condition score (BCS) due to starvation, with no underlying disease but willing and able to consume food, require a food reintroduction plan. See Figure 24.1. Patients with weight loss due to a chronic disease, for example, parasitism, neoplasia, hepatic, adrenal insufficiency, and dental, renal, and debilitating injuries, require a specialized ration (25). Horses with low BCS, regardless of cause, that are unwilling or unable to eat require assisted feeding techniques.

BCS is related but does not directly measure body fat (BF) content and does not include an assessment of muscle mass. Unlike other companion species, the optimal BCS in horses may not be the median (5) on a scale of 1 to 9/9, and the relationship between BCS and %BF may not be linear [4]. However, in the horse, as true of all animals, in the face of deficient calorie intake and decreasing fat stores, skeletal and visceral muscle is catabolized for energy. As protein catabolism increases and synthesis decreases, low serum albumin concentrations in the absence of protein-losing enteropathy, renal or liver disease would indicate inadequate feed intake for many weeks, given the half-life of albumin in the horse is about 19 days.

Measurements of body weight (BW) and BCS do not provide sufficient evidence of emaciation. Muscle wasting in the absence of body fat is a better assessment of malnutrition and the extent of suboptimal nutrient intake [5, 6]. The extent of muscle loss is the primary determinant of survival because without treatment, as seen in several species, a greater than 25–30% loss of body protein compromises cardiac and pulmonary muscle strength [7]. Muscle scoring has been introduced into the physical examination (PE) of dogs and cats, which is assessed by visualization and palpation of the spine, scapulae, skull, and wings of the ilia. Muscle loss

Equine Clinical Nutrition, Second Edition. Edited by Rebecca L. Remillard.

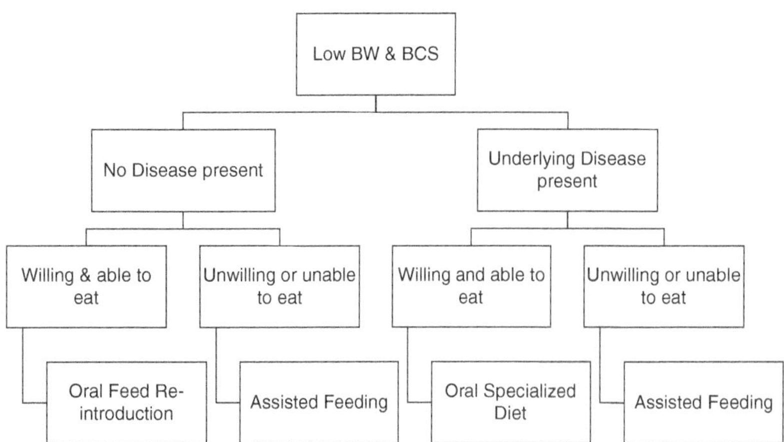

Figure 24.1 Feeding horses with a low BCS algorithm.

is typically first noted in the epaxial muscles on each side of the spine; muscle loss at other sites can be more variable and is graded as normal, mild, moderate, or severe loss [8]. A standardized muscle scoring system does not yet exist for horses; however, the BCS and assessment of muscle wasting are important when triaging cases because about 20% of severely malnourished (BCS 1/9) horses will die regardless of treatment efforts due to extensive muscle wasting [9, 10].

24.1.1 Energy Requirement

There are several different equations by which to estimate a patient's daily energy need. The mammalian basal metabolic rate (BMR) measured across a range of species and body sizes, from mouse to elephant, universally fit the equation [$70 \times (\text{kg BW})^{0.75}$ [11]. The BMR estimates the calories needed to maintain minimal cellular metabolism, vascular circulation, and respiration, and historically was related to body surface area but is now more closely related to BW or fat-free mass [12–14]. BMR measurements in people are done after a 12-hr fast with no previous exercise. Subjects are placed under a canopy hood in a relaxed, supine position but awake in a thermoneutral environment for a 20-min respiration calorimetry measurement [15]. Respiration calorimetry is the measurement of oxygen consumed versus carbon dioxide produced, which estimates the metabolic rate at that moment. Resting metabolic rate or requirement (RER) measurements are completed on individuals who have fasted for 3-4 hrs with no prior activity restrictions and are about 10-20% higher than BMR.

The universal BMR equation is applicable to horses, however, measuring metabolic rates in horses is inherently more difficult in that horses consume feed throughout the day, and the majority of time is spent standing with some ability to move, and controlling the animals' alertness is limited. A minimal metabolic rate has been measured in a study of four adult horses using a series of 30-min masked respiratory calorimetry measurements while standing in a straight metabolic stall and fed 50% of the daily ration [16]. From this work, 21.28 (kg BW) + 975 estimates the caloric need (kcal/d) of stall-confined horses with low feed intake which best approximates resting metabolism and is 75% min DE_m in horses. In human surgical patients, there was little additional benefit to increasing intake once half of the RER of the patient had been consumed [18]. The daily energy requirement for healthy adult horses at maintenance on full feed is greater than BMR and RER because the energy demands of digestion, metabolism, and routine physical activity (without exercise/training) are included. The minimal digestible energy at maintenance (min DE_m) for healthy horses is estimated at 3.04 Mcal/100 kg BW [17]. See Figure 24.2. Conversely, overfeeding a patient risks the occurrence of metabolic derangements known as refeeding syndrome. Meeting the energy requirement of debilitated and hospitalized equine patients, regardless of feeding method (oral, tube, or parenteral), is an estimation that should begin conservatively and increase only based on the patient's response.

For the majority of disease states, the patient's daily energy requirement will be between BMR and min DE_m, and the current, not optimal, BW should be used. Feeding greater than min DE_m is rarely warranted and increases the risk of additional metabolic complications. Feeding for weight gain or growth should not be attempted until the patient is metabolically stable, has recovered from the disease, and has a normal functioning gastrointestinal (GI) tract and microbiota. Most healthy but chronically (months) underfed or starved patients (BCS 1-2/9) can initially be refed at the calculated BMR using current BW. The majority of short-term (weeks) underfed BCS (2-3/9) horses can initially be refed at RER or 75% of min DEm using current BW (19). Initially feeding patients between BMR and RER is a rational and safe recommendation that decreases the probability of metabolic complications with the understanding that actual energy requirements may be slightly greater and will increase with recovery. Regular

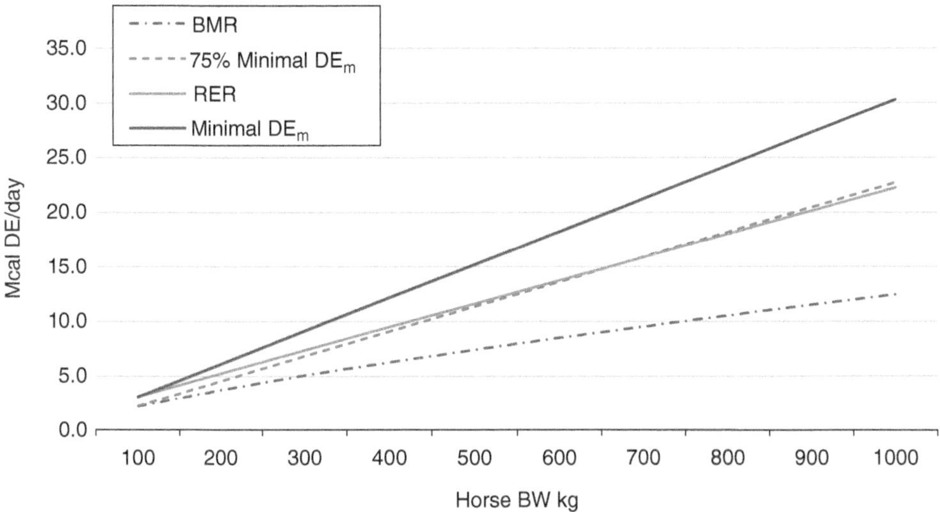

Figure 24.2 Calculated daily energy need at various metabolic rates: (BMR = 70 (kg BW)$^{0.75}$; RER = 21.28 (kg BW) + 975; Minimal DE$_m$ = 3.04 Mcal/100 kg BW) over the range of horse body weights (BW) [12, 16, 17].

nutritional assessments of the patient are used to make adjustments to the food and feeding rates. See Figure 2.1.

24.1.2 Intestinal Recovery

The small intestine (SI) is dependent on intraluminal nutrition and, within days without food, will show evidence of compromise [20]. As seen in other species, by day 7 of no food, intestinal changes will include a 22% decrease in small bowel weight and decreases of 28% mucosal weight, 35% protein, and 25% DNA compared with day 1, all of which compromises SI function [21]. SI atrophy is characterized by decreases in villus height and crypt depth, surface area, motility, brush border enzymes, secretions, and immunity, which lead to an increased risk of bacteria, endotoxin, and cytokine translocation across the intestinal wall and an increased risk of systemic infection. Conversely, the SI recovers when food consumption restarts. Stem cells mature while migrating from the crypt to the villus tip in approximately 3 days. A relatively healthy SI mucosa may return to full function within 7–10 days, that is, 3–4 epithelial turnovers, after refeeding.

The large intestine (LI) in a mature horse is the primary site of the equid microbiome responsible for digesting most of the dietary fiber and about half of the soluble carbohydrate, then absorbing the resulting nutrients. Microbial protein is also produced, digested, and absorbed from the cecum and colon. When refeeding a malnourished horse, consideration must also be given to refeeding the intestinal microbiome, that is, two patients (host and microbiome). One cannot survive or thrive without the other. Our current understanding of the composition and function of the equine intestinal microbiome is limited, but research has shown the microbiome may be profoundly altered in certain disease states, resulting in deleterious health consequences. The reintroduction of a healthy microbiome is imperative to intestinal recovery. See For example, see Microbiota in Healthy Foals and Young Horses in Chapter 4. Translating these mechanisms of microbial acquisition to adults: horses should be "housed" surrounded by other healthy horses, feeds, dirt, and manure to help restore their microbiome rather than keeping the horse isolated in a frequently cleaned stall.

24.1.3 Protein Calorie Malnutrition

Malnourished horses are at risk of developing protein-calorie malnutrition (PCM) and multiple nutrient deficiencies. Loss of peripheral (skeletal) and central (visceral) proteins can have adverse anatomic and functional consequences in food-deprived animals. These adverse effects include anemia, reduced heart muscle mass and function, decreased pulmonary mechanical function, diminished respiratory drive, altered intestinal morphology, and mildly impaired intestinal absorptive abilities [22]. A deficiency of calories, protein, minerals, or vitamins alters the production of inflammatory cytokines, adversely affects leukocyte function, and decreases host resistance to bacterial infections [23, 24]. Protein calorie malnutrition is detrimental to immune system function, tissue healing, recovery from systemic disease, and surgical recovery as it will alter the expected metabolism of certain drugs, which may increase or decrease the therapeutic effect at recommended dosages. Metabolic processes between the last meal and death due to starvation have been well described [25]. The goal of nutritional intervention is to blunt the development of PCM and the metabolic complications that arise from a lack of nutrition and to promote recovery of a healthy body condition.

Chronically starved horses with no underlying medical disability but that have been offered poor-quality feeds or an insufficient amount of feed for 2–6 mos inevitably develop PCM. In the worst-case scenario, an adult horse will lose 40% of optimal BW due to a complete lack of feed within 60–90 days and will no longer be able to stand, will lie sternal, and then become laterally recumbent. Most severe malnourished horses will die within 72–96 hrs if they cannot rise [9, 26]. The cause of death is usually due to a combination of cardiac and respiratory arrest as a result of the muscle degradation combined with severe electrolyte imbalances. Once 40–45% of optimum BW has been lost, survival is unlikely regardless of aggressive treatment. Most cases of simple chronic starvation are not anorexic but willingness to eat until reaching end-stage starvation. Fortunately, most cases of low BCS in horses have historically received some fraction of an inadequate diet, often of poor quality, for more than 3–4 mos and arrive at humane shelters or rescue leagues before becoming recumbent.

Mild to severe PCM may occur due to poor feed quality. As forage quality decreases, both dietary protein and energy may be deficient despite an adequate intake of forage at 2–2.5% BW. See Sidebar 10.3. PCM may also occur when nutritious feeds are fed in limited quantities. Low feed intake can occur as a consequence of competition among horses, for example, when different age horses are mixed and dominant horses push away older and younger animals from the feed source. Prolonged adverse weather conditions may increase nutrient requirements and limit access to feed which increase the subsequent risk for PCM. Adult horses have an estimated increase in energy need by 2.5% for every degree Celsius below the lower critical temperature. When the hair coat is wet and matted during cold temperatures, the energy requirement may be increased by as much as 50% [17]. See Cold Weather Care in Chapter 6.

Horses in end-stage starvation and horses with low BCS due to a medical condition may not be willing or able to eat. Anorexia, the complete loss of appetite or lack of desire for food, usually occurs secondary to a primary disease and is regulated by cytokines, including interleukin (IL-1) and tumor necrosis factor-alpha (TNF-α) that are released during an inflammatory response. Resolution of the primary disease process usually results in a return to voluntary food consumption. Nutritional therapy for horses or foals experiencing anorexia is an important component of medical care. Therapeutic nutrition is provided to blunt the catabolic response that develops when voluntary feed intake is reduced and can be administered to horses in a field or hospital setting. Diet selection and the route of administration (enteral or parenteral) depend on the horse's current nutritional status, type of disease process, and the estimated duration of nutritional support.

Increased nutrient demands above RER occur with a severe disease processes, for example, sepsis, trauma, and burns, but have not been defined well enough in the equine species to result in specific recommendations. Currently, elevated energy and protein requirements are extrapolated from estimates in humans, laboratory animals, and small animal species. Older published estimates in people indicate that requirements for energy and protein increase 10% above RER after elective surgery, 60% with severe infection or sepsis, and 50–110% with severe burns [27, 28]. These values suggest that in horses, both energy and protein requirements are expected to be elevated and should be addressed when hospitalized horses are managed with therapeutic nutrition. Protein degradation and a negative nitrogen balance are hallmarks of the acute response to infection. Weight loss resulting from protein and lipid catabolism is often observed in septic horses with altered metabolic activity and nutrient requirements.

24.2 Feed Reintroduction to Chronically Starved Horses

Malnutrition in the absence of primary disease resulting in weight loss of more than 30% of ideal BW is common due to adverse environmental conditions in feral horses. However, neglect, ignorance of proper care, and financial difficulties are the more common reasons for malnutrition in domesticated horses. A nutritional rehabilitation plan for low (1 to 3/9) BCS horses as a result of simple (uncomplicated by disease) starvation based on initial BCS and laboratory data is designed to help rescue organizations and shelters assess resources needed to rehabilitate such a patient. Refeeding of severely poor-conditioned (BCS 1/9) horses should be initiated only if the horse is in a stable condition. Severe tachycardia, hypotension, colloid, and fluid deficits should be assessed and corrected before offering food. Electrolyte, acid–base abnormalities, and blood glucose concentrations should be within normal limits because refeeding will further compromise a metabolically unstable patient. A practical objective is to begin a refeeding protocol within 48 hrs of initial assessment with the longer-term goal of safely reversing the ongoing catabolic state. A general feed re-introduction guideline is to offer 25–30% of intended DMI/d at current BW on days 1–3 of refeeding, 50–60% on days 4–6, and 75–100% by day 7–10. The more debilitated patients are fed at the slower rates, and the rate of increasing the daily feed offered depends entirely on patient response.

24.2.1 Animal Assessment

Evaluation of the nutritional status of the equine patient includes a complete PE, laboratory analyses, and a review of the horse's recent diet history to determine nutrient intake. A thorough examination of the horse will help to rule out concurrent diseases or preexisting conditions and the ability to voluntarily consume feed orally, which is important in developing a refeeding plan. Often chronically starved horses with no concurrent disease, still able to stand, are willing and able to consume solid feed, that is, forage and complementary feeds. A refeeding or feed reintroduction plan specific to the case is required. Chronically starved BCS 1/9 horses with or without concurrent disease unwilling to stand or eat will require assisted feeding protocols. See Figure 24.1. Body weight should be accurately recorded using a weigh scale as opposed to weight tapes measurements, which even if done correctly can be off +/−5% BW. Many cases of equine starvation occur through the winter months when hair coats are long, dull, and unkempt, which masks the loss of BF and muscle; hence, proper BCS determinations and assessment of muscle wasting must be completed using physical palpation.

In conjunction with BCS, laboratory data may aid in the decision of whether to treat severely emaciated horses given financial, logistical, and time constraints [10, 29–31]. See Table 24.1. Knowledge of the laboratory findings in emaciated horses is useful in scoring the time frame and extent of emaciation and in establishing a prognosis [32]. Most low-BCS horses will have some degree of protein malnutrition, but diagnosis is difficult using routine biochemical tests because the serum urea nitrogen and albumin often do not decrease below reference concentrations until protein malnutrition is severe. Adult horses maintain blood glucose within a normal range during periods of food deprivation; however, dysregulation should be considered in starved horses with abnormally high blood glucose concentrations. Blood concentrations of FFA, glycerol, total lipids, triglycerides (TG), phospholipids, cholesterol, B-hydroxybutyrate, lactate, bilirubin, and cortisol increase, whereas ionized Mg and Ca, K, and insulin decrease with the severity of starvation. Serum TG concentrations are expected to rise in healthy horses during a 24–48 hrs fast but return to normal with refeeding [33]. Adult horses suffering from PCM often have increased serum TG concentrations (>500 mg/dL).

Unless a horse is affected by severe malnutrition, clinical signs of trace mineral and vitamin deficiencies are usually not observed and rarely assessed. Equine patients with a diet history of little to no feed consumption of more than several weeks are assumed to be deficient in trace minerals and vitamins and will benefit from micronutrient supplementation.

Table 24.1 Initial assessment of low BCS horses[a].

BCS	Assessment	1/9	2/9	3/9
Physical examination	BW % of optimal[b]	75% or less	75–85%	85–95%
	Muscle loss	Severe	Moderate	Mild
Lab data				
Complete blood cell count	Red blood cell Hemoglobin Lymphocytes	Low	Low	Normal
Serum biochemistries	Albumin	Low	Low or normal	Normal
	Globulin alpha 1	High	High	Normal
	BUN/Creatinine	Low	Low	Normal
	Triglycerides	Low	High or normal	Normal
	Bilirubin	High	High or normal	Normal
	Alkaline phosphatase	Low	Low	Normal
Electrolytes[c]	Na, Cl, K, Ca, P, Mg	Below or low normal	Low or normal	Normal
Fluid therapy w/o glucose	Hydration	Repletion	Repletion or maintenance	prn[d]
	Acid–base	Corrective		
	Electrolytes	Repletion		
SI integrity[e]		Poor	Moderately poor	Normal
LI microbiome health[e]		Poor	Moderately poor	Normal
Prognosis		Poor	Guarded	Good

[a] In part originally appeared in: Remillard RL. (2016). How to Refeed Starved, Malnourished Horses - A Work in Progress. In: Proceedings of the 62nd Annual Convention of the American Association of Equine Practitioners. Orlando, Fl: American Association of Equine Practitioners (AAEP). p. 537–43.
[b] See Table 2.3 for estimating ideal BW equations.
[c] Sodium (Na), chloride (Cl), potassium (K), phosphorus (P), magnesium (Mg).
[d] pro re nata: as needed.
[e] Small intestine (SI), Large Intestine (LI).

24.2.2 Ration Assessment

24.2.2.1 Feeds

24.2.2.1.1 Forage

There are only a few studies on the refeeding of starved horses, but feeding a good-quality, e.g. mixed mainly grass (MMG) forage first is a common recommendation. See Table 10.3. A low BCS patient with muscle loss warrants feeding a high-quality, e.g. mixed mainly legume (MML) forage because intake of essential amino acids is required to regenerate a full complement of digestive enzymes, cellular transport mechanisms, and carrier molecules to move nutrients from the intestines and liver to other tissues. In general, legume hays (alfalfa) contain >18% protein, whereas grass hays (timothy, orchard, and fescue) contain <16% protein. A "forage first" plan also refeeds the intestinal microbiome, which in turn is essential to regenerating the GI mucosa and motility, and provides nutrients (energy, protein, and vitamins) to the host.

24.2.2.1.2 Complementary Feeds

Feeding grain is not recommended during the initial one to seven days of refeeding for two reasons. First, the atrophied small intestinal mucosa has lost the diet-inducible enzymes of end-stage carbohydrate digestion, allowing undigested starch and sugars to enter the cecum and colon, which may cause colic, endotoxemia, diarrhea or laminitis, and an abnormal microbial population. Second, a large uptake of glucose resulting in hyperglycemia will shift cellular energy metabolism from a steady state of fat and protein catabolism to carbohydrate metabolism, which obligates cells to uptake phosphorus (P), potassium (K), and magnesium (Mg), potentially lowering blood electrolyte concentrations as observed in the refeeding syndrome [10, 34]. Feeding grain to the malnourished patient increases the risk for an adverse refeeding response that may occur days to weeks after an increased intake of nonstructural carbohydrates (NSC), that is, sugars and starch. NSC is highest in grains such as corn (73%), wheat (66%), and oats (48%). Additionally, these grains are relatively low in protein (8–13%) and crude fiber (2–9%) and, as such, are not suggested during initial refeeding of recovering low BCS horses.

24.2.2.2 Key Nutrients

Water, calories, and protein are key nutrients for refeeding malnourished low-BCS horses. Initial treatment, based on blood work, should include oral rehydration if possible; however, intravenous (IV) correction of dehydration, electrolyte, and acid–base imbalances using fluids without glucose may be necessary before the reintroduction of feed (Table 24.1). A parenteral vitamin B product[1] containing thiamine, riboflavin, niacin, and pyridoxine administered at 10–50 mL/500 kg BW in conjunction with IV fluid therapy is advisable to replete water-soluble vitamins that are essential to energy metabolism. See Figure 9.1.

In chronically underfed horses, the thyroid down-regulates metabolism, and the animal exhibits low levels of activity relative to maintenance adult horses to conserve body stores [30, 35]. A state of metabolic "accommodation" that prolongs survival has been recognized in other species, and a similar state probably exists in chronically starved horses [36, 37]. Accommodation occurs when a lower but constant metabolic rate is established to minimize lean tissue wasting before protein deficiency becomes fatal. In cases of chronically low food intake, a low metabolic rate and protein turnover establish a fragile homeostasis until food becomes available again or new stressors intervene. These animals very often do not survive additional stresses such as trauma, surgery, infection, or tumors, as might be expected of a healthy animal.

Ideally in the first three to five days of refeeding, DE calorie intake should match the current metabolic rate at the current BW. The range of daily energy estimates (BMR, RER, and min DE_m) can be used to calculate the starting calorie intake based on BCS and diet history at presentation (Table 24.2). Initially, the energy (Mcal/d) requirement of low-BCS horses due to starvation with no disease etiology and a history of no food consumption or low food intake for months is best estimated at BMR = 70 $(BW_{kg})^{0.75}$ using current BW. See Figure 24.2. The initial energy requirement of low-BCS horses with a history of chronic underfeeding for days to weeks due to factors unrelated to the horse, that is, poor management or adverse environmental conditions, may be estimated at RER = 21.28 $(BW_{kg})x + 975$ or 75% min DE_m using current, not estimated optimal, BW [30]. When diet history is not available, feeding at the lower energy intake calculation (BMR) is an acceptable conservative approach [13, 35, 38–41]. Feeding malnourished horses at the higher healthy adult DE_m intake (3 Mcal/100 kg BW) and/or using the ideal BW in any calculation will initially overfeed the underweight horse that has accommodated to a lower metabolic rate [31]. Based on the horse's response to the feeding protocol, energy intakes may be increased weekly by 25–50% and must eventually exceed maintenance requirements at current BW to improve BCS. Protein should be provided in proportion to the calories consumed and greater than that recommended for adult maintenance horses if there are no contraindications, that is, liver or renal disease (Table 24.3). Higher protein intakes (>40 g/Mcal DE) may be warranted initially to promote intestinal mucosal repair; synthesis of hepatic, pancreatic, and SI enzymes; and the re-establishment of nutrient transport mechanisms, all of which precede BW gain [30, 42].

Commercial complete feeds containing less than 15% dry matter (DM) hydrolyzable carbohydrate, estimated by NSC, minimize the risk of refeeding syndrome, and 15–25% DM crude fibers, preferably from a mix of soluble and insoluble fiber types, are recommended to begin refeeding the microbiome. Examples of nutritionally complete equine feeds

1 Vitamin B Complex 150 Injection, Henry Schein® Animal Health, Dublin, OH.

Table 24.2 Initial feeding recommendations and ration composition for conservatively refeeding chronically starved horses based on diet history and BCS.[a]

Refeeding Plan[b]	Diet History			
	No food for ≥3 weeks	No food for 1–3 weeks	Inadequate food intake for months	Inadequate food intake for weeks
Animal:				
BCS	1 to 2/9	2 to 3/9	1 to 2/9	2 to 3/9
Feeding method:				
Water	IV and free choice	IV and free choice	IV if needed; free choice	Free choice
DE intake first days of refeeding[c]	BMR	BMR	50–75% min DE_m	70–80% min DE_m
Meals/d	6–10	4–6	6	4
DM intake (% BW)	1.0	1.0	1.5–2.0	1.8–2.3
Ration:				
DE (Mcal/kg DM)	2–2.4	2–2.4	2–2.2	1.8–2.0
Protein (% DM)	15–18	15–18	10–15	8–12
NSC (% DM)	10–15	10–15	10–20	15–20
Fat (% DM)	2–5	2–5	6–10	10
NDF (% DM)	≤50	≤50	≤60	≤60
Electrolytes/Salt	IV/free choice	IV/free choice	IV if needed/free choice	IV if needed/free choice
Progress:				
BW gain (lb/d)	0–1	1–2	1–2	~2
Est wks to 5/9 BCS	40–60	15–30	15–30	4 to 8

[a] In part originally appeared in: Remillard RL. (2016). How to Refeed Starved, Malnourished Horses - A Work in Progress. In: Proceedings of the 62nd Annual Convention of the American Association of Equine Practitioners. Orlando, Fl: American Association of Equine Practitioners (AAEP). p. 537–43.
[b] Body condition score (BCS), Digestible Energy (DE),Dry matter (DM), Nonstructural Carbohydrate (NSC), Neutral Detergent Fiber (NDF), Body Weight (BW).
[c] $BMR = 70\ (BW_{kg})^{0.75}$; minimal $DE_m = 3.04$ Mcal/100 kg BW/d using current, not ideal, BW.

Table 24.3 The recommended minimum intake of nutrients relative to digestible energy intake[a].

Nutrient	units/Mcal DE	Adult	Growth (month of age)				
		min DE_m	4	6	12	18	24
Crude protein	g	35.53	50.30	43.61	45.00	41.61	41.18
Lysine	g	1.5	2.17	1.88	1.94	1.79	1.77
Calcium	g	1.3	2.94	2.49	2.01	1.93	1.96
Phosphorus	g	0.9	1.63	1.39	1.11	1.07	1.09
Magnesium	g	0.5	0.27	0.26	0.29	0.32	0.36
Potassium	g	1.6	0.82	0.84	0.93	1.05	1.18
Sodium	g	0.7	0.32	0.32	0.37	0.42	0.47
Chloride	g	2.6	1.18	1.30	1.41	1.67	1.89
Sulfur	g	1.0	0.47	0.52	0.64	0.76	0.86
Copper	mg	6.6	3.17	3.48	4.27	5.05	5.74
Iron	mg	26.32	15.83	17.42	21.36	25.23	28.69
Manganese	mg	26.32	12.67	13.93	17.09	20.18	22.95
Zinc	mg	26.32	12.67	13.93	17.09	20.18	22.95
Cobalt	ug	32.89	15.04	19.35	21.28	26.04	26.74
Iodine	ug	230.26	112.78	122.58	148.94	177.08	203.21
Selenium	ug	65.79	31.58	34.84	42.55	50.52	57.22
Vitamin A	KIU	0.99	0.57	0.63	0.77	0.91	1.03
Vitamin D	IU	217.1	252.63	278.71	341.49	403.13	458.82
Vitamin E	IU	32.9	25.34	27.87	34.15	40.36	45.88
Thiamin	mg	2.0	0.95	1.05	1.28	1.52	1.72
Riboflavin	mg	1.3	0.63	0.70	0.86	1.01	1.15

[a] Suggested non-energy nutrient intakes relative to DE intake regardless of route of administration: oral, feeding tube or parenteral.
Source: Adapted from NRC [18]; Table 16-3 except Growth Vitamin D (20 kg BW) see pg 292.

for refeeding horses are "lite" feed[2] with 10% NCS or "senior" feed[3] with an NSC maximum of 20%. Products designed for refeeding horses contain high-quality protein ingredients such as alfalfa, soy, and whey, with a mix of fiber types, minerals, and some vitamin B and fat-soluble vitamins. A powdered product[4] containing 11% DM NSC can be offered for voluntary consumption or tube-fed after adding water [43].

Ideally, all essential non-energy nutrients should be fed in proportion to the calories consumed such that no nutrient becomes the first limiting factor to recovery or weight gain. (Table 24.3). Although feeding minerals and vitamins initially to starved horses to replete stores and revive co-factors and co-enzymes of metabolism is necessary, feeding these micronutrients with grains is not advisable in the initial weeks. A better option would be a low NSC, mineral–vitamin ration balancer that complements the forage. See Complementary Feeds in Chapter 17.

24.2.3 Feeding Management

Assuming there are no contraindications to oral feeding such as dental, pharyngeal, or esophageal lesions, feed offered for oral consumption is preferable to tube feeding or parenteral nutrition (PN). A nutritional rehabilitation plan for horses with a low (1 to 3/9) BCS due to simple starvation, uncomplicated by a primary disease, has been outlined in Table 24.2 based on amount and duration of food deprivation. Owners, veterinary technicians, nurses, barn personnel, and whoever may have access to the patient must understand that a slow methodical reintroduction to feed is necessary for the animal's recovery. A safe refeeding program limits feeding the patient only the feeds and amount prescribed. The well-intentioned attendant feeding outside of the prescribed plan may inadvertently initiate the refeeding syndrome, risking possible death of the animal [20, 44].

Additionally, the daily amount of feed should be divided into multiple feedings over 24 hrs, depending on diet history, GI function, and BCS, that is, 4 meals/d for a BCS 3/9 horse vs. 6 to 10 meals/d for a BCS 1/9 horse. The amount of feed consumed (feed-in minus feed-out) should be recorded daily and for each meal, and feed consumption as a %BW should be calculated, that is, total kg of feed consumed/100 kg BW/d, and reviewed daily in the early phases of refeeding. Suggested ration macronutrient concentrations of DE, protein, NSC, fat, and NDF are provided in Table 24.2. Micronutrient concentrations of minerals and vitamins should be proportional to calories consumed (Table 24.3). See Sidebar 24.1.

2 Triple Crown Lite, Triple Crown Nutrition, Inc. Wayzata, MN.
3 SafeChoice Senior Horse Feed, Nutrena, Minneapolis, MN.
4 WellSolve W/G, Purina Mills LLC, St. Louis, MO.

Sidebar 24.1: Feed Reintroduction Example

Animal Assessment: A 14-yr-old Welsh pony mare BW 314 kg, BCS 2/9 with moderate muscle wasting, and diet history of having poor quality forage available daily fed at <50% of min DE_m for at least 5 mos is surrendered to a rescue league. The hay provided was described as musty large round bales of grass hay that had been stored outside for 2 yrs.

The horse had no primary disease. Hydration status was adequate and serum electrolytes were within the normal reference range, but albumin was below normal. The horse was subjectively depressed and mildly interested in her surroundings. The GI function was low/adequate based on abdominal auscultation. The horse was protein calorie malnourished and spent most of the time lying sternal. The metabolic rate had been down-regulated to conserve energy. The estimated optimal BW based on the pony's length and height was 345 kg. See Table 2.3.

- Initial estimates of energy requirement:
  - The BMR estimated at 5.2 Mcal DE/d [70 ($314^{0.75}$]
  - The RER estimated at 7.2 Mcal DE/d [75% (3.14 × 3.04]

Ration Assessment: Forage available at the rehabilitation center was a mixed mainly grass (IFN 1-02-277) moderate quality hay with, NDF 58%, 2 with 2.1 Mcal DE/kg, 17% protein, 2.3% fat, and 12% NSC. See Tables 24.2 and 10.3.

Feeding Recommendations: Based on assessments, feeding began at BMR with 2.5 kg of forage/d divided into 6 feedings (5.2 Mcal DE horse/2.1 Mcal/kg hay) for the first three to four days with daily re-assessments and monitoring of serum electrolytes. Dry matter intake (DMI) = 0.8% BW [2.5/314 × 100] and protein intake = 425 g/d or 82g protein/Mcal DE. See Table 24.3.

- Day 5: The pony had been consuming 2.5 kg of hay daily with no evidence of GI disturbances, gained 3 kg likely due to gut fill, showed increased interest in eating and surroundings, maintained adequate hydration and serum electrolytes, no evidence of refeeding syndrome, and produced normal manure; hence, the daily DE intake was increased to RER = 7.2 Mcal/d. Feeding directions were 3.4 kg forage/d divided into 4 meals for another three to four days. DMI = 1.1% BW [3.4/317 ×100] and protein intake was 578 g/d or 80g protein/Mcal DE. A low NSC micronutrient ration balancer for grass hay forages was introduced at 0.05% current BW (40 g/meal).
- Day 10: The pony weighed 325 kg with no indications of feed intolerance or metabolic disturbances. The daily DE intake was increased to 100% min DE_m = 9.9 Mcal/d

[3.25 × 3.04] and feeding directions were 4.7 kg forage/d divided into 3 meals. DMI = 1.4% BW [4.7/325 × 100] and protein intake was 799 g/d or 81 g protein/Mcal DE. Ration balancer continued at 0.1% BW.
- The horse continued to improve and 10 mos later weighed 350 kg BCS 6/9.

24.2.3.1 Improving Appetite

In tempting a partially anorexic or hypophagic horse to eat, satisfying psychological needs is essential. Horses are a prey species that seek safety (from harm) and comfort (absence of pain, peer dominance or herd separation) over food consumption, and only in a safe and comfortable environment will the patient eat. Often hospitalizing a patient, although most convenient for the veterinary staff, is sufficiently frightening to inhibit food consumption [45]. To improve comfort, the horse may be provided with warmer ambient temperatures, heating lamps or mats, or deep bedding. Unfamiliar sights, sounds, smells, aggressive human behaviors, and forced indoor housing with a limited sightline, all may depress appetite and voluntary feed intake [46]. In most cases, keeping herd mates close-by yet separated to avoid feed competition and to allow for measurement of individual feed intake in relatively open spaces is the best indoor situation conducive to appetite improvement.

In cases where oral lesions inhibit or decrease food consumption, in addition to treating the lesions and analgesics, offering soft green grass or a mash using a nutritionally complete low NSC extruded pellet (not bran) soaked in water may decrease the pain of eating sufficiently to improve intake. Grass pastures have 7–23% protein and 6–20% NSC, while mixed mainly grass (MMG) pastures have 11–25% protein and 7–18% NSC DM basis and hence appropriate for some cases as an appetite stimulant. Systemic fever or pain may also decrease appetite, and in such cases, administering antipyretics and analgesics may improve feed intake [47, 48].

Feeding at least 10–25% of the daily DE goal orally has been shown in Guinea pigs to significantly decrease SI atrophy, which in turn should promote appetite [49]. Offering small amounts (0.1–0.3% BW) of fresh forage, removing discarded feed after a few hours, and replacing the forage frequently are stimulating to most horses in combination with being in the presence of other horses eating. Although some horses will eat lying down, most prefer to be standing, and so the use of a sling or other upright supportive measures may improve feed consumption in recumbent horses. If able to walk, grazing in even dried pasture grasses several times a day may improve the horses' overall feed intake and attitude, as some patients prefer to eat from the ground rather than from a hanging bucket, bin, or rack.

Diazepam administered at low dosages IV may induce a horse to consume feed immediately after treatment but only for 15–20 min without distractions; hence, diazepam as an appetite stimulant is not advisable. Additionally, debilitated horses may become tranquilized and ataxic on diazepam unless low dosages are administered. Repeated dosing does not produce consistent results and should be avoided in patients with hepatic compromise. If not contraindicated, anabolic steroids and corticosteroids do not have an immediate effect but may increase feed intake after several days [50]. Completely anorectic or hypophagic chronically starved horses may initially require assisted feeding techniques such as tube-feeding or PN to meet nutritional requirements.

24.2.3.2 Risks

Horses that are affected by severe and prolonged PCM are at risk of developing refeeding syndrome when NSC, principally glucose, is reintroduced. The syndrome should be suspected in a severely malnourished horse that develops hypophosphatemia, hypokalemia, and hypomagnesemia after a period of refeeding. A rapid systemic influx of glucose following a meal or IV dextrose results in an abrupt release of insulin to move the glucose into cells and an obligatory cellular uptake of P for energy metabolism, K for deposition in newly synthesized cells, and Mg as an enzyme cofactor [40]. The intracellular uptake of these electrolytes results in rapid onset of decreased serum concentrations causing edema, respiratory depression, cardiac arrhythmias, and possibly death [10, 34]. Complications associated with refeeding can be avoided by closely monitoring serum electrolyte concentrations and with a careful gradual reintroduction of feeds with low to moderate NSC content. Treatment of electrolyte abnormalities in a horse with refeeding syndrome includes oral and parenteral electrolytes supplementation in an attempt to maintain adequate serum concentrations.

24.2.3.3 Monitoring

Body weight should be assessed weekly using a weigh scale rather than a weight tape if a scale is available. Weights may decrease or not change during initial refeeding days or may increase due to hydration and gut fill [34, 51]. Several weeks of refeeding are needed before a pattern of BW gain can be discerned. Minimizing energy losses by maintaining the horse in a neutral thermic environment or use of light blankets (rugs) when temperatures are below 60 °F minimizes body heat loss. However, sweating, which results in electrolyte losses, should be avoided. Daily blood work including complete blood cell count (CBC), serum biochemistries with electrolytes is advisable in the first two to seven days of refeeding expecting resolution of initial starvation parameters (BUN, TG, bilirubin) and monitoring for electrolyte shifts in P, K, and Mg. Monitoring thereafter weekly or as needed based on clinical signs is recommended. Recovering horses if overfed may have secondary medical conditions, such as acute laminitis, diarrhea, or colic. Most will initially have some soft feces with refeeding that is temporary and not expected to be dehydrating or debilitating.

Interest in eating should improve, and a subjective improvement in the patient should be noticeable within the first five days of refeeding, such as increased interest in surroundings, interactions with people and horses, and voluntary physical activity [52]. Treat and monitor pressure sores in recumbent horses to not only minimize pain, discomfort and improve appetite but also minimize heat and fluid losses through open sores. Recumbent horses should have deep comfortable bedding available but regularly encouraged to stand, walk, and graze, and horses that resume recumbency should be rotated from side to side to prevent pressure sores. There is a limited number of studies available by which to estimate clinical progress in starved equids. Broad estimates of average daily weight gain and weeks to achieve a BSC of 4 or 5/9 are estimated in Table 24.2 [10, 17, 26, 30].

24.3 Assisted Feeding

Low-BCS horses with concurrent disease, completely anorectic or severely hypophagic, may need to be tube fed to meet all or some nutritional needs. Patients with trauma or systemic disease have similar metabolic changes as those in simple starvation but likely at an accelerated rate because the thyroid does not down-regulate metabolism [19, 35, 53]. The combination of an increase in energy expenditure due to inflammatory cytokines, circulating hormones, and neurotransmitters promote an accelerated catabolic state, causing patients to develop PCM sooner in the time course of anorexia than those in simple starvation.

Multiple research studies have demonstrated that the immune response, tissue repair, and recovery are directly related to the nutritional state of the animal [23, 24, 54]. Although the need for nutritional support is obvious in anorexic horses, such support should not be initiated until the patient is hemodynamically stable as administering nutritional support may further compromise an unstable patient. Severe tachycardia, hypotension, colloid, and volume deficits should be corrected before feeding. Major electrolyte, acid–base abnormalities, and blood glucose concentrations should be within or near normal reference ranges before instituting enteral or PN support. A practical goal is to begin nutritional support within 24–48 hrs of the injury, illness, or presentation. The goal of nutritional support is to slow, rarely reverse, the ongoing catabolic state, minimize lean muscle mass losses, and support cellular and tissue functions by providing energy and essential precursors for recovery. The most effective way to manage the detrimental effects of systemic catabolism in a clinically ill foal or adult horse is to provide supplemental nutrition designed for the individual patient [55].

24.3.1 Animal Assessment

When possible, specialized sickness ethograms for horses should be consulted before an assessment is performed [52]. Where sickness behavior(s) is detected but not diagnostic, steps should be taken to identify the underlying cause of the illness. Evaluation of the nutritional status of the patient includes a thorough PE, laboratory analyses, and a review of the horse's recent diet history.

24.3.1.1 Physical Examination

Within a complete PE, an assessment of a horse's ability to prehend and swallow food is critical in developing a nutritional support plan. Presenting complaints of anorexia or hyporexia should be distinguished from dysphagia, neurologic disease, and mechanical disorders of the mouth and GI tract. Horses that are good candidates for assisted enteral feeding (AEF) have progressive GI motility (no ileus), can tolerate the placement of a nasogastric feeding tube, and can be fed while standing or in sternal recumbency. Contraindications for tube feeding include esophageal disease, abnormalities in the nasal or pharyngeal cavities, lateral recumbency, an inability to maintain the head in an upright position, a risk of aspiration, and severe respiratory disease. When a horse cannot be fed with a liquid enteral diet using a feeding tube, parenteral administration of nutrients should be considered.

The BW is used in the calculation of energy, protein, and other nutrient requirements and is an essential component in the nutritional management of the equine patient. Changes in the total mass of the patient can be documented with regular BW measurements if the horse is managed in a hospital facility with a scale available and if the patient can be moved between the stall and the scale. Alternatively, weight tape or anatomical measurements with weight calculations can provide an estimation of BW. See Tables 2.2 and 2.3.

Horses with a BCS 4 to 6/9 have some endogenous stores of fat and adequate muscling to use as a source of protein and amino acids and can tolerate partial to complete anorexia for 48–72 hrs without severe metabolic complications. Horses with a BCS 1 to 3/9 with PCM at the outset of the disease have difficulty recovering from surgery, sepsis, and systemic infections without early nutritional support. Anorexic BCS 7 to 9/9 horses may have complications associated with insulin dysregulation and are at risk of developing hypertriglyceridemia and other complications from abnormal lipid metabolism.

24.3.1.2 Laboratory Analyses

Most sick horses have some degree of protein malnutrition; however, diagnosis may be difficult using routine biochemical tests. Serum urea nitrogen and albumin are often within reference concentrations until PCM is severe, and decreases must be distinguished from hepatic or GI diseases. Additional tests that can be performed to evaluate the systemic protein balance in a patient include measurements of plasma essential and non-essential amino acids and urinary 3-methylhistidine, a myofibrillar protein produced following degradation of actin and myosin and excreted without further metabolism. These tests are not practical but might be useful diagnostic tests in the diagnosis of mild protein malnutrition in the future [56].

Measurements of blood glucose can be useful in equine neonates, adult horses with sepsis, and patients treated with supplemental nutrition during an illness. Neonates have minimal stores of glycogen, protein, and triglycerides and commonly become hypoglycemic when they are unable to nurse. Critically ill neonatal foals may also develop hyperglycemia before the initiation of therapeutic nutrition and would require an enteral or parenteral diet designed to manage the complication [57]. Adult horses maintain blood glucose within a normal range of 75–115 mg/dL during periods of short- and long-term food deprivation. Dysregulation of glucose metabolism should be considered in horses that have abnormally high blood glucose concentrations or that fail to regulate blood glucose with appropriate nutritional therapy. Horses with equine metabolic syndrome or other endocrine diseases with insulin dysregulation require special care and should be managed with therapeutic nutrition that does not exacerbate hyperglycemia and hyperinsulinemia. See Chapter 27 Endocrine System Disorders.

Adult horses that experience prolonged (>48 hrs) caloric deficits often have increased serum TG concentrations. Horses with above maintenance energy requirements (late gestation, lactation), insulin dysregulation, obesity, and some breeds of equids (Miniature horses, ponies, donkeys) are predisposed to hyperlipemia (TG > 500 mg/dL) during periods of illness. Clinically ill neonatal foals also may develop hypertriglyceridemia before the initiation of nutritional therapy. Neonatal foals with a serum TG concentration >200 mg/dL had a higher mortality rate than foals with lower concentrations [57]. Serum TG concentrations must be evaluated in all patients before nutritional support is initiated such that therapies can be designed to manage and resolve hypertriglyceridemia during administration. Serum electrolytes sodium (Na), K, chloride (Cl), calcium (Ca), Mg, and P may be decreased in anorexia but vary in different disease conditions. Serum ionized Ca and Mg fractions provide an accurate estimate of availability. Electrolyte supplementation in IV fluids is indicated as correction of serum concentrations is advisable before initiating nutritional support [58, 59].

24.3.2 Ration Assessment

A diet history provides insights into potential metabolic complications that may be encountered when the horse requires nutritional support. Owners should be asked to provide the type and weight of forage and complementary feeds the horse was eating before the illness. Dietary supplements should be described because some botanical supplements may interfere with the metabolism of pharmacologic therapies. Clinical decisions about when to start or continue nutrition therapy are based on a patient's voluntary DMI; hence, the type and amount of feed offered and refused should be weighed and recorded in the medical record daily. The nutrient intake can be calculated using nutrient concentrations from text books, lab analyses, and the guaranteed analysis on feed labels. See Rations Analysis in Chapter 10.

24.3.2.1 Products for Tube Feeding

There are several product types used in tube-feeding horses, that is, feed slurries and liquid products designed for people and horses. Each option has disadvantages [43, 60, 61]. Before the formulation of equine-specific commercial enteral diets and complete feeds, human liquid enteral formulations were used to provide enteral nutrition to equine patients. Several studies showed that the fiber-free human products, which typically contain corn maltodextrin or sucrose as a source of dietary carbohydrates, often resulted in a self-limiting diarrhea when administered to healthy horses [47, 60, 62]. Other studies reported that certain liquid enteral diets without fiber could be administered without causing diarrhea in horses with short-term anorexia or feed deprivation [63, 64]. Currently, fiber-free human enteral formulations are not an optimal choice in horses because of the potential for GI complications, the high cost of the products, and the more readily available enteral formulas and complete feeds specifically designed for horses.

Commercial enteral products[5] formulated specifically for horses offer a convenient option. Such products are designed to be mixed with water and can be administered

5 WellSolve W/G Well-Gel Purina Animal Nutrition LLC, Gray Summit, MO, USA and Enteral Immunonutrition Formula Platinum Performance, Inc., Buellton, CA, USA.

Table 24.4 Nutrient composition of common equine feeds and enteral diet ingredients.

Feed	Energy	Crude protein	Crude fat	Crude fiber	Non-structural carbohydrates	Calcium	Phosphorus	Magnesium	Potassium
	kcal/g				% As fed				
Commercial feeds									
Equine senior[a]	2.7	14	6	18	18	0.50	0.40	0.37	1.60
Senior[b]	3.4	14	10	17	12	0.90	0.60	0.37	1.25
Low starch[b]	3.1	13	6	18	14	0.75	0.60	0.50	0.75
Protein sources									
Sodium caseinate[c]	3.7	88.0	1.8	1.0	<1.0	0.04	0.71	0.01	0.01
Soy protein isolate[d]	3.4	88.3	3.4	0	0	0.18	0.78	0.04	0.09
Whey protein[e]	3.9	80.5	5.0	0	3.0	0.55	0.36	0.06	0.54
Forages and fiber sources[f]									
Alfalfa hay or pellets	2.4	18.2	2.5	27.1	10.2	1.47	0.28	0.29	2.22
Oat hay	2.0	8.3	2.3	28.8	22.1	0.30	0.20	0.14	1.66
Bermudagrass hay	2.1	11.0	1.9	28.9	13.2	0.49	0.20	0.21	1.69
Grass hay or pellets	2.0	10.9	2.5	31.4	12.9	0.49	0.24	0.21	1.84
Rice Bran	3.1	14.8	16.8	8.3	25.1	1.76	1.74	0.72	1.34
Wheat Bran	3.3	17.5	4.6	9.7	29.8	0.15	1.08	0.43	1.23
Beet Pulp (dry)	2.6	9.3	1.3	18.7	11.8	1.01	0.09	0.24	0.72
Energy sources									
Vegetable oil[e, d]	8.6	0	100	0	0	0	0	0	0
50% dextrose solution	1.7	0	0	0	100	0	0	0	0
Commercial enterals					% As is[g]				
WellSolve W/G® Well-Gel®[a]	2.2	36	6	14	11	2.4	0.95	0.5	1.66
Enteral Immunonutrition Formula[h]	4.7	16	30	10	34	0.34	0.33	0.38	0.95

[a] Purina Animal Nutrition LLC, Gray Summit, MO.
[b] Triple Crown, Wayzata, MN.
[c] Casein by MCO Proteins, Burlington, NJ.
[d] USDA National Nutrient Database for Standard Reference: Soy protein isolate NDB Number 16122. Oil NDB Number 4582.
[e] Equi-Whey by Platinum Performance, Inc., Buellton, CA.
[f] Equi-Analytical Laboratories Feed Profile Database (accessed 2 February 2019), http://equi-analytical.com/common-feed-profiles/
[g] The product as is before adding water.
[h] Platinum Performance, Inc. Buellton, CA.

through a small diameter nasogastric tube or fed per os as a liquid or powder while transitioning the horse to a standard ration. Another option is blenderizing an equine commercial complete feed, which contains the essential nutrients for an adult horse and is widely available. Feeds with ≤20% NSC are preferred to avoid GI complications that could develop with higher sugar and starch feeds. A simple blenderized diet can be made using hay (grass or legume) pellets fed either alone or combined with a source of powdered protein, oil, and a ration balancer for vitamins and minerals. See Table 24.4.

Protein supplementation of soy, casein, or whey is beneficial for patients that are protein malnourished or when grass hay pellets are used in the feed slurry. There are potential advantages to including glutamine and soluble fiber in liquid tube feeding products. Glutamine, a conditionally essential amino acid, is needed during periods of physiologic stress to stimulate SI DNA synthesis and increases SI mucosal mass early in recovery [48]. Fiber (~5%) modulates intestinal motility by providing intraluminal stimuli to re-establish normal peristaltic action and transit time and also provides non-digestible bulk to buffer toxins and holds water minimizing diarrhea. Vegetable oil provides a source of highly concentrated calories and can be added to the enteral diet if the horse is not hyperlipidemic and has a serum triglyceride <100 mg/dL. Adding oil may not be necessary if the commercial complete feed contains supplemental fat. The omega-3 and omega-6 content of the selected oil should be evaluated to help manage systemic inflammation. If a hay pellet is used, a granular vitamin and mineral supplement should be considered to ensure micronutrient adequacy of the diet. Vitamin and mineral products with herb-like ingredients should be avoided in horses with clinical illness and those recovering from colic surgery due to the potential for nutrient–drug interactions. Adjustments in the nutrient composition of the enteral diet are made based on the horse's response to the dietary therapy.

24.3.2.2 Products for Parenteral Feeding

Parenteral admixture formulations designed to manage specific human disease conditions are usually not appropriate for equids. However, commercial amino acid and dextrose products can be mixed to provide a convenient PN option for adult horses and foals. These admixtures can be specifically formulated to contain amino acids (2.75–5.0%), dextrose (5–25%), and electrolyte concentrations tailored to patient needs. The caloric density (0.28–1.05 kcal/mL) and osmolarity (665–1900 mOsm/L) of the formulations can be adjusted as needed. Admixtures with osmolarity >900 mOsm/L are not suitable for infusion through small-diameter peripheral (cephalic, lateral thoracic) veins. Individual solutions providing dextrose, lipids, amino acids, minerals, and vitamins can be designed to meet specific nutritional goals for equine patients (Table 24.5).

Table 24.5 Parenteral nutrition ingredients and commercial mixtures.

Macronutrient additives	Manufacturer	Amino acids (g/mL)	Soybean oil (%)	Dextrose (%)	pH	Osmolarity (mOsmol/mL)	kcal/mL	mEq/mL
Energy solutions								
Intralipid® 20%	Baxter[a]		20		8	0.26	2	
Nutralipid® 20%	B. Braun[b]		20		7	0.39	2	
Dextrose, 50%				50	4	2.55	1.7	
Amino acid solutions								
8.5% Aminosyn® w/ Electrolytes	Pfizer[c]	0.085			5	1.04	0.34	
Sodium								0.065
Potassium								0.065
Magnesium								0.01
Chloride								0.098
Phosphorus								0.03 (mM/mL)[d]
8.5% Aminosyn w/o electrolytes	Pfizer	0.085			5	0.802	0.34	
10% Aminosyn	Pfizer	0.1			5	0.932	0.4	
10% Travasol®	Baxter	0.1			6	0.998	0.4	
15% Clinisol®	Baxter	0.15			6	1.357	0.6	
10% FreAmine® III	B. Braun	0.1			7	0.95	0.4	
Sodium								0.01
Phosphate								0.02
15% Plenamine™	B. Braun	0.15			6	1.383	0.6	
Combination solutions								
Clinimix® 4.25/5	Baxter	0.0425		5	6	0.675	0.34	
Clinimix® 5.0/15	Baxter	0.05		15	6	1.255	0.71	

[a] Baxter Healthcare Corporation, Deerfield, IL.
[b] B. Braun Medical Inc. Irvine, CA.
[c] Pfizer Inc., New York, NY, USA.
[d] mM = millimoles; one mM of phosphorus = 31 mg.

Calories are typically divided between dextrose and lipid in the solution based on the metabolic profile of the horse. Dextrose has a nitrogen-sparing effect and provides a source of energy in PN solutions (50% dextrose has 1.7 kcal/mL). Although 50% dextrose is the most common concentration available at equine hospitals, 70% dextrose solutions are available. The proportion of dextrose is limited by the horse's ability to metabolize glucose. Adding lipid to a PN formulation provides a calorie-dense (20% solution has 2 kcal/mL) and iso-osmolar (330 mOsm/L) solution that is beneficial for horses that can tolerate lipid. The lipid products currently available in the USA include soybean oil as the lipid source and provide both the essential omega-6 linoleic acid and a smaller concentration of omega-3 α-linolenic acid.

Although complications have not been repeatedly identified in horses to date, except for hypertriglyceridemia in neonatal foals treated with PN, concern for lipid overuse in equine PN formulations exists. Newer PN formulations that contain fish oil as a source of omega-3 fatty acids have been used in Europe and have shown promise as alternative lipid solutions with fewer complications [57, 65]. It has been hypothesized that the high linoleic acid concentration promotes a strong inflammatory response when used in critically ill patients. Although lipid solutions with fish oil are currently not available in the USA, this type of lipid ingredient offers promise for an improved way of managing critically ill horses with PN if available in the future.

Commercial amino acid solutions providing essential and non-essential amino acids contain 8.5–10% amino acids have an energy density of 0.34–0.4 kcal/mL, a pH range of 6.0–6.5, and an osmolarity of 810–1144 mOsm/L (Table 24.5). Other solutions with different concentrations of amino acids (3.5, 5, 7, and 15%) are available. Amino acid solutions with and without supplemental electrolytes (Na, K, Mg, Cl, P) can be selected based on the electrolyte needs of the equine patient.

The most effective way to supplement electrolytes in horses is to add those needed to IV fluids that run concurrently with the PN solution. Intravenous fluid supplementation allows for a rapid change in the electrolyte therapy to match the patient's needs without wasting the costly PN formulation. Multiple vitamin[6] and trace mineral[7] products can be added directly to PN solutions. Vitamins vary in their stability when exposed to the plastic admixture bag, IV tubing, and light. When vitamins are added to a PN solution, the admixture bag, and fluid tubing should be shielded from direct natural light. Fluorescent light does not appear to disrupt the structure of the vitamins. All vitamin and mineral supplements should be added to the PN solution only once the macronutrient components have been mixed.

24.3.2.3 Key Nutrients

24.3.2.3.1 Adult Horses

Nutritional support is designed primarily to provide supplemental calories and protein during a period of anorexia or hyporexia [55, 66]. When nutrients are administered IV, the energy provided to the horse is probably similar to other animals, which is 8.5 kcal/g of fat and 3.4 kcal/g for both protein and carbohydrate. Whenever possible and not cost-prohibitive, providing electrolytes, minerals, and vitamins in proportion to the calories is advisable (Table 24.3). Additionally, an enteral diet should contain structural fiber as cellulose or hemicellulose to support the intestinal microbiome and volatile fatty acid production.

It is not possible to measure the metabolic rate in hospitalized or debilitated horses without using "bedside" mask respiration calorimetry. In most cases, the range of daily energy needs is between BMR and minimal DE_m and likely changes with the time course of disease and treatments. Anorexic or hyporexic adult horses affected by some disease processes will likely have a metabolic rate between RER and min DE_m [30, 40, 41]. See Figure 24.2. Studies in sick people and neonatal foals estimate that metabolic rate need ranges between RER and maintenance energy requirements of normal, healthy individuals [67, 68]. Critically ill patients, those with severe sepsis, trauma, burns, or requiring intestinal resection, likely have a metabolic rate closer to maintenance due to inflammatory cytokines, circulating hormones, and neurotransmitters. Bedside calorimetry in people shows that energy requirements can increase above expected RER by 15–20% with trauma, 30–50% with multi-system trauma, and 80–100% relative to the extent of skin damage and surface area exposed in burn patients [69]. The increase in metabolic rate depends on the time course and type of recovery involved [70]. However, feeding to meet the healthy adult average DE_m (3.33 Mcal/100 kg BW) or using the horse's ideal BW in any energy calculation will overfeed most sick horses [19]. Overfeeding a patient runs the risk of creating metabolic derangements and refeeding syndrome, whereas providing 25% to 66% of caloric need may be sufficiently beneficial to support recovery in veterinary patients [1, 18, 68]. Given the metabolic rate of a horse cannot be determined and will likely stay between RER and min DE_m, current recommendations are to initially provide RER in the majority of hospitalized equine patients.

The best estimation of protein requirements for anorexic or hyporexic adult horses is at least the maintenance

6 M.V.I. Adult™, Pfizer Inc., New York, NY, USA and INFUVITE Adult, Baxter Healthcare Corporation, Deerfield, IL.
7 Multitrace®-5, American Regent, Shirley, NY.

protein requirement, 35 g/Mcal, and likely most debilitated horses would benefit from >40 g/Mcal in the short term (Table 24.3) because during illness amino acids are catabolized for energy despite glucose and lipid availability. An estimate of 1.26 g protein/kg BW/d is likely reasonable for horses consuming feed enterally, assuming an average feed digestibility of 46% [17]. Parenteral protein administration estimations for critically ill horses range from 0.5 to 1.5 g/kg BW/d, given the amino acids infused IV do not require digestion. The calorie to nitrogen ratio (kcal : N) should likely be 100–200 for most equine patients [19]. Protein intakes should be tailored lower in patients with renal or hepatic disease but higher for those with protein losses and actively catabolizing protein for energy. Most equine liquid enteral rations contain macro- and trace minerals and vitamins, but these can be added to the formulation if needed. PN solutions should include trace nutrients and water-soluble vitamins. Micronutrients should not be omitted as these are essential in the catabolism of glucose, fatty acids, and protein for energy. See Microminerals in Chapter 8 and Water-soluble Vitamins in Chapter 9.

24.3.2.3.2 Foals

The metabolic rate measured in critically ill foals averaged 1.8 × BMR, which was 25% lower than that in healthy foals measured during the same period, confirming that often ill equine neonates have metabolic rates between basal and comparable healthy cohorts (Figure 24.2) [71]. Neonatal foals requiring nutritional support should be managed with an initial intake of 40–50 kcal/current kg BW/d based on the indirect calorimetry measurements of 1 to 20 day old foals [67, 71]. Older hypophagic foals (2–4 mos) may tolerate 50–80 kcal/current kg BW/d, whereas foals over 4 mos may be fed 75–100 kcal/kg BW/d [71]. Dietary protein requirements for healthy foals at the highest rate of growth is approximately 7 g protein/kg BW/d; however, 2–5 g protein/current kg BW/d is recommended for sick neonatal foals, and the calorie-to-nitrogen ratio should be greater than 100 [19]. Foals with mineral or vitamin deficiencies or electrolyte imbalances require supplemental nutrients in the enteral diet or IV maintenance fluids. Injectable vitamins and minerals, for example, vitamin E and selenium, may be considered based on diet history.

24.3.3 Feeding Management

It is important not to delay nutritional support waiting to see if a patient will develop an appetite or be able to eat in the post-surgical period. Timing has proven important in the prevention of malnutrition-related complications, and early enteral nutrition remains the best tool against cascading problems. A combination of enteral and parenteral feeding introduced by day 4 in those human patients not achieving medical goals or targets of improvement is a valuable adjunct [1]. Some form of caloric therapy should be initiated if (i) food will be withheld for >24 hrs, (ii) the horse has lost >5% of BW, or (iii) the horse has dropped one BCS point or more since the onset of disease or hospitalization. Clinical studies in hospitalized horses have demonstrated an improved recovery after GI surgery in patients supplemented with PN [61]. Although it is possible to meet the daily caloric and amino acid requirements of an adult horse, the technical and financial obstacles are much greater than rehabilitating a low-BCS horse using oral voluntary consumption or tube feeding and hence, PN is rarely implemented in horses under the care of humane shelters or rescue leagues [72, 73].

24.3.3.1 Adult Horses

24.3.3.1.1 Early Therapeutic Nutrition Options

During the first 24–36 hrs of anorexia or hyporexia, or in the early postoperative period following GI surgery, clinicians can begin administering fluids supplemented with dextrose and/or use a "cafeteria feeding" method when appropriate. Intravenous dextrose and cafeteria feeding provide early and simple options for nutritional intervention in adult horses.

Dextrose can be administered along with maintenance IV fluid therapy to provide supplemental calories. Dextrose is added to make a final solution of 2.5 to 10% with an osmolarity ranging from 126 to 505 mOsm/L. When fluids are delivered as a continuous rate infusion (CRI), the patient's renal threshold of glucose (10 mmol/L or 180 mg/dL for adult horses; 12 mmol/L or 216 mg/dL for foals) is usually not exceeded. To avoid complications from hyperglycemia and hyperosmolarity, adult horses are rarely treated with solutions that contain >10% dextrose. The calories provided in dextrose-supplemented fluids (1.7 kcal/L for 50% dextrose) should be calculated and recorded for each 24-hr period. For example, a 450 kg horse treated with IV fluids at a rate of 27 L/d containing 2.5% dextrose will receive 2.3 Mcal/d, approximately 22% of the patient's RER. Dextrose-supplemented fluids can be administered as the sole source of nutrition for 24–48 hrs, but the horse will remain in a protein malnourished state until amino acids are added to the infusion. Horses treated with dextrose should be monitored for the development of hyperglycemia and glucosuria. Care must be taken when any dextrose-supplemented fluids are administered to an equine patient with insulin dysregulation, including horses with pituitary pars intermedia dysfunction or metabolic syndrome.

Cafeteria feeding involves offering a wide variety of highly palatable feeds to a hyporexic or anorexic horse to stimulate voluntary feed intake. Ideal feeds include fresh grass (if available and tolerated), small amounts of highly digestible hay or hay pellets, and complete pelleted feeds that contain ≤20% NSC. Feeds that contain a moderate to high concentration of NSC (>22%) and grain concentrates or individual grains like corn, oats, or barley should be avoided unless they are used in a limited amounts (50–100 g/d) as a top dressing on a fiber-based feed to encourage feed consumption. All feed should be weighed before and after offering to the horse, then discarded and the difference, that is, amount consumed, recorded. Fresh feeds, for example, fresh-cut grass, should be offered every 4–6 hrs to ensure the feed remains palatable. Feeds that have been moistened will spoil and become rancid and should be removed after 2–6 hrs.

If a horse does not tolerate the dextrose infusion and/or does not voluntarily consume enough feed to meet ≥75% of RER and protein requirement, tube feeding or PN should be initiated. The choice between tube feeding and PN depends on the clinical condition of the horse, the resources available for diet preparation and administration in either a field or hospital setting, and the financial limitations of the case.

24.3.3.1.2 Assisted Enteral Feeding

Assisted enteral or tube feeding a liquid or blenderized diet is the preferred form of therapeutic nutrition in any adult horse that can tolerate enteral nutrition because it provides nutrients directly to the intestinal enterocytes and helps to maintain the protective barrier in the GI tract (GIT) [74]. Metabolic disadvantages to tube feeding versus voluntary consumption of the same low-NSC diets have been reported. Adult horses with good BCS consuming a low-NSC feed voluntarily had lower ($P < 0.05$) insulin concentrations at 120 and 140 min and lower blood glucose concentrations at 30 min post-feeding than similar horses receiving the same dose of feed via NG tube [75, 76]. Maintenance of the intestinal microbiome is an important component of therapy and should be managed with enteral nutrition as well as with pre-and probiotics when possible. See The Role of the Microbiota in Chapter 4.

Liquid enteral diets are almost always infused through a nasogastric tube; however, gastroesophageal tubes can be placed in horses that require long-term therapy or in horses that cannot be treated with a nasogastric tube. An equine surgeon should be consulted in the placement of a gastroesophageal tube. Percutaneous gastrostomy tube and jejunostomy tube feeding are not feasible in horses at this time. Equipment requirements for enteral feeding are minimal and limited to a nasogastric tube and an infusion pump or a fluid bag for gravity flow administration. One disadvantage of tube feeding is that some horses become resistant to repeated nasogastric intubation after four to five days and have mild epistaxis if the tube cannot remain in place [26]. Equine enteral formulations are relatively inexpensive, with costs as low as 20 US$/d for diet ingredients. See Sidebar 24.2.

Sidebar 24.2: Assisted Enteral Feeding Worksheet

Patient history: five-year-old Quarter horse mare BCS 4/9 was bright, alert, and active with a painful oral injury resulting in decreased food consumption and 10% BW loss over the last month. A nasogastric feeding tube was placed during surgical correction of the injury with follow-up recommendations of no food per os (NPO), stall confinement, wearing a muzzle, and walking in hand only for another seven days until recheck.

Animal Assessment:

1) Body weight (kg)	450 kg
2) Minimal DE_m (Mcal/d) = 0.03 × (kg BW)	13.5 Mcal
3) RER (Mcal/d) = 75% min DE_m	10.4 Mcal
4) Protein requirement: =1.26 g × (kg BW)	567 g
5) Fluid requirements for maintenance: 60 mL/kg/d	27 L
6) Energy goal between RER and min DE_m based on history	12 Mcal

Ration Assessment:

1) Energy calculation:
   - Feed alfalfa pellets for energy (Table 24.4) 2.4 kcal DE/g
   - Amount to feed to meet DER [12 Mcal/2.4] 5.0 kg/d
2) Protein calculation:
   - 5 kg of alfalfa pellets with 18.2% crude protein [5 kg × 18%] 910 g

Feeding Recommendations:

- In hospital setting, feeding 4 times/d: 5 kg/4 = 1.25 kg alfalfa pellets/feeding.
- If all fluids are provided with enteral nutrition, then 27 L/4 = 6.75 L water/feeding, that is 5 L water can be mixed with the pellets and the remaining 1.75 L used to flush the feeding tube.
- Feed orders: 1.25 kg alfalfa pellet mixed with 5 L water followed by 1.75 L water via NE tube every 6 hrs.
- If NG tube feeding is required beyond 10 days, a mineral vitamin ration balancer pellet should be added to alfalfa meals (0.1% BW/d/4) to achieve a proper balance of micronutrients.

Diet Preparation The total volume of feed that needs to be administered in one day should be determined based on energy and protein calculations for the patient, and the daily volume of feed should be divided into 4–6 meals. If only partial supplementation is required or if a horse is being managed in a field setting, a smaller volume can be administered twice a day. Each meal should be administered within 30 min of preparation to reduce the risk of spoilage and rancidity. Commercial equine complete feeds and hay pellets can be prepared either by grinding dry pellets in a blender[8] and suspending the blended product in water or by soaking the feed or hay pellets in water to create a wet slurry before blending. Commercial feeds that contain beet pulp need to be soaked in more water than alfalfa-based feeds. The total amount of water added to the blenderized diet should be recorded and added to the daily fluid intake measurement for the patient. The maintenance fluid requirements (60 mL/kg BW/d) of a horse can be met if the horse is tube-fed at least four times daily.

Administration The diet and tube combination should be tested by infusing liquid diet or enteral slurry into the tube before the tube is placed in the horse to confirm the tube will not clog with feed. Larger diameter NG tubes (>0.65 cm inner diameter) must be used when fiber is included in the diet. Small diameter NG tubes (18 Fr) require administration of a liquid diet without fiber to ensure the tube will not block. The consistency of the enteral slurry can be adjusted by adding water to the blended ingredients. Tubes that become blocked should be treated with a warm water lavage to clear the tube. Alternatively, infusion of 20–30 mL of carbonated water left in place for up to one hr may be used to disintegrate a food blockage. If the carbonated water fails to dissolve the slurry, the tube should be removed, properly cleaned, and replaced in the patient before the next feeding. If the NG tube remains in place between feedings, the tube should be secured to a leather halter and the horse should wear a muzzle between feedings to prevent removal of the NG tube. A nylon muzzle[9] is well tolerated and easy to clean and causes minimal trauma to the face if the horse rubs the muzzle.

All liquid enteral diets, regardless of type, should be gradually introduced over three to seven days. The total daily volume of the enteral diet should be divided into four to six feedings and administered slowly enough to ensure that the feed does not reflux around the NG tube. No more than 6–8 L, including water flushes, should be administered at one time to an adult horse weighing 450 kg. This volume must be proportionally lowered for ponies and miniature horses and can be increased for draft breeds. Horses with <2 L of residual fluid in the stomach can be given a meal, but if the volume of residual gastric fluid is >2L, the feeding should be delayed for two hrs. Horses with persistent gastric reflux should not be fed enterally, and instead, the clinician should consider parenteral administration. After the diet has been administered, the tube should be flushed with at least 500 mL of water before capping the tube if the tube will remain in place. Excessive distention of the stomach must be avoided. Horses should be offered palatable (<20% NSC) feeds and encouraged to begin voluntary consumption between enteral tube feeding times. The same feeds that are used in the blenderized diet can be offered to the horse during the transition period. Horses should be weaned from tube feeding over two to three days once voluntarily consuming 75% of RER of an appropriate ration.

Monitoring Horses with feeding tubes should be examined twice daily. Elevations in body temperature, pulse, and respiration values beyond the upper normal range require prompt evaluation to identify the cause of the clinical abnormalities. Although a small amount of mucoid nasal discharge is expected with prolonged NG tube placement, purulent nasal discharge, respiratory stridor, tachypnea, and coughing are abnormal and should be evaluated to ensure that the horse has not developed an ulcer or a perforation of the pharyngeal or esophageal tissues [77]. BW should be assessed daily and BCS assessed weekly. Serum values of packed cell volume, total protein, electrolytes, glucose, and triglyceride should be monitored daily until the patient's condition stabilizes; then, the assessment can be every 48–72 hrs.

Serious complications from AEF are rare, and most can be avoided if the liquid enteral diet is introduced slowly and the horse is closely monitored. If complications from ileus or gastric reflux arise during the administration of the enteral diet, the volume and frequency of feeding should be reduced until the horse can tolerate the feedings. Gastric ulcers do not appear to be a common complication with liquid enteral diets for short periods (7–10 days). Mild diarrhea is not a reason to stop tube feeding unless the patient becomes dehydrated, develops colic or colitis, or develops ileus in association with the enteral feeding. Management strategies to help resolve diarrhea should include an increase in the frequency of feedings, a decrease in the volume of feed infused at each meal, and the use of a probiotic supplement. The addition of probiotic products containing *Lactobacillus spp.* or

---

8 Vitamix E310 Vita-Mix Corporation, Cleveland, OH, USA or Blendtec Chef 600 Blendtec, Orem, UT.

9 Best Friend Grazing Muzzle, Best Friend Equine Supply, Inc., Fairfield Glade, TN.

Saccharomyces boulardii may help to restore the natural microbiome in the GIT and may offer some benefit in reducing complications from diarrhea [78, 79].

24.3.3.1.3 Parenteral Nutrition

PN is the preferred form of nutritional therapy in horses that cannot be treated with AEF. Practical limitations to PN use include the need for a dedicated catheter port and intravenous fluid line, CRI delivery, and the necessity of frequent monitoring of serum biochemical parameters which limit therapy to a hospital setting and the cost of PN products.

Formulations can be designed to meet either part or all of the horse's daily energy and protein requirements. A partial parenteral nutrition (PPN) formulation intends to meet ≤50% of the energy and protein needs and includes dextrose and amino acids in addition to IV fluid therapy. A PN formulation intended to meet nearly 100% of the energy, protein, and most of the micronutrients needs will include dextrose, amino acids, lipids, vitamins, and minerals (Table 24.5). Horses with severe PCM are better candidates for full PN; however, the high cost for an adult horse (400–500 US$/d) often prohibits use beyond one wk. The cost of PN can be reduced and the duration of therapy can be extended if the PN is formulated to provide 50–75% of the patient's needs.

In formulating PN or PPN, it is important to design a solution with a nutrient composition that matches the patient's metabolic profile. See Sidebar 24.3. Formulating PN recipes specific for the individual patient rather than using a standard recipe or stock admixtures will often avoid metabolic complications. Horses generally tolerate PN therapy well but will develop hyperglycemia and glucosuria when concentrations of dextrose or the infusion rate is too high [80, 81]. Changes in the recipe or infusion rate may be required during the treatment period to optimize IV administration of protein, lipid, and dextrose. A nutritionist should be consulted in the formulation of a PN solution for a patient with complex metabolic conditions.

Up to 60% of the calories (60% dextrose : 40% lipids) in a PN formula can be provided as dextrose in most horses with normal glucose and insulin regulation. Horses suffering from glucose intolerance or insulin dysregulation should initially be treated with a PN solution that contains <30% of total calories from dextrose (30% dextrose : 70% lipids) as long as the patient does not have concurrent hypertriglyceridemia (>200 mg/dL). These guidelines allow for a wide range of PN formulations to be developed for an individual horse. Judicious use of dextrose will result in better tolerance of the formulation and will minimize the potential complication of hyperglycemia and the need for insulin therapy.

Sidebar 24.3: Partial Parenteral Nutrition Worksheet for Adult Horses

Patient history: five-yr-old Quarter horse mare BCS 4/9 with a painful oral injury that has resulted in decreased food consumption and a 10% BW loss in the last month. A nasogastric feeding tube, during surgical correction, removed after two days due to a sinus infection and PPN was recommended due to financial limitations.

Animal Assessment:

1) Body weight (kg) — 450 kg
2) Min DE_m (Mcal/d) = 0.03 × (kg BW) — 13.5 Mcal
3) RER (Mcal/d) = 75% min DE_m — 10.4 Mcal
4) Decided on 75% of RER based on financial constraints — 7.8 Mcal
5) Protein requirement at 1.26 × (kg BW) — 567 g
6) Fluid requirement for maintenance at 60 mL/kg/d — 27 L

Parenteral Solution Formulation (Table 24.5):

- Volume of 50% dextrose required to meet the energy requirement:
  - 50% dextrose contains 1.7 Mcal/L [7.8/1.7] — 4.6 L[a]
- Volume of 10% amino acids required to meet protein requirement:
  - 10% amino acid solution contains 100 g/L [567 g/100 g] — 5.7 L
- Total PPN volume: — 10.3 L
- Volume of polyionic fluids required to meet fluid requirement:
  - Fluid requirement minus PPN solution [27 L−10.3 L][b] — 16.7 L
- Osmolarity of final solution:
  - Dextrose: 4.6 L × 2550 mOsm/L = 11 730
  - Amino acids: 5.7 L × 998 mOsm/L = 5689
  - Lactated Ringers: 16.7 L × 273 mOsm/L = 4560
  - Total mOsm = 21,978 mOsm
  - Final mOsm/L = 21,978 mOsm/27L — 814 mOsm/L

Feeding orders: administer PPN solution at 1.13 L/hr or 19 mL/min via jugular catheter.

[a] Compare dextrose volume with the fluid requirement. When fluid >dextrose volume, there should be no over-hydration complication.
[b] Dextrose and amino acid solutions can be added to a partially drained bag of polyionic fluids. B vitamins and trace minerals should be added if PPN is needed beyond 3 days.

The osmolarity of the final PN solution should be calculated before compounding to ensure no damage to the endothelium of the catheterized vein. In adult horses, the final osmolarity should be <1200 mOsm/L when using jugular vein catheters or <900 mOsm/L in smaller veins. Strategies to lower the osmolarity of a PN solution include using an amino acid solution without electrolytes, increasing the volume of polyionic fluid or sterile water, decreasing the volume of 50% dextrose, using a lower concentration of dextrose, or increasing the concentration of lipid in the formulation. Calculation of the PN solution osmolarity is the summation of the osmole contribution of each ingredient divided by the total volume (Sidebar 24.3).

Most PN solutions contain at least 50% free water that will be distributed throughout the intracellular and extracellular fluid space. The volume of fluid administered through the PN solution must be calculated into the patient's daily fluid requirement to ensure the horse does not receive an excessive volume of fluid. If the patient has been managed with dextrose-supplemented fluids before the start of PN, the dextrose should be discontinued in the intravenous fluids to prevent complications from hyperglycemia. Most horses, regardless of the duration of therapy, benefit from 1 to 2 mL of B complex vitamins/L of PN solution to facilitate cellular metabolism during a period when intestinal production of B vitamins is reduced [82]. Supplementation of fat-soluble vitamins is recommended if the horse is in a state of severe malnutrition, and trace minerals are recommended if PN therapy will be administered for longer than five days. The normal GI regulation of trace mineral absorption is bypassed during parenteral infusions, and PN concentrations must be lowered as toxicity could develop with IV administration of zinc, copper, iron, and selenium [83]. The daily dose of trace minerals should not exceed 5 mL for a horse that weighs more than 400 kg. Providing macro-minerals, as electrolytes, is routine; however, decreased bone density will occur due to stall confinement, which cannot be avoided [84].

Compounding PN Solutions Parenteral formulations can be compounded by hospital pharmacies or commercial pharmaceutical services.[10] PN solutions can also be compounded within a veterinary hospital using a laminar flow hood or a surgical instrument preparation room with minimal traffic using sterile techniques to ensure aseptic preparation of the formulation.

PN formulations are made by mixing three macronutrients (dextrose, amino acids, lipid) in a compounding container or an infusion bag. Polyionic fluids and sterile water are not typically added to dilute PN solutions. PPN formulas can be made by adding dextrose and amino acids into a bag of polyionic fluids or by adding the amino acid solution to a bag of 5% dextrose. Sterile water is added to admixture bags, carboys, or sterile glass jars to dilute a PPN solution. A variety of container systems are available for PN compounding. All-in-one admixture bags are available in 1, 2, and 3 L sizes and are ideal for in-house compounding of PN solutions using gravity transfer of ingredients.[11] Sterile glass bottles can be used but are not ideal in a large animal hospital setting and are usually reserved for neonatal ICU patients. A sterile carboy can be used for the PN solution, but because carboys are reused, this type of container is the least desirable option and should be used only in an emergency.

The dextrose and amino acid PN ingredients are mixed first. Sterile transfer sets designed for PN compounding are ideal, but if they are not available, the solutions can be transferred using sterile syringes. The lipid solution must be added last to prevent precipitation of the lipid when mixed directly with dextrose. The compounded PN solution should be gently mixed and then inspected for any signs of crystallization or ingredient separation. Vitamin and mineral supplements can be added using sterile syringes once the PN macro ingredients have been mixed. PN solutions, either with or without a lipid additive, should be stable when refrigerated at 35–40 °F for seven days but should be used within 24–48 hrs once the solution has been brought to room temperature (70 °F).

Administering PN solutions Parenteral formulations are almost always infused into a peripheral vein (jugular, lateral thoracic, cephalic, medial saphenous) in adult horses. Whenever possible, a multi-lumen catheter should be used to administer PN to ensure that a dedicated catheter port is available for PN infusion. Blood should not be drawn from a port that will later be used for PN administration. A multiple-site infusion port can be attached to a single lumen catheter if multi-lumen catheters are not available but are not recommended due to the increased risk of sepsis and bacterial contamination. If a multi-port catheter or multiple-infusion port attachment is not available, then a separate intravenous catheter can be placed in another vein for PN administration. Caution should be used if both jugular veins are catheterized in a patient due to the complications that can arise from thrombophlebitis. Patient medications may not be compatible with the PN

10 Central Admixture Pharmacy Services, Inc., a member of the B. Braun Group of Companies and Coram LLC, a CVS Specialty Infusion Services.

11 Baxter Healthcare Corporation, Deerfield, IL, USA and B. Braun Medical Inc., Irvine, CA.

solutions and should be given through a separate line. If a separate line is not available, the PN line should be flushed with saline before and after administration of the medication. Potential drug incompatibilities should be discussed with a pharmacist.

The PN formula should be infused using a fluid pump. The administration should be started at 25–30% of the total infusion rate and maintained for the first six to eight hrs. If the horse tolerates the PN and does not develop hyperglycemia, hypertriglyceridemia, or electrolyte abnormalities, the rate can be gradually increased to the full daily dose over 12–36 hrs. The infusion rate increase may need to be slowed for horses with hyperglycemia or hypertriglyceridemia. Clinicians should not dismiss the use of PN if cost or metabolic intolerance necessitates the provision of less than a full rate as patients still benefit from PPN. The PN solution and infusion lines should be changed every 24 hrs using sterile procedures. Once assembled, the PN infusion line should never be broken. If the horse needs to be moved during the time of PN infusion, the entire PN set should remain connected and should be moved with the horse.

Enteral feeding should begin as soon as the horse can tolerate oral feeds. During the refeeding period, the horse can be fed cafeteria-style or treated with a liquid enteral product to facilitate a return to voluntary food consumption. Once a horse can voluntarily consume or can tolerate infused liquid enteral diet to meet 75% RER, the PN therapy can be discontinued. The rate of PN infusion should be decreased gradually over 24–36 hrs, and therapy can be completely discontinued once the horse is receiving <30% of the total daily infusion volume.

Monitoring Horses treated with PN or PPN should be monitored at least every 8 hrs with a PE, assessment of hydration status, and a close evaluation of the intravenous catheter site. The goal of PN is to prevent the horse from losing additional weight and lean tissue mass. Daily BW measurements using a weight scale are necessary to properly monitor patients on PN. The fecal production in horses treated with PN will decrease, and any horse that develops diarrhea requires an evaluation for pathogenic bacteria. During the first 2–3 days of therapy, total protein, packed cell volume, serum electrolytes, and blood glucose should be measured every 12 hrs and serum triglyceride measured every 24 hrs until the values have stabilized. During the transition period from PN to enteral nutrition, the clinical and biochemical status of the horse should be assessed daily.

If the horse develops hyperglycemia, glucose >180 mg/dL, the rate of PN infusion can be decreased by one-third to one-half and rechecked in 8–12 hrs. If the hyperglycemia has resolved, the PN administration rate can be increased gradually while maintaining normoglycemia. If hyperglycemia persists, the PN solution should be reformulated to reduce the glucose concentration by 30–50%. The calorie deficit can be replaced by lipid in the PN solution if the horse has a serum triglyceride <200 mg/dL. If lipid supplementation is not an option, the PN can be administered as a PPN solution that provides a portion (50–80%) of the RER. The protein requirements can be met using a PPN solution; however, the osmolarity should remain <1200 mOsm/L. Horses that cannot tolerate a parenteral solution with a reduced infusion rate and lowered dextrose concentrations may require a CRI of regular insulin, titrated to effect from a starting rate of 0.01 IU/kg/hr or intermittent treatments of protamine zinc insulin (0.1–0.3 IU/kg BW q12h). During treatment with insulin, the blood glucose concentration must be monitored closely to ensure that the horse does not become hypoglycemic.

It is not uncommon for anorectic horses to have an elevated serum triglyceride at the start of PN therapy. If the nutritional therapy is effective, the triglyceride should decrease within 24 hrs of treatment. Before blood sampling for serum TGs, the PN infusion should be stopped for 15–20 min, allowing liver and peripheral tissues to clear the infused lipids. If the concentration of TGs remains elevated (>200 mg/dL), or if it increases after 48 hrs of therapy, the PN solution should be reformulated to reduce the lipid concentration by 50%.

24.3.3.2 Foals

Foals have minimal energy stores and require supplemental nutrients within 6–12 hrs of losing the ability to nurse. Foals that require supplemental nutrition can be classified into three different categories: (i) healthy neonates that cannot ingest enough milk due to reasons associated with the dam, for example, death, illness, inadequate milk production, foal rejection; (ii) foals that cannot voluntarily or safely consume enough calories to meet requirements; and (iii) critically ill foals unable to nurse or tolerate enteral nutrition due to respiratory, GIT, or neurologic complications. Laboratory evaluation should include CBC, serum biochemistry profile, and IgG concentrations (>800 mg/dL), and nutritional therapy is always used in conjunction with appropriate medical management.

The choice between enteral or parenteral support depends on the competency of the foal's GIT, respiratory tract, and neurologic condition. Enteral nutrition is the preferred feeding method because nutrients are supplied directly to the enterocytes, resulting in an improved mucosal barrier and local immune function. Before initiating therapy, the suckle response should be assessed to determine the safest method of feeding. Foals with a poor suckle response should not be permitted to nurse and should be treated with supplemental nutrition through a nasogastric tube until the suckle response is strong and fully developed. Enteral nutrition is appropriate for all foals that have a healthy GIT. Obtunded foals, foals needing ventilation, and foals showing seizure activity should receive the majority of their nutrients from PN to decrease the risk of milk aspiration during enteral feeding. PN should be administered in conjunction with a small volume of enteral nutrition whenever possible to improve enterocyte integrity and to facilitate the foal's transition to voluntary oral feeding.

24.3.3.2.1 Assisted Enteral Feeding

Mare's milk is the ideal supplemental diet for orphan or critically ill foals and should be used whenever available by hand-milking the dam or with a commercially available milker[12] if the mare and foal pair are hospitalized together or if the foal is fostered to a nurse mare. If mare's milk is not available, a commercial foal milk replacer[13] can be used instead. Vitamins and minerals are provided in the mare's milk and milk replacers. If a foal milk replacer is not available, goat's milk can be fed as a short-term (one to three days) substitute but is not recommended for long-term use because the nutrient profile is different from that of mare's milk and can result in constipation. Cow's milk 2% fat is a poor substitute for mare's milk but can be used for short term in emergencies. If cow's milk is the only available substitute, 20 g of dextrose must be added to each liter of milk to closely approximate the carbohydrate content of mare's milk.

Healthy neonatal foals with normal GIT motility can initially be fed a volume of milk sufficient to meet 10% of BW/d. Critically ill neonatal foals usually require placement of an NG tube for feeding and should be started at a lower volume of milk (2.5–7.5% BW) for the first few days of nutritional therapy to ensure dietary tolerance. The volume of milk fed should be incrementally increased over two to three days until the foal consumes 20% of BW. If the foal is intolerant of the feedings despite a slow introduction to the milk replacer, both the frequency and volume of feeding should be decreased until milk digestion improves. Any foal that cannot tolerate enteral feedings after two to three days despite a reduction in the volume of milk should be placed on PN to ensure energy and protein requirements are met. If appropriate, once a foal is being treated with PN, clinicians should consider administering 5–10 mL of milk/hr via NG tube to provide nutrients directly to the enterocytes. Orphan foals with a suckle reflex should be encouraged to actively ingest and swallow the milk from a pan or bucket to decrease behavioral complications that can develop in bottle-fed foals. Foals that are not ready to transition to a bucket or pan feeding can be fed from a bottle. If a foal is bottle-fed, the nipple should be checked to ensure that milk does not freely flow from the nipple. Improper use of a bottle can result in aspiration pneumonia if the foal does not have a normal swallowing response.

A small diameter NG feeding tube should be placed if the foal does not have a strong suckle reflex to ensure adequate nutrient intake and reduce the risk of aspiration. The NG tube should remain in place until the foal has a strong suckle reflex and can nurse voluntarily. Neonatal foals up to one week of age should be fed every hour as long as the feedings are tolerated, foals that are one to four wks of age should be fed every two hrs, and older foals can have the frequency of feedings gradually extended to every three to four hrs.

24.3.3.2.2 Parenteral Nutrition

The general principles of PN therapy in foals and young horses are the same as in adults. Calories sources are a combination of dextrose and lipid (1–2 g lipid/kg BW/d). Lipid calories should comprise <50% of total calories in a PN formulation but should be omitted in foals with hypertriglyceridemia (TG > 200 mg/dL). Foals that have acute renal failure or severe hepatic disease should be treated with a lower concentration of protein (2–3 g/kg BW/d). Foals receiving PN therapy for >5 days may benefit from increased energy (75–100 kcal/kg BW/d) and protein (6–6.5 g/kg BW/d) intakes. Any significant change in the composition of the PN formulation should be made gradually over 12–24 hrs so the foal can adapt to the new nutrient profile of the solution. Foals treated with PN for longer than three days can be supplemented with 1 mL of B vitamins per liter of PN solution and no more than 1 mL of trace minerals/d. See Sidebar 24.4.

Most PN formulations are hyperosmolar and need to be infused through a central venous catheter, which places a jugular catheter tip in the cranial vena cava for foals. Multi-lumen catheters are preferred, with one port reserved specifically for PN use with a heparin lock if the PN therapy will be delayed. Foals typically have central lines placed for PN administration and can tolerate hyperosmolar PN solutions, but every effort should be made to reduce the PN osmolarity whenever possible. The final osmolarity and dextrose concentration of the PN solution should be calculated and sterile water added to achieve a suitable osmolarity or use 10% or less dextrose in the final PN formulation. Commercial amino acid and dextrose admixtures can also be used in foals and provide a convenient source of energy and protein for short-term administration. When a PN formulation is administered, dextrose in IV fluids should be discontinued.

12 Udderly EZ™ Mare Milker, Humboldt, IA.
13 Mare's Match® Land O Lakes®, Arden Hills, MN; Mare's Milk Plus® MARS Horsecare US, Inc., Dalton, OH; Foal-Lac® Pet-Ag, Inc., Hampshire, IL.

Sidebar 24.4: Parenteral Nutrition Worksheet for Foals

Patient history: Two-day-old Warmblood filly BCS 2/9 with a diagnosis of failure of passive transfer and sepsis has a triple lumen jugular catheter in place and requires PN nutritional support.

Animal Assessment:

1) Body weight (kg) 50 kg
2) RER (Mcal/d)[a] (45–50 kcal/kg BW/d): 50 kg × 50 kcal 2500 kcal
3) Protein requirement (3–5 g/kg BW/d): 50 kg × 3 g/kg 150 g
4) Fluid requirement at 5 ml/kg BW/hr x 24 hr 6000 mL
5) Decided on 60 : 40 dextrose: lipid calorie source

Parenteral Solution Formulation (Table 24.5):

- Volume of 50% dextrose solution (1.7 kcal/mL) providing 60% of calories:
  - 60% of 2500 kcal/1.7 kcal/mL 882 mL
- Volume of 20% lipid solution (2 kcal/mL) providing 40% of calories:
  - 40% of 2500 kcal/2 kcal/ mL 500 mL
- Volume of 10% amino acids (0.10 g/mL) to meet protein requirement:
  - 150 g protein /0.10 g/mL 1500 mL
- Total volume of macronutrient solutions: 2882 mL
  - Add 1–2 mL of B complex vitamins/L of PN 2 mL
  - Add 1 mL of trace minerals/d 1 mL
- Volume of polyionic fluids required to meet fluid requirement:
  - Fluid requirement minus PN solution 6000–2885 mL 3115 mL
- Osmolarity of final solution:
  - Dextose: 882 mL × 2.550 mOsm/mL = 2249
  - Lipid: 500 mL × 0.260 mOsm/mL = 130
  - Amino acids: 1500 mL × 0.998 mOsm/mL = 1497
  - Polyionic fluid: 3115 mL × 0.273 mOsm/mL = 850
  - Total mOsm = 4726 mOsm
  - Final mOsm/L = 4726 mOsm/6 L 788 mOsm/L
- Calories-to-nitrogen ratio:
  - 2500 kcal to 24 g nitrogen[b] = 104

Feeding orders: administer PN solution at 250 mL/hr or 4.2 mL/min via jugular catheter.

The PN should be started at 25% of the final desired infusion rate using a CRI and administered for six to eight hrs, after which time, the foal's physical parameters, serum electrolytes, and blood glucose values should be monitored. The PN infusion rate may then be increased 1–2 mL/hr until achieving 60–70% of the full infusion rate, but again, the foal's physical and serum parameters should be checked. If the PN is well tolerated, the infusion rate may be increased again to achieve the full infusion rate in the next 24 hrs. An initial conservative rate of infusion reduces the risk of hyperglycemic and hypertriglyceridemic complications and enables the clinician to adjust the formulation according to the foal's response to therapy. If the foal cannot tolerate either the lipid or dextrose content of the original PN solution, the rate of infusion should be reduced by a third. The PN solution can be reformulated with a lower concentration of lipid or dextrose, if necessary.

The goal of PN therapy is to maintain the foal's BW. Growth is not an expected outcome but may occur in some foals depending on initial diagnosis and nutritional therapy [57]. If the foal tolerates the infusion but experiences a persistent loss of weight or muscle condition, the energy and protein concentration of the PN can be increased. The foal should be maintained at the full infusion rate for one to two d before the calorie or protein content of the PN is increased and simultaneously be treated with a small volume (10–30 mL) of mare's milk or milk replacer through an NG tube every two to four hrs. Residual gastric fluid should be removed before the milk is infused. As the foal begins to tolerate the milk, the volume should be increased by 10–20 mL feeding. Once the foal can tolerate 5% BW as milk, the PN can be decreased by 1–2 mL/hr and discontinued once the PN infusion rate is below 30% of daily calorie intake. PN solutions contain at least 50% free water and are to be included in the total daily fluid calculation. The foal's IV fluid therapy (4–5 mL/kg/hr) should be adjusted when administering a PN solution to ensure that the total volume of fluids infused plus ingested milk does not exceed fluid requirements.

Management strategies for foals that develop complications from serum electrolyte abnormalities during PN infusion are similar to protocols described for adult horses. Both hyperglycemia and hypertriglyceridemia should first be managed by reducing the PN infusion rate. Continued elevations in serum glucose or triglycerides should be addressed with a reformulation of the PN solution. Omission of the lipid may be necessary if a foal maintains a serum triglyceride above 200 mg/dL for more than 24 hrs. Foals that remain hyperglycemic after the PN has been reformulated should be treated with regular insulin[14] as a CRI to achieve glycemic control. A CRI of insulin allows finer titration to manage blood glucose concentration than intermittent insulin injections. The starting dose rate is

[a] 70–100 kcal/BW kg/d for foals older than 2 mos.
[b] Protein contains on average 16% nitrogen [150 g protein × 16% = 24 g N].

[14] Humulin® R, Eli Lilly, Indianapolis, IN.

0.05 IU/kg BW/hr, which is then carefully adjusted to maintain blood glucose within a narrow range. If a CRI is not possible, administer intermittent insulin (0.1–0.5 IU regular insulin SQ q12h). Blood glucose must be monitored every hour initially when using insulin therapy to prevent complications from hypoglycemia.

24.3.3.2.3 Monitoring

Foals treated with enteral or parenteral therapies should be monitored using the same guidelines as for adult horses. A PE should be performed at least every four to six hrs, including inspection of the NG tube, catheter sites, and fluid lines and measurement of urine and fecal output. Blood glucose and electrolyte concentrations and acid–base balance should be monitored every four to six hrs if the foal is in a critical condition. Monitoring BW and fluid balance is important to prevent complications from over-hydration and pulmonary edema. Urine glucose should be tested when urine is available. A CBC and serum biochemistry panel including TGs should be evaluated daily until the foal's condition stabilizes. As the foal's condition improves, and electrolyte and glucose concentrations normalize, the frequency of assessments can be reduced.

Case in Point

Animal Assessment

A 24-year-old Warmblood gelding weighing 500 kg BCS 4/9 presented with severe abdominal pain of 4-hr duration. Rectal examination revealed a gas distended large colon. Analgesic therapy failed to improve the horse's pain, and an exploratory laparotomy was performed. A mild colon torsion, pelvic flexure impaction, and gas distended cecum and colon were identified and corrected during the surgery[a]. The horse recovered uneventfully from surgery until postoperative day 2 when small and large intestinal ileus became evident with gastric reflux of 84 L in 24 hrs. Postoperative ileus is a common complication resulting in large volumes of gastric reflux in horses that have had colic surgery. Treatment includes restriction of all oral fluids, feeds, and medications with concurrent pain and GI motility therapies. Post-operative PCM will develop without appropriate nutritional support.

1) *How should the horse be managed nutritionally during the period of postoperative ileus?*
2) *A 7 French, 20 cm triple lumen polyurethane catheter was placed in the left jugular vein for PN. What is the goal and composition of the PN solution?*

Complete the following calculations:

Patient Information:

1) Body weight (kg) ___ kg
2) RER (Mcal/d) = 75% minimal DE_m ___ Mcal
3) Protein requirement at 1.0 g/kg BW/d ___ g
4) Fluid requirement at 60 mL/kg BW/d ___ L

Parenteral Solution Formulation to provide RER (Table 24.5):

- Volume of 50% dextrose solution (1.7 kcal/mL) providing 60% of calories:
  - 60% of RER Mcal/1.7 kcal/mL ___ L
- Volume of 20% lipid solution (2 kcal/mL) providing 40% of calories:
  - 40% of RER Mcal/2 kcal/mL ___ L
- Volume of 10% amino acids (0.10 g/mL) to meet protein requirement:
  - g of protein required/100 g/L ___ L
- Total volume of macronutrient solutions: ___ L
  - Add B complex vitamins ___ mL
  - Add trace minerals ___ mL
- Volume of polyionic fluids required to meet fluid requirement:
  - Fluid requirement minus PN solution ___ L
- Osmolarity of final solution:
  - Dextose: 2550 mOsm/L = ___
  - Lipid: 260 mOsm/L= ___
  - Amino acids: 998 mOsm/L = ___
  - Polyionic fluid: 273 mOsm/L = ___
  - Total mOsm = ___ mOsm
  - Final mOsm/L = ___ mOsm/L
- Caloric density of PN solution: ___ kcal/mL
- Calorie to Nitrogen ratio: ___

3) *How should the PN administration be initiated?*

[a] Retrospective studies suggest horses >20-year-old are more likely to develop inappetence and postoperative reflux following colic surgery than 4- to 15-year-old horses [85]. Geriatric horses comprise a unique patient population among critically ill horses that should be managed with some form of early supplemental nutrition following colic surgery.

[b]Protein contains on average 16% nitrogen.

Update:
Gastric reflux continued and the horse developed diarrhea that tested positive for *Clostridium difficile* on hospitalization d 6. By hospitalization d 9, the gelding's clinical condition had improved with medical management for the *C. difficile* infection and gastric reflux volume had decreased to 18 L/d.

4) *How to refeed this horse orally and wean off of PN administration?*

See Appendix A Chapter 24.

References

1 Berger, M.M. and Pichard, C. (2012). Best timing for energy provision during critical illness. *Crit. Care* 16 (215): 661–671.
2 Crane, S.W. (1989). Nutritional aspects of wound healing. *Semin. Vet. Med. Surg. (Small Anim.)* 4 (4): 263–267.
3 Anderson, K.E. (1988). Influences of diet and nutrition on clinical pharmacokinetics. *Clin. Pharmacokinet.* 14 (6): 325–346.
4 Dugdale, A.H.A., Grove-White, D., Curtis, G.C. et al. (2012). Body condition scoring as a predictor of body fat in horses and ponies. *Vet. J.* 194 (2): 173–178.
5 Carroll, C.L. and Huntington, P.J. (1988). Body condition scoring and weight estimation of horses. *Equine Vet. J.* 20 (1): 41.
6 Kronfeld, D. (1998). Clinical assessment of nutritional status of the horse. In: *Metabolic and Endocrine Problems of the Horse* (ed. T.D.G. Watson), 185–217. New York: WB Saunders.
7 Matthews, D.E. and Fong, Y. (1993). Amino acid and protein metabolism. In: *Clinical Nutrition: Parenteral Nutrition*, 2e (ed. J.L. Rombeau), 75–112. Philadelphia, PA: WB Saunders.
8 Tufts University School of Veterinary Medicine (2013). Muscle condition score. WSAVA Global Nutrition Web Site. https://wsava.org/wp-content/uploads/2020/01/Muscle-Condition-Score-Chart-for-Dogs.pdf (accessed 30 September 2021).
9 Finocchio, E.J. (1994). Equine starvation. *Large Anim. Vet.* 49 (2): 6–27.
10 Whiting, T.L., Salmon, R.H., and Wruck, G.C. (2005). Chronically starved horses: predicting survival, economic, and ethical considerations. *Can. Vet. J.* 46 (4): 320.
11 Brody, S. and Lardy, H.A (1946). Bioenergetics and growth. *J. Phys. Chem.* 50 (2): 168–169.
12 Kleiber, M. (1961). *The Fire of Life. An Introduction to Animal Energetics*, 179–222. New York: Wiley.
13 Smil, V. (2000). Laying down the law. *Nature* 403 (6770): 597.
14 Butte, N. and Caballero, B. (2006). Energy needs: assessment and requirements. In: *Modern Nutrition in Health and Disease*, 10e (ed. M. Shils, M. Shike, C. Ross, et al.), 136–148. Baltimore, MD: Lippincott Williams & Wilkins.
15 Mifflin, M.D., St Jeor, S.T., Hill, L.A. et al. (1990). A new predictive equation for resting energy expenditure in healthy individuals. *Am. J. Clin. Nutr.* 51 (2): 241–247.
16 Pagan, J.D., and Hintz, H.F. (1986) and Equine energetics. I. Relationship between body weight and energy requirements in horses. *J. Anim. Sci.* 63 (3): 815–821.
17 National Research Council (2007). *Nutrient Requirements of Horses*. 6th Rev. Animal Nutrition Series, 1–341. Washington, DC: National Academies Press.
18 Elwyn, D.H., Kinney, J.M., and Askanazi, J. (1981). Energy expenditure in surgical patients. *Surg. Clin. North Am.* 61 (3): 545–556.
19 Carr, E.A. (2018). Enteral/parenteral nutrition in foals and adult horses practical guidelines for the practitioner. *Vet. Clin. North Am. Equine Pract.* 34 (1): 169–180.
20 Roberts, P. and Zaloga, G. (2000). Enteral nutrition. In: *Textbook of Critical Care*, 4e (ed. W. Shoemaker, S. Ayres, and A. Grenvik), 875–898. Philadelphia, PA: Saunders.
21 Levine, G.M., Deren, J.J., Steiger, E., and Zinno, R. (1974). Role of oral intake in maintenance of gut mass and disaccharide activity. *Gastroenterology* 67 (5): 975–982.
22 Grant, J.P. (1983). Clinical impact of protein malnutrition on organ mass and function. In: *Amino Acids: Metabolism and Medical Applications* (ed. G. Blackburn, J. Grant, and V. Young), 347–358. Boston, MA: John Wright.
23 Powell, J., Borchers, A.T., Yoshida, S., and Gershwin, M.E. (2000). Evaluation of the immune system in the nutritionally at-risk host. In: *Nutrition and Immunology: Principles and Practice* (ed. M.E. Gershwin, J. German, and C.K. Keen), 21–34. New York: Springer.
24 Sheffy, B.E. and Williams, A.J. (1982). Nutrition and the immune response. *J. Am. Vet. Med. Assoc.* 180 (9): 1073–1076.
25 Engelking, L.R. (2011). Starvation. In: *Textbook of Veterinary Physiological Chemistry*, 2e, 412–432. Amsterdam: Elsevier.
26 Heusner, G.L. (1993). Ad libitum feeding of mature horses to achieve rapid weight gain. In: *Proceedings of the 13th Equine Nutrition and Physiology Society Symposium*, 86–87. Gainsville, FL: Equine Nutrition and Physiology Society.
27 Kinney, J.M. (1980). The application of indirect calorimetry to clinical studies. In: *Assessment of Energy*

Metabolism in Health and Disease (ed. J.M. Kenny), 42–48. Columbus, OH: Ross Laboratories.

28 Long, C.L., Schaffel, N., Geiger, J.W. et al. (1979). Metabolic response to injury and illness: estimation of energy and protein needs from indirect calorimetry and nitrogen balance. *J. Parenter. Enteral Nutr.* 3 (6): 452–456.

29 Barrelet, A. and Ricketts, S. (2002). Haematology and blood biochemistry in the horse: a guide to interpretation. *In Pract.* 24 (6): 318–327.

30 Argo, C.M. (2013). Feeding thin and starved horses. In: *Equine Applied and Clinical Nutrition: Health, Welfare and Performance* (ed. R.J. Geor, P.A. Harris, and M. Coenen), 503–511. Edinburgh: Saunders Elsevier.

31 Jarvis, N. and McKenzie, H.C. (2021). Nutritional considerations when dealing with an underweight adult or senior horse. *Vet. Clin. North Am. Equine Pract.* 37 (1): 89–110.

32 Muñoz, A., Riber, C., Trigo, P., and Castejón, F. (2010). Hematology and clinical pathology data in chronically starved horses. *J. Equine Vet. Sci.* 30 (10): 581–589.

33 Frank, N., Sojka, J.E., and Latour, M.A. (2002). Effect of withholding feed on concentration and composition of plasma very low density lipoprotein and serum nonesterified fatty acids in horses. *Am. J. Vet. Res.* 63 (7): 1018–1021.

34 Witham, C. and Stull, C.L. (1998). Metabolic responses of chronically starved horses to refeeding with three isoenergetic diets. *J. Am. Vet. Med. Assoc.* 212: 691–696.

35 Romijn, J.A. (2000). Substrate metabolism in the metabolic response to injury. *Proc. Nutr. Soc.* 59 (3): 447–449.

36 Bistrian, B.R. (1984). Nutritional assessment of the hospitalized patient: a practical approach. In: *Nutritional Assessment*, 183–205. Boston, MA: Blackwell Scientific Publications.

37 Hoffer, L.J. (1994). Starvation. In: *Modern Nutrition in Health and Disease*, 8e (ed. M. Shils, J. Olson, and M. Shike), 927–949. Philadelphia, PA: Lea & Febiger.

38 Walton, R.S., Wingfield, W.E., Ogilvie, G.K. et al. (1996). Energy expenditure in 104 postoperative and traumatically injured dogs with indirect calorimetry. *J. Vet. Emerg. Crit. Care* 6 (2): 71–79.

39 Ogilvie, G.K., Walters, L.M., Salman, M.D., and Fettman, M.J. (1996). Resting energy expenditure in dogs with nonhematopoietic malignancies before and after excision of tumors. *Am. J. Vet. Res.* 57 (10): 1463–1467.

40 Becvarova, I. and Thatcher, C.D. (2008). Nutritional management of the starved horse. In: *Current Therapy in Equine Medicine*, 6e (ed. N.E. Robinson and K.A. Sprayberry), 53–58. Philadelphia, PA: Elsevier Health Sciences.

41 Kentucky Equine Research Staff (2010). Refeeding malnourished horses. *EquiNews*. https://ker.com/equinews/refeeding-malnourished-horses/ (accessed 13 October 2021)

42 Hoffer, L.J. and Bistrian, B.R. (2016). Nutrition in critical illness: a current conundrum. *F1000Research* 2016: 5. https://doi.org/10.12688/f1000research.9278.1

43 Vineyard, K.R., Gordon, M.E., Williamson, K.K., and Jerina, M.L. (2011). Evaluation of the safety and performance of an enteral diet formulated specifically for horses. *J. Equine Vet. Sci.* 5 (31): 254–255.

44 Solomon, S.M. and Kirby, D.F. (1990). The refeeding syndrome: a review. *J. Parenter. Enteral Nutr.* 14 (1): 90–97.

45 Millman, S. (2007). Sickness behaviour and its relevance to animal welfare assessment at the group level. *Anim. Welf.* 16 (2): 123–125.

46 Broom, D.M. and Fraser, A.F. (2007). Welfare and behaviour in relation to disease. In: *Domestic animal behaviour and welfare*, 4e (ed. D.M. Broom and A. Frazer), 216–225. Oxford: CABI.

47 Naylor, J.M., Freeman, D.E., Kronfeld, D.S. et al. (1984). Alimentation of hypophagic horses. *Compend. Contin. Educ. Pract. Vet.* 6: S93–S99.

48 Ralston, S.L. (1988). Equine clinical nutrition: specific problems and solutions. *Compend. Contin. Educ. Pract. Vet.* 10: 356–363.

49 Remillard, R.L., Guerino, F., Dudgeon, D.L., and Yardley, J.H. (1998). Intravenous glutamine or limited enteral feedings in piglets: amelioration of small intestinal disuse atrophy. *J. Nutr.* 128 (12): 2723S–2726S.

50 Ralston, S.L. and Naylor, J.M. (1991). Feeding sick horses. In: *Large Animal Clinical Nutrition* (ed. J.M. Naylor and S.L. Ralston), 324–445. St. Louis, MO: Mosby.

51 National Research Council (1989). *Nutrient Requirements of Horses*. 5th Rev. Animal Nutrition Series, 1–100. Washington, DC: National Academies Press.

52 Ashley, F.H., Waterman-Pearson, A.E., and Whay, H.R. (2005). Behavioural assessment of pain in horses and donkeys: application to clinical practice and future studies. *Equine Vet. J.* 37 (6): 565–575.

53 Smith, M. and Lowry, S.F. (1999). The hypercatabolic state. In: *Modern Nutrition in Health and Disease*, 9e (ed. M. Shils, J. Olson, M. Shike, and A. Ross), 1555–1568. Baltimore, MD: Lippincott Williams & Wilkins.

54 Naylor, J.M. and Kenyon, S.J. (1981). Effect of total calorific deprivation on host defense in the horse. *Res. Vet. Sci.* 31 (3): 369–372.

55 Preiser, J.-C., van Zanten, A.R.H., Berger, M.M. et al. (2015). Metabolic and nutritional support of critically ill patients: consensus and controversies. *Crit. Care* 19 (1): 1–11.

56 Houweling, M., van der Drift, S.G.A., Jorritsma, R., and Tielens, A.G.M. (2012). Technical note: quantification of plasma 1- and 3-methylhistidine in dairy cows by high-performance liquid chromatography-tandem mass spectrometry. *J. Dairy Sci.* 95 (6): 3125–3130.

57 Myers, C.J., Magdesian, K.G., Kass, P.H. et al. (2009). Parenteral nutrition in neonatal foals: clinical description, complications and outcome in 53 foals (1995–2005). *Vet. J.* 181 (2): 137–144.
58 Garcia-Lopez, J.M., Provost, P.J., Rush, J.E. et al. (2001). Prevalence and prognostic importance of hypomagnesemia and hypocalcemia in horses that have colic surgery. *Am. J. Vet. Res.* 62 (1): 7–12.
59 Toribio, R.E., Kohn, C.W., Chew, D.J. et al. (2001). Comparison of serum parathyroid hormone and ionized calcium and magnesium concentrations and fractional urinary clearance of calcium and phosphorus in healthy horses and horses with enterocolitis. *Am. J. Vet. Res.* 62 (6): 938–947.
60 Buechner-Maxwell, V.A., Elvinger, F., Thatcher, C.D. et al. (2003). Physiological response of normal adult horses to a low-residue liquid diet. *J. Equine Vet. Sci.* 23 (7): 310–317.
61 Geor, R.J. (2001). Nutritional support of the sick adult horse. In: *Advances in Equine Nutrition II* (ed. J.D. Pagan and R.J. Geor), 403–417. Nottingham: Nottingham University Press.
62 Sweeney, R.W. and Hansen, T.O. (1990). Use of a liquid diet as the sole source of nutrition in six dysphagic horses and as a dietary supplement in seven hypophagic horses. *J. Am. Vet. Med. Assoc.* 197 (8): 1030–1032.
63 Hallebeek, J.M. and Beynen, A.C. (2001). Nutrition: a preliminary report on a fat-free diet formula for nasogastric enteral administration as treatment for hyperlipaemia in ponies. *Vet. Q.* 23 (4): 201–205.
64 Golenz, M.R., Knight, D.A., and Yvorchuk-St Jean, K.E. (1992). Use of a human enteral feeding preparation for treatment of hyperlipemia and nutritional support during healing of an esophageal laceration in a miniature horse. *J. Am. Vet. Med. Assoc.* 200 (7): 951–953.
65 Raman, M., Almutairdi, A., Mulesa, L. et al. (2017). Parenteral nutrition and lipids. *Nutrients* 9 (4): 2017; 9(4): 388–399.
66 Singer, P. and Pichard, C. (2013). Reconciling divergent results of the latest parenteral nutrition studies in the ICU. *Curr. Opin. Clin. Nutr. Metab. Care* 16 (2): 187–193.
67 Paradis, M.R. (2001). Caloric needs of the sick foal: determined by the use of indirect calorimetry. In: *Proceedings of the 3rd Dorothy Havemeyer Foundation Neonatal Septicemia Workshop*, Talliores, France.
68 Stapleton, R.D., Jones, N., and Heyland, D.K. (2007). Feeding critically ill patients: what is the optimal amount of energy? *Crit. Care Med.* 35 (9): S535–S540.
69 Mann, S., Westenskow, D.R., and Houtchens, B.A. (1985). Measured and predicted caloric expenditure in the acutely ill. *Crit. Care Med.* 13 (3): 173–177.
70 Souba, W.B. and Wilmore, D. (1999). Diet and nutrition in the care of the patient with surgery, trauma, and sepsis. In: *Modern Nutrition in Health and Disease*, 9e (ed. M. Shils, J. Olson, M. Shike, and A. Rose), 1589–1618. Baltimore, MD: Lippincott Williams & Wilkins.
71 Jose-Cunillers, E., Corradini, I.J.V.I.U., Armengou, L. et al. (2012). Energy expenditure of critically ill neonatal foals. *Equine Vet. J.* 44: 48–51.
72 Furr, M. (2002). Parenteral nutrition. *J. Equine Vet. Sci.* 22 (12): 554.
73 Durham, A.E., Phillips, T.J., Walmsley, J.P., and Newton, J.R. (2004). Nutritional and clinicopathological effects of post operative parenteral nutrition following small intestinal resection and anastomosis in the mature horse. *Equine Vet. J.* 36 (5): 390–396.
74 Magnotti, L.J. and Deitch, E. (2005). Mechanics and significance of gut barrier function and failure. In: *Clinical Nutrition: Enteral and Tube Feeding*, 4e (ed. R. Rolandelli, R. Bankhead, J. Boullata, and C. Compher), 23–31. Philadelphia, PA: Elsevier Saunders.
75 Gordon, M.E., Jerina, M.L., King, S.L. et al. (2007). The effects of nonstructural carbohydrate content and feeding rate on glucose and insulin response to meal feeding in equine. *J. Equine Vet. Sci.* 27 (11): 489–493.
76 Crowell-Davis, S.L., Houpt, K.A., and Carnevale, J. (1985). Feeding and drinking behavior of mares and foals with free access to pasture and water. *J. Anim. Sci.* 60 (4): 883–889.
77 Hardy, J., Stewart, R.H., Beard, W.L., and Yvorchuk-St-Jean, K. (1992). Complications of nasogastric intubation in horses: nine cases (1987–1989). *J. Am. Vet. Med. Assoc.* 201 (3): 483–486.
78 Desrochers, A.M., Dolente, B.A., Roy, M.-F.F. et al. (2005). Efficacy of *Saccharomyces boulardii* for treatment of horses with acute enterocolitis. *J. Am. Vet. Med. Assoc.* 227 (6): 954–959.
79 Stewart, A.S., Pratt-Phillips, S., and Gonzalez, L.M. (2017). Alterations in intestinal permeability: the role of the "leaky gut" in health and disease. *J. Equine Vet. Sci.* 52: 10–22.
80 Hansen, T.O., White, N.A. 2nd, and Kemp, D.T. (1988). Total parenteral nutrition in four healthy adult horses. *Am. J. Vet. Res.* 49 (1): 122–124.
81 Lopes, M.A.F. and White, N.A. (2002). Parenteral nutrition for horses with gastrointestinal disease: a retrospective study of 79 cases. *Equine Vet. J.* 34 (3): 250–257.
82 Shils, M.E. and Brown, R.O. (1999). Parenteral nutrition. In: *Modern Nutrition in Health and Disease*, 9e (ed. M.E. Shils, J. Olson, M. Shike, and A. Ross), 1657–1688. Baltimore, MD: Lippincott Williams & Wilkins.
83 Gabrielson, K.L., Remillard, R.L., and Huso, D.L. (1996). Zinc toxicity with pancreatic acinar necrosis in piglets receiving total parenteral nutrition. *Vet. Pathol.* 33 (6): 692–696.
84 Porr, C.A., Kronfeld, D.S., Lawrence, L.A. et al. (1998). Deconditioning reduces mineral content of the third metacarpal bone in horses. *J. Anim. Sci.* 76 (7): 1875–1879.
85 Gazzerro, D.M., Southwood, L.L., and Lindborg, S. (2015). Short-term complications after colic surgery in geriatric versus mature non-geriatric horses. *Vet. Surg.* 44 (2): 256–264.

25

Musculoskeletal System Disorders

Sarah Dodd and Géraldine Blanchard

KEY TERMS

- Heritability refers to the degree to which a trait is determined by genetics and ranges between 0 and 1, where 1 occurs when all variations in a population are attributed to differences in genotype and there is no environmentally caused variation.
- Free radicals are unstable and highly reactive molecules due to unpaired electrons which leads to damage of bodily tissues.

KEY POINTS

- Prevention of nutrition-related muscular disorders in all ages of horses consists of ensuring adequate daily vitamin E and selenium intake through ration balancing, providing green pasture access, and individual supplementation as needed.
- Antioxidants neutralize free radicals, reducing inflammation and damage to tissues.
- The overarching feeding practices contributing to orthopedic disease in young horses are feeding an imbalanced ration and/or high DE intakes fueling a rapid growth rate.
- Most cases of laminitis seen in private practice are associated with pasture grazing, obesity, and insulin resistance and are not related to a systemic septic condition.

25.1 Muscle Disorders

The antioxidant system includes fat-soluble (vitamin E), water-soluble (ascorbic acid) vitamins, and enzymatic (glutathione peroxidase [GSH-Px]) proteins that function as a group to control the effects of free radicals within the cell. GSH-Px requires the co-factor selenium (Se). The antioxidant protective mechanisms of vitamin E in the cell membrane decrease the formation of lipid peroxides, whereas GSH-Px functions in the intracellular fluid to remove lipid peroxides produced [1]. Se and vitamin E have a sparing effect on each other and should be considered together in meeting animal requirements as optimal amounts of both are necessary to minimize oxidative tissue damage. A vitamin E deficiency may have subclinical effects on immune function and reproduction; however, a severe or sustained deficiency can cause motor neuron disease and myeloencephalopathy in horses. Similarly, Se deficiency can result in myopathies and ischemic necrosis of cardiac and skeletal muscles.

25.1.1 Animal Assessment

Diagnosis and medical treatment options for neuromuscular disorders of horses due to vitamin E and Se deficiencies have been previously detailed [2–4]. The normal range of plasma α-tocopherol (TOC) in horses is 1.1–2 ppm, whereas selenium status is determined from whole blood Se concentration or GSH-Px activity using the appropriate reference ranges specific to the laboratory analyzing the sample [2]. Noteworthy is that in a survey of 331 adult horses, blood selenium and plasma vitamin E concentrations were below optimum in 16.7 and 35.5%, respectively, despite most owners providing supplementation. Less-than-adequate pasture access was associated with vitamin E

Equine Clinical Nutrition, Second Edition. Edited by Rebecca L. Remillard.

deficiency, and selenium deficiency existed even in horses offered Se-containing salt blocks [5].

25.1.1.1 Nutritional Muscular Dystrophy

Nutritional muscular dystrophy (NMD), aka white muscle disease and nutritional myodegeneration, is a non-inflammatory degenerative disease affecting skeletal and cardiac muscles [6]. More severe deficiencies of selenium and/or vitamin E cause myopathies and/or steatitis. Foals may be stillborn or alive but affected at birth with clinical signs of an acute and fulminant disease exhibiting myocardial, diaphragmatic, and respiratory muscle involvement; developing heart failure, dyspnea, and pulmonary edema; and dying within two days of the clinical onset. Foals, normal at birth, become recumbent and have increased heart and respiratory rate, excess salivation, painful subcutaneous swellings under the mane, and desquamation of tongue epithelium within the first weeks of birth. The tongue involvement and difficulties swallowing increase the risk of aspiration pneumonia when suckling. Muscular exertion may initiate the onset of symptoms. Less common, adult Se-deficient horses exhibit a range of signs from subtle trismus, masseter muscle atrophy or swelling, and dropping feed while eating to severe signs of pulmonary congestion, rhabdomyolysis, myoglobinuria, and cardiac failure [4]. Selenium deficiency is a required co-factor for NMD, though not all Se-deficient foals develop the disease, which implicates vitamin E involvement. The concurrent presence of steatitis supports the role of vitamin E deficiency in the disease [6–8].

In NMD cases, striated muscles show irregular fiber degeneration and calcification, which give rise to the characteristic pale-to-white appearance of muscle on postmortem examination [7]. See White Muscle Disease under Selenium deficiency in Chapter 8 and Vitamin E deficiency in Chapter 9. The highly active muscles most severely affected include the heart, pelvic and thoracic limbs, neck, diaphragm, tongue, pharynx, and muscles of mastication [6]. Necropsy lesions include a bilateral pallor and ischemic necrosis of affected cardiac and skeletal muscles, particularly those of the hind legs, neck, and tongue. Most animals respond to an intramuscular injection of 0.055 mg Se/kg BW, but the ration Se and vitamin E concentrations should be checked and balanced if needed. Prognosis is good if treated early with minimal cardiac damage [4].

25.1.1.2 Equine Motor Neuron Disease

Chronic vitamin E deficiency in the broodmare has been associated with the development of equine motor neuron disease (EMND) [9–11]. This disease occurs in older horses with a median age of 10 years and peak risk at 16 years of age [9]. The disease is an acquired neurodegenerative disorder of the somatic lower motor neurons localized in the ventral horns of the spinal cord and brain stem [12, 13]. It is a progressive disease, characterized by weakness, muscle fasciculation, increased recumbency, a camped-under stance, muscle wasting, and weight loss in the face of normal appetite and food intake, due to loss of parental motor neuron cells and degeneration of myelinated axons in the ventral roots, peripheral nerves, and muscles [13–15]. Highly active, and thus oxidative, muscles are more severely affected, such as the postural muscles of the back, neck, and limbs. Chronic vitamin E insufficiency (>18 mos) appears to be required to precipitate clinical signs, and approximately 30% of neurons are lost before signs of EMND are apparent [9, 10].

Diagnosis is based on clinical presentation, low vitamin E concentrations, and elevated muscle enzymes, while electromyography, ophthalmic examination, and biopsy of the sacrocaudalis dorsalis muscle aid in confirmation of the diagnosis [16, 17]. Horses with EMND may have plasma or serum α-tocopherol concentrations <1 ug/mL [18]. Lipopigment deposition, an indicator of increased lipid peroxidation, is reported in endothelial cells of the spinal cord capillaries, retina, and occasionally in the liver and intestine [19, 20]. The prognosis for clinical improvement is poor and neurological dysfunctions are permanent. The horse should not be worked as the risk of relapse is high if the animal is exercised or stressed [10, 17].

25.1.1.3 Equine Degenerative Myeloencephalopathy

A disease that typically affects horses less than one year of age, equine degenerative myeloencephalopathy (EDM) is characterized by diffuse axonal degeneration within the spinal cord and brainstem, resulting in hyporeflexia and symmetrical ataxia and paresis, most pronounced in the pelvic limbs [21–24]. There appears to be a genetic prerequisite for the disease phenotype or a familial predisposition, and a vitamin E deficiency facilitates the manifestation of the disease [22, 25–27]. In a retrospective study of 56 cases, there was a 25-fold higher risk of EDM occurring in siblings of affected foals than non-affected foals [28]. Diagnosis is based on clinical signs and rule-out of other differentials, but definitive diagnosis requires postmortem spinal cord histopathology [27]. As with EMND, a lack of antioxidant activity results in excessive membrane lipid peroxidation, resulting in the accumulation of lipopigment [19]. Characteristic histologic lesions include axonal swelling in the caudal medulla oblongata and cervicothoracic spinal cord [24]. Hypovitaminosis E has not been reported in all affected horses, though supplementation has been shown to improve clinical signs after years of receiving 12 IU/kg BW/d of α-tocopherol acetate, and appropriate supplementation has decreased the incidence of disease in future foal generations [23]. The prognosis is poor because, although deficits may stabilize in two to three years, the debilitation is permanent [4].

25.1.1.4 Primary Vitamin E Deficiency

Horses can present with primary myopathy associated with vitamin E deficiency. Clinical signs are similar to EMND, namely, weakness, recumbency, muscle fasciculation, low head carriage, a camped under-stance, and weight loss but with a normal appetite and food intake, due to muscle atrophy. Sudden death due to cardiac failure may also occur [29]. Horses with primary vitamin E deficiency respond better to therapy than do horses with NMD, EMND, or EDM, and the prognosis for both clinical improvement and return to function is good [16].

25.1.2 Ration Assessment

In addition to the general ration recommendations specific to the life stage of the patient, that is, adult, nursing, or weanling, to maintain adequate body weight (BW) and condition score (BCS) (4–6/9), considerations for horses with muscular or neuromuscular diseases should include increased concentrations of vitamin E and possibly Se [30]. The eight forms of naturally occurring vitamin E vary greatly in biological activity. The TOC is the active form in feeds and the only metabolically active form *in vivo*. See Vitamin E in Chapter 9.

Green growing forages contain 100–450 IU, average quality grass or legume hays 10–60 IU, dehydrated alfalfa pellets 20–80 IU, and cereal grains 5–30 IU vitamin E/kg dry matter (DM). Vitamin E in forages decreases 70–90% with plant maturity, and 30–80% of the activity is lost with the cutting and baling of hay. Preserved forage, regardless of having a “green” color, is unlikely to provide an adequate vitamin E source. Ensuring adequate vitamin E intake year-round as forage options change can be accomplished by feeding a ration balancer with an adequate concentration and form of vitamin E. The ration recommendation is 50 IU for the idle mature horse and 80 IU vitamin E/kg DM for foals, pregnant and lactating mares, and working horses using a synthetic acetate except those on adequate pasture during plant growth. A conservative safe upper limit of dietary vitamin E intake has been suggested at 1 KIU/kg DM [31, 32]. There is an oral water-soluble form of vitamin E that resulted in higher plasma vitamin E concentrations than those of horses fed either synthetic or natural vitamin E acetate [33, 34]. Feeding horses with clinical signs of vitamin E deficiency 10–20 IU/kg BW/d using a liquid micellized natural source of d-α-tocopherol until serum TOC concentrations return to within normal limits is recommended [4].

Cases of EMND are typically seen in horses with no access to fresh forage, such as pasture, but fed old or poor-quality feed and hay, with no other vitamin E source available. However, some animals grazing at pasture have developed EMND; hence, pasture access does not rule out EMND in horses with neuromuscular signs [21, 35–37]. In EMND horses ingesting adequate dietary vitamin E, failure of absorption or retention, potentially due to familial predisposition, intestinal epithelial absorptive dysfunction, for example, eosinophilic enteritis, or dietary factors competing within the intestine, for example, polyunsaturated fatty acids, methionine, selenium, vitamin C, and artificial antioxidants may contribute to low vitamin E bioavailability [37–39]. Thus, while vitamin E deficiency is a significant causative factor, there appears to be individual variation in susceptibility to oxidative stress within a group of horses such that the disease may occur in only one or a few horses on a given farm fed the same ration [22, 36].

Most commercially manufactured horse feeds contain supplemental Se, but animals raised without supplemented feeds are at risk for deficiency, particularly in soil-deficient areas. Se concentration in forages and grain varies 30-fold depending on local soil and weather conditions. Forage analysis for Se is advisable to properly formulate a complete and balanced ration. See Selenium in Chapter 8. A balanced equine ration should have 0.1–0.3 mg Se/kg DM with the safe upper limit of 2.0 mg/kg DM. There are ration-balancing products with selenium and vitamin E at concentrations appropriate for horses with average requirements for both nutrients. See Sidebar 17.2.

25.1.3 Feeding Management

Prevention of nutritional diseases is safer, less costly, and more efficacious than treatment. Prevention consists of ensuring adequate daily vitamin E and selenium intake by horses of all ages through ration balancing, providing green pasture access when possible, and oral supplementation of individuals as needed. Where deficiency has been historically a problem in foals, in addition to providing supplemental vitamin E and selenium to dams, foals should be given a selenium and vitamin E injection at birth. It may not be necessary to repeat this injection, provided the creep feed and weanling diets contain adequate selenium and vitamin E.

25.2 Developmental Orthopedic Disease

A cluster of orthopedic conditions in foals, in particular related to abnormal endochondral ossification, the process of the articular and metaphyseal cartilages maturing to the

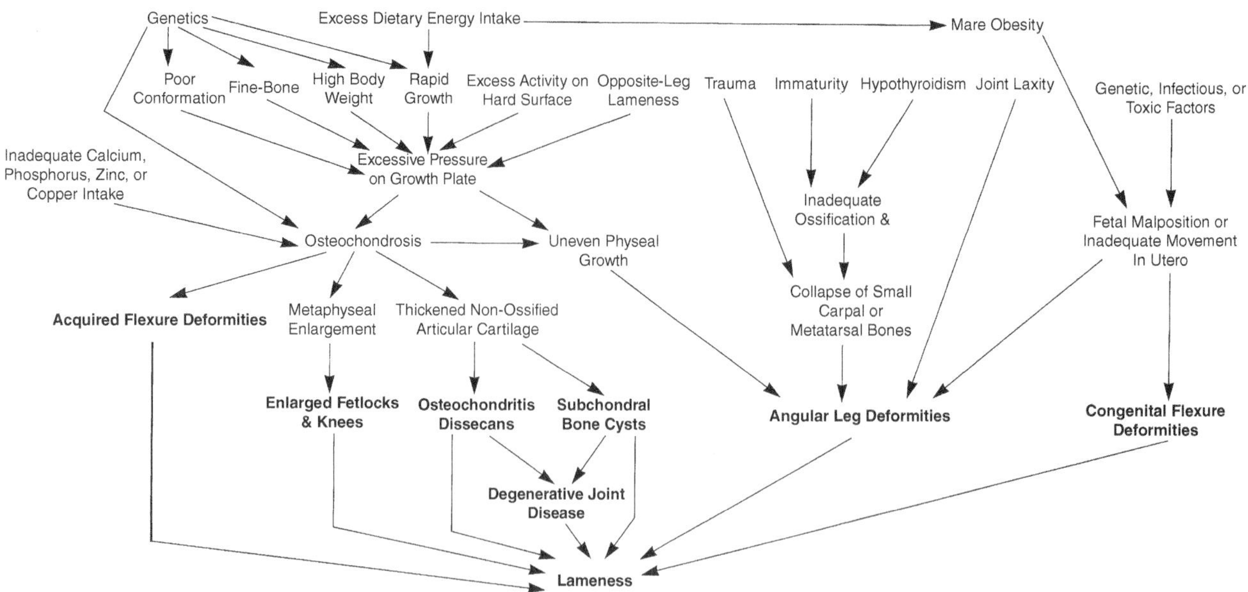

Figure 25.1 Cause and **effect (bolded)** of developmental orthopedic diseases.

bone, has been termed developmental orthopedic disease (DOD) [40]. The term includes osteochondrosis, physeal dysplasia, acquired angular limb deformities, flexural deformities, and cuboidal bone malformations. The definitive cause(s) has not been identified for any of the specific conditions within the DOD cluster, despite active research in horses and other species; however, genetic predisposition is a known factor [41]. Although there is a strong diet association with clinical expression of abnormal endochondral ossification, the direct influence of nutrients likely varies between the different specific abnormalities. Rapid growth, exercise, excessive caloric intake, and/or ration mineral imbalances are thought to be associated with osteochondritis dissecans (OCD), physitis, acquired flexural deformities, and angular limb deformities (Figure 25.1) [40, 42, 43].

25.2.1 Animal Assessment

25.2.1.1 Genetic Predisposition

A genetic predisposition to DOD has been demonstrated in horses. The incidence of tibiotarsal joint osteochondrosis in 325 trotting horses from 9 different stallions ranged from 3 to 30%, yet stallions whose progeny had the highest incidence of osteochondrosis showed no radiologic signs of the disease [44]. Estimates of heritability (h^2) are in the low to moderate range, depending on the type of DOD abnormality, the breed of horse, and joint [40, 41, 44, 45]. Indirectly, young horses with the genetic potential for large body size and high growth rates are predisposed to orthopedic diseases.

25.2.1.2 Rapid Growth

A rapid growth rate is related to genetic capacity, high energy intake, and a compensatory growth spurt as a result of increased feed intake after a dietary deficit. Rapid growth appears to be a major factor in causing DOD. Four to five times more bone aberrations occurred in Quarter horse weanlings gaining 1.05 vs. those gaining 0.67 kg BW/d [46]. Potential final mature height is genetically determined; however, the rate of growth through the first 20 m is not constant [30]. Dutch warmblood foals with osteochondrosis had similar overall growth rates and wither heights to healthy foals; however, those with DOD had a higher average daily gain (ADG) for the 3 m post-weaning compared with normal foals [47]. Growth curves are available on some but limited on most breeds of horses; however, BW at any age can be estimated based on expected mature BW [30]. See Table 21.1.

25.2.2 Ration Assessment

25.2.2.1 Feeds

The complementary grain–mineral–vitamin mix fed to the growing horse must be formulated based on forage analysis. Cereal grains contribute starch energy to ration but have low concentrations of Ca, P, protein, and lysine and 3–20 times more P than Ca. On average,[1] cereal grains contain about 1% phytate, which decreases calcium absorption. Therefore, grains have low concentrations of Ca and P with an inverse

1 Based on a data for accumulated years 2004–2020 from https://www.dairyoneservices.com/feedcomposition/eq.

ratio and decreased Ca availability but provide calories. Legume forages are often fed to growing horses, but with a Ca:P ratio of 5 : 1, the addition of high phosphorus ingredients or supplementation is required to balance mineral intakes. With an average of 2.6 Mcal in legumes vs. 1.98 Mcal DE/kg DM in grass, intake of legumes must be controlled to modulate growth rate. Grass forages may have a 2 : 1 Ca : P ratio but have inadequate concentrations of Ca, P, protein, and lysine to meet growing horse requirements within DMI. A grass forage-based ration generally provides for a slow or moderate growth rate, lowering the risk of DOD, but must be correctly fortified, or mature body size may be reduced as a result of malnutrition. The smaller-sized wild horse is an example of growth moderated by available feeds balanced on the first limiting nutrient [61].

The ration must be formulated to avoid mineral deficiencies relative to the caloric density and/or other competing minerals in the ration that can create mineral imbalances at the site of endochondral ossification. A concentrated feed mix providing energy, protein, vitamins, and minerals should be formulated specifically to complement the forage. Alternatively, a specific caloric density of the ration or creep feed can be formulated using a pelleted combination of grains, oil, fiber, and micronutrients to control the growth rate. However, excessive DE intakes are still possible when consumption of a moderate DE pellet is not controlled.

It has been hypothesized that dietary energy in the form of starch and sugar from cereal grains is more likely to cause osteochondrosis than volatile fatty acids from fiber fermentation, suggesting that insulin was related to DOD [40]. *In vitro*, insulin inhibits chondrocyte apoptosis. In foals, insulin concentrations were higher and insulin sensitivity lower in those adapted to a 40 vs. 12% nonstructural carbohydrate ration [62]. However, the growth rate and incidence of DOD can be as high in weanlings fed high alfalfa vs. high grain ration ad libitum [63, 64]. To date, the relevance of hormone concentrations to the clinical expressions of DOD is absent [40].

25.2.2.2 Key Nutrients

The excessive or inadequate ingestion of several nutrients may predispose an animal to the clinical expression of DOD. Within the dietary recommendations for growing horses, specific attention to caloric density and mineral concentrations is needed to prevent or mitigate the clinical signs of DOD [30]. Nutrients that may be involved for horses include energy, calcium, phosphorus, zinc, and copper. Dietary protein, when excessive relative to requirements, has no impact on DOD if minerals are balanced to caloric density and fall within recommended ratios [48].

25.2.2.2.1 Energy

Clinical signs of OCD were noted in 11 of 12, and histologic signs were found in 12 of 12, 4.5-mo-old foals consuming a ration with 130% of the recommended digestible energy (DE) for 4 m. Whereas postmortem signs of OCD were found in 1 of 12 and histologically in 2 of 12 foals receiving 100% of the recommended amounts of DE, crude protein, calcium (Ca), and phosphorus (P) [49]. ADG, humeral length, and wither height were not significantly different in the foals fed the higher energy ration. However, the number of histological lesions was significantly greater and more severe in the foals fed the higher DE ration compared with foals fed the control. Similar findings were concluded in foals fed a 70, 100, or 130% of recommended DE and protein intakes for 8 m [50, 51]. Excess energy intake can induce DOD lesions within a few months and may not result in taller or heavier foals, but likely histologic abnormalities are present.

The dietary DE consumed by growing horses is first used to maintain current BW and then tissue synthesis, that is, gaining weight. The ADG decreases with age, for example, 0.84 to 0.29 kg/d in 4 vs. 18 month old horses, respectively, but DE required above maintenance per kg BW gained increases, for example, 8.5 to 18.9 Mcal/kg gained in 6 vs. 24 month old horses, respectively. Hence, as the weanling grows, the growth rate declines, but the dietary energy required to gain a kg of BW increases, that is, the conversion of dietary energy to tissue synthesis becomes less efficient. Simultaneously, % dry matter intake (DMI) decreases, for example, 3.5–1.75% BW in nursing and two-year-olds, respectively; however, daily total feed DM consumed increases as BW increases, and the DE required for maintenance (DE_m) decreases; that is, it becomes more efficient [52]. The net effect of these changes during growth; to balance increasing amounts of feed DM consumed daily with decreasing ADG and DE_m/kg BW, the DE ration caloric density should decrease, for example, 3–1.74 Mcal DE/kg DM for weanlings and two-year-olds, respectively [30]. Given a genetic predisposition, continuing to feed a high DE ration and allowing high intakes of calorie fueling growth rate and ADG may promote the clinical expression of DOD [46, 53].

Additionally, non-energy nutrient imbalances occur when these nutrients have not been correctly adjusted as ration DE concentration changes; that is, as ration caloric density increases, non-energy nutrient concentration should also increase (Figure 25.2) [48]. The ration concentration of a non-energy nutrient needed for bone growth depends upon the rate at which growth occurs. Thus, to lower the risk of DOD, the diet must provide the nutrients necessary to support *in vivo* rate of growth. Although a horse is fed adequate quantities of all nutrients thought to be necessary for maximum growth rate, DOD may still occur in some rapidly growing horses likely due to

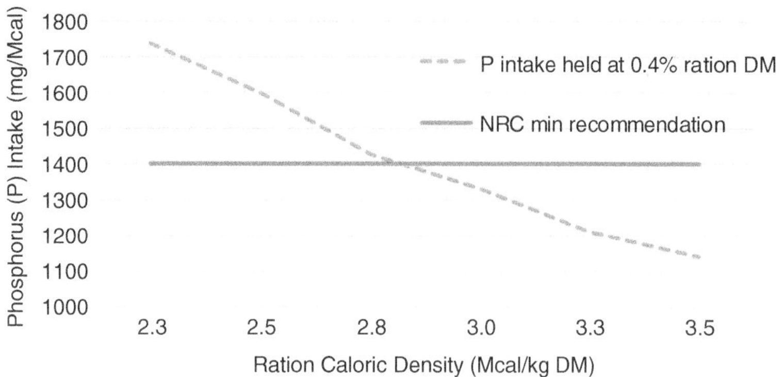

Figure 25.2 Effect of increasing ration caloric density on nutrient intake when [nutrient] is held constant on a DM basis. A deficiency of P will manifest relative to the energy consumed and the rate of bone development [48].

genetics. For some owners, a faster growth rate may be desirable to have a heavier animal for a competitive purpose or by a specific sell date and the ration should be correctly balanced to the higher caloric density and growth rate, although there is no guarantee any DOD condition will be prevented. Horses used for recreation or intended to be sold after maturity can have a lower, less risky growth rate and be fed a ration balanced correctly for lower or moderate ADG.

25.2.2.2.2 Protein

Feeding more protein than the animal needs does not increase the growth rate above that achieved when the diet meets protein requirements [54, 55]. Additionally, high protein intake is unlikely a contributing factor in the occurrence of DOD. In two month old foals consuming a ration containing 100% DE but 125% protein of recommended concentrations for four months, postmortem signs of osteochondrosis were not significantly different from those in the control group consuming 100% of recommended DE and protein concentrations [49]. However, increasing the protein content of a protein-deficient but energy-sufficient ration results in compensatory bone growth, and if the ration does not contain adequate Ca and P to support the subsequent higher rate of bone growth, alterations in endochondral ossification may occur [48, 56].

25.2.2.2.3 Calcium and Phosphorus

Without adequate quantities of Ca or P, endochondral cartilage becomes thickened, bone density and growth decrease, and a DOD condition may occur [57]. The concentration of calcium should be greater than that of phosphorus in the ration, that is, Ca : P of 1–3. Skeletal Ca content in horses is not affected by high Ca intake; however, excessive dietary Ca decreases the intestinal absorption of P and possibly zinc, manganese, and iron as seen in other species [57, 58]. In contrast, diets containing five times the P requirement consistently resulted in osteochondrosis lesions but without signs of nutritional secondary hyperparathyroidism [40, 58].

25.2.2.2.4 Copper and Zinc

Copper (Cu) is a co-factor of lysyl oxidase involved in cross-linking and stabilization of bone collagen. Cu may also have an anti-inflammatory effect within the joint by inhibiting interleukin-1 activity [40]. A copper deficiency impairs these functions. A few studies have suggested the occurrence of osteochondritis, epiphysitis, and limb deformities may be lower in foals fed ration Cu concentrations of 25–55 ppm [59, 60]. Dietary zinc (Zn) concentrations several times those naturally present in feeds may interfere with Cu utilization by horses. There are reported cases of joint disease and lameness in foals consuming excessively high Zn rations, that is, 2% DM or feed contaminated by zinc smelter, which likely resulted in a secondary Cu deficiency [30].

25.2.3 Feeding Management

The risk factors for the clinical expression of DOD are large body size and weight, a high rate of growth due to genetics or growth spurt, and high consumption of calories fueling that growth rate. Providing inadequate amounts of a properly formulated creep feed to the nursing foal, followed by feeding for rapid growth in the weanling, is a common cause for a compensatory growth spurt. In addition to feeding moderate or low DE feeds, controlling feed access or intake effectively lowers energy intakes. Weanling horses voluntarily ingest 2.0–3.5%, whereas yearlings consume 2.0–3.0% BW DM/d [48]. Ad libitum access to a high-DE low-fiber creep feed or overfeeding a concentrate mix at meals and/or unlimited access to high-quality (RFV > 125) legume forages results in high DM and DE intakes and a rapid growth rate.

Quarter horse foals fed a complete and balanced pelleted diet, either free-choice or restricted to 2.2% BW daily, illustrates the benefit of preventing high feed intakes [65]. The ad libitum-fed foals consumed about a third more feed and calories and, at 24 mos of age, were 3.6% taller and 13% heavier than those fed limited amounts of the same feed. The ADG for ad libitum-fed horses was 71% more rapid than for the limit-fed horses between the ages of 18 and 24 mos. There were minimal musculoskeletal abnormalities before one year of age in either group. At 25 mos old, the ad libitum-fed horses had a higher occurrence of conformational and musculoskeletal abnormalities. Six of the nine free-choice-fed colts had developed conformation faults and/or lameness and three were judged sound but had an uncomfortable gait due to a shortened stride, a limited range of motion, and steep angulation of the limbs. In contrast, only two of the nine restricted-fed colts had subtle conformation or gait abnormalities.

In horses showing any clinical signs of DOD, it is recommended that the growth rate be slowed immediately by decreasing dietary energy and that trauma or pressure on the growth plates and articular cartilage be reduced by decreasing physical activity. Feeding a grass hay-based ration, ensuring correct mineral concentrations and ratios, and controlling daily feed intake are necessary to slow growth rate and mitigate ongoing abnormal endochondral ossification.

25.2.4 Summary

Feeding a nutritionally incomplete or imbalanced ration will likely result in the clinical expression of a DOD condition. Allowing ad libitum intake that results in high energy intake fueling a rapid growth rate will also likely result in orthopedic deformities. However, controlled intakes of a nutritionally complete and balanced ration lowers, but cannot eliminate, the risk of DOD, regardless of feedstuffs used, as this is a complex, multifactorial disease that has yet to be unraveled in any species. Ration nutrient profile and feeding methods to manage growth rate are relatively easy to accomplish compared with altering genetic predisposition and avoiding trauma. Bone abnormalities due to moderate nutritional insults will likely not be evident acutely until maturity, so feeding broodmares, suckling foals, weanling, and yearlings specifically to lower the risk of DOD is recommended. See Chapter 20 Feeding Broodmares and Chapter 21 Feeding Growing Horses.

25.3 Osteoarthritis

Osteoarthritis (OA), a common cause of lameness in horses of all ages, aka degenerative joint disease (DJD), is characterized by permanent degeneration of the articular cartilage accompanied by changes in the bone and soft tissues of the joint [66, 67]. In a survey of 467 horses that were ≥20 years of age, approximately 24% reported musculoskeletal problems, and 40% of those were classified as osteoarthritis [68].

25.3.1 Animal Assessment

Most clinical signs of lameness occur in the forelimbs carrying 60–65% BW and must withstand higher load rates than the hind limbs. Trauma related to intensive training or showing is often a contributing factor to the onset of OA in young horses. The initial injury is usually mechanical with an imbalance between the load applied and the tissue capacity to withstand that load. The foreleg fetlock joint has the largest number of degenerative and traumatic lesions in racing horses [69]. Degenerative joint disease has been described in the proximal and distal interphalangeal joint in horses forced to make quick turns and abrupt stops, such as western performance horses, polo ponies, and jumpers [70], whereas degenerative disease in the tarsal joint has been found in Quarter horses, Thoroughbreds, and Standardbreds [71].

Conformation, poor foot care, and acute trauma are other identified risk factors [72–74]. OA is commonly observed in the joints of older horses, and some may be genetically predisposed to developing arthritis in the absence of environmental factors; for example, DJD has been found in wild horses and Icelandic ponies [75, 76]. Most commonly, the carpal, fetlock, proximal interphalangeal, or distal intertarsal/tarsometatarsal joints are afflicted, but in older horses, any articular joint can be impacted, including the spine, hips, and temporomandibular joint (TMJ). The clinical signs include joint effusion and decreased range of motion that deteriorates with time. The horse with OA has signs of lameness described as a shortened stride, uneven gaits, reluctance to pick and maintain or change canter lead, and reluctance to stop or turn while working at higher speeds. These changes lead to poor performance and early retirement for a horse.

25.3.2 Ration Assessment

Given the most likely and varied causes for OA, for example, trauma and genetic predisposition, there are no preventive dietetic options. There are also no validated nutritional or dietary treatment options. In addition to the general ration recommendations for adult horses, maintaining a lower BW and BCS (3–4/9) to minimize joint load is advisable. The patient should be provided a nutritionally complete and balanced ration meeting nutrient requirements, including all vitamins and minerals within 1.5–2.0% BW [30].

Joint supplements are among the most popular equine nutritional products that contain a wide range of ingredients, but evidence of efficacy for most commercially available products is lacking. See Evidence-Based Medicine in Chapter 14. Common oral ingredients include glucosamine (HCl or sulfate), chondroitin sulfate, methylsulfonylmethane (MSM), and hyaluronic acid (HA), while some products may also contain EPA and DHA, collagen peptides, herbal ingredients, anti-oxidants, vitamins, and minerals. See Joint Disease in Chapter 18. In summary, there is some clinical evidence suggesting a benefit to horses with osteoarthritis; however, rigorous randomized, controlled clinical studies are needed.

25.3.3 Feeding Management

Providing predominately forage-based ration helps to manage BW and BCS and can be used to motivate the horse to walk or move about throughout the day. OA horses become stiff, appear uncomfortable after resting, and need time to warm up muscles and joints. Placing hay in various areas within a pasture, paddock, or drylot using small hay nets and placing these at a distance from the water encourage the horse to move about at a comfortable pace. If feeding in a herd, the OA horse may not be able or willing to compete at the feeding station and probably should be fed separately but near herd mates. Consider finding the best height, for example, chest-high vs. ground level, for watering buckets and hay nets for horses with OA in the spine or TMJ [77].

25.4 Laminitis

In a retrospective review of the literature from 1950 to 2010, possibly a third of horses will be afflicted in their lifetime with a debilitating, life-threatening disease affecting the dermal and epidermal tissues of the foot [78, 79]. Inflammation of the laminae binding the hoof wall to the distal phalanx is, however, more likely to be just the most prominent clinical sign of a systemic disease [80]. Of the many observed, suggested, and cited causes of laminitis, there are three related to diet, nutrition, and the feeding of horses [81, 82]. The most common form in North America and Europe has a progressive subclinical onset due to insidious endocrinopathies, for example, insulin dysregulation (ID), hence referred to as endocrinopathic laminitis. The second is likely an acute onset associated with a precipitating systemic inflammatory response syndrome referred to as SIRS-related laminitis. Least are occurrences due to poisonings of hoary alyssum (*Berteroa incana*) contaminating hay or the rare ingestion of black walnut. See Chapter 12 Toxic Plants. Understanding the etiology of laminitis directs dietetic treatment, management, and preventive measures.

25.4.1 Animal Assessment

Historically, laminitis was associated with an inflammatory process as a common sequela of systemic sepsis, for example, enteritis, strangulating colics, pneumonia, metritis, and gut dysbiosis, that is, history of grain overload [83]. However, a 2000 USDA survey indicated that the majority of cases were not related to a septic condition but that most cases seen in private practice were associated with pasture grazing, obesity, and insulin resistance [80, 84, 85].

Most horses or ponies presenting with an acute onset of lameness upon physical examination are found to have long-standing pathology, that is, an acute on chronic presentation: findings of abnormal growth rings on the external hoof wall, flat soles, separation of the hoof wall from the underlying laminae at the white line, and radiographic evidence of an abnormal relationship between the dorsal hoof wall and the distal phalanx indicate chronicity. Many, not all, animals are over 10 years old, overweight or obese, and have a dietary history that includes grain concentrates and/or pasture. In general, insulin sensitivity decreases with age in horses; hence, these animals are likely to have some degree of ID. Additionally, pituitary pars intermedia dysfunction (PPID), a neurodegenerative disease occurring in 15–30% of aged horses, may also be a complicating factor [86].

25.4.2 Ration Assessment

In addition to the general complete and balanced ration recommended for adult horses to maintain adequate BW and BCS 4 to 6/9, the major nutrients of concern for horses predisposed or have a history of laminitis are caloric density and the concentrations of non-structural carbohydrates (NSC), which specifically are sugars, starch, and fructans [30]. Pasture forage NSC content may approach 40% DM at times and should be avoided in susceptible animals [87, 88]. Grass hay (long stem, chopped, cubed, or pelleted) with <12% NSC and very restricted or no access to pasture is recommended.

Horses requiring weight loss (BCS > 6/9) should be fed a predominately dried grass forage ration with <12% NSC and 1.7–2.0 Mcal DE/kg DM at 1.5% BW initially and their weight reassessed in four wks. Feeding at 1.25% BW and replacing a portion of the forage with straw may be necessary in weight-resistant animals. Balancing a low-calorie ration for weight loss may be difficult, and seeking the expertise of a veterinary nutritionist is advisable. While obesity or regional adiposity is the most prevalent phenotype, there are BCS 4 to 5/9 laminitic animals. Feeding a

≥2.0 Mcal DE/kg DM predominately dried forage ration at a DMI of ≥2.0% BW but altering the form of the calories to minimize NSC intake to <12% DM and using fat calories in the form of fat or oil is needed for weight maintenance. See Insulin Dysregulation in Chapter 27 and Chapter 28 Metabolic Syndrome.

Other nutrients of concern for the hoof are protein, copper, zinc, and biotin [89]. Protein content at 7–10% DM using a high-quality protein such as soybean, oilseed, or alfalfa meals ensures intake of sulfur-containing cysteine and methionine and commonly first limiting lysine and threonine amino acids at recommended concentrations. Copper and zinc are essential trace minerals for normal hoof growth, and the ration concentration should be checked and corrected as needed to meet recommendations. Biotin supplements are often toted to support hoof growth; however, there is little data to support such claims; on the other hand, as a water-soluble vitamin, there is no known toxic dose.

25.4.3 Feeding Management

It still is difficult to successfully treat and manage laminitis once the clinical signs are apparent. Xenophon (380 BCE) has been reported to have written "diseases are easier to cure at the start than after they have become chronic and have been wrongly diagnosed" [82]. Therefore, understanding the etiologies and proactively identifying horses and ponies at risk before the first clinical episode of laminitis is the most effective measure.

For SIRS-related laminitis, given the frequent association with septic insults from the GIT, (enteritis, colic, and diarrhea), emphasizing the dietary recommendations concerning feed hygiene and slow feed transitions is prudent. At the onset of laminitis, removing and halting the primary disease is needed, that is, the surgical correction and antibiotics, and providing systemic support, that is, fluid and pain therapies, is essential to minimizing damage to the lamellae [79]. Follow-up dietary recommendations include minimizing and monitoring the starch and fructans intake, as % NSC of ration DM and g starch/kg BW/meal, similar to the horse with endocrinopathic laminitis.

Identifying those animals at risk for endocrinopathic laminitis based on age, breed, BCS, and dietary history and implementing a monitoring plan for insulin and PPID testing for those >10 years of age is prudent [86]. Given obesity and ID represent the most common metabolic and endocrinopathic predispositions for laminitis in horses, the mainstay of prevention and treatment is weight control and managing NSC intake to minimize postprandial hyperinsulinemia [83]. Managing NSC intake includes controlling sugar and starch intake as a percent of ration DM and the absolute quantity of starch consumed per meal from complementary feeds or pasture. Pasture laminitis may be related to high sugar intake and subsequent hyperinsulinemia, or a hindgut dysbiosis related to starch or fructans by-passing small intestinal digestion. Specifically feeding a laminitic horse on pasture is inherently more difficult to quantify and control. Seeking the advice of a veterinary nutritionist may be necessary. See Insulin Dysregulation and Pituitary pars intermedia Dysfunction in Chapter 27 and Chapter 28 Metabolic Syndrome.

Case in Point

A six-mo-old weanling 216 kg BW (500 kg mature BW) is consuming 6.5 kg DM/d (3%BW) of an alfalfa-based ration with 1.0% calcium (Ca) and 0.40% phosphorus (P) DM basis. The weanling has been growing at 1 kg/d, and there are some early signs of joint disease. Based on laboratory analysis, the ration currently fed has 3.5 Mcal DE/kg DM. The ration recommendation for a moderate growth rate (0.72 kg/d) in this case is a 2.87 Mcal DE/kg (Table 21.4).

	Ration DE (Mcal/kg DM)	Average daily gain (kg/d)	DE intake (Mcal DE/d)	P intake (mg/Mcal)
NRC[a]	2.87	0.72	15.5	1387
Current intake	3.50	1.0	22.75[b]	1143[c]

[a] Recommended ration [30] Table 16-3.

[b] 6.5 kg DM/d x 3.5 Mcal/kg DM = 22.75 Mcal/d

[c] 6.5 kg DM/d × 0.4% P = 26 g P/22.75 Mcal = 1143 mg P/Mcal/d.

1) *A phosphorus deficiency exists relative to the energy consumed and the rate of bone development. Calculate the necessary phosphorus concentration in the 3.5 Mcal DE/kg ration to meet the weanling's requirement consuming 6.5 kg DM/d?*
   a) *What is the weanling's daily DE intake?*
   b) *The recommendation is ~1400 mg P per Mcal DE consumed* (Table 24.3) [30]. *How many g P is recommended/d for this weanling consuming the higher calorie ration?*
   c) *What must then be the P concentration in the higher calorie ration to meet P recommendation?*
2) *What is the Ca:P ratio in the current ration and new ration after the phosphorus content has been increased per recommendations, and does the calcium concentration also need to be adjusted?*

See Appendix A Chapter 25.

References

1 Buettner, G.R. (1993). The pecking order of free radicals and antioxidants: lipid peroxidation, a-tocopherol, and ascorbate. *Arch. Biochem. Biophys.* 300 (2): 535–543.

2 Valberg, S.J. (2018). Disorders of the musculoskeletal system. In: *Equine Internal Medicine*, 4e (ed. S.M. Reed, W.M. Bayly, and D. Sellon), 542–579. Elsevier.

3 Nout-Lomas, Y. (2018). Equine neuroaxonal dystrophy/ equine degenerative Myeloenchephalopathy. In: *Equine Internal Medicine*, 4e (ed. S.M. Reed, W.M. Bayly, and D.C. Sellon), 636–640. Elsevier.

4 Urschel, K.L. and McKenzie, E.C. (2021). Nutritional influences on skeletal muscle and muscular disease. *Vet. Clin. North Am. Equine Pract.* 37 (1): 139–175.

5 Pitel, M.O., Mckenzie, E.C., Johns, J.L., and Stuart, R.L. (2020). Influence of specific management practices on blood selenium, vitamin E, and beta-carotene concentrations in horses and risk of nutritional deficiency. *J. Vet. Intern. Med.* 34 (5): 2132–2141.

6 Löfstedt, J. (1997). White muscle disease of foals. *Vet. Clin. North Am. Equine Pract.* 13 (1): 169–185.

7 Dodd, D.C., Blakely, A.A., Thornbury, R.S., and Dewes, H.F. (1960). Muscle degeneration and yellow fat disease in foals. *N. Z. Vet. J.* 8 (3): 45–50.

8 de Bruijn, C.M., Velduis Kroeze, E.J.B., and Sloet van Oldruitenborgh-Oosterbaan, M.M. (2006). Yellow fat disease in equids. *Equine Vet. Educ.* 18 (1): 38–44.

9 Mohammed, H.O., Divers, T.J., Summers, B.A., and de Lahunta, A. (2007). Vitamin E deficiency and risk of equine motor neuron disease. *Acta Vet. Scand.* 49 (17). https://doi:10.1186/1751-0147-49-17.

10 Weber Polack, E., King, J.M., Cummings, J.F. et al. (1998). Quantitative assessment of motor neuron loss in equine motor neuron disease (EMND). *Equine Vet. J.* 30 (3): 256–259.

11 Divers, T.J. (2005). Equine motor neuron disease. *J. Equine Vet. Sci.* 25 (5): 238.

12 Cummings, J.F., de Lahunta, A., George, C. et al. (1990). Equine motor neuron disease; a preliminary report. *Cornell Vet.* 80 (4): 357–379.

13 Valentine, B.A., de Lahunta, A., George, C. et al. (1994). Acquired equine motor neuron disease. *Vet. Pathol.* 31: 130–138.

14 Divers, T.J., Mohammed, H.O., Cummings, J.F. et al. (1994). Equine motor neuron disease: findings in 28 horses and proposal of a pathophysiological mechanism for the disease. *Equine Vet. J.* 26 (5): 409–415.

15 Husulak, M.L., Lohmann, K., Gabadage, K. et al. (2016). Equine motor neuron disease in 2 horses from Saskatchewan. *Can. Vet. J.* 57: 771–776.

16 Bedford, H.E., Valberg, S.J., Firshman, A.M. et al. (2013). Histopathologic findings in the sacrocaudalis dorsalis medialis muscle of horses with vitamin E-responsive muscle atrophy and weakness. *J. Am. Vet. Med. Assoc.* 242: 1127–1137.

17 Divers, T.J., Mohammed, H.O., and Cummings, J.E. (1997). Equine motor neuron disease. *Vet. Clin. North Am. Equine Pract.* 13 (1): 97–105.

18 Johnson, A.L., Divers, T.J., and de Lahunta, A. (2014). Nervous system. In: *Equine Emergencies Treatment and Procedures*, 4e (ed. J.A. Orsini and T.J. Divers), 339–378. St. Louis, MO: Elsevier.

19 Cummings, J.F., de Lahunta, A., Mohammed, H.O. et al. (1995). Endothelial lipopigment as an indicatory of a-tocopherol deficiency in two equine neurodegenerative diseases. *Acta Neuropathol.* 90: 266–272.

20 Finno, C.J., Kaese, H.J., Miller, A.D. et al. (2017). Pigment retinopathy in warmblood horses with equine degenerative myeloencephalopathy and equine motor neuron disease. *Vet. Ophthalmol.* 20 (4): 304–309.

21 Secombe, C.J. and Lester, G.D. (2012). The role of diet in the prevention and management of several equine diseases. *Anim. Feed Sci. Technol.* 173 (1–2): 86–101.

22 Mayhew, I.G., Brown, C.M., Stowe, H.D. et al. (1987). Equine degenerative Myeloencephalopathy: a Vitamin E deficiency that may be familial. *J. Vet. Intern. Med.* 1 (1): 45–50.

23 Miller, M.M. and Collatos, C. (1997). Equine degenerative myeloencephalopathy. *Vet. Clin. North Am. Equine Pract.* 13 (1): 43–52.

24 Aleman, M., Finno, C.J., Higgins, R.J. et al. (2011). Evaluation of epidemiological, clinical, and pathological features of neuroaxonal dystrophy in Quarter Horses. *J. Am. Vet. Med. Assoc.* 239: 823–833.

25 Blythe, L., Hultgren, B., Craig, A. et al. (1991). Clinical, viral, and genetic evaluation of equine degenerative myeloencephalopathy in a family of Appaloosas. *Eur. Am. Vet. Med. Assoc.* 198 (6): 1005–1013.

26 Finno, C.J., Higgins, R.J., Aleman, M. et al. Equine degenerative Myeloencephalopathy in Lusitano horses. *J. Vet. Intern. Med.* 25 (6): 1439–1446.

27 Finno, C.J., Bordbari, M.H., Valberg, S.J. et al. (2016). Transcriptome profiling of equine vitamin E deficient neuroaxonal dystrophy identifies upregulation of liver X receptor target genes. *Free Radic. Biol. Med.* 101: 261–271.

28 Dill, S., Correa, M., Erb, H. et al. (1990). Factors associated with the development of equine degenerative myeloencephalopathy. *Am. J. Vet. Res.* 51 (8): 1300–1305.

29 Barigye, R., Dyer, N.W., and Newell, T.K. (2007). Fatal myocardial degeneration in an adult quarter horse with Vitamin E deficiency. *J. Equine Vet. Sci.* 27 (9): 405–408.

30 National Research Council (2007). *Nutrient Requirements of Horses*. 6th Rev. Animal Nutrition Series, 1–341. Washington. DC: National Academies Press.

31 Kronfeld, D.S. (1989). Vitamin E. In: *Vitamin and Mineral Supplementation for Dogs and Cats: A Monograph on Micronutrients*, 92–95. Santa Barbara, CA: Veterinary Practice Publishing Company.

32 National Research Council (1987). *Vitamin Tolerance of Animals*, 1–108. Washington, DC: National Academies Press.

33 Fiorellino, N.M., Lamprecht, E.D., and Williams, C.A. (2009). Absorption of different oral formulations of natural vitamin E in horses. *J. Equine Vet. Sci.* 29 (2): 100–104.

34 Brown, J.C., Valberg, S.J., Hogg, M., and Finno, C.J. (2017). Effects of feeding two RRR-a-tocopherol formulations on serum, cerebrospinal fluid and muscle a-tocopherol concentrations in horses with subclinical vitamin E deficiency. *Equine Vet. J.* 49: 753–758.

35 de la Rua-Domenech, R., Mohammed, H.O., Cummings, J.F. et al. (1997). Association between plasma vitamin E concentrations and the risk of equine motor neuron disease. *Br. Vet. J.* 154: 203–213.

36 Divers, T.J., Cummings, J.F., de Lahunta, A. et al. (2006). Evaluation of the risk of motor neuron disease in horses fed a diet low in vitamin E and high in copper and iron. *Am. J. Vet. Res.* 67: 120–126.

37 McGorum, B.C., Mayhew, I.G., Amory, M.H. et al. (2006). Horses on pasture may be affected by equine motor neuron disease. *Equine Vet. J.* 38 (1): 47–51.

38 Díez de Castro, E., Zafra, R., Acevedo, L.M. et al. (2016). Eosinophilic enteritis in horses with motor neuron disease. *J. Vet. Intern. Med.* 30 (3): 873–879.

39 Mohammed, H.O., Divers, T.J., Kwak, J. et al. (2012). Association of oxidative stress with motor neuron disease in horses. *Am. J. Vet. Res.* 73: 1957–1962.

40 Vervuert, I. and Ellis, A.A.D.A. (2013). Developmental orthopedic disease. In: *Equine Applied and Clinical Nutrition: Health, Welfare and Performance* (ed. R.J. Geor, P.A. Harris, and M. Coenen), 536–548. Edinburgh: Saunders Elsevier.

41 Metzger, J. (2020). Genetics of equine orthopedic disease. *Vet. Clin. North Am. Equine Pract.* 36 (2): 289–301.

42 Kronfeld, D.S., Meacham, T.N., and Donoghue, S. (1990). Dietary aspects of developmental orthopedic disease in young horses. *Vet. Clin. North Am. Equine Pract.* 6 (2): 451–465.

43 Orsini, J.A. and Kreuder, C. (1994). Musculoskeletal disorders of the neonate. *Vet. Clin. North Am. Equine Pract.* 10 (1): 137–166.

44 Schougaard, H., Ronne, J.F., and Phillipson, J. (1990). A radiographic survey of tibiotarsal osteochondrosis in a selected population of trotting horses in Denmark and its possible genetic significance. *Equine Vet. J.* 22 (4): 288–289.

45 Grøndahl, A.M. and Dolvik, N.I. (1993). Heritability estimations of osteochondrosis in the tibiotarsal joint and of bony fragments in the palmar/plantar portion of the metacarpo-and metatarsophalangeal joints of horses. *J. Am. Vet. Med. Assoc.* 203 (1): 101–104.

46 Thompson, K.N., Jackson, S.G., and Rooney, J.R. (1988). The effect of above average weight gains on the incidence of radiographic bone aberrations and epiphysitis in growing horses. *J. Equine Vet. Sci.* 8 (5): 383–385.

47 van Tilburg, E. and Ellis, A. (2002). *Growth Rates in Dutch Warmblood Horses in Relation to Osteochondrosis*, 158. Cairo: European Association of Animal Science.

48 Ralston, S.L. (2007). Evidence-based equine nutrition. *Vet. Clin. North Am. Equine Pract.* 23 (2): 365–384.

49 Savage, C.J., McCarthy, R.N., and Jeffcott, L.B. (1993). Effects of dietary energy and protein on induction of dyschondroplasia in foals. *Equine Vet. J.* 25 (S16): 74–79.

50 Glade, M.J. and Belling, T.H. Jr. (1986). A dietary etiology for osteochondrotic cartilage. *J. Equine Vet. Sci.* 6 (3): 151–155.

51 Glade, M.J. and Belling, T.H. Jr. (1984). Growth plate cartilage metabolism, morphology and biochemical composition in over- and underfed horses. *Growth* 48: 473–482.

52 National Research Council (1989). *Nutrient Requirements of Horses*. 5th Rev. Animal Nutrition Series, 1–100. Washington, DC: National Academies Press.

53 Lepeule, J., Bareille, N., Robert, C. et al. (2013). Association of growth, feeding practices and exercise conditions with the severity of the osteoarticular status of limbs in French foals. *Vet. J.* 197 (1): 65.

54 Orton, R.K., Hume, I.D., and Leng, R.A. (1985). Effects of level of dietary protein and exercise on growth rates of horses. *Equine Vet. J.* 17 (5): 381–385.

55 Yoakam, S.C., Kirkham, W.W., and Beeson, W.M. (1978). Effect of protein level on growth in young ponies. *J. Anim. Sci.* 46 (4): 983–991.

56 Frape, D.L. (1987). Calcium balance and dietary protein content. *Equine Vet. J.* 19 (4): 265–270.

57 Thompson, K.N., Jackson, S.G., and Baker, J.P. (1988). The influence of high planes of nutrition on skeletal growth and development of weanling horses. *J. Anim. Sci.* 66 (10): 2459–2467.

58 Savage, C.J., McCarthy, R.N., and Jeffcott, L.B. (1993). Effects of dietary phosphorus and calcium on induction of dyschondroplasia in foals. *Equine Vet. J.* 25 (S16): 80–83.

59 Knight, D.A., Weisbrode, S.E., Schmall, L.M. et al. (1990). The effects of copper supplementation on the prevalence of cartilage lesions in foals. *Equine Vet. J.* 22 (6): 426–432.

60 Hurtig, M., Green, S.L., Dobson, H. et al. (1993). Correlative study of defective cartilage and bone growth in foals fed a low-copper diet. *Equine Vet. J.* 25 (S16): 66–73.

61 Ryden, H. (1972). The question of size. In: *America's Last Wild Horses*, 84–90. New York: Ballantine Books.

62 Treiber, K.H., Boston, R.C., Kronfeld, D.S. et al. (2005). Insulin resistance and compensation in Thoroughbred weanlings adapted to high-glycemic meals1. *J. Anim. Sci.* 83 (10): 2357–2364.

63 Cymbaluk, N.F. and Christison, G.I. (1989). Effects of dietary energy and phosphorus content on blood chemistry and development of growing horses. *J. Anim. Sci.* 67 (4): 951–958.

64 Cymbaluk, N.F. (1989). Effects of dietary energy source and level of feed intake on growth of weanling horses. *Equine Pract.* 11 (9): 19–33.

65 Cymbaluk, N.F., Christison, G.I., and Leach, D.H. (1990). Longitudinal growth analysis of horses following limited and ad libitum feeding. *Equine Vet. J.* 22 (3): 198–204.

66 McIlwraith, C.W. and Vachon, A. (1988). Review of pathogenesis and treatment of degenerative joint disease. *Equine Vet. J.* 20: 3–11.

67 Cruz, A.M. and Hurtig, M.B. (2008). Multiple pathways to osteoarthritis and articular fractures: is subchondral bone the culprit? *Vet. Clin. North Am. Equine Pract.* 24 (1): 101–116.

68 Brosnahan, M.M., Paradis, M.R., and Paradis, D.M.R. (2003). Demographic and clinical characteristics of geriatric horses: 467 cases (1989–1999). *J. Am. Vet. Med. Assoc.* 223 (1): 93–98.

69 Pool, R.R. and Meagher, D.M. (1990). Pathologic findings and pathogenesis of racetrack injuries. *Vet. Clin. North Am. Equine Pract.* 6 (1): 1–30.

70 Dyson, S. (2000). Lameness and poor performance in the sports horse: dressage, show jumping and horse trials (eventing). In: *Proceedings of the 46th Annual Convention of the American Association of Equine Practitioners*, 308–315. San Antonio, TX: American Association of Equine Practitioners (AAEP).

71 Schlueter, A.E. and Orth, M.W. (2004). Equine osteoarthritis: a brief review of the disease and its causes. *Equine Comp. Exerc. Physiol.* 1 (4): 221–231.

72 Dubuc, J., Girard, C., Richard, H. et al. (2018). Equine meniscal degeneration is associated with medial femorotibial osteoarthritis. *Equine Vet. J.* 50 (1): 133–140.

73 Brommer, H., Laasanen, M.S., Brama, P.A.J. et al. (2010). Functional consequences of cartilage degeneration in the equine metacarpophalangeal joint: quantitative assessment of cartilage stiffness. *Equine Vet. J.* 37 (5): 462–467.

74 Brommer, H., Weeren, P.R., Brama, P.A.J., and Barneveld, A. (2010). Quantification and age-related distribution of articular cartilage degeneration in the equine fetlock joint. *Equine Vet. J.* 35 (7): 697–701.

75 Cantley, C.E.L., Firth, E.C., Delahunt, J.W. et al. (1999). Naturally occurring osteoarthritis in the metacarpophalangeal joints of wild horses. *Equine Vet. J.* 31 (1): 73–81.

76 Axelsson, M., Björnsdottir, S., Eksell, P. et al. (2001). Risk factors associated with hindlimb lameness and degenerative joint disease in the distal tarsus of Icelandic horses. *Equine Vet. J.* 33 (1): 84–90.

77 Jarvis, N.G. (2009). Nutrition of the aged horse. *Vet. Clin. North Am. Equine Pract.* 25 (1): 155–166.

78 Wylie, C.E., Collins, S.N., Verheyen, K.L.P., and Newton, J.R. (2012). Risk factors for equine laminitis: a systematic review with quality appraisal of published evidence. *Vet. J.* 193 (1): 58–66.

79 Leise, B.S. and Fugler, L.A. (2021). Laminitis updates: sepsis/systemic inflammatory response syndrome-associated laminitis. *Vet. Clin. North Am. Equine Pract.* 37 (3): 639–656.

80 Patterson-Kane, J.C., Karikoski, N.P., and McGowan, C.M. (2018). Paradigm shifts in understanding equine laminitis. *Vet. J.* 231: 33–40.

81 Heymering, H.W. (2010). 80 causes, predispositions, and pathways of laminitis. *Vet. Clin. North Am. Equine Pract.* 26 (1): 13–19.

82 Heymering, H.W. (2010). A historical perspective of laminitis. *Vet. Clin. North Am. Equine Pract.* 26 (1): 1–11.

83 Johnson, P.J., Wiedmeyer, C.E., LaCarrubba, A. et al. (2010). Laminitis and the equine metabolic syndrome. *Vet. Clin. North Am. Equine Pract.* 26 (2): 239–255.

84 Coffman, J.R. and Colles, C.M. (1983). Insulin tolerance in laminitic ponies. *Can. J. Comp. Med.* 47 (3): 347.

85 Jeffcott, L.B., Field, J.R., McLean, J.G., and O'Dea, K. (1986). Glucose tolerance and insulin sensitivity in ponies and Standardbred horses. *Equine Vet. J.* 18 (2): 97–101.

86 Grenager, N.S. (2021). Endocrinopathic laminitis. *Vet. Clin. North Am. Equine Pract.* 37 (3): 619–638.

87 Bamford, N.J., Potter, S.J., Baskerville, C.L. et al. (2019). Influence of dietary restriction and low-intensity exercise on weight loss and insulin sensitivity in obese equids. *J. Vet. Intern. Med.* 33 (1): 280–286.

88 Harris, P.A. (2017). Nutritional management for avoidance of pasture-associated laminitis. In: *Equine Laminitis* (ed. J.K. Belknap), 436–441. West Sussex: Wiley.

89 Burns, T.A. (2021). "Feeding the foot": nutritional influences on equine hoof health. *Vet. Clin. North Am. Equine Pract.* 37 (3): 669–684.

26

Digestive System Disorders

Nicolás C. Galinelli, Andy E. Durham, and Rebecca L. Remillard

KEY TERMS

- Dysbiosis is the reduction in microbial diversity and a decrease in beneficial microbes.

KEY POINTS

- Feeding horses with oral disease or esophageal obstruction most likely requires a change in feedstuff particle size and/or texture and, in some cases, an increase in ration caloric density.
- Feeding horses with gastric ulcers does require a change in the form of energy, i.e., ration starch and fiber content, and feeding protocol.
- Abrupt dietary changes increase the risk of colic or diarrhea associated with dysbiosis.

26.1 Introduction

With a 50 gal gastrointestinal tract (GIT) comprising 45% body weight (BW), the horse has been said to be 55% "heart" and 45% "guts." GIT disturbances and diseases are of primary concern to owners and veterinarians [1]. The diagnosis and medical management for dental and digestive tract disorders of horses have been previously detailed [2, 3].

26.2 Oral Disorders

Routine dental care is a necessary aspect of proper health care for horses. A good understanding of oral and dental anatomy with aging is necessary when assessing the horse's ability to prehend, masticate, and swallow feed [4, 5].

26.2.1 Animal Assessment

An oral examination of the lips, tongue, cheek, teeth, and oropharynx is essential when investigating problems related to feeding, maintaining BW and body condition score (BCS), or abnormal behaviors. Visible abnormal eating behavior includes eating slowly, reluctance to drink cold water, a decrease in feed intake, tilting the head when chewing, wallowing the feed around in the mouth before swallowing, slobbering grain, or quidding forages. Swallowed but improperly chewed feed may cause intestinal impactions and colic. A decrease in feed intake, if sufficient, will cause weight loss, poor physical condition, and impaired performance. Mouth pain can result in behavioral changes, such as non-acceptance of the bit, tongue lolling, abnormal head carriage, head tossing, tail wringing, bucking, and a change in temperament or disposition. With the use of proper instruments and following a consistent step-by-step plan, an oral examination is essential to the diagnosis of problems related to feed consumption [6].

As a greater number of horses reach older ages, the importance of good dental care cannot be underestimated. Teeth are living structures that respond to external stimuli and are continually changing due to a cycle of eruption and wear [7]. The most common cause of a sore mouth is irritation or lacerations of the cheeks, tongue, or gums by sharp edges, hooks, or protuberances on permanent or retained deciduous cheek teeth. The upper cheek teeth extend one-half the width of a tooth outside the lower cheek teeth, and chewing

Equine Clinical Nutrition, Second Edition. Edited by Rebecca L. Remillard.

creates points or edges on the outside of the upper cheek teeth and the inside of the lower cheek teeth, particularly in 2 to 5-yr-old horses. See Mastication in Chapter 3, Figure 3.4. Loss of a tooth may also cause problems because the opposing tooth may become too long which then hinders proper occlusion of incisors for prehension and molars for chewing. Identifying serious complications, e.g., tooth root fractures and equine odontoclastic tooth resorption and hypercementosis requires dental radiographs [8].

26.2.2 Ration Assessment

Feeding horses with oral disease, if the problem cannot be corrected, does not necessarily require a nutrient profile different from that recommended based on life stage, BW, and BCS [9–11]. Changes are more likely needed in the ration feedstuffs, particle size, or texture, and may require some trial and error before finding a successful feed form for a particular horse. Equine dentition is uniquely adapted to reducing the particle size of forages and maximizing the surface area for hydrolysis and fermentation in the lower digestive tract. Long-stem forage, i.e. grass and hay, are normally reduced from >50 to <2 mm size particles.

Changes to the form of forage to accommodate the decreased ability to chew are most often needed. Prepared feeds that have undergone some form of grinding during processing require minimal chewing before deglutition. Mechanical shortening of the fiber length in chopped, cubed, or pelleted forages may be required for the horse to maintain adequate fiber digestibility. See Forms of Hay in Chapter 11. Mechanically processed grains undergo grinding, cracking, or crimping, which decreases particle size and increases surface area which improves digestibility. See Manufacturing Processes in Chapter 13.

26.2.3 Feeding Management

It is important to minimize feed bunk competition and anxiety for horses with oral disease by feeding them separately, but near herdmates, which also allows for quantifying individual animal feed intake. Having forage available frequently or *ad libitum* and allowing more time to consume a meal may be necessary for horses with dental disease to maintain BCS. Softening the forage with water may be needed in the absence of adequate saliva lubrication due to decreased chewing time.

Changes to the caloric density of the ration are likely needed in cases where the oral disease has resulted in BW >15% below ideal, loss of 2 or more BCS units, and/or the existence of other complications. Feeding a complementary feed with higher-fat content, e.g., 5–10%, increases calorie intake. Adding vegetable oil will not only lubricate the feed ingredients, but also effectively increase the ration caloric density without having to change feedstuffs or increase feed DM intake. The addition of oil to the ration should be increased gradually over 7–10 days starting 0.25 mL/kg BW fed once or twice daily up to 1 mL/kg BW/d or 2 cups/1000 lb horse.[1]

26.3 Esophageal Obstruction

26.3.1 Animal Assessment

Simple intraluminal esophageal feed impaction, also known as choke, is the most common equine esophageal disease, although occasionally extraluminal obstructions are also seen associated with mediastinal or cervical masses. The intraluminal esophageal obstruction could involve stricture, dysmotility, or foreign body, but most commonly, it is simply due to ingestion of certain high-risk feedstuffs while exhausted or dehydrated, e.g., after strenuous exercise, or muscle weakness due to chronic disease and sedation increases the risk [12]. A retrospective study of esophageal disease indicated a predisposition in ponies and Friesian horses where megaesophagus appears commonly associated with muscular hypertrophy of the caudal esophagus [13–15]. There is a relationship between dental problems or poor dentition and inadequate mastication as a cause of esophageal obstruction, e.g., horses eating too quickly and swallowing before food is chewed properly or not chewing feed completely due to missing or painful teeth and/or sharp points. Partial obstruction of the esophagus is possible due to tumors or scarring from old injuries. Most esophageal obstructions resolve successfully, although horses >15 yrs of age were six times more likely to develop complications than younger adult horses [16]. A possible risk factor is a relationship between esophageal microbiota and disease. In people, a different microbiome was found between healthy vs. those with esophagitis or esophageal neoplasia [17–20]. However, there is little information at present in horses regarding the esophageal microbiome [21].

26.3.2 Ration Assessment

Feeding horses with an esophageal disease, in general, does not require a nutrient profile different from that recommended based on life stage, BW, or BCS, but rather changes are likely needed in the ration feedstuffs and feeding protocol [11]. Ingestion of poorly masticated carrots or apples and rapid ingestion of dry pellets, cubes,

1 Oil, corn and canola (USDA Food database NDB# 42289) provides 1980 kcal/224 g (8 vol-oz cup) with near 100% digestibility coefficient [11], 2 Mcal DE/cup is commonly used in equine nutrition.

or long stem forages increase the risk of esophageal impaction [22, 23]. The most common causes of intraluminal esophageal obstruction reportedly were a mix of different feeds, dry sugar beet pulp, dry grass nuts, lawn clippings, whole carrots and apples, dry pellets, and a single large bite of grass [12]. Alternatively when soaking the feed before feeding has been recommended, commercially prepared feeds made of small extruded particles require less time. Vegetable oil lubricates and passes easily through the esophagus, and would provide additional calories, if needed, to maintain BCS.

26.3.3 Feeding Management

Horses with a history of choking are prone to recurrent episodes and therefore strict adherence to a feeding plan minimizing the risk of esophageal obstruction is necessary [24]. Feeding protocol following clearance of an esophageal obstruction varies with the etiology, presence, and severity of secondary problems in the esophagus. Initially, preparation of a soft, water-soaked ration with small particle sizes is likely to be beneficial. Horses without mucosal ulceration should be fed water-soaked, nutritionally complete extruded or pelleted feed for at least 12–24 hrs to minimize the likelihood of repeat obstruction. Gradual reintroduction to grass is preferred to dried forage with a gradual return to a previous ration over 7–21 days.

Horses with mucosal ulceration often require a longer and more gradual refeeding protocol. Circumferential ulceration increases the likelihood of a slowly progressive stricture and affected horses should be fed a ration of softened feeds for approximately 60 days followed by endoscopy to evaluate the extent of the mucosal ulceration and stricture. Those horses with esophageal stricture have a high risk of re-obstruction. Some horses with chronic or recurrent esophageal obstruction require a permanent change to a softened, small-particle ration. Where chronic problems persist, feeding horses from an increased height using a raised platform for front feet may aid the aboral transit of ingesta through the esophagus (Figure 26.1). For feeding after surgical procedures, including wounds involving the esophageal wall. See Assisted Feeding in Chapter 24.

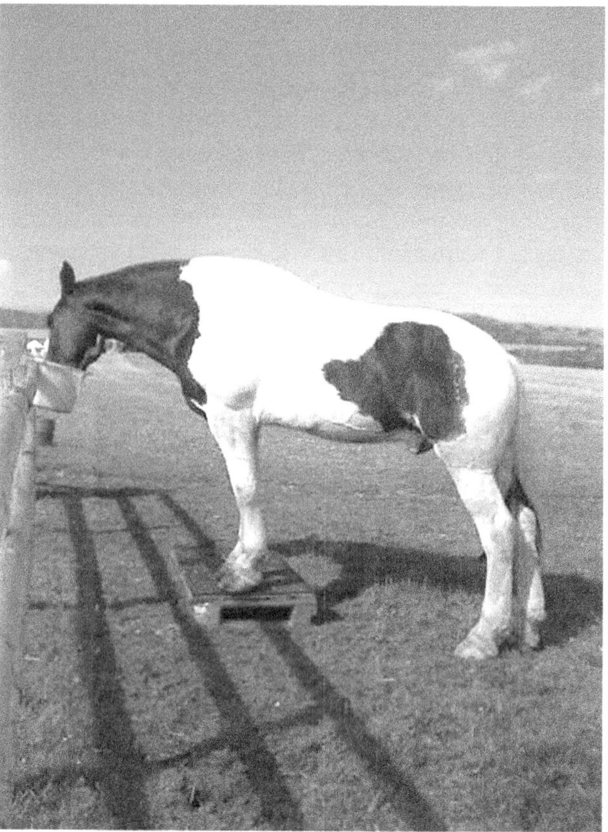

Figure 26.1 Feeding a horse that has suffered recurrent esophageal obstruction from an elevated position to maintain a dorsoventrally gradient to the esophagus.

26.4 Stomach

26.4.1 Ulcers

26.4.1.1 Animal Assessment

Equine gastric ulcer syndrome (EGUS) describes the disease complex associated with ulceration of the esophageal, gastric, or duodenal mucosae. Given marked dissimilarity between the diseases affecting the squamous versus glandular mucosae, the terms equine squamous gastric disease (ESGD) and equine glandular gastric disease (EGGD) are currently used to distinguish the main subtypes of EGUS. The diseases are common in horses of all types and occupations, although there is a general association between disease prevalence and degree of athletic exertion. Clinical signs vary but often include poor exercise performance, poor coat and appetite, nervous or aggressive temperament, abdominal pain, and sensitivity to girthing. Interesting to note is that lesions appeared to be chronically progressive in Thoroughbreds during training but regressed after retirement [25].

The gastric squamous mucosa has little defense against gastric acid and is susceptible to injury whenever comes in contact with unbuffered gastric secretions. Thus, factors that allow gastric juice to contact the mucosa proximal to the margo plicatus lead to ESGD. In contrast, the etiopathogenesis of EGGD is unclear and may include influences, such as impaired mucosal blood flow, prostaglandin inhibition, and factors disrupting the surface mucus layer. Nevertheless, both conditions appear to demonstrate there are important dietary risk factors to be considered in the prevention and management of these diseases.

26.4.1.2 Ration Assessment

Feeding horses with gastric ulcers does not require a different essential nutrient profile from that recommended based on life stage, BW, or BCS, but rather changes are recommended in the form of energy, i.e. ration starch and fiber content, and feeding protocol [11].

26.4.1.2.1 Complementary Feeds

Dietary starch is an important risk factor for EGUS in that feeding >1 g starch/kg BW/meal more than doubles the risk for squamous gastric disease [26]. This may be for several reasons, including less mastication and salivation associated with cereal vs. forage feeds and also a prolonged gastrin secretory response. The gastric squamous mucosal microbiome produces volatile fatty acids (VFAs) and lactate when exposed to dietary starch. The VFAs produced are likely to be harmful to the gastric mucosa when protonated in a low-pH environment and lipophilic below a typical pKa of 4, allowing transit across epithelial cell membranes, consequently intracellular acidification and cell death [27, 28]. Thus, the harmful effects of high-starch intakes can be mitigated with buffering.

26.4.1.2.2 Harvested Forage

When forage intake is limited, the gastric contents are likely to be more fluid and acidic. Although duodenal reflux might buffer gastric acid, higher bile salt concentrations in gastric juice have been shown to adversely affect squamous mucosa *in vitro* [29]. The glandular mucosa may be affected given the presumed higher bile salt exposure in the gastric regions closest to the duodenum. Conversely, a stomach filled above the margo plicatus with saliva-soaked forage is less likely to suffer significant acidic contact with the squamous mucosa due to a stable, non-fluid, pH-stratified gastric digesta. An additional means by which continual forage feeding may protect gastric mucosae is the constant transpyloric aboral flow of feed material. The lower prevalence of EGUS in feral horses also supports the value of constant access to dietary fiber.

Consistent with these mechanisms, studies have demonstrated a significant association between EGUS and forage feeding intervals of greater than 6 hrs. Circadian variability in gastric pH has been noted with more acidic conditions present in the squamous mucosa during the nighttime compared to daytime, which is likely due to relative differences in feed intake, salivation, and gastric filling. A stomach containing acidic fluid with no absorbent and pH-stratified feed mass might be at high risk of ESGD when combined with exercise, which further promotes mixing, agitation, and proximal movement of the fluid gastric content [30]. The effects of forage access on EGGD are less clear as loss of pH stratification is unlikely to harm the ventral glandular mucosa. Nevertheless, the pyloric antrum is likely to experience the highest bile salt concentrations during duodenal reflux, which is consistent with the most prevalent location for EGGD.

Quality of forage may also be an important factor in gastric health. When horses were fed either bromegrass hay (RFV 80) or alfalfa hay (RFV 154) with grain, the latter ration was unexpectedly associated with decreased number and severity of ulcers [31]. Analysis of gastric juice post-feeding indicated that despite the inclusion of grain in the diet of the alfalfa-hay-fed horses, gastric pH was higher in this group, indicating a buffering effect of the alfalfa hay. Statistical modeling of variables predictive of ESGD revealed low gastric pH as well as higher concentrations of propanoic, butanoic, and pentanoic acids in gastric juice to be the most important factors. The alfalfa/grain-fed group had higher VFA concentrations in gastric juice, although the potentially harmful effect of these acids was mitigated by the higher pH. A further investigation of potential benefits of feeding alfalfa hay examined exercising horses that were fed a concentrate ration alongside either alfalfa or coastal bermudagrass hays [32]. Alfalfa hay feeding demonstrated a significantly beneficial effect on both preventing new ulcer development and the healing of existing ulcers. It is not clear whether these rations were nutritionally equivalent or complete. Nutritional properties of alfalfa forage speculated to benefit gastric mucosal health are the relatively high protein, protein quality, and calcium content. However, other studies have failed to find a benefit of alfalfa vs. grass hay on the prevalence of ESGD [33].

The physical nature of the alfalfa may be important with some research suggesting that alfalfa chaff, but not pelleted, might promote EGGD due to physical abrasion. Rough and abrasive forage was also suggested as a possible reason why horses fed straw had greater than four times the risk for ESGD compared with horses fed hay or haylage [26]. Feeding different forage types inherently varies fiber content consumed, i.e. acid detergent fibers (ADF), neutral detergent fibers (NDF) and lignin. Highly lignified forages are less absorbent of liquids compared to higher-quality forages and less capacity to absorb liquid acidic gastric juices which then allows the liquid to move and flow within the stomach and contact the upper squamous mucosa.

26.4.1.2.3 Pasture

Intuitively, encouraging turnout seems to represent a good management approach to reducing gastric ulcer risk [34]. Stall confinement has indeed been shown to exert ulcerogenic effects when compared with pasture turnout in some studies, although contrasting results reported bringing horses into stables from pasture decreased EGUS scores. Several studies have indicated that in horses ESGD lesions can sometimes develop and worsen while moving from stable to pasture. A high prevalence of ESGD has been found in broodmares kept on permanent pasture, and a study of racehorses in New Zealand found no association between EGUS prevalence and time spent at pasture or with pasture quality [35]. Overall, the effects of grazing on EGUS are frequently disappointing suggesting that any assumed benefits are relatively minor and easily overwhelmed by additional adverse factors. It is also possible that fresh grass non-structural carbohydrate (NSC) content and gastric VFA production may play a role similar to cereal grain feeding.

26.4.1.2.4 Other Dietary Factors

Evidence for a beneficial effect of feeding corn oil remains equivocal with evidence of decreased gastric acid output and increased prostaglandin E_2 production in one study, whereas another failed to show any beneficial effects on gastric pH or the development of ulcers [36, 37]. Concentrated electrolyte solutions that may be administered orally to endurance horses have been shown to increase both the number and severity of ESGD lesions following eight hourly doses [38]. Free access to water also appears to be important in gastric defense against EGUS, possibly due to the dilutional effects of consumed water on harmful components of gastric juice. In a mixed population of Danish horses, those without access to water in the paddock were at more than double the risk of having EGUS [26].

26.4.1.3 Feeding Management

Effective medical treatments exist for ESGD and to a lesser extent for EGGD. However, once healed, it is then important to implement a longer-term dietary protocol to minimize the likelihood of recurrence. Such a strategy can also be used in a preventive fashion in horses judged to be at particular risk of developing EGUS. In contrast to what we know about dietary interactions with ESGD, there is little specific evidence on which to base dietary recommendations to help prevent EGGD and in the absence of obvious differences in risk factors, it would appear reasonable to apply similar tactics for the prevention of both diseases.

Horses should ideally have access to at least good-quality preserved forage, preferably constantly available or at least offered every 4–6 hrs [39]. Alfalfa hay may be optimal, although the effects of alfalfa chaff require further evaluation. Feeding straw and forage with high stem-to-leaf ratios should be avoided. Forage quantity should equate to no less than 1.25–1.5% BW dry matter intake (DMI), although less may be necessary for horses on weight-loss programs. Pasture turnout should be encouraged for overall GIT health benefits, although there is little evidence to support grazing as a beneficial factor for EGUS.

Cereal starch should only be fed when necessary and calories should preferably be provided by fiber sources, e.g., beet pulp, coconut meal, almond hulls, or oil. If cereal starch is fed, then <1 g starch/kg BW/meal is advisable and feeding after or with alfalfa hay or antacid supplements may mitigate the adverse effects of starch fermentation. Avoidance of green-growing pastures is advisable due to possible high-starch content under particular environmental conditions [40]. Water should always be available with several sources offered if the horse is turned out into a large area.

26.4.2 Impaction

26.4.2.1 Animal Assessment

Gastric impaction is poorly defined and the time taken for a normal horse to empty the stomach of solid material is highly diet dependent, as well as individually variable. Horses receiving low-forage diets will generally have only gastric juice remaining after 6–12 hrs of fasting, although horses with free access to forage may require 12–24 hrs of fasting before all solid material leaves the stomach. Impaction may be suspected when the stomach remains distended by solid material beyond these periods, especially when foul-smelling fermentative gasses are noted during the gastroscopic examination. Case reports of gastric impactions typically describe horses showing signs of inappetence and recurrent colic episodes [41, 42]. Inherent gastric motility dysfunction, for unknown reasons or as a result of hepatic encephalopathy, may result in secondary gastric impactions. Many horses with gastric impaction do not have access to pasture and dental disease is common, suggesting poor mastication and salivation may play a role in these cases [41].

26.4.2.2 Ration Assessment

The only well-characterized dietary causes of gastric impaction are persimmon fruits (*Diospyros virginiana*) and mesquite beans (*Prosopis sp.*), which may form a hard conglobate mass within the stomach. Sugar beet pulp when ingested dry may also form a progressively enlarging gastric impaction, although esophageal impaction is more commonly seen with beet pulp [43].

26.4.2.3 Feeding Management

Following the resolution of gastric impaction, recommendations are to feed a better quality, smaller particle size foods. A better quality forage has a lower ADF and NDF content, and cubed or pelleted forms of forage have reduced fiber particle sizes compared with fair-quality long stem hay or pasture (Table 10.3). Adding water to the meals may reduce the risk of re-impaction given enteral fluid therapy was of value in treating impacted horses [41]. Finely chopped straw, if needed to provide bulk and decrease calorie intake, can be fed, but it should be water-soaked to help prevent re-impaction.

26.5 Intestines

26.5.1 Colic

Horses adapted to subtropical forest plants transitioned to temperate Great Plains grasses over a 50 million year period. See Alimentary System Changes in Response to a Changing Food Supply in Chapter 1. Present-day dietary changes in feral horses grazing native forages occurs over many weeks due to slowly progressive changes in weather and seasons affecting plant species, quantity, quality, and availability [44]. Feeds fed to domesticated horses are, relative to those consumed throughout evolution, energy dense, high carbohydrate, low fiber, and possibly higher in fat [45]. Additionally, for domesticated horses, time spent feeding has been shortened from grazing ~16 hrs/d to <10 hr/d and the meal feeding of concentrated processed forms of feed. Additionally, the plethora of commercial feeds, supplements, and treats readily available to owners contributes to ill-conceived dietary changes made often or too rapid for GIT adaptation increasing the risk of disturbances.

26.5.1.1 Animal Assessment

Colic has been reported to occur in 4.2 cases/100 horses/yr with 80–85% having responded to medical management or resolved spontaneously with no identifiable cause, whereas 1.4% of colic events required surgery. Additionally, 10–15% of horses having one episode will have one or more episodes subsequently [46]. Colic in horses represents a multitude of different disease processes resulting in abdominal pain. This includes a diverse group of conditions that may have different, or even opposite, dietary risk factors. In the majority of instances, stretching of the intestine and/or mesentery causes colic signs, although alternative causes include muscular spasm, mural thickening, intraluminal obstruction with food or other materials, gaseous distension, or entrapment and strangulation of the intestine; or sometimes non-enteric disease. Thus, although some general dietary advice can be offered for colic-prone horses, refinement is required according to the precise nature of the underlying cause; although it should be acknowledged that a large proportion of colic cases seen in practice may remain of undetermined etiology. In cases where colic reoccurs, dietary modification specific to the type of colic may reduce the frequency.

26.5.1.2 Ration Assessment

Feeding colic-prone horses, in general, does not require an essential nutrient profile different from that recommended based on life stage, BW, or BCS, but rather changes are likely needed in the ration feedstuffs, i.e. forage quality or forage-to-grain ratio, and feeding protocol [11]. Many horses are intolerant of abrupt dietary changes and several studies have indicated an increased risk of colic following the introduction of new rations, i.e. dry forage, pastures, or concentrates with grain, or changing the timing and frequency of feeding hay or concentrate. Interestingly, the greatest changes in grass carbohydrate content occur in the spring and autumn seasons, coincident with seasonal increases in colic cases. Anecdotally, increases in numbers of colic cases frequently follow abrupt weather changes, i.e. warm to cold and dry to wet, which are usually accompanied by changes in barometric pressure and pasture nutrient content in the short term; however, no definitive association has been found [47]. Where dietary changes were associated with an increased incidence of colic, the hazard appears to subside after about 2 wks suggesting dietary adaptation. Given a stable and sustained microbiome benefits GIT health, changing feed digestibility and macronutrient profiles over a short (<2 wks) time frame would be intuitively adverse and attempts should be made to provide uniform nutrient rations in colic-prone horses.

26.5.1.2.1 Complementary Feeds

Equids are adapted to assimilate nutrients from hindgut fiber fermentation indicating the major importance of the cecal–colonic microbiome and decreased reliance on small intestinal enzymatic digestion. Throughout evolution, the horse consumed low-starch feeds and maintains a limited ability to digest and assimilate simple carbohydrates compared with other species [48]. Small bowel intolerance of high-NSC feeds results in starch and sugars entering the large bowel, cecal–colonic acidosis, and destabilization of the microbiome.

Approximately 20% of the ingested starch at 1 g/kg BW may appear in the caecum with likely adverse consequences [49]. A significant increase in the risk of colic was seen when >2.5 kg concentrate DM was fed daily to a varied group of horses and poines. [50]. Although the 'concentrate' portion of the ration was highly variable and starch concentrations were not known, this roughly equates to 1–2 g starch/kg BW/d, and the risk was not mitigated by dividing the ration into multiple meals/d.[2] The causal association between concentrate or cereal feeding with colic is compelling given the positive linear association (Figure 26.2). Particular causes of colic, such as duodenitis–proximal jejunitis in horses, appear to be associated with high concentrate rations. Conversely, enterolithiasis is perhaps the only specific cause of colic where cereal feeding does not appear to be adverse and might even be protective via mild colon acidification impairing enterolith formation.

---

2 Commercial 'concentrate' formulations will have different types and proportions of cereal grains and different starch concentrations. Starch content is not required on an equine feed label (Figure 15.1) unless a specific claim about starch is made. Cereal grains commonly fed to horses range between 40-85% starch (Table 13.1) whereas commercial 'concentrate' products commonly range between 10-25% starch.

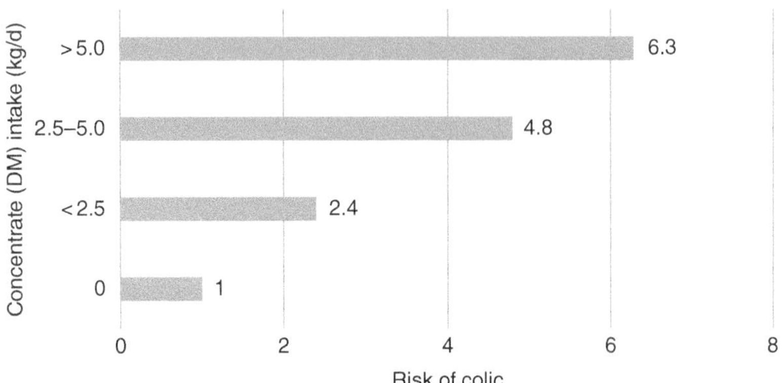

Figure 26.2 The risk of colic increases as the quantity of concentrate consumed per day increases. *Source:* Adapted from Tinker et al. [50].

26.5.1.2.2 Harvested Forage

Forage plays an important role in colic risk, although the influence may vary between specific causes of colic. A change in the type of hay fed was the only significant dietary modification that differed between 1030 pairs of horses with and without colic [51]. Risk factors for colic related to forage in the ration were changes in the batch of hay, feeding bermudagrass: coastal variety, from round bales, and decreased availability of pasture [52]. Hay feeding has also been shown to increase the risk of colon volvulus compared with grazing or feeding haylage [53].

Changes in forage type and nutritional content, i.e. fructan, fiber, and lignin, can result in changes to the colonic pH, VFA production, and microflora, conceivably predisposing to intestinal function disorders resulting in colic. Regardless of nutrient content, the hygienic quality of the hay has also been identified as a risk factor [54]. Dried forages should contain no more than 20% moisture to avoid microbial growth, overheating, and decreased nutritional quality [55]. Anecdotally feeding of highly lignified forages appears to increase the risk of impaction colic. The colon is a common site for simple impaction and, although the introduction of forage is associated with colon impaction, this may be due more specifically to a reduction in grazing time and exercise following stable confinement [56]. Bermudagrass hay (variety: coastal), is a clear risk factor for ileal impaction compared with timothy and alfalfa hays. Other studies have found Bermudagrass hay helps prevent colic caused by duodenitis–proximal jejunitis and that feeding alfalfa hay increases the risk of other colic types, such as small intestinal strangulation and enterolithiasis [57–60]. See Hygienic Quality of Hay in Chapter 10.

26.5.1.2.3 Pasture

As might be expected, free access to grazing has generally been found to be protective against colic in horses and may have further non-nutritional benefits, such as voluntary exercise, which appears to promote intestinal motility, and reduction in stereotypic behaviors, which have also been linked to colic [52]. Grazing appears to be especially protective against colic attributable to colon impactions, colon volvulus, and enterolithiasis. Pasture turnout may also be associated with reduced risk of epiploic foramen entrapment in horses either directly or via reduction of stable-associated stereotypic behaviors. Contrary, grazing has been found to increase the risk of duodenitis–proximal jejunitis and equine grass sickness in Europe. Pastures are heterogeneous varying markedly in starch, fructan, and fiber content depending on the plant type and species, weather, and season affecting growth [45]. This may help explain the contrasting findings in studies examining colic risk factors with pasture turnout.

26.5.1.3 Feeding Management

An important basic principle for feeding colic-prone horses is to maintain the stability of the microbiome, avoid abrupt dietary changes, and provide water [54]. Rations should be nutritionally complete and balanced appropriate for the life stage, BW, BCS, and ensuring at least 1% DM as forage/BW/d. Although forage intake may be voluntarily decreased throughout a 24-hr period, providing forage for at least 20 hrs/d, preferably pasture turnout >12 hrs/d, is recommended for GIT health. Where the dietary change is unavoidable, concentrate feeds and new batches of forage should gradually replace the previous ration over a time course of no less than 2 wks [51]. See Sidebar 26.1.

26.5.1.3.1 Complementary Feed Transitions

Where increased dietary energy is required above that provided by forage alone, initial consideration should be given to high-energy, low-NSC feeds, such as non-molassed beet pulp, alfalfa meal, soy hulls, rice bran, or vegetable oil, although one study suggested an increased risk of colon volvulus in horses fed beet pulp [53].

Sidebar 26.1: Suggested Transition Schedule Between Feeds[a]

Transition day	1	4	8	12	16
			% Dry Matter Intake (DMI)		
Old feed	90	75	50	25	0
New feed	10	25	50	75	100

[a] Ensure horse receives at least >1% BW in forage DM daily.

Examples:

1) A 1000 lb BW adult horse eating 2% DMI is consuming 20 lb DM/d. Transition from old to new hay eating 22 lb as fed/d assuming both hays are 90% DM with no change to ration balancer intake (20 lb DM/0.9 = 22 lb as fed.)

Transition day	1	4	8	12	16
			lb/d as fed		
Old hay	20	17	11	6	0
New hay	2	6	11	17	22
Total hay	22	22	22	22	22

2) A 500 kg BW horse eating 2% DMI as 8 kg hay and 2 kg concentrate DM/d. Transition from 5.5% to 8% fat concentrate feed (both 90% DM) with no change to hay (2 kg concentrate DM/0.9 = 2.2 kg as fed.)

Transition day	1	4	8	12	16
			kg/d as fed		
Low fat	2.0	1.6	1.1	0.6	0
High fat	0.2	0.6	1.1	1.6	2.2[b]
Total concentrate	2.2	2.2	2.2	2.2	2.2

[b] When increasing fat intake, ensure <1 g fat/kg BW/d. When increasing NSC intake, ensure <1 g starch/kg BW/meal. New concentrate has 21% starch and 8.5% fat as fed. Feeding 2.2 kg in one meal provides 0.9 g starch and 0.4 g fat/kg BW.

3) A 1000 lb BW adult horse eating 2% DMI is consuming 20 lb DM/d. Transition from old hay (90% DM) to new pasture (35% DM) with no change to ration balancer intake.

Transition day	1	4	8	12	16
			lb/d as fed		
Old hay	20	17	11	6	0
Pasture	6	14	28	43	57
			lb/d DM		
Total DMI	20[c]	20	20	20	20

[c] [20 lb hay x 0.9 = 18 lb DM] + [6 lb pasture x 0.35 = 2 lb DM] = 20 lb DM/d.

If increasing dietary starch is necessary, intake should be maximized at 1 g/kg BW/meal using a cereal grain that has been heat-processed to improve starch digestibility. Meal feeding of a complementary feed with a higher-NSC content should be introduced over a 2 wks time course mixed with a chopped forage to minimize intraday fluctuations. However, avoidance of cereal starch is especially important in the prevention of duodenitis–proximal jejunitis and, in contrast, some starch intake might be beneficial in horses at risk of enterolithiasis. Adding fat to the ration for additional calories as rice bran or vegetable oil effectively and efficiently increases ration caloric density. Total intake of oil should be limited to 1 mL or g/kg BW, e.g., 2 cups oil/500 kg BW/d, as higher amounts may reduce the cellulolytic capacity of the hindgut. When calories are needed above recommendations to maintain BCS, and the caloric density of the ration increases, the formulation should be reviewed and balanced by an equine nutritionist.

26.5.1.3.2 Forage Transitions

When introducing pasture grazing to a colic-prone horse, time on pasture should be initially limited, in hand or with a grazing muzzle, and gradually increased over 2–3 wks, preferably during a time when pasture plant changes are minimal. Using temporary fencing to limit or control access to pasture is advisable. Pasture-grazing schedule should consider the temporal and climatic variations in NSC concentrations, i.e. highest during the day and in late spring/early summer, highest when temperatures are cool and the sunlight is bright. Long-term pasture management includes fertilization, mowing, and forage reseeding with cool-season vs. warm-season grasses vs. legumes [40]. Pasture turnout should be encouraged and generally helpful in reducing the risk of epiploic foramen entrapment, impactions, and colic in horses with crib-biting or wind-sucking behaviors. However, all-day grazing should be discouraged in horses with duodenitis–proximal jejunitis or where equine grass sickness has occurred previously.

When changing dried or preserved forages, laboratory analysis of structural and NSCs is essential to making a better-informed transition protocol. Generally, avoidance of highly lignified forages should help limit impaction colic, and alfalfa feeding should be limited to less than 50% of the forage intake in geographic regions where enteroliths are known to be prevalent. Haylage may be a preferable forage source to hay where colon volvulus is deemed to pose a particular risk, although colic in crib-biting and wind-sucking horses appears to be doubled when haylage rather than hay is fed. Controlling forage intake throughout a 24-hr period can be accomplished using the various sizes and single vs. doubling of hay nets, containing a mix of forages through the 2-wk transition period [61–64].

26.5.2 Diarrhea

26.5.2.1 Acute

26.5.2.1.1 Animal Assessment

Diarrhea resulting from dietary components is often suspected anecdotally although rarely defined in horses. In most cases of diarrhea in both foals and adults, the precise etiology is not identified. Nutritional factors were not taken into consideration by some large studies of diarrhea in adult horses as there is a far greater research interest in infectious causes [65–67]. Sudden dietary changes intuitively carry some risks, such as colic or diarrhea associated with dysbiosis. Although in most equine cases of colitis, the etiologic agent(s) remain(s) undetermined, marked differences in the microbiome are often found in comparison with healthy horses [68]. This suggests colitis may often be a disease of intestinal dysbiosis rather than simply being an overgrowth of a specific infectious pathogen.

26.5.2.1.2 Ration Assessment

Dietary factors known to produce diarrhea in horses include toxins, such as selenium, raw linseed oil, propylene glycol, castor beans, and acorns. The water source should be considered as diarrhea has been associated with a blue-green algae contamination. An outbreak of severe diarrhea has been reported in horses following ingestion of poor-quality water with a high-salinity and sulfate content [69]. Furthermore, sand ingestion is well known as an inflammatory factor in the intestines that can produce diarrhea, and overfeeding complete liquid enteral diets may cause diarrhea in hospitalized horses. See Assisted Feeding in Chapter 24.

Experimentally, high intakes of starch and oligofructose consistently induce diarrhea in horses, sometimes with systemic inflammatory response syndrome following endotoxin translocation across a compromised cecal–colonic mucosal barrier. Indeed, starch arriving in the hindgut after having exceeded the limited small intestinal digestive capacity, i.e. grain or carbohydrate overload, is among the most important causal factors to consider in the association between diet and diarrhea. Moreover, increased grazing is anecdotally recognized as a common cause of diarrhea, again perhaps following limited pre-cecal digestion of readily fermentable carbohydrates, i.e. simple sugars, fructans, and starches. The equine small intestine is relatively low in alpha-amylase with a limited capacity to digest starch [48]. Furthermore, all mammals lack enzymes capable of degrading fructans, although some pre-cecal bacterial fermentation of fructans is still possible owing to the gastric and small intestinal microbiome.

On the other hand, the normal and crucial fermentative efficiency of the equine large bowel is dependent on fibrolytic bacterial species, which ferment structural carbohydrates to VFAs, mainly acetate, propionate, and butyrate as the major source of energy to forage-fed horses. The composition and stability of these vital fermentative processes are key in helping to maintain intestinal health. High-cereal diets are likely to significantly increase hindgut delivery of starch, which will be hydrolyzed by amylolytic bacterial species resulting in rapid cecal–colonic acidification. Decreased pH will have an effect on hindgut microbiota further increasing amylolytic species and decreasing cellulolytic populations and, as a consequence, fiber digestibility and VFA absorption by the colon will decrease. A further effect of low pH is disruption of the normal intestinal mucosal barrier integrity leading to systemic absorption of bacterial lipopolysaccharide, exotoxins, and vasoactive amines.

26.5.2.1.3 Feeding Management

There is little specific evidence on which to base feeding advice to minimize the risk of diarrhea or to manage horses already affected by diarrhea. However, as dietary changes are strongly suspected in the etiology of many cases, optimizing the current diet must be considered alongside attempts to minimize sudden changes to the diet that the horse is currently receiving. Although temporary withholding of feed is sometimes advocated in cases of diarrhea, a lack of oral alimentation for more than 48 hrs can cause intestinal mucosal atrophy and loss of integrity that may contribute to a worsening of diarrhea or decreased ability to recover from diarrhea. Thus, except in cases where signs of colic coexist with diarrhea, withholding feed is not advisable.

Diarrhea is generally regarded as a disease of the large intestine and therefore dietary management should have the primary aim of promoting recovery and stability of the microbiome residing in the caecum and colon. Good-quality forage, RFV > 100, ingestion promotes VFA production, which, along with the amino acids glutamine and aspartate, is the primary source of nutrition for colonic enterocytes. Thus, initially, ad libitum access to good-quality hygienically clean grass or alfalfa hay is recommended. Where additional calories are considered important in horses that are markedly underweight or have increased caloric demands, e.g., lactation, a source of readily fermentable fiber, such as non-molassed sugar beet pulp, psyllium, or soy hulls, may be fed. NSC entering the large bowel would be likely due to the rapid intestinal transit times associated with diarrhea and therefore supplementary feeds with >5% starch should be avoided, or at least restricted to <0.5 g starch/kg BW/meal, until diarrhea has resolved. For similar reasons, temporary avoidance of grazing high-NSC grasses is advisable to facilitate stabilization of the cecal–colonic microbiome, although an occasional handful of grass, mixed in with chopped hay, may be useful to stimulate the appetite of anorexic horses.

Probiotics have been used in cases of diarrhea with varying results. Overall, more benefits for intestinal health have been reported with the use of yeasts than bacterial cultures. Yeast supplements, *Saccharomyces sp.*, administered to horses have been found by some to enhance fiber digestion and the number of anaerobic bacteria and some studies have indicated a beneficial clinical effect on diarrhea. However, despite widespread availability and use, good scientific evidence supporting commercial probiotic formulations in horses remains limited, several studies have shown no beneficial effects and sometimes an increased risk of diarrhea. Interference and manipulation of the microbiome to recreate a stable and diverse healthy microbial population through the simple addition of a single microbial species into a large and complex population are unlikely to provide a corrective effect to any disease process.

The administration of donor stool via enema or by nasogastric tube has been reported to be effective in controlling diarrhea associated with *Clostridium difficile* infections in humans. While there are no published studies in horses, anecdotal reports suggest that this form of therapy might also be effective in horses with acute colitis or chronic diarrhea [67, 70]. Although fecal transfaunation in horses may be associated with a risk of transmission of infectious disease, this could be avoided by testing the donor horse's feces before transfaunation. An important factor to consider in performing fecal transfaunation is the administration of oral antacids before the procedure to minimize microbial death in the acidic gastric environment.

26.5.2.2 Chronic

26.5.2.2.1 Animal Assessment

Chronic inflammatory bowel disease (CIBD) is a term used to include a group of intestinal diseases associated with chronic inflammatory infiltrates that produce similar clinical signs [71]. In adult horses, there are several subtypes of CIBD recognized, including granulomatous enteritis (GE), sarcoidosis, lymphocytic-plasmacytic enteritis, diffuse eosinophilic enteritis, focal eosinophilic enteritis, and multisystemic eosinophilic epitheliotropic disease (MEED). Additionally, other diseases with similar clinical presentation and consequences should be considered alongside CIBD, including parasitism, cyathostominosis in particular, non-steroidal anti-inflammatory drugs (NSAID) toxicity (right dorsal colitis), sand enteropathy, and infection with the obligate intracellular bacterium, *Lawsonia intracellularis*. The latter leads to the proliferation of crypt epithelial cells (proliferative enteropathy) primarily in weanlings, although it is occasionally seen in older horses.

Clinical signs of these conditions may include weight loss, diarrhea, colic, poor appetite, anemia, and dependent edema due to hypoalbuminemia. When diseases are restricted to the small intestine, e.g., *Lawsonia intracellularis* causing Equine proliferative enteropathy (EPE), the signs are most likely to include chronic weight loss, colic, and protein-losing enteropathy. However, diseases of the large intestine, e.g., parasitism, NSAID toxicity, some cases of CIBD, usually result in diarrhea, weight loss, and protein-losing enteropathy. Ultrasonography and absorption tests allow evaluation and a degree of classification of malabsorptive cases, although firm diagnosis relies on histological examination of biopsies. Although full-thickness jejunal, ileal, cecal, or colon biopsies are preferred, rectal and duodenal pinch biopsies can be collected more easily, although diagnostic power is limited relying on a distal and proximal extension of disease, respectively. In cases of systemic involvement, such as MEED, GE, and sarcoidosis, diagnostic samples, including biopsies, could also be taken from other affected organs, such as the liver, lungs, or skin.

Maldigestion and malabsorption of carbohydrates, protein, fat, mineral, and vitamins can have clinical and subclinical consequences. While malabsorption of carbohydrates is the best-recognized component due to the clinical use of oral glucose or xylose absorption tests, there are different clinical consequences associated with the malabsorption of other nutrients. In the case of fat malabsorption, absorption of fat-soluble vitamins is likely to be decreased with possible clinical consequences. Although intestinal inflammation might well lead to reduced vitamin E absorption, interestingly, the deficiency of selenium and vitamin E has been reported as a cause of eosinophilic enteritis in rats [72].

The etiology of CIBD in horses is unknown; however, some factors could be considered in association with the inflammatory reaction. It has been suggested that the disease process in human CIBD, a recognized delayed hypersensitivity reaction, and canine and feline CIBD, is mediated by hyper-reactive innate immune cells. Similarly, some authors have suggested hypersensitivity reactions as an important mechanism in the development of equine CIBD, although there is very little evidence concerning dietary hypersensitivities in horses [73, 74]. Gluten hypersensitivity is a well-recognized condition in humans and is worthy of consideration in horses also given the presence of wheat derivatives in many commercial equine feeds. However, thus far, although anti-gluten antibodies have been detected in some equine CIBD cases, similar findings exist in healthy horses fed a high-gluten diet.

Changes in the microbiota characterize CIBD cases in several species. Such changes may have consequences on immune reactivity within the enteric mucosa leading to mucosal reactive inflammatory responses to abnormal microbes as opposed to benign ignorance of the normal flora. However, it is also evident that mucosal inflammation and malabsorption might also affect the microbiota in both local and distant parts of the alimentary tract as nutrients are not processed and assimilated normally. For example, simple carbohydrates may reach the large colon in greater amounts following small intestinal maldigestion and malabsorption with obvious downstream consequences on microbial populations, pH, and fermentation leading to a higher risk of colic and diarrhea.

26.5.2.2.2 Ration Assessment

An important first goal in horses with malabsorption is to improve nutrient assimilation and maintain or improve BCS. See Feeding for Weight Gain in Chapter 23. Feeding horses with chronic diarrhea, in general, does not require an essential nutrient profile different from that recommended based on life stage, BW, and BCS [11]. However, due to decreased absorption, dietary concentrations may need to be increased and feed composition, forage-to-concentrate ratio, may be adjusted to improve digestibility. The precise nutritional plan will vary between cases and will be influenced by the anatomic area(s) of the intestinal tract that is affected. For example, where large intestinal disease predominates, a greater caloric reliance may be placed on nutrients likely to be digested in the small bowel, such as simple sugars and starches, protein, and fats. However, excessive provision of NSC in cases of small bowel malabsorption will result in hindgut dysbiosis as undigested, nutrient-rich chyme arrives in the caecum. Thus, a careful balance is required between different energy sources based on the dysfunctional vs. functional segments of the small and large intestines.

Key nutrients include those affected by intestinal inflammation and poor absorption. For example, an association between CIBD and equine motor neuron disease has been described suggesting that intestinal disease-causing malabsorption of vitamin E may trigger this neuromuscular condition [75]. Alternatively, omega-3 fatty acids have been shown to have anti-inflammatory properties in several species, including feeding docosahexaenoic acid (DHA) to horses [76–78]. Although a benefit on equine CIBD has not been investigated, there is potential merit in feeding omega-3 marine- or algae-derived DHA sources.

26.5.2.2.3 Feeding Management

An absolute minimum roughage DM requirement for any horse is 1% BW, whereas horses with healthy colons will ingest at least 2% BW. In horses with large bowel disease where maximal use of small intestinal digestive and absorptive processes is desirable, care should be taken to only supply NSC in amounts and frequency that match the digestive capacity of the small intestine. The recommendation is to feed not more than 1 g/kg BW sugar and starch per meal and no more frequently than every 6 hrs. This recommendation works out to a maximum of 1.1 kg of oats, a cereal grain providing energy, protein and fiber (Table 13.1), per meal to a 500 kg adult horse. Feeding such a meal of oats two times a day would provide 7.1 Mcal or 44% of the 16 Mcal DE required daily. The grain concentrate would have to be complemented with vitamins and minerals to meet dietary requirements and the remaining portion of the ration would be forage (5–8 kg/d). The forage-to-concentrate ratio would be adjusted as tolerated by the patient to accommodate large bowel dysfunction and subsequent recovery. Small intestinal digestion can be exploited further using highly caloric fat products, such as vegetable oil or rice bran. Any oil addition must be introduced gradually while feces are monitored for steatorrhea as this indicates fat is escaping digestion. Horses can digest rations containing as much as 20% fat DM when properly adapted [11, 79]. However, most diets contain 5–10% fat; hence, a gradual introduction of over 7–10 d of added fat is required. Additional vitamin E (alpha) at 1–1.5 IU/g fat added should be supplemented to limit the consequences of increased oxidative products.

In cases of small intestinal malabsorption, NSC and fat absorption would likely be compromised. Starch bypassing the small intestine to the large bowel favors rapid fermentation of starch and the proliferation of *Lactobacillus spp.*, which disrupts the microbial and pH balance, e.g., grain overload, and increases the risk of colic and laminitis. Fat bypassing the small intestine has been shown to further impair hindgut fiber fermentation presumably due to the generation of toxic organic acids following fat arrival in the caecum and colon. The recommendation would be to feed as little NSC and fat as tolerated by the patient, e.g., <10% NCS (0.1–0.5 g NSC/kg BW/meal) and <5% fat of ration DM. High-quality grass hay (RFV > 125) should be available ad libitum complemented with the meal feeding of a low-NSC–low-fat ration balancer providing vitamins, minerals, and protein or amino acids as required to meet nutritional requirements recommended based on life stage, BW, and BCS.

Case in Point

The owner of seven Tennessee Walking horses has requested help in improving his feeding program because, within the last 3 yrs, four horses have been treated for colic, one of which has had two episodes. The episodes of colic mostly have occurred in late winter and all horses were managed medically at his barn. He does show a few of these horses during the spring show schedule.

Animal Assessment

All horses have a BCS 3 or 4/9, range in age from 6 to 18 yrs old, and run together as a herd on about 20 acres year-round with a more than adequate sized three-sided run-in-shed available as shelter. All horses are dewormed regularly and are seen by a dental practitioner every 2 yr. Other than the episodes of colic, there have been no other medical problems. Physical examination of the horses revealed no concerns.

Ration Assessment

The pasture was reasonably maintained containing a mix of grass types with an estimated 10% weed invasion. The owner does chain-harrow the manure piles several times a year and does spray for weeds twice a year. There were two functioning water sources and white salt blocks in the run-in-shed. When the horses are "look'n dull," a scoop of of a sweet feed (7 lb) with vitamins and trace minerals is meal-fed once daily about a month before the show season.

The pasture could not support seven horses year-round even with rotational grazing. Hay is provided when the pasture is inadequate usually winter and summer. Large round bales, 900 lb/each, of mostly fescue are purchased locally and stored on gravel in a three-sided shed until needed. Of the hay remaining in the shed, 15% were sampled using a hay corer and submitted for laboratory nutrient analysis. The nutrient profile of the fescue bales on a DM basis was as follows:

DM	DE	CP	ADF	NDF	NSC
%	Mcal/kg	%	%	%	%
88	2.27	10.8	34.2	57.3	16.8

Feeding Management

When the horses do need some grain, the herd is fed together using 7 buckets hanging from the walls in the run-in-shed. When the pasture is inadequate, one fescue round bale at a time is placed in the open field lasting about 4–7 days, depending on the weather.

1) *Calculate relative feeding value (RFV) and nutritional quality of the forage.*
2) *What subjective information about the hay would be helpful?*
3) *What additional information about the feeding of the sweet feed would be helpful?*
4) *Given there are several possible reasons for the episodes of colic in this case, what dietary recommendations would lower the risk of colic reoccurrence?*

See Appendix A Chapter 26

References

1 Murray, J.M.D., Bloxham, C., Kulifay, J. et al. (2015). Equine nutrition: a survey of perceptions and practices of horse owners undertaking a massive open online course in equine nutrition. *J. Equine Vet. Sci.* 35 (6): 510–517.

2 Easley, J., Dixon, P.M., and Schumacher, J. (eds.) (2010). *Equine Dentistry*. 3e, 1–410. Edinburgh: Saunders Elsevier.

3 Sanchez, L.C. (2018). Disorders of the gastrointestinal system. In: *Equine Internal Medicine*, 4e (ed. S.M. Reed, W.M. Bayly and D.C. Sellon), 709–842. Elsevier.

4 USDA APHIS (2020). Equine Teeth and Aging. https://www.aphis.usda.gov/aphis/ourfocus/animalhealth/nvap/NVAP-Reference-Guide/Appendix/Equine-Teeth-and-Aging (accessed 5 January 2022).

5 Jacobs, R.D., Gordon, M.E., Jerina, M.L., and Fenton, J. (2021). 95 Equine chewing is influenced by dental intervention. *J. Equine Vet. Sci.* 100: 103558.

6 Easley, J. and Tremaine, W. (2010). Dental and oral examinations. In: *Equine Dentistry*, 3e (ed. J. Easley, P.M. Dixon, and J. Schumacher), 3e, 185–198. Philadelphia: Elsevier Health Sciences.

7 Whittle, B.P. (2021). Equine oral anatomy: what a veterinarian needs to know. *Southwest Veterinary Symposium*, San Antonio, TX.

8 Limone, L.E. (2020). Update on equine odontoclastic tooth resorption and hypercementosis. *Vet. Clin. N. Am. Equine Pract.* 36: 671–689.

9 Ralston, S.L., Foster, D.L., Divers, T., and Hintz, H.F. (2001). Effect of dental correction on feed digestibility in horses. *Equine Vet. J.* 33 (4): 390–393.

10 Carmalt, J.L. and Allen, A. (2008). The relationship between cheek tooth occlusal morphology, apparent

digestibility, and ingesta particle size reduction in horses. *J. Am. Vet. Med. Assoc.* 233 (3): 452–455.
11 National Research Council (2007). *Nutrient Requirements of Horses*. 6th Rev. Animal Nutrition Series, 1–341. Washington, DC: National Academies Press.
12 Duncanson, G.R. (2006). Equine oesophageal obstruction: a long term study of 60 cases. *Equine Vet. Educ.* 18 (5): 262–265.
13 Komine, M., Langohr, I.M., and Kiupel, M. (2014). Megaesophagus in Friesian horses associated with muscular hypertrophy of the caudal esophagus. *Vet. Pathol.* 51 (5): 979–985.
14 Broekman, L.E. and Kuiper, D. (2002). Megaesophagus in the horse. A short review of the literature and 18 own cases. *Vet. Q.* 24 (4): 199–202.
15 Fubini, S.L. (2002). Esophageal obstruction. In: *Manual of Equine Gastroenterology* (ed. T.S. Mair, T.J. Divers, and N.G. Ducharme), 92–93. London: W.B. Saunders.
16 Chiavaccini, L. and Hassel, D.M. (2010). Clinical features and prognostic variables in 109 horses with esophageal obstruction (1992–2009). *J. Vet. Intern. Med.* 24 (5): 1147–1152.
17 Di Pilato, V., Freschi, G., Ringressi, M.N. et al. (2016). The esophageal microbiota in health and disease. *Ann. N. Y. Acad. Sci.* 1381 (1): 21–33.
18 Benitez, A.J., Hoffmann, C., Muir, A.B. et al. (2015). Inflammation-associated microbiota in pediatric eosinophilic esophagitis. *Microbiome* 3: 23.
19 Harris, J.K., Fang, R., Wagner, B.D. et al. (2015). Esophageal microbiome in eosinophilic esophagitis. *PLoS One* 10 (5): e0128346.
20 Narikiyo, M., Tanabe, C., Yamada, Y. et al. (2004). Frequent and preferential infection of *Treponema denticola*, *Streptococcus mitis*, and *Streptococcus anginosus* in esophageal cancers. *Cancer Sci.* 95 (7): 569–574.
21 Meyer, W., Kacza, J., Schnapper, A. et al. (2010). A first report on the microbial colonisation of the equine oesophagus. *Ann. Anat.* 192 (1): 42–51.
22 Hillyer, M. (1995). Management of oesophageal obstruction ("choke") in horses. *In Pract.* 17 (10): 450–457.
23 Feige, K., Schwarzwald, C., Fürst, A., and Kaser-Hotz, B. (2000). Esophageal obstruction in horses: a retrospective study of 34 cases. *Can. Vet. J.* 41 (3): 207–210.
24 Craig, D.R., Shivy, D.R., Pankowski, R.L., and Erb, H.N. (1989). Esophageal disorders in 61 horses. Results of nonsurgical and surgical management. *Vet. Surg.* 18 (6): 432–438.
25 Hammond, C.J., Mason, D.K., and Watkins, K.L. (1986). Gastric ulceration in mature Thoroughbred horses. *Equine Vet. J.* 18 (4): 284–287.
26 Luthersson, N., Nielsen, K.H., Harris, P. et al. (2009). Risk factors associated with equine gastric ulceration syndrome (EGUS) in 201 horses in Denmark. *Equine Vet. J.* 41 (7): 625–630.
27 Nadeau, J.A., Andrews, F.M., Patton, C.S. et al. (2003). Effects of hydrochloric, acetic, butyric, and propionic acids on pathogenesis of ulcers in the nonglandular portion of the stomach of horses. *Am. J. Vet. Res.* 64 (4): 404–412.
28 Nadeau, J.A., Andrews, F.M., Patton, C.S. et al. (2003). Effects of hydrochloric, valeric and other volatile fatty acids on pathogenesis of ulcers in the nonglandular portion of the stomach of horses. *Am. J. Vet. Res.* 64 (4): 413–417.
29 Berschneider, H.M., Blikslager, A.T., and Roberts, M.C. (1999). Role of duodenal reflux in nonglandular gastric ulcer disease of the mature horse. *Equine Vet. J.* 31 (S29): 24–29.
30 Lorenzo-Figueras, M. and Merritt, A.M. (2002). Effects of exercise on gastric volume and pH in the proximal portion of the stomach of horses. *Am. J. Vet. Res.* 63 (11): 1481–1487.
31 Nadeau, J.A., Andrews, F.M., Mathew, A.G. et al. (2000). Evaluation of diet as a cause of gastric ulcers in horses. *Am. J. Vet. Res.* 61 (7): 784–790.
32 Lybbert T, Gibbs P, Cohen N, et al. (2007). Feeding alfalfa hay to exercising horses reduces the severity of gastric squamous mucosal ulceration. In: *Proceedings of the 53th Annual Convention of the American Association of Equine Practitioners*. 525–526. Orlando, FL: American Association of Equine Practitioners (AAEP).
33 Le Jeune, S., Nieto, J., Dechant, J., and Snyder, J. (2009). Prevalence of gastric ulcers in Thoroughbred broodmares in pasture: a preliminary report. *Vet. J.* 181 (3): 251–255.
34 Luthersson, N. and Nadeau, J.A. (2013). Gastric ulceration. In: *Equine Applied and Clinical Nutrition: Health, Welfare and Performance* (ed. R.J. Geor, P.A. Harris, and M. Coenen), 558–567. Edinburgh: Saunders Elsevier.
35 Bell, R.J.W., Kingston, J.K., Mogg, T.D., and Perkins, N.R. (2007). The prevalence of gastric ulceration in racehorses in New Zealand. *N. Z. Vet. J.* 55 (1): 13–18.
36 Cargile, J.L., Burrow, J.A., Kim, I. et al. (2004). Effect of dietary corn oil supplementation on equine gastric fluid acid, sodium, and prostaglandin E2 content before and during pentagastrin infusion. *J. Vet. Intern. Med.* 18 (4): 545–549.
37 Frank, N., Andrews, F.M., Elliott, S.B., and Lew, J. (2005). Effects of dietary oils on the development of gastric ulcers in mares. *Am. J. Vet. Res.* 66 (11): 2006–2011.
38 Holbrook, T.C., Simmons, R.D., Payton, M.E., and MacAllister, C.G. (2005). Effect of repeated oral

administration of hypertonic electrolyte solution on equine gastric mucosa. *Equine Vet. J.* 37 (6): 501–504.

39 Reese, R.E. and Andrews, F.M. (2009). Nutrition and dietary management of equine gastric ulcer syndrome. *Vet. Clin. Equine Pract.* 25 (1): 79–92.

40 Watts, K. (2010). Pasture management to minimize the risk of equine laminitis. *Vet. Clin. North Am. Equine Pract.* 26 (2): 361–369.

41 Vainio, K., Sykes, B.W., and Blikslager, A.T. (2011). Primary gastric impaction in horses: a retrospective study of 20 cases (2005–2008). *Equine Vet. Educ.* 23 (4): 186–190.

42 Bird, A.R., Knowles, E.J., Sherlock, C.E. et al. (2012). The clinical and pathological features of gastric impaction in twelve horses. *Equine Vet. J.* 44: 105–110.

43 Kentucky Equine Research Staff (2018). Benefits of beet pulp for horses. *EquiNews*. https://ker.com/equinews/benefits-beet-pulp-horses (accessed 20 January 2022).

44 Pratt-Phillips, S.E., Stuska, S., Beveridge, H.L., and Yoder, M. (2011). Nutritional quality of forages consumed by feral horses: the horses of Shackleford banks. *J. Equine Vet. Sci.* 31 (11): 640–644.

45 Durham, A. (2013). Intestinal disease. In: *Equine Applied and Clinical Nutrition: Health, Welfare and Performance*. 568–581. (ed. R.J. Geor, P.A. Harris, and M. Coenen), 568–581. Edinburgh: Saunders Elsevier.

46 Traub-Dargatz, J.L., Kopral, C.A., Seitzinger, A.H. et al. (2001). Estimate of the national incidence of and operation-level risk factors for colic among horses in the United States, spring 1998 to spring 1999. *J. Am. Vet. Med. Assoc.* 219 (1): 67–71.

47 Tinker, M.K. (1995). A farm-based prospective study for equine colic risk factors and risk associated events. Ph.D. thesis. Virginia Polytechnic Institute and State University.

48 Dyer, J., Fernandez-Castano Merediz, E., Salmon, K.S. et al. (2002). Molecular characterisation of carbohydrate digestion and absorption in equine small intestine. *Equine Vet. J.* 34 (4): 349–358.

49 Potter, G.D., Arnold, F.F., Householder, D.D. et al. (1992). Digestion of starch in the small or large intestine of the equine. *Pferdeheilkunde* 1 (4): 107–111.

50 Tinker, M.K., White, N.A., Lessard, P. et al. (1997). Prospective study of equine colic risk factors. *Equine Vet. J.* 29 (6): 454–458.

51 Cohen, N.D., Gibbs, P.G., and Woods, A.M. (1999). Dietary and other management factors associated with equine colic. *J. Am. Vet. Med. Assoc.* 215 (1): 53–60.

52 Hudson, J.M., Cohen, N.D., Gibbs, P.G., and Thompson, J.A. (2001). Feeding practices associated with colic in horses. *J. Am. Vet. Med. Assoc.* 219 (10): 1419–1425.

53 Suthers, J.M., Pinchbeck, G.L., Proudman, C.J., and Archer, D.C. (2013). Risk factors for large colon volvulus in the UK. *Equine Vet. J.* 45 (5): 558–563.

54 Kaya, G., Sommerfeld-Stur, I., and Iben, C. (2009). Risk factors of colic in horses in Austria. *J. Anim. Physiol. Anim. Nutr. (Berl).* 93 (3): 339–349.

55 Ball, D., Hoveland, C., and Lacefield, G. (2007). Forage quality. In: *Southern Forages. Modern Concepts for Forage Crop Management*, 4e, 136–145. Norcross, GA: International Plant Nutrition Institute.

56 Hillyer, M.H., Taylor, F.G.R., Proudman, C.J. et al. (2002). Case control study to identify risk factors for simple colonic obstruction and distension colic in horses. *Equine Vet. J.* 34 (5): 455–463.

57 Little, D. and Blikslager, A.T. (2002). Factors associated with development of ileal impaction in horses with surgical colic: 78 cases (1986–2000). *Equine Vet. J.* 34 (5): 464–468.

58 Cohen, N.D., Toby, E., Roussel, A.J. et al. (2006). Are feeding practices associated with duodenitis-proximal jejunitis? *Equine Vet. J.* 38 (6): 526–531.

59 Morris, D.D., Moore, J.N., and Ward, S. (1989). Comparison of age, sex, breed, history and management in 229 horses with colic. *Equine Vet. J. Suppl.* 7: 129–132.

60 Hassel, D.M., Aldridge, B.M., Drake, C.M., and Snyder, J.R. (2008). Evaluation of dietary and management risk factors for enterolithiasis among horses in California. *Res. Vet. Sci.* 85 (3): 476–480.

61 Rochais, C., Henry, S., and Hausberger, M. (2018). "Hay-bags" and "slow feeders": testing their impact on horse behaviour and welfare. *Appl. Anim. Behav. Sci.* 198 (1): 52–59.

62 Glunk, E.C., Hathaway, M.R., Grev, A.M. et al. (2015). The effect of a limit-fed diet and slow-feed hay nets on morphometric measurements and postprandial metabolite and hormone patterns in adult horses. *J. Anim. Sci.* 93 (8): 4144–4152.

63 Glunk, E.C., Pratt-Phillips, S.E., and Siciliano, P.D. (2013). Effect of restricted pasture access on pasture dry matter intake rate, dietary energy intake, and fecal pH in horses. *J. Equine Vet. Sci.* 33 (6): 421–426.

64 Glunk, E.C., Sheaffer, C.C., Hathaway, M.R., and Martinson, K.L. (2014). Interaction of grazing muzzle use and grass species on forage intake of horses. *J. Equine Vet. Sci.* 34 (7): 930–933.

65 Love, S., Mair, T.S., and Hillyer, M.H. (1992). Chronic diarrhoea in adult horses: a review of 51 referred cases. *Vet. Rec.* 130 (11): 217–219.

66 Mair, T.S., de Westerlaken, L.V., Cripps, P.J., and Love, S. (1990). Diarrhoea in adult horses: a survey of clinical cases and an assessment of some prognostic indices. *Vet. Rec.* 126 (19): 479–481.

67 Feary, D.J. and Hassel, D.M. (2006). Enteritis and colitis in horses. *Vet. Clin. North Am. Equine Pract.* 22 (2): 437–479.

68 Costa, M.C., Arroyo, L.G., Allen-Vercoe, E. et al. (2012). Comparison of the fecal microbiota of healthy horses and horses with colitis by high throughput sequencing of the V3-V5 region of the 16s rRNA gene. *PLoS One* 7 (7): e41484.

69 Burgess, B.A., Lohmann, K.L., and Blakley, B.R. (2010). Excessive sulfate and poor water quality as a cause of sudden deaths and an outbreak of diarrhea in horses. *Can. Vet. J.* 51 (3): 277–282.

70 Mullen, K.R., Yasuda, K., Divers, T.J., and Weese, J.S. (2016). Equine faecal microbiota transplant: current knowledge, proposed guidelines and future directions. *Equine Vet. Educ.* 30 (3): 151–160.

71 Schumacher, J. (2009). Infiltrative bowel diseases. In: *Current Therapy in Equine Medicine*, 6e (ed. E.N. Robinson and K.A. Sprayberry), 439–442. Saint Louis, MO: W.B. Saunders.

72 Hong, C.B. and Chow, C.K. (1988). Induction of eosinophilic enteritis and eosinophilia in rats by vitamin E and selenium deficiency. *Exp. Mol. Pathol.* 48 (2): 182–192.

73 Lindberg, R., Persson, S.G.B., Jones, B. et al. (1985). Clinical and pathophysiological features of granulomatous enteritis and eosinophilic granulomatosis in the horse. *Zentralbl. Veterinärmed. A* 32 (1–10): 526–539.

74 Sanford, S.E. (1989). Multisystemic eosinophilic epitheliotropic disease in a horse. *Can. Vet. J.* 30 (3): 253–254.

75 Díez de Castro, E., Zafra, R., Acevedo, L.M. et al. (2016). Eosinophilic enteritis in horses with motor neuron disease. *J. Vet. Intern. Med.* 30 (3): 873–879.

76 Nogradi, N., Couetil, L.L., Messick, J. et al. (2015). Omega-3 fatty acid supplementation provides an additional benefit to a low-dust diet in the management of horses with chronic lower airway inflammatory disease. *J. Vet. Intern. Med.* 29 (1): 299–306.

77 Christmann, U., Hancock, C.L., Poole, C.M. et al. (2021). Dynamics of DHA and EPA supplementation: incorporation into equine plasma, synovial fluid, and surfactant glycerophosphocholines. *Metabolomics* 17 (5): 1–10.

78 Elzinga, S.E., Betancourt, A., Stewart, J.C. et al. (2019). Effects of docosahexaenoic acid–rich microalgae supplementation on metabolic and inflammatory parameters in horses with equine metabolic syndrome. *J. Equine Vet. Sci.* 83: 102811.

79 Kronfeld, D.S., Holland, J.L., Rich, G.A. et al. (2004). Fat digestibility in Equus caballus follows increasing first-order kinetics. *J. Anim. Sci.* 82 (6): 1773–1780.

27

Endocrine System Disorders

Nicholas Frank, Elizabeth M. Tadros, and Rebecca L. Remillard

KEY TERMS

- Starch is a polysaccharide found primarily in the seed (grain) and/or root (tuber) portions of plants and can be estimated using a laboratory starch analysis procedure.
- Ethanol-soluble carbohydrate (ESC) is a laboratory procedure to estimate the monosaccharides, disaccharides, oligosaccharides, (sugars) and a small fraction of (short-chain) fructans in plant material.
- Water-soluble carbohydrate (WSC) is a laboratory procedure to estimate all of ESC components plus all fructans in plant material.
- Non-structural carbohydrate (NSC) is *calculated* as WSC plus starch. See Figure 6.2.

KEY POINTS

- Insulin dysregulation (ID) is a metabolic derangement that manifests as any combination of fasting and/or postprandial hyperinsulinemia, exaggerated insulin responses to oral/intravenous sugar, tissue insulin resistance (IR), and dyslipidemia [1].
- Equine metabolic syndrome (EMS) is a constellation of abnormalities, including generalized obesity and/or regional adiposity, and clinical or subclinical endocrinopathic laminitis; a less common, lean phenotype is also recognized [2].
- Pituitary pars intermedia dysfunction (PPID) is a neurodegenerative disease that occurs in 15–30% of aged horses causing loss of dopaminergic inhibitory input to the melanotropes of the pars intermedia and subsequent hormonal dysregulation [3].
- Equine hyperlipemia (EH) results from elevated serum lipid concentrations secondary to negative energy balance and excessive mobilization of fatty acids from adipose resulting in organ failure due to excessive fat infiltration.

27.1 Insulin Dysregulation

ID is of importance because it is the shared pathophysiological abnormality underlying laminitis in both EMS and PPID. ID is central to the pathogenesis of EMS and affects 30–60% of horses with PPID [1, 3, 4]. The most devastating complication of both PPID and EMS is endocrinopathic laminitis. This crippling form of lameness occurs when hormonal abnormalities damage the laminae attaching the hoof capsule to the underlying bone. Weakened laminar tissues are unable to withstand the mechanical forces associated with locomotion, resulting in laminar disruption and displacement, with rotation and/or sinking of the distal phalanx within the hoof capsules. Preventing laminitis is of utmost importance because there is currently no cure for the condition; resultant pain can end a horse's athletic career and, sometimes, become severe enough to necessitate euthanasia.

27.1.1 Introduction

27.1.1.1 Functions of Insulin in Macronutrient Metabolism

Insulin is one of the central regulators of macronutrient metabolism, primarily through actions on the liver, skeletal muscle, and adipose tissues.

27.1.1.1.1 Insulin Signaling

The insulin receptor is a dimer composed of two α-subunits and two β-subunits. The α-subunits are on the extracellular face of the cell membrane, while the β-subunits span the membrane and have cytosolic portions that possess tyrosine kinase activity. Insulin binds to the α-subunits, inducing a conformational change in the β-subunits and subsequent autophosphorylation of the β-subunits on three tyrosine residues. The β-subunits then acquire tyrosine kinase activity and phosphorylate downstream adaptor proteins, including insulin receptor substrate (i) in muscle

Equine Clinical Nutrition, Second Edition. Edited by Rebecca L. Remillard.

and adipose tissues and insulin receptor substrate; (ii) in the liver, leading to phosphoinositide; and (iii) kinase activation. This post-receptor pathway is most important for glucose metabolism because it is required for glucose GLUT4 transporter translocation from intracellular storage vesicles to the cell membrane following ingestion of glucose, as well as regulation of metabolic enzymes. In the unstimulated state, GLUT4 is largely sequestered in intracellular vesicles, with only about 4–10% cycling to the cell surface at any given time [5]. It can therefore be appreciated that abnormalities in post-receptor signaling pathways will reduce insulin mobilization of GLUT4 to the cell surface, as well as reducing the ability to phosphorylate and regulate metabolic genes. Synthesis and catabolism for a given macronutrient are generally regulated in tandem. This is often accomplished through phosphorylation or changes in gene expression of key pathway enzymes. Hormones, such as insulin, can promote activity in one pathway, e.g. synthesis, while concurrently inhibiting the opposing pathway, e.g. catabolism.

27.1.1.1.2 Insulin's Role in Metabolism

Insulin secretion increases following a meal, and insulin plays the dominant role in regulating glucose metabolism in the fed state. Rising blood glucose concentration is detected by pancreatic β-cells and stimulates β-cell insulin secretion. Secretion of glucagon, which raises blood sugar, from pancreatic α-cells also declines as blood glucose concentrations rise. Insulin promotes GLUT4-mediated glucose uptake into adipose and skeletal muscle tissues. Glucose is then either oxidized or converted in muscle to glycogen. In adipose tissue, glucose is either oxidized for energy or partially oxidized to obtain a 3-carbon glycerol backbone and with esterified fatty acids form triglycerides (TG). In the liver, insulin promotes glycogen synthesis, while inhibiting glycogenolysis. It also promotes the activity of hexokinases, including glucokinase, thereby increasing glycolysis while glucose is abundant. Insulin restrains hepatic gluconeogenesis.

In general, insulin promotes the storage of fat by increasing the activity of lipoprotein lipase and dietary fats are taken into body's storage depots. Insulin also decreases the activity of hormone-sensitive lipase and inhibits lipolysis. These effects occur primarily not only in adipose tissue, but also in muscle since myocytes store lipids as intramyocellular TG. Hepatic fatty acid synthesis is enhanced in response to insulin's actions. Insulin has mild effects on amino acid metabolism. In conjunction with growth hormone, acting through insulin-like growth factor-1 (IGF-1), protein synthesis is promoted while catabolism is inhibited. Inhibition of protein catabolism is the main mechanism through which insulin is anabolic and promotes growth. Insulin may also enhance the uptake of amino acids by increasing the activity of amino acid transporters, although this is only a minor function of the hormone.

27.1.1.1.3 The Enteroinsular Axis

Pancreatic insulin responses are enhanced when glucose is absorbed enterally, as opposed to when administered parenterally. This is due to the influence of the enteroinsular axis, which consists of neuronal and hormonal factors released by the intestine under conditions of hyperglycemia that augment postprandial insulin secretion by stimulating pancreatic β-cells [6]. When luminal glucose concentration increases above a threshold, this is detected by endocrine cells of the intestinal wall. Hormones called incretins are then secreted and interact with receptors on pancreatic β-cells to stimulate insulin secretion. The two incretins of biological importance are glucose-dependent insulinotropic polypeptide, which is synthesized and secreted by K cells of the upper small intestine, and glucagon-like peptide-1 (GLP-1), which is synthesized and secreted by L cells of the lower small intestine and colon. Once released into circulation, incretins are rapidly degraded by the dipeptidyl peptidase-4 enzyme and excreted by the kidneys; this renders the effects transient, with half-lives of 2 and 5 min for GLP-1 and glucose-dependent insulinotropic polypeptide, respectively, in humans [6].

27.1.1.2 Pathogenesis of Insulin Dysregulation

Disruption of normal insulin homeostasis can occur on multiple levels, from abnormalities in pancreatic insulin release to tissue IR. Insulin resistance refers to the failure of insulin-sensitive tissues to respond to insulin; the skeletal muscle, adipose, and liver are primarily affected. Consequences of IR result from the failure of insulin to elicit normal physiological effects, including impaired tissue uptake of glucose, increased hepatic gluconeogenesis, and increased lipolysis resulting in higher circulating free fatty acid concentrations. Metabolism of macronutrients can be affected by ID, with the most profound effects on carbohydrate and lipid metabolism.

Clinically, the most important components of ID in the horse are hyperinsulinemia, hyperglycemia, and dyslipidemia. Hyperinsulinemia can develop because of enteroinsular axis overactivity or as a compensatory mechanism by the pancreas to override peripheral tissue IR with enhanced insulin output. Hyperglycemia is most often encountered in horses with EMS and PPID when the hyperinsulinemic state is unable to control blood glucose concentration, known as uncompensated IR. Although uncommon, overt type 2 diabetes mellitus also occurs, particularly in horses with PPID. In these cases, pancreatic insulin output declines due to β-cell exhaustion, and glycemic control is lost.

Horses with ID are predisposed to EH, often precipitated by a state of negative energy balance, such as anorexia during illness. If the affected animal develops severe hepatic lipidosis, the clinical prognosis is poor, with death sometimes occurring due to either fulminant hepatic failure or liver rupture and hemorrhage [7]. Because liver enzyme activity is sometimes elevated in ID-affected equids without overt hepatic failure, chronic mild hepatic lipidosis and resultant dysfunction might also impair hepatic clearance of insulin from circulation, thereby contributing to hyperinsulinemia [8, 9].

27.1.1.2.1 Genetic and Environmental Interactions

The development of ID is the culmination of interactions between genetic, physiological, and environmental risk factors. A horse with underlying genetic risks may avoid developing ID if the environment is optimal. However, decompensation and overt ID occur when at-risk individuals experience multiple factors that negatively affect metabolism. The genetics of ID and EMS are currently under investigation. Predisposing traits likely include “thrifty” genes that promote metabolic efficiency [10]. Surviving on limited nutritional resources was historically advantageous. However, modern management conditions, where food is plentiful and exercise is in short supply, put thrifty individuals at risk of becoming obese and developing ID.

Breed differences in innate insulin sensitivity have been demonstrated. For example, insulin sensitivity is lower and insulinemic responses to carbohydrate challenges (oral and intravenous) are higher in ponies and Andalusians compared to Standardbreds [11]. Insulin resistance and compensatory hyperinsulinemia are more easily triggered in these animals. Genetic differences may also promote heightened incretin responses to oral carbohydrates. Breeds, such as ponies and Andalusians, secrete more GLP-1 after oral carbohydrate ingestion than Standardbreds and this correlates positively with higher postprandial insulin concentrations [12]. There is also evidence that abnormally exaggerated GLP-1 responses might be responsible for postprandial hyperinsulinemia in ponies with ID [13]. The innate function of the enteroinsular axis may therefore predispose at-risk individuals to hyperinsulinemia and laminitis, particularly if they are fed diets relatively high in sugar and starch. In these cases, hyperinsulinemia can develop in the absence of tissue IR [13].

As an individual's genetic predispositions and threshold for developing ID are unknown, it is prudent to preemptively eliminate controllable factors that exacerbate ID, particularly in high-risk breeds. Obesity is better avoided through good husbandry than treated. NSC content should routinely be minimized in the rations of animals at risk of developing hyperinsulinemia. Certain situations are unavoidable, including the development of concurrent illnesses that disrupt glucose and insulin metabolism; the most common of these are PPID, systemic inflammation, and sepsis. However, awareness that these conditions exacerbate ID is important because measures, such as routine PPID screening and close attention to energy homeostasis during systemic illness, can help mitigate the development of severe metabolic derangements.

27.1.1.2.2 The Role of Obesity in Equine Metabolic Syndrome and Insulin Dysregulation

The classic triad of abnormalities defining EMS includes (i) generalized obesity and/or regional adiposity; (ii) ID, hyperinsulinemia, IR, and/or exaggerated insulin responses to oral or intravenous starch and sugars; and (iii) clinical or subclinical endocrinopathic laminitis [2]. While the majority of affected animals are obese, there is recognition of a lean phenotype; such animals appear physically normal but might have increased adiposity of less visible internal fat depots that adversely affects metabolism. Although abnormal adiposity and ID are associated, their relationships to each another are complex and incompletely understood in equids. The degree to which obesity induces or exacerbates ID likely depends on interactions between each individual's underlying genetic predispositions, environment and physiological factors [1].

Obesity was once viewed as central to EMS pathophysiology, but a recent paradigm shift has focused attention on ID as the fundamental abnormality. In other species, obesity-induced adipocyte dysfunction creates a systemic pro-inflammatory state, with resultant disruption of post-receptor insulin signaling, IR, and compensatory hyperinsulinemia [14]. The role of inflammation in equine obesity remains controversial, as abnormal basal inflammatory states are inconsistently identified; however, EMS-affected animals experience exaggerated systemic inflammatory responses to an oral sugar administration and an immunological challenge [15, 16]. Because inflammation is a variable finding, it is possible that other mechanisms, such as abnormal adipokine release, play a more important role in obesity-related ID in horses. In the obese state, secretion of the insulin-sensitizing adipokine adiponectin is reduced; some studies suggest that hypoadiponectinemia is more closely associated with IR than the degree of obesity [17]. If obesity leads to intrahepatic fat accumulation and mild liver dysfunction, this could decrease insulin clearance and also contribute to hyperinsulinemia.

Animals that become obese do not invariably develop ID [17, 18]. The reason why some individuals tolerate being overweight better than others likely depends on whether they have underlying genetic predispositions toward metabolic derangements or concurrent exposure to additional risk factors, such as a high-sugar ration. Improved understanding of these relationships will enable better customization of nutritional plans. Because weight loss is difficult to achieve and requires a substantial commitment on the part of caretakers, it may be helpful to identify those animals that would benefit most from losing weight in addition to reducing dietary hydrolyzable carbohydrate intake. While horses can lose weight and experience improvement in ID, poor owner compliance is a major factor in treatment failure and success often relies on sufficient veterinary guidance and support [19, 20]. Furthermore, some animals are weight loss resistant and require severe caloric restriction before losing body condition [21]. In certain situations, emphasizing owner compliance with dietary recommendations and eliminating sugar, e.g. molasses, and starch, e.g. cereal grains, may improve ID even in the absence of substantial weight loss.

While obesity and/or regional adiposity is the most prevalent phenotype, lean animals can also suffer from ID. These metabolic abnormalities are sometimes related to PPID, but ID can occur as an isolated abnormality in phenotypically normal equids. It can also persist in formerly obese equids that have lost weight [22]. The focus of managing such cases is lowering the sugar content of the ration while meeting the animal's caloric requirement using low NSC forages or rations supplemented with vegetable oils, beet pulp, rice bran, or commercial fat products.

27.1.1.2.3 The Role of Pituitary Pars Intermedia Dysfunction in Insulin Dysregulation

There remains debate about the relationship between PPID and ID, as not all equids with PPID are affected by ID [23]. One possibility is that these are independent conditions that can occur either individually or concurrently; identifying them together may simply represent the coexistence of two common endocrinopathies in the same animal. Given the prevalence of obesity, it is inevitable that some of these metabolically unhealthy animals also develop PPID with age. Alternatively, PPID may induce or exacerbate ID and hyperinsulinemia, particularly in animals with predisposing genetic or environmental risk factors.

In the past, hyperinsulinemia in equids with PPID was attributed to the antagonistic effects of hypercortisolemia on insulin sensitivity. However, an improved understanding of PPID led to the conclusion that cortisol excess is not the dominant feature of the disease in most animals [3]. While hypercortisolemia might play a role in some cases, pathologically high pituitary hormone concentrations are likely the more important drivers of ID. For example, corticotropin-like intermediate lobe peptides and other adrenocorticotropic hormone (ACTH) fragments act as insulin secretagogues in pancreatic β-cells [24, 25]. Heterogeneity in the severity of pituitary lesions, as well as individual variability in the specific proopiomelanocortin-derived peptide profile secreted by the diseased pars intermedia, might explain why PPID induces ID in a subset of affected animals. The presence of mild hepatic dysfunction due to either PPID-associated dyslipidemia or steroid hepatopathy could further exacerbate hyperinsulinemia in some animals by decreasing insulin clearance.

27.1.1.2.4 Aging and Insulin Dysregulation

As in other species, insulin sensitivity decreases with age in horses, and insulin responses to oral and intravenous glucose challenges are exaggerated [26, 27]. Therefore, it is important to consider the effect of pathological conditions that induce hyperinsulinemia superimposed on the normal age-related decline in insulin sensitivity. Mechanisms implicated in causing age-related IR include inflammation, oxidative stress, mitochondrial dysfunction, increased visceral adiposity, decreased lean muscle mass, and reduced physical activity [28]. Because geriatric horses may have heightened insulin responses, pathological conditions that exacerbate ID might increase the risk of developing hyperinsulinemia and endocrinopathic laminitis.

27.1.1.2.5 Hyperinsulinemia and Endocrinopathic Laminitis

Hyperinsulinemia and ID are established risk factors for laminitis and evidence is mounting for hyperinsulinemia as the causative factor of endocrinopathic laminitis in both EMS and PPID [1, 29, 30]. Of all ID components, chronic hyperinsulinemia appears to be the most detrimental, as insulin administration at supraphysiological doses to healthy ponies and Standardbred horses induced laminitis within 48–72 hrs [31, 32]. Pathologically high circulating insulin concentrations are believed to aberrantly activate the laminar epidermal epithelial cell IGF-1 receptor, which shares close structural homology with the insulin receptor and is responsive to supraphysiological insulin concentrations [33]. The IGF-1 receptor is multifunctional and regulates cell growth, adhesion, proliferation, differentiation, and apoptosis. Aberrant activation causes alterations in tissue growth and repair due to abnormal laminar keratinocyte proliferation and maturation, cytoskeletal dysfunction, and changes in the extracellular matrix. This leads to laminar weakening, stretching, and disadhesion of the basal epithelium from the basement membrane. Laminar histological lesions include elongation and widening of the primary epidermal laminae; increased tapering and fusion of primary and secondary epidermal laminae; the presence of mitotic figures in secondary epidermal laminae; apoptotic cells; and proliferation, keratinization, and separation of the epidermis from the underlying dermis. A central role for the IGF-1 pathway is supported by the fact that IGF-1 receptors, but not insulin receptors, are present in laminar epithelial cells and are abundant in laminar tissue [34, 35]. Recently, IGF-1 signaling pathway events have been described in laminar epithelial cells in response to dietary sugar content and hyperinsulinemia [36].

27.1.2 Animal Assessment

Insulin deregulation can be assessed using either static or dynamic tests [1, 37]. Static tests include measurement of resting glucose and insulin concentrations; these represent a snapshot of the animal's endocrine status at a single time point. Dynamic tests involve the administration of either oral glucose, intravenous glucose, or intravenous insulin challenge, followed by an assessment of the physiological endocrine response. While fast and easy to perform, static tests are at best a screening tool because resting glucose and insulin concentrations represent the endpoint of complex metabolic pathways subject to extensive regulation, diurnal and seasonal variation, and the effects of stress and illness. Static tests lack sensitivity and can be normal in animals with ID. By contrast, dynamic tests are designed to perturb the glucose and insulin system, which can improve diagnostic sensitivity by overwhelming any compensatory homeostatic mechanisms attempting to maintain blood glucose and insulin concentration within the resting state reference ranges [2]. Use of dynamic tests is recommended when possible, particularly in cases where the practitioner suspects mild ID. Clinical experience suggests that false-negative test results occur more commonly than false-positive test results in testing for ID when resting insulin concentrations are used alone. See Sidebar 27.1.

27.1.2.1 Static Tests of Insulin Dysregulation

Resting or basal insulin concentration is frequently used as a screening tool and hyperinsulinemia is suggestive of ID [2]. For results to be most reflective of the horse's ID status, it is recommended that samples be collected in the non-fasted state, with the animal receiving either the usual hay or pasture turnout. However, samples should not be collected for at least 4 hrs following a grain meal. It should be remembered that insulin concentrations vary throughout the day, so resting insulin concentration can fall within the normal range at the time of sampling in horses with ID. Insulin concentration is also affected by factors, such as stress, pain, systemic illness, and ration; therefore, a result is more likely to represent a true positive the further it falls outside the reference range. Insulin reference ranges[1] and the cutoff values indicating ID must be

Sidebar 27.1: Medical Management of ID

Diagnosis and treatment options for ID have been previously detailed [38]. Medical management centers on two concepts: (i) direct management of ID with medications and (ii) treatment of concurrent diseases that might exacerbate ID. It must be emphasized that drug therapy is not a substitute for proper dietary modification; it serves only as an adjunct therapy and will not be sufficient to manage ID if the diet remains inappropriate. Two drugs are used to help control ID. Levothyroxine sodium (0.1 mg/kg BW orally every q24 hrs) is administered at supraphysiological doses to induce a state of mild iatrogenic hyperthyroidism and promote weight loss for 3–6 mos. This is particularly useful in horses that cannot exercise due to laminitis pain and in those animals that are resistant to weight loss despite calorie restriction. In horses that are exquisitely sensitive to dietary carbohydrates, metformin hydrochloride (30 mg/kg BW orally every q8–12 hrs) may help block enterocyte glucose absorption and blunt postprandial glucose and insulin spikes. A new class of drugs is also being explored for managing ID in horses. Sodium-glucose co-transporter 2 (SGLT2) inhibitors decrease renal glucose reuptake from the glomerular filtrate via inhibition of transport proteins in proximal renal tubular cells, thereby promoting glucosuria and lowering blood glucose and insulin concentrations [39, 40]. Drugs in this class are expensive and only sold for use in humans at present, but it is hoped that an SGLT2 inhibitor developed for horses will be available in the future.

The second aspect of medical management is addressing any concurrent illnesses that might exacerbate ID. The most common of these is PPID. Treatment consists of inhibiting hormonal secretion from the *pars intermedia* with the dopamine agonist pergolide mesylate. While pergolide is not a direct therapy for ID, improving the overall metabolic state of a PPID-affected animal may help normalize glucose, insulin, and fat metabolism. The other common scenario in which ID may be exacerbated is during systemic illness. Systemic inflammation reduces insulin sensitivity, and this might be particularly deleterious in an animal with pre-existing ID. Should a horse with ID become systemically ill or anorectic, meeting nutritional requirements must remain a priority during treatment. If allowed to lapse into negative energy balance, insulin-dysregulated animals can develop life-threatening hyperlipemia and hepatic lipidosis. Transient type 2 diabetes mellitus can also occur during systemic illness and sometimes requires exogenous insulin therapy.

1 Using the IMMULITE® 2000 immunoassay, Siemens Medical Solutions USA, Inc.

determined by each clinical laboratory. In general, resting blood insulin >50 μU/mL confirms the presence of ID, while concentrations between 20 and 50 μU/mL are highly suggestive, and <20 μU/mL is non-diagnostic. Dynamic testing is suggested if clinical suspicion of ID remains or results are inconclusive.

Most equids with ID are normoglycemic. Hyperglycemia, identified on occasion, indicates a loss of glycemic control and may progress to type 2 diabetes mellitus. Hyperglycemia can be seen in conjunction with hyperinsulinemia, termed partially uncompensated IR, where compensatory hyperinsulinemia is unable to maintain normoglycemia. Hyperglycemia with normoinsulinemia, termed uncompensated IR, occurs due to pancreatic β-cell exhaustion and reduction in insulin output. Factors, such as stress, pain, diet, and drug administration, can cause hyperglycemia and hence, these must be taken into account when interpreting test results.

27.1.2.2 Dynamic Tests of Insulin Dysregulation

The most commonly used dynamic tests for ID in the clinical setting are summarized in Table 27.1 [41–44]. Dynamic testing can unmask abnormalities in glucose and insulin homeostasis that are not evident when resting samples are assessed, and additional metabolic function parameters can be obtained. The most commonly used procedure is the oral sugar test (OST). Other tests include oral glucose tolerance, intravenous glucose tolerance, intravenous insulin tolerance, and combined glucose–insulin tolerance, along with hyperinsulinemic–euglycemic clamp procedures, hyperglycemic clamps, and the insulin-modified frequently sampled intravenous glucose tolerance test with minimal model analysis. These tests are interpreted by comparing parameters, such as the area under the curve values for glucose or insulin, peak and trough glucose and insulin responses, and the return of insulin and glucose concentrations to baseline. As an example, a glucose challenge that elicits an abnormally high insulin peak, delayed return of insulin concentrations to baseline, or an increased area under the insulin curve value could indicate increased β-cell responsiveness to glucose or decreased insulin clearance. During the same test, delayed return of glucose concentrations to baseline and an increased area under the glucose curve value could indicate peripheral IR since glucose is not cleared as rapidly as expected. Because ID is a multifactorial condition, hyperinsulinemia and tissue IR

Table 27.1 Recommended diagnostic tests for ID.

Test	Oral sugar test	In-feed oral glucose test	Insulin tolerance test	Combined glucose–insulin tolerance test
	Assesses postprandial insulin response, including the enteroinsular axis		Assesses peripheral tissue insulin sensitivity	
Procedure	After a 3–8 hrs fast, collect a baseline blood sample and then administer 0.15 mL/kg BW corn syrup orally. Collect blood at 60 and 90 min for measurement of insulin and glucose.	After an overnight fast, collect a baseline blood sample and then administer either 0.5 or 1.0 g/kg BW dextrose powder in non-glycemic feed. Collect blood at 2 hrs for measurement of insulin and glucose.	Do not fast before testing. Collect blood at baseline, followed by administration of 0.10 IU/kg BW regular (soluble) insulin intravenously. Collect a sample at 30 min for measurement of glucose.	Collect a baseline blood sample. Then, concurrently administer 150 mg of dextrose and 100 mIU/kg BW of regular (soluble) insulin intravenously. Collect a sample at 45 min for measurement of insulin and glucose.
Interpretation	Insulin response >45 μU/mL is positive. Assess glucose to detect diabetes mellitus.	Insulin response >68 μU/mL for 0.5 g/kg BW or >85 μU/mL for 1.0 g/kg BW is positive. Assess glucose to ensure that the meal was consumed and to detect diabetes mellitus.	Glucose response <50% decrease from baseline is consistent with insulin resistance.	Failure of glucose concentration to return to baseline by 45 min or an insulin concentration over 100 μU/mL at 45 min is indicative of insulin resistance.
Potential complications	None	None	Hypoglycemia (rare) – if this occurs, immediately administer 0.1–0.2 mL/kg BW of a 50% dextrose solution intravenously	Hypoglycemia (rare) – if this occurs, immediately administer 0.1–0.2 mL/kg BW of a 50% dextrose solution intravenously

can occur either independently or concurrently. Dynamic tests involving administration of an oral glucose challenge incorporate evaluation of the enteroinsular axis, while intravenous glucose challenges and the intravenous insulin tolerance test evaluate only peripheral tissue insulin sensitivity. To obtain a comprehensive picture of the animal's endocrine status, both types of tests may be performed concurrently.

While dynamic tests offer several advantages, the limitations of each test must be recognized. Oral glucose tolerance tests are affected by gastric emptying time, small intestinal absorption rates, hepatic glucose uptake, and pancreatic β-cell responsiveness. Intravenous glucose challenges assess insulin sensitivity by providing information on the functional turnover rate of glucose; however, exaggerated peak glucose concentration or delayed return to baseline may be due to either impaired insulin secretion or decreased insulin sensitivity. Insulin tolerance tests assess the glycemic response to exogenous insulin and may be confounded by endogenous insulin secretion. It is therefore important to consider potential confounders when performing these procedures.

27.1.3 Ration Assessment

Opportunities to prevent and treat ID are possible through dietetics and feeding management when predisposed horses and dietary triggers have been identified [29]. Ration digestible energy (DE) of 1.5–1.8 Mcal/kg dry matter (DM) is suitable for adult horses with ID to maintain adequate body weight (BW) and body condition score (BCS) of 4 to 6/9. Horses should be provided a complete and balanced ration, meeting the energy and nutrient requirements within 1.5–2.0% BW DM intake (DMI) [45].

27.1.3.1 Feeds

Most ID-affected horses should be fed primarily a dried low-NSC grass ration. Forages with relative feeding values (RFV) of 85–115 are recommended for healthy BW horses with ID (Table 10.3). Complementary feeds containing cereal grains (oats, sorghum, corn, barley) with 40–70% DM starch or grain mixes plus molasses (sweet feeds) with 40–50% DM NSC are major sources of sugar and not recommended for ID-affected horses [46]. Manufactured feeds[2] (>$4/d) containing 5–10% fat and <12% NSC using unmolasses sugar beet, soy hulls, or alfalfa meal fibers and fortified with vitamins and minerals, in addition to a low-NSC forage, would be a suitable ration [47]. Alternatively, feeding a low-NSC vitamin–mineral ration balancer ($0.75/d) with a low-NSC forage may be more cost-effective and simplify feeding protocols. See Sidebar 27.2.

Sidebar 27.2: "Low-Sugar" and "Low-Starch" Feed Claims

A word of caution when recommending a commercial "low-sugar" or "low-starch" complete feed. In the United States, a carbohydrate claim is allowed on any commercial horse feed if a guaranteed maximum percent sugar and dietary starch are stated on the label because the values are verifiable by laboratory testing. However, no agreement or regulation dictates a minimum or maximum for horses and "low" has not been defined. See "Labeling Claims" in Chapter 15. Horse owners will require specific guidance on the maximum percent sugar and dietary starch when veterinarians recommend a dietary change to a "low-sugar" or "low-starch" commercial feed, e.g. dietary starch maximum 11% and sugar maximum 4%.

Knowledge of factors affecting pasture NSC is essential to managing ID-affected horses with access to pasture. The NSC content of forage is affected by plant genus and species, light intensity and duration, temperature, nutrient and water status, stage of growth, and grazing management [48]. Pasture forage NSC concentrations fluctuate but may approach 40% DM under certain conditions. Ingesting high-NSC forage increases the risk of laminitis [49]. Due to daily and weekly weather changes, analysis of pasture forages is difficult, fraught with pitfalls, and does not reliably reflect NSC content. In cases of severe ID, pasture access should be avoided; in mild cases, limit pasture turnout to when NSC concentrations are lowest [49–51].

27.1.3.2 Key Nutrients

The essential dietary modification necessary to successfully manage horses with ID is the reduction of sugar and starch intake, as low-NSC diets minimize episodes of postprandial hyperinsulinemia and reduce the risk of laminitis. NSCs are intracellular plant sugars, starches, and fructans. While fructan digestion in the proximal bowel of the horse is considered minimal and unlikely to contribute to hyperinsulinemia, high-fructan intake is related to laminitis via detrimental changes to the large bowel microbiome, similar to a grain overload [52]. Accurate accounting of all feeds and forages is imperative to ensuring a low-NSC[3] ration (≤12%NSC DM). See Figure 6.2. Additionally, providing

2 Example: Purina® WellSolve L/S®, Land O'Lakes, Arden Hills, MN.

3 Where NSC is calculated using wet chemistry laboratory analysis of WSC + starch concentrations. https://dairyone.com/download/forage-forage-lab-analytical-procedures. Near Infrared (NIR) analysis of feeds may not be sufficiently accurate for managing ID.

dietary sources of nutrients that support hoof growth and quality, antioxidants and chromium may also be helpful[4] [53].

Weight loss should be implemented for obese horses with ID to improve insulin sensitivity and glucose tolerance [54, 55]. A low-NSC, low-calorie ration, i.e. 1.7–1.9 Mcal DE/kg DM, RFV of 75–100, promotes weight loss in addition to managing hyperinsulinemia. See Table 10.3. While the major factor stimulating muscle synthesis is exercise, the diet must provide sufficient amino acids to support muscle mass [56]. Feeding a protein–mineral–vitamin ration balancer with an essential amino acid source, e.g. oilseed meals, is recommended in weight loss rations. See Sidebar 28.1.

Some horses with ID are underweight, such as those with PPID or the lean phenotype of EMS. The ration for weight gain in underweight horses must be adequate in calories, i.e. >2 Mcal DE/kg DM while still limiting sugar and starch to less than 12% DM. Vegetable oil[5] and commercial fat supplements[6] effectively increase ration caloric density without adding sugar or starch. See Fat Sources in Chapter 13 and Table 13.4. Palatable corn oil is commonly used but should be introduced over 7–14 d into the ration preferably divided into 2–3 meals/d to allow intestinal adaptation. Fat and oil added to the ration are 76–94% digestible by horses in amounts as high as 20% DM [57]. Another option is stabilized rice bran with 20–25% fat as oil, which also provides several B vitamins but more phosphorus than calcium; hence, the calcium to phosphorus ratio must be corrected in the final ration [58]. See Feeding for Weight Gain in Chapter 23.

27.1.4 Feeding Management

Estimates of small intestinal starch digestion in the horse range 0.2–0.4% BW but <1 g/kg BW/meal has been recommended in ID-affected horses [59, 60]. In older animals with age-associated IR, an intake of 0.5 g NSC/kg BW/meal may manage postprandial insulin responses [61]. Horses with severe ID require further restriction to ≤0.1 g NSC/kg BW/meal to minimize the postprandial insulin response. In some cases, a low-NSC (10–15% DM) ration balancer fed in multiple meals/d is required to manage insulin response [62]. In difficult-to-manage cases, it may be necessary to assess the individual horse's insulin responses to specific forages and feeds.

Various methods, including the use of slow-feeder hay nets and grazing muzzles, can be employed to slow feed consumption and limit the stress of prolonged fasting periods. Barley, wheat, rye, or oat straw can replace ≤50% of the hay in a weight loss ration to extend feeding time [63, 64]. The straw must be harvested as intended for feed and free of pathogenic fungi, mesophilic bacteria, and actinomycetes. A gradual introduction of straw into the ration up to 50% over several weeks with *ad libitum* water will reduce the risk of gastrointestinal impactions and gastric ulcers [65, 66]. See Sidebar 26.1.

Soaking hay in water can reduce WSC content by 40%, although net losses are variable [67, 68]. Ideally, the procedure should start with low-NSC mature grass hay with soaking used to reduce the WSC further. There is also a 20% loss of DM with soaking, which should be accounted for when recommending the amount of hay to be soaked before feeding. Other nutrients lost include protein, vitamins, and macro and micro minerals [67–70]. The water temperature and length of soaking affect the extent of WSC and DM loss, and microbial contamination [67, 71, 72]. Soaking grass hay for 15–30 min is recommended to remove sufficient NSC fractions while minimizing DM losses [68]. Longer periods of immersion will remove more NSC but can lead to contamination with bacteria and mold [73]. The liquid remaining after soaking should not be fed to horses.

27.2 Pituitary Pars Intermedia Dysfunction

Frequently referred to as equine Cushing's disease, PPID occurs more commonly in middle-aged and older horses [74]. Clinical signs of PPID develop when melanotropes within the pars intermedia of the pituitary gland secrete excessive amounts of hormones derived from the prohormone proopiomelanocortin (POMC). In the pars intermedia of a healthy horse, the end-products of the POMC pathway are alpha-melanocyte-stimulating hormone (αMSH), beta-endorphin, and corticotropin-like intermediate peptide (CLIP). When PPID develops, secretion of αMSH and CLIP increases and other hormones derived from POMC are released, including ACTH, which is the primary product of the POMC conversion pathway in the pars distalis. Secretion of ACTH, CLIP, and other POMC products from the pars intermedia induces a form of hyperadrenocorticism as hormone secretion becomes unregulated. It is worth noting, however, that PPID is not a straightforward example of hyperadrenocorticism, as in canines or people, because plasma total cortisol concentrations are rarely increased in affected horses and adrenal hyperplasia has only been

---

4 Example: Empower® Topline Balance® Diet Balancer, Nutrena, Cargill, Inc., Minneapolis, MN.

5 One "cup" (8 vol-oz or 244 mL) of corn/canola oil ~2 Mcal DE.

6 Example: Cool Calories® 100, Manna Pro Products, LLC, Chesterfield, MO.

detected in a subset of cases [75, 76]. The pars intermedia secretes only small amounts of ACTH under normal circumstances and is not under negative feedback control by the hypothalamic–pituitary–adrenal axis. Secretion of hormones by melanotropes of the pars intermedia is controlled instead by dopamine. This neurotransmitter is secreted by dopaminergic neurons that have cell bodies within the paraventricular nuclei of the hypothalamus and extend down to the pars intermedia. These dopaminergic neurons degenerate with age as a result of oxidative damage. Presumably, exaggerated degeneration of dopaminergic neurons occurs in horses with PPID, leading to pituitary hyperplasia, hypertrophy, and the formation of functional pituitary adenomas [77, 78]. Horses and ponies with EMS might be predisposed to PPID and, anecdotally, have been observed to develop pituitary dysfunction at a younger age.

27.2.1 Animal Assessment

The most common clinical signs of PPID are laminitis, hypertrichosis, abnormal body fat distribution, polyuria, and polydipsia. Weight loss was reported in 15% of PPID horses [79]. Accurately assessing BCS can be challenging since skeletal muscle mass is reduced particularly along the topline, and an abnormal fat distribution occurs in 15–30% of cases [3]. The muscle loss or sarcopenia, most notable in the epaxial and gluteal muscles, which progresses to more generalized muscle wasting over time, is assumed to be related to the action of excess cortisol on skeletal muscles (Figure 27.1). Horses in the most advanced stages of PPID may be weak because of severe muscle loss and sometimes exhibit gait abnormalities similar to neurological disease.

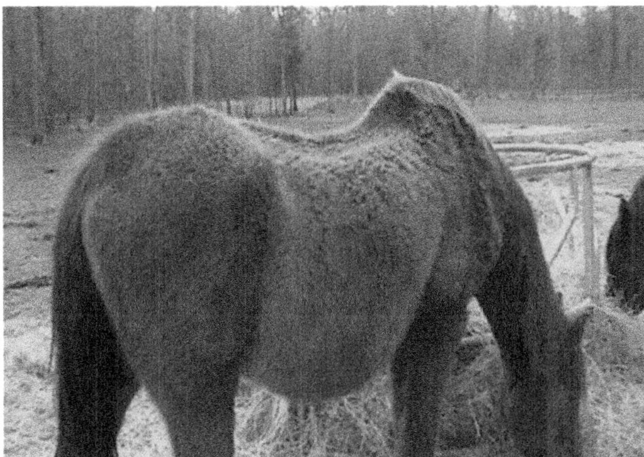

Figure 27.1 Advanced-stage PPID in a 24-yr-old Morgan mare with muscle wasting in the epaxial and gluteal muscles.

Horses and ponies with early PPID may be obese, show signs of muscle loss along the topline, and have haircoat changes. As PPID progresses, muscle mass decreases, but regional adipose deposits located above the eyes in the supraorbital fossa, along the crest of the neck, over the tail head, and in the sheath or mammary region typically become apparent [3]. Loss of muscling along the neck accentuates regional adiposity and a "cresty neck" becomes more apparent, which may explain why this physical characteristic is associated with PPID. Whether fat deposition occurs as a result of PPID or fat accumulation predisposes an animal to the development of PPID is not clear.

The reported association between hyperinsulinemia and PPID in earlier studies led initially to the assumption that all horses with PPID suffered from ID [80]. However, horses with PPID and normal insulin status have been identified providing evidence of two subpopulations of PPID horses: those with ID and those with normal insulin function [23, 81]. Therefore, dynamic testing is strongly recommended to fully assess each PPID patient before making dietary changes. Horses with normal insulin status may be provided feeds that have NSC >15% DM. It is not necessary to make changes to feeding regimens if the PPID horse with normal insulin status is faring well and maintaining appropriate BCS. This is particularly important to consider when managing underweight horses requiring more calories or horses that refuse low-NSC feeds.

Some horses with PPID develop laminitis. Horses with repeated bouts of laminitis should undergo testing for endocrine disorders, even in the absence of phenotypical characteristics [82–84]. Evidence is mounting to support the hypothesis that laminitis develops in PPID horses with ID, whereas those without ID have a low risk of laminitis [81]. Insulin resistance, defined by static fasting hyperinsulinemia, was present in 60% of PPID horses [3]. Although ID is likely to be the main determinant for laminitis, PPID might play other roles in this multifactorial disease. Some laminitic horses may appear sound if pain responses are inhibited by excess production of beta-endorphins. Alternatively, poor tissue healing may delay recovery from laminitis in horses with advanced PPID.

27.2.1.1 Early Stages

Presenting complaints about early PPID include poor performance and reduced activity, loss of muscle mass, delayed shedding of winter hairs body wide or only over certain regions of the body, and development of a slightly coarser, duller, or thicker haircoat. Early haircoat changes are subtle, with longer hairs retained over the palmar and plantar aspects of the legs, under the mandible, or behind the elbow, i.e. regional hypertrichosis. Owners may not have noticed the gradual onset of haircoat abnormalities. PPID must therefore be considered when examining any middle-aged or older horse after changes in activity level or appearance are reported, with an evaluation of the ration and parasite control regimen. Reproductive performance might also be affected by PPID because dopamine inhibition is involved in the regulation of the seasonal anovulatory period, although definitive studies are lacking in this area [85].

27.2.1.2 Advanced Stages

Advanced PPID is easily recognized and presumptively diagnosed based on history and physical examination. As PPID progresses, horses move from delayed haircoat shedding and regional hypertrichosis to year-round retention of the winter haircoat and generalized hypertrichosis. The long curly haircoat detected in horses with advanced disease was previously referred to as hirsutism and considered a pathognomonic clinical sign for PPID. It should be noted, however, that protein–calorie malnutrition and medical conditions causing severe weight loss, such as inflammatory bowel disease and neoplasia, may result in similar changes in BCS and haircoat. Other clinical findings of advanced PPID include rounding of the abdomen, polyuria, polydipsia, recurrent bacterial infections, persistent neutrophilia and lymphopenia, infertility, and inappropriate lactation.

It is important to select the correct diagnostic test for the stage of disease and the time of the year when testing is performed (Table 27.2). As PPID progresses, resting ACTH concentrations rise above the upper limit of the reference interval and this becomes a useful diagnostic test for horses with advanced disease. Seasonally adjusted reference intervals must be applied when interpreting results since ACTH concentrations normally increase in the late summer and fall. It was previously thought that the late summer and fall should be avoided when testing horses for PPID, but the opposite approach is now recommended. Measuring plasma ACTH concentrations when hormonal systems are stimulated may increase the likelihood of detecting early PPID.

27.2.2 Ration Assessment

Feeding horses and ponies with PPID must be tailored to the individual because affected horses are often older individuals ranging from 15 to 40 yrs old with varying degrees of sarcopenia, may be over or underweight, and may or may not have ID and/or recurrent laminitis.

Horses with PPID in good BW and BCS 4 to 6/9 with no evidence of ID or laminitis can be fed the same as a healthy adult horse [45]. Rations with 1.8–2.0 Mcal DE/kg DM are suitable but must be nutritionally complete and balanced when fed within 1.5–2.0% DMI. Rations are predominately dried or fresh forage of moderate quality with RFV ranging from 85 to 115 as needed for weight maintenance [45, 86]. As PPID progresses, adjustments to the calorie intake are needed to manage weight gain or loss. Additionally, nutrients of concern are those supporting muscle mass, i.e. protein, essential amino acids, vitamin E, and selenium. No significant difference was found in the presence of positive or negative regulators of protein synthesis, or positive regulators of protein breakdown between horses with and without PPID [87]. Therefore, feeding an adequate quantity of

Table 27.2 Recommended diagnostic tests for pituitary pars intermedia dysfunction (PPID).

		Thyrotropin-releasing Hormone (TRH) stimulation test		
Early PPID	**Non-Fall** Mid-November to mid-July	Negative Plasma ACTH <110 pg/mL at 10 min	Equivocal Plasma ACTH 110–200 pg/mL at 10 min	Positive Plasma ACTH >200 pg/mL at 10 min
	Fall Mid-July to mid-November	Reference intervals are not available at this time		
		Resting Adrenocorticotropic Hormone (ACTH) concentration		
Advanced PPID	**Non-Fall** Mid-November to mid-July	Negative Plasma ACTH < 30 pg/mL	Equivocal Plasma ACTH 30–50 pg/mL	Positive Plasma ACTH >50 pg/mL
	Fall Mid-July to mid-November	Negative Plasma ACTH < 50 pg/mL	Equivocal Plasma ACTH 50–100 pg/mL	Positive Plasma ACTH >100 pg/mL

Source: Adapted from the 2017 Equine Endocrinology Group Recommendations on Diagnosis and Management of Pituitary Pars Intermedia Dysfunction in Horses (http://sites.tufts.edu/equineendogroup).

high-quality protein ingredients, i.e. supplying essential amino acids in a highly digestible form, e.g. oilseed meals, may slow muscle losses. See Protein Sources in Chapter 13 and Table 13.2. Feeding a protein–mineral–vitamin ration balancer is needed to meet essential micronutrient requirements.

Horses with PPID and ID or laminitis with BCS 4 to 6/9 can be fed the same range of DE rations as adult horses. The dietary modification for PPID horses is low-sugar and low-starch concentrations to prevent episodes of postprandial hyperinsulinemia and reduce the risk of laminitis. Pasture, cereal grains (Table 13.1), textured or sweet feeds containing >3% molasses and ≥15% NSC will likely result in postprandial hyperinsulinemia [88]. Recommendations for horses with PPID and ID are the same as those for horses with ID, i.e. a dried grass forage ration containing <12% DM starch and sugar, and limiting NSC to 0.1–0.5 g/kg BW/meal.

Overweight or obese horses at the time of PPID diagnosis should be fed a weight-loss ration, and underweight animals should be fed a ration to regain BW. Underweight PPID horses with ID require >2.0 Mcal DE/kg DM ration for weight gain using oil or fat for additional calories rather than a cereal grain or sweet feed. See Fat Sources in Chapter 13 and Table 13.4.

27.2.3 Feeding Management

Given the likelihood of comorbidities as the horse ages, caretakers should monitor BW and BCS every 4–6 wks and make small appropriate ration adjustments when needed. PPID horses specifically dental and hoof care, regular dietary and nutritional reviews, and parasite control as the disease is progressive with no cure. See Sidebar 27.3.

Sidebar 27.3: Medical Management of PPID

Diagnosis and treatment options for PPID have been previously detailed [38]. Pergolide mesylate is a dopamine agonist that controls PPID by inhibiting the secretion of hormones. The US Food and Drug Administration-approved drug Prascend[7] is available for use in horses at a starting dosage of 0.002 mg/kg BW, which is equivalent to one tablet/d (1 mg each) orally for a 500 kg horse. Some horses develop transient anorexia when treatment is initiated so gradual introduction of the drug is recommended: 0.5 tablet every other day for three doses, 0.5 tablet daily for 3 d, and then 1 tablet daily. Short-term responses to pergolide treatment include increased activity level and performance. Muscle mass returns to normal after several months of pergolide treatment if the appropriate dose is administered and haircoat shedding may also improve the following spring.

7 Boehringer Ingelheim Vetmedica, Inc., St Joseph, MO.

Many PPID horses are polyuric and polydipsic; hence, access to clean, palatable water should be readily available at all times. Those not able to chew hay may do better fed chopped forage, soaked hay cubes, or pelleted hay in multiple (4–6) small meals/d with appropriate complementary feed for comorbidities. Horses with decreased appetite-related PPID treatment with pergolide may consume more on pasture. Underweight PPID horses with normal insulin function will likely consume more feed when water is available, out on pasture with herdmates, or with small frequent meals of complementary cereal grains or sweet feeds. See Chapter 16 Feeding and Drinking Behaviors. The use of slow-feeder hay nets and grazing muzzles can be employed to slow feed consumption in overweight PPID horses or replace a portion of the ration with straw to reduce the caloric density. See Sidebar 28.1. However, PPID horses with ID may not tolerate pasture forage depending on pasture conditions, forage type, weather, season, and the severity of ID. Hay analysis is necessary to determine the NSC content of the forage and soaking before feeding may be necessary to reduce NSC concentration <10% DM. A low sugar, low starch complementary ration balancer will also be required to complete the nutritional profile of the ration.

27.3 Hyperlipemia

27.3.1 Introduction

Equine hyperlipemia is a metabolic disorder of horses, Miniature horses, ponies, and donkeys. Affected animals exhibit anorexia and depression, and have high circulating TG concentrations. Hyperlipidemia is a term used to describe laboratory results when plasma TG (hypertriglyceridemia) or cholesterol (hypercholesterolemia) concentrations exceed reference intervals. EH occurs when horses become stressed and enter negative energy balance, which stimulates the mobilization of body fats for energy. Often, EH is a secondary condition to other diseases [89]. For example, systemic illnesses or pain associated with laminitis can induce a stress response, which depresses appetite and subsequently increases lipid mobilization. High serum lipid concentrations then further suppress appetite.

Diagnosis and treatment options for hyperlipemia in horses have been previously detailed [90]. Hypertriglyceridemia can be detected in advance of EH clinical signs and signals a state of negative energy balance. The potential for EH should be anticipated in stressed patients not consuming sufficient calories to meet resting energy needs. The clinical signs of severe hypertriglyceridemia, defined as a plasma TG concentration >500 mg/dL, are anorexia, depression, and alterations in organ function [7].

These patients require nutritional support, in addition to medical management, to reverse metabolic starvation.

There are also several reports of severe hypertriglyceridemia occurring in equids that are eating well and maintaining normal liver and kidney function [91]. These cases of hypertriglyceridemia are detected when routine blood tests are performed for other reasons, as the patients are tolerant of severe hypertriglyceridemia for reasons not understood. These clinically normal animals do not require treatment but should be regularly monitored for decompensation.

27.3.1.1 Associated Conditions

An association exists between PPID, diabetes mellitus, and hypertriglyceridemia in older horses. Equids with hyperlipidemia should be evaluated for diabetes mellitus by measuring blood glucose concentrations or testing urine for glucose. Type 2 diabetes mellitus is defined by persistent hyperglycemia with inappropriately low-insulin concentrations. Measured insulin concentrations may either be high or fall within the reference interval, but are inappropriately low to maintain normoglycemia.

It is advisable to test for PPID in older horses with EH and initiate pergolide treatment if indicated. However, results of PPID testing should be interpreted with care in systemically ill animals with EH, as severe illness can cause false-positive results due to metabolic stress [89, 92]. Clinical signs of PPID should be used to guide treatment decisions. Blood glucose and TG concentrations should be measured in PPID horses, and exogenous insulin may be required if hyperglycemia and EH develop. Insulin secretion is suppressed in PPID animals, and exogenous insulin may be necessary, at least initially, to control hyperglycemia and hyperlipidemia. However, PPID-associated inhibition of insulin secretion appears to be reversible because affected horses often respond positively to pergolide treatment. Once treatment is initiated or the pergolide dosage has been increased, insulin secretion increases to restore normoglycemia and suppress lipid mobilization. Hypertriglyceridemia may resolve and insulin treatment can usually be discontinued.

27.3.1.2 Pathophysiology

Obesity is an important risk factor for EH because affected animals may liberate excessive quantities of fatty acids from adipose tissues in response to a negative energy balance when energy expenditure exceeds energy intake. Obese animals have larger amounts of stored TG and often suffer from ID, which is a predisposing factor for EH because hormone-sensitive lipase (HSL) activity is not suppressed by insulin in the ID state. HSL is stimulated when fats are needed for energy and catalyzes the hydrolysis of TG to free fatty acids and glycerol. The activity of HSL increases during negative energy balance, e.g. between meals or with starvation, and decreases after feeding when glucose and other nutrients are abundant and the body is storing energy. Glucagon, cortisol, epinephrine, and growth hormone stimulate HSL and these hormones are released during starvation. In contrast, HSL is inhibited by insulin because this hormone is secreted in response to feeding and signals the body to store energy. Insulin lowers HSL activity because body fat is stored, not mobilized, after feeding. These normal processes are disrupted in the animals with ID because the inhibitory effects of insulin on HSL activity are reduced and responses to negative energy balance can be excessive and unregulated. Lipid mobilization from adipose tissues can occur on a massive scale in obese animals with ID.

When an animal enters a negative energy balance, glucagon and stress hormones stimulate HSL, and stored TG is hydrolyzed to produce glycerol and fatty acids. Glycerol is used for gluconeogenesis and fatty acids are converted into acetyl coenzyme A through beta-oxidation. This process occurs within mitochondria, which are abundant within the liver. Plasma-free fatty acids or non-esterified fatty acids (NEFAs) increase as TG is hydrolyzed within adipose tissues. This process is accelerated in ID animals due to the lack of insulin control. In cases of EH, some NEFAs entering the liver are used for energy via beta-oxidation, but metabolic pathways become overwhelmed and fatty acids are re-assembled into TG. The accumulation of TG within hepatocytes stimulates very-low-density lipoprotein (VLDL) synthesis and secretion providing the liver an export pathway for TG. As negative energy balance continues and EH progresses, more fatty acids are released from adipose tissues, plasma NEFA concentrations continue to rise, hepatic production of VLDL increases as a consequence, and plasma TG concentrations rise. EH is a disorder of elevated VLDL concentrations, but the root cause is an excessive mobilization of fatty acids from adipose tissues. As EH progresses, fatty acids are re-assembled into TG within several other tissue types, leading to steatorrhea, renal failure, and hepatic lipidosis. Clinical signs progress as these organs fail and the animal develops azotemia and hepatic encephalopathy. This metabolic disorder follows a vicious cycle as organ failure continues to suppress appetite. Mortality rates are reported to be greater than 60% for EH primarily due to organ failure [93, 94]. Awareness of EH and more aggressive medical management of this condition has markedly lowered mortality rates in the last decade; however, the prognosis is only fair, even with aggressive treatment.

27.3.2 Animal Assessment

Hyperlipemia is seen most commonly in ponies and Miniature horses, and less frequently in standard-sized adult horses unless the animal is overweight or has a pre-existing endocrinopathy. The clinical signs of EH are vague and often subtle at the outset. The patient at risk will have a diet history of anorexia or reduced feed intakes for several or more days, as a result of a primary disease process or an environmental condition, e.g. decreased access to feed or water. Quintessential to the development of EH is a negative energy balance. EH is most commonly seen in obese animals, but not exclusively. The condition develops and worsens when energy deficits increase, as in late-term pregnancy, lactation, or systemic disease. Systemic inflammation increase resting energy requirements (RER) but also suppress appetite, therefore, TG concentrations should be monitored in horses with inflammatory disease processes until voluntary feed intake resumes that meets or succeeds daily caloric need. While the focus of treatments is on the primary medical condition(s), EH can become a secondary life-threatening problem for the patient. Advanced EH patients may exhibit steatorrhea and clinical signs consistent with liver or kidney failure, with profound depression, icterus, and neurological signs consistent with hepatic encephalopathy. Voluntary water intake may also decrease in depressed patients.

Dietary history of decreased or no feed intake for several days should raise concern over the potential presence of EH. Moderate hypertriglyceridemia with plasma TG > 65 mg/dL will typically progress to EH unless addressed. Severe hyperlipidemia with plasma TG > 500 mg/dL may be detected by the appearance of milky opaque serum in a tube of clotted blood left standing for 30 min. Other laboratory abnormalities include increased plasma enzyme activities consistent with hepatic lipidosis and azotemia. Gamma-glutamyltransferase activity increases as lipids accumulate within hepatocytes and slow bile outflow. Sorbitol dehydrogenase and aspartate aminotransferase activities increase with hepatocellular damage. Increased creatinine concentrations are often detected, caused either by dehydration and prerenal azotemia or secondary to renal lipidosis and dysfunction.

27.3.3 Ration Assessment

Access to nutritionally adequate, hygienically clean feeds and a normal appetite prevents negative energy balance. Insufficient feed intake or poor feed quality, particularly when energy demands are high, e.g. late pregnancy or early lactation, classically result in EH. Consider the animal's ability to obtain feed as several barriers may exist, e.g. animal, physical, or environmental limitations, herd dynamics, and amount of feed available. Assessing animal appetite is done by offering a small number of various forage types and forms, and a choice of complementary feeds, e.g. oats or sweet feed. If a feed is consumed, the animal's ability to prehend, chew, and swallow can be assessed.

Secondly, assess the quality and hygiene of the feeds as the amount of forage consumed is directly related to quality. Most horses will consume old and dusty hay, and will eat around weeds and foreign material, but will refuse to consume moldy, spoiled hay. The forage offered must be palatable in odor and texture to ensure an adequate DMI [95]. A ration of forage with RFV > 100 and a sweet or oat-based complementary feed is normally highly palatable to horses and relatively easy to nutritionally complete as needed for the patient's life stage, ideal BW, and BCS [45].

27.3.4 Feeding Management

Key nutritional concepts for EH include recognizing causes of an energy deficit and supporting the patient until a positive energy balance has been restored. Once EH has developed, the appetite may be suppressed by high blood NEFA and TG concentrations. Animals with EH should be encouraged to eat by offering a variety of feeds and textures. Although ID is a concern in many patients with EH, anorexia and negative energy balance are critical issues, the encouragement of voluntary feed consumption takes precedence and small quantities of sweet feed, applesauce, and molasses may be necessary on a short-term basis. Once interest in food has returned, the horse can be gradually transitioned to a low-NSC ration.

If all feeds are refused, corn syrup (103 kcal DE/30 mL) or applesauce (18 kcal DE/30 mL) administered by mouth using a dose syringe will raise blood glucose concentrations. In addition to providing some calories, this treatment can raise insulin concentrations and suppress HSL activity, decreasing the rate of lipolysis within adipose tissue. There are anecdotal reports of successfully managing EH at home by having owners administer corn syrup or applesauce hourly along with hand-feeding the horse. Intravenous dextrose and insulin are recommended to control hyperlipidemia in severely affected animals, recognizing that treatment costs will increase due to the need for hospitalization. The feeding goal is to provide at least RER, which is 75% of the minimum DE for maintenance (min DE_m). Assisted feeding is an option in those horses not voluntarily consuming at least RER. Monitoring feed intake is essential through quantification of feed offered minus feed refused. Parenteral nutrition (PN) has been used successfully to manage severe EH [7, 91, 96]. A partial PN lipid-free admixture composed of 1 : 1 volumes of (50%) dextrose and (15%) amino acid solutions providing 65–75% of RER and protein successfully resolved hyperlipemia in six animals [96]. If hyperglycemia and glucosuria develop during PN, exogenous insulin may be necessary to maintain blood glucose concentrations below 200 mg/dL. See Assisted Feeding in Chapter 24.

Case in Point

A 14 yr old Arabian gelding is evaluated in early June as part of an annual wellness examination. The horse is used for ranch work; moving cattle 3–4 hrs/wk, comparable to moderate exercise (Table 18.1).

Animal Assessment

The horse BW was 465 kg with a BSC 8/9, with increased adiposity within the nuchal crest and tail head regions, and a cresty neck score of 3/5 [81]. An estimate of ideal BW was 400 kg based on ideal body weight equations (Table 2.3). Physical examination reveals longer hairs on the palmar and plantar aspects of the lower limbs and these hairs are lighter in color than the other hairs of the legs (Figure 27.2). The owner reports that the horse took longer than normal to shed his winter haircoat this past spring. She thinks the longer hairs on his legs were retained from the previous year and that the horse has lost muscle mass along the topline.

Physical characteristics of obesity and increased adiposity within the neck region are consistent with EMS but clinical signs of PPID are also evident with longer hairs and loss of epaxial muscle mass space. An oral sugar test (OST) and thyrotropin-releasing hormone (TRH) stimulation test are performed, and both tests yield positive results, confirming the diagnoses of ID and PPID, respectively. When the OST is performed, plasma insulin concentrations measured at 60 and 90 min after oral administration of corn syrup (0.15 mL/kg BW) were 72 and 98 μU/mL, respectively. Insulin concentrations of 45–60 μU/mL are considered likely positive while results >60 μU/mL are strongly positive for ID.

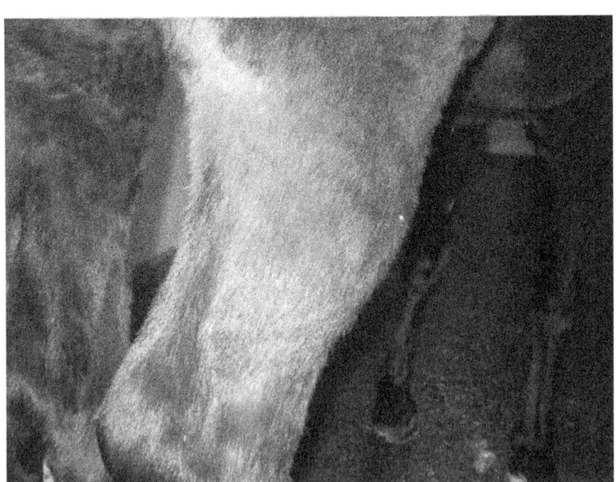

Figure 27.2 Longer and lighter in color hairs on the palmar and plantar aspects of the lower limbs of a horse with early stage PPID.

Ration Assessment

The owner feeds "1/3 bale" of mixed mainly grass (MMG) hay and one "scoop" of sweet feed twice daily. The horse is on pasture during the day and brought into a stall at night. Water and a white salt block were available ad libitum. After weighing the bale and a "scoop" of feed, approximate intakes were 25 lb MMG hay and 4 lb sweet feed as fed (AF) daily.

Based on laboratory analysis, nutrients on DM basis were as follows[a]:

Feeds	DM	DE	CP	ESC	WSC	Starch
	%	Mcal/kg	%	%	%	%
MMG hay	90	1.9	12.4	6.8	10.6	1.7
Sweet Feed	88	3.5	13.0	14	19	6

[a] Dry matter (DM), Digestible energy (DE), Crude protein (CP), Ethanol soluble carbohydrate (ESC), Water soluble carbohydrate (WSC).

The horse began pergolide treatment to manage PPID and a feeding plan was designed to address obesity and ID. The changes should include removing cereal grains from the ration thereby reducing NSC intake to manage postprandial hyperinsulinemia. Daily exercise was to include trotting or cantering for a minimum of 15–20 min on a hillside to promote weight loss.

Feeding Recommendations

1) *What is the current DE intake vs. DE requirement for this patient doing moderate work at ideal BW?*
2) *What is a reasonable weight loss protocol and initial daily DE intake for this patient? Consider the options in Table 23.2.*
3) *Can the owner continue to feed this hay or is a different forage needed?*
4) Owner agrees to replace the sweet feed with a low-starch, low-calorie, vitamin–mineral–protein ration balancer appropriate for weight loss fed at 0.5 g/kg BW twice daily.[8] *How much of the MMG hay/d should the owner feed?*
5) *Are there additional recommendations for this horse while out on pasture?*

See Appendix A Chapter 27.

8 Example: Purina® Enrich Plus®, Land O'Lakes, Arden Hills, MN.

References

1 Frank, N. and Tadros, E.M. (2014). Insulin dysregulation. *Equine Vet. J.* 46 (1): 103–112.

2 Frank, N., Geor, R.J., Bailey, S.R. et al. (2010). Equine metabolic syndrome. *J. Vet. Intern. Med.* 24 (3): 467–475.

3 McFarlane, D. (2011). Equine pituitary pars intermedia dysfunction. *Vet. Clin. Equine Pract.* 27 (1): 93–113.

4 Schott, H.C. (2002). Pituitary pars intermedia dysfunction: equine Cushing's disease. *Vet. Clin. Equine Pract.* 18 (2): 237–270.

5 Ishiki, M. and Klip, A. (2005). Minireview: recent developments in the regulation of glucose transporter-4 traffic: new signals, locations, and partners. *Endocrinology* 146 (12): 5071–5078.

6 de Graaf-Roelfsema, E. (2014). Glucose homeostasis and the enteroinsular axis in the horse: a possible role in equine metabolic syndrome. *Vet. J.* 199 (1): 11–18.

7 McKenzie, H.C. (2011). Equine hyperlipidemias. *Vet. Clin. North Am. Equine Pract.* 27 (1): 59–72.

8 Toth, F., Frank, N., Martin-Jimenez, T. et al. (2010). Measurement of C-peptide concentrations and responses to somatostatin, glucose infusion, and insulin resistance in horses. *Equine Vet. J.* 42 (2): 149–155.

9 de Laat, M.A., Van Haeften, J.J., and Sillence, M.N. (2016). The effect of oral and intravenous dextrose on C-peptide secretion in ponies. *J. Anim. Sci.* 94 (2): 574–580.

10 Lewis, S.L., Holl, H.M., Streeter, C. et al. (2017). Genomewide association study reveals a risk locus for equine metabolic syndrome in the Arabian horse. *J. Anim. Sci.* 95 (3): 1071–1079.

11 Bamford, N.J., Potter, S.J., Harris, P.A., and Bailey, S.R. (2014). Breed differences in insulin sensitivity and insulinemic responses to oral glucose in horses and ponies of moderate body condition score. *Domest. Anim. Endocrinol.* 47: 101–107.

12 Bamford, N.J., Baskerville, C.L., Harris, P.A., and Bailey, S.R. (2015). Postprandial glucose, insulin, and glucagon-like peptide-1 responses of different equine breeds adapted to meals containing micronized maize. *J. Anim. Sci.* 93 (7): 3377–3383.

13 de Laat, M.A., McGree, J.M., and Sillence, M.N. (2016). Equine hyperinsulinemia: investigation of the enteroinsular axis during insulin dysregulation. *Am. J. Physiol. Metab.* 310 (1): E61–E72.

14 Shoelson, S.E., Herrero, L., and Naaz, A. (2007). Obesity, inflammation, and insulin resistance. *Gastroenterology* 132 (6): 2169–2180.

15 Elzinga, S.E., Rohleder, B., Schanbacher, B. et al. (2017). Metabolic and inflammatory responses to the common sweetener stevioside and a glycemic challenge in horses with equine metabolic syndrome. *Domest. Anim. Endocrinol.* 60 (July): 1–8.

16 Tadros, E.M., Frank, N., and Donnell, R.L. (2013). Effects of equine metabolic syndrome on inflammatory responses of horses to intravenous lipopolysaccharide infusion. *Am. J. Vet. Res.* 74 (7): 1010–1019.

17 Bamford, N.J., Potter, S.J., Baskerville, C.L. et al. (2016). Effect of increased adiposity on insulin sensitivity and adipokine concentrations in different equine breeds adapted to cereal-rich or fat-rich meals. *Vet. J.* 214 (August): 14–20.

18 Ungru, J., Coenen, M., Vervuert, I. et al. (2012). Effects of body weight reduction on blood adipokines and subcutaneous adipose tissue adipokine mRNA expression profiles in obese ponies. *Vet. Rec.* 171 (21): 528.

19 Gill, J.C., Pratt-Phillips, S.E., Mansmann, R., and Siciliano, P.D. (2016). Weight loss management in client-owned horses. *J. Equine Vet. Sci.* 39 (4): 80–89.

20 Morgan, R.A., Keen, J.A., and McGowan, C.M. (2016). Treatment of equine metabolic syndrome: a clinical case series. *Equine Vet. J.* 48 (4): 422–426.

21 Argo, C.M., Curtis, G.C., Grove-White, D. et al. (2012). Weight loss resistance: a further consideration for the nutritional management of obese Equidae. *Vet. J.* 194 (2): 179–188.

22 Tadros, E.M., Frank, N., De Witte, F.G., and Boston, R.C. (2013). Effects of intravenous lipopolysaccharide infusion on glucose and insulin dynamics in horses with equine metabolic syndrome. *Am. J. Vet. Res.* 74 (7): 1020–1029.

23 Mastro, L.M., Adams, A.A., and Urschel, K.L. (2015). Pituitary pars intermedia dysfunction does not necessarily impair insulin sensitivity in old horses. *Domest. Anim. Endocrinol.* 50: 14–25.

24 Marshall, J.B., Kapcala, L.P., Manning, L.D., and McCullough, A.J. (1984). Effect of corticotropin-like intermediate lobe peptide on pancreatic exocrine function in isolated rat pancreatic lobules. *J. Clin. Invest.* 74 (5): 1886–1889.

25 Beloff-Chain, A., Morton, J., Dunmore, S. et al. (1983). Evidence that the insulin secretagogue, β-cell-tropin, is ACTH 22–39. *Nature* 301 (5897): 255–258.

26 Liburt, N.R., Fugaro, M.N., Malinowski, K. et al. (2012). The effect of age and exercise training on insulin sensitivity, fat and muscle tissue cytokine profiles and body composition of old and young Standardbred mares. *Comp. Exerc. Physiol.* 8 (3–4): 173–187.

27 Malinowski, K., Betros, C.L., Flora, L. et al. (2002). Effect of training on age-related changes in plasma insulin and glucose. *Equine Vet. J.* 34 (S34): 147–153.

28 de Tata, V. (2014). Age-related impairment of pancreatic Beta-cell function: pathophysiological and cellular mechanisms. *Front. Endocrinol. (Lausanne)* 5: 138.

29 Treiber, K.H., Kronfeld, D.S., Hess, T.M. et al. (2006). Evaluation of genetic and metabolic predispositions and

nutritional risk factors for pasture-associated laminitis in ponies. *J. Am. Vet. Med. Assoc.* 228 (10): 1538–1545.

30 Carter, R.A., Treiber, K.H., Geor, R.J. et al. (2009). Prediction of incipient pasture-associated laminitis from hyperinsulinaemia, hyperleptinaemia and generalised and localised obesity in a cohort of ponies. *Equine Vet. J.* 41 (2): 171–178.

31 de Laat, M.A., de McGowan, C.M., Sillence, M.N., and Pollitt, C.C. (2010). Equine laminitis: induced by 48 h hyperinsulinaemia in Standardbred horses. *Equine Vet. J.* 42 (2): 129–135.

32 Asplin, K.K.E., Sillence, M.M.N., Pollitt, C.C.C., and McGowan, C.M. (2007). Induction of laminitis by prolonged hyperinsulinaemia in clinically normal ponies. *Vet. J.* 174 (3): 530–535.

33 Treiber, K.H., Kronfeld, D.S., Hess, T.M. et al. (2005). Use of proxies and reference quintiles obtained from minimal model analysis for determination of insulin sensitivity and pancreatic beta-cell responsiveness in horses. *Am. J. Vet. Res.* 66 (12): 2114–2121.

34 Burns, T.A., Watts, M.R., Weber, P.S. et al. (2013). Distribution of insulin receptor and insulin-like growth factor-1 receptor in the digital laminae of mixed-breed ponies: an immunohistochemical study. *Equine Vet. J.* 45 (3): 326–332.

35 Kullmann, A., Weber, P.S., Bishop, J.B. et al. (2016). Equine insulin receptor and insulin-like growth factor-1 receptor expression in digital lamellar tissue and insulin target tissues. *Equine Vet. J.* 48 (5): 626–632.

36 Lane, H.E., Burns, T.A., Hegedus, O.C. et al. (2017). Lamellar events related to insulin-like growth factor-1 receptor signaling in two models relevant to endocrinopathic laminitis. *Equine Vet. J.* 49 (5): 643–654.

37 Bertin, F.R. and de Laat, M.A. (2017). The diagnosis of equine insulin dysregulation. *Equine Vet. J.* 49 (5): 570–576.

38 Toribio, R.E. (2018). Disorders of the endocrine system. In: *Equine Internal Medicine*, 4e (ed. S.M. Reed, W.M. Bayly, and D.C. Sellon), 1029–1138. Elsevier.

39 Meier, A., Reiche, D., de Laat, M. et al. (2018). The sodium-glucose co-transporter 2 inhibitor velagliflozin reduces hyperinsulinemia and prevents laminitis in insulin-dysregulated ponies. *PLoS One* 13 (9): e0203655.

40 Meier, A., de Laat, M., Reiche, D. et al. (2019). The efficacy and safety of velagliflozin over 16 weeks as a treatment for insulin dysregulation in ponies. *BMC Vet. Res.* 15 (1): 1–10.

41 Schuver, A., Frank, N., Chameroy, K.A., and Elliott, S.B. (2014). Assessment of insulin and glucose dynamics by using an oral sugar test in horses. *J. Equine Vet. Sci.* 34 (4): 465–470.

42 Smith, S., Harris, P., and Menzies-Gow, N. (2016). Comparison of the in-feed glucose test and the oral sugar test. *Equine Vet. J.* 48 (2): 224–227.

43 Bertin, F.R. and Sojka-Kritchevsky, J.E. (2013). Comparison of a 2-step insulin-response test to conventional insulin-sensitivity testing in horses. *Domest. Anim. Endocrinol.* 44 (1): 19–25.

44 Eiler, H., Frank, N., Andrews, F.M. et al. (2005). Physiologic assessment of blood glucose homeostasis via combined intravenous glucose and insulin testing in horses. *Am. J. Vet. Res.* 66 (9): 1598–1604.

45 National Research Council (2007). *Nutrient Requirements of Horses.* 6th Rev. Animal Nutrition Series, 1–341. Washington DC: National Academies Press.

46 Geor, R.J. and Harris, P.A. (2013). Laminitis. In: *Equine Applied and Clinical Nutrition: Health, Welfare and Performance* (ed. R.J. Geor, P.A. Harris, and M. Coenen), 469–486. Edinburgh: Saunders Elsevier.

47 Gordon, M.E., Jerina, M.L., King, S.L. et al. (2007). The effects of nonstructural carbohydrate content and feeding rate on glucose and insulin response to meal feeding in equine. *J. Equine Vet. Sci.* 27 (11): 489–493.

48 Watts, K.A. (2004). Forage and pasture management for laminitic horses. *Clin. Technol. Equine Pract.* 3 (1): 88–95.

49 Harris, P.A. (2017). Nutritional management for avoidance of pasture-associated laminitis. In: *Equine Laminitis* (ed. J.K. Belknap), 436–441. West Sussex: Wiley.

50 Longland, A.C. (2013). Pastures and pasture management. In: *Equine Applied and Clinical Nutrition: Health, Welfare and Performance* (ed. R.J. Geor, P.A. Harris, and M. Coenen), 332–350. Edinburgh: Saunders Elsevier.

51 Watts, K. (2010). Pasture management to minimize the risk of equine laminitis. *Vet. Clin. North Am. Equine Pract.* 26 (2): 361–369.

52 Longland, A.C., Ince, J.C., Moore-Colyer, M.J.S., and Harris, P.A. (2012). Degradation of grass and grass fructan by equine gastrointestinal digesta in vitro. In: *Forages and Grazing in Horse Nutrition* (ed. M.T. Saastamoinen, M.J. Fradinho, A.S. Santos, and N. Miraglia), 107–108. Wageningen: Wageningen Academic Publishers.

53 Spears, J.W., Lloyd, K.E., Siciliano, P. et al. (2020). Chromium propionate increases insulin sensitivity in horses following oral and intravenous carbohydrate administration. *J. Anim. Sci.* 98 (4): 1–11.

54 Bamford, N.J., Potter, S.J., Baskerville, C.L. et al. (2019). Influence of dietary restriction and low-intensity exercise on weight loss and insulin sensitivity in obese equids. *J. Vet. Intern. Med.* 33 (1): 280–286.

55 Delarocque, J., Frers, F., Huber, K. et al. (2020). Weight loss is linearly associated with a reduction of the insulin response to an oral glucose test in Icelandic horses. *BMC Vet. Res.* 16 (1): 1–8.

56 Graham-Thiers, P.M. and Kronfeld, D.S. (2005). Amino acid supplementation improves muscle mass in aged and young horses. *J. Anim. Sci.* 83 (12): 2783–2788.

57 Kronfeld, D.S., Holland, J.L., Rich, G.A. et al. (2004). Fat digestibility in *Equus caballus* follows increasing first-order kinetics. *J. Anim. Sci.* 82 (6): 1773–1780.

58 Kentucky Equine Research Staff (1999). Stabilized rice bran–just the facts, please. *EquiNews*. https://ker.com/equinews/stabilized-rice-bran-just-facts-please (accessed 19 December 2021).

59 Dunnett, C. (2013). Ration evaluation and formulation. In: *Equine Applied and Clinical Nutrition: Health, Welfare and Performance* (ed. R.J. Geor, P.A. Harris, and M. Coenen), 405–424. Edinburgh: Saunders Elsevier.

60 Harris, P.A., Coenen, M., and Geor, R.J. (2013). Controversial areas in equine nutrition and feeding management. In: *Equine Applied and Clinical Nutrition Health, Welfare and Performance* (ed. R.J. Geor, P. Harris, and M. Coenen), 455–465. Edinburgh: Saunders Elsevier.

61 Jacob, S.I., Geor, R.J., Weber, P.S.D. et al. (2018). Effect of age and dietary carbohydrate profiles on glucose and insulin dynamics in horses. *Equine Vet. J.* 50 (2): 249–254.

62 Macon, E.L., Harris, P., Bailey, S. et al. (2022). Postprandial insulin responses to various feedstuffs differ in insulin dysregulated horses compared with non-insulin dysregulated controls. *Equine Vet. J.* 54 (3): 574–583.

63 Ellis, A.D., Thomas, S., Arkell, K., and Harris, P. (2005). Adding chopped straw to concentrate feed: the effect of inclusion rate and particle length on intake behaviour of horses. *Pferdeheilkunde* 21 (Suppl): 35–37.

64 Dosi, M.C.M., Kirton, R., Hallsworth, S. et al. (2020). Inducing weight loss in native ponies: is straw a viable alternative to hay? *Vet. Rec.* 187 (8): e60.

65 Luthersson, N., Nielsen, K.H., Harris, P. et al. (2009). Risk factors associated with equine gastric ulceration syndrome (EGUS) in 201 horses in Denmark. *Equine Vet. J.* 41 (7): 625–630.

66 Jansson, A., Harris, P., Davey, S.L. et al. (2021). Straw as an alternative to grass forage in horses – effects on post-prandial metabolic profile, energy intake, behaviour and gastric ulceration. *Animals* 11 (8): 2197.

67 Longland, A.C., Barfoot, C., and Harris, P.A. (2011). Effects of soaking on the water-soluble carbohydrate and crude protein content of hay. *Vet. Rec.* 168 (23): 618.

68 Martinson, K., Jung, H., Hathaway, M., and Sheaffer, C. (2012). The effect of soaking on carbohydrate removal and dry matter loss in orchardgrass and alfalfa hays. *J. Equine Vet. Sci.* 32 (6): 332–338.

69 Bochnia, M., Pietsch, C., Wensch-Dorendorf, M. et al. (2021). Effect of hay soaking duration on metabolizable energy, total and prececal digestible crude protein and amino acids, non-starch carbohydrates, macronutrients and trace elements. *J. Equine Vet. Sci.* 101 (June): 103452.

70 Argo, C.M., Dugdale, A.H.A., and McGowan, C.M. (2015). Considerations for the use of restricted, soaked grass hay diets to promote weight loss in the management of equine metabolic syndrome and obesity. *Vet. J.* 206 (2): 170–177.

71 Longland, A.C., Barfoot, C., and Harris, P.A. (2014). Effect of period, water temperature and agitation on loss of water-soluble carbohydrates and protein from grass hay: implications for equine feeding management. *Vet. Rec.* 174 (3): 68.

72 Moore-Colyer, M.J.S., Lumbis, K., Longland, A., and Harris, P. (2014). The effect of five different wetting treatments on the nutrient content and microbial concentration in hay for horses. *PLoS One* 9 (11): e114079.

73 Kentucky Equine Research Staff (2014). Thoughts on soaking hay for horses. *EquiNews*. https://ker.com/equinews/thoughts-soaking-hay-horses (accessed 20 December 2021).

74 McGowan, T.W., Pinchbeck, G.P., and McGowan, C.M. (2013). Prevalence, risk factors and clinical signs predictive for equine pituitary pars intermedia dysfunction in aged horses. *Equine Vet. J.* 45 (1): 74–79.

75 Hart, K.A., Wochele, D.M., Norton, N.A. et al. (2016). Effect of age, season, body condition, and endocrine status on serum free cortisol fraction and insulin concentration in horses. *J. Vet. Intern. Med.* 30 (2): 653–663.

76 Miller, M.A., Pardo, I.D., Jackson, L.P. et al. (2008). Correlation of pituitary histomorphometry with adrenocorticotrophic hormone response to domperidone administration in the diagnosis of equine pituitary pars intermedia dysfunction. *Vet. Pathol.* 45 (1): 26–38.

77 McFarlane, D., Dybdal, N., Donaldson, M.T. et al. (2005). Nitration and increased α-synuclein expression associated with dopaminergic neurodegeneration in equine pituitary pars intermedia dysfunction. *J. Neuroendocrinol.* 17 (2): 73–80.

78 McFarlane, D. (2007). Advantages and limitations of the equine disease, pituitary pars intermedia dysfunction as a model of spontaneous dopaminergic neurodegenerative disease. *Ageing Res. Rev.* 6 (1): 54–63.

79 Donaldson, M.T., Lamonte, B.H., Morresey, P. et al. (2002). Treatment with P-pergolide or cyproheptadine of pituitary pars intermedia dysfunction (equine Cushing's disease). *J. Vet. Intern. Med.* 16 (6): 742–746.

80 McGowan, C.M., Frost, R., Pfeiffer, D.U., and Neiger, R. (2004). Serum insulin concentrations in horses with equine Cushing's syndrome: response to a cortisol inhibitor and prognostic value. *Equine Vet. J.* 36 (3): 295–298.

81 Karikoski, N.P., Patterson-Kane, J.C., Singer, E.R. et al. (2016). Lamellar pathology in horses with pituitary pars intermedia dysfunction. *Equine Vet. J.* 48 (4): 472–478.

82 Donaldson, M.T., Jorgensen, A.J.R., and Beech, J. (2004). Evaluation of suspected pituitary pars intermedia dysfunction in horses with laminitis. *J. Am. Vet. Med. Assoc.* 224 (7): 1123–1127.

83 Karikoski, N.P., Horn, I., McGowan, T.W., and McGowan, C.M. (2011). The prevalence of endocrinopathic laminitis among horses presented for laminitis at a first-opinion/referral equine hospital. *Domest. Anim. Endocrinol.* 41 (3): 111–117.

84 Wylie, C.E., Collins, S.N., Verheyen, K.L.P., and Newton, J.R. (2012). Risk factors for equine laminitis: a systematic review with quality appraisal of published evidence. *Vet. J.* 193 (1): 58–66.

85 Burns, T.A. (2016). Effects of common equine endocrine diseases on reproduction. *Vet. Clin. Equine Pract.* 32 (3): 435–449.

86 Swinker, A.M. (2014). Hay quality for different classes of horses. Pennsylvania State Extension Service. https://extension.psu.edu/hay-quality-for-different-classes-of-horses (accessed 2 July 2021).

87 Mastro, L.M., Adams, A.A., and Urschel, K.L. (2014). Pars intermedia dysfunction. *Am. J. Vet. Res.* 75 (7): 658–667.

88 Waldridge, B. and Pugh, D. (2017). Feeding horses with pituitary pars intermedia dysfunction. In: *Nutritional Management of Equine Diseases and Special Cases* (ed. B. Waldridge), 195. Wiley Blackwell.

89 Dunkel, B., Wilford, S.A., Parkinson, N.J. et al. (2014). Severe hypertriglyceridaemia in horses and ponies with endocrine disorders. *Equine Vet. J.* 46 (1): 118–122.

90 Divers, T.J. and Barton, M.H. (2018). Disorders of the liver. In: *Equine Internal Medicine*, 4e (ed. S.M. Reed, W.M. Bayly, and D.C. Sellon), 871–874. Elsevier.

91 Dunkel, B. and McKenzie, H.C. (2003). Severe hypertriglyceridaemia in clinically ill horses: diagnosis, treatment and outcome. *Equine Vet. J.* 35 (6): 590–595.

92 Durham, A.E., Hughes, K.J., Cottle, H.J. et al. (2009). Type 2 diabetes mellitus with pancreatic β cell dysfunction in 3 horses confirmed with minimal model analysis. *Equine Vet. J.* 41 (9): 924–929.

93 Mogg, T.D. and Palmer, J.E. (1995). Hyperlipidemia, hyperlipemia, and hepatic lipidosis in American miniature horses: 23 cases (1990–1994). *J. Am. Vet. Med. Assoc.* 207 (5): 604–607.

94 Watson, T.D., Murphy, D., and Love, S. (1992). Equine hyperlipaemia in the United Kingdom: clinical features and blood biochemistry of 18 cases. *Vet. Rec.* 131 (3): 48–51.

95 van den Berg, M., Giagos, V., Lee, C. et al. (2016). The influence of odour, taste and nutrients on feeding behaviour and food preferences in horses. *Appl Anim. Behav. Sci.* 184: 41–50.

96 Durham, A.E. (2006). Clinical application of parenteral nutrition in the treatment of five ponies and one donkey with hyperlipaemia. *Vet. Rec.* 158 (5): 159–164.

28

Metabolic Syndrome

Patricia Harris and Simon R. Bailey

KEY TERMS

- Tissue insulin resistance is the pathophysiological state in which cells fail to respond normally to insulin.
- Insulin dysregulation (ID) reflects the presence of one or more of the following: basal or fasting hyperinsulinemia; tissue insulin resistance; exaggerated insulin response to ingested non-structural carbohydrate (NSC), i.e. starch, simple sugars, and fructans; and/or exaggerated insulin response to intravenously provided simple sugars.

KEY POINTS

- The main consistent feature of equine metabolic syndrome (EMS) is the presence of ID. Lean as well as obese animals may have ID.
- Whilst obesity does not automatically mean an animal has EMS with its associated increased risk of laminitis, obesity itself is a cause for concern. Regular monitoring is needed to prevent unwanted weight gain, and a weight-loss program should be initiated in overweight and in particular obese, (i.e. body condition score ([BCS] ≥ 7/9), animals.
- Different weight-loss programs are required based on the cause of obesity, the facilities, pasture available, and possibly other constraints.
- Weight-loss programs must be practical and feasible for the caretaker. Monitoring is key, and options need to be regularly reassessed.
- Key practical nutritional management strategies for obese/overweight animals include promoting weight loss and improved insulin sensitivity via dietary restriction, restricted NSC intake and, where possible, increased physical activity.
- Cereal-based rations are unlikely to be suitable in the feeding program for ID animals or those prone to laminitis.

28.1 Defining Equine Metabolic Syndrome (EMS)

The association between excessive weight and laminitis had been suspected for centuries and thought to be a direct consequence of excessive adiposity until the early 1980s [1]. A link between insulin resistance and laminitis was suggested based on the observation that obese ponies, which were more prone to laminitis, were less sensitive to the effects of insulin, leading to the hypothesis of endocrinopathic laminitis [2–6]. Additional studies found that obese animals were more likely to be tissue insulin resistant compared with non-obese horses [7], laminitis-prone ponies tended to have decreased tissue insulin sensitivity [6]; and healthy body weight (BW) ponies infused with high doses of insulin developed clinical and histological signs of laminitis [8]. Hence, tissue insulin resistance was linked with obesity and a predisposition to laminitis. Various terms were used initially, e.g. EMS, pre-laminitic metabolic syndrome, and peripheral Cushing's syndrome [7, 9–11]. The various strands of work led to EMS becoming the more commonly used terminology; perhaps given the similarities with the human metabolic syndrome which was a collection of risk factors that help to predict the occurrence of coronary artery disease and type 2 diabetes mellitus [12]. However, the term EMS was not without controversy [13].

In 2010, a consensus statement of the American College of Veterinary Internal Medicine recommended the use of the term "equine metabolic syndrome" to describe the phenotype of an animal with obesity and insulin resistance

Equine Clinical Nutrition, Second Edition. Edited by Rebecca L. Remillard.

with a predisposition toward laminitis [14]. The EMS phenotype for the majority of affected equids would include:

1) Increased adiposity overall (obesity) or in specific locations (regional adiposity).
2) Insulin resistance characterized by hyperinsulinemia or abnormal glycemic and insulinemic responses to oral or intravenous glucose or insulin challenges.
3) Clinical or subclinical laminitis has developed in the absence of recognized causes, such as grain overload, colic, colitis, or retained placenta.

There was a recognition that while obesity was observed in the majority of cases, some affected equids were overall lean but with regional adiposity, whereas others did not show overall or regional adiposity. It was also recognized that a variety of other hormones and systemic markers, such as increased leptin and triglycerides, might be linked with EMS and an increased risk of laminitis. Increasingly and erroneously, the term EMS was used to describe any overweight animal.

Since 2010, further work has shown the risk of laminitis is more closely associated with insulin response to the oral ingestion of digestible or hydrolyzable carbohydrates, i.e. starch, simple sugars, and possibly fructans, leading to the increased use of the term ID [15, 16]. The term covers basal hyperinsulinemia and tissue insulin resistance, as well as an abnormal response to oral ingestion of starch and water-soluble carbohydrates (WSC) [17, 18]. The insulin response to the oral ingestion of simple sugars may be considerably greater than the response to the same amount of glucose administered intravenously, due to the effect of intestinal incretin hormones and stimulated pancreatic beta cells. Increased incretin production may be one component of ID [19, 20]. However it is very important to consider that obese animals are not necessarily all insulin dysregulated. A lean animal may have ID, and diet may be an important influencing factor [21, 22]. The actual risk of laminitis results from a complex interaction between genetics and the environment, i.e. epigenetics [23].

Many animals with ID may show fasting or basal hyperinsulinemia, but other individuals do not. This has led to the recommendation that dynamic testing procedures, e.g. the oral sugar test, be completed in those horses suspected of being insulin dysregulated with normal resting insulin concentrations [17, 24–26]. See Insulin Dysregulation in Chapter 27. This led to a subtle but important change in the definition of EMS. The recent consensus statement of the European College of Equine Internal Medicine emphasizes that ID is a key consistent feature of EMS with an increased risk of laminitis and the variable presence of obesity or other metabolic alterations [1, 27].

Therefore, an obese horse or pony cannot be diagnosed with EMS based on BW or BCS alone. Until there is a confirmation of ID, the animal should be considered simply overweight or obese. However, being overweight or obese in itself is a major welfare issue due to a variety of associated adverse consequences, including orthopedic disease, hyperlipemia, hyperthermia, infertility, and poor performance [28, 29]. A pasture-associated laminitis study concluded that overweight animals that develop laminitis tend to have more severe signs than those of optimal weight, and when laminitis does occur, overweight animals are more likely to die of the disease than ideal weight counterparts [30]. Additionally, recent weight gain is a risk factor for laminitis [31]. Obesity also remains a very important risk factor for ID and is therefore implicated in laminitis risk regardless of whether obesity is included in the core definition of EMS or not [32].

28.2 Animal Assessment

28.2.1 Obesity

There must be an appreciation that obesity is a welfare issue and that appropriate nutritional and management changes will need to be made. See Feeding for Weight Loss in Chapter 23. Effective weight-loss programs firstly require the recognition that the animal is overweight and needs to lose weight. Correctly identifying overweight animals visually is difficult for many people [33, 34]. Stable isotope methods accurately assess total body fat in living Equidae, but these are not yet feasible in practice [35]. Ultrasound determined rump and rib fat depth may in fact increase in obese horses and ponies losing weight during the winter [36]. Body mass index (BW/[length × height]) estimates correlated poorly with the % body fat, whereas BCS, completed by experienced investigators, correlated well up to BCS 7/9 and currently is the best practical method for monitoring purposes [37]. Any animal with a BCS ≥7/9 should be considered obese noting that the % body fat to BCS relationship is curvilinear above 7/9 [29, 38].

In addition, it can be very difficult to promote weight loss in certain individual horses or ponies once obese, and in "obesogenic environments" where making changes is challenging [33, 36, 39]. The best way to manage an obese horse or pony is obesity prevention and therefore regular communication with those feeding the animals regarding BW and BSC is key. Discussing weight and condition should be part of any visit using language that encourages interest and action. Ration and management plans require regular monitoring and reviewing, and these plans should be targeted to the individual animal and environmental circumstances and facilities. Once a target BW has been achieved, an ongoing program of weight maintenance will be required.

28.2.2 Insulin Dysregulation

The at-risk groups for being ID are:

- All overweight/obese animals.
- All animals that have had laminitis.
- All animals with pituitary pars intermedia dysfunction (PPID).
- All animals whose breed and lifestyle increase the risk of laminitis.

However, it is important to note that animals are not consistently either ID or non-ID; many factors affect ID status, including age, season, diet, pasture type and quality, and exercise level [15, 40]. This means that, ideally, regular monitoring is required of the above risk groups.

Although insulin response to an oral sugar load may indicate a risk of laminitis, the insulin concentration, duration, or frequency that leads to laminitis is not known. Following a single high glycemic index meal of 1 g of glucose/kg BW, serum insulin concentrations often exceeded 300 μIU/mL in ID ponies without causing clinical laminitis. However, one experimental study in horses caused laminitis within 48 hrs with a continuous infusion of insulin achieving serum concentrations of 300–500 μIU/mL [41]. Furthermore, when fed a high-NSC diet (12 g/kg BW/d) divided into three meals/d for 18 days, ponies with laminitis exhibited postprandial serum insulin concentrations between 300 and 500 μIU/mL [16]. These studies would suggest either a continuous exposure to high concentrations of insulin or repeated peaks of insulin without sufficient time to re-establish low concentrations between feedings may precipitate severe lamellar damage and clinical signs of laminitis. Two prospective studies identified elevated serum insulin concentrations as a major risk factor for laminitis [42, 43]. That said many equines with ID do not develop laminitis despite exhibiting extremely high insulin concentrations. These animals may have subclinical changes; hence, other factors may play a role in leading to structural lamellar failure and clinical signs, including physical factors, such as BW, the surface area of lamellar attachment, or the susceptibility of the lamellar tissues to insulin. It is also important to recognize that individuals with low insulin concentrations can still develop laminitis although their risk is lower than those with higher insulin concentrations [43].

The primary aim in the feeding management of horses and ponies with ID (obese or non-obese) is the avoidance of high-NSC feeds, i.e. starches, simple sugars, and/or fructans. Consumption of NSC increases the risk of laminitis, either by the exacerbation of hyperinsulinemia or possibly via disturbances to the hindgut microbial community that may trigger events leading to laminitis. An essential goal in obese, insulin-dysregulated animals is to promote weight loss [44], and increase exercise when appropriate [45]. Similarly in underweight animals the goal is to promote weight gain using feed stuffs that do not promote high insulin concentrations. Further work, however, is needed concerning insulin-sensitizing agents and dietary supplements that reduce the risks associated with ID in horses.

28.3 Ration Assessment

28.3.1 Grain Concentrates

- Omit grain and sweet complementary feeds which are high in starch and/or sugars from the ration. Provision of these feeds to insulin-resistant equids is likely to exacerbate hyperinsulinemia.
- Recommend low intakes of NSC per meal:
  - Severely ID animals at high risk for laminitis should be restricted to ≤0.1 g NSC/kg BW/meal for a very low insulin response [40].
  - In most older animals with age-associated increases in insulin responses, concentrations could be increased to ~0.5 g NSC/kg BW/meal [46].
  - *Responses are highly variable and not all the nutritional triggers for exaggerated insulin responses are known. Assessing a particular individual's insulin response to a specific meal may be necessary.*

28.3.2 Forages

- Recommend restricted or no access to pasture depending on the pasture type (locally relevant nutrition advice is recommended) and time of year. At certain times of the year, pasture forage NSC content in cool season grasses for example may approach 40% dry matter (DM). In susceptible animals, ingestion of this NSC-rich forage will increase the risk for laminitis [45, 47].
  - NSC intake over a relatively short period can be high when allowed access to a plentiful supply of grass with even a moderate (15–20%) NSC concentration.
  - Zero grazing with suitable forage alternatives may be required if an at-risk horse requires minimal NSC intake or during a weight-management program. However, in many management situations, some periods on pasture cannot be avoided. Therefore, several important points must be considered concerning turnout, which needs to be adjusted to the individual circumstances, e.g. forage species, local environmental conditions, and laminitis risk [47, 48].

- Recommend a grass forage diet based on long-stem or chopped, cubes or pellets with <12% and ideally <10% NSC DM basis. See Figure 6.2.
  - Nutrient analysis[1] of forage is essential for optimal ration formulation and estimating the NSC intake.
  - Assessing a particular individual's insulin response to a specific forage may be necessary.
  - Haylage, more commonly fed in Europe, may promote a greater insulin response for a given concentration of consumed NSC in ID animals [49].
  - Feed well-harvested, cleaned[2] barley or oat straw, chopped long or short, to slow the rate of feed intake, extend meal feeding time, and delay NSC intestinal absorption. Straw can replace up to 50% hay and may promote weight loss, e.g. in native ponies [50, 51].
    - The risk of equine gastric ulcer syndrome (EGUS) increases when straw is the main forage [52]; however, in a small study, no effect on EGUS was seen when straw was fed at 50% of the ration [53].
    - A slow introduction of straw may reduce the risk of *gastrointestinal impactions, although this remains a significant risk with certain breeds, e.g. thoroughbreds, and certain individuals.*
    - Consider steam treatment using commercial steamers before feeding to help improve hygienic quality. See Sidebar 10.2.
  - Hay soaking can result in a variable loss of WSC content (from around 10-40%) but can be a useful adjunct to managing both overweight animals and those prone to laminitis [54, 55].
    - Ideally, choose low-NSC hay and use soaking to reduce NSC further. Steaming is not effective at reducing WSC.
    - Hay-to-freshwater ratio of ~1 : 12 to 14 (w/w) is required for each soak.
    - Soak for >6 hrs in cold water or ~1 hr in >60 °F (16 °C) water. It is not practical to analyze soaked hay (although this is ideal). Water temperature and length of soak influence WSC loss, level of microbial contamination, and extent of DM loss [54, 56, 57]. Post-soak liquid is effluent and must not be consumed by horses.
    - Soaking hay results in a loss of DM, as a guide allow for 20% loss with soaking, as well as loss of some soluble protein, vitamins, and minerals [54, 55, 58, 59]. The ration therefore needs to take into account these losses, e.g. consider the need for a ration balancer.

---

1 Authors recommend that wet chemistry is preferable to NIRS (near-infrared spectroscopy) for WSC analysis. See Ration Analysis in Chapter 10. In Editor's experience in the USA, NIRS WSC analysis of single specie forages correlates well with wet chemistries.

2 See Common Manufacturing Processes: Cleaning in Chapter 13.

28.3.3 Complementary Feeds

- Recommend a forage ration balancer. A mature grass forage-only diet typically does not provide adequate minerals or vitamins and may not provide sufficient quality protein. These deficits become important when ration DM intakes are limited as in weight-loss programs. Additionally, animals will lose muscle mass as well as fat, and therefore where possible an exercise program coupled with a balancer providing essential amino acids, vitamins, and minerals is recommended.
  - Low-NSC forage balancers (typically fed at ~1 g/kg BW/d) should ideally be fed in divided amounts throughout the day [40].
  - Ensure an adequate (0.02–0.03 g/kg BW/d) intake of magnesium. There is no current evidence to suggest that high concentrations of magnesium will be protective or reduce the risk of laminitis.
  - Providing a biotin supplement to help support optimal hoof growth and quality may be helpful.
  - Feeding wheat bran mashes is contraindicated particularly for animals unaccustomed to bran. Bran can be an irritant to the gastrointestinal tract, has an inverse Ca : P ratio, and nutritionally is deficient in many key nutrients, such as lysine.
  - Providing antioxidant vitamin E at 3–4 IU/kg BW to laminitis-prone horses has been recommended [2].

28.4 Feeding Management

- Recommend feeding for maintenance of optimal BW and BCS. Regular evaluation of BW and BCS is the best way to assess the adequacy of energy intake.
  - If optimal BCS, check ration nutrient profile, and balance as needed, to maintain BCS, with particular attention to NSC intake.
  - If underweight, feeding additional energy is required
    - Increase forage digestibility by feeding less mature grass hay but recommend avoid feeding haylage/silage to animals that are prone to laminitis. Hays with NSC >12% DM should be avoided. Some horses may require provision of forages with <10% NSC DM.
    - Utilize highly digestible fiber sources in the ration, e.g., sugar beet pulp without added molasses, and soak to further reduce WSC or soy hulls.
    - If there are no contraindications, feeding vegetable oil effectively increases energy intake. Corn and soy oils are commonly used in equine rations, but need to be fresh, non-rancid, and incorporated gradually into the ration over 7–10 days. Vegetable oils provide

about 2 Mcal DE/244 mL (cup)[3]; ½ to 1 cup of oil can be fed once or twice daily up to a maximum of 1 mL oil/kg BW without requiring a ration reformulation if the base ration is balanced and fortified. Supplemental antioxidant at 1-2 IU vitamin E/mL added oil should be provided. Some animals may not tolerate oil supplementation.

- Stabilized, low starch, rice bran with ~20% fat is another option for increasing the energy density of the diet, providing the calcium: phosphorus ratio of the final ration is checked.
- Consider a low-starch, low-WSC commercial feed containing vegetable oil and highly digestible fibers, e.g., sugar beet or soy hulls, fed in multiple small meals/d. Ideally, use a product shown to produce low postprandial glucose and insulin response in ID animals or monitor response in the patient.
- For all horses cereal grains, other than oats, should be cooked, e.g., steam flaked or micronized to increase starch digestibility, thereby reducing the risk of starch overload into the large bowel. The introduction of grains should be transitioned. See Sidebar 26.1. Restrict cereal grain meal size to <0.3kg/100 kg BW and check starch intake/meal, e.g. <1g/kg BW/meal to reduce the risk of gastric ulcers. Importantly, cereal-based rations are unlikely to be suitable in the feeding program for ID animals or those prone to laminitis.

- If obese, initiate a weight loss program. See Sidebar 28.1. Improved insulin sensitivity and glucose tolerance have been reported in obese animals after weight loss (45).
  - Increasing free and/or structured exercise, based on veterinary advice, may help limit muscle loss associated with calorie-restricted diets, have an anti-inflammatory effect, and at relatively low intensities and duration, e.g., working trot for 15 mins, promote improved insulin sensitivity (29,45).
  - Consider increasing the number, length, or intensity of exercise occasions, changing the type of structured activity, e.g., riding, lunging, as well prolonging free activity in the paddock.
  - Track, paddock, pasture system, or similar may be a solution for some but consideration of land suitability is required (60).

Sidebar 28.1: Weight Loss Plan for Overweight EMS Horses [44]

An overweight animal may begin the weight loss plan at point A, B, or C depending on clinical assessment, the severity of clinical signs, and current feed intake. It is essential to monitor body weight frequently (ideally weekly) and adjust intakes based on BW accordingly.

It is essential to ensure that all personnel providing care to the animal agree that:

- The animal is overweight and this is detrimental.
- Weight loss is necessary to improve quality of life and possible longevity.
- Weight-loss plans may take months and require consistent efforts to achieve their objectives.

I) Understand exactly what is currently being fed:
  a) Know weights, not volumes, of each feed, including forages offered to the horse and calculate actual consumption after weighing all leftover, spilled and discarded feeds (i.e. orts).
  b) Understand the personnel and facilities available, as well as any constraints present.
  c) Agree on an individually tailored feeding plan and monitoring process.

II) Plan A Weight Loss:
  a) Replace "straight" grain or the manufactured feed with a lower-energy density, i.e. a high-fiber, low-starch, and low-sugar feed, preferably one that has been specifically formulated to help promote weight loss yet maximize the time spent chewing.
  b) Check the analysis of the current forage; if necessary, change to one with a lower-energy density, such as mature hay. Aim for <12% NSC on DM basis. Avoid potentially high-energy forages, such as alfalfa or haylage, as well as highly indigestible forages. A low-calorie hay replacer may be useful. Consider restricting or managing pasture access based on forage type and season.
  c) Increase exercise if possible by increasing the number, length, or intensity of exercise sessions, or changing the type of activity, e.g. riding vs. lunging. Consider prolonging free activity in the paddock, including methods to promote movement, e.g. grazing tracks.
  d) If there are insufficient decreases in heart and belly girth, rump width, and BW, then go to plan B.

---

3 Corn oil USDA Food database (NDB# 42289) and ~90% digestibility [61].

III) Plan B Weight Loss:
   a) Restrict access to grass, but if possible provide some drylot (or similar) turnout to maintain exercise and social interactions.
   b) Reduce or omit energy-providing complementary feed and provide a measured amount (1.5–2% BW DMI) of low-energy (<2.0 Mcal/kg DM) forage with minimal intake of grass. Provide an amino acid–vitamin–mineral ration balancer.
   c) Increase exercise if possible.
   d) If there are insufficient decreases in heart and belly girth, rump width, and BW, then go to plan C.

IV) Plan C Weight Loss:
   a) Provide lower-energy hay (1.8–2.0 Mcal/kg DM) with NSC < 10% DM (especially if prone to laminitis or ID) initially at 1.25–1.5% current BW DMI with subsequent reductions if required, but no less than 1.0% BW DMI. Animals should not be fed ≤1.25% BW DMI without veterinary advice and monitoring. Allow for a 20% DM loss if soaking hay. Consider how to extend foraging time.
   b) Divide ration throughout the day and consider strategies to prolong feed intake time, e.g. double small holed hay nets in multiple positions. Consider feeding a good-quality straw (1.7 Mcal/kg DM) as part of the ration. Introduce straw gradually into the ration and monitor GI function.
   c) Take measures to avoid the consumption of bedding materials, including wood shavings.
   d) Maintain a good-quality protein intake to help prevent unwanted muscle loss and provide vitamin and mineral support, e.g. low-energy, low-NSC ration balancer.
   e) Severely ID animals with a high risk of laminitis should be restricted to ≤0.1 g NSC/kg BW/meal if a very low insulin response to meal feeding is required – but it may be needed to monitor the individual response to the ration.

V) Once target BW and BCS are reached, monthly assessments are recommended, particularly with changes in the season and when changes in the feeding management or exercise regimen have been made.

Case in Point

In May, an owner presented a 13-yr-old Welsh pony mare with BW 340 kg and BCS 8/9 that had been showing signs of laminitis. The pony had been kept at pasture and the grass at this time of year appeared lush and green. The animal had been ridden regularly in previous years in a children's Pony Club, but not in the last 2 yrs since the child had advanced to a larger horse. Initially, the pony was walking with a stiff, stilted gait and was reluctant to walk on hard ground. The pony no longer had access to the pasture, but was stabled in a 12′ × 12′ stall, and a colleague from the veterinary practice had initiated treatment by prescribing phenylbutazone and applying frog support pads. The pony's lameness greatly improved with treatment, but at the follow-up visit 10 d later the owner asked for advice regarding feeding and ongoing management. There was an outdoor fenced 24′ × 24′ drylot area on the property, as well as stalls and grass paddocks.

Animal Assessment

Physical examination was unremarkable apart from the obese BCS, including a cresty neck and some faint founder rings noted on the front hooves. The pony was now more comfortable at the walk but was slightly short striding on hard ground, particularly when turning either to the left or the right. A blood sample was taken for serum biochemistry and basal insulin. A dynamic test for ID was not performed at this stage since the pony was still recovering from laminitis and pain or stress can affect the result. However, the basal insulin concentration was 60 μIU/mL, whereas normal for the laboratory used was <20 μIU/mL. The resting hyperinsulinemia indicated this pony was most likely insulin dysregulated. Plasma adrenocorticotropic hormone (ACTH) was 22 pg/mL, which suggested that this animal was unlikely to have PPID. The recent episode of laminitis, accompanied by ID and obesity, was consistent with a diagnosis of EMS.

The pony was moved to the 24′ × 24′ drylot, and an older obese companion pony was also put in a next-door lot, to avoid the stress of isolation as cortisol antagonizes insulin and strongly augments glucose-dependent insulin release, which could make laminitis worse.

1) *What are the dietary management goals in this case?*

Ration Assessment

Current DE intake on pasture could not be calculated but the nutrient profile (DM basis), analyzed by wet chemistry, of the hay was available as follows:

DM	DE	CP	ADF	NDF	NSC
%	Mcal/kg	%	%	%	%
85	2.19	13.3	42.1	62.5	9.8

Dietary Recommendations

The hay was considered to be of fair-quality based on ADF and NDF values (Table 10.3) with a 9.8% NSC which was appropriate for this pony. The owner was advised to feed forage at 1.25% BW DM at current BW.

2) *What is the recommended daily intake of hay on a DM basis?*
3) *What is the recommended daily intake of hay on an as fed basis?*

However, the owner said that she could soak the hay thereby reducing the NSC further.

4) *How much hay as fed (kg/d) should be weighed before soaking to account for the DM losses?*

After weighing the unsoaked hay, for practical reasons, the daily ration was soaked in warm water for 60 min and then divided into portions to be fed in three meals/d. Hay portions were kept cool until feeding. A hay net with small holes (1 inch^2) was used to slow forage intake, i.e. >2 hrs to eat 2 kg of soaked hay.

5) *What is an estimate of the pony's minimum DE_m at 340 kg?*

Although the hay was providing a restricted but acceptable amount of fiber and energy, a complementary feed to ensure adequate dietary protein, (especially essential amino acids), vitamins, and minerals was required. The owner agreed to feed a low-NSC, fiber-based proprietary amino acid–vitamin–mineral ration balancer divided into two meals/d. For weight loss, the total daily ration, forage plus ration balancer, provided 9.3 Mcal, which was 90% of the estimated daily DE_m at current BW (Table 23.2 Protocol #5.). Water and a white salt block were made available at all times.

6) *What are your monitoring recommendations?*

See Appendix A Chapter 28.

References

1 Harris, P.A., Bamford, N.J., and Bailey, S.R. (2020). Equine metabolic syndrome: evolution of understanding over two decades: a personal perspective. *Anim. Prod. Sci.* 60 (18): 2103–2110.

2 Geor, R.J. and Harris, P.A. (2013). Laminitis. In: *Equine Applied and Clinical Nutrition: Health, Welfare and Performance* (ed. R.J. Geor, P.A. Harris, and M. Coenen), 469–486. Edinburgh: Saunders Elsevier.

3 Coffman, J.R. and Colles, C.M. (1983). Insulin tolerance in laminitic ponies. *Can. J. Comp. Med.* 47 (3): 347–351.

4 Field, J.R. and Jeffcott, L.B. (1989). Equine laminitis – another hypothesis for pathogenesis. *Med. Hypotheses* 30 (3): 203–210.

5 Jeffcott, L.B., Field, J.R., McLean, J.G., and O'Dea, K. (1986). Glucose tolerance and insulin sensitivity in ponies and Standardbred horses. *Equine Vet. J.* 18 (2): 97–101.

6 Harris, P.A. and Geor, R.J. (2010). Recent advances in the understanding of laminitis and obesity. In: *The Impact of Nutrition on the Health and Welfare of Horses* (ed. A.D. Ellis, A.C. Longland, M. Coenen, and N. Miraglia), 215–233. Wageningen: Wageningen Academic Publishers.

7 Hoffman, R.M., Boston, R.C., Stefanovski, D. et al. (2003). Obesity and diet affect glucose dynamics and insulin sensitivity in thoroughbred geldings. *J. Anim. Sci.* 81 (9): 2333–2342.

8 Asplin, K.K.E., Sillence, M.M.N., Pollitt, C.C.C., and McGowan, C.M. (2007). Induction of laminitis by prolonged hyperinsulinaemia in clinically normal ponies. *Vet. J.* 174 (3): 530–535.

9 Johnson, P.J. (2002). The equine metabolic syndrome: peripheral Cushing's syndrome. *Vet. Clin. North Am. Equine Pract.* 18 (2): 271–293.

10 Treiber, K.H., Kronfeld, D.S., Hess, T.M. et al. (2005). Use of proxies and reference quintiles obtained from minimal model analysis for determination of insulin sensitivity and pancreatic beta-cell responsiveness in horses. *Am. J. Vet. Res.* 66 (12): 2114–2121.

11 Treiber, K.H., Kronfeld, D.S., Hess, T.M. et al. (2006). Evaluation of genetic and metabolic predispositions and nutritional risk factors for pasture-associated laminitis in ponies. *J. Am. Vet. Med. Assoc.* 228 (10): 1538–1545.

12 Wisse, B.E. (2004). The inflammatory syndrome: the role of adipose tissue cytokines in metabolic disorders linked to obesity. *J. Am. Soc. Nephrol.* 15 (11): 2792–2800.

13 Kronfeld, D.S., Treiber, K.H., Hess, T.M., and Boston, R.C. (2005). Insulin resistance in the horse: definition, detection, and dietetics. *J. Anim. Sci.* 83 (Suppl 13): E22–E31.

14 Frank, N., Geor, R.J., Bailey, S.R. et al. (2010). Equine metabolic syndrome. *J. Vet. Intern. Med.* 24 (3): 467–475.

15 Borer, K.E., Bailey, S.R., Menzies-Gow, N.J. et al. (2012). Effect of feeding glucose, fructose, and inulin on blood glucose and insulin concentrations in normal ponies and those predisposed to laminitis. *J. Anim. Sci.* 90 (9): 3003–3011.

16 Meier, A.D., De Laat, M.A., Reiche, D.B. et al. (2018). The oral glucose test predicts laminitis risk in ponies fed a diet high in nonstructural carbohydrates. *Domest. Anim. Endocrinol.* 63 (Apr): 1–9.

17 Bertin, F.R. and de Laat, M.A. (2017). The diagnosis of equine insulin dysregulation. *Equine Vet. J.* 49 (5): 570–576.

18 Frank, N., Bailey, S., Bertin, F.-R. et al. (2020). Recommendations for the diagnosis and treatment of equine metabolic syndrome (EMS). http://sites.tufts.edu/equineendogroup (accessed 20 March 2021).

19 Bamford, N.J., Baskerville, C.L., Harris, P.A., and Bailey, S.R. (2015). Postprandial glucose, insulin, and glucagon-like peptide-1 responses of different equine breeds adapted to meals containing micronized maize. *J. Anim. Sci.* 93 (7): 3377–3383.

20 de Laat, M.A., McGree, J.M., and Sillence, M.N. (2016). Equine hyperinsulinemia: investigation of the enteroinsular axis during insulin dysregulation. *Am. J. Physiol. Metab.* 310 (1): E61–E72.

21 Bamford, N.J., Potter, S.J., Baskerville, C.L. et al. (2016). Effect of increased adiposity on insulin sensitivity and adipokine concentrations in different equine breeds adapted to cereal-rich or fat-rich meals. *Vet. J.* 214 (Aug): 14–20.

22 Bamford, N.J., Potter, S.J., Harris, P.A., and Bailey, S.R. (2016). Effect of increased adiposity on insulin sensitivity and adipokine concentrations in horses and ponies fed a high fat diet, with or without a once daily high glycaemic meal. *Equine Vet. J.* 48 (3): 368–373.

23 McCue, M.E., Geor, R.J., and Schultz, N. (2015). Equine metabolic syndrome: a complex disease influenced by genetics and the environment. *J. Equine Vet. Sci.* 35 (5): 367–375.

24 Knowles, E.J., Harris, P.A., Elliott, J., and Menzies-Gow, N.J. (2017). Use of the oral sugar test in ponies when performed with or without prior fasting. *Equine Vet. J.* 49 (4): 519–524.

25 Jocelyn, N.A., Harris, P.A., and Menzies-Gow, N.J. (2018). Effect of varying the dose of corn syrup on the insulin and glucose response to the oral sugar test. *Equine Vet. J.* 50 (6): 836–841.

26 Macon, E.L., Harris, P.A., Partridge, E. et al. (2021). Effect of dose and fasting on oral sugar test responses in insulin dysregulated horses. *J. Equine Vet. Sci.* 107 (Sept): 103770.

27 Durham, A.E., Frank, N., McGowan, C.M. et al. (2019). ECEIM consensus statement on equine metabolic syndrome. *J. Vet. Intern. Med.* 33 (2): 335–349.

28 Geor, R.J. and Harris, P.A. (2013). Obesity. In: *Equine Applied and Clinical Nutrition: Health, Welfare and Performance* (ed. R.J. Geor, P.A. Harris, and M. Coenen), 487–502. Edinburgh: Saunders Elsevier.

29 Rendle, D., McGregor Argo, C., Bowen, M. et al. (2018). Equine obesity: current perspectives. *UK-Vet. Equine* 2 (5): 1–19.

30 Menzies-Gow, N.J., Stevens, K., Barr, A. et al. (2010). Severity and outcome of equine pasture-associated laminitis managed in first opinion practice in the UK. *Vet. Rec.* 167 (10): 364–369.

31 Wylie, C.E., Collins, S.N., Verheyen, K.L.P., and Newton, J.R. (2013). Risk factors for equine laminitis: a case-control study conducted in veterinary-registered horses and ponies in Great Britain between 2009 and 2011. *Vet. J.* 198 (1): 57–69.

32 Vick, M.M., Adams, A.A., Murphy, B.A. et al. (2007). Relationships among inflammatory cytokines, obesity, and insulin sensitivity in the horse. *J. Anim. Sci.* 85 (5): 1144–1155.

33 Morrison, P.K., Newbold, C.J., Jones, E. et al. (2020). The equine gastrointestinal microbiome: impacts of weight-loss. *BMC Vet. Res.* 16 (1): 1–18.

34 Furtado, T., Perkins, E., Pinchbeck, G. et al. (2021). Exploring horse owners' understanding of obese body condition and weight management in UK leisure horses. *Equine Vet. J.* 53 (4): 752–762.

35 Dugdale, A.H.A., Curtis, G.C., Milne, E. et al. (2011). Assessment of body fat in the pony: part II. Validation of the deuterium oxide dilution technique for the measurement of body fat. *Equine Vet. J.* 43 (5): 562–570.

36 Argo, C.M., Curtis, G.C., Grove-White, D. et al. (2012). Weight loss resistance: a further consideration for the nutritional management of obese Equidae. *Vet. J.* 194 (2): 179–188.

37 Dugdale, A.H.A., Curtis, G.C., Harris, P.A., and Argo, C.M. (2011). Assessment of body fat in the pony: part I. Relationships between the anatomical distribution of adipose tissue, body composition and body condition. *Equine Vet. J.* 43 (5): 552–561.

38 Dugdale, A.H.A., Grove-White, D., Curtis, G.C. et al. (2012). Body condition scoring as a predictor of body fat in horses and ponies. *Vet. J.* 194 (2): 173–178.

39 Furtado, T., Perkins, E., Pinchbeck, G. et al. (2021). Hidden in plain sight: uncovering the obesogenic environment surrounding the UK's leisure horses. *Anthrozoos* 34 (4): 491–506.

40 Macon, E.L., Harris, P., Bailey, S. et al. (2022). Postprandial insulin responses to various feedstuffs differ in insulin dysregulated horses compared with non-insulin dysregulated controls. *Equine Veterinary Journal* 54 (3): 574–583.

41 Rahnama, S., Vathsangam, N., Spence, R. et al. (2020). Effects of an anti-IGF-1 receptor monoclonal antibody on laminitis induced by prolonged hyperinsulinaemia in Standardbred horses. *PLoS One* 15 (9): e0239261.

42 Menzies-Gow, N.J., Harris, P.A., and Elliott, J. (2017). Prospective cohort study evaluating risk factors for the

development of pasture-associated laminitis in the United Kingdom. *Equine Vet. J.* 49 (3): 300–306.
43 Knowles, E., Elliott, J., Harris, P. et al. (2022). Predictors of laminitis development in a cohort of non-laminitic ponies. *Equine Vet. J.* https://doi.org/10.1111/evj.13572
44 Shepherd, M., Harris, P., and Martinson, K.L. (2021). Nutritional considerations when dealing with an obese adult equine. *Vet. Clin. Equine Pract.* 37 (1): 111–137.
45 Bamford, N.J., Potter, S.J., Baskerville, C.L. et al. (2019). Influence of dietary restriction and low-intensity exercise on weight loss and insulin sensitivity in obese equids. *J. Vet. Intern. Med.* 33 (1): 280–286.
46 Jacob, S.I., Geor, R.J., Weber, P.S.D. et al. (2018). Effect of age and dietary carbohydrate profiles on glucose and insulin dynamics in horses. *Equine Vet. J.* 50 (2): 249–254.
47 Harris, P.A. (2017). Nutritional management for avoidance of pasture-associated laminitis. In: *Equine Laminitis* (ed. J.K. Belknap), 436–441. West Sussex: Wiley.
48 Longland, A.C. (2013). Pastures and pasture management. In: *Equine Applied and Clinical Nutrition: Health, Welfare and Performance* (ed. R.J. Geor, P.A. Harris, and M. Coenen), 332–350. Edinburgh: Saunders Elsevier.
49 Carslake, H.B., Argo, C.M., Pinchbeck, G.L. et al. (2018). Insulinaemic and glycaemic responses to three forages in ponies. *Vet. J.* 235: 83–89.
50 Ellis, A.D., Thomas, S., Arkell, K., and Harris, P. (2005). Adding chopped straw to concentrate feed: the effect of inclusion rate and particle length on intake behaviour of horses. *Pferdeheilkunde* 21 (Suppl): 35–37.
51 Dosi, M.C.M., Kirton, R., Hallsworth, S. et al. (2020). Inducing weight loss in native ponies: is straw a viable alternative to hay? *Vet. Rec.* 187 (8): e60.
52 Luthersson, N., Nielsen, K.H., Harris, P. et al. (2009). Risk factors associated with equine gastric ulceration syndrome (EGUS) in 201 horses in Denmark. *Equine Vet. J.* 41 (7): 625–630.
53 Jansson, A., Harris, P., Davey, S.L. et al. (2021). Straw as an alternative to grass forage in horses – effects on post-prandial metabolic profile, energy intake, behaviour and gastric ulceration. *Animals* 11 (8): 2197–2212.
54 Longland, A.C., Barfoot, C., and Harris, P.A. (2011). Effects of soaking on the water-soluble carbohydrate and crude protein content of hay. *Vet. Rec.* 168 (23): 618.
55 Martinson, K., Jung, H., Hathaway, M., and Sheaffer, C. (2012). The effect of soaking on carbohydrate removal and dry matter loss in orchardgrass and alfalfa hays. *J. Equine Vet. Sci.* 32 (6): 332–338.
56 Longland, A.C., Barfoot, C., and Harris, P.A. (2014). Effect of period, water temperature and agitation on loss of water-soluble carbohydrates and protein from grass hay: implications for equine feeding management. *Vet. Rec.* 174 (3): 68.
57 Moore-Colyer, M.J.S., Lumbis, K., Longland, A., and Harris, P. (2014). The effect of five different wetting treatments on the nutrient content and microbial concentration in hay for horses. *PLoS One* 9 (11): e114079.
58 Bochnia, M., Pietsch, C., Wensch-Dorendorf, M. et al. (2021). Effect of hay soaking duration on metabolizable energy, total and prececal digestible crude protein and amino acids, non-starch carbohydrates, macronutrients and trace elements. *J. Equine Vet. Sci.* 101 (June): 103452.
59 Argo, C.M., Dugdale, A.H.A., and McGowan, C.M. (2015). Considerations for the use of restricted, soaked grass hay diets to promote weight loss in the management of equine metabolic syndrome and obesity. *Vet. J.* 206 (2): 170–177.
60 Furtado, T. (2021). Optimised environments for horse health and wellbeing: the use of alternative grazing. *UK-Vet. Equine* 5 (5): 190–194.
61 Kronfeld, D.S., Holland, J.L., Rich, G.A. et al. (2004). Fat digestibility in *Equus caballus* follows increasing first-order kinetics. *J. Anim. Sci.* 82 (6): 1773–1780.

Appendix

A: Case in Point Answers and Outcomes

Chapter 1

1) *What aspects of meal feeding pelleted feeds and grain concentrates likely relate to ESGD?*
   The gastrointestinal tract (GIT) of horses evolved grazing on low starch, high fiber, long-stem forages for 12–15 hrs/d. Meal feeding horses high starch, low fiber, small particle sized (pelleted) feeds twice daily does not match their GIT design, hence there are bound to be physiological consequences. See Chapter 26.4.1.
2) *What are the total daily intakes of feed (lb/d), energy (Mcal/d), and starch (g/kg BW/meal)?*
   - Daily feed intake is 26 lb/d which is 2% [= 26/1300] of the horse's current body weight and is appropriate.
   - Daily energy intake is 34.75 Mcal/d which is high according to the 2007 NRC pg 300 [1] where a 600 kg horse doing moderate work requires 28.0 Mcal DE/d.
   - Daily starch intake is ~2 g/kg BW/meal [2.4 kg starch/ 591 kg BW/2 meal/d] which is higher than the current recommendation of 1g starch/kg BW/meal [2].
3) *What would be a sound recommendation to the owner regarding the feeding management of this horse to prevent future ulcers?*
   Continue with free access to pasture and water with herd mates.
   To have the ration formulated to:
   - reduce the starch intake to <1 g starch/kg BW/meal [3],
   - reduce daily caloric intake to match caloric expenditure to reduce orts (feed waste),
   - reduce the intake of pelleted hay and offer long-stem hay 15–20 hrs/day,
   - offer grain concentrate divided into 3 or 4 meals/d as needed to manage ulcers, and consider feeding a buffer (calcium carbonate) with each meal.
   - if needed, increase the fat content to maintain caloric intake while reducing the starch.
4) *What is the rationale for these feeding recommendations?*
   The horse evolved as a social herbivore with cecal digestion of fiber, i.e., well suited to a high fiber, low starch diet, and would naturally spend up to 18 hrs/d foraging and would rarely fast voluntarily for more than 2–4 hrs at a time in part due to the constant production of gastric acids.
   - Digestion of starch in the stomach results in volatile fatty acid production, in conjunction with HCl acid, which has been shown to damage squamous mucosal cells.
   - Long stem hay increases chewing time and increases buffering saliva to the stomach.
   - Increased fat intake reduces starch content, the total volume of feed needed and increases calorie intake, if needed.
   - Feeding small meals of concentrate with hay or buffers may also minimize gastric acid damage to squamous mucosal cells.
   - Continue access to herd mates, water, and pasture *ad libitum* to reduce psychological stressors of herd separation. Management systems that allow for voluntary movement with herd mates best match their biological need for a social structure and ability to flee which are, after 50 million years of evolution, intrinsic requirements for their survival, welfare, and psychological comfort [4].

Chapter 2

1) *What was the mare's daily energy intake based on the ration assessment?*
   The mare's DE intake was 35.1 Mcal/d.
2) *What was the mare's recommended daily energy intake at her current BW doing light work?*
   According to the 2007 NRC pg 302 [1], a 900 kg horse doing light work requires 36.0 Mcal DE/d, therefore proportionally an 1800 lb or 818 kg horse doing light work should consume 32.7 Mcal DE/d.

Equine Clinical Nutrition, Second Edition. Edited by Rebecca L. Remillard.

3) *What was the mare's recommended daily energy intake at her ideal BW doing light work?*
   Proportionally a 1700 lb or 772 kg horse doing light work should consume 30.9 Mcal DE/d.
4) *How would you explain to the owner why the mare has a high BCS?*
   Energy intake is 35 Mcal DE/d compared to energy needs of 31 Mcal DE/d) was likely the cause of the mare's excessive BW and BCS.
5) *What recommendations would you suggest to the owner?*
   To achieve weight loss, energy intake can be reduced, energy use can be increased by an increase in work, or a combination of both strategies can be used. In this case, the mare's level of work was maximal for what could be achieved at the ranch, so weight loss was focused on the alteration of the mare's ration.

Ration Recommendations:
After the ranch-grown hay was analyzed, a new ration was formulated to 31.7 Mcal DE/d, which reduced dietary energy by 9.6% or 3.37 Mcal DE/d, by replacing the commercial complete feed product with 2.25 lbs of a commercial ration balancer designed to meet all nutrient requirements when fed with the hay.

Feed	1b fed/d	Mcal/1b	Mcal/d
Hay	30	0.93	27.9
Ration Balancer product	2.25	1.7	3.8
Total	32.3		31.7

The mare was transitioned to the new ration over 6 days by reducing the complete feed by 2 lb/d every 3 days and then replacing the last 2 lb on day 7 with 2.25 lb of a ration balancer. A gradual loss of weight was desired to prevent complications associated with hypertriglyceridemia and hepatic lipidosis that could develop from rapid weight loss in an obese horse. Routine examinations were scheduled every 1–2 mos to evaluate the mare's condition. Additional ration changes with greater energy restriction were planned, if needed, to promote continued weight loss until the mare achieved her ideal weight of 1700 lbs.

Progress Notes:
Over the next 6 mos, BW and BSC gradually decreased while the mare consumed the recommended ration. Once the mare's BW reached 1750 lbs, her weight stabilized for 2 mos so additional calorie restriction was recommended by reducing the volume of hay by 2 lb/d which further reduced daily energy intake to 29.8 Mcal DE/d.

Feed	1b fed/d	Mcal/1b	Mcal/d
Hay	28	0.93	26.04
Ration Balancer product	2.25	1.7	3.8
Total	30.3		29.8

Weight loss resumed and continued until the mare reached a BW of 1710 lbs and BCS of 6/9. At that time, her weight stabilized and the recommendation was made to continue feeding the mare 28 lbs of hay per day with the ration balancer until the next routine visit.

Chapter 3

3) *Summarize the problem(s) for the owner, suggest next steps and general dietary recommendations.*
   It appears this geriatric horse was in good health except for some tooth loss, and oral pain associated with several loose teeth and impending cardiac failure. The recommendations were to 1) consult with an equine dentist regarding the loose teeth as soon as possible, 2) change the form of the feed to accommodate the horse's decreased ability to chew, and 3) increase the caloric density of the ration provided.
4) *What specific changes to the ration could be made to provide more digestible calories to this horse?*
   New Ration: A cubed forage was offered at 1.0% BW twice a day to provide a shorter length of fiber to reduce the need for mastication. The cubes were soaked in water to reduce the chance of choking because excessively dry boluses of feed are to be expected secondary to the reduced chewing time and saliva production. A higher fat (10%) complete pelleted ration was fed at the rate of 0.5% BW twice a day. The horse was stalled individually at feeding time for each meal but otherwise was turned out with herd mate and allowed free access to hay.

   Follow-up:
   The horse regained weight to BCS 5–6/9 over the next 6 mos and was able to maintain a good body condition when fed appropriate feedstuffs for another eight years.

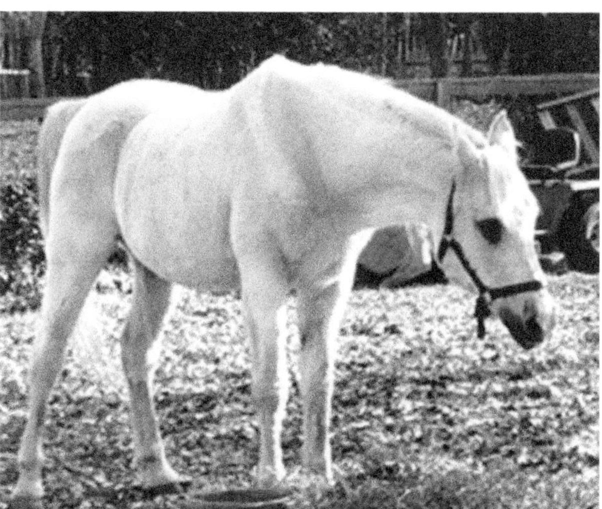

The gelding at 31 yrs old at the time of humane euthanasia due to severe congestive heart failure, unrelated to nutrition.

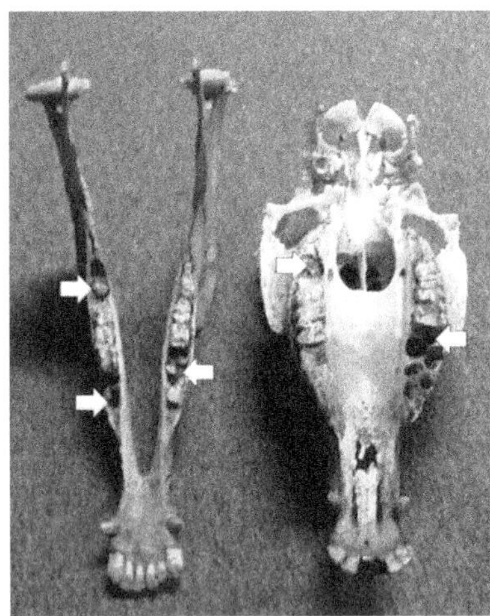

Postmortem mandible and maxilla of the same horse showing the extent of molar loss (arrows).

Chapter 5

1) *How does the water sample analysis compare with water quality guidelines for livestock?*
   The water report was interpreted using the general livestock guidelines in Tables 5.3 and 5.4, and the new well water, if the sample is representative, is above the acceptable limits of sulfates with a marginal TDS value. Although some consider horses tolerant of this TDS concentration, this may not be true for working horses.
2) *How might the water analysis explain the clinical signs exhibited by the cattle?*
   The signs of water refusal by the cattle and horses are consistent with a high TDS concentration. The facial and ear twitching and separation of some cows from the herd are possibly early clinical signs of polioencephalomalacia (PEM) associated with high sulfur intake. Sulfur-related PEM in cattle appears to be due to excessive sulfide gas production by ruminal microbial reduction of ingested sulfur. Although non-reduced forms of sulfur, such as sulfate and elemental sulfur, are relatively nontoxic, sulfide gas is a highly toxic substance that interferes with cellular energy metabolism. The central nervous system is dependent on a high concentration of energy production and the cattle-associated signs of sulfide gas in cattle may be related to an interrupted supply of energy [5].
3) *What are the options for improving the quality of water from this well?*
   The rancher considered several options to improve his water. He inquired into the cost of a water conditioner to remove sulfates and TDS using reverse osmosis but decided the cost was too high. Diluting the well water with good quality water was discounted as being impractical. He inquired if a mineral mix would help correct the situation and was advised that while it might help prevent copper deficiency secondary to high sulfates it would not improve the overall situation. The rancher decided not to pipe the water from this well to a water trough and instead drilled for water at another location.

Chapter 6

How to make a ration recommendation?
A reasonable conservative recommendation, given dietary history is unknown, would be to start feeding minimum daily DE_m at the current low BW and then increase if the animal had no feeding complications.

1) *Assess the animal requirement:*
   The minimum adult DE_m requirement is 11 Mcal/d [365 kg × 30.3 Kcal/kg BW] using current BW. Estimating an ideal BW using equations in Table 2.3 or Appendix E indicates the mare is about 25 kg underweight. She would require about 12 Mcal DE/d [390 kg × 30.3 Kcal/kg BW] at ideal BW and condition. A reasonable recommendation would be to feed at current BW for 5 days (11 Mcal/d), and if there are no clinical problems, increase energy intake to ideal BW DE_m (12 Mcal/d).
2) *Assess the available feeds:*
   Checking book values for timothy hay (IFN 1-04-883), this feed has a DE for horses of 2.00 Mcal/kg and contains 8.1% protein and 2.3% fat as fed [6].
3) *Make a feeding recommendation by matching the feed available to animal requirement:*
   A reasonable feeding recommendation would be to initially offer 5.5 kg of timothy hay daily divided into three feedings [11 Mcal/2 Mcal/kg]. If well tolerated for 5 days, feed 6.0 kg of hay divided into 2 feedings/d for another 5 days. The protein intake would be 0.5 kg/d (6.5 kg × 0.081) which approximates the suggested protein requirement of an average 400 kg mature adult horse. See NRC pg 296 [1]. If no problems occur in 5 days then, add 1 kg of a grass ration balancer pelleted product, containing less than 5% starch, twice a day to meet the mare's vitamin, macro, and trace mineral requirements. Offer clean, palatable water and white salt *ad libitum*. Reassess BW and BCS in 30 days.

Chapter 7

1) *How much of each feed (as fed basis) in the chart below will be required daily to meet the NRC suggested intake of 630 g protein?*

Feedstuff	Protein (%)	Feed* (kg/d)	Lysine (%)	Lysine** (g/d)
Grass hay (good quality)	8	7.9	0.4	31.6
Soybean meal (44%)	45	1.4	2.9	40.6
Sunflower meal (44%)	45	1.4	1.6	22.4

* [0.630 kg protein / % CP = kg feed/d]
** [Daily feed intake × % lysine × 1000 = g lysine/d]

2) *Which feeds fed at the calculated daily rate to meet CP intake will also meet the NRC [1] suggested intake of 27 g lysine/d?*
The grass hay and soybean meal fed to meet the protein requirement also would meet the lysine requirement. Sunflower meal has the same %CP as soybean meal but not the same lysine concentration and, when fed to meet protein requirement, does not meet the lysine requirement.

Chapter 8

1) *Does feeding 15 kg/horse/d (500 kg BW × 3%) of mature Timothy hay and 2 lb of the grain mix meet the crude protein, calcium, and phosphorus requirements of late gestation mares?*

Feed source	Protein	Ca	P
	g/d	g/d	g/d
Timothy hay IFN 1-04-881 [6]	2550	99	51
Grain mix	150	7	4
Total daily intake	2700	106	55

Yes, the crude protein, calcium, and phosphorus intake exceed the requirements of late gestation and early lactating mares (NRC 2007 pg 298) [1].

2) *The foal sent to the ICU was euthanized, and on necropsy was found to have histological changes consistent with thyroid hyperplasia. What is now the primary nutrient of concern?*
Iodine (I) is now the primary nutrient of concern, however, it is not clear if this is a case of iodine deficiency or toxicity.
3) *What are the next steps to determine the imbalance in the mare's ration?*
Estimate iodine intake from the hay and grain mix to determine the iodine intake of the mares.

Feed source	Iodine
	mg/d
Timothy hay IFN 1-04-893 [210]	0.6
Grain mix	0.1
Total daily intake	0.7
Mare requirements	
Mare, 11-mos gestation	4.0
Mare, 1-mos lactation	4.4

The calculation indicates the mares are receiving less than 20% of their iodine requirement (NRC 2007 pg 299) [1]. A free choice TM salt block with 70 mg/kg iodine alone may not suffice for some mares during pregnancy and lactation due to variability in voluntary salt consumption. In this case, each mare would have to consume ~60g TM salt/d (> 3 Tbsp/d) to meet their iodine requirement [4.0 mg I/d needed to be divided by 70 mg I/kg in TM salt = 57g/d of TM salt] [7].

4) *What would be the recommendation for next year?*
Provide a grain mix with at least 4 mg/kg or 0.0004% iodine.

Feed source	Iodine	Amount fed	Iodine
	mg/kg	Kg/d	mg/d
Timothy hay IFN 1-04-893	0.04	15	0.6
NEW Grain mix	4	1	4
Total daily intake			4.6

Chapter 9

1) *What would be your 'next step' recommendation to the owner?*
Poor performance refers to the inability to exercise or perform at a level previously observed or at a level that can be reasonably expected based on the horse's physical characteristics and life stage. The specific cause of 'poor' performance can be a diagnostic challenge. In a retrospective assessment of 200 cases presented to an equine hospital for poor performance, researchers found that 77% suffered from a musculoskeletal issue [8]. Based on the subjective nature of the owner complaint, in the face of a normal PE, negative lameness exam, laboratory data within normal limits, a nutrient profile assessment of the ration was recommended. A vitamin imbalance related to normal muscle physiology was suspected because the ration description lacked a source of vitamins, such as a ration balancer, vitamin supplement or fresh forage.
2) *What vitamins are of greatest concern for potential deficiencies in this horse?*
This case presentation is non-specific, with no pathognomonic signs to pinpoint a single vitamin deficiency. A failure to perform to expectations could result from poor energy metabolism due to B vitamin deficiencies (Figure 9.1), muscular or neuromuscular conditions (vitamins A and E), or skeletal pain (vitamin D). Poor muscle condition could likewise result from suboptimal

muscle development (vitamin A), a failure in protein metabolism (folate, cobalamin, pyridoxine), or nutritional myodegeneration (vitamin E). A poor hair coat is a sign common to almost all vitamin deficiencies and aids little in narrowing the diagnosis. Thus, presenting signs alone does not give much indication of how to proceed. The diet history is more useful in this instance. Vitamins degrade over time with the storage of feed, some at faster rates than others, and while under cover. Given the history of fed hay cut ~18 m prior, "straight" whole oats (no other ingredients), and provision of a white (no cobalt) salt block, this horse's intake of vitamins A, E and B vitamins may be below recommended intake.

3) *How could a suspected vitamin deficiency be diagnosed and treated?*

   There are three possible options in how to approach this case: one could perform computer analysis of the feeds to identify likely deficiencies, submit samples of the hay and oats for laboratory vitamin analysis, or add a source of the suspected deficient vitamins and observe for a response. While veterinarians are trained to make definitive diagnoses before proceeding with treatment, vitamin analyses are expensive, and testing a feed source for an array of multiple vitamins is cost-prohibitive for most clients. Computer analysis can be economical and some practitioners have ration-balancing software. When non-life-threatening nutritional imbalances are suspected, following clinical suspicion is a reasonable first step and recommending a specific change to the ration targeting the suspected deficiencies.

Outcome:

In this case, given changing the hay was not possible in the short term, the whole oats were discontinued and a commercially formulated 'ration balancer' pellet containing the vitamins of concern was fed at the daily rate (0.5 kg/d) recommended by the manufacturer. Three months after the ration change, the owner reported the horse's summer coat was growing well, skin and hair were healthy-looking. The horse had more energy and was more willing under saddle. After the sessions, the horse often rolled and appeared more comfortable moving about in the stall, and had been more interactive with the other geldings in the paddock.

Given the hay portion of the ration was not changed, comparing the concentrations and daily intake of the vitamins of concern (shaded rows) in whole oats to the commercial ration balancer illustrates the notable differences in vitamin intake. The vitamin deficiency (or deficiencies) in the original ration remains unknown.

	Unit per g as fed		Intake unit per day	
Nutrient (units)	**Oats**	**Pellets**	**1 kg Oats**	**0.5 kg Pellets**
Energy (kcal)	3.8	3.5	3800	1750
Protein (g)	0.13	0.32	130	160
Fat (g)	0.065	0.05	65	25
Vitamin A (IU)	0	19	0	9500
Beta-carotene (mg)	0	0.015	0	7.5
Thiamine (mg)	0.005	0.12	5	60
Riboflavin (mg)	0.002	0.0001	2	0.05
Niacin (mg)	0.011	0.037	11	18.5
Pantothenic Acid (mg)	0	0.007	0	3.5
Pyridoxine (mg)	0.001	0.014	1	7
Biotin (mg)	0	0.08	0	40
Folate (mg)	0.00032	0.02	0.32	10
Cobalamin (ug)	0	0.001	0	0.5
Vitamin C (mg)	0	0.004	0	2
Vitamin D (IU)	0	6	0	3000
Vitamin E (IU)	0.42	1.3	420	650
Vitamin K (mg)	0.002	0.012	2	6

Chapter 10

Scenario 3: *What should the caloric density of the ration be to meet the daily energy need of 15 Mcal DE/d within a DMI of 2% BW for a 454 kg adult horse at maintenance?*

1) The horse's DMI at 2% BW is 9.1 kg ration DM/d [454 kg × 2.0%].
2) Ration caloric density needed to meet energy need within the DMI [15 Mcal DE/9.1 kg] is 1.6 Mcal DE/kg DM.

Chapter 11

1) *What should be next investigated?*
   a) Offer the pony a small amount of palatable grain and note appetite and ability to prehend, masticate and swallow the feed: the pony shows great interest in the grain mix and has no observable difficulties eating the grain mix.
   b) Investigate the current feeding method: all horses, including the pony, are fed *ad libitum* hay from a 5 × 4 ft round bale (900 lb/bale) of fescue hay fed undercover (Figure 11.10) with eight feeding stations for 10 horses. Daily each horse is separately (Figure 10.1) fed 0.5-1 lb of a commercial low fat, low starch ration balancer of vitamins and minerals

designed to complement grass hay. According to the owner, the pony did not appear to have any issue getting to the covered hay, and was regularly seen eating contentedly with the rest of the horses.

c) Inspect the hay: the hay was predominately fescue harvested 9 m previously from the same farm and stored properly in a new metal barn. The remaining bales contained no mold, weeds, were yellow on the outside but the interior hay was still pale green, however the leaf to stem ratio appeared to be low.

2) *Given appetite appears to be good, and the pony had no physical problems eating the sample grain mix, and reportedly has no problems eating hay from the group feeder, what would be the next step in the investigation?*
Determine the pony's daily intake of hay and calculate daily DE. Given the pony is group-fed, it is not possible to determine this individual animal's daily DM or DE intake. At the pony's ideal BW of 400 lb (181 kg), the recommended average DE_m would be 6.1 Mcal/d
   - 6.06 Mcal DE/d from NRC 2007 pg 294) [1] adjusted for 181 kg BW or.
   - 6.05 Mcals DE/d from Table 17.1 [3.34 Mcal × 1.81].
3) Hay DM analysis became available: DE 0.91 Mcal/lb, 9% CP, ADF 41.6% and NDF 69.1% and a calculated RFV of 76. *Could this information explain the weight loss in this pony?*
Based on the hay analysis, the ADF and NDF concentrations indicate the forage was harvested later than optimal and is of fair-quality (Table 10.3).
At ideal BW of 400 lb, needing 6.1 Mcal DE/d, the pony would have to eat 6.7 lb forage/day [6.1 Mcal DE/0.91 Mcal/lb] or 1.7% of ideal BW [6.7 lb forage/400 lb BW x 100] to meet maintenance energy need with no consideration yet for the winter environment. Consuming 1.7% BW is reasonable for adult ponies (1.5-2.0% BW) so possibly the old pony is having difficulty gaining access to a sufficient quantity of hay, i.e. the hay feeder, due to competition. Protein intake at 9% of 6.7 lb forage [274 g/d] is adequate for this pony requiring 228 g/d.
In summary, the pony's estimated daily DE requirement was likely greater than 6 Mcal. Given the fair-quality and low DE concentration of the forage, the pony could not consume enough forage to meet DE intake during winter months when energy needs would have been increased to maintain body temperature. The inability to consume enough calories due to the fair-quality of the forage resulted in the pony drawing on body fat stores. This most likely explains the chronic weight loss.
4) *What would be your feeding recommendations for this pony?*
Given the pony will continue feeding on the baled fescue with the herd and the horses are separated once daily and fed a vitamin-mineral supplement, it would be logistically simple to offer this pony additional calories while fed separately. A reasonable first recommendation would be to provide the DE deficit as hay cubes or pellets while feeding separated from the herd. Then re-evaluate BW and condition in 30 days. Hay pellets can be consumed in a relatively short period and will provide the additional DE in a smaller volume than feeding additional long-stem hay. The owner should be sure the pony is eating all the grass pellets offered and if not, then a more concentrated form of DE will have to be offered. At the 30-day re-evaluation, a further adjustment could be made to the ration based on the pony's response and assessing the availability of spring pasture.

Chapter 12

1) *The initial diagnosis is radiation-induced dermatitis. How would you determine if this was primary or secondary photodermatitis?*
Normal mentation, absence of icterus, anemia, and hemoglobinuria would be suggestive of primary photodermatitis. Liver disease is the underlying cause for secondary photosensitivity and therefore assessing liver function by measuring serum sorbitol dehydrogenase (SDH) and gamma-glutamyltransferase (GGT) which reflect hepatic injury would also assist in differentiating primary from secondary photosensitization.
2) *In taking a diet history, specifically what information would help confirm a primary vs. secondary photodermatitis diagnosis?*
Determining the source of the toxin would aid in the diagnosis because certain plants are known to cause primary photosensitization. If the horse had been on pasture for days to weeks before the first lesions appeared, then a walk through the pasture to identify the weeds present would help confirm the diagnosis. If the horse had been fed hay, then a physical examination of the hay, again identifying any weed fragments present would aid in confirming a diagnosis.
3) *The presence of which weeds in the pasture or hay would refine the diagnosis?*
The finding of either buckwheat or St. John's wort in the pasture or hay would suggest a primary photosensitization. Finding plants containing pyrrolizidine alkaloids would raise the suspicion for hepatopathy and secondary photosensitization.
4) *What is your suggested initial treatment?*
Treatment of dermatitis due to photosensitization, whether primary or secondary, is to keep the animal confined undercover, completely out of the sun. Sunlight through a glass window is not harmful, as ultraviolet rays are filtered out by the glass. Gentle daily

cleaning of the skin with a mild organic iodine solution will aid recovery. Appropriate systemic antibiotic therapy based on bacterial antibiotic sensitivity is indicated if there is secondary bacterial dermatitis.

5) *What is the prognosis for primary vs. secondary photodermatitis?*
The prognosis for primary photodermatitis is good to excellent once the horse no longer is consuming the toxic weed. The prognosis for secondary photodermatitis, however, is guarded to poor due to irreversible liver damage.

Chapter 13

Examples of calculating feed cost per head. Given the following factors, calculate the cost per horse per day and per month:

Example #1

8-yr-old BW 450 kg BSC 5/9 average temperament Paint gelding used for team penning. Current feeding regimen is:

- Hay
  - Cost is $60 fescue hay/400 kg bale = $0.15/kg hay
  - Fed 8 kg/d = $1.20/d for fescue hay
- Ration balancer
  - Cost is $25/20 kg bag = $1.25/kg ration balancer
  - Fed 1 kg/d = $1.25/d for ration balancer
- Rice bran
  - Cost is $36/18 kg bag = $2.00/kg rice bran
  - Fed 0.25 kg/d = $0.50/d for rice bran
- Flax seed
  - Cost is $24/4 kg bag = $0.006/g flax seed
  - Fed 60 g/d = $0.36/d for flax seed

Total cost/d = $1.20 + $1.25 + $0.50 + $0.36 = $3.31
Total cost/30 d = $3.31 × 30 = $99.30.

Approximately 75% of the cost is related to providing hay, vitamins and minerals, and 25% is related to feeding specialized fat supplements.

Example #2

3-yr-old BW 500 kg BCS 4/9 elevated temperament Thoroughbred stallion in race training. Current feeding regimen is:

- Hay
  - Cost is $15 timothy hay/25 kg bale = $0.60/kg hay
  - Fed 4 kg/d = $2.40/d for timothy hay
  - Cost is $540 alfalfa hay/metric ton (1000 kg) = $0.54/kg hay
  - Fed 2 kg/d = $1.08/d for alfalfa hay
- Sweet feed
  - Cost is $18/20 kg bag = $0.90/kg sweet feed
  - Fed 6 kg/d = $5.40/d for sweet feed
- Joint Supplement
  - Cost is $120/1.5 kg bag = $0.08/g joint supplement
  - Fed 30 g/d = $2.40/d for joint supplement
- Electrolytes
  - Cost is $22/2 kg bucket = $0.011/g electrolytes
  - Fed 60 g/d = $0.66/d for electrolytes

Total cost/d = $2.40 + $1.08 + $5.40 + $2.40 + $0.66 = $11.94.
Total cost/30 d = $11.94 × 30 = $358.20.

Approximately 74% of the cost is related to providing hay, vitamins and minerals, and 26% is related to feeding specialized performance supplements.

Chapter 14

1) *What feeding recommendations should be made to regain the weight lost?*
A recommendation was made to increase daily caloric intake by 30–50% using fat because lipid metabolism results in lower CO_2 concentrations per calorie consumed than metabolizing carbohydrates (CHO) (16 vs. 23 L CO_2/100 kcal CHO), and blood CO_2 concentration drives respiratory rate. A 30% fat supplement[1] with 1.2 Mcal DE/lb and antioxidants (vitamins A and E, selenium, zinc, and copper) was suggested. After transitioning the pony onto this supplement and feeding an additional 5 Mcal/d over the calculated DE_m of 18 Mcal/d for one month, the pony regained weight to 400 kg (BCS 4/9) which was maintained thereafter feeding the fat supplement at 2.5 Mcal/d in addition to the ration.

2) *What dietary supplement could be considered as adjunctive therapy in this pony?*
The benefit of feeding fish oil to horses with recurrent airway obstruction was explained to the owner [9]. The addition of oil with omega-3 fatty acids was recommended using a product[2] that had been clinically demonstrated to increase EPA and DHA in horse serum and red blood cells [9,10]. After a 2-week transition period, the pony was consuming 25 mL marine-based oil and 15 mL clenbuterol PO q12 hrs. The oil-soaked into alfalfa cubes well and was readily consumed. As daytime averaged 85 °F daily, the respiratory rate and effort remained reasonably comfortable for the pony per owner assessment [11]. The clenbuterol dose was then decreased to 10 mL and marine oil was increased to 30 mL q12 hrs. One month later, the owner reported the pony was still comfortable with 30–35 b/min and mild to moderate abdominal effort while environmental

1 Amplify. Purina Mills. Gainesville, GA.
2 EO3. Kentucky Equine Research. Lexington, KY.

temperatures averaged 90 °F daily. The clenbuterol was discontinued and the marine oil was continued at 30 mL twice daily.

Outcome:
Reassessment one year after the first presentation, the pony (BCS 4/9) was maintaining weight consuming 25 Mcal/d with 30 mL/d of the marine-based oil q 12 hrs, had an average 35–40 b/min respiratory rate without clenbuterol, and was considered to be comfortable. No additional treatment changes were made thereafter. The pony died of cardiac arrest 15 mos after the onset of clinical signs.

Chapter 17

1) *Calculate relative feed value (RFV) and determine the nutritional quality of the forage.*
   Calculated digestible dry matter (DDM), DMI and RFV values:
   - %DDM = 88.9 − (0.779 × %ADF) = 59.5% dry matter digestibility.
   - %DMI = 120 / %NDF = 2.0% BW.
   - RFV = %DDM × %DMI × 0.775 = 92 moderate-quality (Table 10.3).
2) *Based on the calculated DE_m requirement, how much hay (lb as fed) should this horse consume daily?*
   - DE_m requirement is 3.04 Mcal/100 kg BW/d × 5 = 15.2 Mcal/d (Table 17.1).
   - 15.2 Mcal requirement divided by hay 2.1 Mcal/kg = 7.2 kg hay DM/d.
   - Check DMI: 7.2 kg hay DM intake/500 kg BW = 1.4% BW.
   - The horse should be offered 8 kg hay as fed/d or 17–18 lb hay as fed/d [7.2/0.9 × 2.2] to meet min DE_m requirement.

   The owner is currently feeding 1/2 (60 lb) bale = 30 lb hay/d. The horse has an ideal BCS so most likely is leaving / wasting hay.
3) *Does feeding an adequate amount of this hay/d meet the horse's protein, calcium, and phosphorus requirements?*
   Method #1 using absolute nutrient intakes (Table 17.1):
   - CP requirement is 540 g/d [108 g/100 kg BW/d × 5]; 7.2 kg hay DM/d × 8.8% = 634 g/d.[3]
   - Ca requirement is 20.0 g/d [4.0 g/100 kg BW/d × 5]; 7.2 kg hay DM/d × 0.31% = 22.3 g/d.
   - P requirement is 14.0 g/d [2.8 g/100 kg BW/d × 5]; 7.2 kg hay DM/d × 0.29% = 20.1 g/d.

   Yes. Crude protein (CP), calcium (Ca), and phosphorus (P) intakes will be adequate:
   Method #2 using % DM (Table 17.3):
   - Recommended CP is 5.4%; forage contains 8.8% CP.
   - Recommended Ca is 0.20%; forage contains 0.31% Ca.
   - Recommended P is 0.14% P; forage contains 0.29% P and Ca:P ratio = 1.1:1.

   If a sufficient quantity of hay is consumed, the CP, Ca, and P needs should be met. Method #2 is appropriate when there are no problems with feed consumption, i.e. daily DM intake.
4) *The owner asks: "Is my horse fat and how much hay should I be feeding him per day?" What are your nutritional recommendations?*
   Nutritional Recommendations:
   The horse has an ideal BCS of 5/9. The owner is providing more hay than needed to the horse and likely there is soiled hay on the ground in the feeding area that the horse will not ever eat. The dietary recommendation should be to weigh out and feed 8 kg (17–18 lb) as fed hay/d divided into 2 or 3 feedings. A slow-feed hay net can be utilized to extend feeding time. Continue water and offer trace mineralized salt ad libitum as well. Weight tape and record BW of the horse monthly. Consider feeding a ration balancer at the manufacturer's recommended feeding rate. Call if the horse loses or gains more than 25 kg (5% BW).

   Outcome:
   Six months later, the owner reported the horse has remained at ~500 kg BW. The owner feeds 10 lb hay using a hay net 2x/d and the horse does finish all that is offered within 24 hrs. The owner is buying less hay and has less waste to clean up in the dry lot area. She has look at several ration balancer products but is not certain which one to use and would like your opinion.

Chapter 18

1) *Calculate relative feed value (RFV) and determine nutritional quality of the forage.*
   Calculated digestible dry matter (DDM), DMI and RFV values:
   - %DDM = 88.9 − (0.779 × %ADF) = 64.4% dry matter digestibility.
   - %DMI = 120 / %NDF = 2.4% BW.
   - RFV = %DDM × %DMI × 0.775 = 120 good-quality (Table 10.3).
2) *Based on the calculated DE requirement, how much hay (lb as fed)/d should be offered to this horse? First determine the work load (Table 18.1).*

3 Note: Although the crude protein requirement has been met, the essential amino acid lysine should also be checked. Lysine requirement is 27.0 g/d: 8 kg hay DM/d × 0.35% = 28.0 g/d.

- BW = 1200/2.2 = 545 kg. DE requirement is 4.66 Mcal/100 kg BW/d × 5.45 = 25.4 Mcal/d (Table 18.2).
- 25.4 Mcal requirement divided by hay DE of 2.3 Mcal/kg = 11 kg hay DM/d.
- Check DMI: 11 kg hay DM intake/545 kg BW = 2.0% BW.
- The horse should be offered 12 kg hay as fed daily or 26 lb hay as fed daily [11 kg DM/ 0.94 × 2.2] to meet DE requirement.
- The owner is currently feeding 1/4 (80 lb bale) = 20 lb as fed and the horse has a low BCS.

3) *Based on nutrient concentrations (Table 18.4), could this hay meet the ration protein (CP), calcium (Ca), and phosphorus (P) recommendations for this horse?*
   Yes. Crude protein, calcium, and phosphorus intakes will be adequate.
   - Crude protein requirement is ~7.0%; forage contains 13.3% CP.
   - Calcium requirement is 0.31%; forage contains 0.8% Ca.
   - Phosphorus requirement is 0.19%; forage contains 0.31% P and Ca:P ratio = 2.6:1.
4) *Does feeding an adequate amount of this hay/d meet the horse's lysine, copper (Cu), and zinc (Zn) requirements? (Table 18.2).*
   The lysine intake will be adequate but there is a Cu and Zn deficiency.
   Horses requires 36 g lysine [6.6 g/100 kg BW/d × 5.45], 123 mg Cu and 491 mg Zn/d.
   Fed 11 kg hay DM/d from previous calculation:
   - 11 kg forage DM × 0.6% lysine = 66 g lysine/d is adequate.
   - 11 kg forage DM × 9.0 Cu ppm = 99 mg Cu is a 24 mg deficit [123 – 99]/d.
   - 11 kg forage DM × 25.0 Zn ppm = 275 mg Zn is a 216 mg deficit/d.
5) *Does feeding the suggested vitamin-mineral ration balancer with copper (100 ppm) and zinc (850 ppm) at the suggested 1 lb/d dose fulfill the Cu and Zn requirements?*
   Yes however less than 1 lb/d will fulfill the Cu and Zn requirements.
   - 24 mg Cu deficit/100 ppm = 240 g supplement/d is needed.
   - 216 mg Zn defcit/850 ppm = 254 g supplement/d is needed.

   Feeding 250 g daily (~1/2 lb costing $0.5/d) will meet the copper and zinc requirements.
   Caution: When feeding less than the manufacturer's recommendations, meeting the vitamin requirements should be checked.
6) *The owner asks "is this a good idea and how much to feed/d?" What is your nutritional recommendation?*
   Nutritional recommendation: Yes, the horse does need a mineral supplement, and this one suggested can be used. Increase the hay daily feeding to 12 kg (26 lb) as fed divided into 3 feedings and feed at least 0.5 lb of this supplement once daily. Consider feeding at manufacturuer's recommended dose. Continue water and white salt ad libitum as well. Weight tape the horse monthly. The horse has a low BCS and should gain 1 BCS point with a BW gain of 60 lb [1 BCS point is about 5% body fat].

Outcome:
Eight weeks later, the owner reported the horse BW as 1250 lb per weight tape. The horse is fed ~10 lb hay three times/d which does not interfere with the daily workout schedule. Subjectively, the owner comments the horse looks and just feels better, and now wants to ask about preventative joint supplements.

Chapter 19

1) *What is the recommended DE for a non-breeding stallion weighing 455 kg?*
   Table 19.1 16.6 Mcal DE/d [4.55 × 3.64] therefore, overfeeding was likely the cause of the increased BW and BCS.
2) *What dietary and management recommendations should be made for this stallion?*
   The new ration composed of a protein-mineral-vitamin ration balancer pellet and grass hay can meet the nutrient recommendations for a non-breeding stallion at 455 kg BW. Additionally, free access to a salt block and water were recommended, monitoring BW and BCS monthly and minimal imposed exercise, e.g., walking in hand, were suggested.
3) The stallion achieved a BW of 466 kg (BCS 5/9) in 6 mos. *What was the %BW loss per week?*
   0.45%/wk [(523 – 466)/523/24 wks × 100]

Outcome:
By the start of the next breeding season, the stallion had regained the ability to mount a phantom for semen collection several times a week.

Chapter 20

1) *What is the recommended DE for an 11 month pregnant mare at BW of 535 kg (Table 20.1) and how much fescue hay should be fed per day?*
   DE = 23 Mcal DE/d [5.35 × 4.28]
   23 lb fescue hay/d [23 Mcal DE/1.0 Mcal DE/lb AF]
   The recommendations were a ration of 23 lb of mature fescue hay fed daily with 1 lb of a protein-mineral-vitamin ration balancer. The hay and supplement feeding were to be divided into at least two, preferably three, equal daily feedings. Water and a salt block were to be

available ad *libitum*. BW and BCS were to be assessed monthly estimating 2 to 3 months to achieve BSC 5/9 although difficult to predict while pregnant, with parturition pending and then lactation.

2) *What is the recommended DE for a mare during first month of lactation at BW of 535 kg?* (Table 20.2).
   DE = 34 Mcal DE/d [5.35 × 6.34].
   A ration comprising 34 lb of mature fescue hay, 1.5 lb of 30% crude protein/mineral/vitamin ration balancer, *ad libitum* water and salt was recommended for continued weight loss.
3) *What was the %BW loss per week overall?*
   0.25%/wk [574-540/574 × 100 = 5.9% total weight lost /24 wks]

Chapter 21

1) *What are the filly's daily DE requirement and feed DM intake using 3% DMI? (Table 21.2).*
   12.4 Mcal DE [3.10 Mcal/100 kg BW × 4 (given adult BW = 400 kg)].
   5.3 kg Feed DM [3% × 175 kg BW]
2) *Using a 30:70 forage to concentrate ratio, what is the approximate weight of forage DM and concentrate DM recommended for this filly?*
   5.3 kg feed × 30% = 1.6 kg forage DMI which is ~1% DMI as forage
   5.3 kg feed × 70% = 3.7 kg concentrate DMI which is ~2% DMI as concentrate
3) *Can the pasture be used as forage for the filly?*
   Calculated digestible dry matter (DDM), DMI and RFV values:
   - %DDM = 88.9 - (0.779 × %ADF) = 62.1% DDM
   - %DMI = 120 / %NDF = 2.0% BW.
   - RFV = %DDM × %DMI × 0.775 = 96 moderate-quality (Table 10.3).

   The NDF is high and the RFV is low compared with forage recommendations for weanlings (Table 10.3). Therefore, the pasture can be utilized but a complementary growth feed will be needed to meet the full nutritional recommendations for this 6-mo-old pony.
4) *How much DE will the filly derive from consuming a minimum of 1% BW as pasture? And then how many Mcal of DE from the concentrate will be needed to meet daily DE requirement?*
   Pasture: 3.9 Mcal DE [175 kg × 1% x 2.2 Mcal DE/kg]
   Concentrate: 8.5 Mcal DE [12.4 Mcal/d DE requirement - 3.9 Mcal from pasture]
5) *What does the caloric density of the concentrate need to be to meet the filly's DE requirement?*
   The concentrate calorie density must be at least 2.3 Mcal DE/kg DM [8.5 Mcal DE/3.7 kg of concentrate DMI].
6) *The pasture consumed at 1% of BW will not provide sufficient protein, calcium, or phosphorus for the filly. What are your feeding recommendations?*
   A growth concentrate feed providing energy, protein, macro and trace minerals is needed if using this pasture as forage. Specific instructions:
   - Feed an appropriate commercial (protein, lysine, mineral) grain mix divided into 2 or 3 feedings daily fed separately from other horses. Vitamin intake from green pasture should be adequate.
   - The filly should be able to consume 1% BW [3% DMI × 30% forage] in forage DM if allowed sufficient time on pasture and if ample growth and acreage are available.
   - Although the water content of pasture is high (>70%) and concentrate contains salt, continue to offer water and white salt *ad libitum*
   - Monitoring BW and BCS every two weeks is advisable.
   - Monitor pasture quality and availability through the fall and winter. Fall growth of cool season grasses will slow as cold weather approaches and the grass will go dormant in the winter. Providing a high-quality (RFV 125) mixed mainly legume hay will be necessary during the winter months (Table 10.3).

Chapter 23

1) *How to begin a weight loss program?*
   Collecting information on the feeds and feeding method would be the next step. With feed information, the current total daily DE intake can be estimated and compared with DE intake recommendations for the ideal BW.
2) *What is the DE intake from the concentrate?*
   6.5 Mcal/d from the concentrate [4 × 0.454 kg × 3.58 Mcal/kg].
3) *Assume ad libitum consumption is 2.1%BW, what is the DE intake from the hay?*
   23.5 Mcal/d from hay [540 kg × 2.1% × 2.07 Mcal DE/kg]
4) *What is the total daily DE intake?*
   30 Mcal DE/d.
5) *How would you summarize the current total DE intake compared with DE intake recommended for the ideal BW?*
   DE_m at optimal BW for this horse using the DE minimum equation because the horse is undergoing stall rest is 13.9 Mcal DE/d [460 kg × 30.3 Mcal DE/kg BW]. In summary, the horse requires approximately 14 Mcal DE/d but has been fed 30 Mcal DE/d for 5 mos which does explain the 17% increases in BW and 2 BCS units.
6) *What are your initial feeding recommendations for weight loss, expected rate of weight loss, and timeline to optimal BW? There are 7 plausible weight loss protocols in Table 27.2.*
   It would be reasonable to suggest decreasing DE intake while energy expenditure increases with the re-start of

training, and monitoring BW and BCS monthly. See Table 23.2 protocol #7. Given the Owner has 4 more months of hay on hand, feeding a reduced quantity of the same hay to the estimated optimal BW DE_m of 14 Mcal/d and replace the concentrate with a low-fat ration balancer at the recommended 0.5 kg/d for horses at maintenance would be advisable.

Initial Feeding Recommendations: Feed current hay available at 6.8 kg/d [14 Mcal/2.07 Mcal/kg] divided into 5-6 feedings. Monitoring BW weekly as exercise increases because the changes in BW cannot be predicted accurately. Inform the owner that the desired rate of weight loss would be at least 1%/wk or 5 kg/wk [540 × 0.01] for this horse. Given the horse needs to lose 80 kg BW, at the rate of 5 kg/wk, the horse should be approaching ideal BW in 16 wks.

It must be emphasized that individual results may vary from these calculations and the intensity of the exercise will play a major role in the rate of weight loss, hence weekly monitoring is highly recommended. You offer to teach the owner how to measure BW, girth, neck and belly circumference and suggest the data be sent to you for review.

Chapter 24

1) *How should the horse be managed nutritionally during the period of postoperative ileus?*
The recent colic surgery, ileus, and inability to consume nutrients enterally made the horse a candidate for parenteral nutrition (PN).
2) *A 7 French, 20 cm triple lumen polyurethane catheter was placed in the left jugular vein for PN.*
What is the goal and composition of the PN solution?
The PN goal was to provide adequate energy to meet the patient's estimated RER and protein requirement until oral food consumption was possible.
Complete the following calculations:
Patient Information:

1. Body weight (kg)	500 kg
2. RER (Mcal DE/d) = 75% min DE_m	11.4 Mcal
3. Protein requirement: 1.0 g/kg BW/d	500 g
4. Fluid requirement: 60 mL/kg/d	30 L

Parenteral Solution Formulation to provide RER (Table 24.5):
- Volume of 50% dextrose solution (1.7 kcal/mL) providing 60% of calories:
  - 60% of 11.4 Mcal/ 1.7 kcal/ mL 4.0 L
- Volume of 20% lipid solution (2 kcal/mL) providing 40% of calories:
  - 40% of 11.4 Mcal/ 2 kcal/ mL 2.3 L
- Volume of 10% amino acids (0.10 g/mL) to meet protein requirement:
  - 500 g protein/100 g/L 5.0 L
- Total volume of macronutrient solutions: 11.3 L
  - Add 1 mL of B complex vitamins/L PN 11.0 mL
  - Add 5 mL of trace minerals/d 5.0 mL
- Volume of polyionic fluids required to meet fluid requirement:
  - Fluid requirement minus PN solution 30 L - 11.3 L 18.7 L
- Osmolarity of final solution:
  - Dextose: 4.0 L × 2550 mOsm/L = 10200
  - Lipid: 2.3 L × 260 mOsm/L = 598
  - Amino acids: 5.0 L × 998 mOsm/L = 4990
  - Polyionic fluid: 18.7 L × 273 mOsm/L = 5105
  - Total mOsm = 20893 mOsm
  - Final mOsm/L = 696 mOsm/L
- Caloric density of PN solution:
11.4 Mcal/30 L 0.38 kcal/mL
- Calorie to Nitrogen ratio:
  - 11400 kcal to 80 g nitrogen 143

3) *How should the PN administration be initiated?*
PN day 1 started at 30% RER (3.8 Mcal in 10 L/d or 416 mL PN/hr). PN administration was increased to 60% RER on PN day 2 (7.6 Mcal in 20 L/d or 833 mL PN/hr) while the clinician closely monitored the horse for signs of intolerance. PN day 3, the horse received the full infusion rate (11.4 Mcal in 30 L/d) with no complications.
Update: Gastric reflux continued and the horse developed diarrhea that tested positive for *Clostridium difficile* on hospitalization day 6. By hospitalization day 9, the gelding's clinical condition had improved with medical management for the *C. difficile* infection and gastric reflux volume had decreased to 18 L/d.
4) *How to refeed this horse orally and wean off of PN administration?*
The horse was offered small quantities of alfalfa hay (2 lbs q 6 hrs) on PN day 5. On PN day 6, the horse consumed 50% RER in a ration of alfalfa, grass hay, and a complete feed with 12% NSC, and passed formed feces. Appetite continued to improve, manure production normalized the horse consumed 80% RER orally on PN day 7. The PN infusion was reduced to 30% RER on day 8 and discontinued day 9. Recovery progressed uneventfully, and the horse was discharged from the hospital on day 17 with a BW of 448 kg and a BCS of 3.5/9.

Chapter 25

1) *A phosphorus deficiency exists relative to the energy consumed and the rate of bone development. Calculate the necessary phosphorus concentration in the 3.5 Mcal DE/kg ration to meet the weanling requirement consuming 6.5 kg DM/d?*

a) *What is the weanling's daily DE intake?* 6.5 kg DM/d × 3.5 Mcal DE/kg DM = 22.75 Mcal DE/d.
b) *The recommendation is ~1400 mg P per Mcal DE consumed [1]. How many g P is recommended per day for this weanling consuming the higher calorie ration?*
   1400 mg P/Mcal × 22.75 Mcal/d = 31.85 g P/d.
c) *What must then be the P concentration in the higher calorie ration to meet P recommendation?*
   32 g P/d in 6.5 kg DM/d = 0.49% P in ration DM. The previous ration provided 26 g P/d [6.5 kg DM/d × 0.4%] which was about 20% less P than recommended on an energy basis.

2) *What is the Ca: P ratio in the current ration and new ration after the phosphorus content has been increased, and does the calcium concentration also need to be adjusted?*
   Current ration: Ca: P ratio is 1% to 0.40% = 2.5:1.
   P corrected ration: Ca: P ratio is 1% to 0.49% = 2:1.
   No, 1:1 to 3:1 is the recommended range.

Chapter 26

1) *Calculate relative feed value (RFV) and nutritional quality of the forage.*
   Calculated digestible dry matter (DDM), DMI and RFV values:
   - %DDM = 88.9 − (0.779 × %ADF) = 62% dry matter digestibility.
   - %DMI = 120 / %NDF = 2.09% BW.
   - RFV = %DDM × %DMI × 0.775 = 101 good-quality (Table 10.3).
   - The hay quality is appropriate for light working adult horses although %NDF is slightly higher than suggested (<53%) for working horses but appropriate for adult horses.
2) *What subjective information about the hay would be helpful?*
   The nutritional quality of the hay is more than adequate for these horses, however, large round bales fed out in the open field over several days during bad weather grow mold and yeast. Close examination of the hay looking and smelling for spoilage or asking for a laboratory mold and yeast count is needed. In this case, there was spoilage and high mold counts from a bale in the open field [12]. Bales in the barn had no evidence of spoilage and low mold counts. See Hay: Subjective assessments in Chapter 10.
3) *What additional information about the feeding of the sweet feed would be helpful?*
   Ideally observing how the sweet feed is fed out by the owner to the herd and the horses' interactions while the grain mix is available would be helpful. Likely based on the herd hierarchy, without some constraints or barriers between the 7 buckets, it is likely that some horses are getting more grain than others. Feeding 3 kg concentrate in one feeding does increases the risk of colic (Figure 26.2).
4) *Given there are several possible reasons for the episodes of colic in this case, what dietary recommendations would lower the risk of colic reoccurrence?*

Dietary Recommendations:

1) Feeding the large round bales undercover from weather and using a round bale feeder to keep the bales off the ground, would minimize hay spoilage. Fescue is a cool-season grass, relatively low in starch, but relatively high sugar (fructan) concentration. Additionally feeding the hay using a round bale hay net would moderate hay consumption and fructan intake through the day similar to pasture grazing, and would minimize hay waste. Figures 11.2, 11.5 and 11.10.
2) When transitioning from pasture to hay in the fall and from hay to pasture in spring, given the hay is fed in the pasture, a temporary fence placed between the hay and pasture should be used to control access to the 'new' feed increasingly so over a 2-wk period. See Forage Transitions in Chapter 26, Sidebar 26.1 and Figure 11.9.
3) A ration of hay or pasture and occasionally a sweet feed is not a nutritionally complete or balanced diet. All horses should receive a low NSC vitamin and mineral ration balancer designed to complement the forage at approximately 0.1–0.3% BW/d. Each horse should be fed the complementary feed individually which can be done in an open area with training [13]. See Figure 10.1.
4) Meal feeding sweet feed for weight gain allows large amounts of starch and sugar to bypass the small intestine resulting in large bowel dysbiosis. Additionally, feeding horses a grain mix as a group most likely allows the more dominant horses to consume a larger grain meal than intended. Starch intake should be limited to 1 g/kg BW/meal. The recommendation is to individually meal feed underweight horses a complementary 5-8% fat product with a fiber source (beet pulp or soy hulls) to achieve the 'shine and glow' BCS desired for the show circuit.

Chapter 27

1) *What is the current DE intake vs. DE requirement for this patient doing moderate work at ideal BW?*
   - Assuming horse eats all feed offered; 25 Mcal DE/d = [hay (10.2 kg DM × 1.9) + sweet feed (1.6 kg DM × 3.5)]. Note: 25 lb hay AF/2.2 × 0.9 = 10.2 kg DM/d and 4 lb concentrate AF/2.2 × 0.88 = 1.6 DM/d.
   - The DE requirement may be calculated using ave DE_m with moderate work which is 18.7 Mcal DE/d at ideal BW using Table 18.2 or NRC 2007 [1] eq 1-7b pg 26 or Table 16-2 pg 296 [400 kg × 0.0334 × 1.4 for work] ..... however .....

- The horse is overweight/obese BCS 8/9. The calculated DE requirement at ideal BW using min DEm is 17 Mcal DE/d with moderate work [400 kg × 0.0304 × 1.4 for work].
- Conclusion: Can not know which equation is accurate for this horse but the horse is consuming (min to max) 6 to 8 Mcal DE/d more than required at an ideal BW of 400 kg.

2) *What is a reasonable weight loss protocol and initial daily DE intake for this patient? Consider the options in Table 23.2.*
Table 23.2, Protocol #7, initially fed 17 Mcal DE/d because the horse is already doing regular work/exercise.
3) *Can the owner continue to feed this hay or is a different forage needed?*
Based on hay analysis, the NSC of the forage was 12.3% [WSC 10.6 + starch 1.7: see Figure 6.2] close to the ideal recommendation so this hay can be continued for now. Soaking hay to lower NSC could also be implemented now if the owner is willing.
4) *Owner agrees to replace the sweet feed with low-starch, low-calorie, vitamin–mineral–protein ration balancer appropriate for weight loss fed at 0.5 g/kg BW twice daily. How much of the MMG hay per day should the owner feed?*
21 lb (as fed) of the same MMG hay/d [17 Mcal/d /1.9 Mcal/kg DM / 0.9 × 2.2 lb/kg]
5) *Are there additional recommendations for this horse while out on pasture?*
The horse should wear a grazing muzzle while on pasture for the next 30 days. Recheck BW and BCS at that time, and re-assess the feeding recommendations based on the animal's response.

Outcome:
After one month, BW was 453 kg with no change in BCS. Recommendations were to continue the feeding regimen and reassess ID and PPID status through laboratory testing. The owner found the feeding program logistically manageable and less expensive than expected. However, initially, the horse learned to remove the grazing muzzle while on pasture but with some adjustments, the muzzle mostly stayed in place during pasture turnout.

Dietary recommendations must account for all factors involved; obesity, ID, and PPID as in this case, as well as, the owner's ability to follow the feeding plan. The nonstructural carbohydrate content of the feeds must be <12% DM to lower the risk of laminitis. Weight loss will help resolve obesity and manage ID, and the medical therapy of PPID may also help manage ID.

Chapter 28

1) *What are the dietary management goals in this case?*
   a) Since sustained high insulin concentrations are known to increase the risk of endocrinopathic laminitis, the first goal is to feed a low NSC diet that does not stimulate a high insulin response. Since spring pasture may have a WSC content of 25-30% DM, access to pasture should not be allowed. The nutritional recommendation is a calorie-restricted, low NSC (<10% DM) ration.
   b) Immediate BW reduction is necessary because excess weight is likely to put additional strain on the lamellar tissues, and because the loss of weight in an obese animal tends to be associated with an improvement in insulin dysregulation. The pony is thought to be insulin dysregulated based on a high resting serum insulin concentration although an oral sugar test would be required to support the diagnosis.
2) *What is the recommended daily intake of hay on a DM basis?*
340 kg BW × 1.25% = 4.25 kg hay DM/d
3) *What is the recommended daily intake of hay on an as fed basis?*
4.25 kg DM/0.85 = 5.0 kg hay as fed/d
4) *How much hay as fed (kg/d) should be weighed before soaking to account for the DM losses?*
As a guide, allow for a 20% loss in DM with soaking. The pre-soaked as fed weight of hay should be 6.25 kg/d [5.0/0.80].
5) *What is an estimate of the pony's minimum DEm at 340 kg?*
340 kg BW × 0.0304 = 10.3 Mcal DE/d.
6) *What are your monitoring recommendations?*

The owner was taught how to measure BW, girth, and belly circumference, and data were recorded and forwarded for review. Once the pony was established on the low-NSC diet, 2 wks later, blood was drawn for basal insulin and an oral sugar test was performed administering 0.15 mL/kg BW of corn syrup. Basal insulin was 20 μIU/mL, but 90 min after the corn syrup, the insulin was 60 μIU/mL, suggesting that the pony was still insulin dysregulated. It was recommended that the test should be repeated in 2–3 mos by which time weight loss should be apparent. Every 1–2 wks, an adjustment in the hay fed was made based on maintaining DMI at 1.25% BW. It was emphasized that forage WSC was variable and hence new sources or deliveries of hay ideally should be analyzed using the same laboratory using wet chemistry.

By week 4, the pony was sound at a trot and the treating veterinarian suggested an increase in structured exercise. The owner agreed to exercise the pony in hand initially three times a week on a soft surface in a round pen, building up to 15 min at a trot with 5 min walking to warm up and warm down. This would be beneficial in improving insulin sensitivity and help support muscle mass retention and general health, as well as increasing the metabolic rate and aiding weight loss.

By week 12, the girth and belly circumference measurements had decreased by 10 cm and the weight tape indicates that the pony had lost approximately 25 kg. Confirming BW using a calibrated scale would have been preferable but not possible. The cresty neck was visibly reduced and the BCS was 6/9. The average %BW/wk was calculated at (25 kg/340 kg/12 wks × 100) 0.6%, which was within the acceptable range of 0.5–0.75% BW/wk.

Next options were therefore discussed with the owner as:

a) In some obese ponies during the initial weight loss, there may be a delay in BCS decrease most likely due to initial loss of internal visceral fat.
b) Many insulin-dysregulated ponies can be weight-loss resistant and may require further DMI restriction (1–1.2% BW), or substituting some of the hay with good-quality straw.
c) Weight tapes only provide an estimate of weight and therefore the pony may have lost more (or less) weight.

With the owner's agreement, in this case, the restricted hay diet was recommended for at least another 4 wks.

Outcome

In September, the pony remained sound at the trot, but the owner was advised not to turn the pony out onto pasture at this time of year as there had been a recent growth of grass (cool season grass). However, it was advised to repeat the oral sugar test and if normal, the pony might be allowed onto pasture during winter months with access to ad libitum hay and individually fed a vitamin–mineral balancer. The advice was given to continue to monitor serum basal insulin regularly after 60 min of turnout or at a set time of day. It was recommended that the pony should ideally be off pasture before the spring grass growth.

In the long term, it was recommended that BW and BCS should be monitored each spring and fall with an OST and lameness check. If the pony could be maintained at BCS 5–6/9 while being fed a <12% DM NSC hay, ideally ad libitum or at least a DMI of between 1.5 and 2% BW, plus a ration balancer and possibly with short periods on low nutritional quality winter and summer pastures, this could be an adequate solution. However, if BCS became >6/9 with diagnostic indications of ID, feeding restricted quantities of low-NSC forage might be required in the long term.

References

1 National Research Council (2007). *Nutrient Requirements of Horses*. 6th Rev, Animal nutrition series, 1–341. Washington D.C.: National Academies Press.

2 Luthersson, N., Nielsen, K.H., Harris, P. et al. (2009). Risk factors associated with equine gastric ulceration syndrome (EGUS) in 201 horses in Denmark. *Equine Vet J.* 41 (7): 625–630.

3 Luthersson, N., Bolger, C., Fores, P. et al. (2019). Effect of Changing Diet on Gastric Ulceration in Exercising Horses and Ponies After Cessation of Omeprazole Treatment. *J. Equine Vet Sci.* 83: 102742.

4 Waran, N.K. and Van Dierendonck, C.M. (2016). Ethology and welfare aspects. *Veterian Key.* https://veteriankey.com/ethology-and-welfare-aspects/.

5 Lévy, M. (2018). Overview of Polioencephalomalacia Etiology, Pathogenesis, and Epidemiology. In: *Merck Manual Veterinary Manual*. Kenilworth: Merck Sharp & Dohme Corp. https://www.merckvetmanual.com/nervous-system/polioencephalomalacia/polioencephalomalacia-in-ruminants.

6 National Research Council (1982). *United States-Canadian Tables of Feed Composition: Nutritional Data for United States and Canadian Feeds*. 3rd rev. Washington, DC: The National Academies Press.

7 Schryver, H.F., Parker, M.T., Daniluk, P.D. et al. (1987). Salt consumption and the effect of salt on mineral metabolism in horses. *Cornell Vet.* 77: 122–131.

8 Kentucky Equine Research Staff (2019). Poor Performance in Sport Horses. *EquiNews*. https://ker.com/equinews/poor-performance-sport-horses/

9 Nogradi, N., Couetil, L.L., Messick, J. et al. (2015). Omega-3 fatty acid supplementation provides an additional benefit to a low-dust diet in the management of horses with chronic lower airway inflammatory disease. *J. Vet. Intern. Med.* 29 (1): 299–306.

10 Pagan, J.D.D., Lawrence, T.L.L., and Lennox, M.A.A. (2010). Fish oil and corn oil supplementation affect red blood cell and serum eicosapentaenoic acid (EPA) and docosahexaenoic acid (DHA) concentrations in Thoroughbred horses. In: *Proceedings of the 1st Nordic Feed Science Conference Sveriges Lantbruksuniversitet*, 116–118.

11 Gerber, V., Schott, H.C., and Robinson, N.E. (2011). Owner assessment in judging the efficacy of airway disease treatment. *Equine Vet. J.* 43 (2): 153–158.

12 Martinson, K., Coblentz, W., and Sheaffer, C. (2011). The Effect of harvest moisture and bale wrapping on forage quality, temperature, and mold in Orchardgrass Hay. *J Equine Vet Sci.* 31 (12): 711–716.

13 Lawrence L. (1995). Equine Feeding Management ASC-148. University of Kentucky Cooperative Extension Service. http://www2.ca.uky.edu/agcomm/pubs/asc/asc143/asc143.pdf.

B: Nutrition Resources

Academy of Veterinary Nutrition Technicians	http://nutritiontechs.org
American Academy of Veterinary Nutrition	https://www.aavnutrition.org /
American College of Veterinary Internal Medicine	https://www.acvim.org/
American Society for Parenteral & Enteral Nutrition	https://www.nutritioncare.org/
American Society of Clinical Nutrition	http://www.nutrition.org/
Amino Acid Laboratory, University of California, Davies	http://www.vetmed.ucdavis.edu/vmb/labs/aal/
Association of American Feed Control Officials	http://www.aafco.org/
Consumerlab.com	http://www.consumerlab.com/
European Society of Veterinary & Comparative Nutrition	https://esvcn.org/
FDA Center for Food Safety and Applied Nutrition	http://www.fda.gov/Food/default.htm
	http://www.fda.gov/AboutFDA/CentersOffices/OfficeofFoods/CFSAN/
FDA Center for Veterinary Medicine	http://www.fda.gov/AnimalVeterinary/
FDA Recall List	http://www.fda.gov/AnimalVeterinary/SafetyHealth/RecallsWithdrawals/default.htm
NIH National Center for Complementary and Alternative Medicine	http://nccam.nih.gov
NIH Office of Dietary Supplements	http://dietary-supplements.info.nih.gov
United State Pharmacopeia Dietary Supplement Verification Program	http://www.usp.org/verification-services

C: Nutrition Competencies of Equine Veterinarians[4]

Assess the Horse

1) Estimate body weight either using a weight tape calibrated for horses or with morphometric measurements. Describe the limitations of both methods.
2) Know where to find appropriate growth rates for foals of different breeds.
3) Assign a body condition score (BCS) using a 5-point scale (Carroll and Huntington 1988 *Eq Vet J* 20[1]:41-45) or 9-point scale (Henneke *et al.* 1983 *Eq Vet J* 15[4]: 371-372). Recognize thin vs. ideal vs. overweight and how it may vary based on use.
4) Recognize how the physiological state of the horse or herd alters nutritional requirements (i.e. adult maintenance, working/athletes, geriatric, gestation, lactation, and growth). Contrast key nutritional factors of various physiological states.
5) Recognize that breed differences exist relative to feed efficiency and risk of specific metabolic diseases. Determine if the horse or herd has a nutritionally-responsive condition.
6) Recognize classic clinical signs of common nutrient deficiencies or toxicities and select appropriate diagnostic tests.
7) Describe risk factors for and clinical signs of common feed-related toxicoses/contaminants.

Assess the Feeds

1) Obtain accurate details about what the horse(s) is/are fed, including any relevant changes that may affect the health of the horse or herd.
2) Visually distinguish grass vs. legume forage; contrast the general nutrient profile of these two classes of forages.
3) Visually distinguish pasture forage vs. hay vs. haylage vs. straw; contrast the general dry matter content and nutrient differences between these forms of forage.
4) Make a general estimate of forage quality using visual, olfactory, and tactile senses. Describe how plant maturity at the time of harvest influences forage quality.
5) Describe how to obtain representative water and feed samples for quality and nutrient analysis.
6) Describe how to identify an appropriate feed analysis laboratory.

4 2015 American College of Veterinary Nutrition. Reprinted with permission from the American College of Veterinary Internal Medicine, inc.

7) Conduct an assessment of forage from a forage nutrient analysis with an emphasis on digestible energy, crude protein, acid detergent fiber, neutral detergent fiber, water-soluble carbohydrates, ethanol-soluble carbohydrate, starch, and minerals.
8) Describe methods of detection of common feed-related toxicoses/contaminants.
9) Understand feed labels; differentiate marketing claims from information pertinent to the patient.
10) Evaluate the current diet/ration, including forage, concentrates, and supplements. Compare estimated nutrient needs (per National Research Council [NRC] or Kentucky Equine Research [KER]) to what is provided by the diet/ration. Ability to use NRC or similar software for dietary evaluation. Recognize deficiencies, excesses, toxicities, and/or redundancies.
11) Describe the energy density and relative digestibility of commonly fed grains (corn, oats, and barley). Contrast energy density and non-structural carbohydrate content of commonly fed grains.
12) Describe how food processing (i.e. pelleting, extruding, crimping) influences nutrient availability of feeds.

Assess the Feeding Management

1) Obtain accurate details on how water and feeds are presented (i.e. volume/weight per meal, number of meals per day, and feeding system[s]), including any pertinent changes in the last 3 mos.
2) Determine environmental factors that may impact nutrient requirements and water and feed accessibility.
3) Determine an appropriate total daily dry matter intake as a percent of body weight. Describe acceptable ranges, on a percent body weight basis, for forages and concentrates.
4) Describe the principles of good pasture management for grazing including stocking density, grazing muzzles, and rotational grazing.
5) Generally describe diurnal variation in pasture forage non-structural carbohydrates (NSC) and identify general daytimes and circumstances when NSC could be high and low.
6) Describe adequate and inadequate feed management practices, including volume/weight per meal, number of meals per day, and feeding system(s) to clients.
7) Describe how to transition a horse or herd to a new ingredient or ration.
8) Outline management plan for foals from birth to weaning, including recommendations for creep feeding, time of weaning, and weaning strategy.
9) Describe a weaning plan for mares.
10) Describe strategies that can be used to improve appetite in the sick and inappetent horse.
11) Describe appropriate storage of feeds relative to the local environment.

Recommendations and Monitoring

1) Describe how to evaluate label claims of commercial products.
2) Formulate a nutritional plan/ration for the physiological state of the horse(s), including water, forages, commercial feeds/concentrates, vitamin-mineral products, and/or milk replacer.
3) Recognize indications for and routes of assisted feeding in the sick horse.
4) Describe a monitoring plan to determine an individual horse or herd's response to nutritional management.
5) Describe an alternative ration should the recommended ration not provide the results you expect.
6) Describe appropriate resources for equine nutrition recommendations.

D: Feed Glossary - selected feed-related terms and terminology commonly utilized in equine feed manufacturing[5]

Additive An ingredient or combination of ingredients added to the basic feed mix or parts thereof to fulfill a specific need. Usually used in micro quantities and requires careful handling and mixing.

Balanced A term that may be applied to a diet, ration, or feed having all known required nutrients in proper amount and proportion based upon recommendations of recognized authorities in the field of animal nutrition, such as the National Research Council, for a given set of physiological animal requirements. The species for which it is intended and the functions such as maintenance or maintenance plus production (growth, fetus, fat, work, etc) shall be specified.

5 Official Publication of Association of American Feed Control Officials, Inc. 2021.

Blocks (Physical form) Agglomerated feed compressed into a solid mass cohesive enough to hold its form and weighing over two pounds, and generally weighing 30–50 pounds.

Bran (Part) Pericarp of grain.

Brand name Any word, name, symbol or device or any combination thereof identifying the commercial feed of a distributor and distinguishing it from that of others.

Bricks (Physical form) Agglomerated feed, other than pellets, compressed into a solid mass cohesive enough to hold its form and weighing less than two pounds. (See blocks.)

By-product Secondary products produced in addition to the principal product.

Carriers An edible material to which ingredients are added to facilitate uniform incorporation of the latter into feeds. The active substances are absorbed, impregnated or coated into or unto the edible material in such a way as to physically carry the active ingredient.

Chaff (Part) Glumes, husksor other seed covering together with other plant parts separated from seed in threshing or processing.

Chopped, chopping (Process) Reduced in particle size by cutting with knives or other edged instruments.

Cleaned, cleaning (Process) Removal of material by such methods as scalping, aspirating, magnetic separation, or by any other method.

Cleanings (Part) Chaff, weed seeds, dust, and other foreign matter removed from cereal grains.

Commercial feed As defined in the *AAFCO Model Bill*, all materials except unmixed whole seeds or physically altered entire unmixed seeds, when not adulterated, which are distributed for use as feed or for mixing in feed.

Common foods Common foods are commercially available and suitable for use in animal food but are not defined by AAFCO, including but not limited to certain whole seeds, vegetables, or fruits. Common food for animals may include common human foods that are known to be safe for the intended use in animal food. Manufacturers are responsible for determining whether a common food is safe and has utility for its intended use prior to commercial distribution as animal food.

Common or usual feed ingredient name The common or usual name of a feed ingredient shall accurately identify or describe, in as simple and direct terms as possible, the basic nature of the ingredient or its characterizing properties. The name shall be uniform among all identical or similar ingredients and may not be confusingly similar to the name of any other ingredient that is not reasonably encompassed within the same name. Each ingredient shall be given its own common or usual name that states, in clear terms, what it is in a way that distinguishes it from other ingredients. Some feed ingredients may be a common food; in this case the common or usual name should abide by the principles as provided in this feed term.

Complementary feed[6] The EU definition is a compounded feed with a high concentration of certain nutrients to be fed in conjunction with forages.

Complete feed A nutritionally adequate feed for animals other than man; by specific formula is compounded to be fed as the sole ration and is capable of maintaining life and/or promoting production without any additional substance being consumed except water.

Concentrate A feed used with another to improve the nutritive balance of the total and intended to be further diluted and mixed to produce a supplement or a complete feed. *Also may generically refer to the non-forage components of the ration*[6].

6 Not an AAFCO definition.

Conditioned, conditioning (Process) Having achieved pre-determined moisture characteristic and/or temperature of ingredients or a mixture of ingredients prior to further processing.

Cooked, cooking (Process) Heated in the presence of moisture to alter chemical and/or physical characteristics or to sterilize.

Cracked, cracking (Process) Particle size reduced by a combined breaking and crushing action.

Crimped, crimping (Process) Rolled by use of corrugated rollers. It may curtail tempering or conditioning and cooling.

Crumbled, crumbling (Process) Pellets reduced to granular form.

Crumbles (Physical form) Pelleted feed reduced to granular form.

Crushed, crushing (Process) see *rolled, rolling*.

Cubes (Physical form) Agglomerated feed formed by compacting and forcing through die openings by a mechanical process, often larger size than pellets > 1cm.

Cull Material rejected as inferior to the process of grading or separating.

Culture Nutrient medium inoculated with specific microorganisms which may be in a live or dormant condition.

Cultured, culturing (Process) Biological material multiplied or produced in a nutrient media.

Customer-formula feed Consists of a mixture of commercial feeds and/or feed ingredients each batch of which is manufactured according to the specific instructions of the final purchaser.

D-activated, D-activating Plant or animal sterol fractions which have been vitamin D activated by ultra-violet light or by other means.

Degermed (Process) Having had the embryo of seeds wholly or partially separated from the starch endosperm.

Dehulled, dehulling (Process) Having removed the outer covering from grains or other seeds.

Dehydrating, dehydrated (Process) Having been freed of moisture by thermal means.

Diet Feed ingredients or mixture of ingredients including water, which is consumed by animals.

Dietary starch (Nutrient) An alpha-linked-glucose carbohydrate of or derived from plants, animals and/or microbes from which glucose is released through the hydrolytic actions of purified alpha-amylases and amyloglucosidases that are specifically active only on alpha-(1-4) and alpha-(1-6) linkages in samples that have been gelatinized in a heated, mildly acidic buffer. Its concentration in feed is determined by enzymatically converting the alpha-linked-glucose carbohydrate to glucose and then measuring the liberated glucose. This definition encompasses plant starch, glycogen, maltooligosaccharides and maltose/isomaltose.

Digested, digesting (Process) Subjected to prolonged heat and moisture, or to chemicals or enzymes with a resultant change in decomposition of the physical or chemical nature.

Drug (as defined by FDA as applied to feed) A substance (a) intended for use in the diagnosis, cure, mitigation, treatment or prevention of disease in man or other animals or (b) a substance other than food intended to affect the structure or any function of the body of man or other animals.

Dry-milled (Process) Tempered with a small amount of water or steam to facilitate the separation of the various component parts of the kernel in the absence of any significant amount of free water.

Dust (Part) Fine, dry pulverized particles of matter usually resulting from the cleaning or grinding of grain.

Ensiled (Process) Aerial parts of plants which have been preserved by ensiling. Normally the original material is finely cut and blown into an airtight chamber as a silo, where it is pressed to exclude air and where it undergoes an acid fermentation that retards spoilage.

Environmental nutrition The role of nutritional factors in altering animal impacts on the environment.

Enzymatic activity The catalytic activity required to convert a given amount of assay substrate to a given amount of product per unit time under the standard conditions set forth in the assay procedure.

Enzyme A protein made up of amino acids or their derivatives, which catalyzes a defined chemical reaction. Required cofactors should be considered an integral part of the enzyme.

Enzyme product A processed, standardized enzyme-containing material which has been produced with the intention of being sold for use in animal feed and feed ingredients.

Expanded, expanding (Process) Subjected to moisture, pressure, and temperature to gelatinize the starch portion. When extruded, its volume is increased, due to abrupt reduction in pressure.

Extracted, mechanical (Process) Having removed fat or oil from materials by heat and mechanical pressure. Similar terms: expeller extracted, hydraulic extracted, "old process".

Extracted, solvent (Process) Having removed fat or oil from materials by organic solvents. Similar term "new process".

Extruded (Process) A process by which feed has been pressed, pushed, or protruded through orifices under pressure.

Fat (Part) A substance composed chiefly of triglycerides of fatty acids, and solid or plastic at room temperature.

Fatty acids (Part) Aliphatic monobasic acids containing only the elements carbon, hydrogen, and oxygen.

Feed(s) Material consumed or intended to be consumed by animals other than humans that contributes nutrition, taste, or aroma or has a technical effect on the consumed material. This includes raw materials, ingredients, and finished product.

Feed grade Material that has been determined to be safe, functional, and suitable for its intended use in animal food, is handled and labeled appropriately, and conforms to the Federal Food, Drug, and Cosmetic Act unless otherwise expressly permitted by the appropriate state or federal agency (suitable for use in animal feed).

Feedstuff See *feed(s).*

Fermented, fermenting (Process) Acted upon by yeasts, molds, or bacteria in a controlled aerobic or anaerobic process in the manufacture of such products as alcohols, acids, vitamins of the B-complex group, or antibiotics.

Fiber (Nutrient) Any of a large class of plant carbohydrates that resist digestion hydrolysis.

Fines (Physical form) Any materials which will pass through a screen whose openings are immediately smaller than the specified minimum crumble size or pellet diameter.

Flakes (Physical form) An ingredient rolled or cut into flat pieces with or without prior steam conditioning.

Flaked, flaking (Process) See *rolled.*

Flour (Part) Soft, finely ground and bolted meal obtained from the milling of cereal grains, other seeds, or products. It consists essentially of the starch and gluten of the endosperm.

Fodder (Part) The green or cured plant, containing all the ears or seed heads, if any, grown primarily for forage.

Food(s) When used in reference to animals, in synonymous with feed(s). See *feed(s).*

Formula feed Two or more ingredients proportioned, mixed and processed according to specifications.

Free choice A feeding system by which animals are given unlimited access to the separate components or groups of components contributing the diet.

Fresh (Process) Ingredient(s) having not been subject to freezing, treatment by cooking, drying, rendering, hydrolysis, or similar process, to the addition of salt, curing agents, natural or synthetic chemical preservatives or other processing aids, or to preservation by means other than refrigeration.

Fructans (Nutrient) Polysaccharides and oligosaccharides in which fructose is the major constituent and glucose is the minor constituent. Glucose content is 33% or less.

Gelatinized, gelatinizing (Process) Having had the starch granules completely ruptured by a combination of moisture, heat and pressure, and in some instances, by mechanical shear.

Germ (Part) The embryo found in seeds and frequently separated from the bran and starch endosperm during the milling.

Gluten (Part) The tough, viscid nitrogenous substance remaining when the flour of wheat or other grain is washed to remove the starch.

Gossypol (Part) A phenolic pigment in cottonseed that is toxic to some animals.

Grain Seed from cereal plants.

GRAS Abbreviation for the phrase "Generally Recognized as Safe." A substance which is generally recognized as safe by experts qualified to evaluate the safety of the substance for its intend use.

Groats (Part) Grains from which the hulls have been removed.

Ground, grinding (Process) Reduced in particle size by impact, shearing, or attrition.

Hay (Part) The aerial portion of grass or herbage especially cut and cured for animal feeding.

Heads (Part) The seed or grain-containing portions of a plant.

Heat processed, heat processing (Process) Subjected to a method of preparation involving the use of elevated temperature with or without pressure.

Hulls (Part) Outer covering of grain or other seed.

Human grade Every ingredient and the resulting product are stored, handled, processed, and transported in a manner that is consistent and compliant with regulations for current good manufacturing proctices (cGMPs) for human edible foods.

Husks (Part) Leaves enveloping an ear of maize; or the outer coverings of kernels or seeds, especially when dry and membranous.

Hydrolyzed, hydrolyzing (Process) Complex molecules having been split to simpler units by chemical reaction with water, usually by catalysis.

Ingredient, feed ingredient Means a component part or constituent of any combination of mixture making up a commercial feed.

Iodized, iodized (Process) To treat with iodine or an iodide.

Kernel (Part) A whole grain. For other species, dehulled seed.

Kibbled, kibbling (Process) Cracked or crushed baked dough or extruded feed that has been cooked prior to or during the extrusion process.

Laboratory method A technique or procedure of conducting scientific experiment, test, investigation or observation according to a definite established logical or systematic plan.

Leached (Process) The conditionof a product following subjection of the material to the action of percolating water or other liquid.

Leaves (Part) Lateral outgrowths of stems that constitute part of the foliage of a plant, typically a flattened green blade, and primarily functions in photosynthesis.

Lecithin (Part) A specific phospholipid. The principal constitute of crude phosphatides derived from oil-bearing seeds.

Malt (Part) Sprouted and steamed whole grain from which the radicle has been removed.

Mash (Physical form) A mixture of ingredients in meal form. Similar term: *mash feed.*

Meal (Physical form) An ingredient which has been ground or otherwise reduced in particle size.

Medicated feed Any feed which contains drug ingredients intended or presented for the cure, mitigation, treatment, or prevention of diseases of animals other than man or which contains drug ingredients intended to affect the structure of any function of the body of animals other than man. Antibiotics included in a feed growth promotion and/or efficiency levels are drug additives and feeds containing such antibiotics are included in the foregoing definition of "Medicated Feed".

Micro-ingredients Vitamins, minerals, antibiotics, drugs, and other materials normally required in small amounts and measured in milligrams, micrograms or parts per million (ppm).

Middlings (Part) A by-product of flour milling comprising several grades of granular particles containing different portions of endosperm, bran, germ, each of which contains different level of crude fiber.

Mill by-product (Part) A secondary product obtained in addition to the principal product in milling practice.

Mill dust (Part) Fine feed particles of undetermined origin resulting from handling and processing feed and feed ingredients.

Mill run (Part) The state in which a material comes from the mill, ungraded and usually uninspected.

Mineralize, mineralized (Process) To supply, impregnate, or add inorganic mineral compounds to a feed ingredient or mixture.

Mixing (Process) To combine by agitation two or more materials to a specific degree of dispersion.

Molasses (Part) The thick, viscous by-product resulting from refined sugar production or the concentrated, partially dehydrated juices from fruits.

Natural A feed or ingredient derived solely from plant, animal or mined sources, either in its unprocessed state or having been subject to physical processing, heat processing, rendering, purification, extraction, hydrolysis, enzymolysis or fermentation, but not having been produced by or subject to a chemically synthetic process and not containing any additives or processing aids that are chemically synthetic except in amounts as might occur unavoidably in good manufacturing practices.

Nutrient A feed constituent in a form and at a level that will help support the life of an animal. The chief classes of feed nutrients are proteins, fats, carbohydrates, minerals, and vitamins.

Offal (Part) Material left as a by-product from the preparation of some specific product, less valuable portions and the by-products of milling.

Oil (Part) A substance composed chiefly of triglycerides of fatty acids, and liquid at room temperature.

Organic (Process) A formula feed or a specific ingredient within a formula feed that has been produced and handled in compliance with the requirements of the USDA National Organic Program.

Part A subcomponnet of an original material. A "part" feed term can be used in an ingredient name if the ingredient part has gone through a recognized review process.

Pearled, pearling (Process) Dehulled grains reduced by machine brushing into smaller smooth particles.

Pelleted, pelleting (Process) Having agglomerated feed by compaction and forced through die openings.

Pellets (Phyical form) Agglomerated feed formed by compacting and forcing through die openings by a mechanical process.

Pellets, soft (Physical form) Similar term: High Molasses Pellets. Pellets containing sufficient liquid to require immediate dusting and cooling.

Physical form Shape, appearance or structure of a feed based on size, texture, particle size, density, hardness, moisture/dryness or other physical characteristics. Physical form may be used to further describe an ingredient name.

Polished, polishing (Process) Having a smooth surface produced by mechanical process usually by friction.

Pomace (Part) Pulp from fruit or vegetables. See *pulp*.

Popped, puffed (Process) To expand whole or cracked processed grains or non-grains by heat with or without high pressure. Examples of grains are corn, rice, wheat, millet, barley, buckwheat. Example of non-grain is soybean.

Powder, powdered (Process) Pulverizing a feed or feed ingredient into fine or very small particle size or atomization and drying of liquids.

Precipitated, precipitating (Process) Separated from suspension or a solution as a result of some chemical or physical change brought about by a chemical reaction, by cold or by any other means,

Premix A uniform mixture of one or more micro-ingredients with diluent and/or carriers. Premixes are used to facilitate uniform dispersion of the micro-ingredients in a large mix.

Premixing (Process) The preliminary mixing of ingredients with diluents and/or carriers.

Preservative A substance added to protect, prevent or retard decay, discoloration or spoilage under conditions of use or storage.

Pressed, pressing (Process) Compacted or molded by pressure; also meaning having fat, oil or juices extracted under pressure.

Process A method used to prepare, treat, convert or transform materials into feeds or feed ingredients. A "process" feed term can be used to further describe an ingredient name as long as the ingredient is not nutritionally altered from the original.

Product (Part) A substance produced from one or more other substances as a result of chical or physical change.

Protein (Nutrient) Any of a large class of naturally occurring complex combinations of amino acids.

Pulp (Part) The solid residue remaining after extraction of juices from fruits, roots, or stems. Similar terms: *Bagasse* and *Pomace.*

Pulverized, pulverizing (Process) See *ground, grinding.*`

Range cubes (Physical form) Large pellets designed to be fed on the ground.

Ration The amount of the total feed which is provided to one animal over a 24-hour period.

Raw Food in its natural or crude state not having been subjected to heat in the course of preparation as food.

Residue Part remaining after the removal of a portion of its original constituents.

Rolled, rolling (Process) Having changed the shape and/or size of particles by compressing between rollers. It may entail tempering or conditioning.

Roasted (Process) Cooked, dried or browned by exposure to heat.

Roots (Part) Subterranean parts of plants.

Scalped, scalping (Process) Having removed larger material by screening.

Screened, screening (Process) Having separated various sized particles by passing over and/or through screens.

Seed (Part) The fertilized and ripened ovule of a plant.

Self fed A feeding system where animals have continuous free access to some or all component(s) of a ration, either individually or as mixtures.

Separating (Process) Classification of particles by size, shape, and/or density.

Separating, magnetic (Process) Removing ferrous material by magnetic attraction.

Shorts (Part) Fine particles of bran, germ, flour, or offal from the tail of the mill from commercial flour milling.

Sifted (Process) Materials that have been passed through wire sieves to separate particles in different sizes. The separation of finer materials than would be done by screening.

Solubles Liquid containing dissolved substances obtained from processing animal or plant materials. It may contain some fine suspended solids.

Solvent extracted (Process) A product from which oil has been removed by solvents.

Spray dried (Process) Material which has been dried by spraying or atomizing into a draft of heated dry air.

Stabilized (Process) When an ingredient which may deteriorate has been processed to improve stability, the expression "stabilized," "stability improved" or "with improved stability" may appear following the ingredient in the statement of ingredients The process used is to be specified, e.g., heat stabilized.

Stalk(s) (Part) The main stem of a herbaceous plant often with its dependent parts as leaves, twigs and fruit.

Starch (Part) A white, granular polymer of plant origin. The principal part of seed endosperm.

Steamed, steaming (Process) Having treated ingredients with steam or alter physical and/or chemical properties. Similar terms: steam cooked, steam rendered, tanked.

Steep-extracted, steep-extracting (Process) Soaked in water or other liquid (as in the wet milling of corn) to remove soluble materials.

Steepwater Water containing soluble materials extracted by steep-extraction, i.e., by soaking in water or other liquid (as in the wet milling of corn).

Stem (Part) The coarse, aerial parts of plants which serve as supporting structures for leaves, buds, fruit, etc.

Sterols (Part) Solid cyclic alcohols which are the major constituents of the unsaponifiable portion of animal and vegetable fats and oils.

Stillage (Part) The mash from fermentation of grains after removal of alcohol by distillation.

Stover (Part) The stalks and leaves of corn after the ears, or sorghum after the heads have been harvested.

Straw A feed composed of plant residue remains after separation of the seeds in threshing including chaff.

Sugars (Nutrient) The sum of all free disaccharides and monosaccharides such as: sucrose, lactose, maltose, glucose, fructose and galactose or others digestible by enzymes found in an animal's digestive tract.

Sun-cured (Process) Material dried by exposure in open air to the direct rays of the sun.

Supplement A feed used with another to improve the nutritive balance or performance of the total and intend to be: (1) Fed undiluted as a supplement to other feeds, or, (2) Offered free choice with other parts of the ration separately available; or (3) Further diluted and mixed to produce a complete feed.

Syrup (Part) Concentrated juice of a fruit or plant.

Tallow (Part) Animal fats with titer above 40 °C.

Tempered, tempering (Process) See *conditioned, conditioning*.

Titer A property of fat determined by the solidification point of the fatty acids liberated by hydrolysis.

Toasted (Process) Browned, dried, or parched by exposure to a fire, or to gas or electric heat.

Trace minerals Mineral nutrients required by animals in micro amounts only (measured in milligrams per kilograms or smaller units).

Treat A food provided occasionally for enjoyment, training, entertainment, or other purposes, and not generally intended or represented to be a complete feed or supplement.

Tubers (Part) Short, thickened fleshy stems or terminal portions of stems or rhizomes that are usually formed underground, bear minute scaled leaves, each with a bud capable under suitable conditions of developing into a new plant, and constitutes the resting stage of various plants.

Twigs (Part) Small shoots or branches, usually without leaves, portions of stems of variable length or size.

Uncleaned (Physical form) Containing foreign material.

Unsaponifiable matter (Part) Ether soluble material extractable after complete reaction with strong alkali.

Vines (Part) Any plant whose stems require support, or lie on the ground.

Vitaminize, vitaminized (Process) To provide or supplement with vitamins.

Vitamins Organic compounds that function as parts of enzyme systems essential for the transmission of energy and the regulation of metabolisms of the body.

Wafered, wafering (Process) Having agglomerated a feed of a fibrous nature by compressing into a form usually having a diameter or cross section measurement greater than its length.

Wafers (Physical form) A form of agglomerated feed based on fibrous ingredients in which the finished form usually has a diameter or cross section measurement greater than its length.

Water extract The aqueous phase containing dissolved materials resulting from the treatment (e.g. by mixing or boiling) of a solid with water. All or part of the solid matrix may be dissolved in the extract.

Weathered (Process) A material which has been subjected to the action of the elements.

Wet (Physical form) Material containing liquid or which has been soaked or moistened with water or other liquid.

Wet-milled (Process) Steeped in water with or without sulfur dioxide to soften the kernel in order to facilitate the separation of the various component parts.

Whey (Part) The watery part of milk separated from the curd.

Whey solids (Part) The solids of whey (proteins, fats, lactose, ash, and lactic acid).

Whole (Physical form) Complete, entire.
Whole pressed, whole pressing (Process) Having the entire seed to remove oil.
Wilted (Physical form) A product without turgor as a result of water loss.
Wort (Part) The liquid portion of malted grain. It is a solution of malt sugar and other water-soluble extracts from malted mash.

E: Average body weight and heights of horses[7]

Horse breeds:	Weight (lbs)	Height (in)	Weight (kg)	Height (cm)
Albino, American	1003	56–60	455	142–152
Andalusian	1201-1301	60	545-590	152
Appaloosa	1003–1301	56–60	455–590	142–152
Arabian	904–1102	56–59	410–500	142–150
Belgian, American	1896–2205	60–71	860–1000	152–180
Belgian, Ardennais	1400–1598	56–60	635–725	142–152
Cleveland Bay	1201–1499	64	545–680	162
Clydesdale	1598–1797	63–67	725–815	161–170
Cream draft, American	1598–1995	60–67	725–905	152–170
Criollo	1201–1301	60	545–590	152
Dutch Warmblood	1201–1301	63–67	545–590	160–170
Flemish	1797–2403	59–71	815–1090	150–180
Hackney	904–1201	60	410–545	153
Hanoverian	1201–1400	64	545–635	162
Irish Draught	1301–1499	63–67	590–680	160–170
Lipizzaner	904–1201	59–64	410–545	150–160
Morgan	904–1201	56–60	410–545	142–152
Oldenburg	1201–1499	64–68	545–680	162–172
Orlov Trotter	1003–1301	60–67	455–590	152–170
Paso	1201–1301	55–60	545–590	140–152
Percheron	1896–2105	63–68	860–955	160–172
Quarter horse, American	1003–1301	56–67	455–590	142–170
Saddlebred, American	1003–1201	59–63	455–545	150–160
Selle Francais	1003–1201	63	455–545	160
Shire	1698–2701	64–71	770–1225	162–180
Spanish Mustang	805–1003	48–56	365–455	122–142
Standardbred, American	1201	60	545	152
Suffolk	1698–1896	63–67	770–860	160–170
Tennessee Walker	904–1400	59–60	410–635	150–152
Thoroughbred	1003–1301	63–67	455–590	160–170
Trakehner	1201–1499	63–68	545–680	160–172
Walkaloosa	1003–1301	56–60	455–590	142–152

7 https://equi-analytical.com/resources/typical-body-weights. This list is not intended to be all inclusive.

Pony breeds[8]	Weight (lbs)	Height (in)	Weight (kg)	Height (cm)
Caspian	595	39–47	270	100–120
Connemara	805–1003	51–56	365–455	130–142
Dulmen	705–805	48	320–365	123
Exmoor	595–805	48	270–365	123
Halflinger	1201–1301	56	545–590	142
Virginia Highlander	1201–1400	51–56	545–635	130–142
Icelandic	705–904	47–55	320–410	120–140
Norwegian Fjord	1201–1400	51–5	545–635	130–142
Shetland	298–595	37–42	135–270	95–106
Welsh Pony	452–750	47–52	205–340	120–132
Welsh Pony, Cob	595–1003	53	270–455	135
Welsh Pony, Mountain	397–705	47	180–320	120
Miniature Horse, American[9]	198–496	24–35	90–225	60–90

F: Abbreviations

3MH	3-methylhistidine
%DM	% dry matter
ac	acre
ADF	acid detergent fiber
ADG	average daily gain
AF	as fed
aka	also known as
BCS	body condition score
bpm	beats per minute
BW	body weight
CBC	complete blood cell count
cm	centimeter
d	day(s)
DDM	digestible dry matter
DE	digestible energy
DE_m	digestible energy for maintenance
dL	deciliter
ave DE_m	average digestible energy for maintenance 3.34 Mcal/100 kg BW
elv DE_m	elevated digestible energy for maintenance 3.64 Mcal/100 kg BW
DMI	dry matter intake as %BW or kg DM/d or g/kg BW
g	gram
gal	gallon
GI	gastrointestinal
GIT	gastrointestinal tract
HR	heart rate
hr(s)	hour(s)

8 Mature ponies are generally breeds under 56″ at the withers.
9 Mature Miniature horses are generally under 38″ at the withers.

IFN	International feed number has a 5 digit format: x-xx-xxx
in	inch
IM	intramuscular
IU	International Units
IV	intravenous
Kcal	Kilocalorie
Kg	Kilogram
kg/H/d	Kilogram/horse/day
L	liter
lb	pound
LCT	lower critical temperature
meter	meter
Mcal	megacalorie = 1000 kilo (kcal) = 1,000,000 calories
min	minute(s)
min DE_m	minimum digestible energy for maintenance 3.04 Mcal/100 kg BW
mL	milliliter
MMG	mixed mainly grass
MML	mixed mainly legume
m	meter(s)
mm	millimeter
mos	month(s)
mph	miles per hour
mya	million years ago
NA	North America
NDF	neutral detergent fiber
ppm	parts per million
q12hr	every 12 hrs
RFV	relative feeding values
SC	subcutaneous
sec	second(s)
tbsp	tablespoon
tsp	teaspoon
TNZ	thermoneutral zone
UCT	upper critical temperature
wk(s)	week(s)
yr(s)	year(s)

Index

Equine Clinical Nutrition, Second Edition. Edited by Rebecca L. Remillard.

d

e

g

n